THE ESSENTIALS OF ROENTGEN INTERPRETATION

THIRD EDITION

LESTER W. PAUL, M.D.
Professor of Radiology
The University of Wisconsin Medical School

JOHN H. JUHL, M.D.
Professor of Radiology and
Chairman of the Department of Radiology,
The University of Wisconsin Medical School

1323 Illustrations

Medical Department
Harper & Row, Publishers
Hagerstown, Maryland
New York, Evanston, San Francisco, London
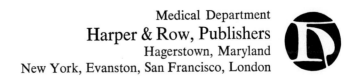

THE ESSENTIALS OF ROENTGEN INTERPRETATION

Copyright © 1958, 1965, 1972 by Harper & Row, Publishers, Inc. All rights reserved. No part of this book may be used or reproduced in any manner whatsoever without written permission except in the case of brief quotations embodied in critical articles and reviews. Printed in the United States of America. For information address Medical Department, Harper & Row, Publishers, Inc., 2350 Virginia Avenue, Hagerstown, Maryland 21740

Third Edition

STANDARD BOOK NUMBER: 06-142142-1

LIBRARY OF CONGRESS CATALOG CARD NUMBER: 79-190485

THE ESSENTIALS OF
ROENTGEN INTERPRETATION

CONTENTS

Preface to Third Edition   vii
Preface to Second Edition   ix
Preface to First Edition   xi
Introduction   1

Section I

THE OSSEOUS SYSTEM

1. Disturbances in Skeletal Growth and Maturation   15
2. The Osseous Dysplasias   28
3. Miscellaneous Skeletal Anomalies and Syndromes   66
4. Metabolic, Endocrine, and Related Bone Diseases   104
5. Traumatic Lesions of Bones and Joints   128
6. Inflammations and Infections of Bone   171
7. Bone Tumors and Related Conditions   191
8. Miscellaneous Conditions   232
9. Diseases of the Joints   261
10. The Superficial Soft Tissues   303

Section II

THE BRAIN AND SPINAL CORD

11. Intracranial Diseases   337
12. The Spinal Cord and Related Structures   386

Section III

THE ABDOMEN AND GASTROINTESTINAL TRACT

13. The Abdomen — 411
14. The Gallbladder — 466
15. The Esophagus — 487
16. The Stomach — 515
17. The Duodenum — 553
18. The Mesenteric Small Intestine — 569
19. The Colon — 596

Section IV

THE URINARY AND FEMALE GENITAL TRACTS

20. The Urinary Tract — 645
21. Obstetric and Gynecologic Roentgenology — 716

Section V

THE CHEST

22. Methods of Examination, Anatomy, and Congenital Malformations — 741
23. Acute Pulmonary Infections — 780
24. Bronchial Diseases — 799
25. Pulmonary Tuberculosis — 808
26. Fungus Diseases and Other Chronic Inflammations — 826
27. Diseases of Occupational, Chemical, and Physical Origin — 847
28. Circulatory Disturbances — 866
29. Tumors of the Lungs and Bronchi — 881
30. Miscellaneous Pulmonary Conditions — 902
31. Diseases of the Pleura, Mediastinum, and Diaphragm — 942
32. The Cardiovascular System — 971

Section VI

THE FACE, MOUTH, AND JAWS

33. The Orbit and Eye — 1047
34. The Sinuses and Mastoids — 1056
35. The Teeth, Jaws, and Facial Bones — 1078

Index — 1099

PREFACE TO THIRD EDITION

Advances in diagnostic radiology, as in other medical disciplines, have been continuous and extensive. The progress made in radiology since the publication of the second edition has necessitated our presenting this, the revised third edition. Our basic aims in writing this book have not changed significantly from those cited in the Preface to the First Edition. In order to satisfy these aims, we have given special attention to the updating of the material presented in the second edition and to the addition of new material corresponding to new developments.

To cover the advances in the last decade in angiography, we are now placing more emphasis on this procedure, particularly the indications for the more common uses and the basic roentgen observations. The references at the end of each chapter have been updated to include some of the recent literature. Most of the new entries are from books and journals available in the average departmental or hospital library.

The osseous dysplasias have been placed in a separate chapter which has been largely rewritten. All other chapters have been revised to bring them up to date. Those most extensively rewritten include Chapter 4—metabolic and endocrine diseases of bone; Chapter 8—miscellaneous conditions—bone and joint; Chapter 16—the stomach; Chapter 18—the small intestine; Chapter 19—the colon; Chapter 20—the urinary tract; Chapter 28—circulatory disturbances; Chapter 29—miscellaneous pulmonary conditions; Chapter 34—teeth, jaws and facial bones.

In addition many sections covering individual diseases or groups of diseases have been rewritten completely or extensively revised. A number of new illustrations have been added.

Newly described conditions include: spondyloepiphyseal dysplasia, cartilage-hair dysplasia, metatropic dwarfism, the mucopolysaccharidoses, pycnodysostosis, dyschondrosteosis, thanatophoric dwarfism, asphyxiating thoracic dystrophy, Apert's syndrome, trisomy 13–15 syndrome, Turner's syndrome, rubella syndrome, angiography of pancreas and liver, sclerosing cholangitis, percutaneous transhepatic cholangiography, arteriography in gastrointestinal bleeding and other gastrointestinal lesions, Crohn's disease of the stomach and duodenum, Zollinger-Ellison syndrome, nodular lymphoid hyperplasia, scleroderma of the small intestine and colon, intestinal lymphangiectasis, hypoproteinemia and intestinal edema, dis-

vii

accharidase deficiency, segmental ischemia of the small intestine and colon, necrotizing enterolitis.

Vascular impressions in intravenous urography, emphysematous and xanthogranulomatous pyelonephritis, congenital multicystic disease and medullary cystic disease of the kidneys, pararenal pseudocyst, renal polyarteritis nodosa, renal angiomyolipoma, squamous metaplasia of the renal pelvis, schistosomiasis of the urinary bladder, vas deferens calcification, intrauterine fetal transfusion, laryngography, pulmonary angiography, azygography, the atypical myobacterial pulmonary infections, diffuse pulmonary aspergillosis, interstitial pulmonary edema, Wilson-Mikity syndrome, nitrofurantoin sensitivity, desquamative interstitial pneumonia (DIP), near drowning, mediastinal lipomatosis caused by steroids, inversion of the left diaphragm secondary to pleural effusion, accessory diaphragm, sialography, and classification of maxillary fractures.

We wish to call attention to some of the newer facets of book production employed in this edition. The book is being printed offset, reflecting the current trend toward this faster, cleaner, and more economical method. We are using a special paper which is less bulky, but without sacrificing strength. This has allowed us to add more than 100 pages and keep the additional weight and thickness within reasonable limits. The paper has a softer appearance than the high-gloss paper used in previous editions, resulting in a reduction of glare, particularly under artificial lighting.

We wish to express our appreciation to our colleagues who have given us invaluable assistance, particularly in the selection of new illustrative material. These include Drs. Richard Blank, George Wirtanen and Margaret Winston; Dr. Andrew B. Crummy furnished most of the new abdominal angiograms; Dr. Justin J. Wolfson did the same for some of the pediatric case material. Dr. Crummy also reviewed the chapters on The Urinary Tract and The Cardiovascular System. Others have been cited in the appropriate figure legends.

As with previous editions the photography has been done by Mr. Homer Montague and the secretarial work by Miss Lorena Carmichael. To them we again extend our sincere thanks. We would be remiss if we did not acknowledge the many courtesies extended to us by the staff of Harper & Row and our appreciation for their skillful guidance which made the finished work possible.

L.W.P.
J.H.J.

PREFACE TO SECOND EDITION

Continued advances in the field of roentgen diagnosis and the acceptance accorded the first edition have made it advisable to issue this second edition. We have been guided by criticism and advice from many of our colleagues and to them we are deeply grateful.

Much of the recent research interest and development has been in the field of opacification of vessels and organs and cannot be included in a book of this kind which is devoted primarily to the basic fundamentals of roentgen diagnosis. Nevertheless advances have been made in practically all aspects of roentgenology and we have attempted to include as many as possible in this edition.

The basic format of the book has not been changed. The title of Chapter 3 has been changed from "Demineralization of the Skeleton" to "Metabolic and Related Bone Diseases." Otherwise the chapter headings remain the same.

All chapters have been revised to bring them up to date. Considerable revisions have been made in many chapters. New material in this edition includes the following: Crouzon's disease, trigonocephaly, Treacher-Collins syndrome, trisomy 17–18 syndrome, diastrophic dwarfism, congenital indifference to pain, juxtacortical chondroma, massive osteolysis, chondromyxoid fibroma, osteoblastoma, chondrocalcinosis, transient synovitis of the hip, cytomegalic inclusion disease, subclavian steal syndrome, gas in the portal veins, congenital absence of the spleen, cinefluorography, calcification in gastric and colonic carcinomas, intraluminal duodenal diverticulum, intramural hematoma of the duodenum, carcinoid of the small intestine, villous adenoma, inflammation of the appendices epiploicae, nephrotomography, renal angiography, renal cortical necrosis, medullary sponge kidney, renovascular hyptertension, retroperitoneal fibrosis, the megacystis syndrome, vesicoureteral reflux, diagnostic pneumomediastinography, extralobar sequestration, pertussis pneumonia, pneumocystis carinii pneumonia, pulmonary paragonimiasis, diatomite pneumoconiosis, idiopathic unilateral hyperlucent lung, Goodpasture's syndrome, pulmonary alveolar proteinosis, cirrhosis of the lung, neurenteric cyst, corrected transposition of the great vessels, kinking of the aortic arch and pulmonary artery coarctations.

In addition to the considerable revisions made throughout the text, there are 128 new illustrations. Some of these replace previous illustrations but most are completely new.

While we have been able to eliminate some material, the addition of new matter and illustrations has made it necessary to increase the number of pages.

As in the first edition the photographic work has been done by Mr. Homer Montague and the typing by Miss Lorena Carmichael and to them we express our thanks. We are also grateful to the publisher, Mr. Paul B. Hoeber, for his continued interest and support.

L.W.P.
J.H.J.

Madison

PREFACE TO FIRST EDITION

In preparing this volume, it has been our aim to organize and to set down as concisely as possible what we consider to be the basic facts of roentgen interpretation. Designed to bridge the gap between the elementary text and the multiple-volume reference work, it will, we believe, serve equally well as a review source for the practicing physician and surgeon, for those taking postgraduate training in one of the specialties, and as a textbook for the undergraduate medical student.

We have discussed briefly the roentgen anatomy of the various divisions of the body. The descriptions of disease processes are concise, with discussions of clinical and pathologic features limited to the information necessary to clarify the roentgen observations. The emphasis necessarily is restricted to roentgen diagnosis. All the common and most of the unusual conditions and diseases with positive roentgen findings are included. Roentgen differential diagnosis has been emphasized in the more common diseases. Methods of roentgen examination are described, particularly those dealing with the more complicated diagnostic procedures such as bronchography and myelography. The care of the patient before and after such investigations is important, and the referring physician should have some idea of what the examination entails and the way in which it is conducted. Technical methods are likely to vary somewhat from one institution to another; those described here are used by us at University Hospitals and give a general concept of the procedures and what they entail.

Descriptions of technical procedures, comments on differential diagnosis, and discussions of rare entities or those of lesser importance have been set in smaller type. We have avoided discussions of controversial matters, indicating only either the existence of controversy or the present lack of knowledge about some subjects.

Because of the variable patterns and the changing character of disease processes, often from day to day, it is possible only to illustrate the signs most frequently encountered. The illustrations have been chosen to present as many facets as possible, but the reader should be aware that only infrequently can a single roentgenogram portray all of the possible variants.

References have been selected carefully to direct the reader to a wide range of literature;

books and articles have been chosen that contain more extensive bibliographies than it would be advisable to include in a book of relatively restricted size such as this.

We have been fortunate in having a group of associates who have been willing to give freely of their time to aid us in many ways. Chapters 1 and 3 have been reviewed by Dr. Edgar S. Gordon and valuable criticisms offered. Dr. D. Murray Angevine has done the same for Chapter 8 dealing with diseases of the joints. Dr. Theodore C. Erickson kindly read Chapters 10 and 11 covering diseases of the brain and spinal cord, Dr. Helen Dickie reviewed the chapters dealing with diseases of the lungs, and Dr. Richard H. Wasserburger, Chapter 31, the cardiovascular system. To these and many others who gave us advice and encouragement go our most heartfelt thanks.

Dr. Margaret Winston prepared the drawings for Figures 252, 253, 274, and 276. Dr. Arthur Chandler, Jr., prepared those for the chapters dealing with diseases of the cardiovascular system and the lungs. Other members of our staff who aided us in many ways during the preparation of the manuscript and the selection of illustrative material include Drs. Charles Benkendorf, Robert F. Douglas, Joyce Kline, Lee A. Krystosek, M. Pinson Neal, Jr., and John F. Siegrist. The photographic work has been under the supervision of Mr. Homer Montague who has personally prepared most of the illustrations. To him goes the credit for the faithful reproduction of the roentgenograms. The typing has been done by Miss Lorena Carmichael with assistance from Mrs. Charlotte Helgeson. Their careful workmanship has made our tasks easier.

Finally we wish to thank the publisher, Mr. Paul B. Hoeber, for his many courtesies and the excellent co-operation we have received at all times. In particular, Mrs. Eunice Stevens of the publisher's staff deserves our gratitude. Her enthusiasm and her skillful guidance have been invaluable aids.

L.W.P.
J.H.J.

Madison

THE ESSENTIALS OF
ROENTGEN INTERPRETATION

INTRODUCTION

DISCOVERY OF ROENTGEN RAYS

The discovery of roentgen rays (x-rays) by Wilhelm Conrad Roentgen, Professor of Physics at the University of Würzburg, Germany, on November 8, 1895, marked the beginning of a new era in medical science. For the first time it became possible to "see through" the intact skin and superficial tissues and to visualize the bones and deeper structures of the body. Improvements in the crude equipment of the early days followed and with the tremendous interest generated throughout the world by the news of the discovery, it was only a short time before methods became available for the study of the body cavities and the visceral structures. The fascinating story of Professor Roentgen's discovery and of the many other scientific advances that preceded it and made it possible is beyond the scope of this book; they have been the subject of numerous articles and books and every student is urged to read the complete story. Following shortly after Roentgen's contribution came the discovery of the radioactivity of uranium by Becquerel and the isolation of the element, radium, by the Curies. Thus was completed the birth of a new science. Radiology, the name applied to this science, is one of the youngest of the medical specialties and yet in the 77 years since its origin it has completely revolutionized the diagnosis and treatment of many diseases, established entirely new concepts of living anatomy and physiology, and has become a tool of research in many phases of scientific endeavor, often in fields remote from the practice of medicine.

The rays that Professor Roentgen discovered he called x-rays after "x," the unknown. It was only a short time, however, before investigations by Roentgen himself determined some of the fundamental properties of the rays and, combined with the investigations of many others through the years, they no longer belong in the category of the unknown. Because of this and to honor their discoverer it has become common usage to refer to them as roentgen rays rather than x-rays and this term will be used throughout this book.

DEFINITION

Roentgen rays are a form of electromagnetic energy of very short wave length (0.5 to 0.06 Å or less). An angstrom unit (Å) is a measure of length, one angstrom being 10^{-8} cm (one hundred-millionth cm). The place of roentgen rays in the electromagnetic spectrum is shown in the accompanying diagram (Fig. 1). Because of their short wave lengths they have the ability to penetrate matter and it is this characteristic that makes them of use in the study of body tissues. In order to understand some of the fundamental properties of roentgen rays it is advisable to review briefly the ways in which they are formed.

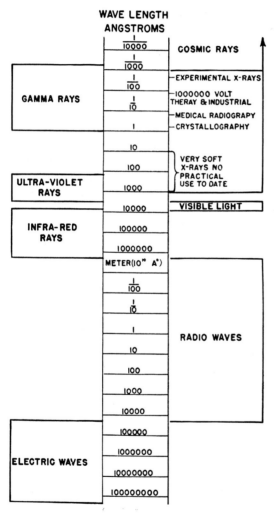

Fig. 1. Diagrammatic representation of the electromagnetic spectrum illustrating the relative position of roentgen rays (x-rays) in relation to the other forms of electromagnetic energy. (*Courtesy General Electric X-ray Corporation, Milwaukee, Wisc.*)

PRODUCTION OF ROENTGEN RAYS

Roentgen rays are formed by the sudden stopping of high-speed electrons. This is accomplished by passing a high-voltage electric current across the terminals situated within a highly evacuated glass bulb (Fig. 2). One of the terminals is called the cathode and it consists essentially of a tungsten wire filament that can be heated to incandescence by a separate current, and a focusing collar around the filament to direct the electron beam toward the other terminal, called the anode. The anode consists of a heavy rod or bar of copper on the face of which is set a small button of tungsten. The face of the anode is called the target. The basic principle of operation of a modern roentgen-ray tube depends upon the fact that metals when heated to incandescence give off free electrons. When the filament in the tube is heated in this manner a cloud of electrons forms about it. When a high-voltage current is applied to the terminals of the tube so that a negative charge is applied to the heated filament and a positive charge to the anode, the electrons will be repelled from the cathode and forced toward the anode. The electrons travel at very high speed and the stream continues as long as the current is applied. These high-speed electrons are known as cathode rays. The focusing collar around the filament focuses the stream of electrons so that they strike the button of tungsten set in the face of the target. This face is set on a slant of approximately 20° from the long axis of the anode stem. The area where the electron beam impinges on the target is called the focal spot and it is here that the roentgen rays are emitted. The size of the focal spot varies in different tubes but usually measures from one to several millimeters in diameter. The velocity of the electrons in the beam depends upon the voltage applied to the terminals. The number of electrons available at the filament depends upon its heat. The cathode-ray output of the filament therefore can be regulated easily by controlling the heat of the filament. When high-speed electrons are stopped by the tungsten target the major por-

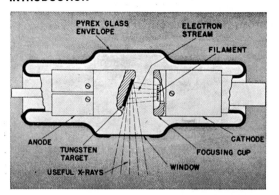

Fig. 2. Diagram of a fixed-focus type of diagnostic roentgen-ray tube. (*Courtesy General Electric X-ray Corporation, Milwaukee, Wisc.*)

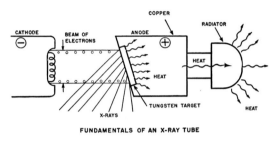

Fig. 3. Diagram illustrating the basic operating principles of a roentgen-ray tube. (*Courtesy General Electric X-ray Corporation, Milwaukee, Wisc.*)

by the electron beam, successive areas of metal along the rim of the disc are brought into the beam and its effect therefore is distributed around the edge of a circle instead of at a single point. The voltages used in diagnostic roentgenology vary from about 35,000 to 150,000 volts (35 to 150 kV). In therapeutic radiology voltages as low as 85,000 are used in the treatment of superficial lesions but for the therapy of lesions involving the deeper structures of the body much higher voltages are employed, and these vary from 200,000 to those in the multimillion volt range.

The majority of the cathode rays striking the target are slowed down gradually and their energies are transformed into heat. Only a relatively small percentage of the total electrons in the beam are stopped suddenly; it is these that have their energies transformed into roentgen rays. Because some of the radiation is produced below the surface of the target, it may be absorbed by the tungsten before it can be radiated into space. Actually, about half of the radiation produced at any given time is absorbed in this manner. The remainder is emitted from the face of the target through an arc of 180°. Because roentgen rays cannot be focused, only a small portion of this beam can be utilized; this portion is confined to a rather

tion of their energy is transformed into heat and only a small part, less than 1 per cent, into roentgen rays. One of the reasons why tungsten is used in the target is because of its relatively high melting point. Copper is used for the stem of the anode because of its heat-transmitting properties (Fig. 3). Various methods are used to dissipate the heat including circulating water, radiator fins attached to the outside of the anode stem, and immersion and cooling of the tube with oil. Most diagnostic roentgen-ray tubes now are of the oil-immersed and oil-cooled type. In order to increase the operating capacity of the tube and keep the focal spot size at a minimum, rotating anode tubes are commonly used (Fig. 4). The anode consists of a disc that is rotated during the exposure. The beam of electrons is focused within a small area along the rim of the disc. Since the disc is rotating during the time that it is being struck

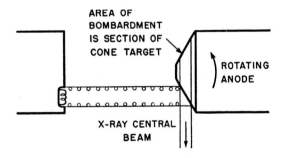

CONSTRUCTION OF A ROTATING ANODE TUBE

Fig. 4. Diagram to illustrate the operation of a rotating target tube. The electron beam from the cathode is focused on a small area of the rotating anode so that the area of bombardment is a circular band on the slanted face of the target. By this means heat is distributed over a fairly wide area, allowing the focal spot to be kept small. (*Courtesy General Electric X-ray Corporation, Milwaukee, Wisc.*)

narrow windowlike opening in the metal cover housing the roentgen-ray rube. The beam often is further reduced in size by the use of metal diaphragms or cones.

CHARACTERISTICS

Roentgen rays travel in straight lines at the speed of light. When a beam of rays passes through matter its intensity is reduced by absorption. This is true even for a gas such as air although the amount of absorption is small. The denser the matter the greater the amount of absorption. Roentgen rays also cause ionization of the substances through which they pass and it is this property, the ionization of gas, which is utilized to measure the intensity of a given beam. In addition to being able to penetrate matter and to be absorbed by it, there are several other characteristics of this form of radiation that make it useful in the study of the body structures.

PHOTOGRAPHIC EFFECT

A photographic film is affected by roentgen rays the same as it is by visible light. The sensitized silver emulsion turns black when it has been exposed to the radiation and the film subsequently processed by development and fixation. When a film protected from light is placed beneath an object, for example a hand, and a beam of roentgen rays of suitable intensity and wave length is passed through it, an image will be produced in the emulsion and brought out by the developing process that will be an accurate representation of the variable densities of the tissues through which the beam has passed. Thus the bones, because they absorb more of the radiation than the soft tissues covering them, will appear as light areas surrounded by the darker soft tissues. The density of the bones is not uniform and, cortex being more compact than the cancellous bone in the medullary cavity, appears lighter on the film. It is this selective absorption by the body tissues that results in an image of the part on the film.

This is, in effect, a two-dimensional representation of the structures within a three-dimensional object. All variations in density overlying a single point will appear as a single composite shadow.

FLUORESCENCE

Another important property of roentgen rays is the ability to cause fluorescence of certain crystalline substances, such as barium platinocyanide, zinc sulfide, and calcium tungstate, or in other words the energy is transformed into visible light. This property is used in fluoroscopy. A fluoroscopic screen consists of a piece of cardboard coated with a thin layer of one of the fluorescent materials such as calcium tungstate in finely divided form. When a part of the body is placed between a tube emitting roentgen rays and such a screen, an image of the part is formed by visible light on the surface of the screen. In contrast to the shadows produced on a film, the denser structures appear the darkest since they absorb more of the rays and prevent them from striking the screen. In radiography, fluorescent screens are used to intensify the effect of the roentgen ray beam. This is done by enclosing the photographic film in a hinged holder known as a cassette. The part of the cassette that will face the roentgen-ray tube is made of a substance such as aluminum or bakelite, which absorbs very little radiation. A fluorescent screen is mounted on the inner surface of each of the leaves of the cassette and the film is placed between them. When the cassette is closed the screens are brought into close contact with the film. The film used in roentgenography differs from ordinary photographic film in that the celluloid base is coated with sensitized emulsion on both sides. When the loaded cassette is exposed to roentgen rays, not only is there a direct effect of the rays upon the film but the image also is registered by means of the visible light from each of the screens. By using intensifying screens the blackening effect of the radiation is increased on the order of 20 times that obtained without screens.

SCATTERING

When roentgen rays pass through matter, not only is some of the radiation absorbed but the character and quality (wave length) of the emergent beam are altered. Some of the rays are deflected and have their directions altered; also, new radiation is produced within the substance. The total effect is known as scattering. Scattered rays may be projected in any direction. Scattered radiation strikes the fluoroscopic screen or the photographic film from many directions other than that of the primary beam. The result is a more or less uniform blackening of the film emulsion with a consequent loss of sharpness and detail of the images. Scattered radiation serves no useful purpose in diagnostic roentgenology and every effort is made to eliminate it or reduce its intensity. This is accomplished by the use of a device known as the Potter-Bucky grid. This consists of a thin grid made of alternating strips of lead and wood set on edge. These are arranged so that they lie in the radii of a circle, the center of which will be the focal spot of the tube. When the grid is placed between the part being examined and the film, only that radiation traveling in a straight direction from the focal spot of the tube can pass through the spaces between the lead strips (Fig. 5). Radiation arising in the body tissues or elsewhere and traveling in any direction but in a line between the focal spot and the film will be absorbed by the metal strips. When the grid is stationary the metal strips cause lines on the film. To eliminate these the grid is kept in motion during the exposure; this blurs the shadows of the lines and they become invisible. Fog also can be reduced by limiting the beam of radiation to as small an area as possible. This is done by means of lead diaphragms placed close to the window of the tube or by means of metal cylinders or cones that limit the size of the beam. For some uses, such as with portable equipment at the bedside, a very thin "wafer" grid is available. The lead strips are so fine that the lines on the film are not objectionable. Stationary thin grids of this type are not

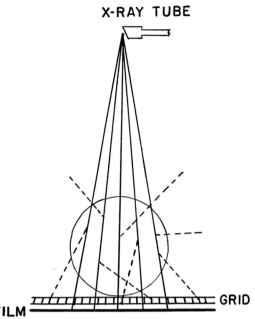

Fig. 5. Diagram illustrating the principles of a grid used to absorb secondary radiation arising in the structure being examined. The vertical lead strips (*solid black lines*) are separated by wood spacers. The lead strips are placed so that only radiation arising at the target of the tube (primary radiation) or traveling in the same direction as the primary beam can pass through the grid to affect the film emulsion. The scattered radiation (*broken lines*) will be absorbed by the lead strips. Lead is very effective in absorbing radiation while wood absorbs very little. Properly constructed grids are very effective in removing unwanted radiation. When a beam of roentgen rays is passed through matter the effect is much the same as when ordinary light passes through fog. The scattering of the radiation causes a blurred image and loss of detail.

as efficient in eliminating scatter as the movable grids but they do clean up fog sufficiently to make their use worthwhile.

BIOLOGIC EFFECTS

The effect of radiation upon living cells has received intensive study; it is this property that makes them useful in the treatment of malignant tumors and other conditions, a subject entirely beyond the scope of this book. It is emphasized that roentgen rays can be lethal to normal tissues, that dangers arise not only from the absorption of relatively large amounts of radiation over a short period of time but also from cumulative effects of very small amounts received over a period of months or years. In diagnostic roentgenology certain exposure limits have been devised that should not be exceeded. Roentgen rays, being a form of ionizing radiation, can add measurably to the total amount of radiation to which the population, as a whole, may be exposed. The fears expressed by geneticists and others concerning the long-range effects of exposure to small amounts of radiation from atomic sources need to be kept in mind but should not unduly influence the use of this valuable procedure when property indicated for the diagnosis and treatment of disease. Anyone who uses roentgen-ray equipment should be familiar not only with the operating characteristics of it, particularly the intensity of radiation emitted under given conditions, but should be fully aware of the hazards of overexposure and the ways to prevent it. (See page 10.)

EQUIPMENT

Modern roentgen-ray generators and the accessories required in diagnostic roentgenology often are complicated devices but the basic principles of construction and operation are not difficult to understand. Only these simplified features will be discussed in this section (Fig. 6).

ELECTRICAL CIRCUITS

The essentials of a roentgen-ray generating circuit consist of the following:

1. A source of alternating current. Usually this is 220 volt, 60 cycle current, although portable units are designed to operate at the bedside on standard 110 to 120 volt circuits. Alternating current is necessary in order that it may be stepped up by means of a transformer to the high voltages needed to produce roentgen rays.

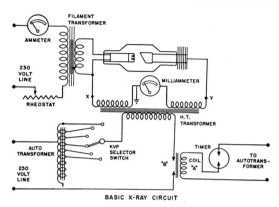

Fig. 6. Diagram of a basic x-ray generating circuit. In this diagram alternating current is supplied to the terminals of the roentgen-ray tube, which acts as its own rectifier (see text). This type of circuit is used in most portable units that operate from ordinary 110 to 120-volt circuits. Most other roentgen-ray generators use rectifying tubes between the secondary of the high-tension transformer and the roentgen-ray tube to change the alternating current to direct current. The autotransformer is used to control the voltage supplied to the high-tension transformer and this, in turn, will determine the voltage in the secondary circuit of the transformer. The filament transformer controls the current that heats the filament of the roentgen-ray tube and this determines the quantity of electrons available for bombardment of the target. (*Courtesy General Electric X-ray Corporation, Milwaukee, Wisc.*)

2. A method for regulating the voltage. This is usually done by a device called an autotransformer by means of which the voltage supplied to the high-tension transformer can be altered without changing the amperage to any great extent.

3. A step-up transformer to increase the voltage of the secondary circuit into the 35 to 130 kV range.

4. A means of rectifying the high-voltage current. A roentgen-ray tube acts most efficiently when direct current is used to energize it. The tube itself can act as its own rectifier and this is done in many portable units. As long as the anode does not become heated to incandescence, the flow of current between the terminals will be, to a large extent, unidirectional since the only source of electrons to allow current flow is at the cathode end. For

greater efficiency, however, it is desirable to have the high-tension alternating current rectified to direct current before it is supplied to the tube. This is done by special rectifying vacuum tubes often called valve tubes because they allow passage of electrical current in only one direction.

5. A means for controlling the quantity of the current flowing through the tube. As indicated in an earlier paragraph this is accomplished by controlling the heat of the tube filament. The filament circuit is a separate one and usually is operated at a low voltage of 10 to 12 volts.

6. Means for protecting against electrical shock and stray radiation. Because of the high voltages employed in the production of roentgen rays special shockproof cables are used to convey the high-tension current from the transformer to the roentgen-ray tube and the tube is immersed in oil. The tube is made rayproof by a metal casing which encloses it and which allows rays to escape only through a window placed beneath the target.

FLUOROSCOPES

Fluoroscopy consists in viewing the image produced when roentgen rays strike a fluorescent screen. In order to prevent damage to the skin of the patient and because roentgen-ray tubes cannot be operated at high current and voltage values for more than a few seconds at a time, fluoroscopy is done with a low current value, usually on the order of 3 to 4 mA.* The intensity of the screen illumination is so low that the retina must be dark-adapted before adequate visualization is obtained. Normally this requires a period of about 20 minutes in the dark and this waiting period is essential if satisfactory visualization of the fluoroscopic image is to be obtained. Most fluoroscopes are incorporated into tables that can be tilted from the horizontal to the erect position, often through an arc of 180°. The roentgen-ray tube is placed beneath the radiotransparent table

---

* One milliampere (mA) equals $\frac{1}{1000}$ ampere.

top, the latter being made of bakelite or similar material that has a low degree of absorption of roentgen rays. The fluoroscopic screen is mounted in a frame above the table, the screen and tube being attached to one another so that they can be moved in unison from one end of the table to the other. The screen is covered with a panel made of leaded glass to protect the operator from the direct beam of rays. Movable lead shutters are available that can be used to limit the beam to a small area. A device is usually incorporated in the screen mounting that will allow a film cassette to be brought into place between the patient and the screen so that the image may be recorded on film whenever it is desired. Roentgenograms made under fluoroscopic control are often referred to as "spot films."

Photofluorography. It is possible to photograph the image produced on a fluoroscopic screen since it is registered in visible light. This procedure is known as photofluorography. The camera and the fluoroscopic screen are enclosed in a lightproof hood so that only the illumination from the screen can enter the aperture of the camera. Photofluorography has found its greatest usefulness in roentgenography of the chest as a part of mass surveys of large groups of apparently healthy persons. The most commonly used film size is 70 mm. This size is small enough so that the film cost is kept at a minimum, roll film can be used in the camera, and the films can be viewed with little or no magnification. Photofluorography of the chest is essentially a screening procedure. When abnormal changes are found in the miniature film further investigation, including the use of standard size roentgenograms, usually is desirable. While the method was devised to assist in tuberculosis case finding, experiences during World War II when millions of persons were examined by the method showed that many other abnormalities of the lungs and cardiovascular system could be identified. Photofluorography of the thicker and denser parts of the body, particularly of the abdominal viscera, has not been very successful until recently because of the long exposure times required. Cameras now are available that are sufficiently "fast" so that the method can be used for radiography of the stomach and intestinal tract as well as other abdominal viscera.

IMAGE INTENSIFICATION. The faint illumination of the fluoroscopic screen requires a period of dark adaptation on the part of the examiner and once adapted to the dark, vision is by means of the retinal rods rather than the cones. Rod vision enables the retina to detect the low intensities of light but detail is poor; this is a function of the retinal cones. To enable fluoroscopy to be done in a lighted room without adaptation to the dark requires a considerable amplification of the fluoroscopic intensity. There is now available a device known as an image intensifier, which is capable of increasing the intensity of the fluoroscopic illumination from 200 to 1000 or more times. This is accomplished by means of electronic amplification using a special electron vacuum tube. In most current models the scanning area of the tube is limited to a field of from 5 to 9 inches in diameter. The larger tube has come into use recently and is of a satisfactory size for fluoroscopy and cinephotography. The unit also is rather bulky and the reduced image at the eyepiece of the tube needs to be magnified by lenses and mirrors before it can be viewed with comfort. The degree of amplification of the illumination is such, however, that fluoroscopy can be done in a lighted room without any adaptation whatsoever. In fact, in order to obtain the benefit from cone vision, adaptation is to be avoided. Fine structures are visualized that are difficult if not impossible to recognize by standard fluoroscopy. Pulsation of vessels in the thorax and of the cardiac chambers can be seen to better advantage. The image can be recorded directly on movie film by attaching a standard movie camera to the eyepiece of the image amplifier tube, and even "slow motion" movies can be made. It is also possible to televise the image substituting a television camera for the movie camera. The image then can be viewed on a monitor by a number of persons at one time, either in the same room as the fluoroscope or, by means of a closed circuit, transmitted to television receivers in distant class or conference rooms.

At the present time the image intensifier finds its greatest usefulness in certain phases of gastrointestinal roentgenology, in cardiac catheterization, in angiographic examinations, and in research investigations on certain physiologic actions where motion plays a part (the act of swallowing, the study of gastric peristalsis, and similar phenomena). Image intensification has exerted a profound influence on the practice of diagnostic roentgenology.

FURTHER OBSERVATIONS

MAGNIFICATION AND DISTORTION

It is important for the student beginning the study of the use of roentgen rays in diagnosis to realize that certain laws dealing with light with which he is familiar also hold true for this type of radiation. There is always some magnification of the object being examined, depending upon its distance away from the film. The farther it is away from the film and the closer to the tube the greater the magnification of its image on the film. Only when a relatively thin part such as a finger is placed in close contact with the film is there absence of appreciable magnification. Because roentgen rays obey the inverse square law (the intensity varies inversely with the square of the distance from the source) the tube-film distance must be kept within certain limits, otherwise the length of exposure must be prolonged unduly. Thus doubling the distance of the tube from the film requires a fourfold increase in roentgenray intensity to achieve the same degree of film blackening. For most parts of the body this distance varies from 30 to 40 inches and the part to be examined must be kept as close to the film as possible. Chest radiography is done routinely at a distance of 6 feet because it does not require very much radiation to penetrate the air-filled lungs and by using the longer distance a more accurate representation of cardiac size is obtained. The image of an object often is distorted because not all parts of it are at the same distance from the film.

Because roentgen rays are not produced at a point source, the farther an object is from the film the more unsharp will its borders become. In a previous paragraph it has been pointed out that the focal spot where roentgen rays are emitted in the tube must be of a measurable size, usually on the order of 1 to 2 mm, because of the intense heat generated at the point where the cathode rays strike the target. Other factors being equal, the tube with the smallest focal spot will produce film images with the greatest detail; also the capacity of such a tube (the amount of current that can be passed through it and therefore the quantity of roentgen rays that can be produced before damage is caused to the tube) will be curtailed correspondingly (Fig. 7).

TERMINOLOGY

The terms roentgenogram, radiograph, x-ray film, and x-ray negative are synonymous but the first is preferred. These terms refer to the finished film that has been exposed to roentgen rays and then records in black and white or in varying shades of gray the structures through which the roentgen-ray beam has passed. The commonly used term "x-ray plate" has no place in modern terminology since it refers to the early days of roentgenology when glass photographic plates rather than flexible cellulose films were used as the recording media.

STANDARD POSITIONS

For most examinations it is essential that at least two views be obtained, preferably at right angles to each other. The observation of any object is facilitated by observing it from more than one vantage point. The two-dimensional character of the roentgen-ray image makes it possible for a dense structure to overlie a less dense part and thus completely obscure it. The size and shape of an object and the relationship of one object to another cannot be appreciated from a single projection. Standard positions usually consist of frontal and lateral views. If for the frontal projection the anatomic structure of greatest interest lies closest to the posterior surface of the body, the part is placed so that its posterior surface is closest to the film holder. This is done to improve detail of the object being examined. Since the beam of roentgen rays will pass through the body traveling in an anteroposterior direction, such an exposure is described as an anteroposterior view (AP view), the designation indicating the di-

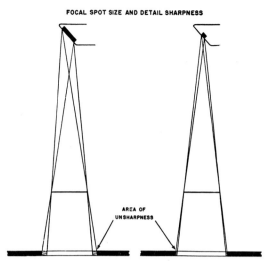

FOCAL SPOT SIZE AND DETAIL SHARPNESS

AREA OF UNSHARPNESS

Fig. 7. Diagram illustrating the effect of focal spot size on detail sharpness. This is known as the penumbra effect. For a given focal spot size, detail also will be influenced by the distance of the object being examined from the film. (*Courtesy General Electric X-ray Corporation, Milwaukee, Wisc.*)

rection taken by the roentgen ray beam in relation to the body surfaces. Lateral views are designated as right or left lateral, depending upon which side is nearer to the film. Oblique positions (usually 45° of obliquity) also are in frequent use and these are described according to the relation of the body surface to the film. Thus in a right anterior oblique view of the chest the patient would be facing toward the film holder with the tube behind him and with the right anterior surface of the body against the film holder.

At times it is impossible to obtain satisfactory projections except in one plane and some anatomic parts are difficult to examine in more than one direction. For the study of complicated anatomic structures, such as the base of the skull or other portions of the cranial vault, it often is advisable to make stereoscopic roentgenograms. Stereoscopy is a method whereby a three-dimensional image may be visualized from a two-dimensional film. The method consists of making two exposures of a part, the two films being in the same relative position to the part at the times of exposure but the tube being shifted a distance approximately equal to the interpupillary distance of the eyes. These films are viewed in a stereoscope, which consists of two viewing boxes and a set of mirrors so arranged that one eye sees one film while the other eye sees only the second film. Since the films were exposed from slightly different angles, the eyes view the film images from different points of view and the brain registers the composite image as one with depth, or in other words as a three-dimensional object. The principle of roentgen-ray stereoscopy does not differ in any way from that with which most individuals are familiar when dealing with photography.

RADIATION HAZARDS IN DIAGNOSTIC ROENTGENOLOGY

The use of roentgen rays for diagnostic purposes has increased at a rapid rate since their discovery by W. C. Roentgen in 1895. Radiologists have long been aware of the hazards of ionizing radiation, and protective measures have been developed and used for years. The National Council on Radiation Protection has made recommendations regarding methods of protection and maximum permissible radiation dosage.* The dose has been gradually decreased through the years to the current permissible weekly level of whole body radiation of 100 mR per week, 400 mR per month, 1250 mR per 13 week period and 5000 mR per year for workers for whom radiation is an occupational hazard.

Radiation exposure is measured in roentgens. The roentgen is the amount of radiation that produces a specific amount of ionization in 1 cm^3 of air at standard conditions. The rad is the unit of absorbed energy or dose. One rad is equal to 100 ergs per gram of tissue, and in the discussion of roentgen-ray dosage, 1 rad is equal to 1 R of exposure. The rem is the unit of absorbed dose, which takes into account the relative biologic effect of varying types of ioniz-

* National Council on Radiation Protection, Reports No. 17, 33 & 34. NCRP Publications. P.O. Box 4867, Washington, D.C. 20008

ing radiation; for roentgen rays, 1 rem can be considered equivalent to 1 R.

The effects of radiation usually considered are the somatic and genetic ones because of the difference in doses necessary to produce injury and also because of the importance of genetic effects of radiation on an entire population. The somatic effects may be local or general. Local injuries can be avoided by the proper use of radiographic and fluoroscopic equipment. Very few general effects have been documented in humans as a result of diagnostic x-rays, but there is some evidence that the incidence of leukemia is doubled in children of mothers who during pregnancy have had roentgen pelvimetry and have thus been exposed to small doses of general body radiation. There is some evidence suggesting that the incidence of leukemia in radiologists is higher than in other physicians who are not exposed to as much radiation. Among the survivors of the Hiroshima and Nagasaki atomic bomb explosions, the incidence of leukemia was increased roughly in inverse proportion to the square root of their distance from the hypocenter of the explosion. The great majority of those developing leukemia had complaints referable to radiation exposure; the dose rates were high, far beyond those used in diagnostic roentgenology. There is evidence to suggest an increase in carcinoma of the thyroid in patients who have received therapeutic irradiation of the thymus in infancy.[6] Animal experimentation has shown that whole body irradiation can shorten life, but the doses used have been relatively large. There is no conclusive evidence to show any shortening of the life span even in radiologists who are exposed to much more radiation than would be received by a patient as the result of diagnostic use of roentgen rays.

The genetic hazards must be considered on the basis of the entire population rather than on the basis of individual exposures. The genetic effect of radiation is based on the production of mutations, the majority of which are undesirable. The number of mutations produced is directly proportional to the gonadal dose, regardless of intensity or time lapse between exposures. This means that 100 R delivered in one sitting has the same genetic effect as the same dose given in small amounts over a long period of time.[2] Some recent evidence shows, however, that there may be some gonadal cellular recovery following small doses of radiation. The committee on genetic effects of atomic radiation of the National Academy of Sciences[10] has estimated that a total dose of 30 to 80 R to the gonads of the entire population would be required to double the existing mutation rate in humans. The committee has used a doubling dose of 50 R as a basis for their calculations of long-range genetic effects. It has further suggested that, up to the age of 30, the general public receive no more than 10 R over and beyond the background of radiation from natural causes. It considered this dose to be reasonable, although not entirely harmless. These figures may require revision in later years. In the meantime, it is necessary to use all possible measures to keep the gonadal dosage from diagnostic use of roentgen rays to the lowest possible limit.

Radiation dosage in various roentgen diagnostic procedures has been measured by numerous investigators and has been the subject of a number of reports. Actual dosages recorded vary considerably in these reports. For example, the dose to the female gonads in pelvimetry ranges from 150 mR (1 mR equals 0.001 R) to 7500 mR, and the dose to the fetus during pelvimetry ranges from 2000 mR to 9000 mR or more. In contrast to this, the gonadal dose in a routine posteroanterior examination of the chest ranges from no detectable radiation to 0.36 mR, while the skin dose to the posterior chest wall ranges from 8 to 190 mR.[7] In the Department of Radiology of University Hospitals, where a high kilovoltage technique is used, the average skin dose to the chest is 27 mR. Doses in fluoroscopy are considerably higher and range from 5 to 10 R or more per minute of exposure.

When the hazard of radiation injury is recognized, it is possible to take precautions to decrease the amount of radiation to the patient, particularly to the gonads, since the gonadal effect is of the greatest long-range importance to the entire population. In most planned and definitely indicated radiologic examinations, the benefit to the patient outweighs the potential hazards, so that no procedure should be condemned when there are indications for it. On the other hand, unnecessary procedures should be avoided. For example, routine roentgen pelvimetry cannot be justified, but in a given individual the value of pelvimetry may far outweigh its potential hazard. The physician who uses radiographic or fluoroscopic equipment should know the output of the equipment and should know how to use it.

A number of specific measures can be taken to decrease the amount of radiation:

1. Filtration. A minimum of 2 mm of aluminum filtration should be used on all fluoroscopes and radiographic units. This results in significant reduction in radiation to the skin in the center of the beam.

2. Cones. Cones or collimating devices of various sizes can be used to limit the exposure to the area undergoing examination.

3. Voltage. The highest voltage consistent with good technique is recommended because it reduces the total radiation exposure.

4. Distance. Radiation dose is inversely proportional to the square of the distance from the source (target of x-ray tube). It is therefore important that the maximum distance consistent with good technique be used in radiography and that the tube be at least 18 inches from the nearest part of the patient in fluoroscopy.

5. Protective devices. Various commercial devices are available to protect those parts of the body not in the area of interest. Lead-rubber aprons or sheets can be used to cover most of the body during dental roentgenography or in examination of the extremities. Special leaded strips can be made to cover the female pelvis and male gonads when the hips or adjacent femurs are being examined.

6. Films and screens. High-speed intensifying screens and fast films should be used to reduce dosage.

7. Image amplifiers. These devices are now in general use, and the apparatus now available reduces the dosage significantly.

8. Fluoroscopy. Because of the high dosage to the patient, fluoroscopy should be held to a minimum. The lowest amperage consistent with adequate visualization and the smallest fluoroscopic field compatible with visualization should be used. In addition, the use of a built-in timer with an automatic shut-off device is desirable.

All physicians should be aware of the potential danger of ionizing radiation, although necessary radiographic procedures can often be done with little or no gonadal exposure if proper precautions are taken. The protection of the gonads is particularly important in the population below the age of 30. The pregnant female must also be protected, and procedures that irradiate the fetus in utero should be held to a minimum.

REFERENCES AND SELECTED READINGS

1. CHAMBERLAIN, W. E.: Fluoroscopes and fluoroscopy (Carman lecture). *Radiology 38:* 383, 1942.

2. CROW, J. F.: Genetic considerations in establishing radiation doses. *Radiology 69:* 18, 1957.

3. FILES, G. W.: *Medical Radiographic Technique,* 2nd ed. Springfield, Ill., Thomas, 1951.

4. GLASSER, O.: *Dr. W. C. Röntgen.* Springfield, Ill., Thomas, 1945.

5. GLASSER, O., QUIMBY, E. H., TAYLOR, L. S., and WEATHERWAX, J. L.: *Physical Foundations of Radiology,* 3rd ed. New York, Hoeber, 1961.

6. HODGES, P.C.: Health hazards in the diagnostic use of x-ray. *JAMA 166:* 577, 1958.

7. LAUGHLIN, J. S., MEURK, M. L., PULLMAN, I., and SHERMAN, R. S.: Bone, skin and gonadal doses in routine diagnostic procedures. *Am. J. Roentgenol. Radium Ther. Nucl. Med. 78:* 578, 1953.,

8. LEWIS, E. B.: Leukemia and ionizing radiation. *Science 125:* 578, 1953.

9. MORGAN, R. H.: Protection from roentgen rays. *Am. J. Med. Sci. 226:* 578, 1953.

10. NATIONAL RESEARCH COUNCIL: *The Biological Effects of Atomic Radiation.* Washington, D.C., National Academy of Sciences, 1956.

11. RHINEHART, D. A.: *Roentgenographic Technique,* 4th ed. Philadelphia, Lea & Febiger, 1954.

12. SANTE, L. R.: *Manual of Roentgenological Technique,* 13th rev. ed. Ann Arbor, Mich., Edwards, 1946.

Section I

THE OSSEOUS SYSTEM

1

DISTURBANCES IN SKELETAL GROWTH AND MATURATION

OSSIFICATION OF THE SKELETON

At birth the shafts of the long tubular bones are ossified but the ends, with a few exceptions, consist of masses of cartilage, the *epiphyses*. Cartilage is relatively radiolucent as compared to bone and has the same general density as the soft tissues. Thus at birth the ends of the bones are separated by radiolucent spaces representing the cartilaginous epiphyses. At variable times after birth, one or more ossification centers appear in the epiphyses (*epiphyseal ossification centers* or EOC). The exceptions occur in the distal femoral and proximal tibial epiphyses where ossification centers appear during the last 1 or 2 months of intrauterine life. The short tubular bones are similar to the long except in having an epiphysis at only one end. The carpal bones are cartilaginous at birth. In the tarsus, normally, ossification centers are present at birth for the calcaneus, navicular, and talus. The other tarsal bones are cartilaginous. For the vertebrae three ossification centers are present, one for the body and two for the arch. Shortly after birth the two halves of the lamina fuse, beginning first in the lumbar area and ascending to the cervical. Union of the arches to the bodies begins in the third year of life and is completed about the seventh year. Here fusion begins in the cervical area and is completed in the lumbar. The cranial bones have ossified but remain separated by fibrous tissue sutures. The individual pelvic bones are present but separated by cartilaginous plates or epiphyseal masses.*

The few epiphyseal ossification centers present at birth, particularly that for the distal femur, are useful indicators of skeletal maturity and since these often can be recognized in roentgenograms of the mother's abdomen during the last month of gestation they also serve as valuable indicators of fetal maturity.

The process of bone formation in cartilage is known as endochondral ossification. The bones grow in length by this means. Some bones are formed in membrane; the bones of the cranial vault are principal examples of this process. In the mandible and clavicle ossification occurs both in cartilage and in membrane. The tubular bones grow in their transverse diameters by bone formation by the osteogenic cells of the inner layer of the periosteum. This is a form of bone formation in membrane. Since the cortices of the bones are formed in this way and

---

* Only the briefest résumé of this important subject will be given here in order to define some of the terms that are used in describing the bones during the developmental period. For a more complete discussion the references listed at the end of the chapter should be consulted.

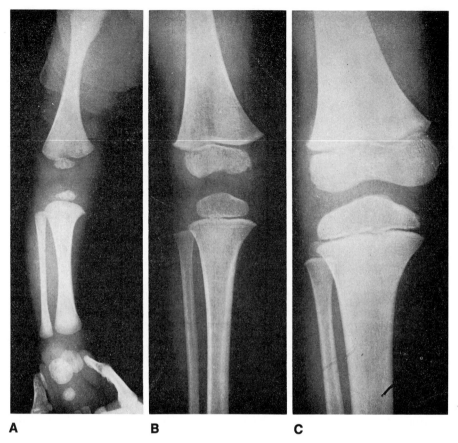

A   **B**   **C**

Fig. 1-1. Normal ossification at the knee. *A,* One-month-old infant. The epiphyses at the knee are largely cartilaginous but ossification centers have formed for the femur and tibia. The apparent "space" between the ends of the bones is occupied by the cartilaginous component of the epiphyses. The radiographic density of cartilage is similar to that of muscles and ligaments, therefore the margins of the cartilaginous epiphyses cannot be clearly identified. *B,* Child 2 years of age. The ossification centers have grown. Note the white transverse zones marking the ends of the shafts. This is the zone of provisional calcification. A few fine, transverse lines are visible in the shafts, the so-called growth lines (see text). *C,* Child 5 years old. The epiphyses have developed to a point where the ends of the bones resemble those of an adult so far as shape is concerned. A cartilaginous plate remains between the epiphysis and metaphysis, the epiphyseal plate.

the cortex makes up the bulk of a tubular bone, it can be appreciated that much of the mass of the skeleton is formed in membrane.

THE BONES IN INFANCY AND CHILDHOOD

After an epiphyseal ossification center appears at or near the center of the epiphysis it gradually enlarges and takes on the shape which is distinctive for the end of that particular bone. In some areas there is more than one ossification center and they may appear at different times (e.g., the distal humerus). The ossified epiphysis remains separated from the shaft by a cartilaginous disc or plate known variously as the epiphyseal plate, growth plate, or physis. The epiphyseal plate gradually be-

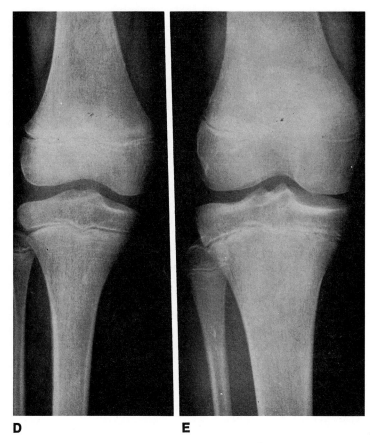

D   **E**

Fig. 1-1 (Continued). *D,* The patient is 8 years old. The epiphyseal plate remains distinct. When the plate becomes this thin it often is referred to in roentgen terminology as the epiphyseal line. There are a few growth lines in the upper end of the tibial shaft. *E,* The patient is 12 years old. The epiphyses have ossified almost completely but thin epiphyseal plates remain. Longitudinal growth can continue until these plates disappear and the epiphyses fuse to the shafts. (Figures *A* through *E* are of different individuals but are shown in true proportions to one another to illustrate growth in size of the bones as well as ossification of the cartilages.)

comes thinner as growth proceeds until it finally ossifies, the epiphysis fuses to the shaft and growth in length is complete (Fig. 1-1).

The times of appearance of the various epiphyseal ossification centers are good indicators of the skeletal age of the individual during infancy and early childhood. Similarly, the times of fusion of the epiphyses can be used as indicators of skeletal age during late adolescence.

The end of the shaft of a tubular bone is bounded by a thin radiopaque line or zone, the *zone of provisional calcification.* This is the area where mineral salts are deposited temporarily around the degenerating cartilage cells. Subsequently blood vessels grow into the lacunae left by the degenerated cartilage cells bringing with them the osteoblasts. These are a specialized connective tissue cell, one of whose main functions is the production of osteoid. Osteoid is the organic matrix in which mineral salts are deposited to make bone. Osteoid also is relatively radiolucent and any large amount of it will cause the bones to appear more translucent than is normal. As osteoid is formed, the zone of provisional calcification, which has acted as a framework for bone formation, disappears on the shaft side and is replaced by trabecular bone. It is replaced on the epiphyseal side so that, normally, it never disappears until the epiphysis fuses to the shaft. It is seen in roentgenograms as a narrow radiopaque line or zone marking the end of the shaft. The area at the end of the shaft where active bone formation is taking place is known as the metaphysis and includes the zone of provisional calcification. It is rather frequent during childhood to see one or more thin opaque lines crossing the shaft near its ends. These are commonly known as "growth lines" and while there may be other causes for them, it is probable that in most cases they indicate a temporary cessation of orderly ossification brought about by one or more episodes of systemic illness.

In summary, the following are definitions of some of the terms used in describing the bones during infancy and childhood:

1. Diaphysis—the shaft of a tubular bone.
2. Epiphysis—the cartilaginous end of a bone.
3. Epiphyseal ossification center (EOC—the ossified portion of an epiphysis).
4. Metaphysis—the end of the shaft of a tubular bone where active bone formation takes place.
5. Epiphyseal plate—the cartilaginous plate separating the EOC from the metaphysis. It also is known as the growth plate or the physis. When it has become thin as a result of growth it sometimes is called the epiphyseal line.
6. Zone of provisional calcification—the layer or zone of deposition of mineral salts at the end of the shaft which serves as a framework for the deposition of osteoid. It is seen in roentgenograms as a thin white line or narrow zone.
7. Osteoid—the organic matrix formed by the osteoblasts and which, when mineralized, becomes bone.
8. Endochondral ossification—the process whereby bone is formed from cartilage.
9. Intramembranous ossification—the process whereby bone is formed from membrane without a cartilaginous stage.

DISTURBANCES IN SKELETAL GROWTH AND MATURATION

The relationship of the endocrine glands to the growth and maturation of the skeleton is a very important one. Roentgen examination of the growing skeleton may give valuable information concerning the presence or absence of disturbances of these glands, particularly the thyroid, pituitary, and gonads. Delay in the times of appearance of epiphyseal centers, in their growth and their fusion, may result from deficient secretion by one or more of these glands. Hypersecretion accelerates these processes.

The times of appearance and fusion of the more important ossification centers are given in the accompanying tables. Because there is a significant difference in the rate of development in males and females, separate tables are given for the sexes. The rate of ossification is more rapid in females and maturation of the skeleton occurs sooner than it does in males. In the literature there is some variation in the times given for the appearance and fusion of many of the ossification centers. More information is available concerning the development of the hand and wrist than of other areas. Because most of the centers for the phalanges, metacarpals and carpal bones appear between the time of birth and the age of 6 years, a more accurate idea of the skeletal age can be obtained during this period than is possible during later childhood and adolescence. Because of the more accurate information available concerning the hand and wrist, centers for these bones are listed separately in Tables 1-1 and 1-2. Figures in parentheses after the name of the center indicate the normal variation in time of appearance. After the ages of 13 to 15 years, when epiphyseal fusions begin, the occurrence of such fusions can be used as additional indicators of skeletal maturity. For detailed study and an analysis of the more critical indicators of skeletal development in the hand and wrist the text by Greulich and Pyle[5] should be consulted. This is an atlas illustrating the development of the bones of the

TABLE 1-1. Ossification Time Table (Females)

Centers present	Hand and wrist	Fusion (in yr)	Other bones	Fusion (in yr)
At birth	Capitate (birth to 3 mo)		Distal femur	17
	Hamate (birth to 3 mo)		Proximal tibia	16 to 17
			Proximal humerus (occasionally)	17½ to 20
			Calcaneus	
			Talus	
			Cuboid	
End of 1 yr	Prox. phalanges II, III, IV	15	Coracoid, scapula	14 to 16
	Metacarpal II, III	15	Capitellum	14 to 15
	Distal radius (9 to 12 mo)	17	Proximal femur (1 to 6 mo)	16 to 17
			Distal tibia (1 to 7 mo)	16 to 17
			Distal fibula (1 to 7 mo)	15½ to 17
			Cuneiform III (3 mo)	
End of 2 yr	Triquetrum (18 to 24 mo)		Metatarsals	17 to 20
	Prox. phalanges I, V	15	Prox. phalanges toes 1 to 2½ yr)	18
	Mid. phalanges II, III, IV	14½	Mid. phalanges toes	
	Dist. phalanges I, III, IV, V	13½	(½ to 2½ yr)	18
	Metacarpals I, IV, V	15		
End of 3 yr	Dist. phalanx II	13½	Proximal fibula (2 to 4 yr)	17½ to 20
	Mid. phalanx V	15	Cuneiform I, II (½ to 2½ yr)	
	Lunate (30 to 36 mo)		Tarsal navicular (1 to 3 yr)	
			Dist. phalanges toes (1½ to 4 yr)	18
			Greater trochanter (1½ to 3 yr)	16
End of 4 yr	Greater multangular (36 to 42 mo)		Med. epicondyle humerus	
	Lesser multangular (42 to 50 mo)		(2 to 5 yr)	20
	Navicular (42 to 50 mo)		Patella (2 to 3½ yr)	
End of 6 yr	Distal ulna	16½	Proximal radius (3 to 5½ yr)	14 to 15
End of 8 yr	Pisiform (variable and unreliable)		Trochlea humerus (7 to 9 yr)	14
			Second. calcaneal (5 to 12 yr)	12 to 22
End of 10 yr			Less. trochanter (9 to 14 yr)	16
			Tibial tuberosity (10 to 13 yr)	19
			Olecranon (8 to 11 yr)	14 to 15
End of 13 yr			Lat. epicondyle humerus	
			(11 to 14 yr)	20
End of 15 yr			Inner border scapula	20
			Secondary centers pelvis	21+
End of 17 yr			Medial end clavicle	25

NOTE: Figures in parentheses indicate range of normal variation in time of appearance.

hand and wrist from birth to maturity. Direct comparison of the roentgenogram of the hand of the patient with the illustrations aids in rapid determination of skeletal age. The charts by Camp and Cilley[1] also are useful and give information about times of appearance and of fusion of all ossification centers.

The more important endocrine conditions that may alter the rate of skeletal growth are considered briefly in the paragraphs to follow

TABLE 1-2. Ossification Time Table (Males)

Centers present	Hand and wrist	Fusion (yr)	Other bones	Fusion (yr)
At birth	Capitate (birth to 3 mo) Hamate (birth to 3 mo)		Distal femur Proximal tibia Proximal humerus (occasionally) Calcaneus Talus Cuboid	18 to 19 18 to 19 21
End of 1 yr	Distal radius (12 to 15 mo)	18	Coracoid, scapula Capitellum, humerus Proximal femur (2 to 8 mo) Distal tibia (1 to 7 mo) Distal fibula (1 to 7 mo) Cuneiform III (6 mo)	14 to 16 14 to 15 18 17½ to 19 17½ to 19
End of 2 yr	Prox. phalanges II, III, IV, V Mid. phalanges III, IV Dist. phalanx I Dist. phalanges III, IV Metacarpals II, III, IV	17 16 to 17 15 15½ 17	Prox. phalanges toes (1 to 2½ yr)	17 to 18
End of 3 yr	Triquetrum (24 to 32 mo) Mid. phalanx II Prox. phalanx I Metacarpal I Metacarpal V Lunate (24 to 36 mo)	16 17 15½ 17	Metatarsals Mid. phalanges, toes (1 to 4 yr) Cuneiform I, II (1 to 3½ yr)	18 to 20 18
End of 4 yr	Mid. phalanx V Dist. phalanges II, V Greater multangular (40 to 48 mo)	16 15½	Great. trochanter (2½ to 4 yr) Prox. fibula (2½ to 5 yr) Tarsal navicular (1½ to 5½ yr)	16 19
End of 6 yr	Lesser multangular (60 to 66 mo) Navicular (60 to 66 mo) Distal ulna (60 to 66 mo)	17½	Medial epicondyle (5 to 7 yr) Patella (2½ to 6 yr) Dist. phalanges, toes (3½ to 6½ yr) Prox. radius (3 to 5½ yr)	20 18 15
End of 8 yr	Pisiform (variable and unreliable)		Trochlea, humerus (7 to 9 yr)	14
End of 10 yr			Less. trochanter (9 to 13 yr) Olecranon (8 to 11 yr) Secondary calcaneus (5 to 12 yr)	16 14 to 15 12 to 22
End of 13 yr			Tibial tuberosity (10 to 13 yr) Lat. epicondyle, humerus (11 to 14 yr)	19 20
End of 15 yr			Secondary centers, pelvis Inner border scapula	21+ 18 to 20
End of 17 yr			Medial end clavicle	25

NOTE: Figures in parentheses indicate range of normal variation in time of appearance.

and the ways in which roentgen examination can be useful are described.

HYPOFUNCTION OF THE THYROID GLAND

CRETINISM

Deficiency of thyroid secretion on a congenital basis and present at birth is known as cretinism. It is characterized roentgenologically by the following:

1. The time of appearance of ossification centers is greatly delayed and growth of them, once they appear, is slow. No other disorder causes as severe a delay in ossification as cretinism (Fig. 1-2).

2. The centers that do ossify often are malformed and irregular in shape.

3. Certain epiphyses, notably those for the proximal ends of the femurs, show a tendency to ossify from numerous small irregular centers rather than from a single one as they normally should. The epiphysis does not grow properly and the femoral head develops a flattened shape (Fig. 1-3). It may resemble rather closely the flattened and fragmented epiphysis of osteochondrosis (Legg-Perthes' disease) or that seen in cases of Morquio's disease, and in

dysplasia epiphysialis multiplex. These conditions are discussed in Chapter 2. Roentgen examination also is useful in the follow-up study of cretins who are under treatment and the progress of skeletal development is a good index of the efficacy of therapy.

4. Dental defects, delay in the development and eruption of the teeth, tend to parallel the delay in ossification of the skeleton. The teeth that do erupt are structurally abnormal and subject to caries.

5. Stunting of growth may not be very obvious during infancy but, as the child becomes older, the thyroid deficiency if not treated will result in dwarfism.

6. Other findings that have been noted in cretinism include (a) increased thickness of the bones of the cranial vault with a brachycephalic shape, (b) shortening of the skull base, (c) the fontanelles may remain open for an abnormally long time and wormian bones along the sutures may be present, (d) in severe involvement, some degree of flattening of the vertebral bodies may be noted and a thoracolumbar gibbus with forward slipping of one vertebra on another may occur, (e) slipping of a capital femoral epiphysis (Fig. 1-4), (f) underpneumatization of the sinuses and mastoids, and (g) prognathous jaw.

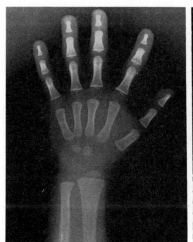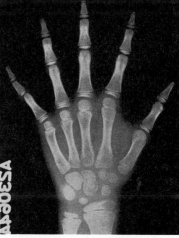

Fig. 1-2. Cretinism. *Left,* Hand of an 8-year-old cretin shows delay in ossification. Compare with (*right*) the hand of a normal 8-year-old child.

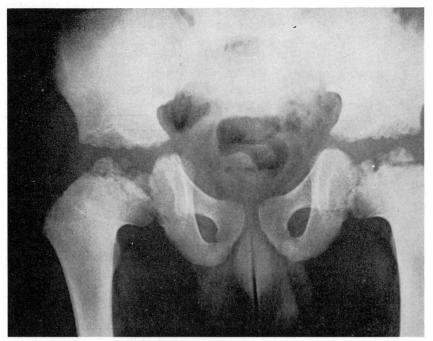

Fig. 1-3. Cretinoid epiphyses. The epiphyses for the femoral heads are ossifying from multiple centers. The femoral necks are broadened.

In many adult cretins little or no residual skeletal deformity persists even though insufficient or no treatment was given.

JUVENILE HYPOTHYROIDISM

When the thyroid deficiency occurs after birth as an acquired disease, the process usually is less severe than it is in cretinism. The term, juvenile hypothyroidism, is used to designate this form of the disease. The roentgen signs will usually be limited to some degree of delay in ossification. In determining the significance of alterations in skeletal age it must be remembered that there is a considerable range of normal variation, and that there is a difference according to sex, females maturing more rapidly than males. It is good practice to allow a variation of 3 months, plus or minus, during the first year of life, and up to 1 year at the end of puberty before considering the skeletal age to be abnormal. This will prevent the unnecessary treatment of children with potent prepara-

tions for supposed hormonal deficiency when none exists.

In chronic cases the metaphyses may appear irregular, somewhat suggestive of rickets. Slipping of the capital femoral epiphyses has been observed (Fig. 1-4). In more severe cases, the roentgen findings may be similar to cretinism.

HYPERFUNCTION OF THE THYROID GLAND

Hyperthyroidism occurring during childhood will cause some acceleration of skeletal development but it seldom is a striking alteration and frequently the skeletal age will remain within or close to the normal range. In chronic cases, particularly in older children, there often is generalized demineralization of the skeleton.

HYPOFUNCTION OF THE PITUITARY GLAND

Decreased function of the pituitary gland during childhood leads to generalized disturb-

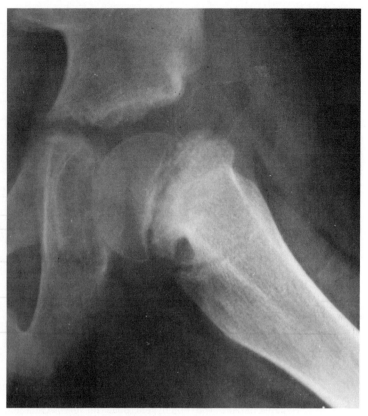

Fig. 1-4. Slipped capital femoral epiphysis in a patient with juvenile hypothyroidism. Note irregularity of metaphysis.

ance in bone growth and maturation since the pituitary is concerned with bone growth both directly and indirectly through the thyroid and the gonads. The epiphyseal centers are slow in appearing and delayed in uniting; at times union may never take place (Fig. 1-5). Since epiphyseal closure is closely related to gonadal function this is generally considered to be an indication of secondary hypogonadism. The bones do not grow normally in length or breadth so that the patients are small in stature, usually well proportioned and with normal mentality, but sexually immature. This condition is known as the Lorain type of pituitary dwarfism.

In many patients there is delay in eruption of the teeth which tend to become impacted because their size is not affected. Since the arrest of skeletal growth occurs during child-hood when the cranial vault is relatively large compared to the facial structures, this disproportion may persist into adulthood. Patients with the clinical signs of hypopituitarism and normal or increased heights have been reported. Slipping of the capital femoral epiphysis has occurred in some patients with the disease.

Decrease in sellar size has been noted in some patients but there still is uncertainty about the significance of the "small" sella particularly when only measurements of the height and anteroposterior diameter are made on a lateral view of the skull. If the width also is measured, then volume determinations can be made and the results may be more meaningful. It should be noted that small sellas have also been found in some other types of dwarfism.

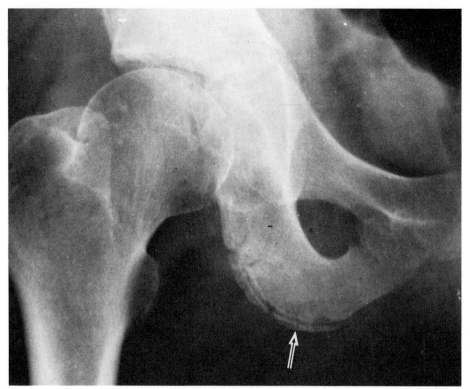

Fig. 1–5. Hypopituitarism. The epiphyseal plate for the ischial tuberosity (**arrow**) has not fused in this 30-year-old female pituitary dwarf.

HYPERFUNCTION OF THE PITUITARY GLAND

Increased secretion by the eosinophilic cells of the anterior lobe of the pituitary gland, either as a result of an adenomatous tumor or from simple hyperplasia, leads to acceleration of bone growth. If this condition develops before growth has ceased it will result in gigantism. If it begins after adulthood has been reached it causes acromegaly.

ACROMEGALY

Increase in length of the bones does not occur in acromegaly, at least to any significant degree, if the disease develops after endochondral bone growth has ceased. Certain well-defined skeletal changes to appear, however, which are characteristic of the disease.

Skull

The cranial bones become thickened and of increased density. The diploë may be obliterated and the cranial bones have the density and appearance of cortical bone. Hyperostotic thickening may develop on the inner table causing the internal surface of the vault to appear shaggy. The nasal accessory sinuses become enlarged and the mastoids overpneumatized. The prognathous jaw, one of the obvious clinical features of acromegaly, can be demonstrated. There may be enlargement of the external occipital protuberance. The sella turcica may or may not be enlarged. In most patients some enlargement is noted and this is caused by pressure erosion from the eosinophilic adenoma that is present. The increase in sellar size seldom is as pronounced as that caused by chromophobe adenoma of the pituitary. The characteristic changes of acromegaly in the cranial bones are shown in Figure 1-6.

Long Bones

While not increased in length the long bones often become enlarged at their ends. This is demonstrated to best advantage in the hands and feet. The heads of the metacarpals and metatarsals become enlarged with irregular bony thickenings along their margins. Diaphyseal width usually remains normal. In some younger patients, however, the shafts of the short tubular bones are narrowed from accentuated growth in length and abnormal resorption along the shafts. The terminal tufts of the distal phalanges enlarge, forming thick bony tufts with pointed lateral margins. These curve proximally and may actually impinge against the phalangeal shafts. Hypertrophy of the soft tissues leading to the typical square, spade-shaped hand can be visualized. Measurement of the heel-pad thickness has been used as an indicator of the increase in soft tissues.[7, 11] This distance is measured from the inferior surface of the os calcis to the nearest skin surface. In the normal this should not exceed 21 mm. However more recent observations indicate that in many obese individuals, heel-pad thicknesses over 21 mm will be found and the same is true of some other persons not overweight. It cannot, therefore, be considered as a completely specific sign. In some patients there is widening of the joint spaces owing to hypertrophy of the articular cartilages. This is best demonstrated in the metacarpophalangeal joints. Degenerative changes in the joints manifested by marginal spurring and sclerosis of articular margins may be seen even in relatively young patients. The general texture of the bones becomes coarsened (Fig. 1-7).

Spine

Calcific spurs may form along the margins of vertebral bodies particularly in the thoracic region and this may be very extensive. The

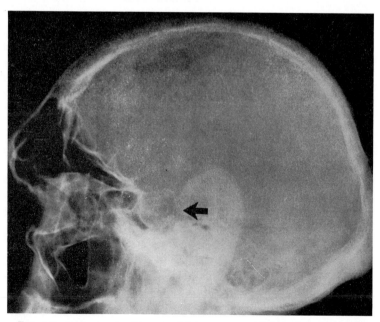

Fig. 1-6. Acromegaly. The cranial bones are thickened and the nasal sinuses enlarged. The sella turcica is moderately enlarged because of an eosinophilic adenoma if the pituitary gland (**arrow**).

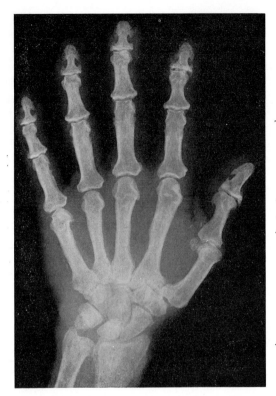

Fig. 1-7. Acromegaly. In the hand, the terminal tufts of the distal phalanges are enlarged. There are spurs at the ends of the bones and they are of generally coarse texture.

HYPOGONADISM

Deficiency of gonadal secretions occurring before skeletal growth has ceased results in delay of epiphyseal closure, therefore the long bones become elongated and slender. The most familiar clinical condition in which this is seen is that which follows surgical removal of the gonads, or atrophy of them from disease, and which is known as eunuchoidism. Delayed fusion of the epiphyses is seen in hypopituitarism and is believed to be caused by secondary hypogonadism in these instances. In contrast to the appearances in eunuchs, the bones in hypopituitarism are small and short, leading to dwarfism.

ACCELERATED MATURATION OF THE SKELETON

Acceleration of skeletal maturation usually is associated with general precocious development and early puberty. Among the conditions in which this is found are the following:

ALBRIGHT'S SYNDROME. This syndrome consists of widespread osseous lesions of fibrous dysplasia and pigmented areas (*café au lait* spots) in the skin. In females there may be precocious sexual development, rapid skeletal growth, and early fusion of the epiphyses. As a result the patients usually show some degree of dwarfism. These latter changes do not occur in males. Fibrous dysplasia is discussed more fully in Chapter 2.

GRANULOSA CELL TUMOR OF THE OVARY. This tumor causes precocious puberty and the skeletal system responds by early closure of the epiphyses.

PINEAL TUMOR. Tumors of the pineal gland may cause precocious puberty in males. Skeletal maturation is accelerated.

HYPERFUNCTION OF THE ADRENAL CORTEX IN CHILDHOOD. This may affect both sexes. In females it causes virilism; in males, sex characteristics are intensified and puberty develops early. The epiphyses fuse prematurely and the patients tend to be dwarfed.

vertebral bodies may actually increase in size. There frequently is an increase in the thoracic kyphosis causing an increase in the anteroposterior diameter of the chest. There is a compensatory accentuation of the lumbar lordosis. The intervertebral discs may be of increased height owing to overgrowth of cartilage.

GIGANTISM

The roentgen features of gigantism are essentially those of an excessively large skeleton because skeletal growth is accelerated and this happens before closure of the epiphyses. Additionally there usually are the signs of acromegaly and if the disease continues to be active after adult life is reached the acromegalic aspects increase. Enlargement of the sella may or may not be present.

REFERENCES AND SELECTED READINGS

1. CAMP, J. D., and CILLEY, E. I. L.: Diagramatic chart showing time of appearance of the various centers of ossification and period of union. *Am. J. Roentgenol. Radium Ther. Nucl. Med. 26:* 905, 1931.

2. DOYLE, F. H.: Radiologic assessment of endocrine effects on bone. *Radiol. Clin. North Am. 5:* 289, 1967.

3. FOLLIS, R. H., JR., and PARK, E. A.: Some observations on bone growth, with particular respect to zones and transverse lines of increased density in the metaphysis. *Am. J. Roentgenol. Radium Ther. Nucl. Med. 68:* 709, 1952.

4. GIRDANY, B. R., and GOLDEN, R.: Centers of ossification of the skeleton. *Am. J. Roentgenol. Radium Ther. Nucl. Med. 68:* 922, 1952.

5. GREULICH, W. W., and PYLE, S. I.: *Radiographic Atlas of Skeletal Development of the Hand and Wrist,* 2nd ed., Stanford, Cal., Stanford University Press, 1959.

6. JACKSON, D. M.: Heel-pad thickness in obese persons. *Radiology 90:* 129, 1968.

7. KHO, K. M., WRIGHT, A. D., and DOYLE, F. H.: Heel-pad thickness in acromegaly. *Br. J. Radiol. 43:* 119, 1970.

8. LANG, E. K., and BESSLER, W. T.: The roentgenologic features of acromegaly. *Am. J. Roentgenol. Radium Ther. Nucl. Med. 86:* 321, 1961.

9. LeMAY, M.: The radiologic diagnosis of pituitary disease. *Radiol. Clin. North Am. 5:* 303, 1967.

10. STEIN, I., STEIN, R. O., and BELLER, M. L.: *Living Bone in Health and Disease.* Philadelphia, Lippincott, 1955.

11. STEINBACH, H. L., and RUSSELL, W.: Measurement of the heel-pad thickness as an aid to diagnosis of acromegaly. *Radiology 82:* 419, 1964.

12. WEITERSEN, F. K., and BALOW, R. M.: The radiologic aspects of thyroid disease. *Radiol. Clin. North Am. 5:* 255, 1967.

2

THE OSSEOUS DYSPLASIAS

The osseous dysplasias consist of a group of disorders characterized by an abnormality in the growth of cartilage or bone or of both.[1] The classification developed by Rubin[27] has received wide acceptance. It was based upon the division of growing bone into four zones, epiphysis, physis or growth plate, metaphysis, and diaphysis. It was considered that the basic disturbance in most of the dysplasias occurred in one of these zones. Each group of dysplasias, epiphyseal, physeal, etc., was further subdivided into hypoplastic and hyperplastic types. McKusick[17] has emphasized the hereditary nature of many of these diseases. More recently Aegerter and Kirkpatrick[1] have presented a classification based largely on the morbid physiology of the cells involved.

It should be noted that in many of these diseases considerable change in the roentgen appearances may occur from infancy to adulthood. Also, many have congenita and tarda types so that a description of the abnormal findings at one age period may not be correct for another.

In the discussions to follow a classification is not attempted but, in general, the listing as given by Aegerter and Kirkpatrick[1] is used with some additions and changes to accommodate more recent information.

STIPPLED EPIPHYSES

Other names applied to this dysplasia include *punctate epiphyseal dysplasia, dysplasia epiphysealis punctata, chondrodystrophia calcificans congenita, Conradi's disease,* and *chondroangiopathia calcarea seu punctata.* Some authorities consider stippled epiphyses to be the *congenita* form of multiple epiphyseal dysplasia and others have commented on the possible relationship of this disorder and multiple epiphyseal dysplasia, spondyloepiphyseal dysplasia, and epiphyseal hyperplasia. Infants frequently are stillborn or die within the first year of life of associated anomalies or of intercurrent disease. The disease is genetically transmitted as autosomal recessive. / dominant -

The characteristic roentgen finding is the presence of numerous small, round, opacities in the unossified epiphyseal cartilages (Fig. 2-1). In some patients, the spots appear to extend into the adjacent soft tissues. They also have been found in other cartilages such as the nasal septum, larynx, and trachea. Stippling of the vertebral cartilages is common in the more severe cases. The extremities may be dwarfed and flexion deformities also may be present. The femur and humerus are most likely to be shortened. In many patients there have been

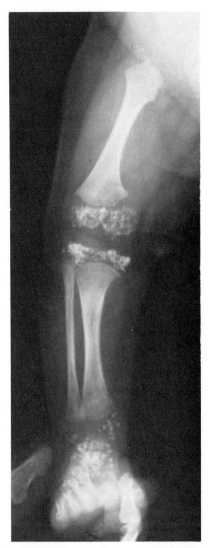

Fig. 2-1. Stippled epiphyses. There are numerous tiny dense foci throughout the cartilages of the skeleton. This figure shows the dwarfed right lower extremity where the foci are most numerous. (Reproduced with the permission of the Editor and Publisher of the American Journal of Roentgenology and Radium Therapy.)

years,[23] dwarfing was severe in the right lower extremity and stippling was extensive throughout the cartilages of the body. The spots gradually disappeared. Normal appearing ossification centers formed which seemed to have no relationship to the abnormal foci. Eventually the epiphyses developed an essentially normal shape. An exception was the proximal femoral epiphysis in the dwarfed right lower extremity. This center was late in appearing and when it did appear it remained small and malformed. Also a left convex thoracic scoliosis developed owing to failure of growth of the right sides of the midthoracic vertebrae. In addition, the fingers and toes may be short and stubby. The carpal and tarsal bones may be normal or show some irregularity in shape.

Chondrocalcification similar to that seen in this disorder also has been noted in the rare *cerebrohepato-renal syndrome,* except that the calcified foci are most marked in the patellae and may be limited to these bones. Other findings in this syndrome as listed by Poznanski and associates[25] include (*1*) marked flaccidity, (*2*) abnormal facies, (*3*) cataracts, (*4*) flexion contractures of the extremities, (*5*) small cortical renal cysts, (*6*) fibrosis of the liver with increased deposits of hemosiderin, and (*7*) abnormality of the cerebrum including lissencephaly and sudanophilic leukodystrophy.

MULTIPLE EPIPHYSEAL DYSPLASIA

The characteristic finding in this dysplasia is the presence of multiple ossification centers for the affected epiphyses giving them a fragmented appearance. The epiphyses may be enlarged and the ends of the long bones may be somewhat flared. The involvement may be limited to a single epiphysis, a pair of epiphyses, or all epiphyses throughout the body. Symmetric involvement of the capital femoral epiphyses is common. Knock-knee or bow-leg deformity may be present and flexion deformities at the knee joint may be seen. The tibias usually are curved. A coronal cleft in the patellas (i.e., "double-layered patella") has

congenital cataracts, saddle nose, hyperkeratotic dermatoses, and failure of proper mental and physical development. If the infant survives it is said that in some cases the foci may ossify and then merge to form a fairly normal epiphyseal center.

In one of our patients, followed for 9

been described[9] as a fairly consistent and characteristic finding in the tarda form.

The vertebrae are usually not involved and the skull is normal. Dwarfing of the extremities, resembling achondroplasia, is present in many and becomes more obvious as the child grows (the pseudoachondroplastic type). The long bones appear to be short and thick. The thickness is an illusion rather than real because of the shortening. An upward sloping, from within out, of the distal articular surface of the tibia is present in about one-half of the patients. The carpal and tarsal bones are often irregular and the digits stubby. In many patients, however, the hands are normal.

The patients usually are brought to the attention of a physician after they begin to walk because of their peculiar waddling gait. Eventually the multiple centers merge and then unite to the shaft. Irregularity of the articular plates frequently persists (Fig. 2-2) and leads to the early development of degenerative joint disease, particularly in the hip joints. At this stage it usually is impossible to determine what the primary disorder was since the other epiphyseal dysplasias may also result in early degenerative joint disease. In mild cases (the *tarda* form of Rubin) the disorder may not be recognized until the arthritic changes bring the patient to the physician. The disease is con-

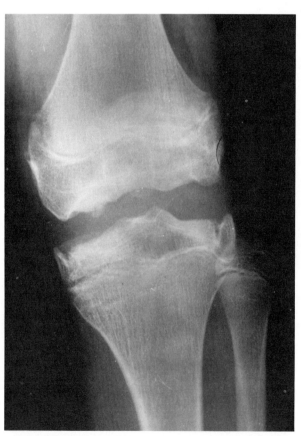

Fig. 2-2. Multiple epiphyseal dysplasia in an adolescent. The other epiphyses for the long tubular bones were affected similarly. The articular surfaces are irregular and will likely lead to the early development of degenerative joint disease.

sidered to be congenital, having a hereditary and familial incidence.

In differential diagnosis, the lack of characteristic changes in the skull and pelvis serves to exclude achondroplasia. The normal vertebrae is significant in excluding Morquio's disease. When the heads of the femurs alone are involved, bilateral Perthes' disease and the epiphyseal dysgenesis of cretinism must be considered.

EPIPHYSEAL HYPERPLASIA

This disorder also has been called *dysplasia epiphysealis hemimelica* (Fairbank) and *tarsoepiphyseal aclasis*. It is essentially an eccentric overgrowth of an epiphysis of a long bone or a small bone of the foot forming an irregular bony mass along one side of the affected epiphysis. Only a single epiphysis is involved; in the great majority it is the talus, followed by the distal femur and distal tibia. Other areas less frequently involved include the upper tibia, upper fibula, lesser trochanter of the femur, and the tarsal navicular and first cuneiform. The bony mass may be attached to the adjacent epiphysis or exist separately. It is usually first noticed during childhood and is asymptomatic until the mass interferes with joint function. Pathologically, the lesion is said to be identical with an exostosis or osteochondroma. However most authorities agree that these latter lesions do not arise from epiphyses.

SPONDYLOEPIPHYSEAL DYSPLASIA

The term, *spondyloepiphyseal dysplasia congenita,* has been used synonymously with Morquio's disease. However, Morquio's disease is now considered to belong to the group of mucopolysaccharidoses. In spondyloepiphyseal dysplasia (SED) growth of extremities and vertebrae is affected and it has been suggested that it is a transitional form between achondroplasia and Morquio's disease. Dwarfism is one of the major features of the childhood form of the disease while precocious degenerative joint disease is the chief finding in adults. The childhood form has also been called *pseudoachondroplastic spondyloepiphyseal dysplasia;* the latent type, *spondyloepiphyseal dysplasia tarda.*

As with many of the other dysplasias, the roentgen signs vary with the age of the patient. In the congenita form, as described in the literature,[32] there is at birth and during early infancy a general delay in ossification. Ossification centers for the distal femurs, proximal tibias, and the calcanei and tali usually are absent and the pubic bones show similar delay. Flattening of the vertebral bodies (i.e., platyspondyly) is present and the posterior parts of the bodies are more decreased in height than anteriorly. The acetabular angles are small. There may be flaring of the anterior ends of the ribs and the thorax is broad and bell-shaped. Lateral bowing of the femurs is frequent. The long tubular bones are shortened with various epiphyseal and metaphyseal abnormalities. In later infancy and early childhood, delay in ossification of the pubis and the femoral heads and necks persists. The vertebral bodies remain flattened and have an ovoid shape in lateral views. Anterior hypoplasia of one or more vertebral segments often is pronounced at the thoracolumbar junction. In the pelvis there is a lack of the normal iliac flare and the ilia appear small in their cephalocaudal dimensions. There is little or no acetabular slant.

In later childhood there is accentuation of the dorsal kyphosis and lumbar lordosis and scoliosis may develop. There is lack of normal ossification of the odontoid process and platyspondyly persists. Ossification of the pubis lags behind the normal, the acetabular roofs are more horizontal than normal and the Y cartilage is wide. Ossification of the femoral heads is still retarded and when they do appear there may be multiple ossification centers.

In the adult there is persisting platyspondyly, hypoplasia of the odontoid, and dysplasia of the proximal femurs with a varus deformity. The hands and feet remain relatively normal. The degree of dwarfism varies from patient to patient and results from both vertebral and long-bone changes.

The most difficult diagnostic problem is that of Morquio's disease. Differentiation is based upon its mode of inheritance, i.e., as a dominant trait, its manifestation at birth, the different roentgen changes, the lack of corneal clouding, and the absence of keratosulfaturia.

In the latent or *tarda form of SED,* the disease often is not recognized until adulthood when precocious degenerative joint disease causes the patient to see a physician. At this stage it may be impossible to recognize the cause of the joint disease as the other epiphyseal dysplasias may lead to similar degenerative changes.

ENCHONDROMATOSIS (OLLIER'S DISEASE)

The basic lesion in this dysplasia is the enchondroma, described as a hamartomatous proliferation of masses of cartilage within the bone.[1] Thus they are radiolucent although spotty areas of calcification within the lesions are common. In some cases the lesions are limited to one extremity or to the extremities on one side of the body. The name, Ollier's disease, has been applied to this form. Even when widely disseminated, the involvement may be more severe on one side of the body. The masses of cartilage and calcified cartilage are found in the ends of the shafts and cause an irregular, club-shaped enlargement of them. The femur and tibia are most often or most severely involved. Stunting of growth of the affected member is common and, at times, a unilateral shortening of one leg has brought the patient to the physician. The epiphyses are not involved. The spine and skull usually are normal. Involvement of the iliac crest and the vertebral border of the scapula has been present in some of the more severe cases.

In the long bones, the lesions may appear as elongated, radiolucent streaks extending in the direction of the long axis of bones and involving the metaphysis and adjacent diaphysis. In the hands and feet, the lesions tend to be globular and cause considerable expansion of the bone (Fig. 2-3). At other times the lesion will involve the entire shaft of one of these short tubular bones.

With growth, the lesions appear to migrate into the shaft. Eventually they may ossify but residual deformity persists.

Maffuci's syndrome consists of a combination of enchondromatosis and multiple cavernous hemangiomas which may be widely distributed throughout the body. The presence of calcified thrombi (phleboliths) may allow roentgen recognition of the vascular lesions. This disease is rare.

Malignant transformation of an enchondroma into a chondrosarcoma can occur, par-

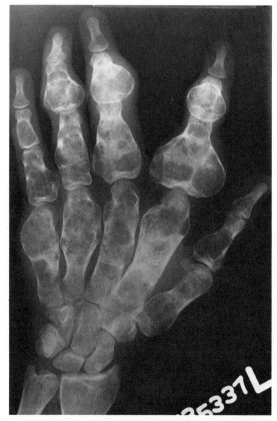

Fig. 2-3. Enchondromatosis involving the hand. The lesions have caused marked expansion of the shafts. Only the terminal phalanges are uninvolved.

ticularly in the lesions in the long tubular bones, and this is one of the common causes of chondrosarcoma in later life.

HEREDITARY MULTIPLE EXOSTOSES (OSTEOCHONDROMATOSIS; HEREDITARY DEFORMING CHONDRODYSPLASIA)

This dysplasia is characterized by the presence of numerous osteochondromas at the ends of the shafts of the tubular bones and in other bones preformed in cartilage. The disorder is inherited, the trait usually passing from the father to his children. Males are affected over females about three to one. The lesions are not present at birth but usually are first discovered during childhood and, as a rule, are asymptomatic unless they cause pressure upon other structures. The lesions are most common at the sites of greatest growth, i.e., at the knee, shoulder, and wrist. The number may vary from a few to hundreds but they are usually bilaterally symmetric. Small lesions in the hands and feet are noted in some patients and the metacarpals and metatarsals may be shortened; in others, the hands and feet are normal. Lesions occur in the pelvic bones, the ribs, scapula, vertebrae, and very rarely, in the base of the skull.

The characteristic lesion is a broad-based, bony outgrowth with the apex pointing away from the nearest joint (Fig. 2-4). It consists of a cortical shell surrounding a core of cancellous bone. The cortex of the lesion merges smoothly with the normal cortex of the bone, and the growth is covered by a layer of cartilage which acts as an epiphyseal plate. This is not visible in roentgenograms. Occasionally the lesion is more pedunculated, with a narrow base and a bulbous outer extremity containing lucent areas of cartilage and stippled areas of calcification similar to the solitary osteochondroma (Fig. 2-5). The osteochondromas originate in the metaphyseal region of the long tubular bones and cause the end of the shaft to be thickened and club-shaped.

In about one-third of the patients there is a characteristic deformity of the forearm owing

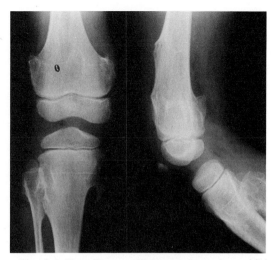

Fig. 2-4. Hereditary multiple exostoses in a child. In the knee area multiple osteochondromas are visualized. The epiphyses are not affected.

to shortening and bowing of the ulna which does not extend far enough distally to take part in formation of the wrist joint. Another characteristic deformity occurs in the necks of the femurs. The neck is grossly thickened, particularly on the undersurface, caused by irregular, bony overgrowth, sometimes likened to candle gutterings (Fig. 2-6). The fibula may be shortened and stunting of growth of other bones is seen in the more severe cases.

Growth of the osteochondromas continues throughout childhood and usually ceases when the nearest epiphysis fuses. Malignant degeneration can occur and is said to have an incidence of about 5 per cent. When an osteochondroma, after a stationary asymptomatic period, begins to enlarge and becomes painful, sarcomatous degeneration should be suspected.

DIASTROPHIC DWARFISM

This dysplasia was first reported by Lamy and Maroteaux in 1960. It is inherited as an autosomal dominant. Characteristics include delay in appearance of the epiphyseal centers, subluxation of various joints, especially the hips, scoliosis, and clubfeet.

The long bones are short and thick with

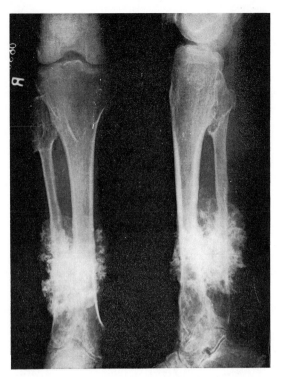

Fig. 2-5. Hereditary multiple exostoses in an adult. An example of the more severe form of the disease with large osteochondromas. In this patient there was some stunting of growth in length but not in breadth so that the bones have some resemblance to the extremities of an achondroplastic dwarf.

widened metaphyses, simulating achondroplasia. In the hands, the bones are short and rectangular, especially the thumb and it may project at a right angle to the other digits ("hitch-hiker's thumb"). The metacarpal of the thumb also may have an ovoid shape. The bones of the feet show changes similar to those in the hands. In addition there is bilateral clubfoot deformity.

The epiphyseal centers are late in appearing and when they do appear, are apt to be flat and abnormal in shape. In most patients, laxity of ligaments and tendons cause subluxation of the joints. Bilateral dislocation of the hips is common. The subluxations are not present at birth but develop after the child begins to walk. Scoliosis also appears at about the same time. Other bones including the vertebrae, the skull,

and the pelvis are normal. The tarsal bones may be distorted because of the equinovarus deformity but otherwise are normal.

The differentiation from achondroplasia, in the average patient, is not difficult if all findings are taken into consideration. The normal appearance of the skull, vertebrae, and pelvis is significant.

THANATOPHORIC DWARFISM

This rare dysplasia was first recognized as a distinct entity in 1967. Previously it probably was mistaken for a severe type of achondroplasia because of its many similar features including dwarfing of the long tubular bones with a relatively long trunk, a prominent forehead with a short skull base and depression of the nasal root, small square iliac wings with horizontal acetabular roofs, a narrow thorax with short ribs, and a decrease from above downward of the interpedicular distances in the lumbar spine. Distinguishing features that have been pointed out[10] include extreme flattening of the vertebral bodies which appear waferlike and with thick intervertebral spaces, very short limb bones with bowing, especially in the lower extremities, and with no reported cases of involvement of other members of the family with the same disorder.

The infants have been stillborn or have died shortly after birth possibly from respiratory failure owing to the short ribs and narrow thorax. However, the cause of death has not been clearly established in most of the patients.

ACHONDROPLASIA

Achondroplasia is an hereditary, congenital, and familial disturbance caused by inadequate endochondral bone formation leading to dwarfism. Bone formation in membrane is not affected. It is the most common form of dwarfism. Achondroplasia has been recognized since antiquity. Many of the affected became court jesters and today many obtain employment in circuses and sideshows as clowns. If an achondroplast marries a person of normal stature there is a 50 per cent chance that their

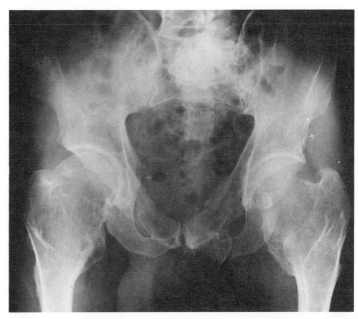

Fig. 2-6. Hereditary multiple exostoses in an adult, illustrating the characteristic appearance of the upper ends of the femurs in this disease. The broad neck with irregular bony overgrowths along the inferior surface has been likened to candle gutterings. There is a large osteochondroma overlying the upper sacrum and another attached to the left pubis.

children will have the disease. If two achondroplasts marry, it is almost a certainty that all of their children will be affected.

Characteristically, the short limb bones contrast with the nearly normal length of the trunk. The facies also is characteristic with a prominent skull vault, saddle nose, and prognathous jaw. Writers frequently comment on the fact that achondroplasts all look as if they belonged to the same family. The following are the most typical changes in the skeleton[1,14,27]:

SKULL. The skull is brachycephalic in shape with a short base and a relatively large vault with frontal bulging. This is owing to the fact that the base is preformed in cartilage while the vault is of membranous origin and thus not affected in growth. Communicating hydrocephalus is said to be common but is seldom severe enough to cause mental retardation. The mandible, also, shows relatively normal growth and thus appears prognathous.

VERTEBRAE. The length of the spinal column may be normal or nearly so but vertebral development is not normal. In infancy the bodies may be quite thin and the intervertebral disc spaces as thick as or thicker than the bodies. The pedicles are short and thick and the posterior surfaces of the bodies are concave. In the lumbar area the interpedicular distances narrow progressively from above downward instead of increasing normally. The net effect is a stenotic spinal canal which, in adult life, may lead to severe neurologic symptoms, especially if herniated disc or degenerative joint disease develops. The lumbar lordosis is increased and the lumbosacral angle becomes more acute than is normal. The sacrum tends to be tilted upwards. One or several vertebrae at the thoracolumbar junction (T-12 to L-3) may be wedge-shaped and crowded backward.

PELVIS. Characteristic changes occur in the pelvis. The ilia are short and square. The sacrosciatic notch is small. The ischial and pubic bones also are short and broad. The acetabular angles are decreased in infancy. The sacrum articulates low on the ilia (Fig. 2-7).

LONG TUBULAR BONES. The shortening of these bones is responsible for the dwarfism. The humerus and femur tend to be relatively more affected than the distal bones of the extremities. The diameter is usually normal but the bones appear thick because they are short. The ends of the shafts are flared. The zone of provisional calcification may be smooth or irregular. At times there is a sizable V-shaped notch in the metaphyses and the epiphyseal

centers may be partially buried in the metaphyses—ball and socket epiphyses (see Fig. 2-10). The fibula often is longer than the tibia causing an inversion of the foot. Bowing of the long bones is common. The distal ends of the femoral shafts tend to be tilted upwards, laterally (Fig. 2-8). Langer[14] has described a rectangular-shaped translucent area in the upper end of the femur caused by an unusual thinning of the bone in its anteroposterior diameter (Fig. 2-9).

SHORT TUBULAR BONES. These bones show changes similar to those in the long bones. They are short and appear thick and the fingers

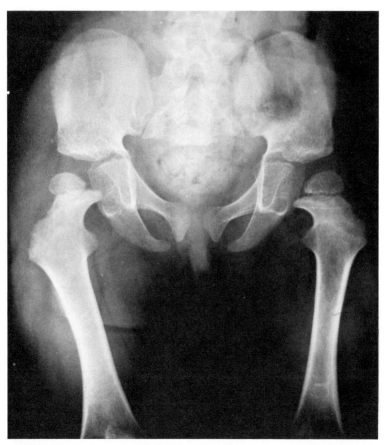

Fig. 2-7. Achondroplasia in a child. Note the short, square-shaped ilia, the short sacrosciatic notches, and pubic bones and the large but shallow acetabula. The sacrum articulates low on the ilia. There is subluxation of the proximal femoral epiphyses and the femurs are short and relatively broad.

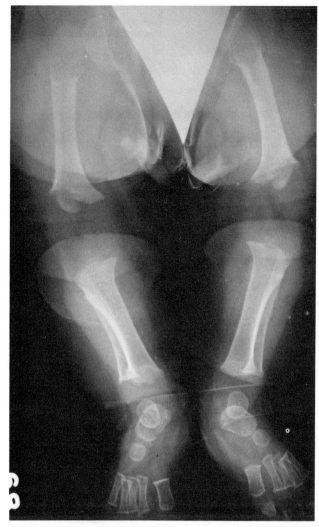

Fig. 2-8. Achondroplasia. Lower extremities of an infant showing short and apparently thick bones. The metaphyses are irregular and the distal femoral metaphyses have an upward outward slant. The thickening is an illusion owing to the decrease in length.

tend to be of similar lengths, i.e., the so-called trident hand (Fig. 2-10). Ball and socket epiphyses are common.

OTHER BONES. The carpal and tarsal bones are normal. The scapula is short and the sternum may be thick and short. The ribs are short causing a decrease in the anteroposterior diameter of the thorax.

In the differential diagnosis of achondroplasia, in addition to the pseudoachondroplastic forms of multiple epiphyseal dysplasia and spondyloepiphyseal dysplasia as described by Rubin,[27] the following entities have been listed by Silverman[29]:

1. Metaphyseal dysostosis (p. 39)
2. Cartilage-hair hypoplasia (p. 38)
3. Hypochondroplasia (p. 38)
4. Ellis-van Creveld syndrome (chondroectodermal dysplasia) (p. 62)

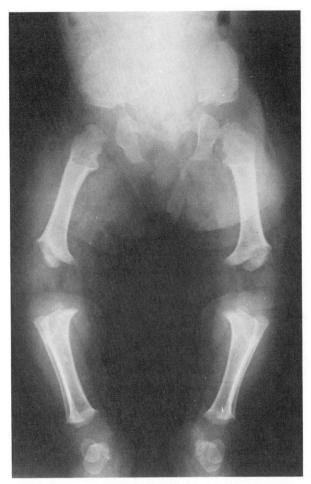

Fig. 2-9. Achondroplasia in an infant. The distal ends of the femoral shafts are tilted upward, laterally and the epiphyses tend to be laterally placed. The bones are short.

5. Asphyxiating thoracic dystrophy (p. 64)

6. Diastrophic dwarfism (p. 33)

7. Dysplasia epiphysealis punctata (stippled epiphyses) (p. 28)

8. Metatropic dwarfism (p. 39)

In addition, thanatophoric dwarfism probably should be included as it is considered by some authors to be a separate disease and not a severe form of achondroplasia. The roentgen changes in these dysplasias, including differential features, have been considered elsewhere in this chapter.

According to some authors, incomplete or mild forms of achondroplasia do not occur. These cases, although uncommon, have been termed *hypochondroplasia* to distinguish them from typical achondroplasia. Thus the skull and pelvis in these patients may be normal or nearly so and shortening of the tubular bones may be less than is seen in achondroplasia.

CARTILAGE-HAIR DYSPLASIA

This dysplasia was found by McKusick[17] among the Old Order Amish of Eastern Pennsylvania and Canada. Dwarfism is noted at birth owing to shortening of the tubular bones of the extremities and it is said that adults seldom exceed 4 feet in height. The epiphyses are normal and the skull is normal, an important point in differentiating this dysplasia from achondroplasia. The hair is fine, sparse, short, and brittle and is said to be char-

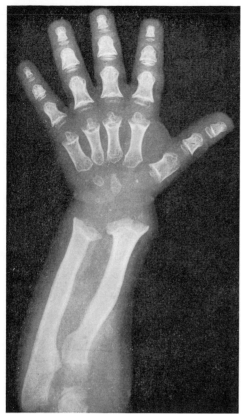

Fig. 2-10. Achondroplasia in a child. The bones of the hand are short and broad and there are "ball and socket" epiphyses at the distal ends of the metacarpals. Note flaring of metaphyses, particularly of the radius and ulna.

acteristic of this dysplasia. Other findings include flexion deformities at the elbows, hyperextensibility of the wrists and fingers, an excessively long fibula and pes planus. The fingers are greatly shortened. The intelligence is not affected. Genetically the disorder is autosomal recessive. At maturity the roentgen findings at the ends of the bones resemble metaphyseal dysostosis.

METAPHYSEAL DYSOSTOSIS

In 1934, Jansen reported a case of dwarfism which resembled achondroplasia except that the skull and epiphyses were normal. The disorder was characterized roentgenologically by a rachitic rosary, coxa vara, genu valgum, and anterior bowing of the femurs. The growth plates of the tubular bones were thickened and irregular owing to extensions of cartilage into the metaphyses. There were no hereditary features.

In 1949, Schmidt reported patients having similar but much less severe changes. Most writers, including Schmidt, have considered the two types to be variants of the same dysplasia. The Schmidt type is relatively common; 21 cases were reported from our department in 1964.[18] The spine and skull are not affected so that the dwarfism is of the rhizomelic type as seen in achondroplasia. The skeletal changes are not present at birth but appear between 3 and 5 years of age. Dwarfism is relatively mild compared to the Jansen type. Bowing of the legs is marked and patients have a waddling gait. Mild to moderate inhibition of growth of all cylindrical bones is present, there is bilateral coxa vara and a tendency for epiphyseal slipping. The hereditary and familial nature of the disease now is well established. Irregularity of the zones of provisional calcification resembles rickets and is caused by extensions of cartilage into the metaphyses (Fig. 2-11). There has been discussion in the past as to whether these cases actually are atypical examples of vitamin-D refractory rickets. In contrast to rickets, the epiphyseal ossification centers usually are normal and the diaphyses, except for bowing, are roentgenologically normal.

METATROPIC DWARFISM

This is one of the recently defined entities that cause dwarfism and which may have been confused, in the past, with achondroplasia.[16] Roentgen changes are apparent at birth with shortening of the long tubular bones and hyperplastic, greatly flared metaphyses. There is overconstriction of the midshafts so that the bones have a dumbbell shape. Epiphyseal ossification centers are delayed in appearance and when they do appear are deformed. The ribs tend to be short with a narrow chest. Kyphoscoliosis is present and there is some degree of platyspondyly i.e., flattening of the vertebrae. In the pelvis the iliac wings are short,

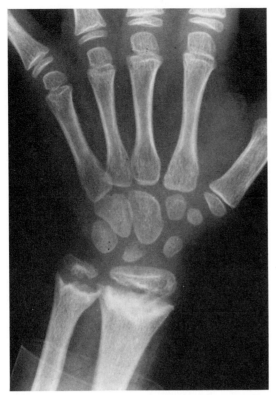

Fig. 2-11. Metaphyseal Dysostosis. The metaphyses of the radius and ulna are concave and irregular. Similar changes are present in the metaphyses of the other long tubular bones. Those of the bones of the hands are not affected.

the sacroiliac notches are short and deep, and the acetabula are horizontal. As the child grows older there is lengthening of the long bones, more than is seen in achondroplasia. However the platyspondyly and the kyphoscoliotic curvature worsen and the child changes clinically from what appears to be achondroplasia to an appearance resembling spondyloepiphyseal dysplasia. In this connection it is to be noted that the base of the skull is not foreshortened and the interpedicular distances in the lumbar spine usually remain normal, findings which aid in differentiating this dysplasia from achondroplasia during infancy.

THE MUCOPOLYSACCHARIDOSES

The mucopolysaccharidoses consist of a group of metabolic diseases. In addition to the skeletal, other tissue systems are involved. Each is characterized by the excretion in the urine of abnormal amounts of one or more mucopolysaccharides and in an abnormality in the elaboration and storage of these substances.[1] Seven types have been defined according to the mucopolysaccharide involved, their mode of genetic transmission, and their clinical and roentgen features.[30]

Type I. Hurler's disease (gargoylism)
Type II. Hunter's syndrome
Type III. SanFilippo's syndrome
Type IV. Morquio's disease
Type V. Scheie's syndrome
Type VI. Syndrome of Maroteaux-Lamy
Type VII. Lipomucopolysaccharidosis

From a roentgen point of view, Morquio's disease and Hurler's disease (gargoylism) are the most important. The others differ one from another chiefly in their nonroentgen manifestations.

MORQUIO'S DISEASE

This dysplasia also has been called *Morquio-Brailsford disease* and *chondro-osteodystrophy.* The term, *spondyloepiphyseal dysplasia congenita,* has been used in the past. The disease is rare and is characterized by dwarfism, kyphosis, and severe disability. The dwarfism is caused primarily by shortness of the spine although some degree of shortening of the long tubular bones is common. Both sexes are affected equally and it is hereditary and familial, the genetic transmission being autosomal recessive. Consanguinity has been noted in some histories.

VERTEBRAE. The most characteristic change is universal platyspondyly, a flattening of the vertebral bodies. The disc margins are irregular and roughened and an anterior, central, tonguelike projection is seen in the thoracolumbar region (Figs. 2-13 and 2-14). Also undergrowth and posterior displacement of one

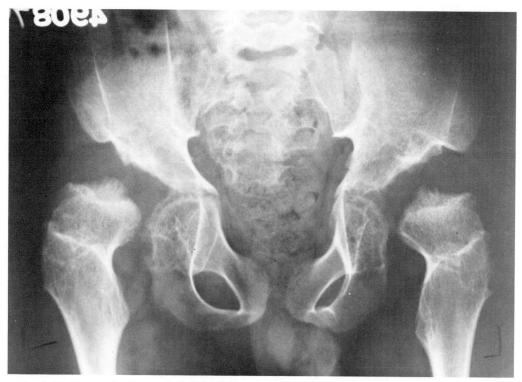

Fig. 2-12. Morquio's disease. Characteristic changes in the pelvis and proximal femurs include the "wine-glass" contour of the pelvis, the large, irregular acetabula, the small, poorly formed femoral epiphyses, and the broad femoral necks. The ilia are flared. The femurs are partially subluxated.

vertebra on another is usually present at the thoracolumbar junction. This results in a sharp angular kyphosis, one of the significant clinical observations. The intervertebral discs may be thick early in life, but later are reduced in height.

LONG TUBULAR BONES. Epiphyseal ossification centers may be multiple and often are irregular. They are late in appearing but mature normally. The degree of dwarfing of the long bones is variable; in some patients they are of normal lengths. The zones of provisional calcification are irregular and the metaphyses are broad. The proximal femur is often the most severely affected. Delay in appearance of the capital epiphysis, fragmentation, flaring, and irregularity of the metaphysis and subluxation

at the hip are common (see Fig. 2-12). The acetabulum has a coarse outline and it may be enlarged and deepened.

SHORT TUBULAR BONES. These bones often are short with irregular epiphyseal ossification centers. The second, third, fourth, and fifth metacarpals often taper at their ends. The metatarsals are affected similarly (Fig. 2-15).

FLAT BONES. The ilia flare laterally and the acetabular cavities are enlarged and have rough margins. Rubin[27] describes the ribs as "canoe paddles," the vertebral end being narrow while the remainder is broad.

OTHER FINDINGS. The skull and facial bones are normal, another significant finding in the

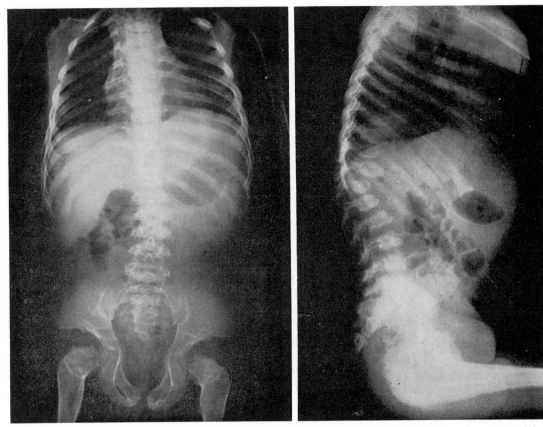

Fig. 2-13. Morquio's disease. *Left,* Anteroposterior and (*right*) lateral view of the spine and pelvis showing the characteristic changes in the pelvis similar to those in Figure 2-12. The vertebrae are flattened (platyspondyly) with a sharp, angular kyphosis at the thoracolumbar junction, hypoplasia of T 12, and forward displacement of T 11 on T 12.

differentiation from achondroplasia. A hypoplastic or absent odontoid process is seen in many patients. The carpal and tarsal bones are late in appearing and, later, may have irregular or angular shapes.

The head appears large in relation to the size of the trunk. The lower extremities are more undeveloped than the trunk and the trunk more so than the head and the upper extremities. The joints appear widened and some of the large joints are hypermobile owing to laxity of muscles and tendons. However flexion deformities also occur at the elbows, hips, and knees caused by the epiphyseal distortions. The hands are held in ulnar deviation. The first symptoms usually are noted at the time that the child begins to sit, stand, or walk. The disorder is due to an abnormality in the elaboration and storage of the mucopolysaccharide (MPS), keratosulfate.

HURLER'S DISEASE (GARGOYLISM)

This disorder is usually first noted after the first year of life. Clinical characteristics include a large, bulging head, flared nostrils, flat nasal bridge, hypertelorism, and corneal opacities leading to blindness. One of the significant clinical findings is hepatosplenomegaly, often of considerable degree. The lips are thick and the tongue large. The teeth are poorly formed.

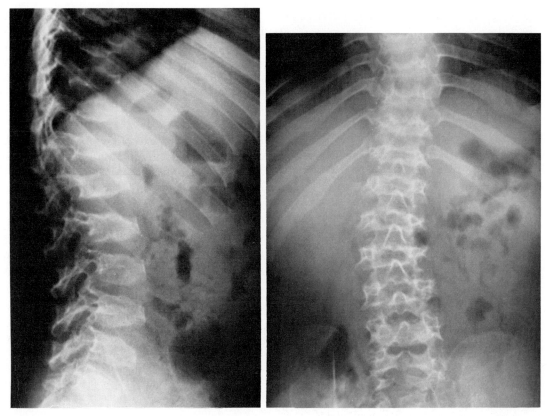

Fig. 2-14. Morquio's disease. Lower thoracic and lumbar spine. The flattening of the vertebrae and irregularity of disc surfaces are evident. The anterior central beaking can be seen in the lower thoracic bodies in the lateral view (*left*). The lower ribs are narrowed at their vertebral ends.

The stature is dwarfed. The facial appearance has been likened to that of a gargoyle, hence the designation, *gargoylism*. The genetic transmission is autosomal recessive. The typical lesion is a distended cell, derived presumably from the fibroblast, and called a "clear cell" or "gargoyle cell" owing to deposition in the cytoplasm of large amounts of the mucopolysaccharides. Correspondingly large amounts of these substances are excreted in the urine. Normally, 20 mg of mucopolysaccharide are excreted daily—in gargoylism the amount usually exceeds 60 mg.[1]

Recently, cases have been reported in which roentgen and clinical findings of Hurler's disease have been present but no abnormal mucopolysaccharide excretion could be demonstrated.[33]

SKULL. The skull often is scaphocephalic owing to premature closure of the sagittal and metopic sutures. The anteroposterior diameter of the sella is lengthened with an anterior depression, described as shoe-shaped or "J-shaped" (Fig. 2-16). The sinuses and mastoids are poorly pneumatized. The mandible is short and thick and the articular surfaces of the condyles are often concave, one of the characteristic findings. Hyperostotic thickening of the frontal and occipital areas may develop but the base does not become sclerotic.

RIBS. The ribs, especially the lower, are broad and flat.

LONG TUBULAR BONES. The upper extremities are more involved than the lower; the latter

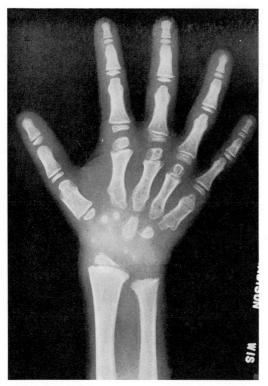

Fig. 2-15. Morquio's disease. Hand and wrist of same patient illustrated in Figure 2-13. There is moderate tapering of the proximal ends of the second, third, fourth and fifth metacarpals. Compare with hand in Hurler's disease as shown in Figure. 2-19.

VERTEBRAE. There is an angular kyphosis or gibbus at the thoracolumbar junction with one or several of the bodies hypoplastic and with an anterior inferior beak (Fig. 2-20). Posterior displacement of one vertebra on the one above or below is often present at the level of T-12 to L-1. The intervertebral disc spaces are intact.

FLAT BONES. The pelvis may resemble achondroplasia during early infancy but in those that survive, its appearance comes to resemble that of Morquio's disease (Fig. 2-21).

OTHER BONES. The carpal and tarsal bones may be late in appearing and then may show irregular or angular contours. The clavicle may be thickened. The teeth are poorly developed.

OTHER MUCOPOLYSACCHARIDOSES

The other mucopolysaccharidoses mentioned above appear to be variants of Hurler's disease. They differ from one another chiefly in their clinical manifestations and the mucopolysaccharide involved, rather than in specific roentgen characteristics. In the *Hunter* syndrome the skeletal changes and mental retardation are less severe than in Hurler's disease. There is no corneal clouding and the genetic transmission is X-linked recessive instead of autosomal recessive as in Hurler's.[30] In the *SanFilippo* syndrome the skeletal changes are mild and there is no corneal clouding. However mental retardation is severe. The genetic transmission is autosomal recessive. In the *Maroteaux-Lamy* syndrome skeletal changes are severe and there is corneal clouding. However the mentality is not affected. In the *Scheie* syndrome bone changes are mild with normal mentality, clouded corneas, and congenital heart disease (aortic regurgitation). In *lipomucopolysaccharidosis* the skeletal changes may be severe and mentality is retarded, but the corneas are clear. The genetic transmission is the same in all of these syndromes, autosomal recessive, except for Hunter's syndrome in which it is X-linked recessive. In Morquio's disease the mucopolysaccharide involved is keratosulfate. In the others it is chondroitin sulfate-A, chondroitin sulfate-B, or heparatin sulfate, alone or in combination.[30]

may be normal. The humerus is short and the shaft widened and a constriction with a coxa vara-like deformity of the humeral neck may be seen (Fig. 2-17). The radius and ulna show similar changes and the distal metaphyseal surfaces tend to be tilted toward one another (Fig. 2-18). The femoral neck is constricted and there is a coxa valga deformity at the hips. The epiphyseal ossification centers are often flattened and irregular.

SHORT TUBULAR BONES. The appearance of the hands usually is characteristic. The bones have a coarse texture with wide shafts and the metacarpals in particular have conical or pointed proximal ends (Fig. 2-19). Similar changes may be seen in the feet or they may be relatively normal.

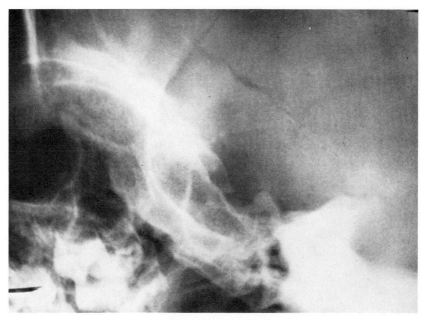

Fig. 2-16. Hurler's disease. Lateral view of skull showing the anterior depression of the tuberculum (J-shaped sella).

OSTEOGENESIS IMPERFECTA (OSTEITIS FRAGILITANS; FRAGILITAS OSSIUM CONGENITA; OSTEOPSATHYROSIS IDIOPATHICA; BRITTLE BONES)

Osteogenesis imperfecta is a rare hereditary disorder characterized by an unusual fragility of the bones leading to multiple fractures often from a trivial cause. It is generally considered to be a congenital form of osteoporosis caused by a deficiency of osteoid. There is failure to produce an adequate amount of normal intercellular substances of certain mesenchymal derivatives, particularly osteoblasts and fibroblasts.[1] This results in fragile bones, thin skin and sclera, poor teeth, and hypermobility of the joints. There are two forms of the disease, (1) osteogenesis imperfecta congenita and (2) osteogenesis imperfecta tarda. In the former, the disorder develops in utero and is noted at birth, the infant being born with multiple fractures. In the tarda type, the disease is first noted during childhood because of the unusual tendency for fractures. The joints are lax, dislocations are frequent, deafness caused by otosclerosis becomes apparent, and the teeth are discolored, fragile, and break easily. Blue sclera also becomes more apparent, evidently owing to the intraocular pigment which shows through the thin sclera.

SKULL. In the congenita type the cranial bones are largely membranous at birth. If the infant survives, ossification progresses slowly leaving wide sutures and multiple wormian bones (*mosaic skull*). Still later the sutures become of normal width. In older children a bulge in the temporal region is said to be characteristic.

LONG BONES. In the congenital form the infant usually is born with multiple fractures of the long bones (Fig. 2-22). The shafts are wide and appear short owing to the multiple fractures and the width of the bones. However, the cortices are thin. In the tarda type the width of the bones is reduced and they appear thin and gracile. The ends appear wide and the zones of provisional calcification may be denser than normal. The trabeculae are diminished in size

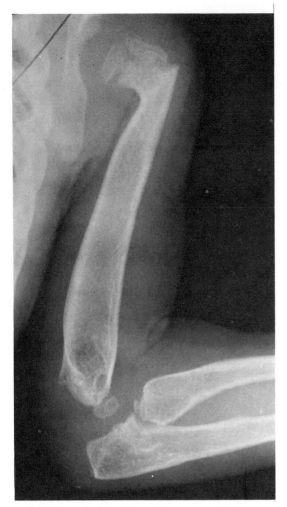

Fig. 2-17. Hurler's disease. The humerus shows a constriction of the neck, a varus deformity, and expansion of the mid and distal portions of the shaft.

and number; the cortices are thin. There often is extensive deformity owing to fractures and previous fractures which have healed (Fig. 2-23). The epiphyses are normal.

SHORT BONES. Fractures involving these bones are less frequent than in the long bones. Otherwise they show similar changes.

VERTEBRAE. Growth of the vertebrae is normal but they are demineralized owing to osteoporosis with thin cortical margins. Compression fractures are frequent and multiple bodies may show biconcave disc surfaces, i.e., fish vertebrae. The intervertebral disc spaces may be widened. Scoliosis is frequent.

FLAT BONES. The pelvis may show changes in shape secondary to the osteoporosis and protrusio acetabuli is common. Fractures of the ribs also are common. Here, as elsewhere, the fractures heal readily, often with exuberant callus.

OTHER FINDINGS. The teeth are often small, deformed, and the pulp chambers and root canals obliterated. Dislocations of the larger joints may occur secondary to the laxity of the ligaments and hypertonicity of the muscles.

Of considerable interest is the tendency for fractures to heal with excessive callus formation (Fig. 2-24). This may be so extensive that a malignant tumor may be suspected.

OSTEOPETROSIS (ALBERS-SCHÖNBERG DISEASE; OSTEOSCLEROSIS FRAGILIS; MARBLE BONES)

This is a rare dysplasia characterized by an unusual density or radiopacity of the bones. Although dense to roentgen rays, the bones are brittle and fracture readily. The disease may be discovered at birth or shortly thereafter, or not until adulthood. As with most of the other dysplasias the earlier the disease is found the more severe it is likely to be. In the infant, all of the bones may be affected, having a uniformly dense, structureless appearance with complete obliteration of normal trabecular architecture. The medullary canal is obliterated by dense sclerosis and merges with the cortex. The density of the bones is thought to be the result of failure of normal removal of old bone while new bone continues to be formed. Growth is often stunted and myelophthisic anemia may become severe and lead to death. Jaundice, hepatosplenomegaly, and cranial nerve palsies are common. Death often occurs within the first year of life. In the infantile (congenita)

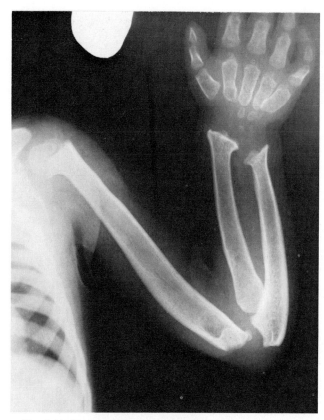

Fig. 2-18. Hurler's disease. Left upper extremity. In addition to the expanded shafts, the distal metaphyses of the radius and ulna are tilted toward one another. Also characteristic changes in the hand. There is delayed ossification of epiphyses at the elbow and wrist and of the centers for the carpal bones.

form the disease has been found in utero and the baby may be stillborn.

In the adult form the disease may first come to attention of a physician because of a fracture of a long bone. Characteristically, these are of transverse type. Or there may be a history of repeated fractures during childhood. Another presenting symptom may be an unexplained anemia. These patients often suffer from carious teeth and dental or jaw infections.

SKULL. The base shows the most marked sclerosis but all of the cranial bones may be involved. The sinuses and mastoids may show complete lack of pneumatization. The cranial foramina are encroached upon leading to various cranial nerve palsies such as blindness and deafness. The teeth are late in erupting and develop caries early. Dental infection may lead to osteomyelitis of the jaw. The lamina dura, the cortical margin of the tooth socket, may be unusually thick and dense and the disease may be suspected from dental roentgenograms.

VERTEBRAE. These bones are uniformly involved by the sclerosis and there may be impingement on the spinal nerves. In the adult or latent type the sclerosis may be limited to the upper and lower surfaces ("sandwich vertebrae"; "rugger jersey spine").

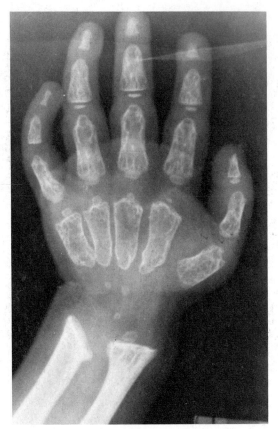

Fig. 2-19. Hurler's disease. Hand and wrist show-ing characteristic changes as described in the text.

OTHER BONES. In the long and short tubular bones the sclerosis is usually uniform in the infantile form. Occasionally there may be alternating bands of sclerotic and normal bone at the ends of the shafts. The trabecular pattern is completely obliterated. The length of the bones is usually normal but is occasionally shortened. Characteristically the ends of the bones are club-shaped owing to failure of nor-mal modeling (Fig. 2-25). The epiphyseal ossification centers are dense but they mature normally. In the adult, the increased density often is limited to bands of sclerosis at the ends, sometimes alternating with bands of normal density. The bones of the hands and feet are involved the same as the long tubular bones. The sternal ends of the clavicles may be widened.

PYCNODYSOSTOSIS

This disease is often confused with osteo-petrosis because of the generalized dense, scle-rotic appearance of the bones.

In the *skull* there is a failure of closure of the cranial sutures and fontanelles and numer-ous wormian bones are present (Fig. 2-26). The skull has a dolichocephalic shape due to bossing. The mandibular rami are hypoplastic with loss of the normal mandibular angle which is characteristic. Sclerosis and thickening

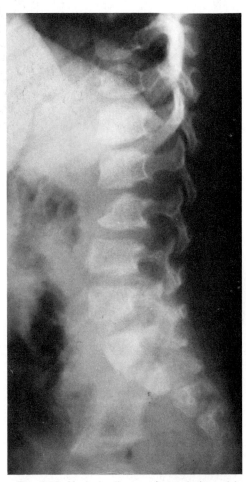

Fig. 2-20. Hurler's disease. Lateral view of lumbar spine shows the anterior inferior beaking of L-3, mild angular kyphosis and malalignment of L-2 on L-3. The vertebrae are moderately flattened, this is better ap-preciated in an anteroposterior view.

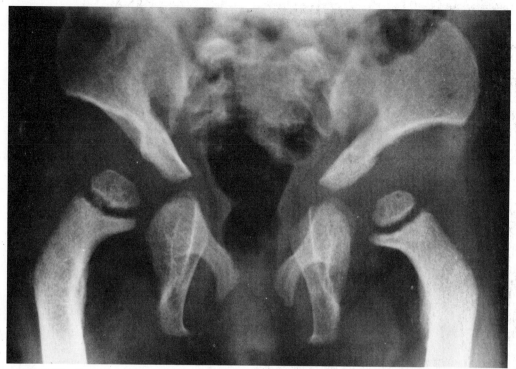

Fig. 2-21. Hurler's disease. The contour of the pelvis resembles Morquio's disease but the femoral epiphyses are better developed. The acetabula are shallow. The femoral necks are moderately constricted. Neither femoral head appears properly seated in the acetabulum.

of the cranial and facial bones may be severe. The sinuses may fail to develop, particularly the frontals, and the mastoids often are not pneumatized. The *hands* are short and stubby with partial agenesis or aplasia of the terminal phalanges (Fig. 2-27). The *vertebrae* are sclerotic and there is a lack of fusion of the neural arches in some. Fractures are extremely common and in the long bones they are of the transverse type. The stature is reduced and deformity from old fractures may lead to further shortening of the long tubular bones. Dental caries occur frequently.

METAPHYSEAL DYSPLASIA (PYLE'S DISEASE; CRANIOMETAPHYSEAL DYSPLASIA)

In this dysplasia the basic disturbance appears to be a failure of modeling of the cylin-

drical bones. The changes are often most noticeable at the lower ends of the femurs and upper ends of tibias leading to a club-shaped enlargement often referred to as having an "Erlenmeyer flask" appearance. The cortices at the ends of the bones are thin and thus the bone is more subject to fracture. The disease is familial and probably hereditary and consanguinity has been noted in the histories of many of these individuals.

The skull is involved. In mild cases this may take the form of sclerosis of the base and vault. In more severe disease there is marked thickening of the base of the skull and of the facial bones (a form of leontiasis ossea), and lesser involvement of the vault. The sinuses and mastoids lack pneumatization. Cranial nerve palsies may result from encroachment on the basal foramina. The eyes tend to be widely spaced (hypertelorism).

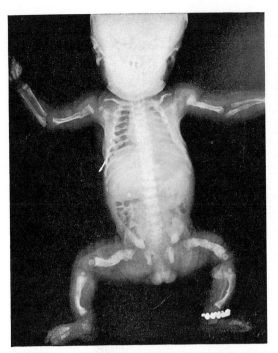

Fig. 2-22. Osteogenesis imperfecta, infantile type. The baby was born with the multiple fractures.

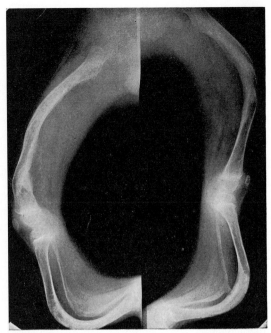

Fig. 2-23. Osteogenesis imperfecta tarda. The misshapen bones have been caused by their abnormal softness and by multiple fractures that have healed.

DIAPHYSEAL SCLEROSIS (ENGELMANN'S DISEASE; PROGRESSIVE DIAPHYSEAL SCLEROSIS)

The major manifestations of this dysplasia consist of symmetric cortical thickening in the mid-diaphyses, particularly of the femur and the tibia. The lesion tends to progress and eventually involve most of the diaphysis. The epiphyses and metaphyses are spared. The disorder may begin in early childhood with a difficulty in walking and a shuffling or waddling gait being the first sign. The cortical thickening begins subperiosteally but with failure of resorption within, the medullary canal may be encroached upon leading to anemia and hepatosplenomegaly. The disease also progresses to involve other bones as the child grows older and, in some, may involve the short bones of the hands and feet as well as the bones of the trunk, skull, and face. The base of the skull may become thick and dense with its subsequent impingement on the cranial nerves.

The vault is seldom involved except for frontal and occipital bossing. The muscles tend to be flabby and weak. Dental caries is often present. In a small percentage of patients the skin has been noted to be thick and dry and the hair scanty. The mentality is not affected.

RIBBING'S DISEASE (HEREDITARY MULTIPLE DIAPHYSEAL SCLEROSIS)

In 1949, Ribbing described the occurrence of a disorder in siblings consisting of a dense diaphyseal sclerosis not unlike that seen in Engelmann's disease. He believed it was a separate entity, however, because of the late onset of symptoms and the familial nature, which had not been recorded in Engelmann's disease. In 1953, one of us (LWP)[22] reported two cases of a similar disease, occurring in brothers (Fig. 2-28). One was asymptomatic. The other complained of aching pain in one leg although there were similar lesions in other bones. Subsequently we examined the father of

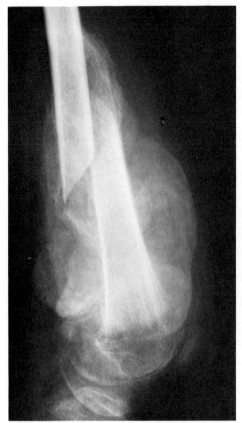

Fig. 2-24. Osteogenesis imperfecta. Excessive callus with spiral fracture of the femur. The calcified callus forms a huge mass around and below the fracture.

these two patients and found mild involvement in some of the long tubular bones, also asymptomatic. Also we later examined the son (age 5) of one of the original patients and found an appearance typical of Engelmann's disease. We believe, therefore, that the two disorders, Engelmann's disease and Ribbing's disease are closely related, the latter probably being the adult or latent type of the former. However, to our knowledge, the familial nature of Ribbing's disease has not been noted in Engelmann's disease.

MELORHEOSTOSIS

This disorder presents as an irregular thickening of the cortex along one side of a bone or the bones

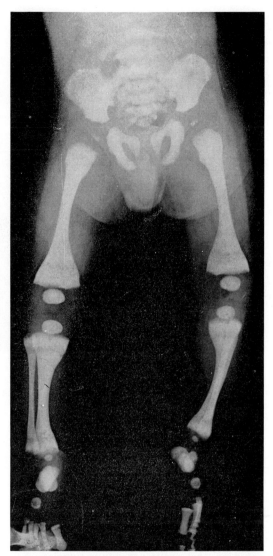

Fig. 2-25. Osteopetrosis (marble bone disease) in an infant. The bones throughout the skeleton are chalky white with loss of trabecular architecture. Translucent bands can be visualized crossing the ends of the shafts, representing periods of more normal ossification as the bones grew in length. The metaphyses are enlarged and club-shaped, owing to a failure of modeling as the bones increased in length.

of one extremity. The thickening may be external, internal, or both (Fig. 2–29). The appearance has been likened to molten wax flowing down the side of a candle. If an extremity is involved the pelvis (or shoulder girdle) on the affected side is likely

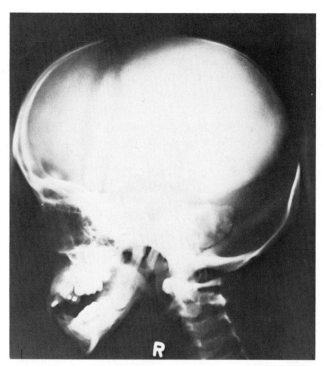

Fig. 2-26. Pycnodysostosis. Lateral view of the skull demonstrates the sclerotic cranial bones, the large unossified areas especially along the lambdoid sutures, and the loss of the mandibular angle.

to show similar thickening. The onset may be in infancy or not until late adolescence, i.e., at age 20. The presenting symptom is pain which may be severe. The disease does not appear to be hereditary. If the disease begins early in life the epiphyses may fuse prematurely causing shortening of the involved extremity. The lesions usually cease progressing when skeletal growth is complete. Regression has not been noted. The disease is rare, less than 50 cases having been reported in the literature.

OSTEOPOIKILOSIS (OSTEOPATHIA CONDENSANS DISSEMINATA)

This is an asymptomatic disorder characterized by the appearance of numerous small, round or oval densities in the ends of the long bones (Fig. 2-30), the small bones of the hands and feet, and in the acetabulum. The lesions are composed of dense, compact bone. They are discovered by chance on roentgen examination for some other condition. The disorder is familial and hereditary and has been discovered in newborns as well as in the fetus in utero. The lesions may increase or decrease in size and number during the period of active bone growth and have been noted to disappear altogether. In the acetabulum when numerous and oval in shape the lesions tend to radiate toward the hip joint. Solitary sclerotic foci of the same nature are common throughout the appendicular skeleton and pelvis and are known as *compact islands*. While usually small an occasional compact island is seen which measures more than a centimeter in diameter. When observed over a period of several years or longer, compact islands have been noted to increase or decrease in size. Such a lesion may be mistaken for a sclerotic focus of metastatic carcinoma.

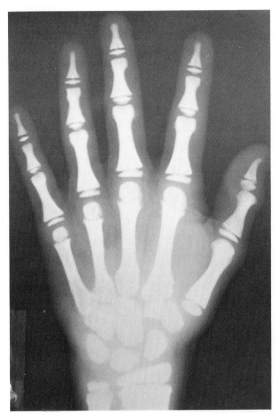

Fig. 2-27. Pycnodysostosis. The bones of the hand and wrist are uniformly increased in density. There is tapering of the distal phalanges with loss of the terminal tufts.

OSTEOPATHIA STRIATA (VOORHOEVE'S LINES)

This process is similar in many ways to osteopoikilosis but instead of rounded foci, consists of striae of dense bone extending toward the nearest joint. In children the striae begin at the epiphyseal line and extend for a short distance into the diaphysis. In the acetabulum the striae have a "sunburst" appearance, fanning outward toward the iliac crest. Any or all of the long bones and the pelvis may be involved. The lesions are asymptomatic and are discovered by chance.

FIBROUS DYSPLASIA

This disease usually begins during childhood and is characterized, pathologically, by re-

placement of normal bone undergoing physiologic lysis by an abnormal proliferation of fibrous tissue.[1] The disease may involve a single bone (monostotic), the bones of one extremity, or be widely distributed throughout the skeleton (polyostotic). There is some predilection for the long bones of the extremities but any bone may be involved. The individual lesions tend to begin in the metaphysis and progress into the shaft. In cases with the more extensive bone lesions, areas of skin pigmentation (*café au lait* spots) having a geographic distribution are common. *Albright's* syndrome consists of the osseous lesions of fibrous dysplasia with precocious sexual development and *café au lait* spots. This occurs only in females.

Roentgen Observations. The individual lesions vary from one to another. In some the appearance is that of a well-defined lucent area or "cyst." The cavity is filled with fibrous tissue rather than fluid so that it does not represent a true cyst (Fig. 2-31). The affected bone may have a "milky" or "ground-glass" appearance with absence of normal trabeculation (Fig. 2-32). The margins often are ill-defined but in the "cystic" variety, a thin sclerotic rim may bound the lesion (Fig. 2-33). The cortex may be eroded from within and the bone locally expanded (Fig. 2-34). This predisposes to fracture. The fracture heals with ample periosteal callus. Recently cases of fibrous dysplasia have been reported showing a sequestrum within an apparent "cavity" in a long bone.[26] In severe and long-standing disease the bones may be bowed or misshapen, some of which is the result of previous fracture. Thus the upper end of the femur characteristically shows a "shepherd's crook" deformity with coxa vara and lateral and anterior bowing of the shaft. Bending also occurs because of the fibrous tissue replacement of normal bone.

In the skull vault the lesion appears as a somewhat multilocular cystlike area involving the diploic space and expanding the tables (Fig. 2-35). The margins are somewhat sclerotic and the boundary of the lesion not sharply defined. When fibrous dysplasia involves the base of the skull and the facial

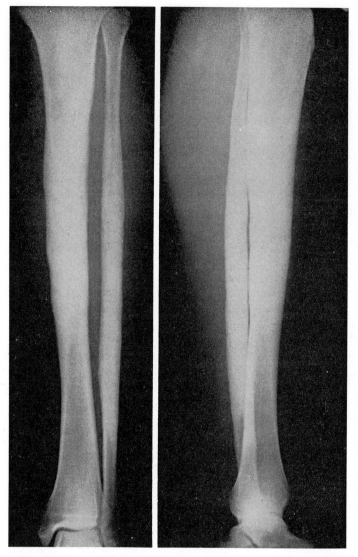

Fig. 2-28. Hereditary multiple diaphyseal sclerosis. The patient had rather similar lesions in both femurs and one radius. His brother and father have similar bone changes, completely asymptomatic. The patient's son (2 years of age) has changes characteristic of Engelmann's disease.

bones, the appearance is different. It causes a marked sclerosis and thickening. The sinuses may be obliterated. In the skull base the similarity to meningioma may cause difficulty in diagnosis and, at times, arteriography or air studies may be necessary. Involvement of the facial bones is similar to that in the skull base with thickening and sclerosis (Fig. 2-36). This

appearance is known as *leontiasis ossea* and while there are other causes for it, fibrous dysplasia is probably the most frequent lesion responsible.

In the differentiation from meningioma, the lack of dilated vascular grooves leading to the area of the bone lesion has been considered a significant finding. However a few cases have

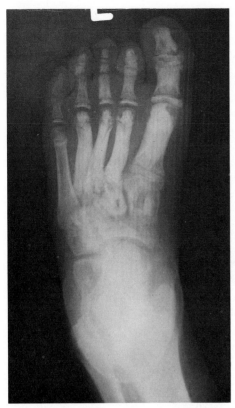

Fig. 2-29. Melorheostosis. Anteroposterior view of left foot showing dense sclerosis particularly of first to fourth metatarsals and phalanges of first toe. Similar changes were present along the inner side of the long bones of this extremity and left side of pelvis.

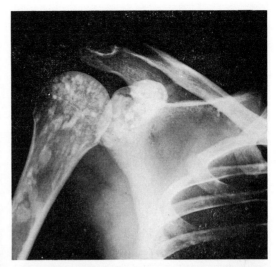

Fig. 2-30. Osteopoikelosis (spotted bones). The islands of dense bone were widely distributed throughout the skeleton in the bones adjacent to joints.

been reported recently where enlarged, tortuous grooves were found in fibrous dysplasia so that the occurrence of dilated vessels cannot be considered entirely specific for meningioma when sclerotic or "mixed" lesions are found. Of greater importance is the lack of involvement of the inner table in fibrous dysplasia and its occurrence in meningioma.

When involvement is extensive there may persist severe crippling and deformity. Solitary lesions or disease of lesser magnitude may cease progression when skeletal growth is complete and may cause little or no permanent disability or deformity. Sarcomatous degeneration has been reported as a complication of fibrous dysplasia but appears to be uncommon.

HEREDITARY FIBROUS DYSPLASIA OF THE JAWS (CHERUBISM)

This condition was first described by Jones in 1933 in four of five siblings. The lesion appears as multilocular, radiolucent, cystic areas expanding the jaw. This causes rounding of the facial features, hence the term "cherubism." The lesions involve the mandible bilaterally with or without posterior maxillary disease. The entire mandible, except the condyles, may be involved. Maxillary involvement is less frequent and less severe than mandibular disease and probably does not occur without lesions in the lower jaw.[5] While the exact etiology is unknown, it has been suggested that the disease represents an hereditary form of fibrous dysplasia.

NEUROFIBROMATOSIS (VON RECKLINGHAUSEN'S DISEASE)

This disease entity was first described by von Recklinghausen in 1882. It is a disease of the supporting tissues of the nervous system. While skin tumors are the most prominent feature of the disorder, it may involve other systems including the endocrine, gastrointestinal, and

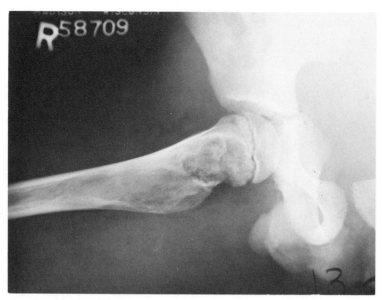

Fig. 2-31. Fibrous dysplasia, monostotic form. While the lesion in the neck of the femur looks cystic, the abnormal bone continues well into the shaft fading gradually into normal appearing bone.

skeletal. The present discussion is concerned chiefly with the latter. In addition to skin nodules, brownish pigmented areas (*café au lait* spots) occur frequently. The extent of the disease may vary considerably but there is a tendency for it to slow or stop when skeletal growth is completed. It is said that about 10 per cent of the lesions may change to a neurofibrosarcoma. There is an increased frequency of meningiomas in patients suffering from von Recklinghausen's disease.

SKELETAL LESIONS. Kyphoscoliosis is common in the spine. The scoliosis is usually a sharp, angular one and its cause often is obscure since associated neurofibromas are not found (Fig. 2-37). The vertebrae often are wedge-shaped at the height of curvature. The ribs often are thin and have been likened to a "twisted ribbon." In the long bones pressure from an adjacent tumor may cause a small local excavation in the cortex, the so-called "pit" or "cave" defect. A neurofibroma may arise within bone causing a sharply outlined area of radiolucency. Another peculiar manifestation of the disease is localized enlargement of a part such as a finger or one extremity (focal giantism). The bone, except for its greater size, appears normal. In the skull, absence of part of the orbital wall may cause unilateral exophthalmos, often pulsating in type. There may be absence of the clinoid processes of the sella on the affected side. As with some of the other bone changes (e.g., scoliosis) an associated tumor need not be present and the loss of bone is not caused by pressure erosion. Localized thinning along the left lambdoid suture has been recently reported. A neurofibroma may affect a cranial nerve, particularly the acoustic, causing enlargement of the corresponding foramen.

Lateral intrathoracic meningocele is found with some frequency in neurofibromatosis. It presents as a rounded mass projecting into the thoracic cavity alongside the spine and is usually associated with considerable deformity of the contiguous vertebrae including kyphosis, scoliosis, and erosions of vertebral bodies, arches, and ribs. Scalloping of the posterior surfaces of one or more vertebral bodies is common in association with other spinal de-

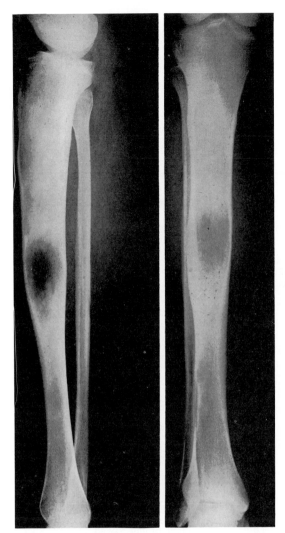

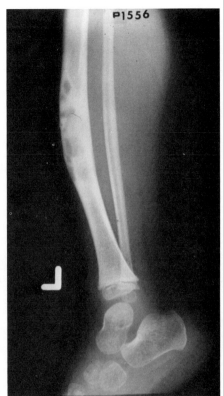

Fig. 2-33. Fibrous dysplasia of the tibia. There is a mixture of cystlike rarefactions and sclerosis in the midshaft. There is anterior bowing of the tibia and local expansion at the site of the disease.

Fig. 2-32. Fibrous dysplasia of the tibia. There is loss of normal trabeculations with a "milky" or "ground-glass" appearance. The central cavity is not a true cyst but is filled with fibrous tissue. The extreme upper end and the lower third of the tibial shaft are uninvolved.

formities. It has been shown that scalloping can occur in neurofibromatosis without there being any associated tumor or other mass to account for it.

A neurofibroma of a spinal nerve root often is of dumbbell shape having intraspinal and extraspinal extensions. This type of tumor is prone to erode the contiguous vertebral pedi-

cles and, in the thoracic area, a paraspinal mass may be seen. A neurofibroma of an intercostal nerve causes a mass density along the thoracic wall and often there is pressure erosion of adjacent ribs and localized widening of the rib interspace (Fig. 7-42). It should be noted that a solitary neurofibroma may occur in many different areas of the body without the other stigmata of von Recklinghausen's disease being present. (See section on Neurofibroma, Chapter 7.)

PSEUDARTHROSIS. During the newborn period (occasionally noted at birth) a pathologic fracture may occur through one of the weight bearing bones, usually the distal one-third of the tibia. The fracture fails to heal, the ends of the fragments become pointed or rounded and smooth

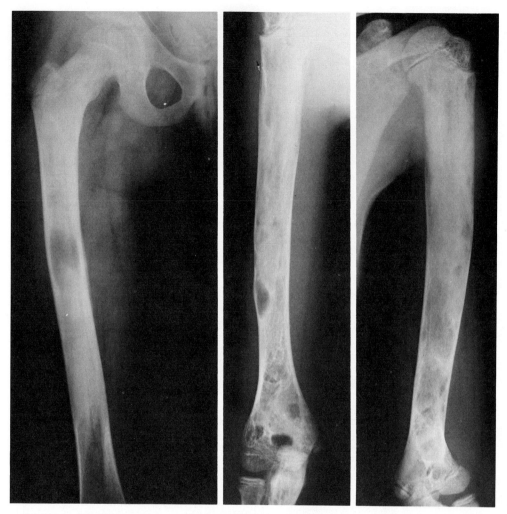

Fig. 2-34. Polyostotic form of fibrous dysplasia. Widespread involvement of the skeleton is present. These three figures show characteristic lesions and demonstrate the variations in the pattern of the disease that may be present, even in a single bone.

and pseudarthrosis results. In about one-half of these patients stigmata of neurofibromatosis, such as *café au lait* spots, may be present. When observed early the lesion appears as a gradual local lysis of bone with failure to replace the deossified bone by normal bone.[1] In some the fracture heals temporarily but refractures when weight bearing is attempted. Some authorities have contended that a neurilemmoma is responsible for the lesion but other investigators believe differently and, at present, the exact pathogenesis of the lesion is obscure (Fig. 2-38).

MISCELLANEOUS DYSPLASIAS

DYSCHONDROSTEOSIS

This entity was first reported by Leri and Weill in 1928. Its major abnormality is at the wrist where a lesion similar to or the same as Madelung's deformity occurs (see "Madelung's Deformity," Chapter 3). Some believe that Madelung's deformity and dyschondrosteosis are one and the same. Others point out that

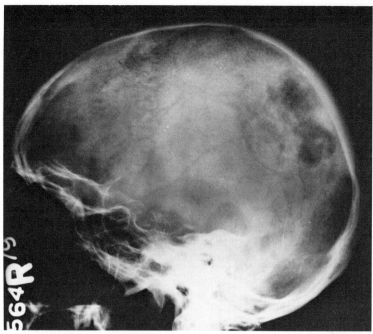

Fig. 2-35. Fibrous dysplasia of the skull. The lesion in the posterior parietal area consists of areas of irregular rarefaction and some sclerosis. In tangential view the lesion involved the diploë with expansion of the tables, chiefly the outer.

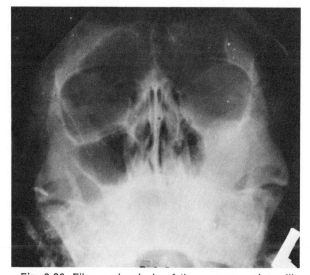

Fig. 2-36. Fibrous dysplasia of the zygoma and maxilla on the left. The marked thickening of the bone has encroached upon the maxillary sinus and floor of the orbit.

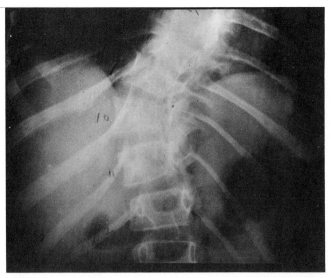

Fig. 2-37. Neurofibromatosis. Anteroposterior view of the lower thoracic spine illustrating the sharp scoliosis and malformed vertebrae. The lower ribs, particularly on the left, are thin.

while the lesion at the wrist corresponds to Madelung's deformity, there also are other findings in most patients.[8] Among these is shortening of the forearms and legs (middle-segment dwarfism). Genu varum is also found and occasionally an exostosis occurs on the tibia. There is a familial tendency.

MARFAN'S SYNDROME (ARACHNODACTYLY)

Marfan's syndrome is a disease of connective tissue caused by an individual's inability to manufacture normal collagen or one of the constituents of collagen.[1] It involves the heart and aorta and one of its common manifestations is aneurysm formation, usually of the ascending aorta and of dissecting type. The affected individuals are tall and slender, usually over 6 feet in height. The muscles are poorly developed with poor tone. Thus the joints may be hypermobile, there may be dislocation of the hips, genu recurvatum, dislocation of the patella and pes planus. Ectopia lentis is common. Of interest is the discovery of an abnormal amino acid in the urine of some patients who have roentgen changes similar to those of

Marfan's disease.[30] This metabolic disorder has been called *homocystinuria*.

The bones are of normal density but long and gracile. The thickness is normal but the increased length gives an illusion of thinness. In the hands, elongation of the bones leads to a characteristic appearance (*arachnodactyly*) described as "spiderlike" (Fig. 2-39). Scoliosis is frequent. The skull often has a dolichocephalic shape owing to increased length of the base. There is a decrease in subcutaneous fat so that the individuals appear emaciated. There often is pectus excavatum. The hereditary nature of the disease has been established in many patients.

CLEIDOCRANIAL DYSOSTOSIS

In most cases of this disorder the skull and clavicles are involved but other structures may be affected as well. The skull usually has a brachycephalic shape. The sutures remain open and numerous wormian bones are present. Permanent patency of fontanelles is usually seen. Often the anterior fontanelle particularly is large and extends forward between the frontal

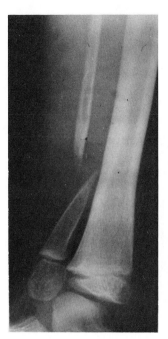

Fig. 2-38. Pseudarthrosis of the fibula in neuro-fibromatosis.

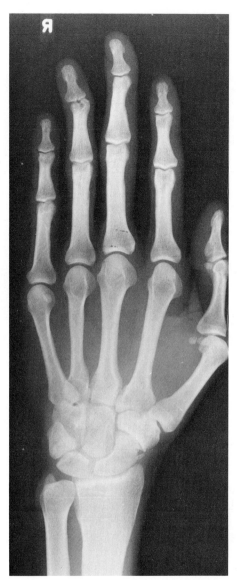

Fig. 2-39. Arachnodactyly (Marfan's syndrome). Note the long slender bones, particularly the proximal phalanges. There is an old posttraumatic deformity of terminal joint of fourth finger.

bones with the metopic suture failing to close (Fig. 2-40). The foramen magnum is large and shows a forward and downward slant. The mandible is prognathous but the maxilla is hypoplastic as are other facial bones. The malar, lacrimal, and nasal bones may be deficient. The palate tends to be narrow with a high arch. The sinuses often are small.

Another major abnormality is deficiency of or absence of the clavicles (Fig. 2-41). Because the clavicle ossifies from three centers, any part may be absent so that there are many variations in the appearance of these bones. Clinically the deficiency of the clavicles allows the individual to approximate the shoulders anteriorly, a significant feature of the disease.

The radius may be short. There may be extra epiphyses for the metacarpals and phalanges. Occasionally the second metacarpal is unusually long with a steplike shortening of the third, fourth, and fifth metacarpals.

In the pelvis the bones are often underdeveloped and the symphysis pubis may be unusu-ally wide. The sacrum and coccyx may be malformed or the coccyx may be absent. Coxa vara is noted at the hips. Changes in the feet are often similar to those noted in the hands. Scoliosis, lordosis, or kyphosis may be seen in the spine and failure of fusion of the arches has been observed.

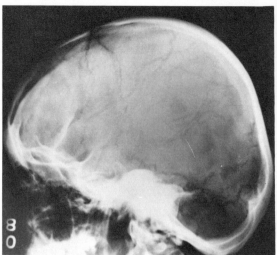
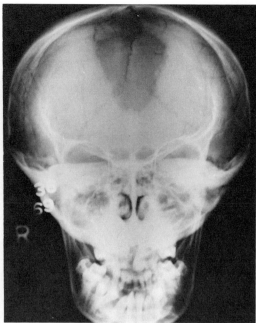

Fig. 2-40. Cleidocranial dysostosis. Same patient as Figure 2-41. The anterior fontanelle remains open and is greatly enlarged. The basal angle of the skull is flat. Note Wormian bones along the lambdoid suture and the malposition of some of the teeth.

The teeth usually are abnormal. There may be retention of deciduous teeth, delay in eruption of permanent teeth, faulty implantation, and dental caries. Dentigerous cysts have been reported in some patients.

CHONDROECTODERMAL DYSPLASIA (ELLIS-VAN CREVELD DISEASE)

This rare disorder has probably been misdiagnosed in the past as achondroplasia. It was first defined as a distinct entity by McKusick[17] who found cases among the Old Order Amish people of Pennsylvania. He considered the disease to be transmitted as an autosomal recessive trait. Cardiac anomalies (atrial septal and ventricular septal defects being the most frequent) have been found in about 60 per cent of patients. The ectodermal component of the syndrome is manifested by small, friable nails, defective dentition and, in a few cases, alopecia.

The changes in the skeleton are usually

characteristic. Fusion of the hamate and capitate bones in the wrist is often present. Polydactyly and syndactyly are almost universal. These changes involve the ulnar side of the hand so that a partially or completely formed sixth metacarpal is fused to the fifth. Its distal

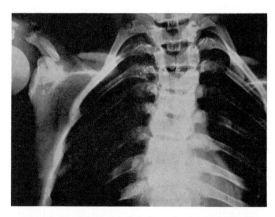

Fig. 2-41. Cleidocranial dysostosis. Defects in ossification of the clavicles are seen. There also are mid-line spina bifida clefts in the arches of the first, second, and third thoracic vertebrae.

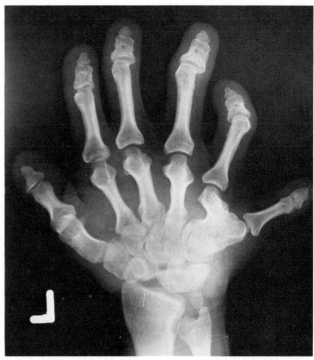

Fig. 2-42. Ellis-van Creveld disease in an adult female. There is progressve shortening distalward of the bones, polydactyly, syndactyly, and carpal fusions. (*Courtesy of Dr. M. Pinson Neal, Jr., Virginia Commonwealth University, Richmond, Va.*)

end, however, is free so that there is a sixth digit (Figs. 2-42 and 2-43). Cone epiphyses are common during childhood (see section on "Peripheral Dysostosis"). Shortening of the long tubular bones characteristically becomes more severe distalward. Thus the tibia and fibula are much shorter than the femur and the distal phalanges more dwarfed than are the proximal. The distal end of the radius and proximal end of the ulna are somewhat enlarged. Also, the radial head may be flared and frequently dislocated at the elbow. The proximal end of the tibia also is widened and the epiphysis offset medially. A small exostosis on the upper inner cortex of the tibia is frequently present. The intercondylar notch of the femur is shallow and the tibial spine is small.

The teeth are delayed in appearance and then are small, defective, and irregularly spaced. In the pelvis the iliac crest tends to be flared but in many cases the pelvis is normal. The same is true of the vertebrae, ribs, and skull.

PERIPHERAL DYSOSTOSIS. This uncommon entity, described by Brailsford in 1948 and also by Singleton, Daeschner and Teng in 1960, has been considered by some to be only a mild form of the Ellis-van Creveld disorder. The characteristic roentgen changes are limited to the short tubular bones of the hands and feet which are short and broad and with cone-shaped or ball and socket epiphyses. The term, *cone epiphysis,* refers to an epiphyseal center which is partially or completely buried in the metaphysis, and usually with the shape of a cone. A *ball and socket epiphysis* is similar except that the center is more rounded than

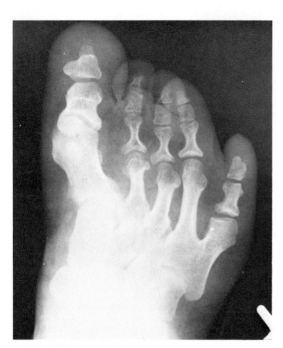

Fig. 2-43. Ellis-van Creveld disease. Foot of same patient illustrated in Figure 2-42.

cone-shaped. The terms, however, are often used interchangeably. Supernumerary epiphyses and pseudoepiphyses are often present. Cone-shaped epiphyses also have been found in a number of other conditions including (1) cleidocranial dysostosis, (2) Ellis-van Creveld disease, (3) tricho-rhino-phalangeal syndrome, (4) osteopetrosis, (5) epiphyseal hyperplasia, (6) Apert's syndrome, (7) pseudohypoparathyroidism, (8) achondroplasia, (9) multiple hereditary exostoses, and (10) no recognizable cause.[21] In the *tricho-rhino-phalangeal syndrome* changes in the hands and feet are similar to those of peripheral dysostosis but there also are retardation of growth, thin, sparse, slow-growing hair, and a characteristic physiognomy with a pear-shaped nose.

The tendency among investigators working in this field is to consider peripheral dysostosis as a symptom rather than a specific entity and one that may be found in association with various abnormalities, the Ellis-van Creveld disease being only one of such syndromes.

ASPHYXIATING THORACIC DYSTROPHY

This dysplasia was first reported by Jeune in 1955 in two infant siblings who died of respiratory distress associated with a small, and relatively immobile, thorax. The major roentgen abnormalities[12,24] consist of very short ribs and a variable degree of shortening of the long tubular bones with metaphyseal notching.

The ribs project horizontally and may be so short as to barely reach the anterior axillary line. The shortened ribs reduce the volume of the thorax and are responsible for the respiratory distress. The cardiac silhouette often appears large but this is probably an illusion because of the smallness of the thorax. In the pelvis, the ilium is shortened in its inferosuperior diameter, the acetabular roof is broad and there may be a deep V-shaped notch in it. The disease frequently is fatal with the infant dying from respiratory complications. Associated renal disease has been reported and in some patients with less severe skeletal changes, renal failure may be the cause of death.

It should be noted that short ribs with a narrow thorax occur in some other dysplasias including achondroplasia and thanatophoric dwarfism and that other changes common to achondroplasia may be seen in asphyxiating thoracic dystrophy and thanatophoric dwarfism (see page 34). Some investigators still believe that these latter two entities may represent only the severe form of achondroplasia in which the infants often die early in life usually owing to respiratory embarrassment.

As case reports of this disease accumulate, it is evident that a number of these infants may survive, some for many years, so that it is no longer considered as uniformly lethal in the neonatal period as formerly believed.

REFERENCES AND SELECTED READINGS

1. AEGERTER, E., and KIRKPATRICK, J. A., JR.: *Orthopedic Diseases,* 3rd ed. Philadelphia, Saunders, 1968.
2. CAFFEY, J.: Chondroectodermal dysplasia (Ellis-van Creveld disease); report of three cases. *Am. J.*

Roentgenol. Radium Ther. Nucl. Med. 68: 875, 1952.

3. CAMPBELL, C. J., PAPADEMETRIOU, T., and BONFIGLIO, M.: Melorheostosis. A report of the clinical roentgenographic and pathological findings in 14 cases. *J. Bone Joint Surg. 50-A:* 1281, 1968.

4. COMINGS, D. E., PAPAZIAN, C., and SCHOENE, H. R.: Conradi's disease. Chondrodystrophia calcificans congenita, stippled epiphyses. *J. Pediat. 72:* 63, 1968.

5. CORNELIUS, E. A., and MCCLENDON, J. L.: Cherubism-hereditary fibrous dysplasia of the jaws. Roentgenographic features. *Am. J. Roentgenol. Radium Ther. Nucl. Med. 106:* 136, 1969.

6. ELMORE, S. M.: Pycnodysostosis. A review. *J. Bone Joint Surg. 49-A:* 153, 1967.

7. FELMAN, A. H., and KIRKPATRICK, J. A.: Madelung's deformity. Observations in 17 patients. *Radiology 93:* 1037, 1969.

8. HENRY, A., and THORBURN, M. J.: Madelung's deformity. A clinical and cytogenic study. *J. Bone Joint Surg. 49-B:* 66, 1967.

9. JUBERG, R. C., and HOLT, J. F.: Inheritance of multiple epiphyseal dysplasia tarda. *Amer. J. Hum. Genet. 20:* 549, 1968.

10. KEATS, T. E., RIDDERVOLT, H. O., and MICHAELIS, L. L.: Thanatophoric dwarfism. *Am. J. Roentgenol. Radium Ther. Nucl. Med. 108:* 473, 1970.

11. KETTLEKAMP, D. B., CAMPBELL, C. J., and BONFIGLIO, M.: Dysplasia epiphysialis hemimelica. A report of 15 cases and a review of the literature. *J. Bone Joint Surg. 48-A:* 476, 1966.

12. KOHLER, E., and BABBITT, D. P.: Dystrophic thoraces and infantile asphyxia. *Radiology 94:* 55, 1970.

13. LANGER, L. O., JR.: Dyschondrosteosis, a hereditable bone dysplasia with characteristic roentgenographic features. *Am. J. Roentgenol. Radium Ther. Nucl. Med. 95:* 178, 1965.

14. LANGER, L. O., JR., BAUMANN, F. A., and GORLIN, R. J.: Achondroplasia. *Am. J. Roentgenol. Radium Ther. Nucl. Med. 100:* 12, 1967.

15. LANGER, L. O., JR., and CAREY, L. S.: The roentgenographic features of the K. S. mucopolysaccharidosis of Morquio (Morquio-Brailsford disease). *Am. J. Roentgenol. Radium Ther. Nucl. Med. 97:* 1, 1966.

16. LAROSE, J. H., and GAY, B. B., JR.: Metatropic dwarfism. *Am. J. Roentgenol. Radium Ther. Nucl. Med. 106:* 156, 1969.

17. MCKUSICK, V.: *Heritable Disorders of Connective Tissue,* 3rd ed. St. Louis, Mo., Mosby, 1966.

18. MILLER, S. M., and PAUL, L. W.: Roentgen observations in familial metaphyseal dysostosis. *Radiology 83:* 665, 1964.

19. NEUHAUSER, E. B. D., et al.: Progressive diaphyseal dysplasia. *Radiology 51:* 11, 1948.

20. NEUHAUSER, E. B. D., et al.: Diastematomyelia: Transfixation of the cord or cauda equina with congenital anomalies of the spine. *Radiology 54:* 659, 1950.

21. NEWCOMBE, D. S., and KEATS, T. E.: Roentgenographic manifestations of hereditary peripheral dysostosis. *Am. J. Roentgenol. Radium Ther. Nucl. Med. 106:* 178, 1969.

22. PAUL, L. W.: Hereditary multiple diaphyseal sclerosis (Ribbing). *Radiology 60:* 412, 1953.

23. PAUL, L. W.: Punctate epiphyseal dysplasia (chondrodystrophia calcificans congenita); report of a case with nine year period of observation. *Am. J. Roentgenol. Radium Ther. Nucl. Med. 71:* 941, 1954.

24. PIRNAR, T., and NEUHAUSER, E. B. D.: Asphyxiating thoracic dystrophy of the newborn. *Am. J. Roentgenol. Radium Ther. Nucl. Med. 98:* 358, 1966.

25. POZNANSKI, A. K., NASANCHUK, J. S., BAUBLIS, J., and HOLT, J. F.: The cerebro-hepato-renal syndrome (CHRS). *Am. J. Roentgenol. Radium Ther. Nucl. Med. 109:* 313, 1970.

26. PRATT, A. D., FELSON, B., WIOT, J. F., and PAIGE, M.: Sequestrum formation in fibrous dysplasia. *Am. J. Roentgenol. Radium Ther. Nucl. Med. 106:* 162, 1969.

27. RUBIN, P.: *Dynamic Classification of Bone Dysplasias.* Chicago, Year Book, 1964.

28. SCHWARZ, E.: Hypercallosis in osteogenesis imperfecta. *Am. J. Roentgenol. Radium Ther. Nucl. Med. 85:* 645, 1962.

29. SILVERMAN, F. N.: A differential diagnosis of achondroplasia. *Radiol. Clin. North Am. 6:* 223, 1968.

30. SILVERMAN, F. N.: "Pediatric Radiology," in *Modern Trends in Diagnostic Radiology—4,* ed. by J. W. McLaren. New York, Appleton-Century-Crofts, 1970.

31. SINGLETON, E. B., DAESCHNER, C. W., and TENG, C. T.: Peripheral dysostosis. *Am. J. Roentgenol. Radium Ther. Nucl. Med. 84:* 499, 1960.

32. SPRANGER, J. W., and LANGER, L. O., JR.: Spondyloepiphyseal dysplasia congenita. *Radiology 94:* 313, 1970.

33. STEINBACH, H. L., et al.: The Hurler syndrome without abnormal mucopolysacchariduria. *Radiology 90:* 472, 1968.

34. TASKER, W. G., MASTRI, A. R., and GOLD, A. P.: Chondrodystrophia calcificans congenita (dysplasia epiphysalis punctata). *Am. J. Dis. Child. 119:* 122, 1970.

3

MISCELLANEOUS SKELETAL ANOMALIES AND SYNDROMES

ACCESSORY BONES AND OSSIFICATION CENTERS

Certain accessory bones and centers of ossification that fail to unite are found rather frequently in the skeleton. An accessory bone represents either a supernumerary ossicle not ordinarily found in the skeleton or a bony process or secondary center for the tip of a process that has failed to fuse and remains as a separate bony structure. An accessory bone may be mistaken for a pathologic condition, particularly a fracture, and a knowledge of their distribution and frequency is of some importance.

DIFFERENTIATION OF ANOMALOUS BONES FROM FRACTURES

A fracture line is ragged along the margin and it is invariably irregular. Anomalous fissures are characterized by smooth margins, rounding of the edges, and a line of cortex along the entire surface. A chip fracture will have an irregular surface at the line of fracture and there is a defect in the adjacent bone corresponding to the avulsed chip. Fresh fractures are always accompanied by swelling of the contiguous soft tissues. Accessory centers

and anomalous bones are commonly bilateral. Examination of the corresponding part of the opposite extremity is helpful in doubtful cases.

THE FOOT AND ANKLE

The foot is a common site for the appearance of accessory bones (Fig. 3-1) and the following are the most frequent:

Os Trigonum. This accessory ossicle occurs in about 10 per cent of individuals. It is a separate center for the posterior process of the astragalus to which the astragalofibular ligament is attached. Its shape varies from a small triangular fragment to one more rounded or oval. The division from the astragalus may be incomplete. A fracture of a long posterior process of the astragalus may resemble an os trigonum. Differentiation depends upon the factors listed in the preceding paragraph.

Os Tibiale Externum. This ossicle represents the unfused tuberosity on the medial proximal side of the tarsal scaphoid (navicular). It is sometimes called the divided scaphoid or an accessory scaphoid. It is a common variation and is usually bilateral.

Os Peroneum (Peroneal Sesamoid). The os peroneum is a small ossicle found in or adjacent

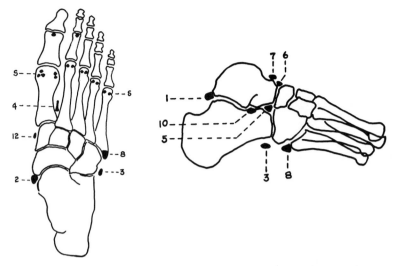

Fig. 3-1. Common accessory ossicles in the foot. **(1)** Os trigonum; **(2)** os tibiale externum; **(3)** os peroneum; **(4)** os intermetatarseum; **(5)** calcaneus secondarius; **(6)** supranavicular; **(7)** secondary astragalus; **(8)** os vesalianum; **(10)** os sustentaculi; **(S)** sesamoid bones (The **small black dots** over the metatarsal heads and proximal phalanges of first and second toes represent the most frequent sites of these sesamoid bones but they may occur in other locations). No. **9** is not included, for purposes of clarity.

to the tendon of the peroneus longus just lateral to and below the os calcis and cuboid (Fig. 3-2). It is found in about 8 per cent of individuals. Occasionally there may be two or even three separate ossicles representing a bipartite or tripartite sesamoid.

Os Intermetatarseum. This is a small bone having the form of a tiny rudimentary metatarsal found between the proximal ends of the first and second metatarsals; its frequency is about 10 per cent.

Calcaneus Secondarius. The secondary os calcis is a small, irregular bony mass found at the upper anterior end of the os calcis where it articulates with the astragalus and navicular. It is seen to best advantage in oblique roentgenograms of the foot; its frequency is about 2 per cent.

Supranavicular (Pirie's Bone). This is a small, triangular bone occurring at the proximal superior edge of the navicular and which articulates with the astragalus and navicular. It is relatively common and can easily be mistaken for a fracture.

Secondary Astragalus. The secondary astragalus is a small rounded bone found just above the head of the astragalus; it is seen only in lateral views of the foot. It should not be confused with the supranavicular, which lies between the astragalus and scaphoid.

Os Vesalianum. This is a rare accessory bone found just proximal to the head of the fifth metatarsal. It should not be mistaken for the lateral epiphysis of the metatarsal head, which is a normal finding (see below).

Epiphysis for the Head of Metatarsal V. This bony center is not an anomaly but is a constant epiphysis that appears about the age of thirteen and unites shortly thereafter. It is a flat bony center found along the lateral side of the proximal end of metatarsal V. It often is irregular in shape but its long axis parallels the long axis of the metatarsal. A fracture in this location is also common but the line of fracture invariably extends across the long axis of the shaft, the fracture surfaces are irregular, the soft tissues overlying the area are swollen, and the proximal fragment often is displaced or rotated.

Os Sustentaculi. This is a rare small wedge-shaped bone that comprises the upper posterior end of the sustentaculum tali.

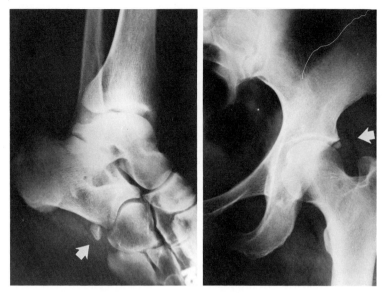

Fig. 3-2. *Left,* Os peroneum; (*right*) os acetabuli.

CUBOIDEUM SECONDARIUM. This is another rare bone, which represents the cuboid divided into two portions.

PARACUNEIFORM. Only a few cases of this bone have been reported. It is a small rounded ossicle lying along the medial aspect of the internal cuneiform and is seen to best advantage in anteroposterior roentgenograms of the foot.

OS SUBTIBIALE. The os subtibiale is a separate ossification center for the tip of the medial malleolus.

OS SUBFIBULARE. Corresponding to the subtibiale, this is a separate center for the tip of the lateral malleolus. It varies from a tiny rounded ossicle to a fairly large triangular fragment. It is best seen in anteroposterior views of the ankle joint. Some of these apparent accessory ossicles around the ankle joint may be old chip fracture fragments that have smoothed off and have united with fibrous rather than bony union. Others may be foci of ossification that have formed as a result of soft tissue injury. It often is impossible to determine the nature of such an ossification in the ankle area from a single roentgen examination. Because of the frequency of injury to the ankle one must always consider the possibility of an apparent ossicle of this type being secondary to injury rather than an anomalous ossification center.

THE KNEE

BIPARTITE PATELLA. The patella may be divided into two or even more segments. The smaller segment or segments are usually located along the upper outer quadrant of the patella. The recognition of this anomaly is important as it may be mistaken for fracture. In approximately 80 per cent of the cases the anomaly is bilateral.

FABELLA. The fabella is a small sesamoid bone very frequently found in the tendon of the lateral head of the gastrocnemius muscle at the level of the knee joint. It may become enlarged and roughened in the presence of degenerative disease of the knee joint.

THE HIP

OS ACETABULI. The os acetabuli is a round or oval ossicle lying along the upper rim of the acetabulum (see Fig. 3-2). This is not the anatomic os acetabuli that forms in the Y-shaped triradiate acetabular cartilage, but is either an ununited epiphyseal center or a sesamoid bone. There is normally an epiphyseal center or centers for the upper rim of the acetabulum that appear at about the age of 13 and that undergo fusion with the acetabulum within a very short time. Failure of this epiphysis to unite results in some cases of this so-called roentgenologic os acetabuli. In other instances a small sesamoid may be found in this area, usually situated more laterally than the epiphysis but called by the same name.

THE SHOULDER

Os ACROMIALE. The os acromiale is the unfused tip of the acromion process. It represents a normal secondary ossification center that fails to undergo fusion. The incidence of this anomaly has been reported as from 1 to 6 per cent but we have seen it infrequently.

THE ELBOW

PATELLA CUBITI. The patella cubiti is a small bony center that forms at the tip of the olecranon process of the ulna. Some authorities contend that there are no proved accessory centers at the elbow and that this is actually an example of osteochondritis dissecans (see Chapter 8).

THE WRIST AND HAND

The variations in the wrist are numerous, Pfitzner listing 33 possible carpal elements. They are less common clinically than those in the foot. The most important ones are listed below (Fig. 3-3).

Os CENTRALE. This is a small ossicle situated on the radial side of the os magnum (capitate). In the embryo this is a frequent cartilaginous center and it may persist into adult life as a separate ossicle. Frequently the cartilaginous os centrale does not ossify but remains as a separate cartilage fragment visible only as a distinct notch or space on the outer side of the os magnum.

DIVIDED SCAPHOID (NAVICULAR). The carpal scaphoid may be found in two parts with a trans-

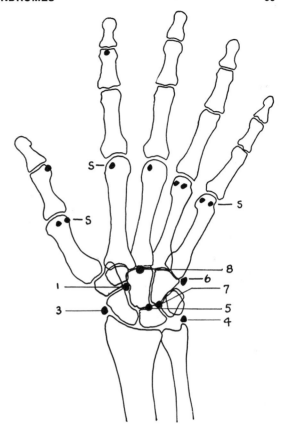

Fig. 3-3. Diagram illustrating the most frequent accessory ossicles in the hand and wrist. **(1)** Os centrale; **(3)** os radiale externum; **(4)** os triangulare; **(5)** epilunatum; **(6)** os vesalianum manus; **(7)** epipyramis; **(8)** os styloideum; **(S)** the most frequent sites for sesamoid bones in the hand; No. **2** is not included, for purposes of clarity.

verse fissure through the center. It may be difficult to determine whether this is an anomaly or an old ununited fracture since fractures of this bone are notorious for their failure to unite with bony union. Eburnation of edges, roughness, and cystlike areas along the line of the fissure favor the diagnosis of an ununited fracture. When the fissure is the result of an anomaly the bone otherwise is normal.

RADIALE EXTERNUM. The radiale externum is an infrequent small ossicle lying just distal to the styloid process of the radius.

Os TRIANGULARE. This is a small bone found at the tip of the ulnar styloid. It can be differentiated from fracture of the styloid process by the fact that the styloid is of normal length without the addition of this fragment.

EPILUNATUM. The epilunatum is a separate center for the dorsal tip of the semilunar (lunate).

OS VESALIANUM MANUS. This is a small bone in the wrist that corresponds to a similar one in the foot and is found at the proximal end of the 5th metacarpal. It is a rare anomaly.

EPIPYRAMIS. The epipyramis is a small ossicle that occurs between the os magnum, unciform, and cuneiform. This is another of the uncommon variants in the wrist.

OS STYLOIDEUM. The unfused styloid process of the third metacarpal is known as the os styloideum. It projects from the dorsal side of the base of the third metacarpal and is usually visualized best in true lateral projections of the wrist. It is a rather frequent anomaly.

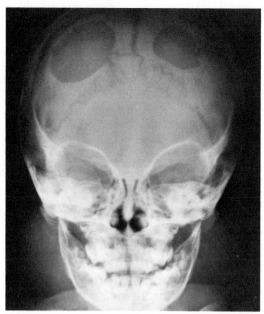

Fig. 3-4. Congenital enlarged parietal foramina. Note wormian bones along the lambdoid suture.

CONGENITAL VARIATIONS IN THE SKULL AND FACIAL BONES

WORMIAN BONES

Wormian bones are small separate ossicles found between the sutures of the skull; they are most frequent near the junction of the coronal and lambdoid sutures (Fig. 3-4). They are of no clinical importance as a rule but are often associated with other anomalies of the skeleton. A particularly large ossicle is occasionally seen forming the superior portion of the occipital bone; this is known as the Inca bone.

SKULL DEFECTS WITH MENINGOCELE

A meningocele of the skull represents herniation of a meningeal sac through a defect in the skull and is of fairly frequent occurrence. The sac may contain only the meninges and cerebrospinal fluid or it may contain a variable amount of brain tissue. The size of the defect in the skull varies greatly and occasionally it may be very large. Meningoceles occur in the midline of the skull and the most frequent situation is in the occipital region. In some cases the defect communicates with the foramen magnum and in others there is absence of one or more of the upper cervical arches (occipitocervical meningocele). Less frequently cranial meningocele occurs in the anterior aspect of the skull in the region of the glabella and, rarely, in the base of the skull.

CONGENITAL PARIETAL FORAMINA

The parietal foramina are two tiny channels in the posterior parts of the parietal bones close to the midline for the passage of the parietal arteries. Rarely, these may be greatly enlarged up to several centimeters in diameter (Fig. 3-4). They may communicate across the midline, forming a dumbbell-shaped defect. There is a distinct hereditary tendency for the occurrence of enlarged parietal foramina. They are of no clinical importance but may be mistaken for trephine holes or for destruction caused by disease.

LACUNA SKULL (LÜCKENSCHÄDEL)

In association with a spinal meningocele and occasionally seen as an isolated defect without meningocele, the cranial bones may show excessively prominent lakelike depressions of the inner table that give the skull a relief map appearance (Fig. 3-5). The skull is thinned in the depths of the depressions, which are surrounded by smooth ridges. There may be complete bony defects in some areas. In addition to the spina bifida and meningocele there often are other skeletal deformities, particularly in the spine and ribs. The cause of the skull changes is unknown; theories that have been suggested include increased intracranial pressure during intrauterine life, and a congenital ossification defect of the cranial bones. In some patients the entire skull is involved. More frequently the changes are confined to the posterior aspect of the vault or at least are the most prominent in this region. If the lacuna skull is an isolated defect and not associated with other

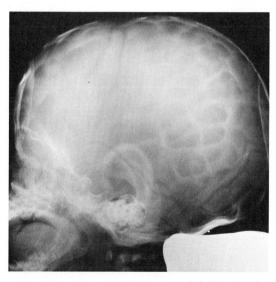

Fig. 3-5. Lacuna skull (lückenschadel). The translucent areas represent thin bone separated by ridges on the inner table. The condition can be distinguished from the "beaten silver" appearance caused by increased intracranial pressure by the normal size of the skull and the presence of normal vault sutures.

lesions that might cause early death, there is a gradual disappearance of the abnormality and the skull, after a period of several years, tends to assume a normal appearance.

PREMATURE FUSION OF THE SUTURES (CRANIOSYNOSTOSIS)

The sutures of the skull usually remain open until middle life or later and may never completely fuse. When they fuse prematurely before growth is complete the skull becomes deformed; if fusion is extensive and occurs early enough in life, increased intracranial pressure may result as the brain continues to grow. Growth of the skull is largely a reflection of growth of the brain and most of this (80 per cent) occurs during the first 3 years of life. The brain is reported to double its weight during the first 7 months of life and to triple it in 30 months. Premature fusion of the sutures developing during the first year of life, therefore, is more significant than a similar occurrence during later childhood. While one or more of the sutures may be fused at the time of birth, it is more frequent to find them open with the fusion occurring some time later. A suture that is going to close prematurely often will show some thickening or heaping up of bone along its edges when the suture is viewed end on. The normal sutures in the newborn are poorly defined with the edges of the bones fading gradually into the suture area. When the margins of the bones are sharply defined and the suture lines easily visualized during very early infancy, the possibility of imminent fusion is considerable. Once a suture has fused, growth proceeds in whatever direction possible unless all sutures fuse simultaneously; then severe signs of increased intracranial pressure are to be expected (Fig. 3-6). It is important to recognize the more severe forms of craniosynostosis during early infancy, preferably during the first year of life, because surgical measures are available that will prevent undue deformity of the skull from developing.

In addition to primary premature closure of

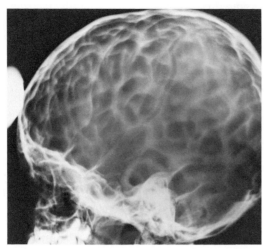

Fig. 3-6. Craniosynostosis. Premature closure of all the vault sutures has caused a deepening of the convolutional impressions on the inner table ("beaten silver" appearance), indicating that there is chronic increase in intracranial pressure. This is caused by growth of the brain within the unyielding skull. Note complete absence of suture lines that normally should be present during childhood.

the sutures, craniosynostosis occurs as a secondary phenomenon in a variety of diseases and dysplasias.[14]

Depending upon which sutures fuse first a number of different types of craniosynostosis can be recognized:

MICROCEPHALY

When all the vault sutures close early and at about the same time there results an abnormally small head with roentgen signs of increased intracranial pressure (deep impressions on the inner table of the skull and erosion of the sella). This type of craniosynostosis is not very frequent and defective development of the brain is a more common cause of a microcephalic skull. As noted above, unless growth of the brain proceeds in a normal manner, enlargement of the skull will not occur. In these patients with defective brain growth the skull is abnormally small but the sutures remain visible. The bones of the vault instead of showing increased convolutional impressions and being unusually thin may actually be thicker than normal. Even under these circumstances the sutures may fuse early, but signs of increased pressure do not develop since there is a failure of the brain to grow.

TURRICEPHALY (OXYCEPHALY; TURRET HEAD)

Turricephaly is a form of craniostenosis characterized by an unusually high vertex and an increased vertical diameter of the skull. As a rule it is caused by an early closure of one or more of the transverse sutures (coronal or lambdoid) so that growth proceeds in an upward direction only. The premature fusion may be limited to the coronal suture, to the coronal and the lambdoid, or it may affect all the vault sutures. When all the sutures are found to be fused and the skull still has a turricephalic shape it usually indicates that the fusion began in the lambdoid and that the other sutures fused at a later date. Increased convolutional impressions are often seen in the frontal area in this condition and they may be widespread in the more severe cases (the impressions probably do not actually correspond to the convolutions of the brain, but the term "convolutional impression" has come into wide use). With more extensive fusion there may be the clinical signs of increased intracranial pressure including exophthalmos, mental retardation, convulsions, headaches, and failing vision. Several cases have been reported in which an abnormal-appearing sella turcica was found in association with an oxycephalic skull leading to the erroneous impression of a pituitary tumor.[22]

SCAPHOCEPHALY

In scaphocephaly the head is long and narrow and the deformity is caused by an early closure of the sagittal suture so that skull growth is predominantly in an anteroposterior direction. This type of skull is called dolichocephalic (see below). When viewed from the front the scaphocephalic skull is triangular in shape with the base of the skull broadened and the vertex more or less pointed (Fig. 3-7).

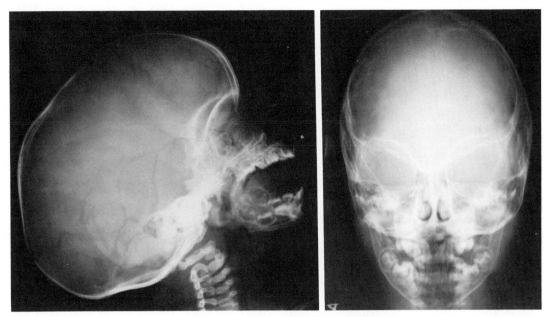

Fig. 3-7. Scaphocephaly. In this defect the head is long and narrow and growth occurs mainly in an anteroposterior direction. This is caused by premature fusion of the major part of the sagittal suture. The lateral vault sutures remain open.

When viewed from the side the appearance sometimes resembles a canoe with upward bulging anteriorly and posteriorly and a central depression.

PLAGIOCEPHALY

Early unilateral closure of one or more of the transverse sutures results in an asymmetrical skull, one side being smaller than the other. This condition is known as plagiocephaly. Few skulls are completely symmetrical and minor degrees of visible asymmetry are moderately frequent. As with other forms of craniostenosis, the significance of these lesser changes is doubtful because lack of growth in one direction can be compensated for in another. It is only when the fusion is present at birth or develops during the first year or two of life that the distortion in shape of the skull may become sufficient to be of clinical importance. When there is unilateral closure of one coronal suture the orbit develops an elliptical shape with an upward slanting of the outer roof (Fig. 3-8).

This is a characteristic finding even when the evidence of sutural closure is not too obvious. There is also elevation of the ipsilateral sphenoid wings and the calvarium becomes flattened on the side of closure. The nasal septum may be directed obliquely upward toward the involved side. Early treatment is aimed at preventing exophthalmos, loss of vision, and to correct cosmetic deformities.

TRIGONOCEPHALY

This is a congenital malformation of the skull in which there is a small pointed forehead. This, together with an increase of the biparietal diameter, gives the skull a triangular or egg-shaped configuration. The cause is unknown but some investigators believe it is the result of premature closure of the metopic (frontal) suture. While the majority of patients with trigonocephaly are otherwise normal, in some there is an associated malformation of parts of the forebrain. In these cases there may be other anomalies such as a deformed nose,

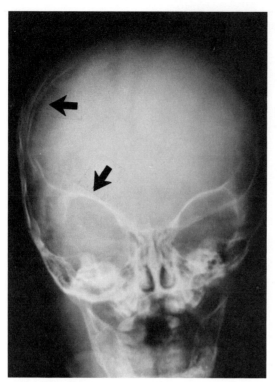

Fig. 3-8. Plagiocephaly. Note elliptical shape of right orbit (**lower arrow**) and piling up of bone along right coronal suture (**upper arrow**).

an undivided nasal cavity, absence of the premaxilla and microcephaly. Hypotelorism, with the orbital cavities close together, is another common associated finding. Trigonocephaly usually is more obvious on clinical inspection than on roentgen examination.

CRUZON'S DISEASE

Cruzon's disease, or craniofacial dysostosis, is a form of craniosynostosis inherited as autosomal dominant. The sutural closure most often affects the coronal leading to a brachycephalic skull. However, other sutures may fuse first so that the skull shape is variable. In some it shows the features of a trigonoscaphocephaly. There is hypoplasia of the facial bones. Hypertelorism, exophthalmos, and a divergent squint are present. The nose is beaked (parrot nose). Mental deficiency has been described in

some patients. (See the section on "Apert's Syndrome.")

CLOVERLEAF SKULL (KLEEBLATTSCHÄDEL) SYNDROME

In this rare syndrome there is premature fusion (before birth) of multiple skull sutures including the coronal, lambdoid, squamous, and sagittal. The result is a bizarre, trilobed or cloverleaf-shaped skull.[1] Additionally there are severe exophthalmos, hypertelorism, and shallow orbits. The nose is beaked with a depressed bridge and the ears are low in position. There is hypoplasia of the maxillae with a relative prognathism of the mandible. Abnormalities of the teeth are frequent and there is macroglossia. Of interest are changes in the appendicular skeleton which resemble achondroplasia and which aid in differentiation from Cruzon's disease. Ankylosis of some of the large joints and bowing of the tibias have been described. Webbing of the toes, an equinovarus deformity and spadelike thumbs have been noted in some. The cause is unknown. Most of the patients have died early in life.

CEPHALIC INDEX

The cephalic index is a useful indicator of skull shape. It is obtained by dividing the maximum width of the skull by its length and multiplying by 100. The normal index varies between 65 and 75. If the cephalic index is above 75 the skull is relatively short for its width and this is called brachycephaly. If the index is below 65 the opposite condition is present and the skull is long for its width; this is known as dolichocephaly. In connection with premature fusion of the sutures, the oxycephalic or turricephalic type of skull is usually a form of brachycephaly since the anteroposterior diameter is short compared to the width. In scaphocephaly, however, the length of the skull is increased for the breadth and thus the skull is of dolichocephalic shape. In addition to being caused by premature closure of the sutures, brachycephalic and dolichocephalic skulls may result from other factors, including racial and hereditary influences. Mentally and physically retarded infants who do not or cannot sit up at the normal time and thus are kept on their backs for months often develop brachycephalic skulls because of molding of the soft cranial bones.

APERT'S SYNDROME (ACROCEPHALOSYNDACTYLISM)

This syndrome consists of abnormalities of the skull, hands and feet. Clinically there is an unusually high-peaked forehead, wide-spaced bulging eyes, and a flat face with a short nose. The skull is brachycephalic in shape with a short anteroposterior diameter, a wide transverse diameter, and a high-peaked skull with maximum height between the anterior and posterior fontanelles caused by premature fusion of the transverse vault sutures. The palate is narrow with a high vault. The other prominent feature of the dysplasia is syndactyly (Fig. 3-9). This may be partial or complete. The synostoses may occur between the metacarpals, metatarsals, or phalanges of various digits. The visual appearance has been called "mitten hands" or "stocking feet" because of the extensive soft tissue fusions. Also there may be

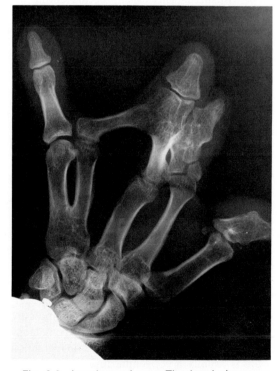

Fig. 3-9. Apert's syndrome. The hand shows extensive fusion anomalies. Similar changes were present in the feet and the skull showed the typical changes of the syndrome.

fusion of two or more segments of the same digit or multiple digits.

OCULAR HYPERTELORISM AND HYPOTELORISM

In *ocular hypertelorism (Greig's syndrome)* the orbital cavities are more widely spaced than normally. The condition is encountered with a variety of associated anomalies including mental retardation, syndactyly, renal hypoplasia, webbing of the neck, congenital heart anomalies, high-arched palate, cleft lip and palate, hypoplasia of the maxilla, macroglossia, microdontia and Sprengel's deformity.[29] Hypertelorism also is seen in various types of craniosynostosis and craniofacial dysostosis. The cause is unknown but it has been suggested that there is overdevelopment of the lesser wings of the sphenoid and a relative underdevelopment of the greater wings. Most cases of hypertelorism can be recognized on frontal roentgenograms of the skull. In borderline cases the measurements devised by Hansman can be used.[23]

Hypotelorism indicates that the orbital cavities are closer together than in the normal.

MANDIBULOFACIAL DYSOSTOSIS (TREACHER-COLLINS SYNDROME)

In this entity there is hypoplasia of the facial bones. The malar bones may be underdeveloped or completely absent (Fig. 3-10). The zygomatic arches are often incomplete. A receding hypoplastic mandible has been present in most of the reported cases and is a distinguishing feature. The palpebral fissures are oblique. Defects of the auricles, stenosis or absence of the external auditory canals and middle ear defects are part of the syndrome in some patients.

GOLDENHAR'S SYNDROME. This entity also is known as *oculoauriculovertebral dysplasia.*[12] There is unilateral hypoplasia or absence of the zygomatic arch, hypoplasia or aplasia of the maxillary sinus on the same side and a low position of the orbit. There is minimal to marked unilateral hy-

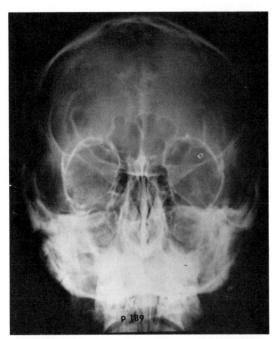

Fig. 3-10. Treacher-Collins syndrome. Note complete absence of both zygomatic arches. Compare with normal right zygoma in Figure 2-36.

poplasia of the mandible and hypoplasia of the temporal bone with decreased development of the mastoid. The unilateral nature of the defects allows differentiation from the Treacher-Collins syndrome. Multiple anomalies of the vertebrae are present including hemivertebrae, fused vertebrae, and spina bifida. The odontoid process may be elongated.

PORENCEPHALY

Porencephaly represents a defect in the cerebral structures, which appears as a cystlike cavity either communicating with the ventricles or separated from them by only a thin layer of tissue. It is found most commonly near the central fissure but may occur elsewhere in the brain. Porencephaly may be either congenital or acquired; the latter usually is the result of trauma occurring at or shortly after birth. In many cases, when the patient has reached late adolescent or early adult life, plain roentgenograms of the skull reveal a unilateral decrease in size of the skull, depressions on the inner table with local thinning of the

diploë, and an overdevelopment of the sinuses, particularly of the ethmoid cells on the side of the cyst. Such changes in the cranial bones always suggest the possibility of an underlying porencephaly but similar findings are observed in unilateral cerebral atrophy without actual cyst formation. During encephalography or ventriculography after gas has been introduced into the subarachnoid space and the ventricular system, the cyst may fill and this type of procedure offers the maximum diagnostic information.

ANENCEPHALY

In anencephaly there is an almost complete absence of the skull and brain and the anomaly is incompatible with life. The cranial bones that are present form an ill-defined mass. The chief importance roentgenologically lies in the detection of this condition in utero and the diagnosis can be made without difficulty on roentgen examination of the mother when ossification of the fetal skeleton has developed sufficiently for the bones to be visualized. This usually occurs during the fifth or sixth month of gestation.

PLATYBASIA

In platybasia the base of the skull is unusually flat. *The normal basal angle* is formed by drawing lines from the nasofrontal suture and the anterior lip of the foramen magnum to the tuberculum sellae. This angle has an upper limit of normal of about 140°. Basal angles above 140° indicate some degree of platybasia. Flattening of the base of the skull in itself is of no importance but it frequently is caused by an invagination of the occiput into the base (basilar invagination). In turn, basilar invagination may be a developmental anomaly or it may be caused by abnormal softening of the bones as a result of disease. Among the conditions that predispose to basilar invagination are Paget's disease (Fig. 3-11) and osteomalacia. In the congenital type of basilar invagination there is usually a congenital fusion anomaly of the first cervical vertebra with the occiput (Fig. 3-12). When either *basilar invagination* or *cervico-occipital fusion* is present, the foramen

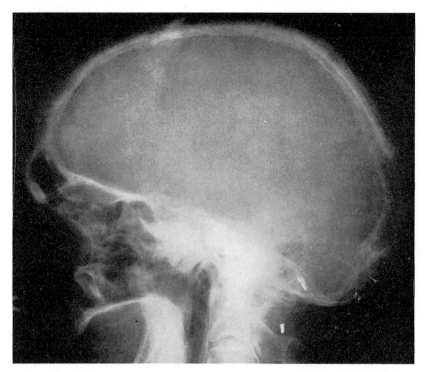

Fig. 3-11. Platybasia caused by Paget's disease of the skull. The basal angle (see text) is nearly 180° (normal is 140°). This is caused by the softness of the cranial bones, which allows the skull to be molded over the upper part of the cervical spine.

magnum may be decreased in size and deformed in shape and thus cause pressure upon the cord or medulla, with the development of clinical signs and symptoms.

SINUS PERICRANII

Occasionally a large vein extends through the skull, forming a localized soft tissue swelling in the scalp. Characteristically the swelling becomes larger when the patient lowers his head or when the intracranial pressure is elevated from any cause such as sneezing or coughing. It decreases in size or disappears when the head is held upright. This condition is known as sinus pericranii. The opening in the skull through which the venous channel extends may be large enough to be visible in skull roentgenograms and then is seen as a smooth, rounded defect. The diagnosis is readily apparent when the clinical signs are elicited.

DERMOID TUMORS

A dermoid tumor of the scalp may have an intracranial extension through a small defect in the cranial bone or the major portion of the tumor may be in the cranial cavity with a small stalk projecting through the skull. Dermoids are found in or very close to the midline. The character of the skull defect is not diagnostic in skull roentgenograms and it may appear similar to the defect of sinus pericranii or that of a small craniocele or meningocele.

PARIETAL THINNING

An area of thinning of the bone is seen infrequently in the superior portion of one or both parietal bones. When viewed tangentially the inner table is seen to be normal but the diploë is absent in the area of thinning and the inter-

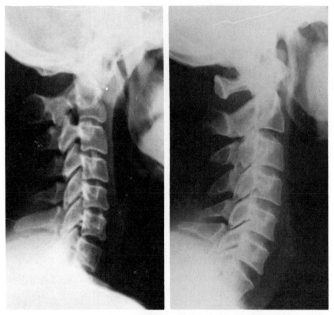

Fig. 3-12. Congenital cervico-occipital fusion (*left*). The first cervical vertebra is fused to the occiput, only a part of its arch being visible. Compare with lateral view of normal cervical spine on the *right*.

nal and external tables are fused. The defect extends in an anteroposterior direction and may be in the form of a distinct groove, which is easily palpated. The condition is of no clinical importance and is not a cause of symptoms.

BATHROCEPHALY

In this anomaly there is an overgrowth of the apex of the occipital bone, superiorly, so that it projects posterior to the parietal bones when viewed from the side. Its only importance lies in the fact that it may be mistaken for a depressed fracture.

CONGENITAL VARIATIONS IN THE SPINE

Many developmental anomalies are found in the spinal column. Because of the important part that the spine plays in weight-bearing,

some of these lead to clinical symptoms while others are only incidental findings and of importance because they may be confused with changes resulting from trauma or disease.

DEVELOPMENT OF THE SPINE

Because of its importance in roentgen interpretation, a summary of the development of the spine as described by Ehrenhaft[15] is given here. The column of cells derived from the entoderm around which the vertebrae develop is called the notochord. During the early weeks of embryonic life this forms a long rounded column extending from the hypophyseal pouch to the lower end of the primitive spine. It is the central structure around which the vertebrae are formed. Without going into the more precise details concerning vertebral development it is sufficient to recall that the mesenchyme surrounding the notochord undergoes segmentation with the formation of zones of densely packed cells called scleromes separated by less dense zones. The scleromes develop processes that form the anlagen for the vertebral bodies, the neural arches, and the transverse processes or ribs. Eventually the notochord is completely surrounded by the processes arising from the scleromes and the primitive vertebrae are formed. With further development the notochord becomes more and more squeezed into the regions that will become the intervertebral discs. The anlage for the vertebral body is divided initially into two lateral halves by an extension of the perichordal sheath. Centers of chondrification begin on either side of the sheath. The cartilage centers fuse but for a time there is left a remnant of the sheath in the center of the cartilaginous body, known as the mucoid streak. This is continuous with the remnants of notochord that come to lie within the disc regions. These masses of notochordal cells with the addition of mucoid material, fibrous tissue, and hyalin cartilage cells form the nucleus pulposus of the fully developed disc. Notochordal cells can be identified in the nucleus until the age of adolescence or even later. During early life and until about the age of 25 to 30 years the nucleus forms a semifluid, noncompressible substance that is of great importance in absorbing shocks and in distributing the stresses to which the spine is subjected. During the period of its development the intervertebral disc is supplied by blood vessels derived from the periosteal vessels as well as by some extending into the disc from the vertebral bodies. The latter vessels penetrate the cartilage plate surrounding the nucleus pulposus. Along with other degenerative changes that begin in the disc shortly after birth, these vessels regress and eventually disappear. Where the vessels penetrated the cartilage plates of the disc, defects in chondrification result and these may persist throughout life. They form weakened areas through which protrusion of disc material into the vertebral body can occur. These herniations are known as Schmorl nodes (Fig. 3-13). The discs become avascular during the third decade of life and the nucleus pulposus gradually is replaced by fibrous tissue.

While the remnants of notochord enclosed within cartilage will disappear as the disc becomes avascular, there are areas where small masses of fetal notochord may persist throughout life. These are found most frequently in the region of the clivus at the base of the skull and in the sacrococcygeal area. It is in these locations where the tumor known as chordoma is prone to develop.

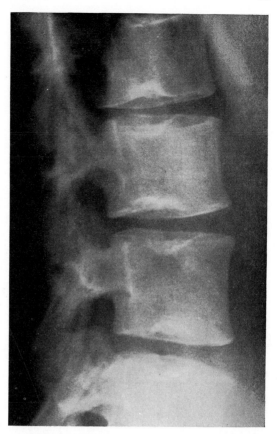

Fig. 3-13. Schmorl nodes. There are shallow, concave defects on the upper and lower disc surfaces of the lumbar vertebrae. These are probably congenital defects.

Remnants of notochord sometimes persist where the mucoid streak entered the disc. These are visible roentgenologically as smooth, cup-shaped or concave defects centrally situated on the disc surface of one or more of the vertebral bodies. Usually the defects are multiple and they are seen most frequently in the lower part of the thoracic and upper part of the lumbar spine. Such defects represent weakened areas with thinning or at times a complete deficiency of the cartilage plates of the disc. They are in effect a congenital or developmental type of Schmorl node. In some instances larger masses of notochordal tissue remain, causing larger defects on the disc surface of the vertebral bodies. As noted above, gaps in chondrification of the disc may form where the cartilage was perforated by vessels arising from the vertebral body. These weak areas predispose to traumatic protrusion of disc material. So long as the herniated material is composed only of cartilage the defect may be difficult or impossible to visualize in roentgenograms. Usually with the passage of time reactive sclerosis forms around the herniated cartilage nodule and it then becomes visible. Traumatic Schmorl nodes usually occur near the center of the disc surface of the body but may be situated eccentrically. The defect is concave and the wall of sclerosis usually is distinct (see Fig. 5-22). Thinning of the intervertebral disc space may or may not accompany herniation of disc material. Thinning of the disc in these cases is caused not so much by the actual loss of disc material as it is by the associated degenerative changes that may either precede or follow the herniation. With degeneration the disc loses turgor and elasticity and its total volume is reduced.

Ossification of the vertebral body begins at 3½ to 4 months of fetal life from two separate centers. These do not correspond to the two centers of chondrification mentioned above but rather are situated dorsally and ventrally to one another. Shortly after their appearance they fuse to form a single center for each vertebral body. The neural arch ossifies from two centers, one for each lateral half. At birth the vertebra consists of three separate ossification areas, one for the body and two for the arch, and these are separated by zones of cartilage. Shortly after birth the two halves of the laminae unite, beginning first in the lumbar area and ascending to the cervical. Union of the arches to the bodies begins during the third year of life and is completed by about the seventh year. In this instance fusion begins in the cervical region and is completed in the lumbar. At the time of puberty secondary ossification centers appear for the tips of each of the vertebral processes and a ringlike epiphyseal plate for the upper and lower edges of the bodies also begins to ossify (Fig. 3-14).

FUSION OF VERTEBRAE

Fusion or partial fusion of two or more vertebral bodies is a frequent occurrence. Usually such fusion can be differentiated from that resulting from disease by the fact that the sum in height of the combined fused bodies is equal to the normal height of two vertebrae less the intervertebral disc space; the bony structure is

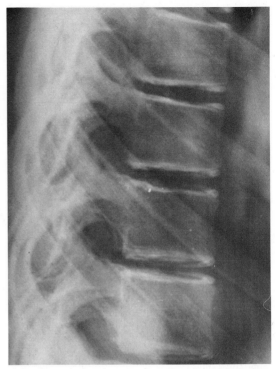

Fig. 3-14. Normal "ring" epiphysis of the vertebrae. Lateral view of midthoracic spine of an adolescent.

normal except for the fusion; in cases of partial fusion it is the anterior aspect that fuses while a rudiment of the disc remains in the posterior portion. This condition sometimes is called *block vertebra* (Fig. 3-15). Clinical symptoms ordinarily are not associated with vertebral fusion except as listed below.

OCCIPITOCERVICAL FUSION

This consists of a fusion or partial fusion of the atlas and the occiput. Associated with this there usually is deformity of the foramen magnum, which is often decreased in size and irregular in shape and frequently a platybasia deformity of the skull. This has been discussed in the section "Platybasia" (see Fig. 3-12). In most normal individuals the upper edge of the odontoid process of the second cervical vertebra lies below a line drawn between the poste-

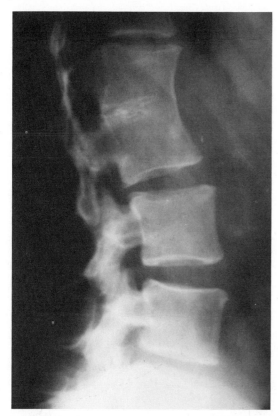

Fig. 3-15. Congenital fusion of two lumbar vertebrae ("block vertebra"). A remnant of the intervertebral disc is present posteriorly.

to the skull but the two mentioned are the most commonly used. In some cases there is almost complete assimilation of the first cervical into the occiput with complete bony fusion of these structures. Because of the narrowing that results in the upper cervical spinal canal and at the level of the foramen magnum, pressure on the cord and medulla may result and these patients often develop symptoms simulating multiple sclerosis, lateral sclerosis, syringomyelia, and other neurologic disorders.

KLIPPEL-FEIL SYNDROME

This syndrome is essentially an extensive fusion of the cervical spinal segments. There is a numerical variation in the cervical vertebrae with more or less complete fusion into one bony mass or with multiple irregular ossified segments present. The upper dorsal vertebrae may be affected in the same way and there often are spina bifida defects as well as other skeletal anomalies (see Fig. 3-31). Males and females are affected equally. The classic physical signs include apparent absence or shortening of the neck with a lowering of the hairline on the back of the neck and limitation of motion of the head. Other signs and symptoms that may be present include torticollis, mirror movements, facial asymmetry, dorsal scoliosis, difficulty in breathing or swallowing, and hearing deficiencies. Klippel-Feil syndrome is sometimes associated with congenital elevation of the scapula (see Fig. 3-31).

HEMIVERTEBRA

Failure or improper development of a lateral half of a vertebral body results in a hemivertebra. Embryologically the fault probably lies in an absence of one of the lateral centers of chondrification. A hemivertebra has a triangular shape when viewed in the anteroposterior roentgenogram and it causes an acute lateral angulation of the spine. A hemivertebra in the thoracic region has only one rib, that on the side of the ossified center. Associated with a hemivertebra there may be numerical variations in the ribs, fusion of two or

rior margin of the hard palate and the posterior rim of the foramen magnum (Chamberlain's line) in a lateral roentgenogram of the skull and cervical spine. At times in the normal the odontoid projects slightly above this level, perhaps as much as 5 to 7 mm; when there is fusion of the first cervical vertebra and the occiput, the odontoid also is situated close to the occiput and will invariably extend above this line. McGregor's line also can be used. This is drawn from the upper surface of the posterior edge of the hard palate to the most inferior part of the floor of the posterior fossa, i.e., the occipital curve. Normally, the tip of the odontoid does not project more than 4.0 mm above this line. There are several other lines that have been proposed to indicate abnormal elevation of the odontoid in its relation more ribs, and rudimentary development of some of the others. Except for the scoliotic deformity that it causes, a hemivertebra is of no clinical importance (Fig. 3-16).

MIDLINE CLEFTS

Rarely the two lateral centers of chondrification for a vertebral body fail to fuse and a cleft persists in the midsagittal plane, dividing the body into two lateral halves. More frequently the cleft is only partial, resulting in a rather characteristic shape that is described as "butterfly vertebra" (Fig. 3-17). Another anomaly consists in a partial or complete cleft in the coronal plane, separating the vertebral body into anterior and posterior portions. Either the anterior or posterior half of a vertebral body may fail to develop and the result is a ventral or a dorsal hemivertebra. A dorsal hemivertebra is more common and because of its wedge shape and absence of normal ossifica-

tion anteriorly there results a sharp gibbus deformity in the spine.

NEURAL ARCH DEFECTS

The presence of a vertical cleft or ossification defect in the midline of a vertebral arch is common in the lumbosacral region or at other transitional areas in the spine, such as the first cervical, the cervicodorsal, or the dorsolumbar junctions. This condition is known as *spina bifida manifesta* when there are associated soft tissue defects or when there is a meningocele; *spina bifida occulta* when no visible soft part malformation exists. The latter is very frequent in the lumbosacral region, affecting either the arch of the fifth lumbar or the first sacral segment. It is doubtful if any symptoms are caused by the defect in most cases. If there is an associated anomalous development of the

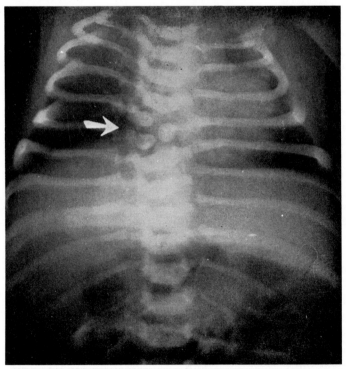

Fig. 3-16. Congenital hemivertebrae in the thoracic spine of an infant. Three hemivertebral segments are visualized. The vertebrae are not fully ossified at this age so that they have not developed the typical triangular shape.

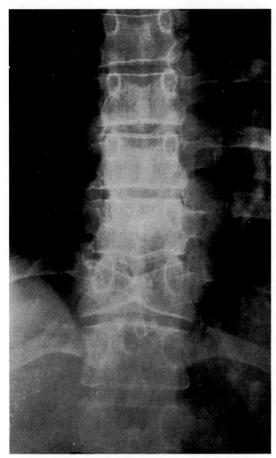

Fig. 3-17. Partial sagittal cleft of the tenth thoracic vertebra ("butterfly vertebra").

articular processes or a partial fusion of adjacent vertebral bodies, such as sacralization of the fifth lumbar or lumbarization of the first sacral segment, it is possible that localized weakness of the spine may result and become manifest after severe exertion. Some orthopedists place more emphasis on this condition than others and its importance as a cause of low back disability is not entirely settled. Cleft formation between the superior and inferior articular processes of a vertebra is frequent, the incidence being reported as from 6 to 7 per cent. The clefts usually are bilateral and they predispose to the forward displacement of one vertebra upon the other. When clefts exist without displacement the condition is known as *spondylolysis.* If displacement is present it is termed *spondylolisthesis* (Fig. 3-18). This

condition is observed most frequently at the lumbosacral joint where the clefts occur in the arch of the fifth lumbar; occasionally the fourth lumbar is affected; only rarely are lateral clefts seen above this level. The amount of displacement varies widely in different cases. Meyerding's classification[35] of the degree of spondylolisthesis is a useful one (Fig. 3-19). In a lateral roentgenogram the superior surface of the sacrum is divided into four equal parts. A forward displacement of the fifth lumbar up to one-fourth the thickness of the sacrum is called a first-degree spondylolisthesis, half the thickness a second-degree spondylolisthesis, etc. Complete displacement of the fifth lumbar on the sacrum with the body of the fifth actually lying in front of the upper sacrum can happen. This is termed a fourth-degree spondylolisthesis. Because the clefts are present between the superior and inferior articular masses, the arch is not attached to the vertebral body by bony support and it is described as a "floating arch." When clefts are present the vertebral body often is decreased in size, particularly in its anteroposterior diameter. The arch may be generally small and poorly developed. Midline spina bifida is sometimes present. Some investigators have been of the opinion that lateral arch defects of this nature are acquired rather than being of developmental origin and have considered birth trauma with a failure of bony union at the sites of the arch fractures as a possible etiologic factor. Also, a chronic stress or fatigue fracture has been implicated in some cases. Anatomists have described these defects as being of developmental origin and consider them to result from the presence of two ossification centers for each side of the arch with subsequent failure of fusion. However, the accumulated evidence indicates an acquired origin, in most cases a stress or fatigue type of fracture.

UNFUSED CENTER FOR ARTICULAR PROCESS

A small, triangular bony mass may be found at the tip of one or more of the inferior articular

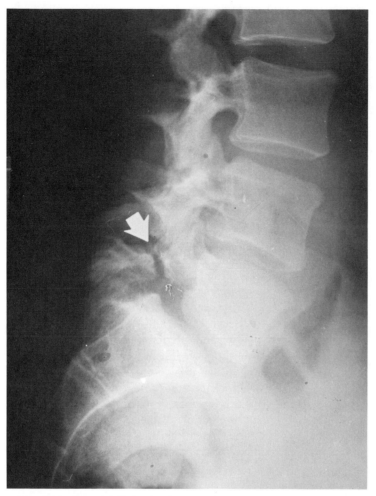

Fig. 3-18. Spondylolisthesis. Lateral view of the lumbosacral area showing a forward displacement of the fifth lumbar vertebra on the sacrum (second-degree spondylolisthesis). Note the clefts in the arch between the upper and lower articular processes (**arrow**). The antero-posterior diameter of *L5* is smaller than that of the other vertebrae and has failed to develop properly; this accentuates the forward offset of this body on the sacrum.

processes of the vertebrae. This represents an un-united ossification center and it can be confused with a fracture. Isolated fracture of this process is very unusual without an associated fracture of the body or neural arch. A similar center occasionally is seen for the superior articular process but is much less frequent.

TRANSITIONAL VERTEBRA

At the junctions of the various major divisions of the spine a vertebra may take on part of the characteristics of both divisions. This is most frequent at the dorsolumbar and the lumbosacral areas. The first lumbar, and rarely the second, may have rudimentary ribs articulating with the transverse processes. The fifth lumbar may be partially sacralized, often with one transverse process fused with the sacrum, the other being free and with only a rudimentary disc between them (Fig. 3-20). The first sacral segment may become partially lumbarized in the same manner. When the transition is complete there will be six lumbar

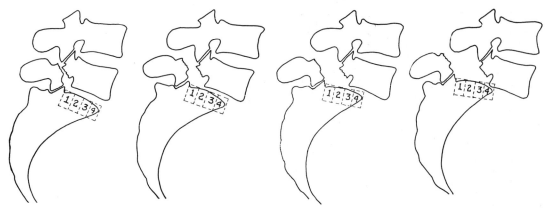

Fig. 3-19. Diagrams illustrating Meyerding's classification of spondylolisthesis. The superior surface of the sacrum is divided into four zones. From *left* to *right* the diagrams illustrate first-, second-, third-, and fourth-degree spondylolisthesis, respectively.

vertebrae or 13 dorsal and four lumbar or various combinations. As a rule an addition of a segment to one division of the spine will be corrected at another level.

The seventh cervical vertebra may have ribs attached to its transverse processes. The ribs may be only short, nubbinlike structures or they may be long enough to articulate with the sternum. Frequently the rib is fused with the first dorsal rib or it forms a pseudarthrosis with it. Even when the rib is short a fibrous band may extend from its tip to the first rib or to the sternum and be a source of pressure upon the brachial plexus or the subclavian artery. There may be only one rib or the condition may be bilateral.

DIASTEMATOMYELIA

This is a rare anomaly of the vertebrae and the spinal cord, usually consisting of a vertical division of the cord or the cauda equina, the two portions being separated by an osseous or fibrocartilaginous septum. This septum is attached anteriorly to one or more of the vertebral bodies. Frequently there is anomalous ossification of the vertebrae; the interpedicular spaces are widened at the site of the defect. Diastematomyelia is found most frequently in the lumbar part of the spine, less commonly in the thoracic region. The lesion is clinically significant and the patient will show evidence sooner or later of impaired innervation to the lower extremities. Dimpling of the skin,

local pigmentation, or excessive hair may be present over the area at birth. Occasionally there is an associated meningocele. Roentgenograms of the spine show widening of the neural canal over several segments and often a fusion or partial fusion of vertebral bodies. Other abnormalities commonly associated include kyphosis, scoliosis, spina bifida, hemivertebrae, abnormal fusion of lamina and narrowing of intervertebral spaces. If the septum dividing the cord is ossified it may be visualized in anteroposterior views as a vertical thin bony plate lying in the midline of the neural canal. When an iodized oil such as pantopaque is injected into the spinal subarachnoid space the defect caused by the septum is readily demonstrated (Fig. 3-21). This procedure of myelography is discussed more fully in Chapter 12.

SACRAL AGENESIS; THE CAUDAL DYSPLASIA SYNDROME

Absence of part or all of the sacrum is an uncommon but not rare anomaly. There is a high incidence of neurogenic bladder in these infants with the complications of vesicoureteral reflux, hydronephrosis, and infection. Occasionally, patients with agenesis of the sacrum or of the lumbar vertebrae or both show a more severe neurologic deficit below the level of the vertebral anomaly and which may be complete. The changes associated with sacral agenesis have been termed the *caudal dysplasia syndrome.*[18] In addition to neurogenic bladder, in the more severe cases there may be abduction and flexion deformities of the

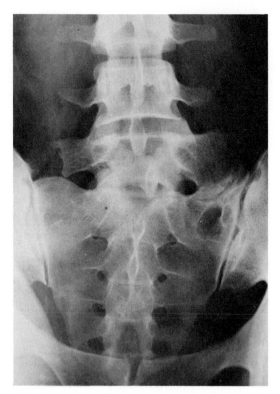

Fig. 3-20. Transitional vertebra. The fifth lumbar has become partially sacralized; its left transverse process is broad and articulates with the sacrum. The right transverse process remains free. In other cases one transverse process will be fused with the sacrum rather than form a joint.

lower extremities with popliteal webbing so that the legs cannot be straightened. The appearance of the lower extremities has been described as "frog-like" or as having a "stuck-on" appearance. Most patients have an equinovarus deformity of the feet and, less frequently, dislocation of the hips. Anomalies in other systems that may be present include renal agenesis, congenital heart disease, imperforate anus, cleft lip or palate, and microcephaly. The upper extremities usually are normal. The increased frequency of this syndrome in infants of diabetic mothers has been commented on in the literature.

MISCELLANEOUS ANOMALIES

Many other variations in development may be found in the spine. The vertebral bodies may be abnormally tall or one or more may show an increased height with the adjacent ones normal. Occasionally a vertebra may be of unusual height in its posterior aspect while the anterior part is normal. This causes it to appear wedge-shaped in the lateral view and to resemble the deformity produced by a fracture. Recognition of the increased height together with the normal texture and appearance of the bone will aid in preventing error. Secondary ossification centers appear at the tips of all the vertebral processes; occasionally one or more of these fail to unite and will persist into adult life as a separate bony fragment. Portions of one or more of the epiphyseal plates for the upper and lower vertebral body surfaces may fail to unite. This results in a triangular bony mass along the anterior border with a corresponding defect in the adjacent vertebral body and is known as *"limbus vertebra"* (Fig. 3-22). The vertebral bodies may be unusually wide for their heights, the condition being termed platyspondyly. This is often associated with other anomalies, particularly of the spinal cord (see section on Diastematomyelia) and in the mucopolysaccharidoses (see Chapter 2).

CONGENITAL VARIATIONS OF EXTREMITIES, THORAX, AND PELVIS

In addition to the ununited ossification centers and supernumerary bones referred to previously, a large number of malformations may involve parts of the skeleton. Many of these are obvious on clinical examination and roentgen study is useful only to make a record of the anatomical changes. Among these are such easily recognized defects as absence of a part, supernumerary digits, etc. A few of these defects deserve mention because they may be confused with acquired disease and others cause significant deformities and interference with functions.

CONGENITAL SYNOSTOSIS

A congenital synostosis consists of a fusion of two or more bones. It is a frequent anomaly in the thorax where there may be a partial fusion of several of the ribs. This may affect

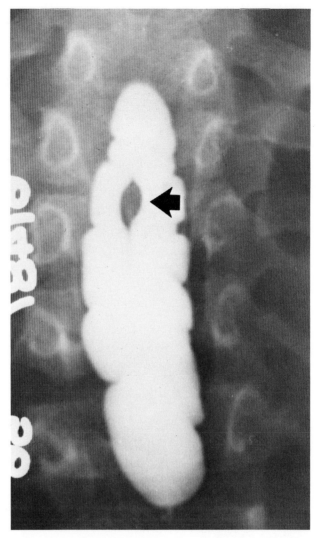

Fig. 3-21. Diastematomyelia. Oil myelogram illustrating the central defect in the oil column caused by the bony spur (**arrow**). Note the widened interpediculate distances of most of the vertebrae at and below the level of the spur. Fusion anomalies also are present.

any part of the rib but is more frequent in the lateral portions and at the vertebral ends. In the latter location the fused ribs may cause a dense shadow along the mediastinum which may, on casual inspection of thoracic roentgenograms, be interpreted as a mass in the mediastinum or the lung.

The proximal ends of the tibia and fibula occasionally are fused. Another uncommon site of fusion is at the proximal ends of the radius and ulna; this results in an inability to supinate the forearm. In some cases there is an associated dislocation of the head of the radius (Fig. 3-23).

Fusion of the vertebral bodies has been discussed in the previous section dealing with the spine.

The *calcaneonavicular bar* is a bony bridge

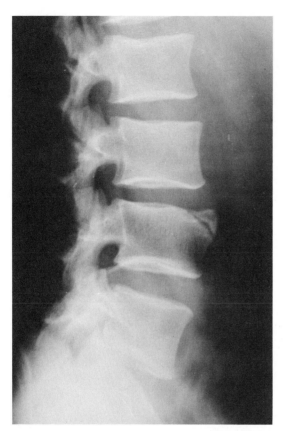

Fig. 3-22. "Limbus vertebra." There is an unfused ossification center along the upper anterior border of the fourth lumbar vertebra. This should not be mistaken for a fracture. It is found most frequently in the lumbar area.

complete or incomplete between the os calcis and the navicular and it may lead to the clinical condition referred to as "peroneal spastic flatfoot" or "rigid flatfoot." The latter term is preferred since the rigidity of the tarsus is the result of bony fixation and not of spasm. The bony fusion may occur at any point between the two bones but is most frequent along the anteromedial aspect. The bony bridge may be incomplete with a fibrous or cartilaginous type of union present. Other tarsal bones may be fused to one another and the general class of these fusion anomalies is known as *tarsal coalition* (Fig. 3-24). Because of the unusual rigidity of the fused joints, clinical complaints of pain may ensue, particularly when unusual stresses are placed upon the foot.

CONGENITAL DISLOCATION

DISLOCATION OF THE HIP

The hip is the most frequent site of congenital dislocation. It is six to ten times as common in females as in males, the left hip is involved more often than the right in the ratio of 3:2, and it is much more frequent in whites than in Negroes. It is unusual for dislocation to be present at birth; rather displacement occurs gradually during the first year of life. Because it has been believed that faulty development of the hip joint and its associated structures was responsible for the dislocation, the term "hip joint dysplasia" has come into common use to denote the conditions that may be present before actual dislocation has developed. However, it is no longer believed by most writers on the subject that the fault lies in lack of proper development or hypoplasia of the bony structures of the hip, particularly the acetabulum. Rather, most investigators consider the fault to be in the supporting soft tissues of the hip joint with the primary abnormality being relaxation of the joint capsule. Shortening or tightening of the muscles which activate motion across the joint is considered by some to be the result rather than the cause of the dislocation. Others, however, consider this to be one of the primary causes along with increased relaxation of the fibrocartilaginous structures, so that when stress is applied dislocation will result. The diagnosis of the predislocation stage during the newborn period is often difficult both clinically and roentgenologically. Caffey and his associates[8] seriously doubt the existence of a dysplastic or predislocation phase, at least in a form that can be recognized by clinical or roentgen examinations.

According to Doberti and Manhood[13] the head of the femur, even though still cartilaginous, will produce a shallow concavity or fossa on the superior wall of the acetabulum through muscular traction and pressure. The floor of the fossa is bounded by a sclerotic margin which aids in identifying it in the neonatal period. Identification of this shallow fossa aids in determining the position of the cartilaginous

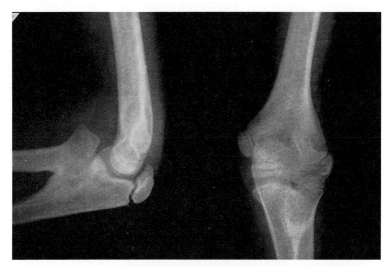

Fig. 3-23. Congenital radioulnar synostosis with congenital dislocation of the head of the radius. There is bony fusion between the dislocated radius and the ulna.

femoral head. If it lies within the inner one-third of the acetabular roof, the head is considered to be in normal position. If situated more laterally, the head is considered to be in abnormal position and the hip dysplastic.

Roentgen examination of the hips for a suspected hip joint dislocation should include an anteroposterior roentgenogram of the pelvis made with the legs straight or slightly flexed at the knee and with the toes pointing forward, and a so-called "frog" view. In this position the thighs are flexed, externally rotated and maximally abducted with the feet brought together in the midline. Careful positioning is necessary to be certain that the hips are symmetrically placed in relation to the film cassette and the roentgen-ray tube so that one side can be compared with the other.

Roentgen Observations

INCREASED ACETABULAR ANGLE. The acetabular angle is in effect a measure of the slope of the upper half of the acetabular wall. The method of determining it is shown in Figure 3-25. For some time it has been considered that the normal acetabular angle for a newborn infant should be approximately 25° with an upper limit of 30°. The acetabular angle as shown in Figure 3-25 is determined by drawing a line along the iliac portion of the acetabular roof to its point of intersection with a line drawn through the centers of both acetabula. An angle above 30° was considered as significant for the presence of hip joint dysplasia that would in turn predispose to hip joint dislocation. Recent observations of Coleman[10] and of Caffey and his associates,[8] based upon the measurement of a large number of infants, indicate that the normal angles vary widely and that the upper limit of normal should be close to 40°. These observations indicate that considerable caution should be exercised in the diagnosis of hip joint dysplasia based only upon the finding of an acetabular angle that measures more than 30°. When only one hip is affected, the acetabular angle is more useful than when both are involved and a definite discrepancy in the angles on the two sides is an important finding. It should be noted in this regard that Caffey's figures indicate that the acetabular angle for the left hip is usually slightly larger than the right. The normal angle decreases considerably between birth and the

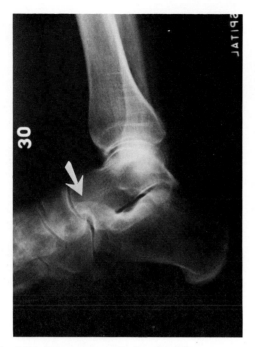

Fig. 3-24. Calcaneonavicular bar (**arrow**).

age of 6 months and to a lesser degree between the ages of 6 months and 1 year.

The iliac angle also can be measured and, when added to the acetabular angle, gives the iliac index. The method for obtaining the iliac angle and index is given in Figures 3-36 and 3-37.

LATERAL DISPLACEMENT OF THE FEMUR. An important finding in many cases is a lateral displacement of the femur in its relationship to the acetabulum. Because the ossification center for the head of the femur is not present at birth and does not appear normally until the age of 3 to 6 months, the neck of the femur must be used for this determination in the newborn. The distance of the upper inner margin of the femoral neck to a fixed point in the acetabulum, such as the inferior edge of the ischial portion, can be measured and, if one hip is normal and the other is displaced, there will be a measurable difference. Perkin's line, as shown in Figure 3-25, is useful when either one or both hips are involved. This consists of a vertical line drawn from the upper outer edge of the

iliac portion of the acetabulum to intersect at a right angle the transverse line drawn through the centers of both acetabula. Coleman found that normally the beak of the femoral neck fell medial to this line in practically every case while in the majority of abnormal hips (60 per cent) the femoral neck was situated lateral to this line.

DISRUPTION OF SHENTON'S LINE. Shenton's line is a smooth, curved imaginary line formed by the inner margin of the femoral neck and the inner surface of the obturator foramen as shown in Figure 3-25. A lateral displacement of the femur may disrupt the smooth curve but usually it requires some degree of upward displacement before a significant break in the curve is seen.

DELAYED OSSIFICATION OF FEMORAL EPIPHYSIS. The ossification center for the head of the femur appears normally between the ages of 3 to 6 months. In the presence of hip joint subluxation or dislocation the center may be delayed in appearance and when it does appear its growth lags behind the normal (Fig. 3-26). In the older infant a disparity in the size of the centers for the femoral heads should be viewed with suspicion as a possible indicator of subluxation on the side of the smaller center. Other signs must be present, however, before this finding can be considered of significance and as a solitary observation it need not be abnormal.

LATER STAGES. In older children and in adults gross displacement usually is present and the diagnosis is made without difficulty (Fig. 3-27). In untreated cases the head and neck of the femur do not develop properly, remaining small and hypoplastic. The acetabular fossa is very shallow, never having accommodated the femoral head. The head often impinges against the outer pelvic wall above and behind the shallow acetabulum and here a shallow pseudo-acetabular cavity may form.

HIP JOINT DYSPLASIA IN THE ADULT. It is still somewhat debatable whether there is such an

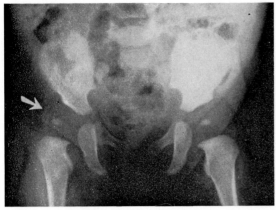
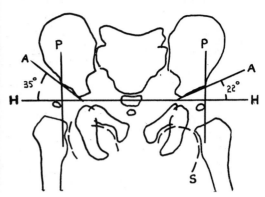

Fig. 3-25. Congenital dislocation of the right hip in an infant. *Left,* Roentgenogram of the pelvis. *Right,* Tracing of roentgenogram. The method for determining the acetabular angle is illustrated. It must be realized that the line **A** drawn along the upper margin of the acetabulum represents the bony roof of the fossa and that at this age the acetabulum is composed largely of cartilage and the cavity of the hip joint actually is not visualized. While the acetabular angle is larger on the right side the amount of difference, in itself, is hardly enough to be diagnostic. The other findings, however, indicate that subluxation is present. The **H** line is drawn through the centers of the triradiate cartilages of the acetabular fossae. The vertical **P** lines are drawn through the outer limits of the bony margin of the acetabular roof on either side so as to be perpendicular to the **H** line. Note that the right femoral epiphysis is situated farther laterally than the left. The curved broken line **S**, or Shenton's line, is disrupted on the right and normal on the left. In most cases of subluxation or dislocation, the roentgen findings are sufficiently definite so that it is unnecessary to construct the lines illustrated; they are used here to emphasize the differences in the two hips.

entity as hip joint dysplasia, that is, underdevelopment or hypoplasia of the acetabulum and partial subluxation of the femoral head. Some support for this opinion is given by the work of Doberti and Manhood referred to earlier.[13] Also, there are some hip joints in adults where the acetabulum is small or shallow and the fit of the femoral head is poor. The early development of degenerative joint disease in these hips is common.

OTHER CONGENITAL DISLOCATIONS

Congenital dislocations affecting joints other than the hip are infrequent. In the elbow joint dislocation of the radial head is seen occasionally. In these cases the radial head is displaced forward on the humerus. In some cases there is an associated congenital fusion of the dislocated radius with the proximal part of the ulna, the latter bone maintaining a normal relationship with the humerus (see Fig. 3-23). This

lesion may be unilateral but more often is bilateral. With the passage of time it will be noted that the head of the radius fails to develop properly and the proximal end of the bone is smaller than the normal.

MISCELLANEOUS ANOMALIES

FORKED RIBS. The sternal end of a rib may be bifid or forked. The third and fourth ribs are most frequently involved.

FENESTRATED FIRST RIB. Fenestration of the first rib consists of a smooth rounded opening in the anterior end of the rib. The significance of this deformity lies in the fact that it may be mistaken for a cavity in the lung in roentgenograms of the chest.

SUPRACONDYLAR PROCESS OF THE HUMERUS. This is a small bony spur found occasionally along the anteromedial border of the distal third of the

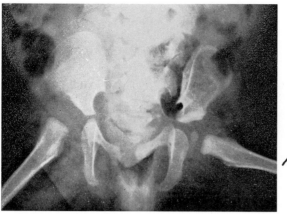 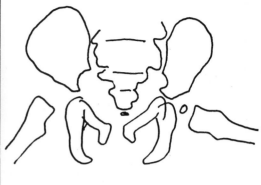

Fig. 3-26. Congenital hip joint dislocation, illustrating the "frog" position with the thighs abducted and externally rotated. Note absence of an ossified center for the right femoral epiphysis and the poorly developed acetabular roof on this side (increased acetabular angle). The position of the femoral neck clearly indicates that the femur is subluxated even though the femoral head is not visible. Patient also has extensive spina bifida malformation in the lumbar spine. *Left,* Roentgenogram of the pelvis; (*right*) tracing of roentgenogram.

humerus. It is directed distally and may form a foramen as in some of the lower animals.

RHOMBOID FOSSA OF THE CLAVICLE. Occasionally a well-marked concave depression is seen on the undersurface of the sternal end of the clavicle.

This is a fossa for the attachment of the rhomboid ligament.

PSEUDOEPIPHYSES FOR THE METACARPALS AND METATARSALS. These are partial cartilaginous clefts appearing in the proximal ends of one or

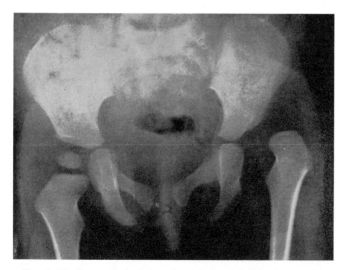

Fig. 3-27. Congenital dislocation of the left hip in an older child. The femoral epiphysis has not developed an ossification center. The acetabulum is hypoplastic, having never accommodated the femoral head.

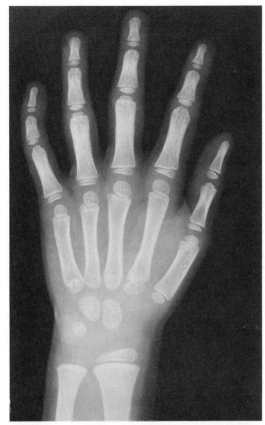

Fig. 3-28. Pseudoepiphyses and supernumerary epiphyses. The former are represented by incomplete clefts in the distal ends of the proximal phalanges and proximal end of the fifth metacarpal. The latter are present at the proximal end of the second metacarpal and distal end of the first metacarpal.

more of the lateral four or the distal end of the first metacarpal or metatarsal where normally no epiphyses are found. Less frequently the cleft is complete; these are termed supernumerary epiphyses (Fig. 3-28). It has been suggested that pseudoepiphyses and supernumerary epiphyses, especially when occurring in more than one bone, indicate the likely presence of other congenital stigmata or of disease acquired early in life. Some evidence has been presented to indicate that malnutrition during infancy or early childhood is important in the causation of these defects.

KIRNER'S DEFORMITY (CLINODACTYLY). This deformity is an anterior and radial curvature of the shaft of the terminal phalanx of the fifth finger associated with a widening of the epiphyseal plate and partial dorsal displacement of the shaft on the epiphysis.[45] The epiphyseal margin adjacent to the growth plate is irregular. The entire distal phalanx may be shortened. The deformity may occur as an isolated defect, usually bilateral, or as a part of a more generalized growth disorder or dysplasia. It is more common in females (occurring in 66 per cent of cases as reported in the literature).

PHYSIOLOGIC BOWLEGS OF INFANCY. During early infancy a mild degree of bowleg deformity is physiological. In addition to an actual bowing of the bones, the bowed appearance is accentuated by the distribution of fat. It has been suggested that this bowing is the result of the normal internal tibial torsion that occurs during intrauterine life. Occasionally this bowing is accentuated to the point where it may be considered abnormal (Fig. 3-29) and the result of disease, particularly rickets or Blount's tibia vara (see Chapter 2). Differentiation from rickets can be made with assurance in most cases because the metaphyses are well ossified and none of the other findings seen in active rickets are present. It may not be possible to exclude a healed rickets but, since this type of bowing usually comes to the attention of the physician during the first months or year of life, there seldom will have been time for rickets to have been present and to have undergone complete healing. Differentiation from Blount's tibia vara may be more difficult. Holt, Latourette, and Watson[24] call attention to the fact that in tibia vara the deformity is an angular one centered at the junction of the proximal metaphysis and epiphysis of the tibia, there is a broad beaklike projection of the inner side of the metaphysis within which are small islands of cartilage, and the tibial epiphysis tends to be triangular with the apex pointing medially. In physiologic bowing both the tibia and femur are affected, the femur often showing more deformity than the tibia. Both the upper metaphysis of the tibia and the lower metaphysis of the femur show medial beaks but they are pointed rather than blunt. This type of bowleg deformity tends to correct itself and usually the legs have become perfectly straight by the time the child has reached the age of 4 to 5 years.

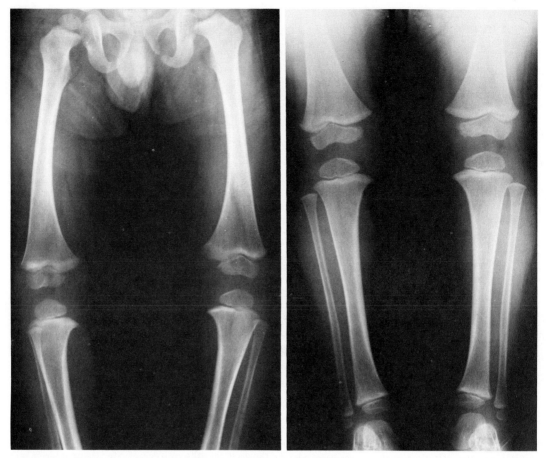

Fig. 3-29. Physiologic bowlegs. Initial views (*left*) demonstrate moderate bowleg deformity in an infant. *Right,* Approximately 1 year later the bowing has largely disappeared. Note that bowing involves both femur and tibia.

MADELUNG'S DEFORMITY

Madelung's deformity is a chondrodysplasia of the distal radial epiphysis. Some investigators believe that this deformity is a part of the dysplasia known as dyschondrosteosis (see Dyschondrosteosis, Chapter 2); others believe that it can occur as a separate deformity without other osseous stigmata. It causes a curvature of the shaft of the radius, giving a bayonet-shaped deformity of the hand at the wrist somewhat as though there were an anterior dislocation of the hand. The reverse type also is seen but is very rare. The lesion usually is bilateral and the deformity is first noticed at about the beginning of adolescence. The characteristic roentgen findings include:

1. The radius is shortened in comparison to the length of the ulna.

2. There is lateral and dorsal curvature of the radius.

3. There is early fusion of the radial epiphysis on the internal side. This results in a tilting of the radial articular surface so that it faces internally and anteriorly more than normal. The epiphysis develops a triangular shape.

4. Because the radius fails to grow properly in length there develops a subluxation of the radioulnar articulation and the lower end of the ulna projects posterior to the radius.

5. The deformity of the radial articular surface leads to a derangement in alignment of the carpal

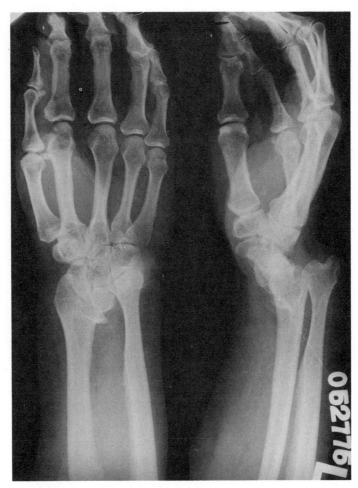

Fig. 3-30. Madelung's deformity.

bones. The carpus assumes the form of a pyramid with the apex pointing toward the radius and ulna and the base being formed by the carpo-metacarpal articulations (Fig. 3-30).

SPRENGEL'S DEFORMITY

Sprengel's deformity also is known as congenital high scapula or congenital elevation of the scapula. The scapula is small, high in position, and rotated so that the inferior edge points toward the spine. The deformity may be unilateral or bilateral. A fusion of the cervical and upper thoracic vertebrae, the Klippel-Feil syndrome, is present in practically all cases (Fig. 3-31). This fusion anomaly may exist, however, without elevation of the scapula. In some cases there is a bony connection between the elevated scapula and one of the vertebrae, usually the fifth or sixth cervical. This bony connection is known as the *omovertebral bone* and it may join the scapula and the vertebrae by either bony or fibrous union (Fig. 3-32).

OSTEOCHONDROSIS DEFORMANS TIBIAE (TIBIA VARA; BLOUNT'S DISEASE)

Blount's disease is an infrequent cause of bowlegs during infancy and childhood. Its cause is uncertain but it often is classified with the osseous

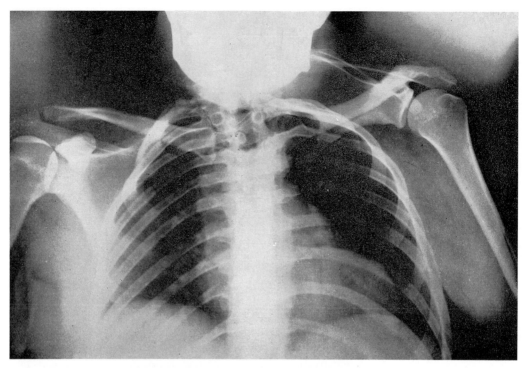

Fig. 3-31. Sprengel's deformity. The left shoulder is affected. There is an associated abnormality of ossification of the cervical and upper thoracic vertebrae with irregular segments fused together (Klippel-Feil deformity). These deformities frequently coexist.

dysplasias. The possibility of ischemic necrosis as a causative factor has been considered by some investigators. Clinically there is a progressive non-rachitic outward bowing of the legs. Roentgenographically, the upper tibial metaphysis is broadened with a blunt medial beaklike projection within which small islands of cartilage may cause irregular translucent defects. The upper tibial epiphysis often is triangular in shape with the apex pointing medially. The deformity actually is an angular one rather than a curved bowing, and is centered at the junction of the proximal tibial epiphysis and metaphysis (Fig. 3-33). For differential considerations see discussion of "Physiologic Bowlegs of Infancy."

HEREDITARY ARTHRODYSPLASIA AND DYSTROPHY OF THE NAILS

This rare condition is a complex disorder characterized by abnormalities of the fingernails, absence or hypoplasia of the patellae, defects in the head of the radius, discoloration of the iris, and bony processes along the posterior surfaces of the iliac bones (iliac horns) (Fig. 3-34). Not all features of the syndrome need to be present in the individual case. The disorder affecting the nails varies from unusual thinning and small size to a complete absence of one or more of the nails. The thumb is involved most frequently and severely. The patellae are absent or small and hypoplastic. The femoral condyles, particularly the medial, may be unusually prominent and there may be a valgus deformity. In the elbow, the head of the radius is poorly formed; in some cases the radius is abnormally long so that the head projects behind the joint when the forearm is flexed. Less frequently other bones show deformity in size and shape. The iliac horns are not a constant feature and in some cases appear to be the only abnormality. Fong[17] was the first to report a case of this nature. The lesions consist in bilateral pointed bony projections or exostoses extending posteriorly from the iliac bones.

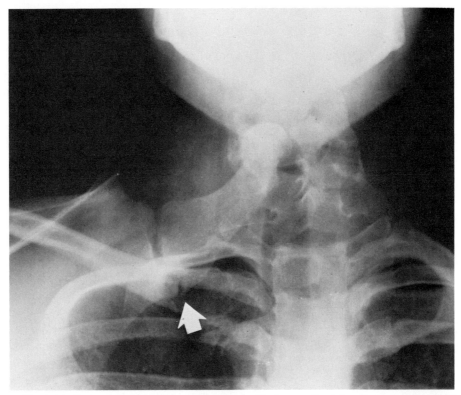

Fig. 3-32. Omovertebral bone in association with Sprengel's deformity and Klippel-Feil syndrome. The bone forms an articulation with the scapula (**arrow**) and the arch of one of the cervical vertebrae.

PROGERIA

Also known as the *Hutchinson-Gilford syndrome* this is, essentially, premature senility developing in a child.[34] The infants appear normal at birth but the typical features become evident within the first few years of life. The appearance has been likened to that of "a wizened old man." There is loss of subcutaneous fat, alpoecia, and atrophy of the muscles and the skin. The facies show a receding chin, beaked nose, and exophthalmos. There is premature arteriosclerosis in the coronary arteries and other vessels which leads to death during late childhood or early adolescence. The patients are dwarfed. Roentgen findings include hypoplastic facial bones, open cranial sutures and fontanelles, and dwarfism. The long bones are apt to be short, thin, and osteoporotic, and there is coxa valga which may be marked. A significant feature is acro-osteolysis of the terminal digits of the fingers and toes.

CHROMOSOMAL ABNORMALITIES

The normal human cell contains 22 pairs of somatic chromosomes, called autosomes, numbered from one through 22, and two sex chromosomes, XX in the female and XY in the male, for a total of 46. The somatic chromosomes are usually placed into seven groups: Group A, numbers one through three; group B, 4 and 5; group C, 6 through 12; group D, 13 through 15; group E, 16 through 18; group F, 19 and 20; and group G, 21 and 22. The addition of a chromosome to one of the autosomal groups leads to one of the trisomy syndromes, the most common locations being the 13–15, the 16–18 and 21–22 groups. Of the entities caused by abnormality of the sex chromosomes, Turner's syndrome is most apt to have significant roentgen findings.

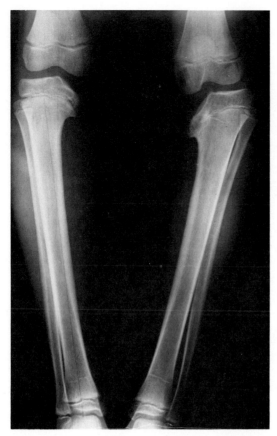

Fig. 3-33. Blount's disease. There is bilateral involvement with an angular deformity at metaphyseoepiphyseal junction. The tibial shafts are straight and the femurs uninvolved.

TRISOMY 21 SYNDROME; MONGOLISM; DOWN'S SYNDROME

Mongolism is the result of an autosomal trisomy of chromosome 21. A number of skeletal stigmata have been described in mongolism, some of which are fairly specific and aid in recognition of the disease when clinical findings are equivocal, that is, during the early months of life. Among the skeletal anomalies that have been described are the following:[2,4,9,19]

1. In the pelvis during infancy the acetabular angles are flattened, the iliac bones large and flared and the ischia elongated and tapering (Fig. 3-35). The iliac index is decreased. The iliac index is said to be more significant

than the acetabular angle in the diagnosis of mongolism. This index consists of the sum of the acetabular and iliac angles on both sides, divided by two. The method for determining the index is shown in Figures 3-36 and 3-37. In the newborn the normal iliac index has a mean value of 81° with a range of 68 to 97°. In mongolism the index has a mean value of 62° with a range from 49 to 87°. According to Astley[2] if the index is under 60°, mongolism is very probable; if it is over 78° the child probably is normal. These changes are most significant during the first 6 to 12 months of life.

2. Shortening of the middle phalanx of the fifth finger.

3. The manubrium sterni may ossify from two or three centers instead of one as in the normal. This can be identified in a lateral view of the chest.

4. The lumbar vertebrae may be small in the anteroposterior diameter and increased in height.

5. Dental defects with anomalies of the teeth and delay in eruption have been noted frequently.

6. Coxa vara may be present.

7. Skull changes include: (a) the sphenoid is rotated up and back in relation to the clivus, (b) the bones of the calvarium are thin, (c) the palate has a high short arch, (d) the nasal sinuses are hypoplastic, (e) the interorbital distance is decreased (hypotelorism), and (f) closure of the cranial sutures may be delayed.

8. Subluxation of the atlas is common. The normal atlanto-odontoid interval in children has an upper limit of 5.0 mm.

9. Visceral anomalies include congenital heart disease, usually atrioventricular commune, an increased frequency of an aberrant right subclavian artery and duodenal obstruction (duodenal atresia or annular pancreas).

TRISOMY 18 SYNDROME

Recent advances in cytogenetics have brought about recognition of several new syndromes of

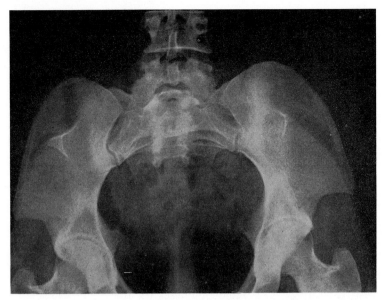

Fig. 3-34. Iliac horns in a patient with hereditary arthrodysplasia. Note the pointed projections along the posterior surfaces of the ilia.

which the trisomy 18 syndrome is one of the most frequent. The abnormalities result from an extra chromosome for number 18. The clinical and roentgen findings include:[28] (*1*) low-set, malformed ears and recession of the chin (man-dibular and maxillary hypoplasia), (*2*) ulnar deviation of the fingers with flexion deformities. When the fingers are forcibly extended the second and third fingers form a V-shaped notch. (*3*) Retarded bone age, (*4*) short, hypoplastic

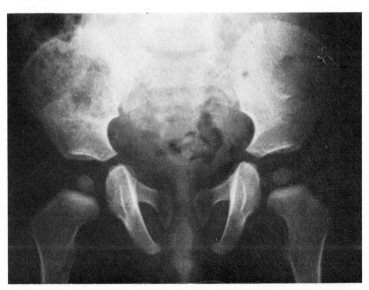

Fig. 3-35. Mongolism. Pelvis of a mongoloid infant showing flaring of the ilia, elongated, tapered ischia, and flattening of the acetabular angles.

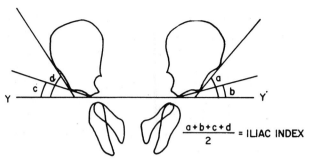

Fig. 3-36. Method for determining the acetabular and iliac angles and the iliac index. This index is the sum of the acetabular angles (**b** and **c**) and the iliac angles (**a** and **d**), divided by 2. The diagram illustrates the proper placement of the lines necessary for determining the various angles. (Reproduced with permission of Dr. E. C. K. Tong and the Editor and Publisher of Radiology.[46])

first metacarpals, (*5*) pseudoepiphyses for the metacarpals, (*6*) equinovarus and "rocker-bottom" feet with hammer-toe deformities, short first toe, and hypoplastic distal phalanges, (*7*) thin ribs and short, undersegmented sternum and an increase in the anteroposterior diameter of the chest, (*8*) narrow transverse diameter of the pelvis owing to anterior rotation of the ilia (antimongoloid pelvis), (*9*) hypoplasia or absence of the medial third of the clavicle, (*10*) hypoplastic dislocated femoral heads and with increased acetabular angles, (*11*) thin cranial bones with a prominent elongated posterior fossa and a shallow, J-shaped sella.

In addition, congenital cardiovascular disease is frequently present, usually a patent interventricular septum (VSD) or patent ductus arteriosis. Eventration of the diaphragm and malformation of the kidneys are relatively

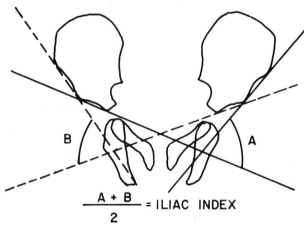

Fig. 3-37. Tong's method for determining the iliac index (**A** and **B** divided by 2). The measurement of the larger angles gives less chance for error than the method shown in Figure 3-36 and is mathematically accurate. (Reproduced with permission of Dr. E. C. K. Tong and the Editor and Publisher of Radiology.[46])

common. The latter defects include double ureters, multicystic kidneys, horseshoe kidneys, and hydronephrosis.

TRISOMY 13–15 SYNDROME

The genetic fault in this syndrome is an extra chromosome for the 13–15 group. It is less common than trisomy 18. The infants are usually small and do not thrive. Death often occurs during the first year of life. The ears are malformed and low set and there is micrognathia. Some of the skeletal stigmata resemble those found in the trisomy 18 syndrome but the major anomalies include craniofacial clefts, polydactyly, and syndactyly together with various anomalies of the viscera. Congenital heart disease is common, usually a ventricular septal defect with or without a patent ductus arteriosis and dextroposition. The skeletal anomalies include:[27] (1) cleft palate, (2) poorly ossified cranial bones with microcephaly, (3) hypoterlorism with small orbits, microphthalmia, and a sloping forehead, (4) polydactyly and syndactyly with narrow distal phalanges, (5) malformed ribs with asymmetry of the thorax, (6) increased interpediculate distance in the cervical spine, (7) the fifth finger overlaps the fourth, and (8) "rocker-bottom" feet.

The visceral anomalies, in addition to heart disease, include: (1) diaphragmatic hernia, (2) genitourinary tract anomalies as seen in trisomy 18, (3) umbilical or inguinal hernias, (4) malrotation of the colon, (5) undescended testes, and (6) mental and motor retardation.

TURNER'S SYNDROME

Of the group of syndromes in which there is abnormal gonadal development, the one which may show significant roentgen findings is Turner's syndrome, or gonadal aplasia.[2,30,44] In this syndrome there is relative shortening of the fourth metacarpal in relation to the third and fifth. The *metacarpal sign* is determined by drawing a straight line tangential to the distal ends of the heads of the fourth and fifth

metacarpals.[5] If this line passes through the head of the third metacarpal, the sign is said to be positive. Normally, the line will pass distal to the head of the third metacarpal. However, a positive sign occurs in some normals and in other growth disturbances so that it is not absolutely specific. The time of appearance of epiphyseal ossification centers is normal but fusion is delayed. Skeletal density is diminished particularly in the wrist and foot. The proximal row of carpal bones assumes an angular configuration somewhat similar to Madelung's deformity with the apex pointing proximally. Various other abnormalities of the bones of the hands also have been described. At the knee, the medial femoral condyle is enlarged and the opposing tibial plateau is flattened or depressed. The medial part of the proximal tibial epiphysis may overhang the metaphysis and in some cases an appearance rather similar to Blount's disease has been noted. In the spine there may be scoliosis and the posterior arch of C 1 may be hypoplastic. An appearance similar to Scheuermanns' disease also has been described. An increased carrying angle at the elbow, cubitus valgus, one of the significant clinical signs, also can be demonstrated radiographically (see Fig. 5-32).

OTHER SYNDROMES

A considerable number of syndromes have been described in the literature, often with eponymic titles, that include skeletal roentgenographic changes. Most of these are decidedly uncommon and limitations of space make it impossible to include them in this chapter. Most are of interest chiefly to pediatric radiologists and descriptions can be found in the more recent radiologic and pediatric literature or in books devoted to the subject.

REFERENCES AND SELECTED READINGS

1. ANGLE, C. R., McINTIRE, M. S., and MOORE, R. C.: Cloverleaf skull: Kleeblattschädel-deformity syndrome. *Am. J. Dis. Child. 114:* 198, 1967.
2. ASTLEY, R.: Chromosomal abnormalities in child-

hood with particular reference to Turner's syndrome and mongolism. *Br. J. Radiol. 36:* 2, 1963.

3. ASTLEY, R.: Trisomy 17–18. *Br. J. Radiol. 39:* 86, 1966.

4. AUSTIN, J. H. M., PREGER, L., SIRIS, E., and TAYBI, H.: Short hard palate in newborn. Roentgen sign of mongolism. *Radiology 92:* 775, 1969.

5. BLOOM, R. A.: The metacarpal sign. *Br. J. Radiol. 43:* 133, 1970.

6. BLOUNT, W. R.: Tibia vara; osteochondrosis deformans tibiae. *J. Bone Joint Surg. 19:* 1, 1937.

7. BROMER, R. S.: Osteogenesis imperfecta. *Am. J. Roentgenol. Radium Ther. Nucl. Med. 30:* 631, 1933.

8. CAFFEY, J., AMES, R., SILVERMAN, W. A., RYDER, C. T., and HOUGH, G.: Contradiction of the congenital dysplasia-predislocation hypothesis of congenital dislocation of the hip through a study of the normal variations in acetabular angles at successive periods in infancy. *Pediatrics 17:* 632, 1956.

9. CAFFEY, J., and ROSS, S.: Mongolism (mongoloid deficiency) during early infancy—some newly recognized diagnostic changes in the pelvic bones. *Pediatrics 17:* 642, 1956.

10. COLEMAN, S. S.: Diagnosis of congenital dysplasia of the hip in the newborn infant. *JAMA 162:* 548, 1956.

11. CONWAY, J. J., and COWELL, H. R.: Tarsal coalition: Clinical significance and roentgenographic demonstration. *Radiology 92:* 799, 1969.

12. DARLING, D. B., FEINGOLD, M., and BERKMAN, M.: Roentgenological aspects of Goldenhar's syndrome: Oculoauriculovertebral dysplasia. *Radiology 91:* 254, 1968.

13. DOBERTI, A., and MANHOOD, J.: A new radiologic sign for the early diagnosis of congenital hip dysplasia. *Ann. Radiol. 11:* 276, 1968.

14. DUGGAN, C. A., KEENER, E. B., and GAY, B. B., JR.: Secondary craniostenosis. *Am. J. Roentgenol. Radium Ther. Nucl. Med. 109:* 277, 1970.

15. EHRENHAFT, J. L.: Development of the vertebral column as related to certain congenital and pathological changes. *Surg. Gynecol. Obstet. 76:* 282, 1943.

16. FELMAN, A. H., and KIRKPATRICK, J. A.: Madelung's deformity. Observations in 17 patients. *Radiology 93:* 1037, 1969.

17. FONG, E. E.: Iliac horns (symmetrical bilateral central posterior iliac processes); case report. *Radiology 47:* 517, 1946.

18. GELLIS, S. S., FEINGOLD, M., TUNNESSEN, W. W., JR., and RAETTIG, J. A.: Caudal dysplasia syndrome (picture of the month). *Am. J. Dis. Child. 116:* 407, 1968.

19. GERALD, B. E., and SILVERMAN, F. N.: Normal and abnormal interorbital distances with special reference to mongolism. *Am. J. Roentgenol. Radium Ther. Nucl. Med. 95:* 154, 1965.

20. GORDON, I. R. S.: Microcephaly and craniostenosis. *Clin. Radiol. 21:* 19, 1970.

21. GORLIN, R. J., COHEN, M. M., JR., and WOLFSON, J.: Tricho-rhino-phalangeal syndrome. *Am. J. Dis. Child. 118:* 595, 1969.

22. GRUNDY, L., GAREE, J. A., and JIMENEZ, J. P.: Oxycephaly in the adult simulating pituitary tumor. *Am. J. Roentgenol. Radium Ther. Nucl. Med. 108:* 762, 1970.

23. HANSMAN, C. F.: Growth of interorbital distance and skull thickness as observed in roentgenographic measurements. *Radiology 86:* 87, 1966.

24. HOLT, J. F., LATOURETTE, H. B., and WATSON, E. H.: Physiological bowing of the legs in young children. *JAMA 154:* 390, 1954.

25. HOPE, J. W., SPITZ, E. B., and SLADE, H. W.: The early recognition of premature cranial synostosis. *Radiology 65:* 183, 1955.

26. JAMES, A. E., JR.: Tarsal coalitions and peroneal spastic flat foot. *Austral. Radiol. 14:* 80, 1970.

27. JAMES, A. E., JR., BELCORT, C. L., ATKINS, L., and JANOWER, M. L.: Trisomy 13–15. *Radiology 92:* 44, 1969.

28. JAMES, A. E., JR., BELCORT, C. L., ATKINS, L., and JANOWER, M. L.: Trisomy-18 syndrome. *Radiology 92:* 37, 1969.

29. KEATS, T. E.: Ocular hypertelorism (Greig's syndrome) associated with Sprengel's deformity. *Am. J. Roentgenol. Radium Ther. Nucl. Med. 110:* 119, 1970.

30. KEATS, T. E., and BURNS, T. W.: The radiographic manifestations of gonadal dysgenesis. *Radiol. Clin. North Am. 2:* 297, 1964.

31. KOONTZ, W. W., JR., and PROUT, G. R., JR.: Agenesis of the sacrum and neurogenic bladder. *JAMA 203:* 481, 1968.

32. LACHMAN, E.: Pseudo-epiphyses in hand and foot. Editorial. *Am. J. Roentgenol. Radium Ther. Nucl. Med. 70:* 149, 1953.

33. LILIEQUIST, B.: Diastematomyelia. *Acta Radiol. (Diag.) 3:* 497, 1965.

34. MARGOLIN, F. K., and STEINBACH, H. L.: Progeria. Hutchinson-Gilford syndrome. *Am. J. Roentgenol. Radium Ther. Nucl. Med. 103:* 173, 1968.

35. MEYERDING, H. W.: Spondylolisthesis as an etiologic factor in backache. *JAMA 111:* 1971, 1938.

36. MORRISON, S. G., PERRY, L. W., and SCOTT, L. P., III: Congenital brevicollis (Klippel-Feil syndrome). *Am. J. Dis. Child. 115:* 614, 1968.

37. POPPEL, M. H., JACOBSON, H. G., DUFF, B. K., and GOTTLIEB, C.: Basilar impression and platybasia in Paget's disease. *Radiology 61:* 639, 1953.

38. RECHNAGEL, K.: Dysplasia epiphysialis hemimelica. *Acta Orthop. Scand. 29:* 237, 1960.

39. SALTER, R. B.: Etiology, pathogenesis and possible prevention of congenital dislocation of the hip. *Can. Med. Assoc. J. 98:* 933, 1968.

40. SHERMAN, R. S., and GLAUSER, O. J.: Radiological identification of fibrous dysplasia of the jaws. *Radiology 71:* 553, 1958.

41. SHOPFNER, C. E., and COIN, C. G.: Genu varus and valgus in children. *Radiology 92:* 723, 1969.

42. SHOUL, M. I., and RITVO, M.: Clinical and roentgenological manifestations of the Klippel-Feil syndrome (congenital fusion of the cervical vertebrae, brevicollis); report of eight additional cases and review of the literature. *Am. J. Roentgenol. Radium Ther. Nucl. Med. 68:* 369, 1952.

43. SILVERMAN, F. N.: "Pediatric Radiology," in *Modern Trends in Diagnostic Radiology—4,* ed. by J. W. McLaren. New York, Appleton-Century-Crofts, 1970.

44. SINGLETON, E. B., ROSENBERG, H. S., and YANG, S. J.: The radiographic manifestations of the chromosomal abnormalities. *Radiol. Clin. North Am. 2:* 281, 1964.

45. STAHELI, L. T., CLAWSON, D. K., and CAPPS, J. H.: Bilateral curving of the terminal phalanges of the little finger. *J. Bone Joint Surg. 48-A:* 1171, 1966.

46. TONG, E. C. K.: The iliac index angle. *Radiology 91:* 376, 1968.

47. VAUGHAN, W. H., and SEGAL, G.: Tarsal coalition, with special reference to roentgenographic interpretation. *Radiology 60:* 855, 1953.

48. VOGT, E. C., and WYATT, G. M.: Craniolacunia (lückenschädel); report of 54 cases. *Radiology 36:* 147, 1941.

49. WITTENBORG, M. H.: Malposition and dislocation of the hip in infancy and childhood. *Radiol. Clin. North Am. 2:* 235, 1964.

4

METABOLIC, ENDOCRINE, AND
RELATED BONE DISEASES

Bone is living tissue with old bone being removed constantly and replaced with new bone. Normally this exchange is in balance and the mineral content of the bones remains relatively constant. Under some conditions and as a result of certain diseases this balance may be disturbed and there will be either demineralization of the skeleton or increased mineralization of it. Decreased ossification may result because of a defect in or deficiency of the osteoblasts which do not produce sufficient organic matrix (osteoid) without which bone cannot be formed. Also it may result from failure of mineralization of osteoid because of insufficient calcium or phosphorus or from other factors such as insufficient vitamin D. Finally, it can result from increased deossification with more old bone being removed than can be replaced. Loss of mineral salts causes bone to become more radiolucent than normal. Increased radiopacity of bone can result from increased formation with new bone being laid down faster than old bone is removed. The same result will occur if there is interference with normal deossification, provided that bone formation continues at a normal rate. Various metabolic and endocrine diseases can cause one or more of these processes including osteoporosis, osteomalacia, and hyperparathyroidism.

OSTEOPOROSIS

Osteoporosis is caused by a defect in or a deficiency of the organic matrix of bone without which there can be no bone formation. It results from decreased activity of the osteoblasts or an increased activity of the osteoclasts. Resultant bone is more radiolucent than normal. It is difficult to recognize lesser degrees of osteoporosis in roentgenograms unless the process is localized and there is normally mineralized bone near by for comparison. When osteoporosis is diffuse and generalized a considerable loss of mineral salts is required before recognition is assured. Overexposed roentgenograms may also give a false impression of demineralization. Because of these difficulties a number of methods have been devised to measure the mineral content of bone *in vivo* more accurately than can be done by observation of roentgenograms. This problem has been of recent concern because astronauts may spend considerable time in space in relative inactivity.[21, 22]

DISUSE OSTEOPOROSIS

To maintain osteoblastic activity at a normal level requires that the bones be subjected to a normal amount of stress and strain and this demands muscular activity. Following fracture of a bone, within a few weeks there begins to be discernible localized demineralization of the affected part. This is more pronounced distal to the site of the injury. The demineralization during childhood and adolescence is most pronounced in the metaphyses, apparently because of the increased blood supply at the sites where active bone growth is taking place. Even in adults it is likely to be most intense along the sites of the previous epiphyseal plates (Fig. 4-1). The cortical margin of the bone involved by the osteoporosis becomes thinned but never disappears completely, an important point in distinguishing disuse osteoporosis from destruction of bone caused by disease. The demineralization is largely the result of inactivity although hyperemia undoubtedly plays a part. Demineralization tends to be uniform with loss of all trabeculae so that when severe or long-standing the bones develop a "ground-glass" appearance. This, combined with the thinned cortices, forms a characteristic pattern for osteoporosis. The same type of osteoporosis may develop following acute infections of the bone or of the soft tissues, or even after simple immobilization. Infrequently, after a relatively minor injury, severe local osteoporosis may develop and lead to a prolonged period of disability and pain. This is known as *Sudeck's atrophy* (Fig. 4-2). This same severe form of osteoporosis may appear during the course of treatment of any fracture in the distal part of an extremity and delay the return of normal function. The cause of Sudek's atrophy is not well understood. It has been suggested that vasomotor disturbances develop following the injury and that this leads to increased loss of calcium from the bones over what might ordinarily be expected as a result of disuse. During

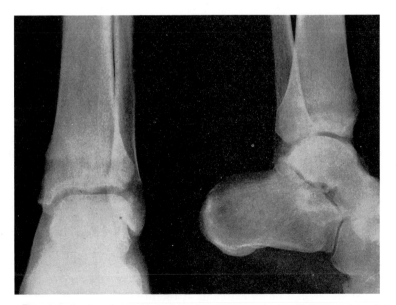

Fig. 4-1. Acute disuse osteoporosis. Anteroposterior (*left*) and lateral (*right*) views of the ankle. Note the bandlike nature of the decreased density of the bones at the sites of former metaphyses. There is a slight demineralization of the tarsal bones but the changes are more easily detected in the tibia and fibula.

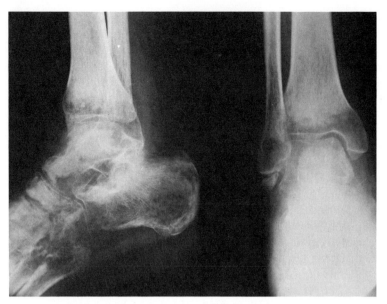

Fig. 4-2. Sudeck's atrophy. Anteroposterior (*left*) and lateral (*right*) roentgenograms of the ankle. There is severe decalcification of the bones, which followed a fracture of the tip of the lateral malleolus. Note the localization of the demineralization to the distal ends of the tibia and fibula and the bones of the foot with the tibial and fibular shafts normal. The thin but intact cortical margins of the affected bones serve to exclude destruction resulting from disease. The patchy and mottled character of the demineralization is characteristic.

the acute stage, the mottled appearance of the bones and the severe demineralization is striking. As the process becomes more chronic, the mottled appearance is lost and the bones assume a ground-glass, uniform loss of density. Sudek's atrophy develops at or distal to the area of injury, never proximal to it. After recovery the bones affected often show persisting coarse structure that may last for several years.

Chronic disuse osteoporosis may develop gradually from a partial limitation of activity or it may be the continuation of an acute osteoporosis. The bones involved show a uniform demineralization with poorly defined trabecular structure and thinning of the cortices. The osteoporosis may be limited to one extremity or part of an extremity if the disuse was limited to such an area or it may be generalized throughout the skeleton if there was total bodily inactivity. When the vertebrae are affected the cancellous structure is lost but the

cortical margins remain distinct ("picture-frame vertebrae").

POSTMENOPAUSAL OSTEOPOROSIS

Following the menopause some individuals develop a chronic osteoporosis that may be sufficiently severe to cause fracture. The vertebral column and the pelvic bones are particularly susceptible to this form of osteoporosis. Because of the pronounced demineralization, compression fractures of one or more vertebrae may result. The bodies in the mid and lower thoracic areas are most frequently affected. Fracture can occur after a very minor injury or even during the course of normal activity. In severe forms of the disease many of the vertebral bodies develop concave superior and inferior disc surfaces, giving what has been called a "fish" contour as seen in lateral roentgenograms (Fig. 4-3). Such deformity is caused by expansion of the intervertebral discs at the expense of the weakened vertebral bodies. An almost constant finding in association with the vertebral changes is the occurrence of calcific plaques in the abdominal aorta.

SENILE OSTEOPOROSIS

The bones lose density with advancing age and this is part of the aging process. They become more brittle, fracture readily, and heal more slowly. Since many elderly persons are likely to be less active and dietary habits may be poor, a combination of factors can lead to severe osteoporosis with compression fractures of the vertebrae similar to those seen in the postmenopausal form. Some pathologists prefer the term, osteopenia, for this form of osteoporosis, limiting the latter designation to the postmenopausal type of the disease. It is obvious that in many persons showing chronic osteoporosis there may be more than one fac-

tor responsible and the dividing line between, for example, a postmenopausal osteoporosis and the senile type of the disease often is not distinct.

OSTEOGENESIS IMPERFECTA

Osteogenesis imperfecta is a congenital form of osteoporosis in which there is a defect or deficiency of osteoblasts. This condition is discussed in Chapter 2.

CUSHING'S SYNDROME

Osteoporosis is one of the skeletal manifestations of Cushing's syndrome whether owing to administration of corticosteroids or to the spontaneous form of the disease. The latter may be caused by adrenocortical hyperplasia, or less frequently by adrenal cortical adenoma or carcinoma.[11] As a result of the demineralization the vertebrae are prone to collapse with

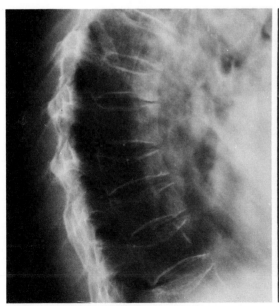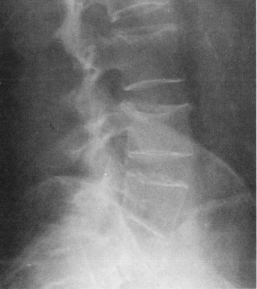

Fig. 4-3. Postmenopausal osteoporosis. *Left,* Lateral roentgenogram of the thoracic spine illustrates the demineralization and multiple compression fractures resulting from the softness of the bones. The cortical margins are thin but stand out clearly as white lines marking the borders of the vertebrae. *Right,* Lateral view of the lumbar spine. Note plaques of calcium in the abdominal aorta.

multiple compression fractures leading to bi-concave contours of the vertebral bodies (Fig. 4-4). Howland et al.[8] have called attention to the fact that there is marginal condensation especially along the upper surfaces of the compressed vertebrae and more than is commonly seen following vertebral compressions from other causes. It has been suggested that this change is a manifestation of attempted repair with excess callus formation.[11] Rib fractures also are present particularly in the anterior segments and exuberant callus often forms around these. As is true with other fractures occurring in this syndrome, the fractures frequently are painless. Fractures of the pubic and ischial rami may occur, also frequently showing heavy callus.

Ischemic necrosis of the head of the femur and in the ends of other bones is another complication of the disease. The exact cause is not known. Because of the osteoporosis the skeletal density is decreased. In the skull this may take the form of a granular rarefaction. Skull roentgenograms also may show an en-

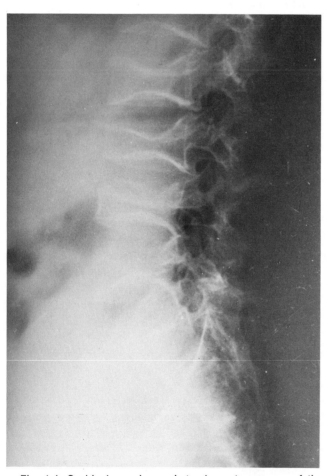

Fig. 4-4. Cushing's syndrome. Lateral roentgenogram of the lumbar spine demonstrates compression of all the lumbar vertebrae. Expansion of intervertebral discs into the softened vertebral bodies causes a characteristic biconcavity of their upper and lower surfaces.

larged sella in the uncommon cases of the syndrome that are secondary to a pituitary tumor. The lamina dura, the cortical margin of the tooth socket, may disappear. In children there may be delay in skeletal maturation.

Nonskeletal roentgen manifestations include excess subcutaneous and intra-abdominal fat and mediastinal widening from excess fat deposits. Extrapleural fat pads and epipericardial fat accumulations also may be seen in chest roentgenograms. Visualization of the enlarged adrenals often may be obtained by suitable techniques (see Chapter 20). In those cases secondary to a carcinoma of the adrenal, calcified deposits have been found in approximately 25 per cent of cases.

MALNUTRITION AND RELATED CAUSES

Since protein deficiency or abnormal protein metabolism can cause osteoporosis, it may develop whenever there is severe malnutrition. Thus, osteoporosis and osteomalacia may both be present after periods of starvation. Osteoporosis may develop in cases of nephrosis as a result of loss of protein. When diabetes is poorly controlled over a long period of time the bones become osteoporotic since these individuals use abnormal amounts of protein to make up for the inability to use glucose.

SCURVY

Infantile scurvy is a form of osteoporosis caused by a deficiency of vitamin C. This vitamin is necessary for normal osteoblastic activity and the organic matrix of bone cannot be laid down without it. Because of the lowered activity of the osteoblasts, the serum alkaline phosphatase usually is low or occasionally normal. The tendency for hemorrhage in this disease is said to be caused by a lack of formation of intercellular cement substance in the capillaries. Scurvy is not a disease of the immediate postnatal period but is most frequent between the ages of 6 months and 2 years.

Roentgen Observations

1. There is a diffuse demineralization of the entire skeleton. The trabecular structure is lost and the cortices of the bone are thinned.

2. Zones of increased density develop at the metaphyses of the long bones and around the margins of the epiphyseal centers. As the cancellous bone of the center becomes more translucent than normal, the dense outer rim gives the appearance of a ring and this is a very significant finding in scurvy. This zone of density, known as the white line of scurvy, represents an abnormally wide zone of provisional calcification and it is caused by a failure of normal proliferation of cartilage cells so that the change from cartilage to bone becomes arrested.

3. On the shaft side of the metaphysis a zone of lessened density develops, forming a transverse band of rarefaction across the shaft. This is the area where active bone formation should be taking place but does not and the balance between bone formation and resorption is disturbed in favor of the latter. This is a weakened part of the bone and it is here that fracture may occur. The epiphysis and the zone of provisional calcification may be displaced because of such fracture. This zone of rarefaction is known as the *scurvy zone* (see Fig. 4-6). The scurvy zone often disappears as the epiphysis together with the zone of provisional calcification become impacted into the shaft. Lateral extension of the zone of provisional calcification into the soft tissues for a short distance, forming spurlike projections, is a common finding (Fig. 4-5).

4. The "corner sign of scurvy" sometimes is an early and fairly characteristic change. It is a small area of rarefaction involving the cortex and spongiosa just proximal to the metaphysis on one or both sides of the shaft and it represents the early development of the scurvy zone (Fig. 4-6).

5. Healing of scurvy is shown first by the calcification of areas of subperiosteal hemorrhage. During the active stage of the disease

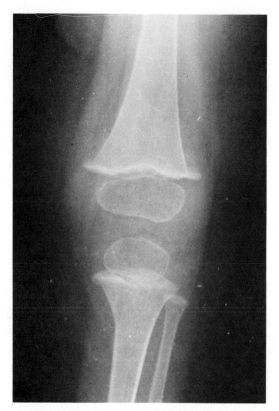

Fig. 4-5. Infantile scurvy. Anteroposterior roentgenogram of the knee. The "white line" of scurvy is particularly distinct in the metaphysis of the femur. Note spurlike projection of the zone of provisional calcification laterally. The translucent scurvy zone is not visible because of impaction of the shaft into the metaphysis.

extensive hemorrhages may develop beneath the periosteum and elevate it. During infancy and childhood the periosteum is loosely attached to the cortex of the bone and it is elevated easily by hemorrhage beneath it. However, it is firmly attached at the end of the shaft and hemorrhage is limited at this point and it is here that the first deposition of calcium salts often occurs. Under adequate treatment calcium is deposited throughout the area of hemorrhage, forming a dense shadow surrounding the shaft (Fig. 4-7). The scurvy zones recalcify. There is a gradual remineralization of the skeleton and the cortices regain normal thickness. As growth proceeds, the thickened zone of provisional calcification appears to migrate into the shaft where it remains as a thin, dense, white line for a long period of time. In like manner a ring of density may be visible within the epiphyseal center as normal bone forms around the edge of the old center ("ghost epiphysis" or "bone-within-a-bone"). The calcified subperiosteal hemorrhages gradually are absorbed. If epiphyseal dislocation did occur, the deformity will be corrected by growth and remodeling over a period of time.

OSTEOMALACIA

Unless adequate amounts of calcium and phosphorus are available, proper calcification of osteoid cannot occur and the process of bone formation is arrested. Because removal of dead or devitalized bone continues, the balance is disturbed in favor of demineralization. When this happens during adult life the condition known as osteomalacia is caused. During childhood the effect on bone already formed is the same as in the adult. In addition, new bone being formed as a part of the process of growth is greatly altered and changes become obvious that are not seen in the adult. This form of osteomalacia is known as rickets. The two diseases, therefore, are essentially the same and the roentgen findings differ only because of the presence or absence of areas of actively growing bone (epiphyses and metaphyses).

The causes of osteomalacia are varied and include an inadequate intake or a failure of absorption of calcium, phosphorus, or vitamin D, singly or in combination. The importance of the first two in the proper mineralization of bone is obvious. The major effect of vitamin D is to increase absorption of calcium and phosphorus from the intestinal tract. It also may have a direct effect on bone. In addition to disturbances in the intake and absorption of calcium and phosphorus, certain renal diseases in which there is tubular insufficiency without glomerular involvement may cause osteomalacia. For details concerning these aspects of osteomalacia the reader should consult one of the texts listed in the "Bibliography" at the end of this chapter.

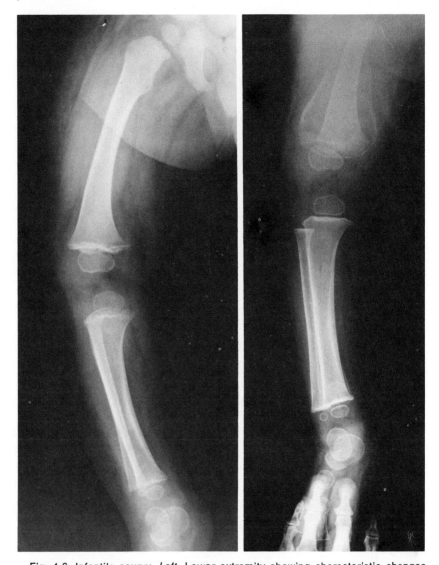

Fig. 4-6. Infantile scurvy. *Left,* Lower extremity showing characteristic changes of scurvy. Note the scurvy zone in the lower metaphysis of the femur. *Right,* Same patient after treatment was begun. Subluxation of the lower epiphysis of the femur has developed but the evidence of beginning healing is indicated by the calcification of a large subperiosteal hemorrhage surrounding the femur.

INFANTILE RICKETS

Infantile rickets is osteomalacia occurring during infancy, usually because of a lack of vitamin D in the diet or of ultraviolet radiation (ultraviolet converts the sterols in the skin into vitamin D). This form of rickets is less prevalent than it used to be. It is found mainly between the ages of 4 and 18 months. It is very uncommon during the first few months of life. The significant roentgen observations include the following:

There is a generalized demineralization of the skeleton, the bones having a coarse texture. In contrast to infantile scurvy, which is a form of osteoporosis, demineralization of the bone

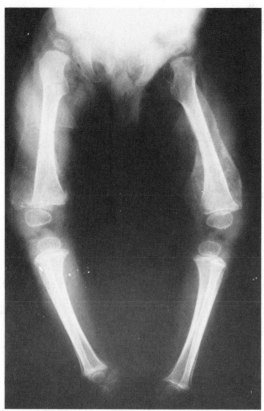

Fig. 4-7. Infantile scurvy. Another patient shortly after the beginning of treatment. Note subluxation of the right lower femoral epiphysis and the large subperiosteal hematomas that are beginning to calcify. The ring contours of the epiphyses are distinct.

irregular appearance, becoming coarse and frayed. This is characteristic of rickets (Figs. 4-8 and 4-9). With failure of proper calcification of the newly formed osteoid in the metaphysis, the distance between the ossified portion of the epiphysis and the end of the shaft is increased. Modeling of the end of the bone, the normal reshaping that occurs as growth in length and width proceeds, is also interfered with and the ends of the shafts become broadened. Typically, a certain amount of cupping or concavity of the metaphysis also develops although this finding is less constant than the others that have been described.

In severe rickets, thin stripelike shadows frequently develop along the outer cortical margins of the long bones. These resemble the periosteal calcifications of inflammatory type but actually represent zones of poorly calcified osteoid laid down by the periosteum, which would normally result in transverse growth of the bones.

Demineralization of the cranial bones occurs and in the young infant the suture margins become indistinct. The bones are soft and the skull is molded readily by pressure. The tendency for a piling up of poorly calcified bone leads to the formation of bosses or prominences, particularly in the frontal bone, and these become noticeable especially when healing has begun.

Also in severe disease, transverse fissurelike clefts may develop in the shafts of the long bones (Fig. 4-10), the axillary borders of the scapulae, the pubic rami and other areas. These are called pseudofractures or Looser zones and are similar to those seen in osteomalacia of adults. The margins of the ossified epiphyseal centers become indistinct and in severe cases the centers may be difficult to visualize or even apparently disappear because of the pronounced decalcification (Fig. 4-9).

The changes noted in the metaphyses of the long tubular bones also develop in the sternal ends of the ribs and lead to the clinical sign of "beading." This is not specific for rickets as beading of the ribs, or the so-called rachitic rosary, is also seen in some other diseases.

trabeculae occurs unevenly and those that remain stand out more prominently than in the normal. Because of the poor mineralization of the bones, bowing of the weight-bearing bones will develop if the infant has begun to stand or walk. Even in the very young infant, fractures of the greenstick variety may occur. However, these are more likely to develop in the older child. If the rickets is very severe, transverse fissurelike clefts may form in the shafts of the long bones similar in all respects to the pseudofractures of osteomalacia in the adult (see section entitled "Osteomalacia" this chapter).

The white line marking the ends of the shafts, the zone of provisional calcification, disappears and the metaphyses develop a very

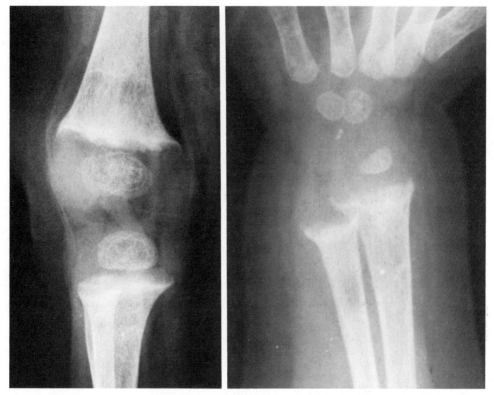

Fig. 4-8. Infantile rickets. *Left,* Anteroposterior roentgenogram of the knee. The poorly calcified, frayed metaphyses, tendency toward cupping and broadening of them, and the coarse texture of the bones are the significant findings. *Right,* Wrist of another infant showing similar changes.

The healing of rickets is shown by recalcification of the zone of provisional calcification. At first this is seen as a broad band of uniform density extending across the end of the shaft. Subsequently this is transformed into trabecular bone. Remineralization of the skeleton is a slow process and may take several months or even longer. The epiphyseal centers gradually regain normal density and sharpness of outline. The subperiosteal, poorly calcified osteoid is transformed into bone and the periosteal stripes disappear. If the bones have become bowed or otherwise deformed during the active stage of disease, the deformities are likely to persist. Thus when rickets has completely healed only the deformities from bowing or fracture will remain as evidence of the previous disease (Fig. 4-11).

OSTEOMALACIA IN ADULTS

The disease, osteomalacia, is the same as infantile rickets, but occurring after bone growth has ceased. In the United States osteomalacia probably is caused most often by faulty absorption of the fat-soluble vitamin D and other substances from the intestinal tract because of the steatorrhoea that occurs in the malabsorption syndromes, of which idiopathic sprue is the most common. Osteomalacia secondary to dysfunction of the proximal renal tubules (renal osteomalacia) is seen less frequently and dietary deficiency, the common cause of infantile rickets, also is infrequent in the United States. The basic roentgen abnormality is a generalized demineralization of the skeleton. The texture of the bones is coarse,

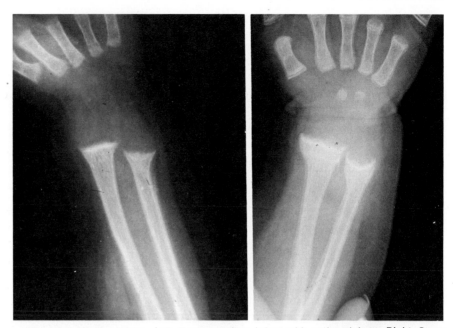

Fig. 4-9. Infantile rickets. *Left,* Forearm of an infant with active rickets. *Right,* Same patient after 2 weeks of therapy. The metaphyses have partially recalcified. The osteoid zones that were invisible before now can be seen as transverse bands of calcification crossing the ends of the shafts. Periosteal "stripes" (see text) are more evident as subperiosteal osteoid is beginning to calcify. Two carpal centers are visible where formerly none could be discerned. Cupping is still evident but will eventually disappear as healing continues.

the same as is noted in rickets. This is caused by an irregular absorption of the bone trabeculae; the total trabecular structure of the bone is decreased but the primary trabeculae that remain stand out more prominently than is normal. In contrast to osteoporosis, the cortical borders of the bones are not very distinct. Osteoporosis is characterized by a uniform demineralization, when long standing, so that a ground-glass appearance results. This, combined with the sharply outlined cortices, aids in distinguishing osteoporosis from osteomalacia. However, in severe osteomalacia there often is an associated osteoporosis so that the type of demineralization may be difficult to evaluate. Because bone growth has ceased, the metaphyseal and epiphyseal changes that form a large part of the findings in infantile rickets are not observed. Pseudofractures are frequent and are highly characteristic of osteomalacia, although

they may be found in a few other conditions. These are fissurelike defects or clefts extending transversely part way or completely through a bone. They represent fracture fissures filled with uncalcified osteoid and fibrous tissue. They are common along the axillary borders of the scapulae, the inner margins of the femoral necks, the ribs, the pubic and ischial rami and the bones of the forearms. These fissures also are sometimes called Looser's zones.

The condition described by Milkman (1930)[12] and known as *Milkman's syndrome* is now considered to represent a mild form of osteomalacia in which the pseudofractures are particularly numerous. Some investigators now consider this syndrome to represent the form of osteomalacia caused by a dysfunction of the proximal renal tubules, either a persistence of Vitamin D-refractory rickets from childhood or the result of some toxic agent such as plasma

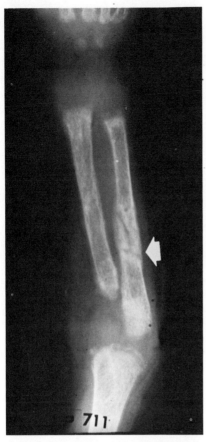

Fig. 4-10. Pseudofractures or Looser zones in active rickets. In addition to a transverse fissure there is an oblique one (**arrow**). The characteristic changes of florid rickets are present including coarse demineralization of the bones and ragged fraying of the metaphyses.

cell myeloma, metal poisoning (including copper—i.e., Wilson's disease), and glycogen storage disease, among others (see below.)[1]

Because osteomalacia causes softening of the bones, they may bend or give way as a result of weight-bearing. In the pelvis there may be an inward bending of the pelvic sidewalls with deepening of the acetabular cavities (protrusio acetabuli) (Fig. 4-12). In the skull, softening of the bones may lead to a downward molding of the skull over the first and second cervical vertebrae. The basal angle of the skull is flattened and the condition is known as platybasia.

HYPOPHOSPHATEMIC VITAMIN D-REFRACTORY RICKETS

This condition has also been called rachitis tarda or late rickets because it is found in older children (beyond the age of 2½ years). It was formerly considered to be due to a high-tissue threshold for the effects of vitamin D since massive doses of the vitamin are necessary to effect a cure. While this may play a part, newer concepts hold that there is a variety of conditions in which the proximal tubules of the kidneys are congenitally unable to reabsorb a number of substances from the glomerular filtrate or in which a number of toxic agents may cause this inability.[1] When phosphorus, or less frequently, calcium is lost as a result of this defect, rickets or osteomalacia will develop, depending on the age of the individual, because there is not enough mineral salts for normal ossification. (The designation, *Fanconi syndrome*, also has been used for this disease because it is a form of renal tubular dysfunction in which rickets or osteomalacia will develop.)

There is no glomerular disease and therefore patients do not develop uremia. The disease has a familial incidence and affects both males and females. Laboratory findings include hyperphosphaturia, hypophosphatemia and an elevated serum alkaline phosphatase. The serum calcium is normal. A number of types of hypophosphatemic vitamin D-refractory rickets have been described.[1]

Type I. Vitamin D-resistant rickets. This is the most common type.

Type II. With aminoaciduria

Type III. With aminoaciduria and acidosis

Type IV. Cystine storage disease

Type V. With hyperglycinuria

Type VI. Lowe's disease (oculocerebro-renal syndrome)

Roentgen Findings

The roentgen findings are those of rickets but as the patients are older, bowing of the

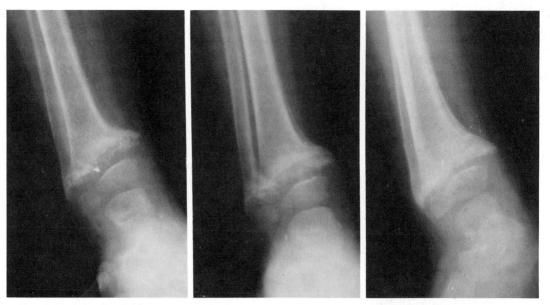

Fig. 4-11. Infantile rickets. Anteroposterior roentgenograms of the ankle of a 2-year-old child with active rickets. *Left,* Appearance at the time of beginning treatment. *Center,* Same patient, 18 days after beginning treatment. The metaphyses are beginning to recalcify. *Right,* Four weeks later healing is well advanced. Because this infant had begun to walk, bowing of the legs has occurred.

Fig. 4-12. Osteomalacia secondary to sprue. The demineralization is so intense it is difficult to portray the osseous structures. There is pronounced inward bending of the pelvic sidewalls, a characteristic deformity in severe osteomalacia.

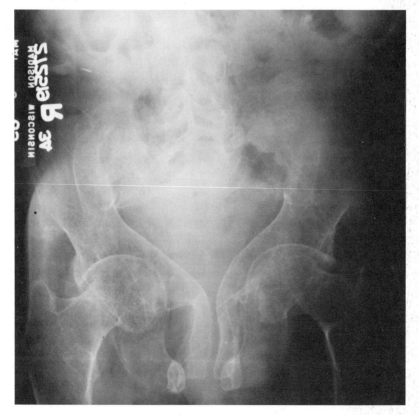

weight-bearing bones is greater and shortening of the long bones leads to some degree of dwarfing (Figs. 4-13 and 4-14). The cupping and fraying of the metaphyses, loss of zones of provisional calcification, and coarse texture of the demineralized bones are the same as those of rickets (Fig. 4-15). When the changes are mild, they are best demonstrated at the knees where widening of the epiphyseal line tends to be greatest on the medial sides of the distal femoral and proximal tibial metaphyses. Pseudofractures or Looser's zones occur with more severe disease. Occasionally, the bones appear sclerotic instead of radiolucent. The disease may be mistaken for achondroplasia because of the dwarfing of the long bones. However, the characteristic changes of rickets and the lack of the typical skull and pelvic changes of achondroplasia should allow differentiation.

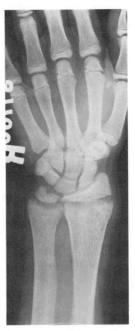

Fig. 4-14. Vitamin-D refractory rickets. Hand and wrist of another patient showing changes similar to those seen in Figures 4-13.

HYPOPHOSPHATASIA

Hypophosphatasia is an inborn error of metabolism characterized by a low level of alkaline phosphatase in the serum and the body tissues. It is probably inherited as an autosomal recessive gene. The lack of adequate amounts of alkaline phosphatase causes failure of proper mineralization of osteoid and the result in the skeleton is an appearance similar to rickets or osteomalacia. The disease may be present at birth and has been discovered in utero in roentgenograms of the mother's abdomen. The earlier the disease is detected the more severe it is likely to be and infants born with it seldom survive more than a year or two. In these patients there is severe demineralization of the metaphyses, the ends of which have a coarse, frayed appearance. The long bones in the newborn tend to be short and thin and with a coarse texture. The bones of the cranial vault are largely unossified, and there is bulging of the anterior fontanelle. Fractures of the long

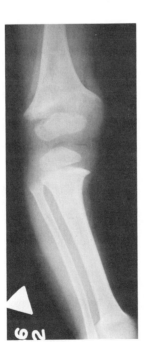

Fig. 4-13. Vitamin-D refractory rickets. The changes are the same as those seen in infantile rickets with the additional findings of bowing of the leg and stunting of the longitudinal growth of the bones.

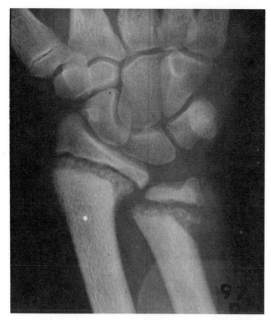

Fig. 4-15. Renal osteodystrophy. Wrist area shows severe rachitic changes in the radial and ulnar metaphyses with subluxations of the epiphyses on the shafts. Subperiosteal erosions were prominent in the phalanges (not shown) so that there were changes both of rickets and hyperparathyroidism.

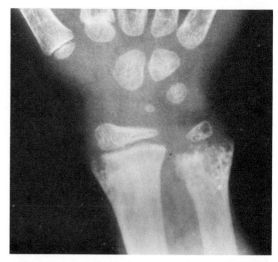

Fig. 4-16. Hypophosphatasia in a child. Wrist area demonstrates the deficient ossification of the radial and ulnar metaphyses with a roughened, frayed appearance, noted particularly in the ulna. The changes resemble those of rickets. The other long bones showed similar changes. This is from a patient with relatively mild involvement. Note the pseudoepiphysis for the second metacarpal.

bones may occur. There is an increased excretion of phosphorylethanolamine in the urine. The mechanism for the formation of this substance is not known but it may be a normal substrate of alkaline phosphatase which accumulates in excess amounts because of deficiency of the enzyme.[1] In older children, the changes are similar but less severe and resemble infantile rickets (Fig. 4-16). If the patient survives and the cranial bones ossify, craniosynostosis often develops. Dwarfism also becomes a feature and a genu valgum deformity is common. Many of these patients improve spontaneously. In its mildest form the disease manifests itself chiefly by an increased tendency to fracture of the bones and a low serum alkaline phosphatase.

HYPERPHOSPHATASIA

Other names applied to this condition according to Rubin[16] are, *juvenile Paget's disease, hyper-*

ostosis corticalis deformans juvenilis, chronic idiopathic hyperphosphatasia congenita. The serum alkaline phosphatase has been elevated in all reported cases. Clinical findings include lateral bowing of the femurs and muscular weakness. The mentality is normal. The disease probably has no relationship to Paget's disease.

Roentgen Findings

The characteristic finding is an extensive thickening of the diaphyseal cortex of all of the bones. The cortex is thickened both externally and internally and may, if severe, obliterate the medullary canal. Both the long and short tubular bones are affected. The bones of the cranial vault are thickened with patches of sclerosis. The pelvic bones may be of increased density. The carpal and tarsal bones have been normal and the vertebrae show only minimal sclerosis. The femurs are bowed laterally.

VAN BUCHEM'S DISEASE. Rubin[16] classified this rare dysplasia as *chronic hyperphosphatasemia tarda.* It also is known as *hyperostosis corticalis generalisata.* However Van Buchem does not believe that the seven cases reported by him are related to chronic idiopathic hyperphosphatasia but instead represent a distinct dysplasia.[16] The onset appears to be later than in the *congenita* form described above, ages of patients ranging from 23 to 52 years. The disease was asymptomatic in the cases described by Van Buchem et al. The major roentgen finding was a symmetrical, diaphyseal, cortical thickening of all of the long tubular bones, chiefly on the internal surface. The short tubular bones were involved in the same way. The femurs were not bowed. The epiphyses were spared. The cranial bones showed marked thickening of both vault and base. The maxillary sinuses and the mastoids were densely sclerotic. The mandible and clavicle were affected. There was diffuse sclerosis of the pelvic bones and the ribs were thickened when there was severe involvement elsewhere. Most of the patients did not show vertebral changes. As with the congenita form, the serum alkaline phosphatase was elevated in all cases with calcium and phosphorus levels being normal.

HYPERPARATHYROIDISM

Hyperparathyroidism is an uncommon, although not rare, disease which results from either an adenoma of one or several of the glands or a diffuse hyperplasia of them. Primary hyperparathyroidism usually is caused by an adenoma; secondary hyperparathyroidism, as in renal osteodystrophy, results from hyperplasia of the glands. Primary disease occurs mainly during middle age although it has been found in the very young and the old. It is about twice as common in females as in males. The increased parathyroid activity leads to excessive secretion of parathyroid hormone which in turn causes (*1*) demineralization of the skeleton, (*2*) the occurrence of focal areas of bone destruction ("brown tumors"), and (*3*) decrease in the serum phosphorus level and increase in the serum calcium level, factors which eventually cause dystrophic and, later, metastatic calcification of the soft tissues, renal stones and nephrocalcinosis and, eventual impairment of renal function.

It is believed that parathyroid hormone acts to increase the number of osteoclasts with resulting deossification of the skeleton. It also may diminish the reabsorption of phosphate from the glomerular filtrate by the proximal tubules causing hyperphosphaturia and hypophosphatemia.[1] These are complex biochemical processes, however, and complete information about them is not available.

When the kidney threshold for calcium is exceeded this substance is excreted in the urine in increased amounts. Eventually renal stones may be formed and calcification of the kidney tubules may develop (nephrocalcinosis). When kidney function has been impaired in this way there is retention of phosphates and further calcium loss. Then the serum phosphorus level may rise to normal or higher and the calcium level falls.

The high serum calcium level may lead to calcification of other tissues which can be visualized roentgenographically, such as the blood vessels and articular cartilages. When the serum phosphorus level rises and the calcium falls as a result of renal impairment, the resulting high ionization product may cause further metastatic soft tissue calcification.

Only about 5 per cent of renal stones are caused by hyperparathyroidism but this disease should be a consideration when renal stones are found since it may be the cause of the presenting symptoms in some cases. Nephrocalcinosis can be caused by a number of different diseases including medullary sponge kidney, chronic pyelonephritis, sarcoid disease, vitamin D poisoning, or any other cause of hypercalcemia. Calcification of the articular cartilages occurs more frequently as a result of senescence or the pseudogout syndrome than it does from hyperparathyroidism but, again, it may be a roentgen clue to the proper diagnosis which might not otherwise be suspected. Calcification in the walls of arteries may be seen even in the very young patient with hyperparathyroidism. The blood chemical findings include a normal or lowered phosphorus level, an elevated calcium level, and an elevated alkaline phosphatase level.

In cases with minimal skeletal disease most of the bony structures may appear quite normal or, at the most, show a slight decalcification. An occasional cystlike lesion may be present and renal stones or nephrocalcinosis may be demonstrated. These findings are not specific enough to allow a diagnosis to be made but they may arouse the suspicion of the disease.

In patients with well-defined skeletal disease, some or all of the following findings will be present.

GENERALIZED SKELETAL DEMINERALIZATION. The trabecular structure of the bones becomes hazy and indistinct, occasionally coarse and prominent. The cortical margins also become hazy and not well defined. In the skull, the bones develop a fine, granular appearance and the tables become indistinct (Fig. 4-17). This type of granular decalcification of the skull is a highly significant finding in this disease. The lamina dura, the cortical margin surrounding the tooth socket, disappears. Normally this is seen as a sharp, thin, white line surrounding

the peridental membrane that attaches the tooth to the bone (Fig. 4-18). Loss of the lamina dura is not pathognomonic for hyperparathyroidism as some degree of it may be seen in osteomalacia and in other diseases. Dental roentgenograms are useful when the question of hyperparathyroidism arises.

SUBPERIOSTEAL RESORPTION. This is a type of decalcification that is seen to best advantage in the phalanges but may be present elsewhere and seems to be a specific sign of the disease (Pugh[15]). It consists of a fine, irregular loss of density along the outer margins of the cortices, especially of the middle phalanges (Figs. 4-19 and 4-20). The roughened surface has been described as lacelike. In advanced disease there may be sufficient resorption to cause a general narrowing in width of the shaft, leaving the ends relatively intact (Fig. 4-21). In the distal phalanges, resorption of the terminal tufts may

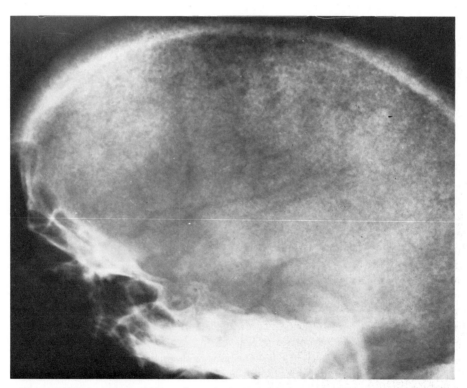

Fig. 4-17. Hyperparathyroidism. Lateral skull roentgenogram illustrating the granular demineralization of the cranial bones.

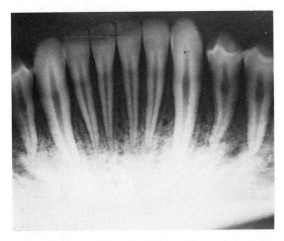

Fig. 4-18. Hyperparathyroidism. The anterior teeth of the lower jaw are shown. There is nearly complete absence of the lamina dura around the roots of the teeth. The trabecular pattern of the mandible is coarsened and demineralized.

be an associated finding. Other areas where subperiosteal resorption may be found include the distal end of the clavicle (Figs. 4-22 and 4-23), the symphysis pubis, and the sacroiliac joints. In these areas there may be considerable loss of bone substance leading to a rough, frayed appearance. Erosions also may be seen at the calcaneal tendon insertions, the ischial tuberosities, and other bony prominences. The lamina dura absorption probably represents the same process.

DESTRUCTIVE LESIONS. Localized destructive cystlike lesions of various sizes are frequent in this disease (Fig. 4-24). They are often referred to as "brown tumors." They are not true cysts but contain fibrous tissue, giant cells, osteoclasts, and decomposing blood.[1] The larger ones may be misinterpreted as giant cell tumors. This tumor is solitary and involves the end of a bone. Brown tumors may occur anywhere in the bone and often are multiple. The jaws, pelvis, and femurs are favorite sites but the lesion may be found in any part of the skeleton.

PATHOLOGIC FRACTURE. Fracture may result from the general weakening of the bone struc-

ture or because of localized destruction caused by a cystic lesion.

TISSUE CALCIFICATION. Calcium deposition in various structures, but particularly the kidneys, is common. Calcium may be deposited in the joint cartilages; however senescence and the pseudogout syndrome are more common causes of articular cartilage calcification. Premature calcification in the walls of the arteries is seen occasionally. Calcium deposition may occur in other tissues such as the pancreas and in the soft tissues around the joints. Calcification of the auricular cartilages has been noted.

ESOPHAGEAL AND TRACHEAL DISPLACEMENT. In some patients the parathyroid tumor is large enough to cause recognizable deformity in outline of the trachea or esophagus or both. This may be found in the lower part of the neck or in the upper mediastinum. Barium study of the esophagus is a useful procedure in the evaluation of patients suspected of having a parathyroid adenoma since it will, at times, localize the lesion, thus facilitating its surgical removal.

OSTEOSCLEROSIS. In some cases, increased density or osteosclerosis may be found. This is seen most often in the subchondral and metaphyseal areas and is more frequent in the secondary form of the disease (renal osteodystrophy). In the spine the upper and lower margins of the vertebral bodies are affected ("rugger-jersey" appearance or "sandwich vertebra").

The differential diagnosis of hyperparathyroidism includes consideration of all the other diseases that cause generalized skeletal demineralization. While the final diagnosis usually rests upon the results of chemical examination of the blood and urine, together with the use of angiography and radioactive isotopes to localize and identify the tumor in some cases, two roentgen signs, when present, are considered to be highly reliable. The one, subperiosteal resorption of the cortices of the phalanges, and other areas such as the distal end of the clavicle, appears to be specific for the disease;[15] the other, loss of the lamina dura around the roots of the teeth, does occur in a few other

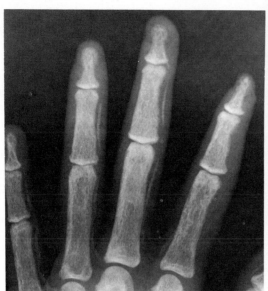 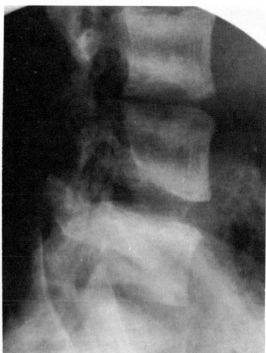

Fig. 4-19. Secondary hyperparathyroidism (renal osteodystrophy) in a female, age 21. The patient had known renal disease since early childhood. *Left,* there is subperiosteal resorption and the bones have a coarse texture with thickened trabeculae. The linear calcific stripes in the soft tissues of the fingers represent calcification in the digital arteries. Calcification also is present in other vessels including the uterine arteries. Patient has clinical signs of vascular insufficiency in the fingers. Note loss of soft tissues in the tip of the index finger owing to dry gangrene. *Right,* same patient shown in left. Lateral view of lumbar vertebrae shows osteosclerosis which is most intense along upper and lower borders ("sandwich vertebrae"). Patient also has considerable sclerosis and thickening of the cranial bones.

conditions but is more distinct in hyperparathyroidism. Renal osteodystrophy (renal rickets) may cause changes identical with those seen in primary disease of the parathyroid glands. This is because of the secondary hyperplasia of the parathyroids and the skeletal changes of hyperparathyroidism become a significant feature of the disease.

RENAL OSTEODYSTROPHY

This disease has been called renal rickets in the past but most investigators believe the term renal osteodystrophy is preferable since much of the skeletal disease which develops is owing to increased parathyroid activity (secondary hyperparathyroidism). The exact pathogenesis is not clear. Recent investigations indicate that the intestinally active metabolite of vitamin D is generated in kidney tissue. As a result of certain renal diseases a decrease in this substance would inhibit the removal of calcium from the intestine causing hypocalcemia. This would, in turn, stimulate the parathyroids and lead to the clinical state hyperparathyroidism. The low serum calcium level causes failure of normal mineralization of newly formed bone and thus the changes of both rickets and hyperparathyroidism develop.

The skeletal disease usually does not become manifest before the age of 2 years. The kidney diseases responsible usually are congenital such as polycystic disease, hypogenesis, or congenital obstructions of the ureters, bladder outlet or

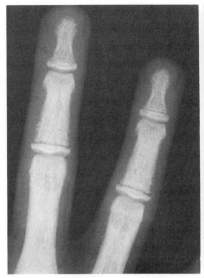
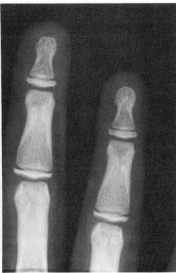

Fig. 4-20. Renal osteodystrophy. *Left,* Fingers of a child with the disease showing subperiosteal resorption along the borders of the phalanges. This causes a fine roughening of the cortical margins. Note frayed appearance of terminal tufts of distal phalanges. These changes are indicative of hyperparathyroidism and aid in distinguishing renal osteodystrophy from vitamin D rickets. *Right,* Fingers of normal child for comparison.

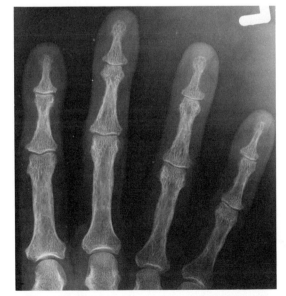

Fig. 4-21. Hyperparathyroidism. Long-standing disease has caused thinning of the midshafts of the phalanges, particularly the middle phalanges owing to subperiosteal resorption. There is fraying of the terminal tufts of the distal phalanges and generalized decreased density of all of the bones.

urethra. Chronic pyelonephritis is frequently superimposed as a result of urinary tract stasis.[1]

Roentgen Findings

The roentgen findings are essentially a combination of those seen in rickets and hyperparathyroidism (Figs. 4-20 and 4-25). The latter include (*1*) subperiosteal resorption (Fig. 4-19), (*2*) generalized demineralization, (*3*) brown tumors, (*4*) loss of lamina dura around the teeth. The rachitic changes are similar to those of infantile rickets (Figs. 4-15 and 4-26) except that epiphyseal subluxations may occur and a genu valgum deformity is common at the knee instead of a varus deformity.

If the disease begins early in life and the patient survives for a number of years significant dwarfism occurs. Calcification in the walls of the arteries may be seen, even in the very young. Nephrocalcinosis may develop but renal stones are uncommon. If the disease develops later in life dwarfism does not occur and the

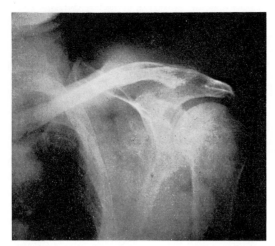

Fig. 4-22. Primary hyperparathyroidism caused by a parathyroid adenoma. The bones are severely demineralized and are difficult to portray in roentgenograms. Note the erosion of the distal end of the clavicle causing an apparent widening of the acromioclavicular joint space.

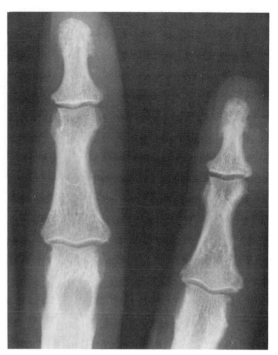

Fig. 4-24. Fingers of patient with parathyroid adenoma. Subperiosteal resorption has led to a thinning of the shafts of the middle phalanges. There is a small "brown tumor" in one proximal phalanx.

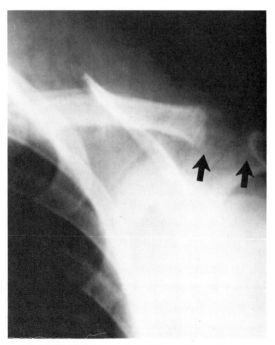

Fig. 4-23. Hyperparathyroidism. There has been considerable loss of bone in the distal end of the clavicle causing apparent widening of the acromioclavicular joint space. **Right arrow** points to the medial side of the acromion process and **left arrow** to the distal end of the clavicle.

bone changes are mainly those of hyperparathyroidism. Osteosclerosis develops in some patients, chiefly at the ends of the bones and the superior and inferior margins of the vertebrae. It is more frequent than in the primary form of the disease. The reason why osteosclerosis develops is not clear. A recently discovered substance elaborated by the thyroid and known as calcitonin is known to lower the serum calcium level and it may do so by preventing the normal removal of calcium from bone.

HYPOPARATHYROIDISM

Hypoparathyroidism usually results from injury or accidental removal of the glands during thyroidectomy. Spontaneous idiopathic hypoparathyroidism occurs but is uncommon. The clinical symptoms are those that result from the hypocalcemia (parathyroid tetany). The serum calcium

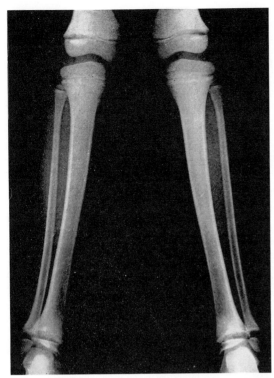

Fig. 4-25. Renal osteodystrophy. The metaphyses show changes resembling those of rickets. Note the knock knee deformity.

is low and the phosphorus elevated. Roentgen changes are relatively few and in some cases the skeletal system is normal. In others the bones have shown increase in density with widening of the cortices of the long bones. Infrequently the bones of the calvarium are thickened. In some patients stippled areas of calcification occur within the brain. These tend to be symmetrically situated in the basal ganglia. This finding is not specific for hypoparathyroidism but is always suggestive of it.

PSEUDOHYPOPARATHYROIDISM (PH) AND PSEUDO-PSEUDOHYPOPARATHYROIDISM (PPH)

Pseudohypoparathyroidism (PH) is a congenital hereditary disorder characterized by a failure of normal response to parathyroid hormone.[20] There is hypocalcemia and hyperphosphatemia as in hypoparathyroidism and little or no response to the administration of parathyroid hormone. Most patients are obese and of short stature with a round facies, corneal or lenticular opacities, brachydactyly and mental retardation.

Usually all of the tubular bones of the hands and feet are short but some, especially the fourth and fifth metacarpals, are shorter than the others. Also they tend to be broad owing to lack of normal constriction of the midshafts. The terminal and middle phalanges tend to be relatively shorter than the proximal. Cone epiphyses are common and the epiphyseal plates are thin or, at times, partially fused at the apex of the cone when they first appear. Accelerated fusion is common in the hands and feet.

Calcified or ossified deposits may be found in the skin or subcutaneous tissues. Stippled calcification is often found in the basal ganglia or elsewhere in the brain, as in hypoparathyroidism. In some, the cranial bones are thickened and the skull has a brachycephalic shape. The interpedicular distances in the lumbar spine may decrease from above downward instead of showing the normal increase. The general skeletal density is decreased apparently owing to osteoporosis and the trabecular structure may be coarse. However, increased density has been reported in some patients and, apparently because of the hypocalcemia, the changes of secondary hyperparathyroidism may develop. In some infants the hands and feet have been normal but become abnormal as the child grows older.

Dentition often is abnormal including defective dentine, excessive caries, delayed eruption, and wide root canals. Other findings have been observed in some patients including coxa vara or valga, bowing of the long bones and an occasional exostosis including one on the inner proximal tibia similar to that seen in the Ellis-Van Creveld syndrome and in Turner's syndrome.

The hereditary nature of PH has been established. It is possible for some members of the family to show roentgen findings characteristic of the disease but with normal blood chemistry and no evidence of tetany. This entity has been called pseudo-pseudohypoparathyroidism (PPH) and is considered to be the partial expression of a disease of which PH is the complete syndrome.[20] Families showing only the characteristics of PPH have been reported and in some members the bone changes have been very minimal such as a shortening of one or more of the metacarpals. There also is a lower incidence of intracranial calcification in PPH.

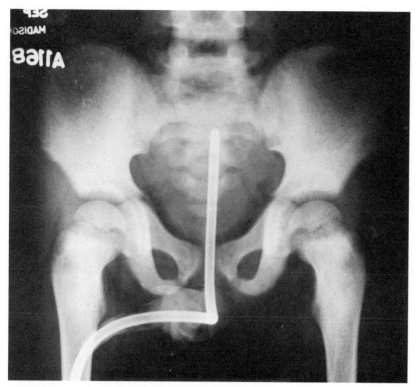

Fig. 4-26. Same case as Figure 4-25. The patient had congenital obstruction of the bladder neck that led to severe renal damage.

Among the entities to be considered in differential diagnosis are, (1) peripheral dysostosis, (2) chondroectodermal dysplasia, (3) multiple hereditary exostosis, and (4) Turner's syndrome.[20] These have, as a rule, other roentgen, clinical, and genetic findings that aid in differentiation. Short metacarpals and metatarsals also occur as isolated defects.

REFERENCES AND SELECTED READINGS

1. AEGERTER, E., and KIRKPATRICK, J. A., JR.: *Orthopedic Diseases,* 3rd ed. Philadelphia, Saunders, 1968.

2. BROMER, R. S.: Rickets. *Am. J. Roentgenol. Radium Ther. Nucl. Med. 30:* 582, 1933.

3. CAMP, J. D.: Osseous changes in hyperparathyroidism. A roentgenologic study. *JAMA 99:* 1913, 1932.

4. DARLING, D. B., LORIDAN, L., and SENIOR, B.: The roentgenographic manifestations of Cushing's syndrome in infancy. *Radiology 96:* 503, 1970.

5. EDEIKEN, J., and HODES, P. J.: *Roentgen Diagnosis of Diseases of Bone.* Baltimore, Md., Williams and Wilkins, 1967.

6. GLEASON, D. G., and POTCHEN, E. J.: The Diagnosis of hyperparathyroidism. *Radiol. Clin. North Am. 5:* 277, 1967.

7. HAFF, R. C., BLACK, W. C., and BALLINGER, II, W. F.: Primary hyperparathyroidism: Changing clinical, surgical and pathologic aspects. *Ann. Surg. 171:* 85, 1970.

8. HOWLAND, W. J., JR., PUGH, D. G., and SPRAGUE, R. G.: Roentgenologic changes of the skeletal system in Cushing's syndrome. *Radiology 71:* 69, 1958.

9. JACKSON, D. M.: Heel-pad thickness in obese persons. *Radiology 90:* 129, 1968.

10. JONES, G.: Radiological appearances of disuse osteoporosis. *Clin. Radiol. 20:* 345, 1969.

11. MCALISTER, W. H., and KOEHLER, P. R.: Diseases of the adrenal. *Radiol. Clin. North Am. 5:* 205, 1967.

12. MILKMAN, L. A.: Pseudofractures (hunger osteopathy, late rickets, osteomalacia). *Am. J. Roentgenol. Radium Ther. Nucl. Med. 24:* 29, 1930.

13. MURRAY, R. O.: Radiological bone changes in Cushing's syndrome and steroid therapy. *Br. J. Radiol. 33:* 1, 1960.

14. PATTON, J. D.: Changes in metabolic bone disease. *Proc. R. Soc. Med. 59:* 1231, 1966.

15. PUGH, D. G.: Subperiosteal resorption of bone. A roentgenologic manifestation of primary hyperparathyroidism and renal osteodystrophy. *Am. J. Roentgenol. Radium Ther. Nucl. Med. 66:* 577, 1951.

16. RUBIN, P.: *Dynamic Classification of Bone Dysplasias.* Chicago, Year Book, 1964.

17. STEIN, I., STEIN, R. O., and BELLER, M. L.: *Living Bone in Health and Disease.* Philadelphia, Lippincott, 1955.

18. STEINBACH, H. L.: The roentgen appearance of osteoporosis. *Radiol. Clin. North Am. 2:* 191, 1964.

19. STEINBACH, H. L., et al.: Primary hyperparathyroidism: A correlation of roentgen, clinical and pathologic features. *Am. J. Roentgenol. Radium Ther. Nucl. Med. 86:* 329, 1962.

20. STEINBACH, H. L., and YOUNG, D. A.: The roentgen appearance of pseudohypoparathyroidism (PH) and pseudo-pseudohypoparathyroidism (PPH). *Am. J. Roentgenol. Radium Ther. Nucl. Med. 97:* 49, 1966.

21. WHEDON, G. D., CAMERON, J. R. (eds.): *Proceedings of the Conference on Progress in Methods of Bone Mineral Measurements.* Washington, D.C., United States Government Printing Office, 1970.

22. WHEDON, G. D., NEWMAN, W. F., and JENKINS, D. W. (eds.): *Progress in Development of Methods in Bone Densitometry. N.A.S.A. Report SP-64.* Washington, D.C., National Aeronautics and Space Administration, 1966.

5

TRAUMATIC LESIONS OF BONES AND JOINTS

While the presence of a fracture often is obvious on clinical examination, roentgenograms are essential to delineate the nature of the injury clearly, and only from roentgen examination can an accurate idea be obtained of the anatomic structures involved and the severity of the injury to them. In a great many instances roentgen examination is necessary to determine whether a fracture exists or not because the clinical findings are not reliable. Conversely, there may at times be clinical evidence to suggest fracture, but roentgenograms fail to reveal it initially. As a general rule, when the slightest doubt exists concerning the presence or absence of a fracture or dislocation, roentgen examination should be performed. After reduction of a fracture roentgenograms are needed to determine the accuracy of reduction, to furnish a record of the status of the fracture and, later, to follow the progress of healing. The frequency of follow-up examinations to determine the degree of healing will vary widely, depending upon such factors as the type of fracture, the bone involved, the method of treatment employed, and the age of the patient, among others, so that no set rules can be given. A fracture being treated by means of skeletal traction may require daily examinations, at least until reduction has been accomplished. A fracture that has been reduced satisfactorily and the part placed in a cast should be examined immediately after the application of the cast and at intervals of several weeks thereafter until healing is sufficiently solid for use of the part. Oblique or spiral fractures need closer observation than transverse or impacted fractures because of the tendency for slipping of the fragments within the cast.

ROENTGENOGRAMS

It is usual in examining the bones for fracture to obtain at least two views made at right angles to one another. These are necessary in order to obtain a true perspective of the spatial relationships of the fragments (Fig. 5-1). At times the fracture line may be visible in only one of several projections and the examiner rarely is justified in saying that a fracture does not exist solely on observation of a single roentgenogram of a part. Even with multiple exposures and technically good roentgenograms, a fine hairline fracture may escape detection until a reexamination some days later will show it clearly. The usual decalcification that occurs along the edges of the fracture

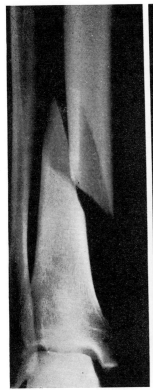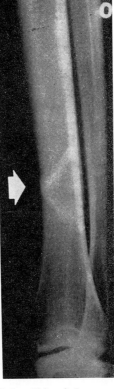

Fig. 5-1. Spiral fracture of the tibia. Anteroposterior (*left*) and lateral (*right*) views of the lower half of the leg. Note the amount of displacement in the anteroposterior view and the lack of it in the lateral. When viewed from the side the fragments overlap so that a fracture line cannot be seen. Instead there is a zone of increased density indicating the overriding (**arrow**). The need for multiple views when examining a bone for fracture is illustrated clearly in this patient.

at the time of the initial examination and only a general survey can be made to indicate the presence and extent of gross fractures. More detailed examination may have to wait until such complications as shock or internal injuries have received attention. In head injuries, the damage to the brain often is of much greater importance than any associated fracture of the cranial bones; the desire to find out the extent of the patient's bone injuries should not influence the judgment of the physician in his care of the patient.

TERMINOLOGY. When describing displacement of fracture fragments it is usual to refer to the displacement of the distal fragment in relation to the proximal, the latter being considered as the stationary part. Thus, one speaks of a posterior displacement of the distal fragment of the tibia on the proximal fragment rather than an anterior displacement of the proximal on the distal. The same method is used in describing dislocations, the distal extremity being considered to be the dislocated one. For example, all dislocations of the elbow joint are displacements of the bones of the forearm on the humerus. In describing angular deformity it also is usual to consider the distal fragment as being angled on the proximal. Unless otherwise modified, the term "medial angulation" refers to an inward angulation of the distal fragment on the proximal. For greater accuracy it is better to describe angulations in terms of convexity and concavity. In the example referred to above, where the lower fragment was turned inward on the proximal, the proper description would be a medial concave angulation of "x" degrees, or if preferred, a lateral convex angulation of "x" degrees. Using the terms "concave" and "convex" will indicate clearly the nature of the deformity.

FLUOROSCOPY

At one time fluoroscopy was widely used to aid in the reduction of fractures because it enabled the orthopedic surgeon to manipulate the fragments under direct fluoroscopic vision. The danger of overexposure to radiation to the person doing the reduction is real. Many physicians in the past have developed severe roentgen ray reactions from repeated or prolonged exposure of

fragments may make the fracture line more readily visible after a short period of time. Such fractures are seen occasionally in the carpal navicular and in the ribs. The term *occult fracture* has been used to denote this lesion, implying a fracture that may give clinical signs of its presence but which cannot be demonstrated roentgenologically until reparative changes have occurred.

Where two right-angle views are impossible to obtain, usually because of the condition of the injured patient, a third-dimensional image can be obtained by the use of stereoscopic roentgenograms. It is often impossible to secure completely satisfactory films of a severely injured patient the hands during the fluoroscopic manipulation of fractures. The danger of overexposure of the skin of the patient during a protracted reduction also must be kept in mind and is a definite hazard. Because of these harmful possibilities, fluoroscopy for this purpose has fallen into disrepute. If it is used, certain precautions are essential: (*1*) the person operating the fluoroscope must be fully aware of the amount of radiation being delivered by the roentgen ray tube and equally aware of methods of protection; (*2*) a timing device should be incorporated in the roentgen-ray circuit to shut off the current automatically after a predetermined amount of time has elapsed; (*3*) all manipulation should be done with the fluoroscope turned off and it should be turned on for quick visual inspection only when the surgeon's hands have been removed from the field of exposure; (*4*) if repeated attempts at reduction become necessary, fluoroscopy should not be used; (*5*) an image intensifier should always be used if available.

TYPES OF FRACTURES

There are several ways in which fractures of the bones of the extremities can be classified. They can be divided into two major groups, open and closed fractures. An open fracture is usually spoken of as a compound fracture and this term is used to denote a perforation of the skin over the fracture. The importance of a compound fracture, of course, lies in the possibility of infection developing because of contamination at the time of injury, and this possibility must be taken into account when progress roentgenograms of a compound fracture are being evaluated. A closed fracture not infrequently is changed into an open one because of the need for surgical reduction, the placement of metal plates, bone grafts, or other fixation devices. While very infrequent with good surgical technique, there is always the possibility of such a fracture becoming infected.

Fractures also can be classified according to the mechanics of the stress that produces them and thus one finds such terms as torsion fractures, bending fractures, and shearing fractures

used in descriptive terminology. While one can frequently suspect the nature of the force that caused the fracture from the roentgen appearances, this is not always the case and in general these terms are not commonly used in roentgenologic descriptions.

The following grouping of fractures is useful for descriptive purposes and the terms are those used in roentgen and clinical evaluation. Some fractures will not fit into a specific group because they show mixed features. For example, a compression fracture may also show evidence of comminution; the line of demarcation between an impacted fracture and a compression fracture is not sharp; a Colles' fracture at the wrist is usually comminuted as well as impacted. These limitations must be kept in mind when one attempts to classify any specific fracture.

COMPLETE, NONCOMMINUTED FRACTURES

This term is used to designate a fracture that has caused a complete dissolution in continuity of the bone with separation of it into two fragments. The fracture is visualized in roentgenograms as a dark line or zone between the fragments and there may or may not be displacement.

OBLIQUE, SPIRAL, AND TRANSVERSE FRACTURES

According to the direction of the fracture line there can be recognized oblique, spiral, and transverse fractures. Spiral and oblique fractures are common in the shafts of the long tubular bones (see Fig. 5-1). Transverse fractures are less frequent but can occur if the force producing the fracture is of the bending rather than the torsion type. A particular type of transverse fracture often occurs through abnormal bone, i.e., a pathologic fracture. The line of fracture often extends directly through the bone at a right angle to the long axis and the ends of the fragments are smooth or at the most show only a moderate irregularity.

Transverse fractures through normal bone are invariably ragged along the line of fracture.

MULTIPLE FRACTURES

When two or more complete fractures involve the shaft of a single bone, they are spoken of as multiple fractures. Multiple fractures differ from comminuted fractures in that each fracture is a complete one leaving a fragment of intact shaft between them. In a comminuted fracture one or more small fragments have been separated along the line of major fracture but these pieces, as a rule, do not represent a complete thickness of the bone.

AVULSION FRACTURES

An avulsion fracture consists of the separation of a fragment of bone that has been pulled away from the shaft. Usually avulsion fractures involve a tuberosity or bony process. Common examples are avulsion of the internal epicondyle of the humerus and avulsion fracture of the greater tuberosity of the humerus (Fig. 5-2). In other cases there may be avulsion of a fragment of cortex as a result of muscle or ligament pull occurring as part of a sprain. These are referred to as cortical avulsions or flake fractures and are frequent in the ankle area in association with severe sprains.

CHIP FRACTURES

A chip fracture resembles an avulsion fracture and is a type of avulsion but the term usually is limited to the separation of a small fragment or chip of bone from the corner of a phalanx or other long bone. They also are sometimes called corner fractures. They are very common in the fingers and the fragments often are very tiny. Chip fracture fragments do not always undergo bony union but fibrous union generally takes place and unless the fragment was displaced considerably or was rather large there is usually little impairment of function.

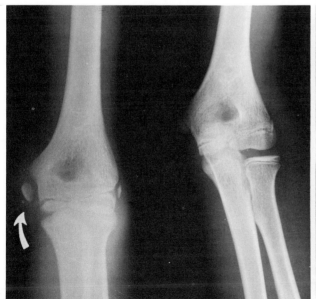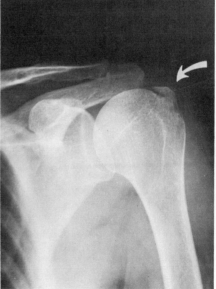

Fig. 5-2. Avulsion fractures. *Left,* Avulsion fracture of the epiphysis for the internal epicondyle of the left humerus (**arrow**). Normal right elbow for comparison. *Right,* Avulsion fracture of the greater tuberosity of the humerus.

COMMINUTED FRACTURES

A comminuted fracture is one in which, in addition to the major line of fracture that extends through the bone, one or more fragments have been separated along the edges of one or both major fragments. Occasionally the bone may be extensively shattered. More often the comminution is less severe and the fracture may follow a fairly distinct pattern. Thus one finds T, V, and Y fractures, the designation indicating the general appearance of the fracture lines. T fractures are frequent in the lower end of the femur with a transverse fracture extending through the bone just above the level of the condyles and a vertical component forming the stem of the T extending into the joint and separating the condyles (Fig. 5-3). A Y fracture is rather similar; it is found occasionally in the lower end of the humerus. V fractures occasionally occur in the midshafts of the long bones.

A crush fracture is a special type of comminuted fracture seen in a distal phalanx and usually results from the finger being crushed in a door or between heavy objects. The terminal tuft often is broken into many small fragments that are spread apart slightly but generally not severely displaced. Crush fractures also may involve the os calcis as the result of a fall from a height, the patient landing on the heels. Usually there is considerable impaction also present and this type of fracture often is a mixture of comminution and impaction.

INCOMPLETE FRACTURES

In an incomplete fracture not all the bone structure gives way. Some of the trabeculae are disrupted completely but others only buckle or bend or remain intact. There may be an angular deformity but there can be little or no displacement.

GREENSTICK FRACTURE

The greenstick fracture is one of the common forms of incomplete fracture (Fig. 5-4).

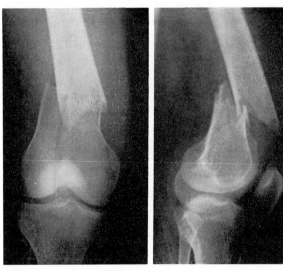

Fig. 5-3. Comminuted T fracture of the lower end of the femur. *Left,* Anteroposterior view. In addition to an irregular transverse fracture through the shaft, there is a vertical component extending through the condyles and into the articular surface. *Right,* Lateral view of same patient.

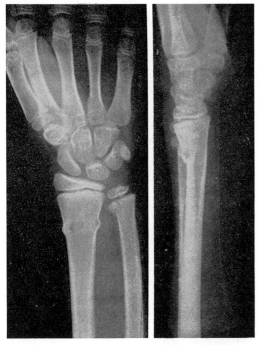

Fig. 5-4. Greenstick fractures of the radius and ulna in a child. There is buckling of the bone with disruption of some of the trabeculae but not all of them, and the fragments are held by remaining trabeculae.

Only a part of the framework structure gives way, allowing a buckling or sharp angulation of the bone. The effect is similar to that obtained by trying to break a green twig in two. The simplest form may show only a slight buckling of the cortex and clinical symptoms may be negligible. Greenstick fractures are found almost exclusively during infancy and childhood. In older persons the bones are more brittle and this type of fracture does not occur. Greenstick fractures heal promptly.

IMPACTED FRACTURE

An impacted fracture usually is incomplete although there occasionally may be a complete disruption at the line of fracture with secondary impaction having occurred. In an impacted fracture the fragments are driven into one another either along the entire line of fracture or only along one side. A radiolucent fracture line is not seen in this type of fracture since the impaction completely obscures it. Instead the line of impaction is denser than normal because of the condensed bony trabeculae within it. In addition, an impacted fracture can be recognized by the disruption of normal bone trabeculae and architecture at the site of impaction, by the sharp angulation of the cortical margin at least on one side of the fracture, and by the general disturbance of normal anatomic relationships. One of the frequent sites for impacted fracture is the neck of the femur. A type of impacted fracture frequent in the vertebrae and that also may involve some of the irregular bones, such as the os calcis, is called a compression fracture. This is essentially the same as an impacted fracture but the latter term is usually limited to fractures occurring in the long bones, while the term "compression fracture" is applied to injuries involving the vertebrae or the bones of the carpus and tarsus.

INFRACTIONS

An infraction is a form of impacted fracture and the term is used to designate an injury of limited extent. Thus an impacted fracture of a metatarsal head in which there is a barely recognizable deformity might be designated as an infraction rather than a fracture. The term also is used to describe a minor localized break in the cortex of a bone that causes only slight local deformity. Local injury to a bone by a blunt object that causes only a small indentation or fragmentation of cortex can properly be called an infraction.

BUCKLING FRACTURE

This term is used for certain fractures that occur almost entirely in demineralized bone, chiefly secondary to severe osteoporosis. The bone breaks only part way through and there results a sharp angular deformity without lateral displacement. The effect can be likened to that obtained by sharply bending a thin rubber tube. Buckling fractures are caused by a bending type of strain. Porotic bone, being softer than normal bone, may give way in this manner. A normal bone suffering the same type of strain might not fracture at all or if it did the fracture would most likely be complete.

PENETRATING FRACTURE

This term is used to indicate the type of bone injury that results from penetration by a sharp object such as a bullet or perforation by a sharp piece of metal. The injury is localized to a relatively small portion of the bone without there being a complete dissolution in con-

tinuity. The fracture therefore is properly included in the group of incomplete fractures but frequently there is comminution with separation of small fragments at the site of injury. Some of these fractures are difficult to classify because they encompass various groups.

EPIPHYSEAL FRACTURES

During childhood a fracture may extend part way or completely through the epiphyseal plate at the end of a long bone and lead to displacement of the epiphysis on the shaft. This type of injury is frequent in the lower end of the

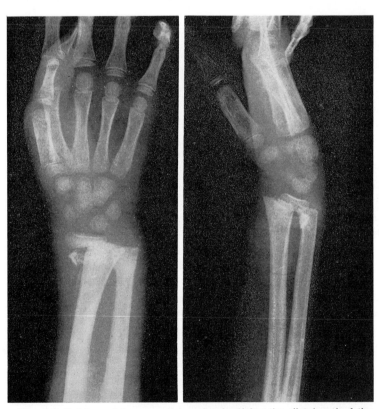

Fig. 5-5. Epiphyseal fracture dislocation involving the distal end of the radius. Anteroposterior (*left*) and lateral (*right*) views of the lower forearm and wrist of a child. The distal epiphysis of the radius together with a corner fragment from the metaphysis has been displaced dorsally and laterally on the shaft. The injury is about a week old and there is beginning periosteal calcification where the periosteum was elevated from the shaft on the outer posterior aspect.

tibia and in the distal end of the radius (Fig. 5-5). If the line of fracture is limited to the cartilage it will not be directly visible and its detection rests upon the evidence of epiphyseal displacement or upon variation in width of the epiphyseal line. In the absence of displacement, detection of a pure epiphyseal plate fracture is difficult; comparison with the opposite extremity is helpful in doubtful cases. In most cases the fracture does not remain confined to the cartilaginous plate but angles sharply into the bone so that a corner fragment of the shaft remains attached to the epiphysis and is carried along with it if the epiphysis becomes displaced. If there is no displacement, the oblique fracture line in the shaft can be recognized and indicates the nature of the injury.

PATHOLOGIC FRACTURES

A pathologic fracture is one occurring through diseased bone. A pathologic fracture may occur in practically any of the forms described in the preceding sections. There are two types, however, which always suggest that a fracture has occurred through diseased bone: (1) A buckling fracture such as described in the third paragraph above. This usually happens when fracture involves osteoporotic bone. This type of fracture is rather frequent in osteogenesis imperfecta, which is a form of osteoporosis. If with healing the angular deformity has not been corrected, the bones become bowed (see Fig. 2-22). (2) A transverse fracture extending at right angles to the longitudinal axis of the bone and with the ends of the fragments smooth or only slightly irregular (Fig. 5-6). In the presence of any fracture, the structure of the bone should be observed carefully for evidence of disease that may have predisposed to the injury. Occasionally a bone cyst, enchondroma, or other benign lesion is discovered because of the fracture. In adults, a pathologic fracture may bring to light a focus

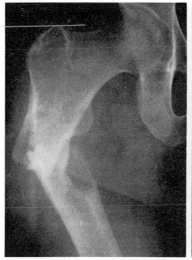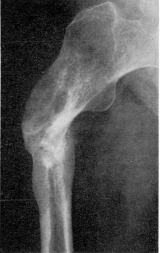

Fig. 5-6. Pathologic fracture of the femur secondary to a focus of metastatic carcinoma (primary carcinoma of the breast). *Left,* Appearance immediately following fracture. The fracture extends transversely through the bone. The translucent area on the inner side represents the metastatic focus that has destroyed the bone and predisposed to the fracture. *Right,* Same patient after roentgen therapy. The fracture has healed and the metastatic lesion also has recalcified. Such a good result is not always obtained but at times a metastatic lesion can be brought under control by treatment and the healing of a fracture promoted.

of metastatic carcinoma or other significant local lesion of bone.

PSEUDOFRACTURES

These are transverse fissurelike defects that extend part way or completely through the bone. They are seen frequently in osteomalacia and are sometimes referred to as the "zones of Looser" or *Umbauzonen*. They are infractions of bone in which osteoid is formed in the defect but with failure of calcium deposition so that a fissure defect persists in the roentgenogram. A failure of proper calcification of osteoid is one of the characteristics of osteomalacia. In this disease, pseudofractures are usually bilateral and symmetrical, being found most frequently along the axillary borders of the scapulae, the inner margins of the femoral necks, and in the pubic rami. Multiple pseudofractures of this type were described by Milkman in 1930 and the condition sometimes is designated as Milkman's syndrome. Most investigators now believe that this represents only osteomalacia in which the pseudofractures happen to be a particularly prominent part of the disease (see Chapter 4, section on "Osteomalacia").

A similar type of fracture is seen in Paget's disease, fibrous dysplasia, and osteogenesis imperfecta. Some authorities contend' that these differ from the pseudofractures of osteomalacia in that they are true fractures that have healed by fibrous or cartilaginous union. Roentgenologically they do not differ from the pseudofractures of osteomalacia but the basic change of the underlying bone disease (e.g., Paget's disease) will be different and will usually lead to the correct diagnosis (Fig. 5-7). A pseudofracture may become complete following an injury and lead to displacement of fragments and the clinical signs and symptoms of fracture (see Fig. 8-25). Pseudofractures are probably very similar to the chronic fatigue fractures that occur in the metatarsals and other bones (see section "Chronic Stress or Fatigue Fracture") and they probably develop in bone that is incapable of withstanding the stresses placed upon it. In normal bone, fissures will heal promptly. In abnormal bone, such as in osteomalacia, healing is delayed and the fissure persists as a roentgenologically visible defect. Steinbach has suggested that the fissure develops directly beneath an artery and that the pulsation of the ves-

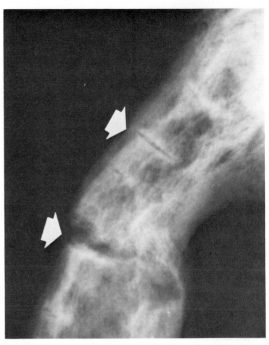

Fig. 5-7. Pseudofractures in Paget's disease. A portion of the shaft of a femur is illustrated with characteristic changes of severe Paget's disease. There are several incomplete transverse fissures (**upper arrow** points to one of them) and a complete fracture has occurred (**lower arrow**) with slight malalignment of fragments.

sel might be responsible for its occurrence. Others, however, have not been able to confirm this.

CHRONIC STRESS OR FATIGUE FRACTURE

This is a type of fracture most frequently found in the metatarsals, particularly the second. It develops as a result of chronic foot strain. Following a brief period of pain and swelling, roentgenograms show a faint hazy fusiform callus shadow near the distal end of the metatarsal shaft (Fig. 5-8). Within a few weeks this callus shadow becomes dense and generally at this time a faint line of fracture can be seen extending transversely through the bone. The lesion is considered to be a simple fracture that occurs in a bone unable to withstand the strains placed upon it but which is otherwise normal. The lesion also can develop as a result of abnormal stresses that have been applied for some time by muscle

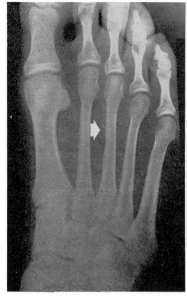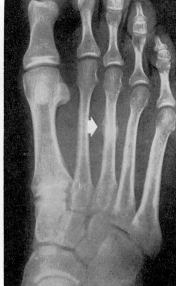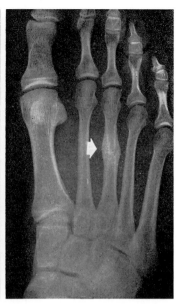

Fig. 5-8. Fatigue fracture of the third metatarsal. *Left,* Appearance of the bone about 10 days after the onset of complaints of aching pain in the foot. In the original roentgenogram there was a suggestion of a faint hairline fissure in the shaft of the third metatarsal. *Center,* Appearance 19 days after figure on the *left.* The area of fracture now is easily recognized because of the fusiform periosteal calcification (callus) that has developed around it. The fracture line itself remains faint. *Right,* Same patient 3 months later. The evidence of break in continuity of the bone is more distinct but there also has been increased callus and solidification of the callus so that healing is well advanced. (**Arrows** indicate the fracture site.)

or ligament pull as part of an activity not ordinarily indulged in by the individual. It received the name *"march foot"* because it was first encountered in recruit soldiers after long marches. The line of fracture does not become visible for a week or two, or until decalcification along the fracture line makes it more prominent. Even then the fracture line may be very faint. The same type of fracture occasionally is found in other bones, particularly the inner upper margin of the tibia. Here the area of fracture may first appear as an incomplete transverse line of increased density with a small amount of periosteal calcification overlying it. This is a manifestation of early repair. In the os calcis the same finding, that of a linear zone of sclerosis, may be the first clue to the diagnosis. These fractures also have been described as occurring in the superior aspect of the femoral neck, the anterior portion of the first rib (Fig. 5-9), the upper end of the fibula, and the superior and inferior pubic rami. We have seen two examples of fatigue fracture involving the inner cortex of the tibia, several inches above the ankle joint, which developed in long-distance

runners. When one finds a transverse line or band of increased density extending part way or completely through the end of either a long bone or one of the small bones, stress fracture should be considered the likely diagnosis.

UNION OF FRACTURES

In order to understand the changes that can be recognized in roentgenograms during the process of fracture repair, a brief résumé of the histology of bone healing is in order. The following is based upon Boyd's description of the healing of fractures in experimental animals.

The repair of bone is carried out entirely by the osteoblasts that lie in the deep layer of the periosteum, the endosteum, and the Haversian canals, because the adult bone cells have lost the power of proliferation and play no part in the regeneration of bone. Osteoblasts are present both in the periosteum and the surface layer of

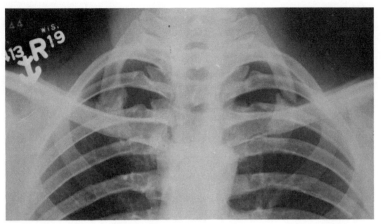

Fig. 5-9. Chronic fatigue fracture of both first ribs. On the right side there is considerable callus and partial union of the fracture in the anterior part of the rib. The fracture involving the left first rib is more recent and there is no callus.

bone, so that repair can occur either with or without the periosteum. The essential function of the periosteum is to supply the outer part of the bone with blood and removal of it or separation of it from bone is apt to be followed by death of this part of the bone. The three major stages of fracture healing are as follows:

1. GRANULATION TISSUE FORMATION. Following fracture, blood and a varying amount of exudate are poured out, between and around the ends of the bone. This clot is invaded by cells and new capillaries and a kind of granulation tissue is produced. The proliferating cells are osteoblasts, derived for the most part from the deep layer of the periosteum. The proliferation of osteoblasts is very rapid.

2. FORMATION OF OSTEOID. After 4 or 5 days the osteoblasts form trabeculae around central spaces that will become Haversian canals. This is osteoid tissue, resembling bone in its structural arrangement but with no calcium salts in its matrix. This osteoid tissue also is known as callus and it becomes increased in amount so that it acts as a splint. It is abundant by the end of the second week.

3. CALCIFICATION. Eventually the osteoid becomes calcified and the ends are knit together by rigid, fully formed bone. Callus forms not only along the external surface of the fracture but directly between the fracture surfaces and internally, filling the marrow cavity.

In the immediate neighborhood of the fracture the bone cells die. Near the fracture the osteogenic cells proliferate and may form cartilage instead of bone. This cartilage formation is most marked when there is movement or separation of the fragments. The new cartilage is invaded and replaced by bone. This is ossification in cartilage as compared with the process just described, which corresponds to ossification in membrane. Changes in the hydrogen ion concentration influence the process. The pH is first acid, favoring decalcification. At the end of a week it changes to the alkaline side with resulting deposition of calcium. About a week later phosphatase is liberated by the osteoblasts; this causes deposition of calcium and phosphorus in the osteoid tissue. If the gap between the fragments is not bridged by osteogenic cells within a certain time, fibroblasts will fill the gap with fibrous tissue, the matrix of which has no special affinity for calcium salts and the result is fibrous union or nonunion.

ROENTGEN EVIDENCE OF BONE UNION

There is a great variation in the rate of healing of fractures and the rapid development of callus as noted in fractures produced in the experimental animal does not always occur in the human. The site of the fracture, the amount of displacement, and the age of the patient are a few of the factors that influence healing. In general, fractures heal at a much more rapid rate in infants and children than they do in adults (Fig. 5-10). There are several aspects of fracture healing noted in the description given in preceding paragraphs that are of interest roentgenologically. The only change in the bones that can be recognized during the first and second stages of repair is the decalcification of bone along the fracture edges. Usually this can be visualized within a week or two in most fractures and because of it, the fracture line may become more prominent than it was immediately after the injury. A hairline frac-

ture that may have been very difficult to visualize initially will usually become more obvious within a week or two. Uncalcified osteoid callus is not visible roentgenologically. If healing progresses normally, this uncalcified callus may be sufficiently solid to prevent motion between the fragments even though roentgenograms fail to show any signs of reformation of bone across the fracture. Failure to visualize calcified callus, therefore, does not necessarily indicate that the fragments are not held together. However, uncalcified osteoid callus is relatively soft and in weight-bearing bones will not allow use of the part; in the nonweight-bearing bones, it may result in bending if support is discontinued. One must wait, therefore, until roentgenograms show calcified callus and, in the weight-bearing bones, this must become

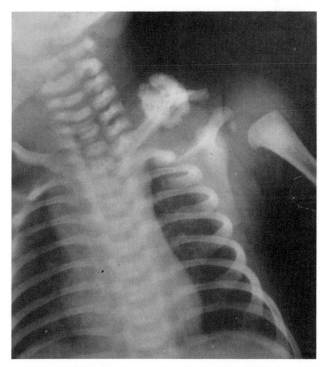

Fig. 5-10. Birth fracture of the left clavicle. The bone was fractured at the time of delivery. This roentgenogram, taken approximately 2 weeks after birth, shows exuberant callus surrounding the fracture in the midportion of the clavicle. In time this callus will be absorbed and there will be little if any residual deformity.

fairly dense and solid before the part can be used (Fig. 5-11).

Satisfactory progress of healing of a fracture is shown in roentgenograms by the following changes.

DECALCIFICATION OF FRAGMENT ENDS

As noted previously, removal of bone along the injured surfaces of the fragments follows the injury within a matter of days. Definite evidence of such removal is sometimes not apparent in roentgenograms, particularly if the fragments are separated or displaced to any appreciable degree. The roentgen demonstration of decalcification of the ends of the frag-

ments, however, is a favorable early sign that healing may take place in a normal manner but its occurrence is no guarantee that bone union will develop.

PERIOSTEAL CALLUS

The most reliable roentgen evidence of beginning bone union is the visualization of calcified periosteal callus. This is seen at first as a faint hazy area of calcium density developing in the tissues adjacent to and directly overlying the borders of the fracture line. When this is sufficient to be visualized as a continuous zone of calcification extending from one fragment to another, it is reliable evidence that solid bone

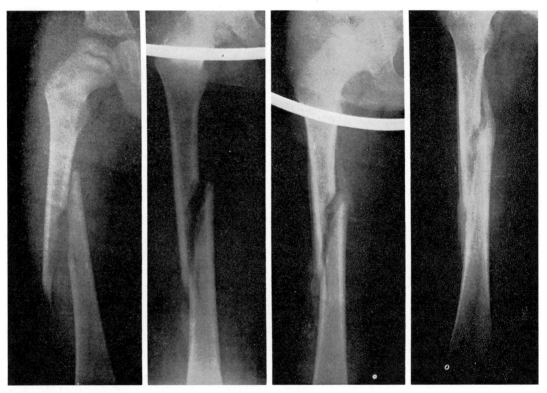

Fig. 5-11. Healing of a spiral fracture of the femur in a child. *Left,* Appearance immediately after injury. *Left center,* Two weeks later hazy periosteal callus is beginning to form around the margins of the fracture. *Right center,* Ten days later the callus is more easily visualized and is beginning to form a solid bridge between the fragments. *Right,* Five weeks later there has been increased solidification of callus, which now forms a solid bridge between the fragments and along the external surfaces representing endosteal and periosteal callus formation. With the passage of time remodeling of the bone will take place and the slight angular deformity will be corrected as growth proceeds. (*Courtesy Dr. Ralph C. Frank, Eau Claire, Wisconsin.*)

union will occur (see Fig. 5-11). With the passage of time, the periosteal callus shadow becomes increased in density and its outer margin more distinct. Eventually the callus becomes as dense as the normal cortex and in time it blends with the cortical margin and no longer remains as a distinct zone of density. The amount of visible periosteal callus varies greatly in different fractures. It is more extensive when there is displacement of fragments than when there has been accurate replacement and a close apposition of fragments. It is more prominent beneath large muscle masses and, in bones that are covered with little or no muscle, periosteal callus will be slight. This is noted in fractures of the phalanges, which often unite with little evidence of periosteal callus. It also is observed in fractures of the tibial shaft where heavy calcified periosteal callus may form along the posterior and outer side of the fracture but with very little over the anterior surface. Fractures occurring through the intracapsular portion of the femoral neck will show no periosteal callus because there is no periosteum covering the bone at this site. Fractures of the skull also do not show periosteal callus because the periosteum does not have osteogenic properties in the bones of the cranial vault.

The amount and character of periosteal callus are satisfactory indicators as to when the part may be removed from traction or casts. Again the site and nature of the fracture must be taken into account. A fracture in an upper extremity that is nonweight-bearing will usually be held firmly enough for some degree of use when roentgenograms show a rather hazy periosteal callus shadow. In the lower extremity, however, such faint calcified callus is not enough and it is usually advisable to withhold any use of the part until the outer margin of the callus shadow has become sharp and continuous across the entire site of fracture. An impacted fracture may not require support as long as one that was not impacted.

While a large amount of periosteal callus may have formed around a fracture in which the fragments were not completely replaced in anatomical relationship, with the passage of time much of this will be absorbed peripherally and, particularly in children, there is a tendency for remodeling of the bone. The callus surrounding shaft fractures in childhood will disappear completely and with growth and remodeling even rather extensive deformity may be completely corrected.

ENDOSTEAL CALLUS

While periosteal callus is forming and calcifying, endosteal callus formation also is taking place. The roentgen visualization of endosteal callus is much less distinct because the early calcified callus is obscured by the bone surrounding it. Thus the fracture line may remain relatively clear even when periosteal callus can be visualized. However, in normal healing the line of fracture eventually becomes hazy and less distinct as calcified callus forms between the ends of the fragments and along the inner surface of the cortex. Eventually the fracture line disappears completely and the dense homogeneous shadow of endosteal callus is gradually replaced by trabecular bone so that a marrow cavity is reformed. In most fractures it is not necessary to wait for roentgen demonstration of recalcification of the fracture line before the part can be used. Occasionally a very accurate replacement of fragments has been accomplished so that even in the immediate postreduction roentgenograms the fracture line can barely be distinguished. In these cases one will find very little periosteal callus developing. Because the fracture line is indistinct from the very beginning, it may be difficult to tell when sufficient endosteal callus has formed to prevent motion. Usually sufficient decalcification will occur along the line of fracture to make it more clearly visible within a few weeks after the injury and the gradual fading of this line and its eventual disappearance are the roentgen indicators of satisfactory healing.

REFORMATION OF TRABECULAR BONE

This is a late manifestation of bony union and represents the end stage of fracture repair.

It indicates that the replacement of calcified callus by true bone has been accomplished. In certain areas, such as in the neck of the femur where there is no periosteal callus formation and where endosteal callus may be difficult to identify, the most certain evidence of bone union is the reformation of trabeculae that can be traced from one fragment to another without loss of continuity. Even in these examples, however, there is as a rule solid enough union before this observation can be made to allow use of the extremity.

EFFECTS OF STRAIN

The demonstration of a lack of motion between fragments in roentgenograms that were made while pressure was being applied in several directions is of considerable value in determining whether there is solid union. This is a useful procedure when routine roentgenograms and the results of clinical examination leave some doubt as to the presence of union. It is important that care be used in applying the pressure so that fresh callus will not be damaged or that precarious and early union be not disrupted.

FURTHER OBSERVATIONS

Fractures occurring through diseased bone often heal surprisingly well. Fracture through a simple bone cyst in a child usually heals promptly and in the course of healing frequently initiates healing of the bone cyst. Even in osteoporotic bone, such as is found in osteogenesis imperfecta, healing may be prompt and often occurs with excessive periosteal callus. Even a fracture occurring through a focus of osteolytic metastatic carcinoma may heal partially with callus in the face of a destructive malignant lesion (see Fig. 5-6). In these cases, of course, union is precarious and as the lesion increases refracture may occur.

Roentgen evidence of healing in fractures of compression type is difficult to evaluate. Because there is no true line of fracture visible initially and because these fractures usually occur in bones where little periosteal callus forms, it is very difficult to establish the progress of healing. This will be considered further in the discussion dealing with vertebral fracture. The healing of

fractures of the cranial bones also will be considered in the section dealing with such fractures.

DELAYED AND NONUNION OF FRACTURES

GENERAL ASPECTS

When the rate of progress of healing of a fracture is slower than is normal for the particular type of fracture under consideration, but with healing eventually occurring, it is spoken of as slow or delayed union. Some of

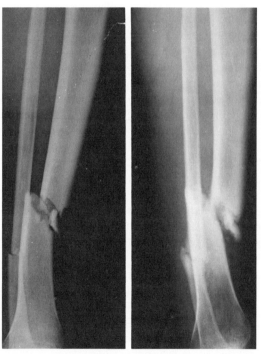

Fig. 5-12. Failure of union of a tibial shaft fracture. *Left,* Lateral view of the leg showing fractures of the tibia and fibula 3 weeks after injury. There is no evidence of callus formation. The fracture in the tibia is comminuted with separation of a fragment along the anterior border. *Right,* Same patient 8 months later. A small amount of periosteal calcification is visible along the ends of the fragments but this does not bridge across and offers no support. There has been no endosteal callus formation. The ends of the fragments have become eburnated. Chronic disuse osteoporosis has become noticeable in the lower ends of the tibia and fibula.

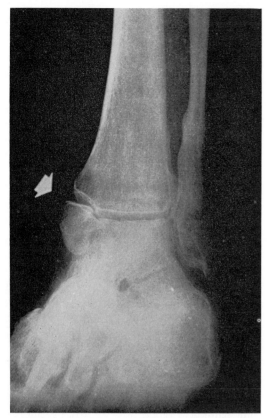

Fig. 5-13. Ununited fracture of the medial malleolus (**arrow**). Anteroposterior view of the ankle. Cortical bone has formed over the fracture surfaces and bony union will not occur without operative intervention. There is a moderate amount of chronic disuse osteoporosis in the bones comprising the ankle joint. There was a fracture of the fibula just above the level of the ankle joint and this has healed solidly with callus leaving only a slight deformity in contour of the bone.

the causes that are operative in production of nonunion of fractures also may be responsible for delay in union but with eventual healing taking place. Fractures unite more slowly in the aged than in younger adults and always heal more slowly in adults than they do in infants and children. The rapidity of callus formation and bone union in fracture occurring during birth is striking. For example, a birth fracture of a clavicle may develop a fusiform area of dense periosteal callus easily visualized in roentgenograms within 5 to 7 days after the injury (see Fig. 5-10). The term "nonunion"

refers to absence of bony union. Some fractures that fail to undergo bony union may unite with fibrous union and in certain areas this may be sufficient for practical purposes. In bone subjected to much use, and particularly in the weight-bearing bones, fibrous union is not adequate (Fig. 5-12). From roentgenograms it is impossible to determine whether solid fibrous union is present or not because the fibrous tissue joining the ends of the bones is relatively nonopaque.

Fractures in certain areas are noted for the frequency with which delayed or nonunion occurs. These include fractures at the junction of the middle and lower thirds of the tibia, the carpal navicular, the central third of the shaft of the humerus, and fractures in the lower third of the ulna.

The causes of nonunion include (*1*) infection, (*2*) distraction of fragments,* (*3*) injury to the blood supply of one or both fragments, (*4*) improper fixation, (*5*) interposition of soft tissues between the fragment ends. Other causes include local bone disease at the site of fracture and, possibly, certain generalized conditions, such as osteomalacia, syringomyelia, and tabes among others.

ROENTGEN OBSERVATIONS

Roentgen evidence of nonunion depends upon the demonstration of one or more of the following changes:

Smoothness of Fragment Ends

A fracture that is not going to unite often shows, as the first evidence, the development of smoothness of the ends of the fragments that formerly were ragged and irregular. This is first noticed along the margins, the sharp corners disappearing and being replaced by rounded borders. Eventually the end of each fragment heals over with cortical bone (Fig. 5-13).

* Distraction refers to a separation or pulling apart of the fragments, leaving a gap between them. It is usually caused by excessive traction.

Abscence of Calcified Periosteal Callus

While visible periosteal callus is not necessary for satisfactory healing of a fracture provided the ends are in close and accurate apposition or when the fracture occurs in an area where the periosteum is absent, such as in the intracapsular portion of the femoral neck, in most fractures some periosteal callus does become visible and its presence is a good indicator that union is commencing. Failure to demonstrate a periosteal callus shadow that is continuous across the external surfaces at the line of fracture should be viewed with suspicion. Not infrequently periosteal spurs form along the margins of both fragments but these do not bridge across the line of fracture; rather an irregular translucent line remains between them, which appears to be an extension of the fracture line. Such periosteal callus is of no value in furnishing support because it does not offer a solid bridge (see Fig. 5-12).

Eburnation of Fragments

The fragment ends may undergo increasing sclerosis and eburnation when bony union fails to take place. The amount of eburnation varies from case to case but often the occurrence of sclerotic density in the fragment ends is the first evidence that bony union will fail to occur. The longer the duration of nonunion, the more eburnated the fragments become. The fracture surfaces also develop a sclerotic appearance relatively early when the fracture has not been properly immobilized.

Motion between the Fragments

When roentgenograms are made with and without the application of pressure, or with pressure applied to one fragment in several directions, if there is lack of bony union, motion can be demonstrated. This is an excellent way to demonstrate absence of union in cases where the clinical examination gives indefinite results. As mentioned in the section "Effects of Strain," care should be exercised when pressure is made in an attempt to elicit

motion so that early callus be not disrupted or that the bone not be refractured.

Pseudarthrosis

Occasionally a false joint is formed between fragments in the presence of nonunion. Usually this occurs as a result of incomplete fixation or with use of the part allowed before union has taken place.

OTHER COMPLICATIONS

DISUSE OSTEOPOROSIS AND SUDECK'S ATROPHY

Simple immobilization of a bone will result in a loss of mineral salts and this is known as disuse osteoporosis (see Fig. 5-12). When there is, additionally, hyperemia, the osteoporosis is intensified at and distal to the level of hyperemia. Occasionally following a fracture and sometimes after relatively minor trauma without fracture there develops a more severe and painful osteoporosis known as Sudeck's atrophy. These conditions also are discussed in Chapter 4 under the heading of osteoporosis (see Fig. 4-2). The roentgen differentiation between a simple disuse osteoporosis and Sudeck's atrophy depends to a large extent upon the severity of the demineralization. Simple disuse osteoporosis seldom causes more than a minimal to moderate degree of increased transparency of the bones that have been immobilized. Often this is more pronounced in the regions of the metaphyses in children, or in adults at the site of the previous epiphyseal plates. This is probably because of increased vascularity of the bone in this region. The demineralization develops gradually and usually can be noticed within several weeks after immobilization. There is a loss in density of the bones which may be uniform or mottled and that will if immobilization is continued develop after a period of time a "ground-glass" type of density. In Sudeck's atrophy, on the other hand, demineralization becomes much more intense and usually is of a patchy or mottled character. It is limited to the bones at and distal to the site of injury and may be a cause of prolonged disability. The cause of Sudeck's atrophy is not completely understood but it apparently represents a combination of disuse osteoporosis, the effects of hyperemia, with an added element of vasomotor disturbance that severely disturbs the normal balance between bone removal and new bone formation.

INFECTION

A compound fracture may become infected. Following surgical procedures for the reduction of fractures infection may develop. The appearances are essentially those of osteomyelitis with the occurrence of periostitis, irregular destruction of bone at the site of infection, and the formation of sequestra. The clinical evidences of infection usually are obvious and roentgenograms serve to establish the extent of involvement and the progress of the disease (see Fig. 6-10).

LATE JOINT CHANGES

When a line of fracture has entered the articular surface of a bone, injury to the articular cartilage results and not infrequently this is followed in time by the development of degenerative changes. This is particularly true in the weight-bearing joints and is seen most frequently in the knee and in the ankle. This condition sometimes is termed "traumatic arthritis" but it represents, essentially, degenerative joint disease that has been initiated by an acute trauma. The reader is referred to Chapter 9, "Diseases of the Joints," for a further consideration of this disease.

FRACTURES OF THE SKULL

The majority of fractures involving the bones of the cranial vault can be identified provided a sufficient number of technically good roentgenograms are obtained. A linear fracture of hairline type may stand out clearly only when the injured area was close to the film

at the time the exposure was made. Such a fine fracture line in a part of the skull at a distance from the film may be completely invisible or nearly so because of the loss of detail that will occur. At times with even the best of technique linear fractures of the cranial vault will escape detection because of the thinness of the fracture line and its failure to be situated in a position where the roentgen beam passes directly through it.

Because many patients with head injuries are in serious condition, clinicians rightfully have stressed that roentgen examination should wait until other necessary emergency care of the patient has been given. The damage to the brain often is more important than the injury to the cranial bones. With some exceptions, and these often are obvious, fractures of the skull may not require immediate surgical treatment. Eventually, however, the individual who has suffered a head injury should have a complete roentgenologic study of the skull. If a fracture exists an effort should be made to determine if there is any depression of bone and the amount of such depression. This is best accomplished by means of tangential views so that the area of fracture is viewed on edge.

TYPES OF SKULL FRACTURE

Linear Fracture

A linear fracture is visualized as a sharp, dark translucent line, often irregular or jagged, and occasionally of branching character (Fig. 5-14). Linear fractures often extend into the base of the skull and their inferior terminations become invisible. A linear fracture must be distinguished from suture lines and vascular grooves. A blood vessel groove usually has a smooth curving course and is not as sharp or distinct as a fracture line. An old fracture of 6 months' duration or longer may resemble a vessel groove very closely and at times it is difficult or impossible to be certain about the nature of such a line. Suture lines generally have serrated edges. Occasionally the sagittal suture will appear as a straight dark line when

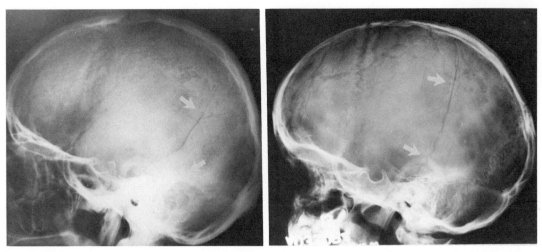

Fig. 5-14. Linear fracture of the skull. Lateral roentgenograms of two patients illustrate the character-istic appearance of a linear fracture. The tendency for branching of the fracture line is shown on the *left.* Compare the sharp translucent line of the fracture (**arrows**) with the appearance of suture lines and blood vessel grooves in the illustration on the *right.* The suture lines are serrated. The blood vessel grooves are wider and less translucent.

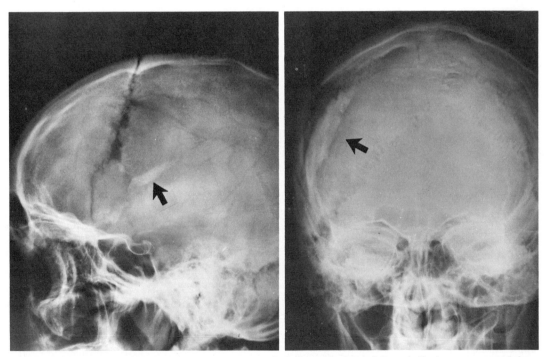

Fig. 5-15. Depressed, comminuted skull fracture. *Left,* Lateral view of the skull shows a ragged frac-ture line more or less following the coronal suture. The fracture branches inferiorly and there is a zone of increased density (**arrow**) indicating an overlap of fragments so that the x-rays have to penetrate a double thickness of bone. *Right,* Posteroanterior view more clearly depicts the extent of the depression and shows a large bone fragment displaced inward at least a centimeter (**arrow**).

viewed end-on in anteroposterior roentgeno-grams. The sutures between the temporal, parietal and occipital bones may also resemble fracture lines. The bilateral and symmetrical nature of the lines and their positions should enable the examiner to recognize them.

Depressed Fracture

After more severe trauma, particularly if the force has been localized to a small area of the skull, one or more fragments of bone may be separated and depressed into the cranial cavity. Such fractures often are stellate with multiple fracture lines radiating outward from a central point and with one or more comminuted pieces present. When viewed *en face* the line of fracture may appear denser than the normal bone because of overlap of fragments, the roentgen rays having to penetrate a double thickness of bone. Tangential views are essential to determine the amount of depression (Figs. 5-15 and 5-16).

Fracture Diastasis

Not infrequently a linear fracture follows a suture along at least a part of its course (Fig. 5-

17). At times the entire fracture follows a suture. Usually there is some spreading of the suture where it is involved by the fracture so that it stands out more clearly than the normal, thus allowing the diagnosis to be made. Occasionally in transverse sutures, such as the coronal or lambdoid, one suture may, normally, appear wider than its mate. This may be caused by a slight tilting of the head from a true anteroposterior plane. The possibility of this normal variant should be kept in mind when fracture diastasis of a suture is a consideration. Even when a fracture does not involve a suture there may be some separation of fracture surfaces from a few millimeters up to a centimeter or even more. This type of fracture is seen most frequently during infancy and childhood and is called a *diastatic fracture.*

Basal Skull Fracture

Fracture limited to the base of the skull may be very difficult to visualize by roentgen examination. While this part of the skull can be shown in suitable projections, the clarity of detail may be poor and the anatomical structures comprising the base add to the difficulty in recognizing fracture lines. Many basal frac-

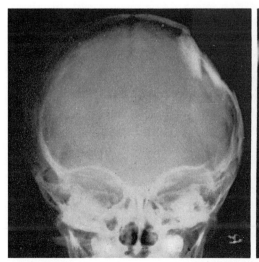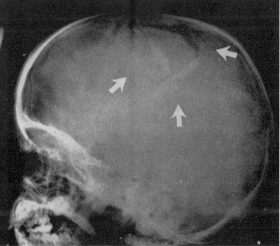

Fig. 5-16. Depressed skull fracture. Posteroanterior and lateral roentgenograms of the skull. The severity of the injury and the degree of depression of the fragments are clearly indicated only when the fracture area is shown tangentially in the illustration on the *left.*

tures will extend into the vault for at least a short distance and a part of the fracture will be visible. The technical procedure of tomography or body-section roentgenography often is useful in identifying a basal skull fracture when routine views fail to show it. Failure to demonstrate a basal skull fracture does not exclude its presence and the clinical signs of such an injury may be more reliable than roentgen examination. A basal skull fracture may extend into the sphenoid sinus. If lateral roentgenograms are made with the patient sitting upright, an air-fluid level may be seen in the sinus. If unable to sit, a lateral view of the skull with a horizontal roentgen ray beam and the film cassette placed alongside the head will demonstrate an air-fluid level if one is present. Clinical signs of injury also must be present, as infection also may cause an air-fluid level in the sinus.

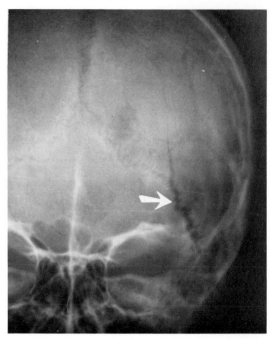

Fig. 5-17. Fracture-diastasis of the skull. The fracture follows the lambdoid suture and then extends into the parietal bone (**arrow**).

HEALING OF SKULL FRACTURES

The time required for the disappearance of a skull fracture is extremely variable. A fracture in a young child usually heals promptly. The fracture line fades gradually and may disappear completely within several months. Fine hairline fractures heal more rapidly than those with a greater separation of surfaces. In older individuals fracture lines tend to remain visible for longer periods of time and in some cases never completely disappear. Usually after several months the sharp edge of bone along the fracture line becomes indistinct. Gradually some recalcification develops with portions of the fracture becoming obliterated. A residual defect may remain more or less permanently as a hazy dark line that is easily mistaken for a vascular groove.

FURTHER OBSERVATIONS

Cerebrocranial Cicatrix. If the dura were torn beneath an area of fracture it may become adherent to the bone along the margins of the fracture and allow the cerebral cortex to come into contact with the bone. An accumulation of cerebrospinal fluid may form in this space and develop into a leptomeningeal cyst. In other instances there are only the adhesions of the cortex and dura to the bone. Either condition predisposes to a gradual erosion of the bone overlying the cyst or cicatrix, apparently caused by the pulsating pressure of the blood vessels along the surface of the cortex. This condition is seen most frequently in infants or young children. It occurs most commonly in the parietal area and following a diastatic type of fracture. The fracture may heal satisfactorily at first but within a few months erosion of bone along the line of fracture becomes apparent (Fig. 5-18). The bone often is destroyed sufficiently for a soft-tissue mass to bulge through the defect and to be obvious to inspection and palpation.

Pneumocephalus. If a fracture has extended through the frontal, ethmoid, or sphenoid sinuses,

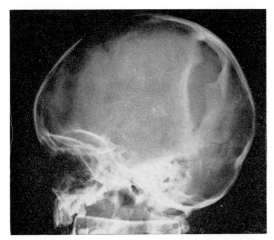

Fig. 5-18. Cerebrocranial cicatrix following fracture in the parietal area. Several months after the injury the child developed a swelling over the region of a previous fracture. At operation the torn dura was found adherent to the margins of the defect. Pulsation of vessels on the surface of the brain in intimate contact with the bone caused the erosion.

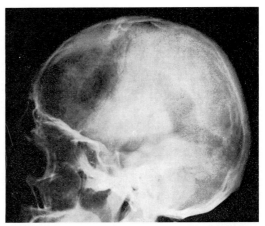

Fig. 5-19. Posttraumatic pneumocephalus. Lateral roentgenogram of the skull following a fracture through the frontal bone that involved the frontal sinuses shows air outlining one of the lateral ventricles. The air is seen as a dark and more translucent zone outlining the lateral ventricle. The roentgenogram was made with the patient recumbent so that only the uppermost ventricle contains gas. The presence of the pneumocephalus indicates that the dura was torn and that air from the frontal sinus has entered the cranial cavity.

or the mastoids, air may enter the skull. If the dura and arachnoid have been torn, the air may find its way into the subarachnoid space and eventually reach the ventricles. This condition is known as posttraumatic pneumocephalus (Fig. 5-19). It is an uncommon but serious complication and can be recognized easily in roentgenograms because of the transparency of the air in contrast to the density of the surrounding brain tissue and cerebrospinal fluid. After a compound-depressed fracture a brain abscess may form at or close to the site of brain injury. If gas-forming organisms are present the abscess may become visible as a gas- and fluid-filled cavity, the gas again offering the contrast needed to demonstrate it.

SUBDURAL AND EPIDURAL HEMATOMA. These conditions have been considered in Chapter 11, to which the reader is referred. A special type of hematoma formation not necessarily associated with fracture is known as *cephalhematoma*. This is found in newborn infants as a result of birth trauma. Usually caused by the application of forceps, injury to the external fibrous tissue covering of the skull is followed by formation of a hematoma beneath it. This forms a localized mass that subsequently undergoes calcification. It is visi-

ble then in roentgenograms as an area of increased density. When viewed tangentially the typical cephalhematoma is visualized as a homogeneous shadow of calcium density showing a sharply demarcated convex outer border, the margins of which merge smoothly with normal bone (Fig. 5-20). The bone beneath the area of calcification usually is normal. With the passage of time, a cephalhematoma tends to undergo gradual decrease in size and may disappear completely if small or at the most leave only an area of slightly thickened bone.

INJURIES INVOLVING THE VERTEBRAE

Any of the vertebrae may be fractured but the most common locations are in the cervical part of the spine and in the mid and lower thoracic regions. The first and occasionally the second lumbar vertebrae also are frequently involved but fractures of the lower lumbar

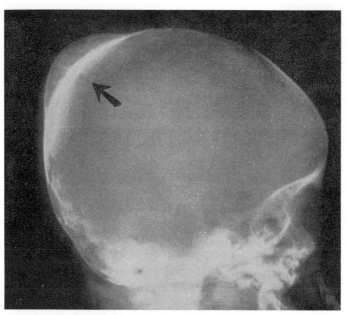

Fig. 5-20. Calcified cephalhematoma following birth trauma. A sub-periosteal hemorrhage occurring during birth has calcified, forming a dense calcified mass over the vertex (**arrow**). In time this will gradually diminish in size and eventually disappear.

bodies are less common unless the bone has been weakened by disease, particularly osteoporosis.

FRACTURES

COMPRESSION FRACTURE

The compression fracture is the most frequent type of injury involving a vertebral body. It is caused by an acute forward flexion of the spine and the damage usually is limited to the upper portion of the vertebral body and particularly to the upper anterior margin. The extent of compression varies, of course, depending upon the severity of the injury, from a very slight infraction of the upper anterior margin to rather extensive and general compression affecting the entire vertebral body (Fig. 5-21). A minor degree of compression is difficult to recognize unless technically good roentgenograms are obtained and such a fracture usually can be seen only in a lateral view. It is visualized then as a slight depression of the upper anterior disc surface coupled with a slight forward bulge of a small portion of the vertebral body along the superior anterior margin. There often is condensation of the bone extending inward from the marginal buckling indicating the compression nature of the injury. The superior disc surface of the affected vertebral body usually is somewhat concave. With a more severe injury the concavity of the disc surface of the vertebra becomes more marked and the loss in height and anterior wedging of the vertebral body is more severe. With the more extensive compression there usually is some loss in height of the vertebral body posteriorly as well as anteriorly although the injury is generally more marked in the anterior aspect because of the lack of bony support at this point. Rather infrequently the injury is limited to the inferior surface of the vertebral body and even less frequently, both surfaces are involved by compressions.

COMMINUTED FRACTURES

With more severe injury one or more vertebral bodies may be extensively crushed and fragmented and there may be associated fractures of the arch or processes (Fig. 5-23). In addition there may be varying degrees of subluxation or dislocation. The term "subluxation" is used to designate displacement that is incomplete, while dislocation is used to indicate a complete displacement of one bone on the other. Subluxations are more frequent in the spine than dislocations (Fig. 5-24). A particularly serious injury is that of a fracture-dislocation involving the odontoid process of

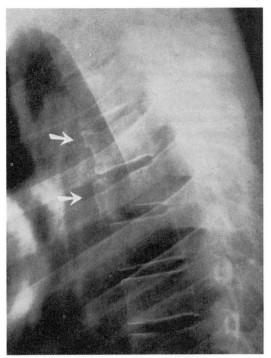

Fig. 5-21. Fractures of the thoracic vertebrae. Lateral roentgenogram of the thoracic spine shows a compression fracture of one vertebra and a comminuted fracture of the vertebra below. The anterior third of the body has been separated and displaced forward. (**Arrows** indicate the fractures.)

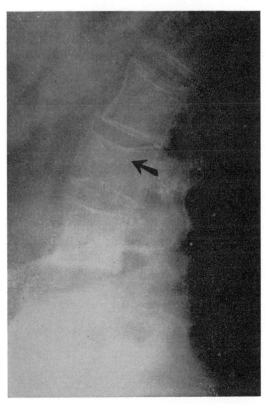

Fig. 5-22. Healed fracture of the third lumbar vertebra. Lateral roentgenogram reveals a moderate loss in height of the body, a concavity of the superior disc surface, and a more localized defect extending into the central part of the body from the superior disc surface (**arrow**). This represents a herniation of disc material into the body and is a posttraumatic type of Schmorl node (see Fig. 3-13).

Because of the damage to the disc surface there is a tendency for expansion of the intervertebral disc at the expense of the softened vertebra that accounts for the usual deformity (Fig. 5-22). The lesser degrees of compression fracture usually show no significant alteration in the spinal curvatures but with a greater degree of compression there may be a definite gibbus deformity. With the more severe injury there often is some bulging of the posterior surface of the vertebral body into the spinal canal and this may be sufficient to produce signs and symptoms of cord compression. In the thoracic region in anteroposterior views one occasionally sees a slight fusiform soft-tissue density adjacent to the fractured vertebral body, which represents a paraspinal hematoma. This seldom is very pronounced and it usually disappears within a short time after the injury.

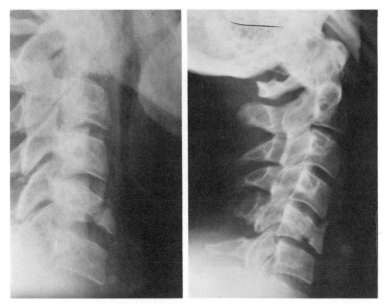

Fig. 5-23. Fracture of the fifth cervical vertebra caused by patient diving into shallow water. *Left,* Lateral roentgenogram of the cervical spine shortly after injury demonstrates fragmentation of the anterior portion of the fifth cervical vertebral body and some compression of it. The upper posterior border bulges into the spinal canal, causing a sharp off-set in the alignment of the posterior surfaces of the vertebrae. *Right,* Same patient 6½ months later and after being in traction. The fragments have united solidly with only small defects on the disc surfaces and a moderate anterior compression. The alignment of the vertebrae is satisfactory for this type of injury.

the second cervical vertebra because of the danger of compression of the upper cervical cord and medulla and the possibility of sudden death. The roentgen diagnosis is established by noting the disturbance in relationship between the odontoid and body of the second cervical.

FRACTURES OF THE VERTEBRAL PROCESSES

These may occur as part of a more severe injury as indicated in the preceding paragraph. Isolated fractures of the vertebral processes are uncommon except in the lumbar region where one or more transverse processes may be fractured. This injury occurs as a result of sudden muscle pull, especially in muscular young men. One must be on guard not to mistake a rudimentary rib attached to the twelfth thoracic

vertebra or to the first lumbar vertebra for a fracture of a transverse process. The margin of the psoas muscle as it crosses the transverse process produces a sharp dark line that may simulate a fracture. Fracture of a spinous process as an isolated injury is infrequent. Normally, a lateral deviation of the spines of some of the vertebrae is common and should not be mistaken for fracture or dislocation. Such deviation often is noted in anteroposterior views of the cervical spine. Isolated fracture of an articular process also is rare.

KÜMMELL'S DISEASE

This is a rare and somewhat equivocal lesion and consists of a gradual compression of a vertebral body developing some time after an injury, there being no evidence of fracture imme-

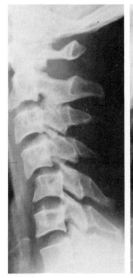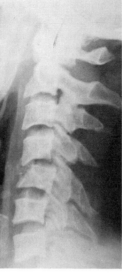

5-24. Subluxation of the fourth on the fifth cervical vertebrae. *Left,* Lateral roentgenogram of cervical spine immediately after injury. *Right,* Same patient 2 months later showing the development of a calcific bridge anteriorly between the vertebrae. This is sufficiently solid so that traction and support can be discontinued. Skeletal traction has failed to reduce the subluxation.

diately after the trauma. It has been considered to be caused by an ischemic necrosis resulting from interference with the blood supply to the vertebra. Some cases probably are actually unrecognized fractures in which no deformity is apparent immediately after the injury but with collapse occurring as a result of continued weight-bearing without support, and it seems likely that most cases of so-called Kümmell's disease belong in this category.

WHIPLASH INJURY

Because of the increased frequency of automobile accidents the whiplash injury of the cervical spine has become of considerable importance. This type of injury follows a sudden deceleration of the body, as when an automobile in which the occupant is riding is stopped suddenly by collision. A similar type of injury may result when a stationary automobile is struck by a moving vehicle from behind, the head being snapped back and then pulled forward rapidly by muscular

contraction. There is a considerable difference of opinion as to the importance of this so-called whiplash injury as a cause for clinical complaints and disability. When a definite compression fracture or subluxation between the lower cervical vertebrae can be identified in roentgenograms, the evidence of injury is obvious. When no fracture exists but with injury to the supporting ligaments, the diagnosis becomes more difficult and it may be impossible to state from roentgen evidence alone if such injury exists or not. Frequently, following a whiplash type of injury, roentgenograms will show a sharp reversal of the normal cerival lordotic curve at the fourth, fifth, or sixth cervical disc level, and at times, a slight forward subluxation of the vertebrae above on the one below the level of gibbus. If lateral views are made with the head in flexion and in extension, the reversed curve may not completely disappear during the maneuver, being increased with flexion and not entirely eliminated with extension of the head. These are suggestive signs of soft tissue injury but they are not specific since a similar type of deformity is seen in association with other lesions that cause cervical muscle spasm. A similar deformity may occur with localized degenerative disease affecting one or more of the mid or lower cervical discs. Minor degrees of reversal of the cervical lordotic curve can be seen in normal individuals. A careful evaluation of the roentgen appearances with a consideration of the age of the patient, the duration of the injury, and the character of the clinical findings and complaints is necessary in cases of this nature.

FRACTURES AND DISLOCATIONS IN SPECIAL AREAS

Most fractures and dislocations are recognized easily in roentgenograms and cause little difficulty in diagnosis. For a detailed analysis of the various types of fractures and dislocations, the mechanical principles involved, the complications, the methods of treatment, and the processes of repair, the reader should consult one of the texts dealing specifically with these problems. Only those features of importance from the standpoint of roentgen examination and diagnosis will be considered in this section.

THE HAND AND THE WRIST

COLLES' FRACTURE

This is the most common fracture in the wrist area and consists of a fracture through the distal 1 inch of the radius. The distal fragment is usually angled backward on the shaft with impaction along the dorsal aspect and with the impaction more severe on the outer side so that the hand tends to be in some degree of radial deviation. There frequently is an associated avulsion fracture of the styloid process of the ulna (Fig. 5-25). There often is comminution along the line of fracture and the distal radial fragment may be considerably fragmented. The injury occurs, as a rule, from a fall on the outstretched hand. The resulting deformity is usually obvious on clinical examination and has been described as a silver fork

or spoon deformity. In reduction of Colles' fracture it is important to reestablish as nearly as possible the normal anatomic relationships. The normal angle formed by the distal radial articular surface with the transverse and longitudinal axes of the bone is shown in the accompanying diagram (Fig. 5-26). Normally the articular surface is tilted anteriorly from the transverse axis of the bone approximately 10 to 15° and it faces toward the ulnar side of the joint approximately 15 to 25° in relation to the longitudinal axis. It is not always possible to reduce a Colles' fracture completely; even when reduction has been complete there is considerable difficulty in some cases in holding the fragments. Maintenance of reduction is favored if the hand is held in palmar flexion and ulnar deviation. A reverse type of Colles' fracture occasionally is encountered but it is rather infrequent; it consists in an anterior dis-

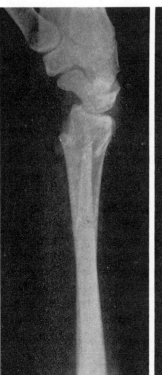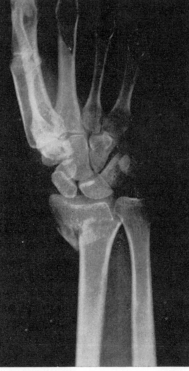

Fig. 5-25. Colles' fracture. A characteristic example of this common injury. There is backward angulation and dorsal and radial impaction of the distal fragment of the radius on the shaft and an avulsion fracture of the styloid process of the ulna. The comminution and impaction results in a typical "silver fork" deformity in the lateral view.

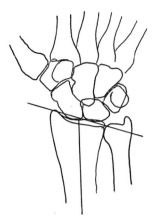

Fig. 5-26. Diagram of an anteroposterior roentgenogram of the wrist showing the usual angle formed by the radial articular surface with the long axis of the bone.

placement and angulation of the distal fragment on the shaft.

FRACTURES OF THE NAVICULAR

Another common fracture in the wrist area is that involving the navicular (scaphoid). This is the most common fracture involving the carpal bones. The fracture usually is transverse in type and occurs through the central part or waist of the bone (Fig. 5-27). Displacement of one fragment on the other may or may not be present. Frequently displacement is slight or absent altogether so that the visualization of the line of fracture may be difficult. Roentgenograms must be of good quality and multiple views may be required. The best projection to demonstrate a fracture through the waist of the navicular is made with the hand and wrist in an oblique position and with the hand placed in as much ulnar deviation as possible. This brings the navicular into profile. Union occurs by endosteal callus only. Nonunion of navicular fractures is common, or at least there is an absence of bony union. Fibrous union, however, may hold the fragments fairly well. After fracture of the navicular the proximal fragment may become avascular because the blood supply of the bone is derived chiefly through the distal portion. Ischemic necrosis of the proximal fragment becomes apparent as disuse osteoporosis develops in the bones around it. They become more transparent as there is a general loss of mineral salts from them while

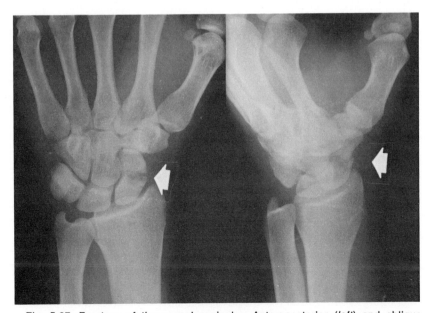

Fig. 5-27. Fracture of the carpal navicular. Anteroposterior (*left*) and oblique (*right*) roentgenograms of the wrist show a fracture through the central part or waist of the navicular (**arrow**). This is the most common site of injury of this bone.

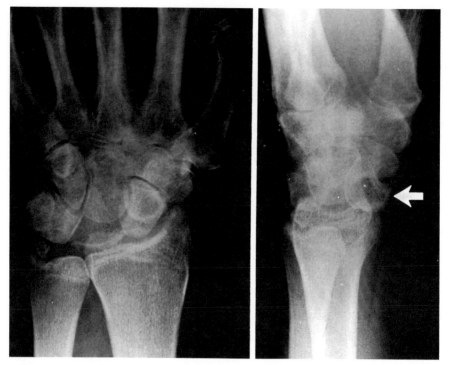

Fig. 5-28. Anterior dislocation of the carpal lunate (**arrow**). In the lateral view (*right*) the bone is seen to be displaced forward and rotated clockwise.

the proximal fragment, having no blood supply, remains of normal density. Thus it stands out as a denser shadow than the viable bone. Subsequently the avascular fragment may undergo compression and fragmentation.

LUNATE AND RETROLUNAR DISLOCATIONS

Dislocations at the wrist joint usually involve the lunate. This bone may be dislocated forward from the radius and from the rest of the carpal bones and the nature of the injury is usually recognized without difficulty in true lateral views of the wrist (Fig. 5-28). Less frequently a retrolunar dislocation of the carpus is seen. In this injury the lunate maintains a normal relationship to the radius but the hand and all the rest of the carpal bones are dislocated backward on the lunate. The nature of this injury is recognized to best advantage only in lateral views of the wrist. There frequently is an associated fracture of the carpal navicular.

BENNETT'S FRACTURE

Of the various fractures involving the metacarpals, one of the important ones is a Bennett's fracture. This consists of a triangular fracture through the proximal end of the first metacarpal with the line of fracture usually entering the articular surface. The triangular fragment consisting of the base of the bone remains in relationship to the multangular bone but the shaft is dislocated outward (Fig. 5-29). Fractures of other metacarpal bones are usually of oblique or spiral type and because of the slanting nature of the fracture line there often is overriding and foreshortening.

ANOMALOUS BONES

In the interpretation of fractures involving the bones of the hand and wrist attention must be paid to the possibility of mistaking an accessory ossification center or ununited epiphysis for a fracture fragment. The various accessory

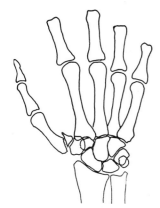

Fig. 5-29. Bennett's fracture of the first metacarpal. Diagram illustrates the characteristic deformity of this fracture.

ossification centers that occur in this region are described in Chapter 3 and the reader is referred to it for further informaton.

THE FOREARM AND ELBOW

MIDSHAFT FRACTURES

When both bones of the forearm are fractured in their midportions a sufficient number of roentgenograms must be obtained so that the width of the interosseous space can be determined. Overriding of fragments is common at either one or both fracture sites and in the presence of overriding or if there is much angular deformity, the fragments of the radius and ulna may come close together. If union occurs with a narrowed interosseous space there will be some limitation of pronation and supination. Occasionally cross union occurs with a bridge of callus forming between the radius and ulna, and when this happens pronation and supination will not be possible.

HEAD OF THE RADIUS

Fracture of the head or neck of the radius is a common lesion and frequently the fracture is of the impacted type. Roentgen evidence may consist only of a slight tilting of the plane of the articular surface of the head in its relation

to the longitudinal axis of the bone plus a slight buckling or sharp angular deformity of the cortical margin of the neck, usually along the outer aspect (Fig. 5-30). With more severe injury the head may be comminuted and there often is a vertical fissurelike cleft extending through the articular surface, separating a small fragment from the outer margin. This may be displaced a variable degree or the line of fracture may be difficult to detect unless the roentgenograms are of good quality. Injury to the ends of the bones forming the elbow joint is accompanied by joint effusion. Normally there is a small accumulation of fat adjacent to the anterior surface of the lower end of the humerus. If the joint capsule is distended by fluid this fat pad will be displaced forward and upward (Fig. 5-31). Recognition of the abnormal position of the fat pad should cause the observer to search carefully for bone injury if it is not readily apparent.[3,6] Occasionally the fat pad cannot be seen in the normal and in emaciated individuals it is not present. There is a similar fat pad along the posterior surface of the humerus but, in the normal, it lies largely within the olecranon fossa and may not be visible in lateral views of the elbow. If the joint capsule is distended by fluid the pad is elevated and displaced posteriorly and then can be visualized. Displaced fat pads are a sign of joint effusion and thus, in addition to trauma, may occur in any disease or condition in which there is synovitis (e.g., rheumatoid arthritis). Dislocation of the head of the radius occurs occasionally, chiefly in infants and children. In the adult, dislocation of the upper end of the radius sometimes occurs along with a fracture in the proximal portion of the ulna. This is known as a Monteggia fracture. The roentgen significance of this lesion lies in the fact that the radial dislocation may be overlooked.

DISLOCATIONS OF THE ELBOW JOINT

Complete dislocations at the elbow joint almost invariably consist in a posterior dislocation of the radius and ulna on the humerus. Frequently small avulsion fractures are present in association with the dislocation or larger

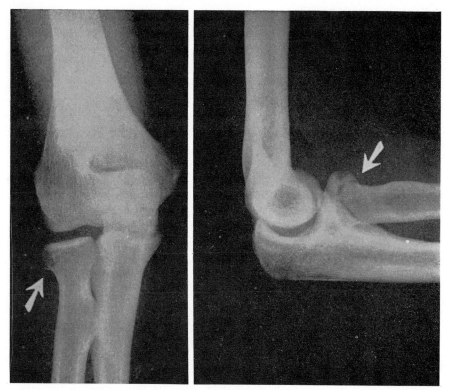

Fig. 5-30. Impacted fracture of the head of the radius. There is a buckling of the cortex on the anterior and lateral sides of the radial head and a slight impaction on the outer side (**arrows**). Note the slight tilting of the plane of the articular surface of the head of the radius in relation to the longitudinal axis in the anteroposterior view (*left*).

fragments may be broken off, particularly of the coronoid process of the ulna. Elbow joint dislocations are often followed by the occurrence of areas of calcification in and around the elbow joint, a posttraumatic myositis ossificans, and this may lead to considerable impairment of function even though anatomic relationships of the bones have been restored.

FRACTURES OF THE ELBOW AREA IN CHILDREN

Because of the numerous ossification centers present in the elbow area during childhood, difficulty in interpretation of fractures is not infrequent. A knowledge of the appearance of the various ossification centers during the developmental period is essential in order to avoid errors. It is always helpful in doubtful cases to obtain roentgenograms of the opposite normal elbow joint and with these available it is usually possible to determine if fracture exists or not (see Fig. 5-2). In the very young infant, when most of the epiphyses at the elbow are still cartilaginous, injuries confined to them may be very difficult to detect until reparative changes develop in the form of periarticular calcification. In these cases, displacement of the fat pads, as noted above, offers a very valuable diagnostic clue at the initial examination.

One of the common fractures of childhood in the elbow region is a supracondylar fracture involving the humerus. This usually is the result of a fall on the outstretched hand with the elbow partially flexed and, typically, there is a

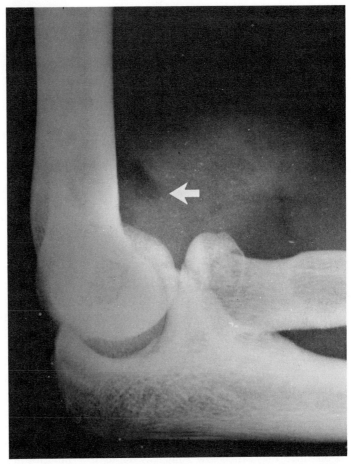

Fig. 5-31. Displacement of anterior fat pad at the elbow (**arrow**) indicates joint effusion secondary to fracture of the head of the radius. Enlarged lateral view of same patient as shown in Figure 5-30.

backward angulation or displacement of the condylar fragments on the humeral shaft. The condyles may be comminuted and the fracture may be of T type with a vertical component extending into the joint separating the condyles. In reduction of fractures involving the lower end of the humerus, an attempt is made to establish a normal carrying angle (Fig. 5-32). This is the angle formed by the longitudinal axis of the forearm in its relationship to the humerus and in the normal is approximately 170° in the male and 160° in the female (the forearm deviating laterally on the arm from 20 to 30°).

THE SHOULDER AREA

DISLOCATIONS

Dislocations at the shoulder are mainly of two types, an anterior and a posterior. In the anterior type, which is much more common, the humerus is displaced forward beneath the coracoid process and anterior to the glenoid of the scapula. It is known as a subcoracoid dislocation (Fig. 5-33). Detection is not difficult in roentgenograms because of the gross distortion of anatomic relationships. Posterior dislocation is much less frequent and more

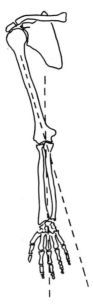

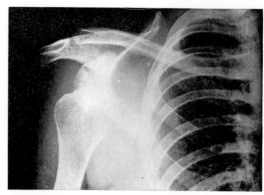

Fig. 5-33. Subcoracoid dislocation of the humerus. The head lies anterior to the glenoid and beneath the coracoid process of the scapula.

Fig. 5-32. Diagram illustrates the method for determining the carrying angle of the elbow joint and the normal angle.

difficult to detect in standard roentgenograms. The humerus is displaced directly backward and in a straight anteroposterior view of the shoulder it may not appear to be in abnormal relationship to the glenoid. Stereoscopic roentgenograms are of value in recognizing this lesion since they will show sufficient depth to establish the fact that the humerus lies posterior to the glenoid. Other views, including a transthoracic projection of the humerus and an axial view in which the film cassette is placed beneath the axilla and the roentgen-ray beam directed downward through the shoulder area, are useful technical procedures to identify this injury.

Approximately 20 per cent of patients with dislocations of the shoulder also have associated fractures. This may consist of an avulsion fracture of the greater tuberosity, a fracture of the neck of the humerus, or an injury to the anterior lip of the glenoid. These should be watched for in any dislocation and roentgenograms always should be obtained after reduction of the dislocation because fractures frequently are more easily seen after normal relationships have been established. In patients

suffering from recurrent dislocations of the shoulder, it is common to observe a groove-like defect on the posterolateral surface of the neck of the humerus directly opposite the lesser tuberosity. This defect is brought out to best advantage when the roentgenogram is made with the arm abducted and internally rotated. There has been some discussion concerning the nature of this defect but it is generally assumed to be the result of an infraction of the bone following previous dislocation with the neck of the humerus having been driven against the anterior margin of the glenoid.

Subluxations or complete dislocations of the acromioclavicular joint are frequent injuries, particularly in athletes, and are caused by a fall on the shoulder. The dislocation may be incomplete and the lesion then is termed a subluxation (Fig. 5-34). When complete, the clavicle is displaced upward on the acromion and the ligaments attaching the clavicle to the coracoid process are ruptured. Incomplete separations may be difficult to detect unless multiple roentgenograms are made with the arm in different positions. Usually a roentgenogram made with the patient sitting or standing and holding a weight in the hand will show subluxation or dislocation if it exists. In evaluating the presence or absence of subluxation, the relationship of the undersurface of the clavicle to that of the acromion is important. The relative thickness of the acromion and clavicle varies in different individuals and the superior borders of these bones cannot be relied upon to indicate normal or abnormal relationships. The inferior surfaces, however, usually lie in the same plane. The width of the acromioclavicular joint space narrows gradually during life and becomes rather thin in the elderly individual because of degenerative changes in the cartilage. As with many other injuries, comparison with the opposite shoulder may be very helpful in determining whether minor deformity exists or not.

FRACTURES OF THE SCAPULA

Fractures of the scapula are not very frequent and are not too difficult to recognize in roentgenograms of the shoulder. There often are multiple fracture lines extending through the bone but healing usually occurs promptly. Unless a fracture extends directly into the glenoid there usually is little residual limitation of motion at the shoulder joint.

FRACTURES OF THE HUMERUS

Fractures of the upper end of the humerus are usually divided into those involving the anatomic neck and those through the surgical neck of the bone. It often is difficult to classify fractures in this area according to this method because many times the fracture involves both the anatomic and the surgical necks. Fractures of the shaft of the humerus are of all varieties and this is one of the areas where delayed union or nonunion is rather common.

FRACTURES OF THE CLAVICLE

Most fractures involving the clavicle occur at the junction of the middle and distal thirds with a downward and forward displacement of the distal fragment on the proximal. Frequently there is separation of one or more comminuted fragments that may come to lie at a right angle to the long axis of the bone. Fracture involving the inner end of the clavicle is very uncommon as is dislocation at the sternoclavicular joint. Fractures occur in the outer end of the clavicle

although they are less common than in the shaft proper. The fractures involving the distal end of the bone are often associated with subluxation of the acromioclavicular joint.

STERNUM AND RIBS

FRACTURES OF THE STERNUM

Demonstration of fracture of the sternum requires technically good roentgenograms, particularly a true lateral projection. Many of these injuries result from automobile accidents, the driver being thrown against the steering wheel column. The fracture may be incomplete with only a slight angular deformity, or it may be complete with separation of the fragments and overriding of them.

FRACTURES OF THE RIBS

Complete fractures of the ribs with some degree of displacement of fragments usually can be identified without difficulty in roentgenograms made to show rib detail. Incomplete or greenstick fractures, occurring during childhood and buckling fractures without displacement are more difficult to recognize. Hairline fractures also occur in the ribs and are very difficult to visualize at times. In some of these patients, reexamination after several weeks will show the presence of cloudy periosteal callus and evidence of a fracture line when none could be clearly identified in roentgenograms made immediately after the injury. Visualization of hairline fractures is facilitated when the exact site of the suspected injury is known at the time the roentgenograms are made so that proper exposures can be obtained.

As a result of repeated and severe coughing spells, one or more fatigue type of fractures may occur in the lower ribs. These usually develop in the axillary arcs of the seventh, eighth, or ninth ribs and may or may not be a cause of pain. They have been discovered in roentgenograms of the chest in patients who have had no complaints referable to the fracture. As with fatigue fractures elsewhere, the line of fracture may be very in-

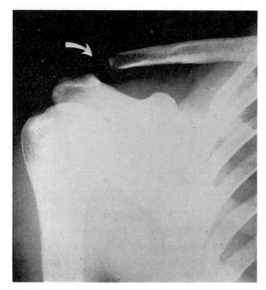 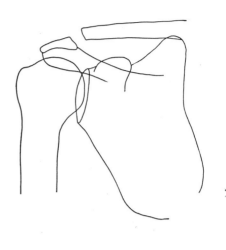

Fig. 5-34. Acromioclavicular separation. Anteroposterior roentgenogram of the shoulder. The acromioclavicular joint space is abnormally wide and the clavicle is displaced upward on the acromion. On the *right* is a line drawing of the roentgenogram shown on the *left.*

distinct at first and only become obvious after several weeks or after periosteal callus begins to form. These are termed "cough fractures."

Fracture in the anterior arc of the the first rib also has been observed as a type of chronic fatigue fracture. As an example this fracture has been found in recruits after long marches carrying heavy packs and is believed to be due to abnormal stresses and strains on the rib with the development of a fatigue fracture very similar to those more commonly found in the metatarsal bones. These have been described earlier in this chapter (see Fig. 5-9).

FRACTURES OF THE PELVIS

Many types of fractures occur in the pelvic bones, depending upon the nature of the injury and the severity of it. The bones most commonly involved are the pubic rami on one or both sides; usually in association with pubic fracture there is a fracture of the sacrum on the same or contralateral side. The deformity of the sacral fracture often is minimal and may be overlooked unless roentgenograms are carefully inspected. Most other pelvic fractures can be identified without difficulty in roentgeno-

grams. In children a green-stick type of fracture is observed and its recognition may be difficult because of the rather minimal deformity that results. The examiner must pay careful attention to the trabecular architecture of the bone and to slight variations in contour of the various portions.

Dislocation of the coccyx on the sacrum is a moderately common injury and can be identified usually without much difficulty in lateral roentgenograms. In some individuals the sacrum is unusually flat and forms a rather sharp angle with the lumbar spine instead of a smooth lordotic curve. In these patients, usually females, the coccyx points directly forward to form a right angle or occasionally even an acute angle with the sacrum. This is developmental and should not be confused with traumatic displacement.

FRACTURES OF THE UPPER END OF THE FEMUR

The various types of fracture affecting the upper end of the femur are shown in the accompanying diagram (Fig. 5-35). Those frac-

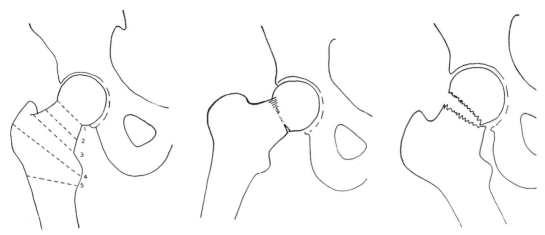

Fig. 5-35. Diagrammatic representations of fractures of the upper part of the femur. *Left,* The usual sites of fracture: **(1)** Subcapital, **(2)** transcervical, **(3)** basocervical, **(4)** intertrochanteric, **(5)** subtrochanteric. *Center,* Abduction fracture illustrates the usual impaction that occurs along the superior part of the fracture in this type of injury. *Right,* Adduction fracture. There is little tendency for impaction in this type, instead the fragments are completely separated.

tures occurring in the subcapital or transcervical area are intracapsular. There is an absence of periosteum in this region so that periosteal callus does not form and union occurs only by endosteal callus formation. Because of this and the poor blood supply in this part of the bone, union often is slow and occasionally nonunion results. Before the advent of modern methods of treatment with fixation devices, nonunion of femoral neck fractures was frequent. It is much less so at the present time. Fractures of the femoral neck may be either of abduction or

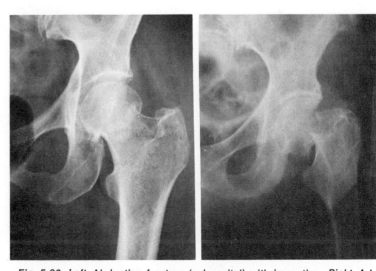

Fig. 5-36. *Left,* Abduction fracture (subcapital) with impaction. *Right,* Adduction fracture (transcervical). The shaft is in a varus position in relation to the head, it is externally rotated, and the fracture surfaces are not in apposition. This is a characteristic example of this type of fracture.

adduction type. The difference is important because abduction fractures frequently are impacted along the superior aspect (see Fig. 5-35). Healing generally occurs without difficulty. Adduction fractures, on the other hand, are almost invariably associated with displacement of fragments. The femur often is held in external rotation so that the fracture surfaces are not in apposition (Fig. 5-36). Fractures through the intertrochanteric area usually heal with bony callus and without delay. Varying degrees of comminution are likely to be present and frequently the lesser trochanter is avulsed as a separate fragment (Fig. 5-37). From the point of view of roentgen diagnosis, femoral neck fractures can be recognized without difficulty, except the minor degrees of abduction-impaction fractures. In such a fracture there may be an absence of a distinct fracture line and the diagnosis depends upon demonstrating an angular deformity between the superior surface of the femoral head and the contiguous neck, some condensation where the bone has been impacted, and a valgus deformity with an increased angle between the neck and head (Fig, 5-36, *left*).

Dislocations of the hip are relatively infrequent lesions and the dislocation is usually a posterior one. It is easily recognized in roentgenograms. As with dislocations affecting other joints, it is important to search for evidence of avulson fractures and it is essential that roentgenograms be obtained after reduction in order to determine the adequacy of reduction and better to demonstrate small avulsion fractures if such be present.

FRACTURES INVOLVING THE KNEE

CONDYLAR FRACTURES OF THE FEMUR

Supracondylar fracture of the femur is a frequent lesion and often there is a vertical fracture associated with the transverse one so that the condyles become separated. It is important to recognize this intra-articular component of the injury. The roentgen diagnosis of these fractures is not difficult (see Fig. 5-3).

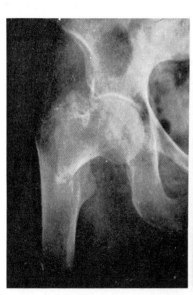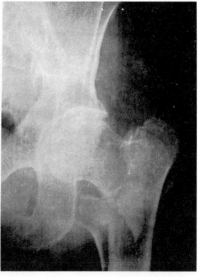

Fig. 5-37. Intertrochanteric fracture of the femur. *Left*, Anteroposterior view showing fracture through the trochanteric portion of the femur with the shaft externally rotated and in moderate adduction on the head and neck. *Right*, Another example of intertrochanteric fracture in which there has been considerably more comminution. The lesser trochanter has been avulsed and fragmented.

UPPER END OF THE TIBIA

Most fractures involving the tibia are demonstrated without difficulty in roentgenograms. Again it is important that any fracture lines extending into the articular surface should be observed and the condition of the articular surface be noted. Fractures of the tibial plateau often result in depression of one of the condyles, leaving an irregular articular surface that predisposes to subsequent development of degenerative joint disease.

As an isolated injury, an avulsion of the tibial spine occurs, particularly in adolescents. It is caused by pull of the anterior cruciate ligament with avulsion of its attachment carrying with it a fragment of the spine. The fragment usually is elevated and rotated.

PATELLA

Most fractures of the patella are transverse and separation of fragments may be severe because of the pull of the quadriceps muscle on the upper fragment (Fig. 5-38). Infrequently the line of fracture is vertical and may be visualized with difficulty unless oblique or tangential views of the bone are obtained. In dealing with injuries to the patella care must be used not to confuse a bipartite or multipartite patella for a corner fracture. This anomaly consists of one or several unfused ossification centers that remain along the upper outer quadrant of the bone. The rounded corners of an anomalous center and the generally smooth cortical borders are in contrast to the irregular edges of a fracture fragment. The condition is bilateral in about 80 per cent of cases.

FRACTURES AND DISLOCATIONS OF THE ANKLE AND FOOT

THE ANKLE

Injuries involving the bones comprising the ankle joint are very frequent and the roentgen diagnosis is made without difficulty in most cases. No attempt will be made here to classify these fractures and dislocations but it may be stated that a wide variety of injuries can occur. The simplest fracture is one involving only the lateral malleolus with or without a slight spreading of the ankle joint mortise (the tibio-

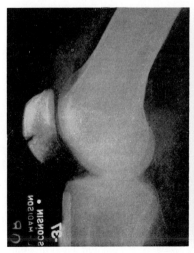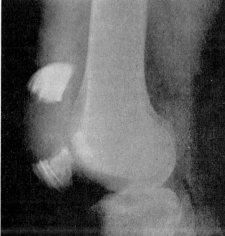

Fig. 5-38. Fracture of the patella. *Left,* Incomplete fracture shown in lateral roentgenogram of the knee joint. *Right,* Complete fracture separating the patella into two fragments. This is the usual type of fracture involving the patella, with a transverse break through the bone and the fragments separated a variable distance because of the pull of the quadriceps muscle.

fibular articulation). More severe injuries lead to fractures of the medial malleolus and the posterior articular process of the tibia; these may or may not be associated with dislocation. When dislocation exists, the foot is usually displaced posteriorly on the leg and the malleolar fragments tend to be carried backward with the foot (Fig. 5-39). As is true in fractures involving other joints, it is important to determine whether fracture lines enter the articular surface; if they do, whether the articular surface has been disrupted to any significant degree. In children, epiphyseal fracture may be difficult to recognize if there has been little or no displacement. As noted under epiphyseal fractures when a line of fracture extends through cartilage and does not affect bone it cannot be visualized readily unless it has caused some displacement of fragments. Usually the fracture does not remain in cartilage throughout its extent but a corner fragment of bone, either of the shaft or of the epiphysis, remains attached to the cartilaginous plate and is displaced along with it. If the fracture is entirely through cartilage, a slight widening of the epiphyseal plate may be apparent. This can be recognized more easily if comparison with the opposite normal foot is available.

THE TARSUS

Fractures of the Os Calcis. For the demonstration of fractures involving the os calcis, an axial view is required in addition to

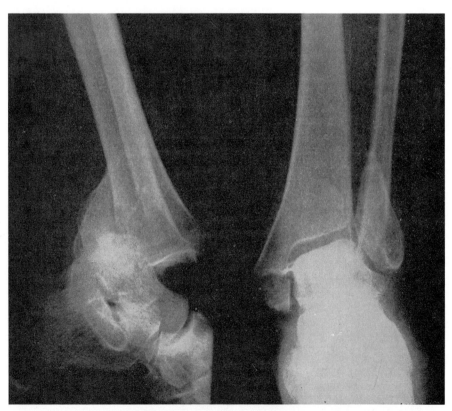

Fig. 5-39. Fracture dislocation of the ankle. This is a common type of injury and these views illustrate the usual deformity. Note that the fractured condyles tend to follow the foot posteriorly. This is frequently described as a trimalleolar fracture dislocation because the posterior process of the tibia is also separated and displaced backward together with the lateral and medial malleoli.

lateral and oblique projections of the bone. The more severe injuries to the bone can be visualized without difficulty because of the crushing and comminution, since most of these occur as a result of a fall from a height with the patient landing on the feet. Slight degrees of compression fracture may be difficult to recognize unless one is completely familiar with the normal appearance of this bone and in some cases it is advisable to compare the injured side with the opposite normal foot. A measurement of value in the examination of fractures of the os calcis consists in determining the tuber-joint angle (Fig. 5-40). This is an angle formed by drawing two lines, one from the anterior superior margin of the bone and the other from the posterior superior margin to the highest point of the articular surface. These lines meet at an angle of 140 to 160° in the normal. The complement to this angle is therefore 20 to 40°. When there is impaction the tuber-joint angle of 20 to 40° is reduced and may become zero or actually reversed (Figs. 5-41 and 5-42). In many fractures involving this bone there is injury to the subastragalar joint surfaces and the later development of a traumatic type of degenerative joint disease.

FRACTURES OF THE ASTRAGALUS. Any part of the astragalus may be involved by fracture and with the more severe injuries there often is accompanying dislocation. A fracture of a long posterior process must be distinguished from an accessory ossicle that occurs in this location, known as the os trigonum. An accessory

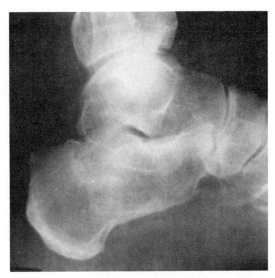

Fig. 5-41. Compression fracture of the os calcis. Lateral view showing loss of the tuber-joint (Boehler's) angle. Compare with normal, Figure 5-42.

ossicle usually has rounded margins, is bounded by cortex around the entire periphery, and is separated from the major part of the bone by a space of uniform width. A fracture of a process, on the other hand, will show irregularity of the margin where the process was separated from the bone, with an absence of cortex at this site, the soft tissues will be swollen around the area of fracture, and the fragment may be definitely displaced away from the bone.

Fractures through the neck of the astragalus are usually of vertical type occurring along the anterior part of its tibial articular surface. Fractures of this type often are followed by an ischemic necrosis of one or both fragments and the development of this complication should be watched for in serial roentgenograms (see Chapter 8).

FLAKE FRACTURES. In association with severe sprains of the ankle area, avulsion of one or more small flakes of cortical bone often occur where a ligament or tendon was attached and partially or completely separated as a result of the injury. The demonstration of such small

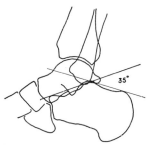

Fig. 5-40. The tuber-joint angle of the calcaneus. Diagram illustrates the method for determining this angle, sometimes called Boehler's angle.

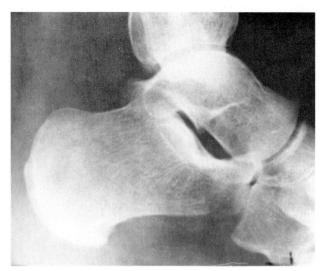

Fig. 5-42. Lateral view of normal os calcis. Compare with Figure 5-41.

cortical flake fractures merely indicates the severity of the soft tissue injury.

FRACTURES OF THE METATARSALS

THE FIFTH METATARSAL. Fractures involving the proximal end of this bone are frequent, usually following an inversion injury to the foot. Characteristically the fracture line extends transversely across the proximal end of the bone with separation of a triangular fragment (Fig. 5-43). This fracture must not be confused with a normal epiphysis that occurs at the proximal end of this metatarsal, appear-

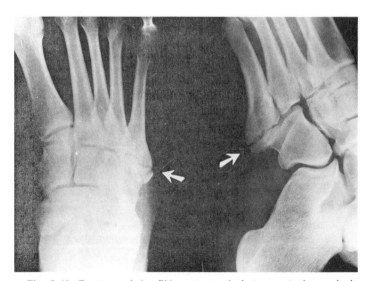

Fig. 5-43. Fracture of the fifth metatarsal. Anteroposterior and oblique roentgenograms of the tarsus demonstrate a transverse fracture through the proximal end of the bone (**arrows**). There is no significant displacement. This is a common injury resulting from inversion of the foot.

ing during adolescence and uniting within a few years. The epiphysis for this bone occurs on the outer side and the long axis of the epiphyseal center lies in the direction of the long axis of the bone. A familiarity with the appearance of this normal epiphysis will aid in preventing error in diagnosis.

FATIGUE FRACTURES OF THE METATARSALS. Chronic insufficiency or fatigue fractures of the metatarsals have been discussed under the heading "Chronic Stress or Fatigue Fracture."

THE BATTERED CHILD SYNDROME

In roentgenograms of the skeletons of infants one occasionally finds bizarre changes that appear to be the result of trauma. These changes may be discovered while examining the infant for some totally unrelated condition and a history of injury may be unobtainable from the parents. In some cases this may be a deliberate misrepresentation; in other cases the low mentality of the parents may account for it. In still others the traumatic episode may not have been noticed by other members of the family. The possibility of deliberate mistreatment of the infant by a psychotic or an alcoholic parent must be borne in mind. The condition has come to be known as the "battered child syndrome."

The infant skeleton responds to trauma more easily and with greater rapidity than the older child or the adult. The lesions vary considerably in their roentgen appearances. There may be separation of one or more small fragments from the corner of a metaphysis. Characteristically the metaphyseal margin of one or more bones may show an irregular or serrated appearance probably representing the effects of previous metaphyseal infractions. Skull fractures may be found in some of these patients and subdural hematoma may be one of the complications. Subluxation of one or more of the epiphyses, extensive subperiosteal calcification, or even a frank shaft fracture showing evidence of callus may all be present in the individual case. Typically, the lesions are likely to be found in multiple bones although there is no particular symmetry to the distribution and they vary a great deal in severity from one area to another. Among the conditions that must be considered in differential diagnosis are infantile scurvy, infan-

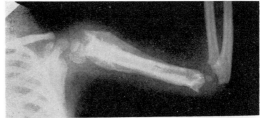
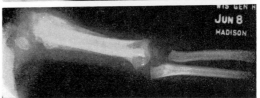

Fig. 5-44. Posttraumatic changes discovered in an infant without a clear history of antecedent injury. While the type of periosteal calcification is not diagnostic of trauma, there is a definite subluxation of the proximal epiphysis of the humerus (the epiphysis is ossifying from two centers). The irregular contour of the distal metaphysis of the humerus probably has resulted from previous infractions. Several other bones in other extremities reveal similar changes. Subsequent investigation revealed that the child had been mistreated by the parents.

tile cortical hyperostosis, osteomyelitis, and bone neoplasms. The proper diagnosis, in the absence of a history of injury, depends upon the irregular distribution of the lesions in the skeleton, the normal density and texture of the bones otherwise, the lack of clinical signs of infection or of other serious disease, the evidence of fragmentation, especially along the metaphyseal borders, and the presence of epiphyseal separations (Fig. 5-44). In some cases the final diagnosis will depend upon the observation of prompt spontaneous regression and eventual healing.

CONGENITAL INDIFFERENCE TO PAIN

This is a rare disorder characterized by a congenital insensitivity to pain. The skeletal lesions are a reflection of this and consist in gross fractures or healing fractures, various forms of osteochondrosis or ischemic necrosis apparently owing to repeated minor traumata, and osteomyelitis in its various phases. In some cases the roentgen evidence of trauma is similar to that noted in the preceding paragraph, with metaphyseal in-

fractions or "corner" fractures and reactive periosteal calcification. The inflammatory lesions are
usually those of an infection of low virulence, with
abscess formation. Necrosis of the distal phalanges
has been reported, evidently the result of persistent cutaneous infections of the fingers. Other
lesions that have been described include hydrar-
throsis and subluxations.

REFERENCES AND SELECTED READINGS

1. BLICKENSTAFF, L. D., and MORRIS, J. M.: Fatigue
   fractures of the femoral neck. *J. Bone Joint Surg.
   48-A:* 1031, 1966.

2. BLOUNT, W. P.: *Fractures in Children.* Baltimore,
   Md., Williams & Wilkins, 1954.

3. BOHRERS, S. P.: The fat-pad sign following elbow
   trauma. Its usefulness and reliability in suspecting
   "invisible" fractures. *Clin. Radiol. 21:* 90, 1970.

4. BOYD, W.: *A Text-Book of Pathology.* Philadelphia, Lea & Febiger, 1953.

5. KEMPE, C. H., SILVERMAN, F. N., STEELE, B. F.,
   DROEGEMULLER, W., and SILVER, H. K.: The bat-
   tered-child syndrome. *JAMA 181:* 17, 1962.

6. KOHN, A. M.: Soft tissue alterations in elbow
   trauma. *Am. J. Roentgenol. Radium Ther. Nucl.
   Med. 82:* 867, 1959.

7. LEVITIN, J., and COLLOFF, B.: *Roentgen Interpretation of Fractures and Dislocations.* Springfield,
   Ill., Thomas, 1956.

8. SALNER, N. P., and PENDERGRASS, E. P.: Roentgenologic considerations in fractures of the neck
   of the femur. A review of pertinent aspects of
   diagnosis and treatment. *Am. J. Roentgenol.
   Radium Ther. Nucl. Med. 67:* 732, 1952.

9. SANDELL, L. J.: Congenital indifference to pain.
   J. Fac. Radiol. 9: 50, 1958.

10. SIEGELMAN, S. S., HEIMANN, W. G., and MANIN,
    M. C.: Congenital indifference to pain. *Am. J.
    Roentgenol. Radium Ther. Nucl. Med. 97:* 242,
    1966.

11. SILVERMAN, F. N.: The roentgen manifestations
    of unrecognized skeletal trauma in infants. *Am. J.
    Roentgenol. Radium Ther. Nucl. Med. 69:* 413,
    1953.

12. WILSON, E. S., JR., and KATZ, F. N.: Stress frac-
    ture. An analysis of 250 consecutive cases. *Radi-
    ology 92:* 481, 1969.

13. WINFIELD, A. C., and DENNIS, J. M.: Stress frac-
    tures of the calcaneus. *Radiology 72:* 415, 1959.

6

INFLAMMATIONS AND INFECTIONS OF BONE

OSTEOMYELITIS

Osteomyelitis caused by pyogenic organisms may affect any bone at any age period. In the young it is usually the result of a hematogenous infection while in adults it is more often secondary to compound fractures, penetrating wounds, or surgical procedures such as the open reduction of fractures. While a variety of organisms can cause the disease, the most frequent is *Staphylococcus aureus*. Since the advent of antibiotics and chemotherapy, osteomyelitis has become a much less serious disease than it formerly was. The incidence of osteomyelitis also has decreased considerably. One of the reasons for this probably is the early treatment with antibiotics of lesions that may cause hematogenous osteomyelitis such as boils, carbuncles, and other localized infections. Frequently the lesion is brought under control at an early stage and roentgen findings may be minimal. However, cases of osteomyelitis, particularly in infants or children, are again being seen, although much less frequently than before, apparently owing to the development of resistant strains of organisms. In most cases the infection is aborted before much damage to bone has developed. Occasionally a small abscess cavity will remain, sometimes containing a sequestrum, indicating the amount of bone that was damaged by the initial assault of the infecting organisms. In any individual case the lesions may be single or multiple. In the child where hematogenous infection is the rule, multiple foci of disease are relatively frequent. Hematogenous foci show a great tendency to develop in or near the metaphysis. The infection often is limited by the epiphyseal plate, but not necessarily so; it may extend through the plate or around the epiphysis into the adjacent joint and cause a pyogenic arthritis (Fig. 6-1).

Chronic osteomyelitis, or chronic bone abscess, is one of the common manifestations of the *neutrophil dysfunction syndromes,* also referred to as *chronic granulomatous disease,* wherein the neutrophils are unable to digest the bacteria which they have ingested.[20] The bone infection in this disease differs somewhat from ordinary osteomyelitis. The causative organisms are usually of low virulence with little soft-tissue swelling or erythema. The most frequent sites of involvement are the small bones of the hands and feet. The course is one of an indolent infection. Later there may be extensive destruction but with the bone eventually returning to a normal appearance. Sequestrum formation is uncommon.

The types of osteomyelitis are: (*1*) acute osteomyelitis, (*2*) chronic osteomyelitis, (*3*) bone abscess (acute, chronic, and Brodie's abscess), and (*4*) Garre's sclerosing osteitis.

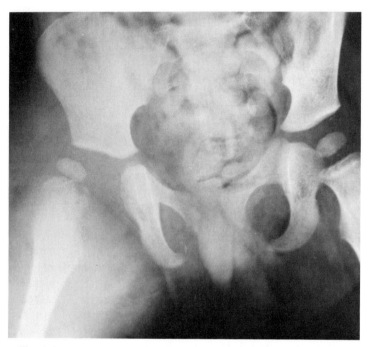

Fig. 6-1. Acute osteomyelitis of the proximal metaphysis of the femur with secondary involvement of the joint. There is irregular loss of bone substance along the inner margin of the metaphysis indicative of osteomyelitis. The femur is displaced laterally out of the acetabulum because of distention of the joint by fluid. There is generalized soft-tissue swelling in the upper thigh and hip region.

ACUTE OSTEOMYELITIS

Normally there is a latent period of a week to 10 days between the time of onset of clinical symptoms of acute osteomyelitis and the development of definite roentgen changes in the bone. Because it is essential that adequate therapy be instituted as early as possible, one should not wait for the development of roentgen signs of bone disease in the presence of an acute virulent infection before instituting treatment.

The first roentgen evidence of the disease is a swelling of the soft tissues. Characteristically this is deep and adjacent to the bone and may be localized or extensive (Figs. 6-2 and 6-3). The early swelling is recognized because of displacement or obliteration of the normal fat planes adjacent to and between the deep muscle bundles.[4] At first the superficial fatty layer is unaffected but its outline soon disappears as the inflammatory reaction spreads. With skin infections, in contrast, the early swelling is superficial and usually a massive deep edema does not develop. The first evidence of disease in the bone usually is an area of indefinite rarefaction in the metaphysis. This is difficult to visualize unless the roentgenograms are of excellent quality (Fig. 6-4). The rarefaction of the bone has a fine granular or slightly mottled appearance. The area of involvement is poorly defined. Associated with this or occasionally preceding it, there will be noted a slight amount of periosteal calcification

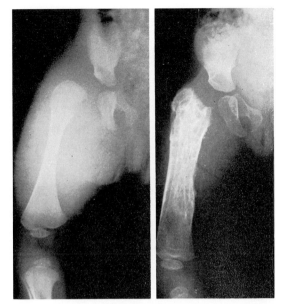

Fig. 6-2. Acute osteomyelitis of the proximal end of the femur in an infant. *Left,* Appearance 7 days after the onset of fever and swelling in the thigh. There is a slight amount of destruction of the inner cortex of the upper end of the right femur, a generalized swelling of soft tissues in the thigh, and lateral subluxation of the femur in relationship to the acetabulum. Serial roentgenograms showed a rapid progression of the lesion in spite of treatment with antibiotics. *Right,* Appearance 3 months later after the infection had been brought under control. Extensive periosteal calcification has formed surrounding most of the shaft of the femur. This involucrum forms the main support. The remnants of the old femoral shaft can be visualized faintly through the density of the involucrum that in time will replace the cortex with new cortical bone. Several irregular cavities can be visualized in the proximal end of the femur representing residues of abscess formation.

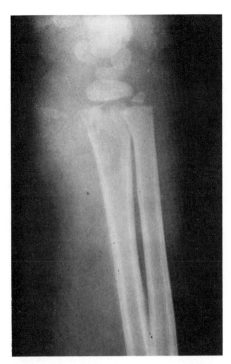

Fig. 6-3. Acute osteomyelitis in the distal end of the radial shaft. Bone destruction in the metaphysis is minimal but there is extensive and deep swelling of soft tissues.

ently normal bone (Fig. 6-8). The periosteal calcification becomes more pronounced and the shaft at the site of the disease may be surrounded by a shell of calcification, known as the involucrum. Unless treated, the disease gradually progresses into the chronic stage.

laid down along the outer side of the cortex and paralleling it (Figs. 6-5, 6-6, and 6-7); swelling of the soft tissues around the involved area can be visualized. The limits of the bone lesion remain poorly defined throughout much of the acute stage and during the early course of the disease the extent of involvement appears much less than it actually is.

Within a short time bone destruction becomes more prominent and this causes a ragged, moth-eaten appearance with foci of destruction intermingled with areas of appar-

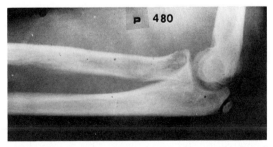

Fig. 6-4. Acute osteomyelitis of the proximal end of the radius. There is a small area of bone destruction in the head and neck of the radius with extensive swelling of soft tissues. Periosteal calcification is minimal.

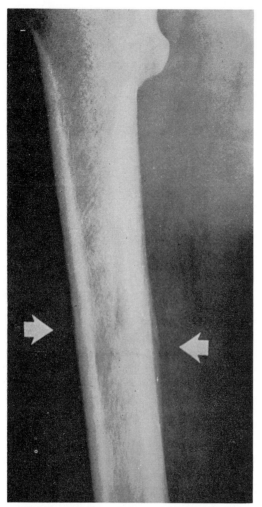

Fig. 6-5. Acute osteomyelitis of the midportion of the femur of an adult. Roentgenogram taken approximately a week after the onset of symptoms shows a slight irregular demineralization of the bone and a small amount of periosteal calcification along the inner side of the area of involvement (**arrows**).

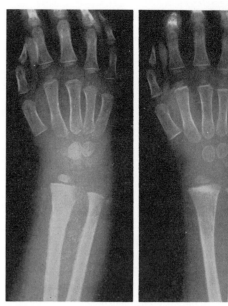

Fig. 6-6. Acute osteomyelitis of the distal end of the radius of a child. *Left,* Appearance several weeks after the onset of symptoms showing ragged loss of bone substance along the inner margin of the radial metaphysis with a diffuse swelling of soft tissues in the wrist and distal part of the forearm. *Right,* Two months later after antibiotic therapy and drainage of superficial abscess in the wrist area. There has been recalcification of the radial metaphysis and return of the bone to nearly normal appearance.

CHRONIC OSTEOMYELITIS

Chronic osteomyelitis is a continuation of the acute stage, there being no sharp line of demarcation between them. The patchy bone destruction becomes more pronounced but the limits of the lesion still remain poorly defined. In untreated cases the infection may extend to involve the entire shaft, the involucrum forming the main support (Fig. 6-2).

Pieces of cortex die and become sequestra. These are evident in the roentgenogram as areas of dense bone surrounded by zones of rarefaction. Because the sequestrum usually has lost its blood supply early in the course of the disease from vascular thrombosis and infarction it remains as dense as normal bone, standing out clearly from the demineralized bone around it (Fig. 6-9). Sequestra usually lie within abscess cavities (Fig. 6-10).

The end result of a chronic osteomyelitis after the infection has subsided is a thickened bone with a sclerotic-appearing cortex and a wavy outer margin. The cortex may become so dense and thickened that the medullary cavity

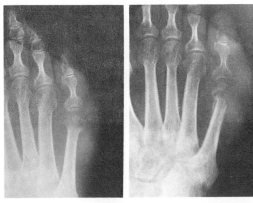

Fig. 6-7. Acute osteomyelitis of the fifth metatarsal. *Left,* There is swelling of soft tissues around the distal end of the fifth metatarsal and involving the toe. The head of the metatarsal shows a slight loss of density. *Right,* Appearance 18 days later. There now is well-defined destruction of the head and neck of the metatarsal and a hazy shadow of periosteal calcification extending proximally into the midportion of the shaft. Soft-tissue swelling has increased. There is a little periosteal calcification forming around the shaft of the proximal phalanx of the little toe.

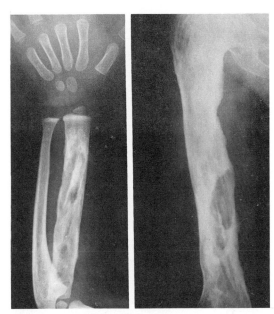

Fig. 6-9. Chronic osteomyelitis. *Left,* Chronic osteomyelitis of the radius of a child. The entire bone has been involved. There are irregular cavities representing chronic abscesses with one large sequestrum lying within a cavity in the lower part of the shaft. The general thickening of the bone is the result of chronic periostitis and the original cortex has been completely replaced (see Fig. 6-2). *Right,* Chronic osteomyelitis of the femur of an adult. The infection is of long duration and the bone is irregularly thickened and sclerotic. A large irregular abscess cavity occupies the lower part of the shaft and within it several linear sequestra can be visualized.

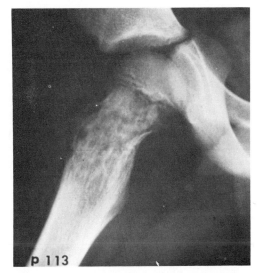

Fig. 6-8. Acute osteomyelitis involving the metaphysis and proximal shaft of the femur of a child. The patchy destruction is characteristic.

may not be apparent. Areas of defect where sequestra have been absorbed or removed surgically add to the general deformity of outline. If the infection becomes reactivated, and this is common, it is shown by the recurrence of deep soft-tissue swelling, by areas of hazy periosteal calcification, and by the development of relatively sharply outlined cavities within the bone representing abscess formation. It often is impossible to determine with any certainty by roentgen examination whether active infection is or is not present in an old osteomyelitis because of the irregular density and the marked sclerosis that may hide even large abscess cav-

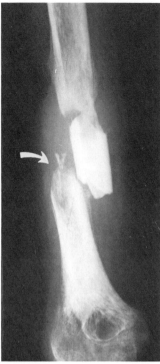

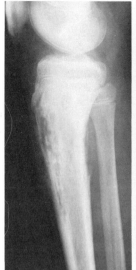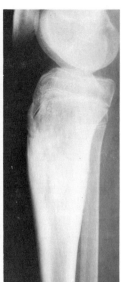

Fig. 6-11. Osteomyelitis of the upper end of the tibia of a child. *Left,* During the acute phase of the disease the bone is irregularly rarefied and there are several linear sequestra forming along the anterior margin of the region of involvement. *Right,* Same patient after the infection has been brought under control. There is localized thickening of the bone from previous periostitis and an irregular sclerosis throughout the area of former involvement. It is always difficult to determine if there are any residual abscesses or sequestra within dense bone of this nature. In this patient there was subsequent reactivation of the infection and the development of an abscess with sequestra.

Fig. 6-10. Infected fracture of the humerus. The bone was fractured in two places and the fracture was compound. Infection developed and the central fragment, having no blood supply, remained of normal density while the proximal and distal fragments have undergone osteoporosis. There are several irregular sequestra in the proximal end of the distal fragment (**arrow**). Periosteal calcification is seen around the ends of the fragments but it does not form a bridge of callus.

ities (Fig. 6-11). It is in these cases that tomography or body-section roentgenography is useful to visualize the interior of the bone to better advantage.

ACUTE BONE ABSCESS

The initial roentgen signs of an acute bone abscess are very similar to those of an acute osteomyelitis. Instead of the lesion extending to involve large areas of bone, it remains localized. The area of destruction becomes walled off by a zone of sclerosis and the lesion gradu-

ally becomes a chronic bone abscess. Acute bone abscess is a more frequent lesion than diffuse osteomyelitis because of the effect of penicillin and the other antibiotics in bringing the infection under control early in its course. The amount of bone destroyed will depend in large measure upon the time interval between the initial involvement by the infecting organisms and the onset of adequate therapy.

CHRONIC BONE ABSCESS

Chronic abscess may develop because the infecting organisms are of low virulence or it may be the continuation of acute abscess that has subsided into a chronic stage. It is characterized by a sharply outlined area of rarefaction of variable size, though often small, surrounded by an irregular zone of dense sclerosis (see Figs. 6-12 and 6-13). Frequently one or more sequestra will be seen lying within the cavity and a dense shell of periosteal calcification often is present surrounding the region of the abscess.

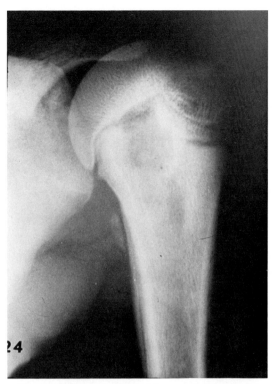

Fig. 6-13. Bone abscess of the proximal end of the humeral shaft. The cavity of the abscess is surrounded by considerable sclerosis. Periosteal calcification extends well down the shaft and away from the area of the abscess.

BRODIE'S ABSCESS

This term has been used to indicate a form of chronic bone abscess of low virulence that has never gone through an acute stage. While such chronic bone abscesses do occur, it is probable that many of the lesions so diagnosed in the past were actually examples of the tumor known as osteoid-osteoma (see Chapter 7). The symptoms may be similar, with intermittent episodes of pain and with little in the way of constitutional reaction. From the standpoint of treatment and prognosis it makes little difference since both lesions can be cured by curettage or local excision.

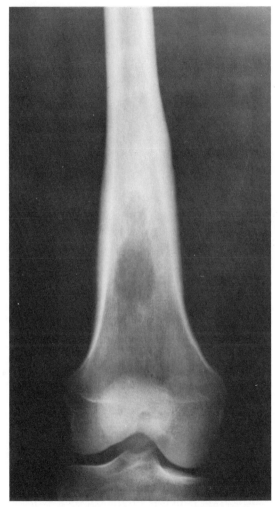

Fig. 6-12. Chronic bone abscess of distal end of femur. The abscess cavity is seen as a well-demarcated area of rarefaction surrounded by sclerotic bone. There is cortical thickening from old periostitis.

GARRE'S SCLEROSING OSTEITIS

As originally described by Garre, this was a peculiar type of osteomyelitis which, after an acute

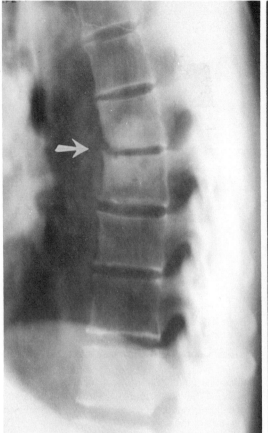

A

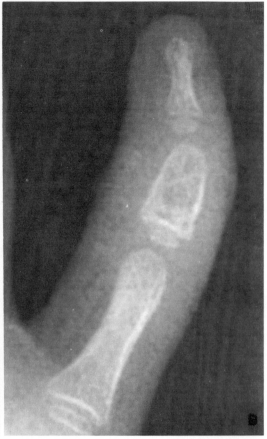

B

Fig. 6-14. *A*, Vertebral osteomyelitis. Lateral tomogram of the thoracic spine. There is erosion of the anterior inferior edge of one body (**arrow**) with considerable sclerosis. The intervertebral disc is narrowed slightly. *B*, Tuberculous dactylitis in a child. The middle phalanx is involved with irregular destruction of the trabecular bone and expansion of the shaft. There is no periosteal calcification.

and virulent onset, subsided without drainage or the formation of sequestra, leaving only a thickened, sclerotic bone. With the passage of time this term has come to be used for a chronic infection of bone of low virulence developing insidiously and leading only to a sclerotic reaction without any bone destruction or sequestration. Such a type of infection of bone is relatively rare and many lesions so diagnosed initially often turn out to be something else. If other entities can be excluded the disease may be termed *chronic sclerosing osteitis.*

OSTEOMYELITIS IN SPECIAL AREAS

FLAT BONES (SKULL, PELVIS). Osteomyelitis of the flat bones is characterized by a patchy type of destruction without sharp demarcation.

In the skull periosteal reaction is absent but a certain amount of sclerosis may be present. In the pelvis periostitis occurs but the periosteal calcification is not as prominent as it is in the long bones. Sequestra form as in other bones and they show the same roentgen appearance.

VERTEBRAE. In pyogenic osteomyelitis of the vertebrae the roentgen changes often are slow in developing and the process may be chronic. The earliest roentgen change usually consists of a roughening or erosion of one surface of a vertebral body, most often along an intervertebral disc surface (Fig. 6-14-A). The sharp cortical outline becomes lost and the edge of the bone has a frayed appearance. Narrowing of an intervertebral disc space is another relatively early finding and sometimes is the first manifestation of the disease. There appears to be a tendency for vertebral osteomyelitis to develop close to the intervertebral disc and, in some cases, the infection may be primary in the disc. In any event spread to the contiguous vertebra is usual. If the disease progresses one or several bodies may develop a moth-eaten type of destruction with intermixed sclerosis. Periosteal reaction occurs fairly early in the disease and is seen as periosteal spurs along the disc edges of the vertebra or along the margins of the body. This reactive change, together with the sclerosis within the vertebral body, is of help in differentiating chronic pyogenic osteomyelitis from tuberculosis. The latter infection is characterized by its destructive nature, with little in the way of sclerotic reaction or periosteal calcification.

NONSPECIFIC SPONDYLITIS. The etiology of this disease is not definitely known but many investigators believe that it is a very low-grade inflammatory process which involves an intervertebral disc and the contiguous surfaces of the adjacent vertebrae. Cultures usually have been sterile and organisms not seen on direct smear although scattered inflammatory cells have been found. Also clinical signs of infection may be absent. The disease occurs both in children and adults and often no precipitating cause is evident. In some patients there has been a history of preceding mild trauma or infection 3 or 4 weeks before the onset of back pain. Roentgen findings resemble those described under Vertebral Osteomyelitis with thinning of an intervertebral disc space followed some weeks later by erosion of the disc surfaces of the adjacent vertebral bodies. In turn this is followed by a dense sclerotic re-action which may involve much of the vertebral body. The disease is self limited and after 3 or 4 months healing usually has taken place with remineralization of the eroded vertebra. Some thinning of the disc may persist although with mild involvement it may return to normal thickness. It seems likely that this disease is similar to the one which develops after lumbar disc surgery or lumbar spinal puncture.

A similar disease is seen infrequently in children and which has been called *juvenile spondylarthritis* or *discitis*. Some investigators believe that it is a distinct entity and while simulating the roentgen changes noted above is not caused by an infection. Alexander[1] considers trauma to be the initiating factor with disruption of the vertebral epiphyseal cartilaginous plate leading to disc thinning and vertebral erosion.

DIFFERENTIAL DIAGNOSIS

BENIGN BONE TUMORS. These lesions, when they arise in the medullary canal, are very likely to cause expansion of the bone with thinning of the cortex. There is no periostitis or sequestration. A great many benign tumors are asymptomatic until fracture occurs through them. A significant exception is the osteoid-osteoma as noted above. Giant cell tumor also is a symptomatic lesion with the occurrence of pain and dysfunction early in the course of the disease. The roentgen appearance of this tumor, however, is not at all suggestive of osteomyelitis. The clinical signs of infection are absent in benign tumors.

MALIGNANT BONE TUMORS. Primary malignant bone tumors destroy bone as they grow. There are no sequestra. Periosteal calcification, if present, is much more irregular with a tendency for spicule formation at right angles to the cortex. Triangular shadows of periosteal calcification at the margins of the lesion, the so-called Codman triangles, are very suggestive of a malignant tumor but can be seen in some infections. Ewing's tumor may simulate infection closely and some of these lesions are extremely difficult to distinguish from infection based solely on the roentgen findings. The clinical history and symptoms should always be taken into consideration in evaluating roentgen changes and this is particularly true in Ewing's tumor. Even then the signs of infection may be mimicked by a neoplastic lesion and the nature of the process must depend upon biopsy. When the slightest doubt exists concerning the possibility of the presence of a malignant tumor biopsy is indicated.

TUBERCULOSIS. A tuberculous abscess of a long bone has very little or no periosteal reaction or sclerosis around it. The abscess cavity has a sharp outline and causes a punched-out defect in the bone. In the vertebrae tuberculosis is predominantly destructive.

FUNGAL INFECTIONS. There are few differential features by which fungal infections can be recognized on roentgen examination. Actinomycosis is a very invasive infection with the development of extensive sinus tracts and with spread occurring without regard to fascial planes. Blastomycosis of bone usually appears as a chronic bone abscess. In the spine it may be destructive, and it also shows a tendency to spread to contiguous vertebral bodies. Draining sinuses are common to most fungal infections.

SYPHILIS. In syphilis of bone periostitis is a prominent feature and the periosteal calcification is very likely to be extremely dense. Sequestration is not common. Multiple lesions are frequent. In congenital syphilis widespread periostitis is the rule.

TUBERCULOSIS

Tuberculosis of the shafts of the long bones is infrequent. However, in tuberculous disease of the joints the initial foci may be in the ends of the bones. This is particularly true of tuberculous joints in children where the initial lesion may be an abscess in the epiphysis or the metaphysis close to the joint. The bone infection is of hematogenous origin and pulmonary involvement is usually demonstrated. The clinical onset of the disease is insidious and the roentgen signs are those of a chronic nonvirulent infection. Tuberculosis may occur as a localized bone abscess or as a more diffuse osteomyelitis; the former is more frequent.

ROENTGEN OBSERVATIONS

TUBERCULOUS OSTEOMYELITIS. This lesion is a low-grade, chronic infection of bone which is difficult to distinguish from pyogenic osteomyelitis on roentgen examination. The lesion is largely a destructive one and periosteal calcification is minimal or sometimes completely absent. The amount of sclerosis surrounding areas of destruction also is slight in degree. Chronic draining sinuses are frequent. Because of these, secondary infection may be added and then the appearance is hardly different from pyogenic osteomyelitis. During infancy or childhood tuberculous dactylitis is occasionally seen; this represents an infection involving one or more of the phalanges. The diseased bone has an expanded appearance with irregular destruction of the bone architecture and absence of periosteal calcification (Fig. 6-14-B). The lesion differs from syphilitic dactylitis, which is also encountered during infancy, in that the affected bone has an expanded appearance while in syphilis the bone is thickened as a result of periosteal calcification, which forms a dense shell around the shaft.

TUBERCULOUS BONE ABSCESS. This is a chronic bone abscess, usually appearing as a sharply outlined cavity within the bone (Fig. 6-15). The most common location is near the end of the shaft and, in children, often involving the epiphysis. In contrast to a pyogenic bone abscess the tuberculous lesion has very little sclerosis around the cavity and there is usually an absence of periostitis. Chronic draining sinuses are often present. Extension of the infection to involve the adjacent joint is a frequent complication and one that leads to the development of a tuberculous arthritis. This disease is considered more fully in Chapter 9. Subsequently the joint changes tend to obscure the lesion in the bone and to become the predominant clinical feature.

OSTEITIS TUBERCULOSA CYSTOIDES. These lesions appear in the form of cystlike areas and were originally thought to be the result of tuberculosis of a low degree of virulence. This condition now is generally considered to be sarcoid disease of

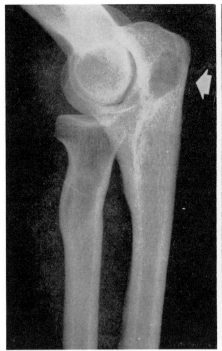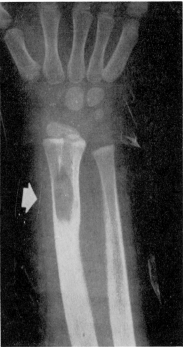

Fig. 6-15. Tuberculous abscess. *Left,* Tuberculous abscess involving the olecranon process of the ulna. Lateral roentgenogram of the elbow and forearm shows a cavity (**arrow**) in the olecranon. There is only a slight amount of sclerotic density marking the boundary of the cavity and no periosteal reaction overlying it. This is in contrast to the usual pyogenic bone abscess in which there is a more pronounced sclerotic wall (see Fig. 6-12). *Right,* Tuberculous abscess in the lower end of the radius of a child (**arrow**). There is a little more sclerotic reaction at the proximal margin of the abscess cavity but no reactive periosteal calcification. There was a draining sinus, which is frequently present in cases of this nature.

bone and is discussed more fully later in this chapter.

FUNGAL INFECTIONS

Fungal infections of bone are infrequent, the most common being blastomycosis, actinomycosis, and coccidioidomycosis. A lesion caused by one of these fungi can hardly be differentiated from other infections of bone. The lesion is likely to be a low-grade chronic infection with formation of a chronic bone abscess and draining sinus. The appearance of the abscess resembles tuberculosis in that it often is found in cancellous bone, is destructive in nature, and with little or no periostitis surrounding it. There also is little tendency for sclerosis to mark the boundary of the abscess in

many cases (Fig. 6-16). Carter has listed some of the findings that are suggestive of mycotic disease: (*1*) Those lesions arising at points of bony prominence such as the edges of the patella, the acromion or coracoid processes of the scapulae, the olecranon process, the styloid processes of the radius and ulna, the condyles of the humeri or the extremities of the clavicles, lesions of the malleoli, lesions arising in the tuberosities of the tibiae. (*2*) Marginal solitary lesions of the ribs. (*3*) Localized destructive lesions of the outer table of the skull. (*4*) Destructive lesions of the vertebrae attacking indiscriminately the body, processes, or neural arch.

Coccidioidomycosis is endemic in certain areas of the country, notably the San Joaquin valley of California and in the arid zones of the Southwest. Blastomycosis is seen chiefly in the North Central

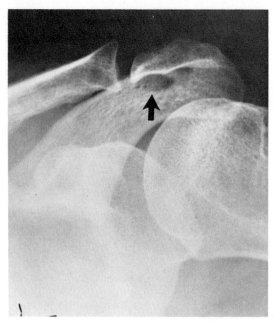

Fig. 6-16. Blastomycotic abscess in the acromion process of the scapula (**arrow**). Note the lack of a sclerotic reaction around the abscess cavity and absence of periosteal reaction.

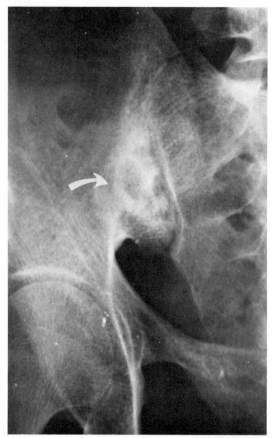

Fig. 6-17. Coccidiodomycosis of the ilium. There are small, irregular abscess cavities surrounded by considerable sclerosis (**arrow**). Injection of radiopaque material into a draining sinus in the anterior abdominal wall showed it to lead directly to the area of disease.

states and actinomycosis has a rather similar distribution. Actinomycosis is noted for the way it extends across muscle and fascial planes, causing the development of deep and extensive sinus tracts. Bone involvement most frequently occurs secondary to soft tissue invasion with a mixed destructive and proliferative reaction. Blastomycosis and coccidioidomycosis resemble one another more closely than they do actinomycosis and are more likely to occur in the form of localized abscesses. The development of chronic draining sinuses is common to all (Fig. 6-17).

SYPHILIS

The incidence of osseous syphilis has decreased considerably in recent years and it has become a rather infrequent lesion in general radiologic practice. In general syphilis has a tendency to form multiple lesions when it involves the bones. No age period is exempt. The lesions are both destructive and proliferative and often the proliferative phase is much more

pronounced than the destructive. Syphilis is usually a disease of the shafts of the bones and it rarely involves the epiphyses or the joints.

CONGENITAL SYPHILIS

PERIOSTITIS

Extensive periosteal calcification is a feature of congenital syphilis. The calcium is laid down parallel to the shafts, forming a thin, shell-like shadow surrounding them (Fig. 6-18). To be of significance for the diagnosis of congeni-

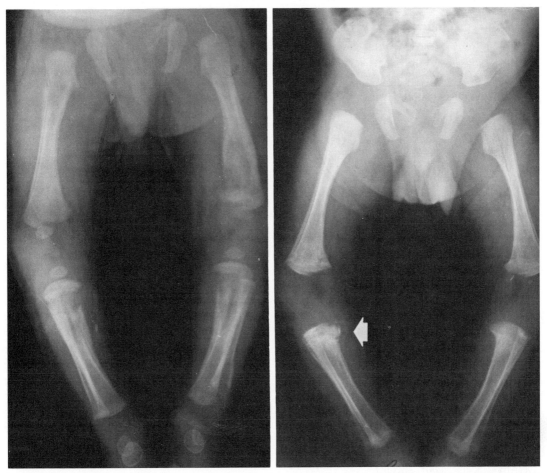

Fig. 6-18. Congenital syphilis. *Left,* Three-month-old infant with congenital syphilis. There is periosteal calcification surrounding the shafts of all the long bones. Areas of osteomyelitis are noted causing foci of destruction in the medial aspects of the upper ends of the tibias and the distal end of the left femur. *Right,* Congenital syphilis in a newborn infant. There are stripelike zones of periosteal calcification along the cortical margins of the bones. The proximal metaphysis of the right tibia is irregular (**arrow**) and there is a lesser degree of this change in the metaphysis of the right femur.

tal syphilis, periostitis must be widespread throughout the skeleton and involve the bones in a symmetrical manner. Unilateral periostitis or disease confined to one or two bones is most often not caused by congenital syphilis. During early infancy there is encountered an appearance that simulates the early periostitis of congenital syphilis and this may be found in perfectly healthy infants. Thin, pencil-line shadows of calcific density will be noted paralleling the outer edges of the cortices of the long bones and separated from the cortices by narrow translucent areas (see Fig. 10-14). The exact mechanism for the production of these shadows is not clear but they are seen in normal and actively growing infants and are believed to represent only a manifestation of active periosteal bone formation. In infantile rickets the deposition of a large amount of uncalcified osteoid beneath the periosteum may simulate the appearance of periostitis. In this disease the other findings characteristic of rickets will ordinarily be quite obvious.

OSTEOMYELITIS

Syphilitic osteomyelitis may develop in localized areas and cause irregular defects in the shafts. Foci of osteomyelitis often are symmetrical in location and one of the favorite sites is along the medial side of the upper end of the tibia. This is seen as a localized area of bone destruction involving cortex and extending into the medullary canal (see Fig. 6-18). Pathologic fracture may occur through such an area because of the amount of bone destroyed.

OSTEOCHONDRITIS

The metaphyses of the long bones may be serrated or irregular and occasionally considerable destruction may be present in these areas. In some cases there is a band of increased density crossing the metaphyses with an adjacent zone of lessened density on the shaft side, which resembles rather closely the changes found in scurvy. However, in congenital syphilis these findings are usually much less pronounced than they are in scurvy, the ring contour of the epiphyseal centers is not present, and the ground-glass demineralization of the bones is not as apparent.

CHANGES IN THE SKULL

The cranial bones may show areas of patchy destruction or localized areas of thickening, which in themselves are not specific of the disease.

DIFFERENTIAL DIAGNOSIS

RICKETS. Cupping, flaring, and fraying of the metaphyses are characteristic of infantile rickets. The serrated ends of the shafts seen in syphilis lack the fine frayed appearance noted in rickets. There are no focal areas of destruction in rickets but bowing is a prominent feature in the weight-bearing bones. Rickets is uncommon before the age of 6 months while congenital syphilis usually is evident at birth or shortly thereafter.

SCURVY. Ground-glass demineralization of the bones with thin cortices is a significant finding in scurvy. The ring contour of the epiphyses, the dense zones of provisional calcification with transverse bands of rarefaction, and the epiphyseal separations are characteristic of scurvy. Scurvy does not develop during the first 6 months of life, while syphilitic changes may be present at birth. Subperiosteal hemorrhages are not found in syphilis but are very frequent in scurvy.

OSTEOMYELITIS. The individual lesions of pyogenic osteomyelitis are more localized than the changes encountered in congenital syphilis. Extensive periostitis in multiple bones is absent. Sequestration is common in pyogenic osteomyelitis and it is one of the diagnostic features of this disease.

LATENT CONGENITAL SYPHILIS

Latent congenital syphilis is manifested by a chronic periostitis and osteitis and is most frequently seen in the tibia. The bone changes are often discovered during late childhood or even during adult life. The affected bone becomes thickened as a result of the chronic periostitis. This is more intense on the anterior aspect and in the tibia leads to a "saber-shin" deformity. Characteristically in this lesion the epiphyses remain normal (Fig. 6-19).

ACQUIRED SYPHILIS

Acquired syphilis assumes a wide variety of roentgen appearances. Generally it occurs in the form of a chronic osteitis and periostitis and multiplicity of lesions is the rule. The periosteal calcification is characterized by its unusual density, which approaches that of normal cortex. The chronic osteitis is manifested by irregular sclerosis of the medullary cavity. Localized areas of destruction simulating a pyogenic osteomyelitis are frequent, usually indicative of gumma formation (Fig. 6-20). Occasionally syphilitic periostitis is seen as a coarsely trabeculated periosteal shadow described as "lacelike." The typical sequestra common to pyogenic osteomyelitis usually are not found in syphilis.

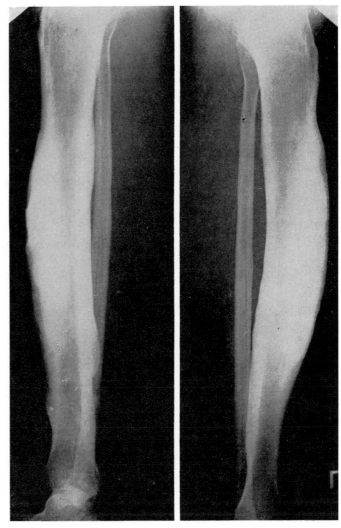

Fig. 6-19. Chronic syphilitic osteoperiostitis of the tibias causing a saber-shin deformity.

INFECTIONS AFTER LOWER URINARY TRACT AND OTHER SURGERY

OSTEITIS PUBIS

"Osteitis pubis" is the term given to an inflammatory condition involving the pubic bones, which seems to develop chiefly after operations on the lower urinary tract, usually suprapubic or retropubic prostatectomy. The disease begins some weeks after the operation with severe pain in the region of the pubis, which is aggravated by motion. A few weeks later roentgenograms reveal beginning rarefaction of the margins of the pubic bones. The affected bone has a washed-out appearance at first; later, complete dissolution occurs in the region of the symphysis (Fig. 6-21). The process may remain confined to this area or it may spread into the pubic rami. After a variable length of time, which usually is at least 3 or 4 months, there is a gradual recalcification of the rarefied or destroyed bone. In cases with slight involvement the bone may return to a fairly normal appearance. In other cases healing is shown by the development of sclerosis; the normal carti-

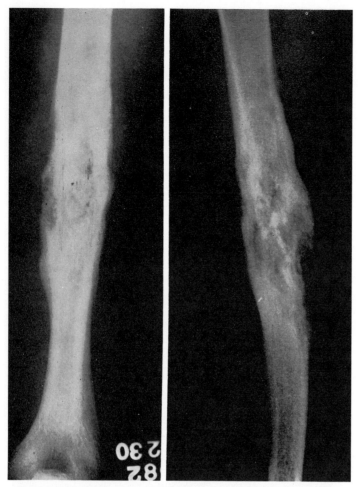

Fig. 6-20. Syphilitic osteomyelitis or gumma involving the humerus of an adult. Anteroposterior (*left*) and lateral (*right*) views. There is a combination of bone destruction and proliferative response. The destruction gives the bone a moth-eaten appearance. The proliferative reaction causes an increased density and an irregular sclerosis. The lesion healed promptly under antisyphilitic therapy.

laginous space in the symphysis becomes thin. In cases with the most severe involvement there will be a permanent loss of bone substance in the body of the pubis adjacent to the symphysis, the margin of the defect being bounded by a zone of sclerosis (Fig. 6–22). The cause of osteitis pubis is unknown but the infectious theory has received considerable support. This presupposes trauma to the periosteum or to the nutrient vessels of the pubic bones and subsequent infection of the injured tissue caused by a spread of urine or infected material from the wound. Steinbach[17] found distended venous channels in the area which produced hyperemia and this, in turn, led to bone resorption with localized thrombophlebitis. He considered these changes to be responsible for the alterations noted in the roentgenogram.

Sclerotic lesions in the pubis with narrowing of the symphysis are fairly common in women who have borne children. Usually they are asymptomatic and found by chance. We prefer to call this lesion *osteitis condensans pubii* (see Chapter 9

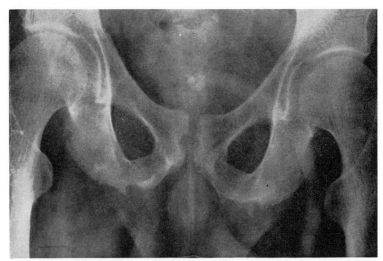

Fig. 6-21. Osteitis pubis following suprapubic prostatic resection. There is irregular loss of bone substance in the pubic bones adjacent to the symphysis and irregular periosteal proliferation along the inferior margins of the inferior pubic rami and ischial tuberosity on the left.

in the section entitled "Osteitis Condensans Ilii") because of its similarity to *osteitis condensans ilii,* which, also, usually is seen in women who have borne children and both the pubic and the iliac lesions may be seen in the same individual. The changes most likely represent a reaction of the bone to chronic stress.

VERTEBRAL OSTEOMYELITIS

Vertebral osteomyelitis is an infrequent complication of prostatic surgery. The spread of infection from the prostatic area evidently is by way of the plexus of vertebral veins described by Batson. These are in direct communication with the prostatic veins. In the cases of vertebral osteomyelitis reviewed by DeFeo,[6] pain in the back was the primary complaint and it began on the average 4 weeks after the operation. Fever and leukocytosis were present. The pain invariably was severe and was aggravated by motion. The average time required for the appearance of bone changes in roentgenograms was 9 weeks after operation. A similar type of vertebral osteomyelitis may develop after genitourinary tract infection. Also, operative procedures on the spine, or even a simple spinal puncture, may be followed by a very similar type of lesion. Many investigators consider

this lesion to be a very low-grade inflammatory process although proof of this is lacking in some cases.

The earliest roentgen evidence in this form of vertebral osteomyelitis consists of narrowing of the intervertebral disc space indicative of cartilage destruction. In most patients there soon develops destruction of adjacent vertebral surfaces, usually along an anterolateral margin (Fig. 6-14). This is followed by a dense sclerosis in the affected portion of the bodies. A paravertebral soft-tissue shadow representative of abscess formation is not seen very often. Any part of the spine may be affected but the most common location is in the region of the thoracolumbar junction. The disease runs a self-limited course. With the milder degrees of involvement, little residual deformity persists except for some thinning of the disc space and some sclerosis in the vertebra. With more severe involvement narrowing of the disc may progress to complete loss and this is usually followed by bony ankylosis of the vertebrae. Immobilization of the spine by means of a plaster jacket combined with antibiotic therapy has been recommended as the most satisfactory method of treatment. For other aspects of vertebral osteomyelitis and nonspecific spondylitis see section on "Osteomyelitis in Special Areas."

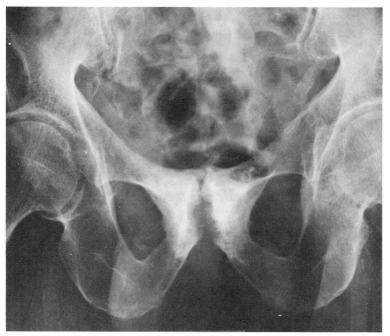

Fig. 6-22. Osteitis pubis. Appearance of another case after the lesion had become quiescent. There is left an irregularity of the pubic bones adjacent to the symphysis and a considerable amount of sclerosis in the bodies of both pubic bones.

SARCOIDOSIS

Sarcoidosis is a chronic, often widely disseminated disease, the cause of which remains unknown. While originally considered to represent a form of tuberculosis of a low degree of virulence, the tuberculous nature of the disease has never been established with any certainty. The opinion has been expressed that sarcoidosis is a nonspecific response of the body tissues to a variety of inflammatory and toxic agents of which the tubercle bacillus may be one. The characteristic histologic lesion of sarcoid is the "hard" tubercle composed of epithelioid cells, giant cells of the Langhans' type, often with central necrosis but without the caseation typical of tuberculosis.

Of interest roentgenologically is the fact that sarcoidosis not only involves the viscera frequently but occasionally the osseous system as well. Osseous lesions are usually associated with involvement of the skin but this is not a necessary prerequisite. The osseous manifestations of sarcoid were described by Jüngling[12] as a manifestation of tuberculosis, which he called osteitis tuberculosa multiplex cystica (cystoides). While multiple chronic cystlike abscesses of tuberculous nature occasionally are found in the skeletal system, they are probably not the same lesions described by Jüngling. Because the tuberculous nature of sarcoid remains to be proved, the term originated by Jüngling probably should be dropped from current terminology since it is a source of confusion. The incidence of bone lesions in patients with cutaneous or visceral sarcoidosis is difficult to determine but has been reported to occur in approximately 15 per cent of cases. The high incidence of osseous involvement in Negroes who have the disease is noteworthy and figures dealing with the incidence of the lesions are probably influenced by this fact. Sarcoidosis is generally a more serious disease in the Negro race than in the white.

The bones most frequently involved are those of the hands and feet, although the lesions have been found in practically all parts of the skeleton. In the hands and feet the distal and middle phalanges are affected somewhat more frequently than the others. There may be single or multiple lesions and they are almost always associated with clinical evidence of pain and swelling. Two types of lesions have been described. In one, the lesion is seen as a sharply marginated cystlike area of rarefaction. A more frequent and more characteristic lesion appears as an area of destruction, having a lacelike pattern (Fig. 6-23). The margins often are not sharply defined and coarse trabeculae remain in the area. In some, there is a fine granular stippled rarefaction involving cancellous and cortical bone. There is no periosteal reaction associated with the lesions of sarcoid

and they do not extend across the joint to involve adjacent bone.

In differential diagnosis one must be careful to exclude the small cystlike areas commonly found in the metacarpal heads or in some of the carpal bones. Some of these follow previous trauma but in many cases these small defects are believed to represent only developmental ossification defects and to have no clinical significance. The marginal erosions of rheumatoid arthritis and the defects caused by gouty tophi usually can be distinguished without difficulty. Such defects occur in or along the joint margins and the other manifestations of these diseases should be present. A rare disorder in which numerous xanthomatous tumors develop in and along the tendon sheaths and known as *xanthoma tuberosa* has caused difficulty because these tumors may erode underlying bone and the type of rarefaction is somewhat suggestive of that

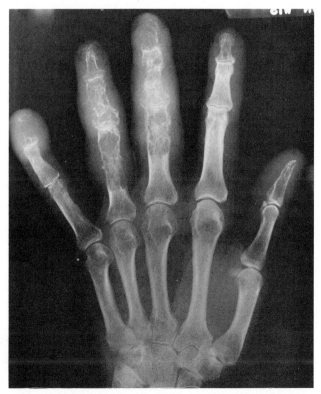

Fig. 6-23. Sarcoid disease involving multiple phalanges. The lacelike destruction is characteristic. The soft tissues in the affected areas are swollen. There are similar, though less extensive, lesions in the opposite hand.

seen in sarcoidosis. Biopsy may be necessary to establish the diagnosis.

LEPROSY

Bone changes in leprosy are found most frequently in the neural type of the disease. The other main clinical form of leprosy, the lepromatous (also known as the cutaneous or nodular) is not often associated with bone changes. The lesions occurring in neural leprosy are similar to those found in a number of other diseases, including scleroderma, Raynaud's disease, syringomyelia, and tabes dorsalis. Occasionally the lesions resemble those of a chronic infection such as is seen in diabetic patients. In some cases of long-standing chronic rheumatoid arthritis the appearances resemble in many ways the absorptive changes that are found in leprosy.

As reported by Faget and Mayoral,[8] the neurotrophic changes of neural leprosy are found in the hands and feet. In the former the changes begin in the distal phalanges with a slowly progressive absorption of bone. The terminal tufts disappear, leading to a "collar-stud" appearance, followed by a gradual disappearance of the bone. The proximal phalanges are the last to disappear. Rarely, the metacarpals are affected but the process does not ascend higher than this. In the feet the absorption of bone begins in the metatarsal heads or in the proximal phalanges. There is a gradual thinning of the shafts and the ends become pointed. Eventually the involved bone may completely disappear. In some of the joints a painless arthropathy resembling the Charcot joint of tabes dorsalis develops with gross disorganization of the articular ends of the bones.

REFERENCES AND SELECTED READINGS

1. ALEXANDER, C. J.: The aetiology of juvenile spondylarthritis (discitis) *Clin. Radiol. 21:* 178, 1970.

2. BAYLIN, G. F., and WEAR, J. M.: Blastomycosis and actinomycosis of the spine. *Am. J. Roentgenol. Radium Ther. Nucl. Med. 69:* 395, 1953.

3. BENNINGHOVEN, C. D., and MILLER, E. R.: Coccidioidal infection in bone. *Radiology 38:* 663, 1942.

4. CAPITINIO, M. A., and KIRKPATRICK, J. A.: Early roentgen observations in acute osteomyelitis. *Am.*

J. Roentgenol. Radium Ther. Nucl. Med. 108: 488, 1970.

5. DAVIS, L. A.: Antibiotic modified osteomyelitis. *Am. J. Roentgenol. Radium Ther. Nucl. Med. 103:* 608, 1968.

6. DE FEO, E.: Osteomyelitis of the spine following prostatic surgery. *Radiology 62:* 396, 1954.

7. DOYLE, J. R.: Narrowing of the intervertebral disc space in children; presumably infectious lesion of disc. *J. Bone Joint Surg. 42-A:* 1191, 1960.

8. FAGET, G. H., and MAYORAL, A.: Bone changes in leprosy: A clinical and roentgenologic study of 505 cases. *Radiology 42:* 1, 1944.

9. GOLD, R. H., DOUGLAS, S. D., PREGER, L., STEINBACH, H. L., and FUDENBERG, H. H.: Roentgenographic features of the neutrophil dysfunction syndromes. *Radiology 92:* 1045, 1969.

10. GRUNOW, O. H.: Radiating spicules, a nonspecific sign of bone disease. *Radiology 65:* 200, 1955.

11. HOLT, J. F., and OWENS, W. I.: Osseous lesions of sarcoidosis. *Radiology 53:* 11, 1949.

12. JÜNGLING, O.: Ostitis tuberculosa multiplex cystica (eine eigenartige Form der Knochentuberkulose). *Fortschr. Geb. Roentgenstr. Nuklearmed. 27:* 375, 1920.

13. LOWMAN, R. L., and ROBINSON, F.: Progressive vertebral changes following lumbar disc surgery. *Am. J. Roentgenol. Radium Ther. Nucl. Med. 97:* 664, 1966.

14. PAJEWSKI, M., and VURE, E.: Late manifestations of infantile cortical hyperostosis (Caffey's disease). *Br. J. Radiol. 40:* 90, 1967.

15. POPPEL, M. H., LAWRENCE, L. R., JACOBSON, H. G., and STEIN, J.: Skeletal tuberculosis; a roentgenographic survey with reconsideration of diagnostic criteria. *Am. J. Roentgenol. Radium Ther. Nucl. Med. 70:* 936, 1953.

16. REEVES, R. J., and PEDERSEN, R.: Fungous infection of bone. *Radiology 62:* 55, 1954.

17. STEINBACH, H. L.: Infections of bone. *Semin. Roentgenol. 1:* 337, 1966.

18. WEAR, J. E., BAYLIN, G. F., and MARTIN, T. L.: Pyogenic osteomyelitis of the spine. *Am. J. Roentgenol. Radium Ther. Nucl. Med. 67:* 90, 1952.

19. WILLIAMS, J. L., MOLLER, G. A., and O'ROURKE, T. L.: Pseudoinfections of the intervertebral disc and adjacent vertebrae. *Am. J. Roentgenol. Radium Ther. Nucl. Med. 103:* 611, 1968.

20. WOLFSON, J. J., KANE, W. J., LAXDAL, S. D., GOOD, R. A., and QUIE, P. G.: Bone findings in chronic granulomatous disease of childhood. A genetic abnormality of leucocyte function. *J. Bone Joint Surg. (Amer.) 51:* 1573, 1969.

7

BONE TUMORS AND RELATED CONDITIONS

In the evaluation of any bone lesion, particularly tumors and tumorlike processes, certain features, as listed below, should be considered. As a result the number of diagnostic possibilities often will be reduced to a relatively few or even to only one.[23] The division of tumors into benign and malignant groups rather than according to cells of origin may be too simplified, as some benign tumors may become malignant, but it is important to be able to do so in any given case, and at times this is as far as the radiologist can go.

1. *Age* and *sex*. 2. *Single* or *multiple* lesions. 3. *Bone* or *bones* involved. 4. *Site within bone* (epiphysis; metaphysis; diaphysis). 5. Probable *site of origin* (medullary canal; cortex; periosteum). 6. *Destructive, reactive,* or *mixed.* If destructive, whether circumscribed (geographic[24]), motheaten (patchy), or granular (permeative). If reactive, whether cancellous sclerosis, endosteal thickening, or periosteal calcification (see Chapter 10). 7. *"Tumor bone"* (only chondro- or osteogenic tumors). 8. Soft tissue involvement.

BENIGN TUMORS

CHONDROMA (ENCHONDROMA; CENTRAL CHONDROMA)

A chondroma is a benign cartilaginous tumore that arises from cartilage cell rests. It is found chiefly in children and young adults. The favorite locations for these tumors are in the small bones of the hands and feet, less frequently in the long tubular bones and in the ribs. Chondroma is one of the most frequent tumors found in the bones of the hands.

Roentgen Features

Chondroma is a central lesion originating within the medullary canal. It is a destructive lesion that grows slowly. As it enlarges it expands the bone locally, thins the cortex, and eventually weakens the bone to a point where fracture may result from very slight trauma (Fig. 7-1). The inner surface of the cortex has a scalloped appearance. There is no soft-tissue involvement and no periosteal reaction except for callus after fracture. In the long tubular bones these lesions may undergo partial calcification, giving them a mottled appearance (see Fig. 8-17). Ollier's disease is a congenital osseous dysplasia characterized by the occurrence of multiple chondromas at the ends of the long bones, usually in one extremity only, or in the extremities on one side of the body (see Chapter 2).

OSTEOCHONDROMA, EXOSTOSIS, OSTEOMA

Osteochondroma is a benign tumor composed of cartilage, calcified cartilage, and bone

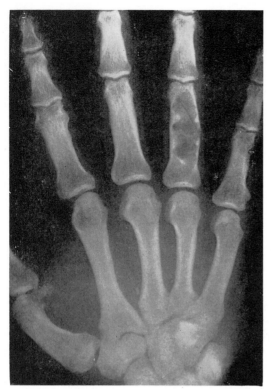

Fig. 7-1. Enchondroma of the proximal phalanx of the fourth finger. The lesion was asymptomatic until a fracture occurred through it following minor trauma. The patient has multiple small exostoses on other bones (note the base of the proximal phalanx of the fifth finger).

in variable amounts. The term "exostosis" is more or less synonymous with osteochondroma. An osteoma is composed only of bone rather than a mixture of cartilage and bone. These tumors begin during early childhood; growth is slow and usually ceases when skeletal growth is complete. Single lesions may appear in any part of the skeleton preformed in cartilage; they occur most frequently in the distal ends of the long tubular bones, particularly the lower end of the femur and the upper and lower ends of the tibia. When multiple practically all the bones will be involved; this condition is known as osteochondromatosis or hereditary multiple exostoses. It is discussed in Chapter 2. As a rule, single lesions are asymptomatic unless the mass becomes large enough

to interfere with the function of the part. Any osteochondroma is capable of becoming malignant, developing into an osteochondrosarcoma. When an osteochondroma, after a period of stationary size, begins to enlarge and become painful, malignant degeneration should be suspected. This has been reported to occur in approximately 15 per cent of cases.[2]

Roentgen Features

The tumor arises from the cortex and grows outward, pointing away from the nearest joint. It usually is pedunculated and cauliflower-shaped, the pedicle merging smoothly with the normal cortex of the bone (Fig. 7-2). The borders of the pedicle are formed of cortical bone; the center has a cancellous texture. The peripheral part of the mass has an irregular density since it is composed of cartilage, calcified cartilage, and bone. The outer margin of the tumor is distinct and usually bounded by a thin rim of calcification or bone. Indistinctness of margin and poor demarcation between the tumor and the contiguous soft tissues always raises the question of sarcomatous degeneration. Occasionally, instead of a pedunculated appearance the lesion is flat and broad but has the other features of an osteochondroma.

SUBUNGUAL EXOSTOSIS

This is a special type of exostosis that develops at the end of the terminal phalanx of a toe, usually the first, and grows upward beneath the nail. Because of its location, pain, swelling, and elevation of the nail result. Trauma or chronic irritation probably is the cause and the lesion is found more often in females than in males. Clinically, it may be mistaken for an infected ingrown nail or even for a malignant tumor.

OSTEOMA

Osteomas are flat, bony growths having the density of cortical bone and thus appearing structureless in roentgenograms. They are fairly common in the skull, usually on the surface of the outer table in the posterior parietal or occipital

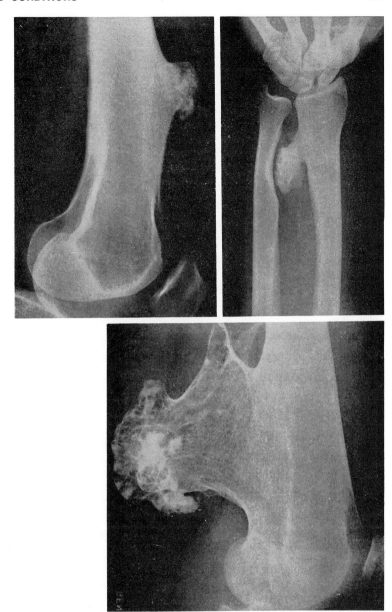

Fig. 7-2. Osteochondroma. *Left,* Lateral roentgenogram of the lower part of the femur. There is a broad-based osteochondroma arising from the anterior cortex of the femur. The pedicle of the lesion is composed of cortical bone that merges and is continuous with the normal femoral cortex. The irregular mottled density in the peripheral part of the bony mass is the result of islands of calcified cartilage. *Right,* Another example of a benign osteochondroma in the distal end of the radius. Growth of the lesion has caused an outward bowing of the ulna. *Below,* Example of a very large osteochondroma arising from the posterior cortex of the lower end of the femur. The periphery of the lesion is sharply demarcated and composed of a mixture of cartilage, calcified cartilage, and bone.

area. Less frequently they arise from the inner table. A similar lesion is seen rather frequently in the nasal sinuses, chiefly in the frontal or ethmoid cells. These tumors show little tendency to enlarge and the small ones are probably of no clinical significance. Occasionally a sinus osteoma may enlarge sufficiently to cause bulging of the sinus wall or, by obstructing the orifice, lead to retention of secretions and the development of sinus infection. These complications are infrequent.

JUXTACORTICAL CHONDROMA

This type of chondroma has a distinctive roentgen appearance. The lesion develops in the periosteum or immediately contiguous tissues. The soft tissue mass is characterized by the presence of multiple mottled calcareous deposits usually without the sharply marginated outer boundary common to the more frequent osteochondroma. The base of the lesion erodes the underlying cortex but is bounded by a sclerotic zone and the tumor does not invade the medullary cavity (Fig. 7-3). Ordinarily the lesion is relatively small, on the order of several centimeters in size.

OSTEOID-OSTEOMA

This peculiar lesion is a benign osteoid-forming tumor that resembles, in many ways, a low-grade chronic bone abscess. Most investigators now consider it to be a true tumor and not an inflammatory lesion. About 75 per cent of cases occur between the ages of 11 and 26. The tibia and the femur are frequent sites of involvement but the lesion may be found in any of the tubular bones as well as in the pelvis and vertebrae. The patient complains of pain, usually of a mild and intermittent character, worse at night, and relieved by simple drugs such as acetylsalicylic acid.

Roentgen Features

Osteoid-osteoma is essentially a lesion of the cortex and is seen, roentgenologically, as a small lucent area or "cavity" surrounded by a dense sclerosis. The "cavity" is often no more than a few millimeters in diameter. Within it a

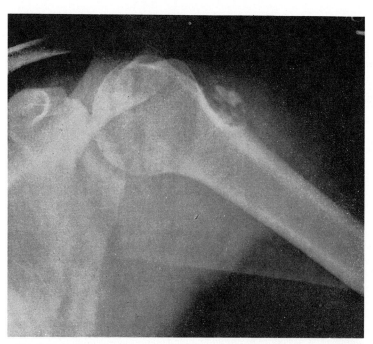

Fig. 7-3. Juxtacortical chondroma. There is mottled calcification within the mass. The base of the lesion is bounded by a zone of sclerosis. There is no pedicle as in the usual osteochondroma.

small, central nidus of increased density may be found at times. The translucent area is bounded by a zone of increased density forming a sclerotic wall. Usually the sclerotic reaction is intense and may be sufficient to obscure the cavity (Fig. 7-4). In the long bones a dense periosteal calcification commonly forms over the lesion and may almost surround the shaft at the level of the lesion. The periosteal reaction, the sclerotic wall, and the normal cortex tend to merge into one another without sharp demarcation. Tomography, or body-section roentgenography, is a useful method for visualizing this lesion and often will demonstrate the cavity when routine exposures fail to show it. In the flat bones, such as the pelvis, a diffuse zone of sclerosis of variable width surrounds the cavity. Because the essential part of the tumor lies within the rarefied area or "cavity," this must be removed completely at the time of surgical excision or the

lesion will recur. It is not necessary to remove the reactive calcification even though this may form the major part of the lesion.

BONE CYSTS

A bone cyst is not a true neoplasm but it may resemble one roentgenologically and clinically and it must be considered in the differential diagnosis of bone tumors. There are a number of lesions that appear as "cysts" in roentgenograms, that is, as sharply outlined cavities in bone, but which are filled with solid tissue rather than fluid. The roentgenographic density of fluid and of the various soft tissues that may occupy such a cavity is the same. These "pseudocysts" are not included in the present discussion. Several varieties of bone cyst can be recognized, each having some fairly characteristic features.

SOLITARY (UNICAMERAL) BONE CYST

A solitary bone cyst is a lesion of childhood and adolescence. A favorite location for it is the proximal end of the shaft of the humerus; next in frequency, the proximal end of the femoral diaphysis. The lesion is asymptomatic unless fracture occurs. Most are recognized only because of a fracture that may have followed a very slight injury. After fracture, some cysts will recalcify and heal; others do not and require surgical curettage and the placement of bone chips within the cavity. Because of the frequency of the lesion during childhood and its rarity in adults, it seems likely that spontaneous healing takes place in some cases.

Roentgen Features

A solitary bone cyst forms an expansile, destructive, centrally situated lesion that appears as a cavity within the bone (Fig. 7-5). According to Lodwick the lesion does not actively expand the bone but it interferes with normal modeling; thus the greatest diameter of the cyst is no larger than that of the epiphyseal plate. The margins of the lesion are well defined

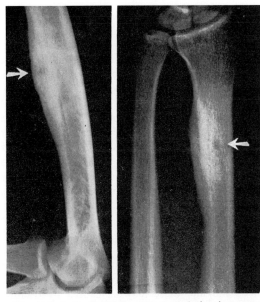

Fig. 7-4. *Left,* Osteoid osteoma of the humerus. The lesion is visualized as a small area of rarefaction within the anterior cortex and it has caused a considerable amount of reactive periosteal calcification forming a thickening of the cortex. *Right,* Osteoid osteoma in the distal shaft of the radius. The small area of rarefaction represents the lesion. The reactive sclerosis and periosteal calcification is a prominent feature.

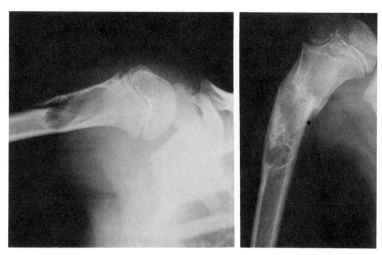

Fig. 7-5. Solitary bone cyst of the humerus. *Left,* The lesion was discovered because of a fracture occurring through it. There had been no symptoms referable to the lesion prior to the injury. *Right,* Same lesion 1½ years later. The initial fracture healed but there was not a complete obliteration of the cystic cavity. A second fracture occurred that also has undergone nearly complete healing and the cyst at the site of the second fracture has completely recalcified. There remains a small residual cystic cavity farther down the shaft representing an area that has not healed. Subsequently this also recalcified. This illustrates the apparent migration of a cyst into the shaft produced by growth of the bone at the metaphysis.

from the normal bone adjacent to it. There is, however, no limiting border of sclerosis except during the healing phase. The lesion gradually thins the cortex, and thus predisposes to fracture. It is located in the shaft and does not cross the epiphyseal plate to involve the epiphysis. Some cysts have a multilocular appearance as though composed of multiple communicating cavities. This is usually the result of ridges along the thinned cortex rather than actual bony septa within the cyst. With healing the expanded appearance of the bone remains for a time but the rarefied appearance of the cyst is replaced gradually by calcium density and, eventually, this is transformed into bone. Because this takes some time and since skeletal growth is continuing, the healing cyst will appear to migrate toward the midshaft. Little or no "scar" remains after healing is complete.

LATENT BONE CYST

A latent bone cyst represents a cyst of childhood that has persisted into adult life, becoming inactive as far as increase in size is concerned, but with a cystic cavity remaining. During its active stage, the cyst is located near or adjacent to the epiphyseal plate. With growth of the bone it appears to migrate toward the midshaft; thus latent bone cysts are found within the shaft but some distance from the epiphyseal plate. An inactive or latent cyst usually has a thin, sclerotic border around the margin and the diameter of the bone is not appreciably increased at the site of the lesion. It is an uncommon cause of cystlike lesions in the adult skeleton.

POSTTRAUMATIC BONE CYST

Small cystic areas are found with considerable frequency in the bones particularly of the wrist and hand and these may be caused by trauma. Such a cyst forms as a result of a localized area of hemorrhage within the bone. Multiple cysts of this type have been reported in workers using pneumatic air drills. Similar cystlike lesions also are found in persons without a history of previous injury. Some of these probably are islands of cartilage that failed to ossify during the course of skeletal growth. A small round cavity or "cyst" of this type is a frequent finding in the neck of the femur; it has no clinical significance. It is to be noted that some pathologists consider the solitary unicameral bone cyst to be the result of intraosseous hemorrhage owing to trauma.

ANEURYSMAL BONE CYST (SUBPERIOSTEAL GIANT CELL TUMOR; GIANT CELL VARIANT OF BONE CYST)

Aneurysmal bone cyst is not a true neoplasm but while a number of theories have been proposed, its pathogenesis remains in doubt. Some pathologists do not believe that it belongs in the category of bone cysts and have noted its occurrence in some cases of giant cell tumor.[3] From a roentgenologic point of view the lesion is important because it can be mistaken for a malignant bone tumor, while actually it is benign and curable by surgical excision or curettage. The lesion occurs chiefly during childhood and adolescence, although it has been found in infancy up to middle age, and

equally in the sexes. It involves the shaft rather than the epiphysis, a feature that aids in distinguishing it from giant cell tumor. It develops most commonly along the external cortical margin of a bone near the metaphysis. While practically any bone in the skeleton can be the site of this lesion, it occurs most frequently in the long bones and in the vertebrae (Fig. 7-6). The clavicle occasionally is involved. In the vertebrae the lesion usually involves the posterior aspect (the arch and spinous process), producing an expanded ballooned-out mass which is characteristic. In the long bones the roentgen features are those of an expansile, cystlike lesion, often with a honeycomb appearance, which involves the cortex and forms a visible mass external to the bone. The outer margin of the mass usually is bounded by a thin shell of periosteal bone but this may be incomplete (Fig. 7-7). Thin layers of calcification may be seen at the junction of the tumor and the normal cortex, somewhat similar to the onion-skin periosteal reaction found in Ewing's

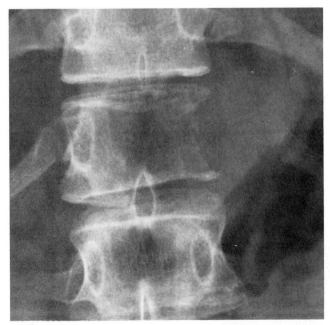

Fig. 7-6. Aneurysmal bone cyst. The lesion involves the left side of the body and arch of T-12 and the adjacent part of the twelfth rib. Note absence of left pedicle. The lesion is purely destructive.

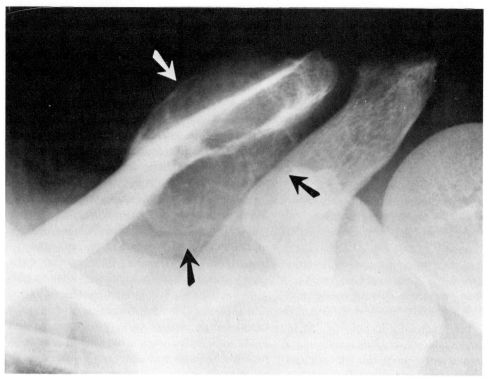

Fig. 7-7. Aneurysmal bone cyst of clavicle. The lesion has a ballooned-out appearance with a thin calcific shell marking the boundaries (**arrows**).

tumor. Symptoms of pain and swelling are noted clinically. Atypical examples of aneurysmal bone cyst are difficult to recognize correctly on roentgen examination. Occasionally the lesion arises within the medullary cavity of the shaft near the metaphysis and causes an expanded rarefied area resembling a solitary bone cyst. In these cases biopsy will be needed to establish the correct diagnosis.

GIANT CELL TUMOR

Giant cell tumor is a rather uncommon tumor of cancellous bone usually considered benign but with malignant degeneration reported in about 10 per cent of cases. Some authorities believe these latter tumors are malignant from the very beginning and thus speak of benign and malignant forms of giant cell tumor. Still others[2] believe that giant cell tumor is essentially always a malignant lesion

although late to metastasize. This opinion would greatly influence the type of therapy used and indicate that surgical resection, or even amputation, in some cases, is preferable to roentgen therapy. It is apparent from the literature that the pathologic diagnosis of giant cell tumor may be difficult and that correlation with roentgen and clinical findings is essential in most cases. The tumor, characteristically, is limited to the ages between 20 and 35 years. It is essentially a lesion of early adult life. The favorite locations for it are the proximal end of the tibia, distal end of the femur, and distal ends of the radius and ulna. It seldom develops in the vertebrae and most of those so diagnosed from biopsy specimens are probably aneurysmal bone cysts. It should be noted that some pathologists[3] believe that the two lesions frequently coexist particularly in those tumors that progress rapidly with extensive destruction of bone. It may originate in the pelvic bones, ribs and mandible. In the latter location it should not be confused with the tumor known as epulis, which is a giant cell tumor arising from the soft tissues of the gum.

Roentgen Features

Giant cell tumor is an expansile destructive lesion situated in the end of a long bone after epiphyseal closure. Thus it is rarely found before the age of 17 years and is uncommon after the age of 35. It arises at the site of the old epiphyseal plate and extends both into the metaphysis and the epiphysis but particularly into the latter so that by the time of the initial examination the lesion often has reached the articular plate. Initially the lesion is eccentric in position but as it enlarges it involves the entire end of the bone. The tumor extends to the articular surface of the bone but does not involve the joint. On the shaft side the destruction is fairly well demarcated from normal bone but there is no sclerotic shell or border (Figs. 7-8 and 7-9). This finding is helpful in differentiating giant cell tumor from other benign tumors such as chondroblastoma and chondromyxoid fibroma of bone. The lesion often has a trabeculated appearance. There is no periosteal calcification unless there has been a fracture. With the larger lesions the cortex may be completely destroyed in areas; a finding which suggests the malignant nature of the tumor. Surgical curettage and the placement of bone chips in the cavity is a favored method of treatment. It has the advantage in that biopsy specimens are available and the histology of the lesion can be determined. A giant cell tumor may recur after initial healing following either roentgen irradiation or surgical curettage. Repeated recurrences or difficulty in obtaining a satisfactory response to the initial treatment are suggestive signs of malignancy.

In differential diagnosis the lack of a scle-

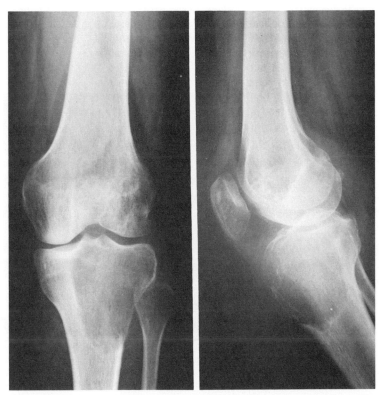

Fig. 7-8. Giant cell tumor of the upper end of the tibia. Anteroposterior (*left*) and lateral (*right*) roentgenograms.

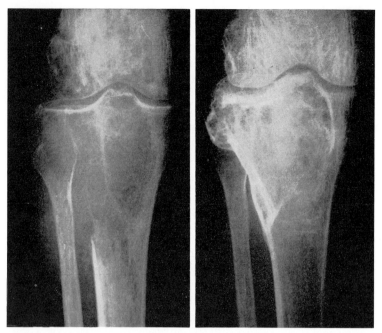

Fig. 7-9. Giant cell tumor of the upper end of the tibia. *Left,* Appearance of the lesion at the time of initial examination. Note the coarse trabecular appearance in areas and the eccentric position of the lesion in relation to the tibial condyles. *Right,* Same patient after surgical curettage and placement of bone chips in the cavity. The lesion has recalcified but the bone remains abnormal in appearance and this is usual following recalcification of a giant cell tumor.

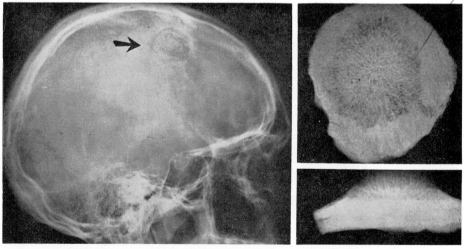

Fig. 7-10. Benign hemangioma of the skull. *Left,* Lateral roentgenogram of the skull shows the lesion as a granular area of rarefaction in the upper anterior portion of the parietal bone. *Upper right,* Roentgenogram of excised specimen. *Lower right,* Roentgenogram of excised specimen seen on edge, illustrates the characteristic linear striated appearance of the bony spicules when the lesion is visualized tangentially. (*Courtesy The Radiological Registry of the Armed Forces Institute of Pathology,* Washington, D.C.)

rotic boundary aids in recognition from a chondroblastoma or chondromyxoid fibroma. The occurrence in an epiphysis and in an adult aids in distinguishing it from a simple bone cyst. It does not have the ballooned-out appearance characteristic of an aneurysmal bone cyst. The absence of periosteal reaction with periosteal spicules or Codman triangles is evidence against an osteolytic osteogenic sarcoma. The "brown tumor" of hyperparathyroidism may cause difficulty in diagnosis if it occurs at the end of a bone. However, other signs of the disease usually are present in the skeleton and there may be multiple tumors; giant cell tumor is a solitary lesion.

HEMANGIOMA OF BONE

Hemangiomas primary in bone are uncommon tumors except in the cranial bones and the vertebrae. They are benign lesions corresponding, histologically, to the more frequent hemangiomas of the skin and subcutaneous tissues. They are infrequently seen in children but are encountered during the remainder of life. Usually there are no symptoms. In the skull the tumor may cause a small palpable bump. In the vertebrae they are usually found by accident. Rarely, the tumor may cause collapse of a vertebral body and result in clinical signs and symptoms of vertebral compression. The rare tumors of the long tubular bones may cause symptoms because of growth of the tumor mass.

ROENTGEN FEATURES

In the skull the lesion appears as a round translucent area of small size and on the order of 1 to 2 cm in diameter. The lesion is most common in the frontal area. The bone within the area has a fine granular appearance. When viewed on edge, the lesion is visualized as a smoothly convex bony mass protruding from the outer table and showing fine vertical striations. This is characteristic and almost diagnostic of the tumor (Fig. 7–10). In the vertebrae, hemangioma produces a coarse vertical striation within the vertebral body. The bony striae are separated by clear zones. The normal trabecular architecture is more or less completely replaced by these alternating vertical trabeculations and the clear spaces between them. The vertebral processes may or may not be affected but they usually are not. Multiple lesions are common in the spine but not elsewhere. In some persons a large number of vertebral bodies will show some features of this pattern, perhaps to only a slight degree. In these cases the changes represent hardly more than an anatomical variation. In the flat bones such as the scapula and pelvis, hemangioma causes a sunburst appearance with radiating spicules of bone somewhat suggestive of an osteogenic sarcoma. In hemangioma, the margin of the tumor usually is sharp and distinct, there is no evidence of soft-tissue invasion, and clinical symptoms are slight or entirely absent. In the long tubular bones the appearance of hemangioma is completely different from that seen in other locations. The tumor causes an expansile, multilocular appearance sometimes described as "soap bubble." It may resemble giant cell tumor rather closely except that the trabeculations are coarser and the location may be in the shaft rather than in the end of the bone.

MASSIVE OSTEOLYSIS (DISAPPEARING BONES)

This is a rare entity which apparently represents an unusual form or variant of angiomatosis. It is characterized by extensive regional loss of bone. It may originate in practically any bone but is more frequent in the shoulder girdle and pelvis. The majority of patients are children or young adults. Multiple contiguous bones are usually involved by the purely lytic process and this is a diagnostic feature of the disease. Early, the lesion resembles osteolysis, owing to other causes, but as the lesion spreads and contiguous bones become involved the diagnosis becomes more apparent. The course cannot be predicted but in most cases there is spontaneous arrest after a few years. In some the disease progresses to a fatal termination.

BENIGN FIBROUS CORTICAL DEFECT AND NONOSSIFYING FIBROMA

A fibrous cortical defect is not a true neoplasm but represents only a localized defect in bone growth. It is found in childhood and tends to disappear as growth proceeds. Usually there are no symptoms referable to the lesion and it is found incidentally during an examination for other reasons. It has been estimated that from 30 to 40 percent of all children will develop one or more such defects during the period of ossification. Favorite locations are the upper or lower third of a long bone. The lower shaft of the femur is a common site and it is generally more frequent in the lower than in the upper extremities. Usually no treatment is required.

The lesion is seen as a small area of rarefaction, sharply marginated, and bounded by a thin shell of sclerosis. It often has a scalloped border and may appear multilocular. It is found in or directly beneath the cortex and may involve the cortex with a slight localized bulging of the thin cortical plate that remains over the defect (Fig. 7-11). Other lesions appear as small dished-out defects involving the outer surface of the cortex.

NONOSSIFYING FIBROMA. According to Jaffe,[19] this represents essentially a benign fibrous cortical de-

fect which continues to enlarge instead of regressing and eventually may reach considerable size. As it does so it may be a cause of clinical complaints. The term *fibroxanthoma* is preferred by some. However, it probably is best to consider benign fibrous cortical defect and nonosteogenic fibroma as essentially the same lesion, differing chiefly in size. Thus it is not considered to be a true tumor, in spite of the name, but rather represents a fault in ossification. Roentgenologically the lesion is seen as a sharply marginated area of translucency bounded by a thin sclerotic shell. It does not differ appreciably from the appearance of a benign cortical defect except for its size. It may extend completely across the shaft (Fig. 7-12).

CHONDROBLASTOMA (CODMAN'S TUMOR)

Chondroblastoma is a rare benign tumor of bone representing a variety of chondroma arising

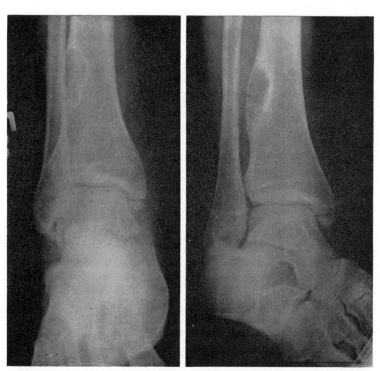

Fig. 7-11. Benign fibrous cortical defect in the lower end of the tibia. The lesion has caused expansion of the cortex both inward and outward and is limited by a thin sclerotic shell. The patient was examined for a fracture of the tip of the medial malleolus and the cortical defect was an incidental finding.

merus, lower femur or upper tibia, lower tibia and upper femur, in that order of frequency.

ROENTGEN FEATURES

The tumor consists of a well-defined area of rarefaction with a fuzzy or mottled appearance, involving the region of the epiphyseal plate of a long bone and extending into the epiphysis and into the shaft to some extent, depending on the size of the lesion; if small it may be limited to the epiphysis. The margins of the lesion are limited by a thin zone of sclerosis. It often extends to the articular surface but does not invade the joint. Mottled areas of calcification often are present within the tumor (Fig. 7-13).

CHONDROMYXOID FIBROMA

Chondromyxoid fibroma is a relatively rare benign tumor of bone first described by Jaffe and Lichtenstein in 1948.[20] It is found chiefly in young adults with a lesser incidence in children and in the older ages. The tibia is the favorite site, being involved in about half of the cases according to Jaffe.[19] In the remaining cases the lesion involves the femur, fibula, metatarsals, or calcaneus. Occasional tumors are found in the humerus, ribs, ilium, and mastoid.

The tumor most frequently involves the end of the shaft of a long bone and occasionally crosses the epiphyseal plate, if still present. Except in the smaller bones, the lesion does not extend completely across the width of the shaft.

Roentgenologically it is seen as a sharply marginated area of rarefaction of rounded or oval shape which causes local bulging and thinning of the overlying cortex. In some cases the cortex may be completely destroyed over the tumor but the lesion usually is contained by a thin shell of cortex. Internally the lesion has a clear-cut margin with a thin sclerotic shell separating it from adjacent normal bone (Figs. 7-14 and 7-15). There is no periosteal reaction.

Differentiation from a simple bone cyst may be difficult in some cases. Location in the upper end of the humeral shaft is a characteristic of this latter lesion and there usually is no sclerotic boundary. Giant cell tumor usually occurs at a later age and involves the epiphyseal end of a bone. It does not have a sclerotic margin separating the tumor from normal bone. Other lesions

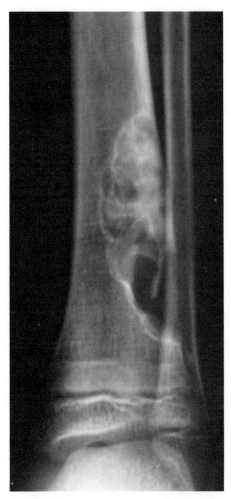

Fig. 7-12. Nonossifying (nonosteogenic) fibroma of bone. The lesion resembles a benign fibrous cortical defect except for its larger size. (The cortical defect on the outer, inferior edge is from previous biopsy.)

in or near the region of the epiphyseal cartilage. It is an essentially epiphyseal lesion although the epiphysis may have fused by the time the tumor is first discovered. The cells making up this tumor are not mature cartilage cells as in chondroma and thus may be confused with chondrosarcoma by pathologists who may not be familiar with the lesion.[19] The age period for this tumor lies between 10 and 25 years. While some consider that the tumor may be malignant occasionally, most believe it never is malignant and does not change from a benign to a malignant course. Treatment should be conservative. Favorite locations for chondroblastoma are the upper end of the hu-

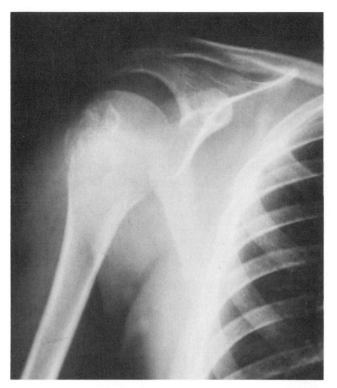

Fig. 7-13. Chondroblastoma of the upper end of the humerus. The lesion is seen as an area of rarefaction involving the outer aspect of the upper humerus, extending across the faint remnants of the epiphyseal line to involve epiphysis and shaft. The interior of the lesion is coarsely mottled, representing areas of calcified cartilage. The boundary of the lesion is marked by a narrow zone of sclerotic density. (*Courtesy Dr. Robert Schmitz, Madison, Wisconsin*)

such as enchondroma, benign chondroblastoma, nonosteogenic fibroma, and aneurysmal bone cyst enter into the differential diagnosis.

OSTEOBLASTOMA
(GIANT OSTEOID OSTEOMA)

This is a relatively rare tumor which occurs chiefly in the 10-to-20-age period. It is found most frequently in the vertebral column, involving the neural arch and pedicles. It is considered by some pathologists to represent the reaction of bone to some type of injury and thus not to represent a true neoplasm. In some cases the lesion is sclerotic and more or less uniformly radiopaque. In others it is seen as a lytic area which tends to expand the overlying cortex and to be bounded by a sclerotic rim. Stippled calcified deposits often are present within the lesion. The lytic type of lesion may be difficult to distinguish from an aneurysmal bone cyst. The lesion also must be differentiated from giant cell tumor, chondroblastoma, and chondrosarcoma. The typical location in a neural arch and the stippled calcification within the lesion are helpful findings.

MALIGNANT BONE TUMORS

OSTEOGENIC SARCOMA

Osteogenic sarcoma is one of the most frequently encountered primary malignant tumors

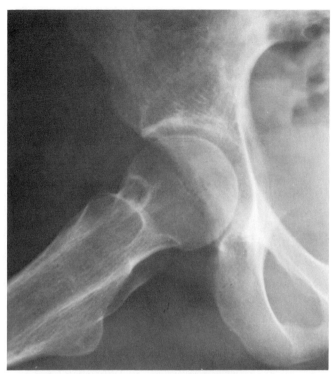

Fig. 7-14. Chondromyxoid fibroma. The lesion is visualized as a cystic-appearing defect in the neck of the femur. A noteworthy feature is the boundary zone of sclerosis.

of bone, apparently arising from the primitive bone-forming mesenchyme. It is more common in males than in females. The greatest incidence is in the age period between 10 and 25. Thus it is essentially a lesion of late childhood and early adult life. Occasional examples are seen above the age of 25 (Fig. 7-16). Some of these originate in bone involved by Paget's disease, especially after the age of 40. However, the lesion occasionally does occur as a primary disease in older adults. Osteosarcoma also may arise from a preexisting osteochondroma. It has also been found in fibrous dysplasia. Heavy doses of roentgen radiation to an area has been followed by the development of osteosarcoma. It has been reported as occurring in persons working with luminous watch dials who had ingested radium and mesothorium in excessive amounts.

The most frequent locations are the lower end of the femur, the upper end of the tibia, and the upper end of the humerus. The tumor is less common in the upper fibula, the iliac bones, the vertebrae, and the mandible. The lesion originates in the end of the shaft near the epiphyseal line. Pain and local swelling are the usual presenting complaints.

If the tumor is growing rapidly there may be weight loss and a secondary anemia. Pulmonary metastases may develop early and a chest roentgenogram should be obtained when osteogenic sarcoma is a diagnostic consideration.

Although it is essentially a solitary lesion, a few examples of multiple tumors in a single individual have been reported. These have been of the sclerotic type. It is undetermined whether these represent multiple primary lesions or metastases from a single primary.

For roentgen descriptive purposes three

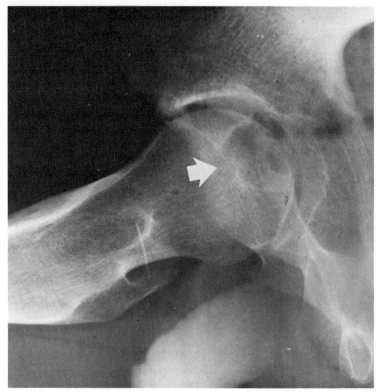

Fig. 7-15. Chondromyxoid fibroma in the head of the femur (**arrow**). There is a thin sclerotic rim around the margin.

forms of osteogenic sarcoma may be recognized depending upon the presence or absence of new bone formation within the tumor and the periosteal reaction about it.

OSTEOLYTIC FORM

The lesion begins as a central area of destruction with little or no new bone formation or periosteal reaction. The margins of the lesion are poorly defined and ragged. The cortex is involved early and is destroyed over the tumor. Extension of the tumor into the soft tissues occurs relatively early and swelling of the soft tissues, sometimes with a well-defined mass, can often be recognized. Where the periosteum is being elevated at the margins of the rapidly growing tumor, triangular shadows of calcification may appear. These are called Codman's triangles (see Fig. 7-18). They are highly sug-

gestive of a malignant tumor whenever encountered in a lesion of bone, although a similar periosteal reaction may be found occasionally with other lesions, mainly infections.

SCLEROSING FORM

The sclerosing form of osteogenic sarcoma also arises within the medullary canal as a rule. Early, there is seen a hazy area of mottled sclerosis. As the cortex becomes involved its outline becomes lost; the sclerotic reaction of the tumor and the dense new bone formation completely cover it. The lesion soon extends into the soft tissues, forming dense spicules of bone. These tend to form at right angles to the surface of the bone. A characteristic of this type of osteogenic sarcoma is the amount and density of the bone formed by the tumor; when the lesion is well developed it produces an irregular

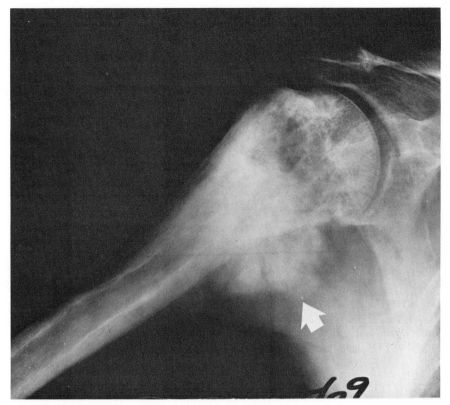

Fig. 7-16. Osteosarcoma developing in Paget's disease of the humerus. Note the thickened cortex of the proximal humerus owing to Paget's disease. The tumor is both destructive and productive with tumor bone formation extending into the soft tissues (**arrow**).

dense mass surrounding the shaft. While there is always a destructive aspect, it is largely obscured by the proliferative reaction.

MIXED FORM

This roentgenologic type of osteogenic sarcoma is the most frequent; it is characterized by a mixture of bone destruction and bone production. One or the other may predominate but in most examples the destructive aspect overshadows the productive. The bone destruction is characteristically ragged and uneven. The tumor extends into the soft tissues early in its development. Codman's triangles are frequently seen at the edges of the tumor where it is elevating the periosteum and stripping it away from the cortex. Spicules of tumor bone

or calcification are present throughout the mass, often arranged at right angles to the cortex, giving what has been described as a sunburst appearance. Right-angle spiculation is not pathognomonic of a malignant bone tumor but it is seen infrequently with other lesions. In some cases there are irregular masses of mottled calcification or bone formation scattered throughout the tumor mass (Figs. 7-17 and 7-18).

METASTASES

Osteogenic sarcoma shows a great tendency to metastasize to the lungs and roentgenograms of the chest should always be obtained when this lesion is a diagnostic consideration. The pulmonary lesions are visualized in roentgeno-

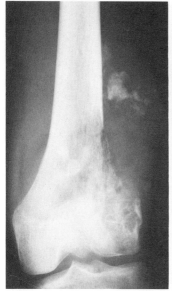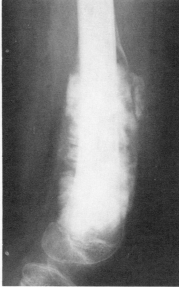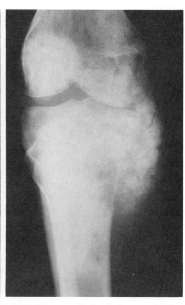

Fig. 7-17. Osteogenic sarcoma. Three different examples of osteogenic sarcoma. *Left,* Anteroposterior roentgenogram shows a destructive lesion involving the outer portion of the shaft and condyle of the femur. There is a large soft-tissue mass and within it areas of calcification or new bone formation. The margins of the area of destruction are poorly defined and this is characteristic of a malignant tumor. *Center,* Lateral roentgenogram of the femur of another patient showing a more productive lesion with a greater amount of calcification and less evidence of destruction. Note the triangular area of reactive calcification along the anterior cortex where the periosteum is being elevated by the growing tumor. This is a characteristic example of a so-called Codman triangle. *Right,* Another example of osteogenic sarcoma in which the productive phase of the lesion tends to obscure much of the destructive. There is, however, evidence of definite loss of bone substance along the inner cortex of the tibia.

grams as discrete, round nodules of variable size, usually multiple, and sometimes partially calcified or ossified.

PAROSTEAL SARCOMA

This lesion has been known as parosteal osteoma and juxtacortical osteogenic sarcoma. Most authorities now believe that it is a malignant neoplasm and thus the terms *parosteal* or *juxtacortical osteogenic sarcoma* are used. The tendency now is to drop the "osteogenic" from the name and call the tumor *parosteal sarcoma* because various mesenchymal tissue types may be found in histologic sections.[3]

The lesion is found in a somewhat older age group than is osteogenic sarcoma, that is, between the ages of 15 and 55 years. About half of the patients are over the age of 30. It is an uncommon tumor. It is most frequently found in the distal end of the femur in the region of the popliteal space (Fig. 7-19). Its growth is slow, but with a pronounced tendency to recur after local excision and, later, to metastasize especially to the lungs. It appears, roentgenologically, as a broadbased, juxtacortical, densely ossified mass. The periphery is somewhat less dense than the base, but is usually sharply demarcated from the surrounding soft tissues and may be somewhat lobulated. The mass is attached to the cortex along a part of its base and it tends to encircle the shaft leaving a narrow clear zone between the tumor and the cortex. Although growth is slow initially, the lesion eventually progresses to cortical destruction and medullary invasion. After excision recurrences are manifested by the development of densely calcified masses in the soft tissues and recurrence of the tumor where it

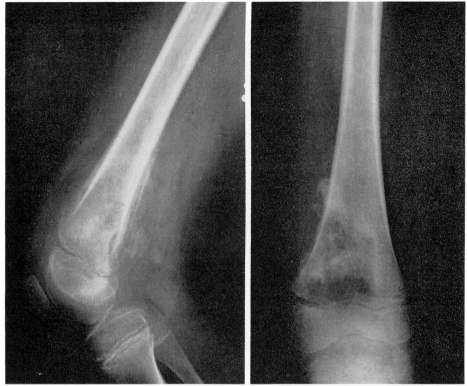

Fig. 7-18. Osteogenic sarcoma of the lower end of the femur. Anteroposterior (*right*) and lateral (*left*) roentgenograms. The irregular destruction is most apparent in the anteroposterior view. The periosteal calcification is somewhat laminated in areas. There is mottled new bone formation in the mass which surrounds the femur. Codman triangles are present.

was attached to bone. Histologically the lesion in its early stages is said to resemble myositis ossificans, but the roentgenologic features are usually sufficiently characteristic that a diagnosis can be made on this basis.

In differential diagnosis *myositis ossificans* usually can be excluded if progress studies are done. The lesion follows trauma or paralysis, and the ossification becomes discrete and laminated with the passage of time. In an *ossifying subperiosteal hematoma,* the lesion follows trauma and is more likely to involve the central shaft of the bone. *Osteochondroma* is attached to the cortex by a broad or narrow pedicle which has the features of normal bone, that is, cortex and medullary cavity. The periphery of the lesion is characteristically mottled, owing to islands of calcified cartilage. *Osteogenic sarcoma* is characterized by rapid growth, pain,

and a systemic reaction. Codman triangles and periosteal spiculation often at right angles to the cortex are characteristic.

CHONDROSARCOMA

Chondrosarcoma is about half as common as osteosarcoma. It develops at a later age period, is more slowly growing and metastasizes later. The age range given by Jaffe[19] is between 11 and 66 years with a median age of 45. Over half the patients were over 40 years and most of the rest between 20 and 40. There is a preponderance of males over females in most reported series.

Chondrosarcoma may be either primary or secondary. In the former instance the tumor originates without a preexisting lesion. In the

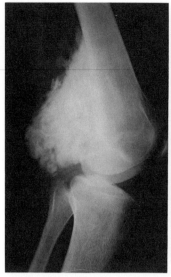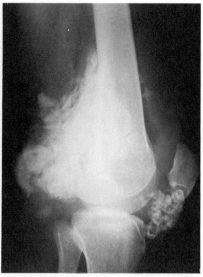

Fig. 7-19. Parosteal sarcoma. *Left,* Lateral roentgenogram of the knee showing a large mass of calcific density along the posterior aspect of the lower femur. The density is more or less amorphous and there is no evidence of trabecular bone within it as is seen in benign osteochondroma. There also is no evidence of bone destruction. *Right,* Same patient after recurrence of the lesion. Local excision of the mass was followed by recurrence and gradual increase in size. There are irregular masses of calcification or bone formation in the anterior joint compartment and the lesion has spread widely in and around the joint.

latter type the tumor develops on the basis of a preexisting lesion, usually an enchondroma or osteochondroma. The tumor also can be classified as central or peripheral depending on its location in the bone. Central chondrosarcomas are found most commonly in the bones of the trunk and the proximal parts of the humerus and femur. Peripheral tumors are more frequent in the bones of the extremities.[3] The bones of the hands and feet are uncommon sites and tumors that develop here usually begin in preexisting enchondromas. Both peripheral and central types may be either primary or secondary.

CENTRAL CHONDROSARCOMA

Many of these tumors arise from enchondromas but by the time the lesion is first examined the original lesion has been destroyed. Chondrosarcoma is reported to occur in about 10 per cent of patients with hereditary multiple exostoses. Solitary enchondromas may become malignant, the potentiality for this change decreasing from the hip or shoulder areas distally to the fingers or toes.[3] Thus the tumor is very uncommon in the small bones of the hands and feet. If examined early the change from benign to malignant tumor may be difficult to recognize. Any enchondroma or osteochondroma that becomes painful or begins to enlarge should be viewed with considerable suspicion.

The average central chondrosarcoma of a tubular bone appears as a radiolucent area within the cancellous bone of the diaphysis and rather poorly marginated from normal bone at either end. It may be situated near the metaphysis or towards the midshaft. The internal surface of the cortex overlying the lesion often is eroded. This combined with external reactive periosteal new bone formation gives an appearance of local expansion (Fig. 7-20). One of the characteristics of chondrosarcoma is the presence of numerous spotty foci or streaks of dense calcification within the tumor. This type of calcification, however, also is seen in benign cartilaginous tumors (i.e., in enchondroma and osteochondroma) and is not specific for malignancy. Eventually, the tumor erodes through the cortex and forms a soft-tissue mass adjacent to the bone lesion. This mass also may show foci of calcification which may be quite extensive.

In a few of our cases the early lesion was seen as a small, rather uneven, area of sclerosis in the medullary canal. The cortex appeared thickened over the lesion owing to reactive periosteal new bone formation and a small soft-tissue mass was present. Evidence of bone destruction was minimal. In the pelvis, large bulky masses containing spotty or streaky calcification, along with variable amounts of bone destruction, are common; the lesion probably arising from an osteochondroma.

At times the extension into the soft parts seems to result from a pathologic fracture through the weakened bone.

PERIPHERAL CHONDROSARCOMA

This type of chondrosarcoma arises adjacent to the external surface of the bone. It probably

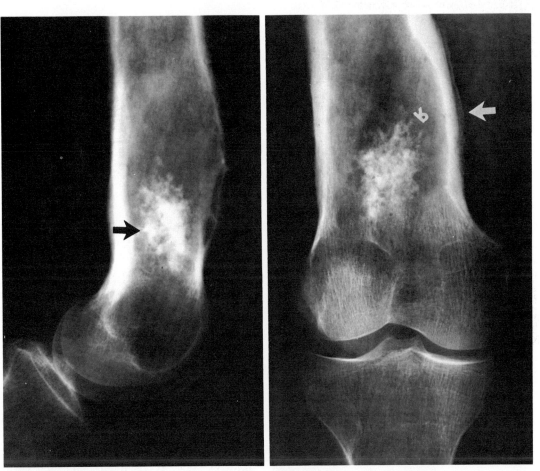

Fig. 7-20. Central type of chondrosarcoma. The malignant tumor probably developed from an enchondroma, the remnant of which is seen as a mottled, calcified density in the medullary canal (**left arrow**). The bone has been expanded locally, the cortex thinned and disrupted in part, and the trabeculae have been largely destroyed around and above the calcified area. There is minimal periosteal calcification (**right arrow**).

began, in most cases, in an osteochondroma
and, if examined early, remnants of the original
lesion may still be present. However, in many,
if there was a preexisting lesion it has been
destroyed by the malignant tumor when first
examined. A soft-tissue mass, often large and
bulky, forms adjacent to the bone. The characteristic spotty and streaky calcifications are
usually present in the mass. The underlying cortex may be intact or show erosion of its external surface. Eventually the cortex is destroyed
beneath the mass and the tumor then invades
the medullary canal.

OTHER PRIMARY MALIGNANT TUMORS

FIBROSARCOMA OF BONE

This is a rare tumor and is not to be confused
with the more common fibrosarcoma of the
periosteum or other soft tissues which may

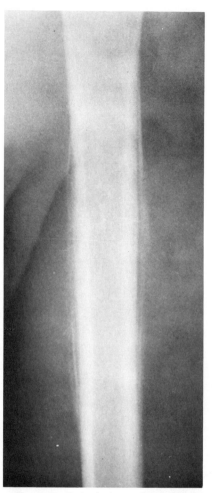

Fig. 7-22. Ewing's tumor involving the midshaft of
the femur of a young adult. Changes in the bone are
minimal but laminated periosteal calcification extends for a considerable distance around the shaft.
This type of lesion is difficult to distinguish from an
inflammatory process. The lamination and poor definition of the outer border of the periosteal calcification are helpful signs of a malignant process.

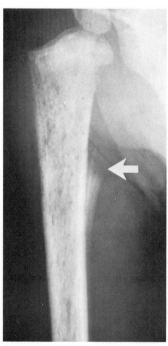

Fig. 7-21. Ewing's tumor involving the proximal
shaft of the humerus of a child. There is a fine,
granular rarefaction of the bone and a well-defined,
laminated Codman triangle (**arrow**).

eventually erode the contiguous bone. This
tumor begins within the interior of the medullary cavity. It produces a fairly well-circumscribed area of radiolucency as the tumor
destroys bone. It eventually thins the cortex,
predisposing to pathologic fracture, and may
then extend into the surrounding soft tissue. The
diagnosis of fibrosarcoma can hardly be made
on the basis of roentgen examination. The

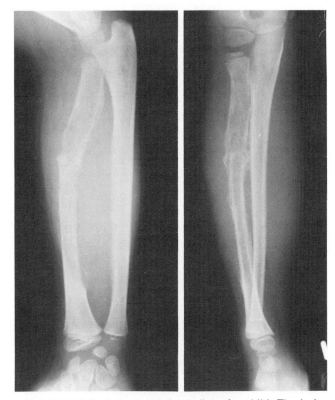

Fig. 7-23. Ewing's tumor of the radius of a child. The lesion involves much of the shaft, sparing only the ends. Although it is predominately destructive in character, the involved area is surrounded by a lacy periosteal calcification. There is swelling of the soft tissues, indicating that the lesion has invaded the soft parts. A pathologic fracture has occurred in the proximal third of the shaft. Characteristic features include the location in the midshaft, the age of the patient, and the destructive nature of the lesion.

lesions we have seen have mimicked a central lytic type of chondrosarcoma or other lytic tumor. Age is variable but most occur in the older ages; growth usually is slow.

MALIGNANT HEMANGIOENDOTHELIOMA OF BONE (ANGIOSARCOMA)

This is another rare tumor of bone which reveals itself mainly as a localized destructive lesion. A diagnosis based on roentgen evidence usually cannot be made and the lesion is most frequently considered to be an osteogenic sarcoma or a focus of metastatic carcinoma. There are relatively few cases on record and knowledge of the lesion is relatively limited.

EWING'S TUMOR

Ewing's tumor is a primary malignant tumor arising in the bone marrow. Some investigators believe that it is closely related to plasma cell myeloma and reticulum cell sarcoma. The clinical symptoms of pain, fever, and leukocytosis may suggest osteomyelitis. Ewing's tumor is most frequent between the ages of 10 and 25 years; males are affected more frequently than females in the ratio of 2:1. Favorite sites of

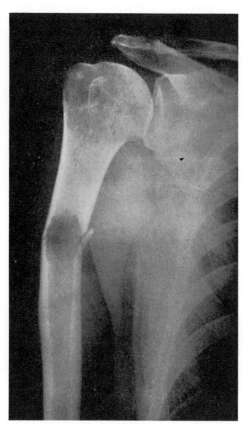

Fig. 7-24. Osteolytic metastasis to the humerus from adenocarcinoma of the kidney. The lesion has caused a fairly localized area of bone destruction and through this there has occurred a pathologic fracture.

involvement are the long bones of the extremities, the femur being most frequently affected with the tibia second. It also is found in the pelvis, ribs, and scapulae. It is relatively common in the vertebrae and in the bones of the foot, particularly the os calcis.

This tumor shows a distinct tendency to metastasize to other bones and thus multiple lesions may be present at the time of the initial study.

Roentgen Features

When it occurs in a long bone the lesion usually involves a considerable length of the shaft (Figs. 7-21, 7-22, 7-23). It begins as an area of central destruction. A variable amount of sclerosis may be present intermingled with the osteolysis. When the tumor perforates the cortex it elevates the periosteum stimulating it to deposit calcium. This often forms in multiple layers, and results in the so-called "onion-skin" appearance. This type of periosteal calcification is always suggestive of Ewing's tumor but is not specific for it (Fig. 7-21). The lesion may have a coarsely mottled appearance because of intermixed destruction and sclerosis. In other instances the tumor is primarily destructive or there may be radiating spicules of bone in the soft tissues resembling those seen in osteogenic sarcoma. A soft-tissue mass is invariably present around the lesion. In the pelvis the tumor often causes a mixture of osteolysis and sclerosis, resulting in a mottled shadow without sharply defined margins. In the vertebrae mixed destruction and sclerosis may be present and one or the other may predominate. The differentiation of Ewing's tumor from osteomyelitis may be very difficult and biopsy should be done if there is the slightest doubt concerning the diagnosis. It may also mimic osteogenic sarcoma and other malignant tumors and require biopsy for differentiation. Most Ewing's tumors are radiosensitive but this cannot be relied upon as a diagnostic test since other tumors may respond as well. The occurrence of a malignant-appearing lesion in the midshaft of a long bone in a patient under the age of 30 should make Ewing's tumor the most likely diagnosis (Fig. 7-23).

METASTATIC CARCINOMA

While any carcinoma may metastasize to bone, the common primary sites are the breast, prostate, kidney, thyroid, and lung. Because of their frequency, cancers of the breast and prostate result in the majority of bone metastases. Spread to the bones from carcinomas of the gastrointestinal tract and the pelvic organs is relatively infrequent. Favorite sites for the appearance of metastatic foci are the red marrow bones, i.e., the spine, pelvis, ribs, skull, upper ends of humerus and femur. Metastatic lesions below the elbow and knee are infrequent but do occur, especially with bronchogenic tumors.

Roentgen Features

OSTEOLYTIC TYPE. The lesion begins in the medullary canal. The bone is destroyed as the tumor grows; it eventually involves the cortex, thus predisposing to pathologic fracture (Fig. 7-24). The margins of the defect are ragged and frayed, seldom sharp and smooth. In some instances the lesion causes only a granular mottled appearance. There is usually no periosteal reaction and no sclerosis around the margins (Fig. 7-25). The most common sources for this type of metastasis are the breast, kidney, and thyroid. Tumors of the kidney are prone to cause a large and apparently single metastatic focus; metastases from breast carcinoma are more often multiple when first seen. Occasionally, metastatic foci from the thyroid result in an expansile trabeculated lesion somewhat resembling a giant cell tumor (Fig. 7-25, *right*).

In the spine there is a tendency for involvement not only of the vertebral bodies, but of the pedicles and neural arches also. In some cases loss of outline of one or more pedicles may be the only or the earliest sign of involvement (Fig. 7-26).

The disease most commonly considered in differential diagnosis is multiple myeloma. At times the differentiation cannot be made on roentgen evidence. In the spine myeloma is less likely to involve a pedicle; an associated soft-tissue mass is more common than in metastatic

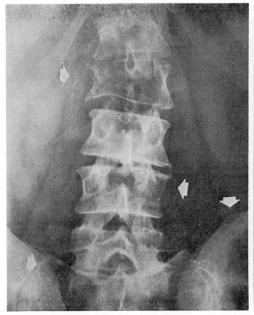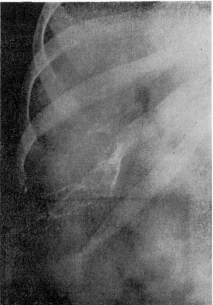

Fig. 7-25. *Left,* Metastasis to the lumbar spine and pelvis from carcinoma of the breast. There is a destructive lesion involving the second lumbar vertebra and causing a partial collapse of the vertebra. There is a smaller lesion on the left side of the body of lumbar four. There is another destructive process involving the upper right portion of the sacrum and a small lesion can be visualized along the upper margin of the left iliac crest. This is an example of the purely osteolytic type of metastatic carcinoma. *Right,* Metastasis to the right eleventh rib from a carcinoma of the thyroid. The lesion has caused a considerable expansion of the bone with a coarsely trabeculated appearance.

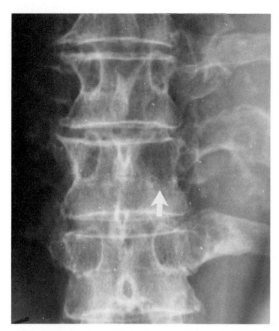

Fig. 7-26. Metastases to the left pedicle (**arrow**) of a thoracic vertebra from carcinoma of the breast. Note absence of the normal ovoid "ring" shadow of the pedicle as compared to opposite side and above and below. Rib lesions are also present.

carcinoma. In the skull the lesions of myeloma are more sharply defined. Also, in myeloma the bones generally may appear quite osteoporotic; in metastatic carcinoma they often are of normal density except for the foci of disease.

OSTEOBLASTIC TYPE (SCLEROTIC). Sclerotic metastatic foci are characterized by their pronounced density. They may occur as more or less isolated rounded foci of sclerotic density or as a diffuse sclerosis involving a large area in the bone and in multiple bones (Figs. 7-27 and 7-28). Within the involved region the normal architecture is lost and the lesion shows a fairly uniform density similar to that of cortical bone. In males this type of metastasis usually is secondary to a primary in the prostate. An increase in the acid phosphatase in the blood serum, often to very high levels, is observed frequently in the presence of prostatic metastases. In females sclerotic metastasis usually is secondary to carcinoma of the breast. Sclerotic metastases also have been observed from primary carcinoma of the gastrointestinal tract, particularly from the pancreas.

MIXED FORM. In the mixed type of metastasis there is a combination of destruction and sclerosis, usually with destruction predominating. The affected bone has a mottled appearance with intermixed areas of rarefaction and increased density. Periosteal calcification sometimes is seen over the lesion (Fig. 7-29). Following roentgen irradiation, destructive metastatic lesions often develop varying degrees of sclerosis, sometimes with complete recalcification of the area. The same response is seen in metastatic carcinoma of the breast after roentgen or surgical sterilization and following hormonal therapy.

METASTATIC NEUROBLASTOMA

Neuroblastoma is a highly malignant tumor arising from the sympathetic nervous tissue and often from the adrenal gland. The tumor is encountered mainly in infants and young children. A palpable mass in the abdomen may be the first evidence of the primary tumor. Calcification in the form of fine granular deposits may be visible within the primary tumor. The shadow of the mass and evidence of downward displacement of the kidney are other roentgen signs of the lesion in the abdomen. The tumor shows a pronounced tendency to metastasize to the skeletal system.

Roentgen Features

1. In the skull, neuroblastoma produces rather characteristic changes. The cranial sutures are spread, owing to plaques of tumor tissue growing along the surface of the brain. There are poorly defined areas of spotty rarefaction causing a finely granular type of osteoporosis. Thin, whiskerlike calcifications are frequently present, extending outward and inward from the tables of the skull. The combination of these findings is highly significant for the diagnosis of metastatic neuroblastoma (Fig. 7-30).

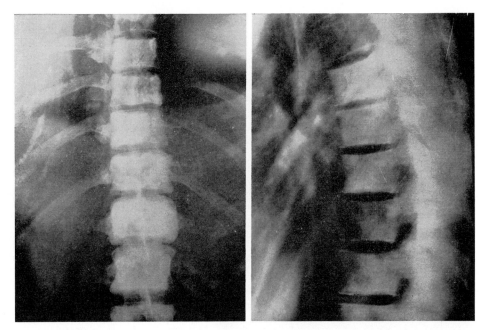

Fig. 7-27. Sclerotic metastasis. Anteroposterior (*left*) and lateral (*right*) roentgenograms of the dorsolumbar portion of the spine. The areas of involvement are manifested by a dense sclerosis that tends to obliterate the normal architecture of the bone. Multiple vertebrae are affected.

2. In the long tubular bones foci of fine granular rarefaction may be seen. The cortex may be eroded in some areas. Such zones of cortical erosion frequently are symmetrical and it is common to find them along the medial surfaces of the proximal metaphyses of the humeri and the distal metaphyses of the femurs (Fig. 7-31). The periosteum may be elevated by tumor tissue and result in hazy shadows of periosteal calcification either parallel to the cortex or, as in the skull, forming whiskerlike spiculations at right angles to the cortex.

TUMORS AND ALLIED LESIONS OF BONE MARROW, LYMPHATIC TISSUE, ETC.

MULTIPLE MYELOMA

Myeloma is a tumor that seems to arise from the hematic cells of the bone marrow, occasionally developing in extraskeletal sites. It is the consensus that the tumor arises from the marrow plasma cells and that it usually is of multicentric origin. Myeloma is found chiefly in the age period between 40 and 60 years. It is somewhat more frequent in males. The bones involved by myeloma are the same as noted in metastatic carcinoma, the spine, ribs, pelvis, skull, proximal ends of the humerus and femur.

Roentgen Features

The lesions of myeloma are, typically, multiple, round, clean-cut areas of destruction with no surrounding sclerosis. In the flat bones such as the pelvis and skull the individual lesions can be seen to best advantage, appearing as numerous small punched-out defects (Fig. 7-32). In the long bones (Fig. 7-33) the lesions may enlarge, coalesce, and lead to pathologic fracture; this is of frequent occurrence in the ribs. Occasionally a myeloma lesion may cause expansion of the cortex or even appear trabeculated or honeycombed. Extension to the surrounding soft tissues is frequent and, in the ribs, these tumor masses may

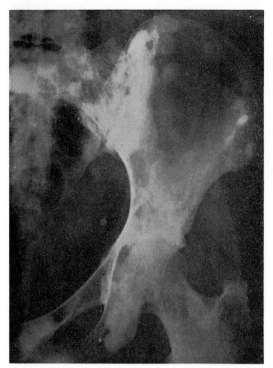

Fig. 7-28. Sclerotic metastasis involving the pelvis. The lesions form fairly discrete rounded areas of increased density with the bone in between them being normal.

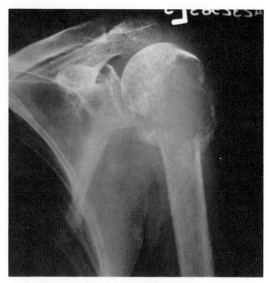

Fig. 7-29. Metastasis to the upper end of the humerus. The primary was an adenocarcinoma of the kidney. The lesion is destructive but there also is reactive periosteal calcification, some of which undoubtedly has been caused by a pathologic fracture resulting from the extensive dissolution of the bony structure.

produce soft-tissue shadows that bulge into the lung fields. In perhaps one-fourth of the cases of multiple myeloma the typical circumscribed defects may be absent during the early phase of the disease. In some patients the bones may be essentially normal. In others there is only a generalized decalcification which, in the spine, may lead to collapse of the vertebral bodies similar to that seen in senile or postmenopausal osteoporosis. Bone biopsy or other studies may be necessary to establish the diagnosis in a case of this type.

Rarely, in myeloma one or more vertebrae will appear unusually translucent, forming a "negative" density as contrasted with the surrounding soft tissues.[36] This is probably caused by extensive deposition of fat in the marrow, since, of the body tissues, only fat is more translucent than water. Also, rare examples of myeloma have been reported in which the foci of disease were sclerotic rather than lytic. These manifestations must be considered as distinctly unusual.

SOLITARY MYELOMA

Infrequently, myeloma occurs as an apparently solitary lesion. Some of these pursue a relatively benign course, remaining as single lesions for years. In the majority of cases, however, the tumor eventually becomes widespread throughout the skeleton and develops into typical multiple myeloma. The average age of patients when solitary myeloma is first detected is 45 years. The tumor is more frequent in males. The favorite sites for it are the spine, upper end of the femur, pelvis, and upper part of the humerus.

Roentgen Features

In the long bones solitary myeloma causes a central area of destruction, usually in the shaft. Expansion and some trabeculation are common

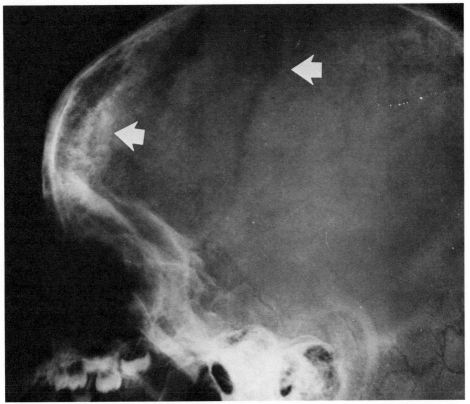

Fig. 7-30. Metastasis to the skull from neuroblastoma. There is demineralization and proliferative response in the frontal bone (**left arrow**) and spreading of coronal suture (**right arrow**).

with little or no periosteal reaction. The lesion resembles giant cell tumor but the location in the shaft rather than in the epiphysis and the age of the patient are important differences. In the pelvis, expansile trabeculated tumors are the rule. In the spine, some lesions show expansion and trabeculation; others are purely destructive, causing collapse of the affected body. A soft-tissue mass surrounding the vertebra is common. The tumor has a tendency to extend around the intervertebral discs to involve contiguous vertebrae. Extension into the vertebral processes is frequent.

LYMPHOSARCOMA

Involvement of bone by lymphosarcoma is not common and when it does happen the lesions usually are of destructive type and resemble metastatic carcinoma of osteolytic form.

HODGKIN'S DISEASE

Hodgkin's disease affects bone more frequently than lymphosarcoma. In many instances the lesions resemble those of metastatic carcinoma very closely and the diagnosis of Hodgkin's disease cannot be made from the roentgen appearance (Fig. 7-34). Sometimes the lesions are purely destructive; at other times they are of mixed destructive and sclerotic type; in still other cases, they are mainly sclerotic. The osteolytic or mixed lesions are more common. Sclerotic lesions tend to be confined to the vertebrae, which are frequent sites of the disease. In some cases there is erosion of the anterior surfaces of one or several contiguous bodies, suggesting that the tumor invaded the bone by direct extension from adjacent lymph nodes. As would be ex-

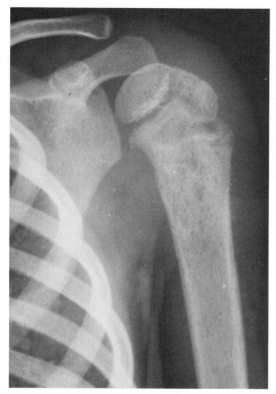

Fig. 7-31. Metastasis to the upper humeral shaft from neuroblastoma of the adrenal. There is a granular type of destruction. A similar process was present in the opposite humerus and in the lower ends of the femurs.

pected, the greatest incidence occurs in the upper lumbar and lower thoracic regions corresponding to the sites of prevertebral nodes. In the pelvis the lesions are of mixed osteolytic and osteoblastic type. Multiple lesions are the rule.

PRIMARY RETICULUM CELL SARCOMA OF BONE

This infrequent tumor now is recognized as a distinct entity. In the past, most cases of reticulum cell sarcoma probably were diagnosed as Ewing's tumor, which it resembles closely. In contrast to Ewing's tumor it occurs mainly in older patients, the average age being about 40 years; it is more common in males than in females, the ratio being 3:1. In about 80 per cent of the cases the lesion

involves a long tubular bone and it is most frequent near the knee. In the upper extremities the proximal humerus is the most common site. The lesion causes ragged destruction of bone; it arises in the medullary cavity but soon involves the cortex. Periosteal proliferation is a variable finding, being absent in some cases, minimal in others, and fairly pronounced in a small percentage. Most authorities consider this lesion as one of the malignant lymphomas and this designation is used to include reticulum cell sarcoma. Since reticulum cell sarcoma resembles, in some cases, osteogenic sarcoma and, in others, Ewing's tumor, it usually is impossible to make a definitive diagnosis from roentgenograms and about all that can be said is that one is dealing with a malignant bone tumor.

ACUTE LEUKEMIA

In the acute leukemias of infants and young children changes in the bones are very common. Occasionally, bone lesions will precede the typical findings in the peripheral blood and roentgen examination may be of considerable value in suggesting the correct diagnosis. One of the early changes consists in the appearance of transverse zones of diminished density crossing the shafts of the long bones adjacent to the metaphyses (Fig. 7-35). These are somewhat similar to the "scurvy zones" seen in infantile scurvy. Fracture may occur through such a weakened area. Similar zones of demineralization are sometimes seen as a manifestation of osteoporosis. Thus, while not specific, especially during early infancy, this finding always suggests the possibility of leukemia, particularly in patients over the age of 2 years.

Another change is the development of areas of fine, patchy, bone destruction. These may be found in any bone and are often symmetric in distribution. Periosteal calcification is frequent (Fig. 7-35). Large areas of destruction and thickening or transverse striations of the ends of the shafts may be seen. In differentiation metastatic neuroblastoma may cause similar findings. Transverse zones of rarefaction are not usual. The primary tumor may be demonstrated on urography. The fine granular foci of bone destruction often are quite similar; at times they

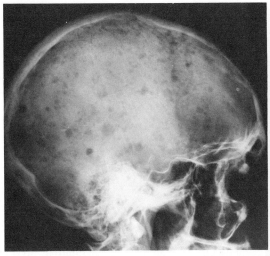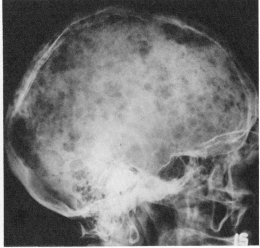

Fig. 7-32. Multiple myeloma. *Left,* Lateral roentgenogram of the skull. There are widely disseminated small rarefied lesions of "punched-out" character. *Right,* Another example of multiple myeloma involving the bones of the cranial vault but more advanced than in the patient shown on the left. The lesions tend to become conglomerate as they have increased in size and merge with one another so that the sharp discrete punched-out defects are not as apparent.

tend to be more distinct and to involve both cortical and medullary bone. Periosteal reaction is common either as calcified shadows parallel to the cortex or as fine, whiskerlike striations perpendicular to the cortex. In the skull, spreading of the sutures, patchy bone destruction, and fine vertical spicules along the surfaces of the tables are seen in neuroblastoma but also can occur at times in leukemia.

CHRONIC MYELOID LEUKEMIA

While involvement of the bone marrow is frequent in myelogenous leukemia, the disease rarely causes distinct roentgen changes other than, perhaps, a nonspecific osteoporosis. Osteosclerosis has been described as occurring in this disease. However, it seems likely that most cases so diagnosed are actually examples of myelofibrosis which terminate with a leukemoid blood picture (see next paragraph). It is not to be expected, therefore, that roentgen examination of the skeleton will yield any significant information in most patients having this disease.

MYELOFIBROSIS WITH OSTEOSCLEROSIS

This is now recognized by most investigators as a separate disease entity, closely related to myeloid leukemia, but not a variant of it. Myelofibrosis runs a relatively benign course and in approximately half of the patients osteosclerosis will develop. The disease is also known as nonleukemic myelosis, agnogenic myeloid metaplasia of the spleen, osteosclerotic anemia, and leukoerythroblastic anemia, to mention only a few. The disease may be of the idiopathic variety, which is the most common, or be secondary to some other disease such as polycythemia vera. It is estimated that from 10 to 20 per cent of cases of polycythemia vera terminate with the picture of myelofibrosis. Clinically there are anemia, a normal, lowered or moderately elevated white blood cell count, the constant presence of immature red and white cells in the peripheral blood, significant enlargement of the spleen and often of the liver. When osteosclerosis is present it is often widely distributed throughout the bones of the trunk and some of the bones of the extremities, particularly the humerus and femur. In smaller bones such as the ribs there may be an even increase in density with loss of much of the trabecular architecture. In larger bones such as the femur the sclerosis is

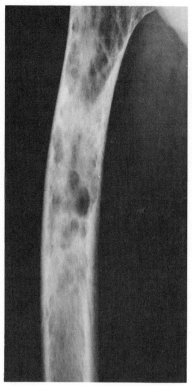

Fig. 7-33. Multiple myeloma. Anteroposterior roentgenogram of the midshaft of the femur, showing the involvement of the bone by multiple myeloma. The individual lesions have enlarged and merge with one another so that they cause a more or less general destruction of the medullary canal.

are known as *Gaucher's cells.* Replacement of the bone marrow by these cells may lead to patchy areas of destruction which may simulate tumors such as myeloma. In some cases there is only a rather generalized demineralization. If the disease has existed for some time, expansion of the lower end of the femur may occur resulting in the so-called "Erlenmeyer flask" appearance. This is suggestive but not diagnostic of Gaucher's disease. In children the disease may cause changes in the femoral head like those of Perthes' disease. In the adult an appearance resembling ischemic necrosis of the head of the femur has been described. Involvement of the vertebrae may lead to collapse of one or more bodies. In the long bones there may be numerous sharply circumscribed osteolytic defects resembling, to some extent, the lesions of metastatic carcinoma or even multiple myeloma. The cortex is thinned and scalloped internally and there may be periosteal calcification over the involved area. Occasionally, sclerotic areas are present. The skull is rarely affected, and the same is true of the hands and feet. A very large spleen and a moderately enlarged liver are clinical features of this disease and roentgen evidence, particularly of the splenomegaly, will be present.

Niemann-Pick disease apparently is a very rare variant of Gaucher's disease occurring in families and almost always in Jews. It, too, is a form of lipid reticulosis, the lipid at fault being sphingomyelin. The effect on the bones is similar to that of Gaucher's disease.

more mottled and patchy in distribution (Fig. 7-36). In the femur the earliest changes can often be recognized in the distal end. When diffuse increase in density of the skeleton is encountered in an adult, one should think first of the possibility of this disease being present. Osteoblastic metastasis is rarely distributed as uniformly. Osteopetrosis (marble bones) is essentially a disease of the young.

GAUCHER'S DISEASE AND NIEMANN-PICK DISEASE

Gaucher's disease is not a tumor but a metabolic disorder characterized by the abnormal deposition of cerebrosides in the reticuloendothelial cells of the spleen, liver, and bone marrow. These develop a characteristic histologic appearance and

AMYLOIDOSIS

Bone lesions are occasionally found in primary amyloidosis. The upper part of the humerus and the proximal femur are the most frequent sites. The lesions are caused by replacement of bone by large deposits of amyloid and appear, roentgenologically, as well-demarcated areas of destruction. This appearance is not specific and the diagnosis is made on other grounds such as the abnormal serum protein patterns.

According to Weinfeld, Stern, and Marx,[40] amyloid lesions may occur in two forms. (*1*) In the first type large deposits of amyloid may occur in and around the major joints; these are visualized roentgenologically as soft-tissue

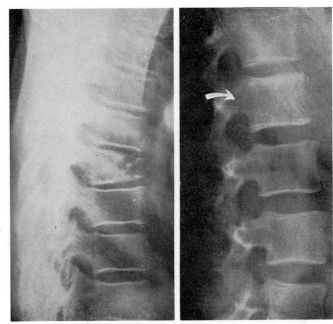

Fig. 7-34. Hodgkin's disease. *Left,* Lateral roentgenogram of the thoracic spine showing involvement of one of the midthoracic vertebrae by Hodgkin's disease. The lesion is predominantly destructive and has caused a moderate anterior collapse of the vertebra. *Right,* Lateral roentgenogram of the lumbar spine of another patient with Hodgkin's disease. One of the vertebrae (**arrow**) shows a coarse mottled increase in density but the anterior surface is irregularly eroded. There is a smaller amount of involvement in the vertebra immediately below.

swellings. The masses may invade contiguous bones causing multiple small erosions. (2) In the second form there is diffuse infiltration of the marrow causing generalized demineralization with collapse of vertebral bodies, resembling multiple myeloma or other diseases causing diffuse demineralization. Or, there may be more localized areas of bone lysis as noted above. They also found ischemic necrosis of the femoral head in one patient caused by the deposition of amyloid in and around the blood vessels of the bone marrow.

HISTIOCYTOSIS X

The terms *reticuloendotheliosis, reticulosis,* or *histiocytosis X* are synonymous and include Letterer-Siwe disease (nonlipid reticulosis),

Hand-Schüller-Christian disease (xanthomatosis), and eosinophilic granuloma, since many investigators believe that these three conditions represent various manifestations of the same disorder. The basic change is a granulomatous proliferation of the reticulum cells in various parts of the body.

In Letterer-Siwe disease the lesions are widely disseminated throughout the body. It is a disease of infants and young children. The course is rapid and death occurs so early that roentgen changes often are not present even though the bone marrow may be extensively involved. There are splenomegaly, hepatomegaly, generalized lymphadenopathy, localized tumors over the bones, a tendency to hemorrhage and a secondary anemia.

Hand-Schüller-Christian disease is a much more benign process and is characterized by

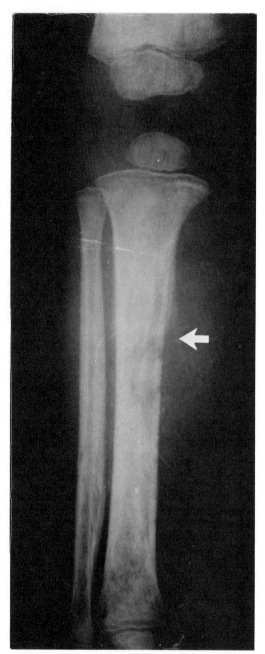

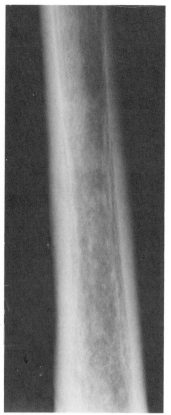

Fig. 7-36. Myelofibrosis with osteosclerosis. Anteroposterior roentgenogram of a portion of the femur of a patient with myelofibrosis. There is a mottled sclerotic increase in density distributed throughout the medullary canal. The cortex is somewhat thickened and there are linear stripelike areas of increased density along the internal cortical margins. This appearance is characteristic of this disease.

Fig. 7-35. Leukemia involving the tibia. There are ill-defined areas of destruction and periosteal calcification that is not continuous (**arrow**). Note the thin, translucent band crossing the upper metaphyses of tibia and fibula and lower femur.

the development of destructive lesions, mainly in the skull and other flat bones. It develops during late childhood, adolescence, or even during early adult life. There may be diabetes insipidus and exophthalmos (depending upon the presence of lesions involving the orbital walls and the sella). The clinical course may extend over a period of years. The lesions usually respond to roentgen therapy. The bones most frequently involved are the skull, pelvis, and scapulae.

Eosinophilic granuloma is the most benign lesion of the group, usually occurring as a solitary process that may respond well to curettage

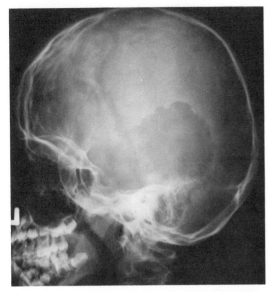

Fig. 7-37. Hand-Schüller-Christian disease. Lateral roentgenogram of the skull of a child. There is a large area of destruction in the posterior inferior parietal area. The margins of the lesion are scalloped but there is no reactive sclerosis.

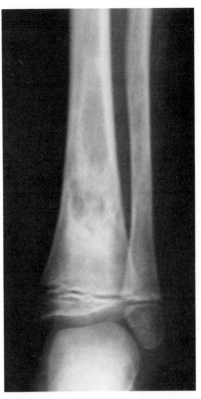

Fig. 7-39. Eosinophilic granuloma of the lower tibial shaft. There is an irregular area of destruction and considerable surrounding sclerosis.

or to roentgen therapy. Spontaneous regression is not unknown. Eosinophilic granuloma is a lesion of childhood or of young adult life. In location, it is widely distributed throughout the skeleton but is most frequent in the skull (in-

cluding the mandible), pelvis, femur, and ribs in that order of frequency. Lesions are infrequent below the knee and the elbow.

Roentgen Features

There are solitary or multiple areas of bone destruction. The edges of the individual lesion are sharply marginated, often slightly scalloped or irregular, and with no boundary zone of sclerosis. When Hand-Schüller-Christian disease involves the skull the lesions may become very large and "maplike" (Fig. 7-37). The lesions of eosinophilic granuloma tend to be small, on the order of 1 to 2 cm in diameter. In the skull, characteristically, the lesion usually involves the diploë and one or both tables, causing a sharply outlined, slightly irregular, translucent defect. The lack of a sclerotic boundary

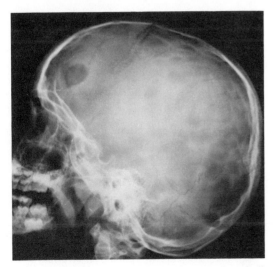

Fig. 7-38. Eosinophilic granuloma of the skull. There is a sharply demarcated destructive lesion in the frontal bone.

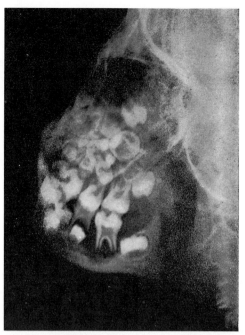

Fig. 7-40. Hand-Schüller-Christian disease. There is a lesion in the left mandible that has caused dissolution of the alveolar bone in the region of the molar teeth. The permanent first molar appears to be suspended in space or floating, being surrounded only by a soft-tissue tumor mass and with its bony socket having been destroyed.

reaction. In the vertebrae eosinophilic granuloma may cause extensive destruction of one vertebral body leading to uniform collapse so that the body appears as a thin, "waferlike" shadow in lateral roentgenograms (Fig. 7-41). Thus this lesion is probably the most frequent cause of *vertebra plana* or *Calve's disease* (see Chapter 8). Visible and palpable soft-tissue masses may be noted in association with the bone lesions. The lesions of eosinophilic granuloma often are tender to pressure. Pulmonary involvement occasionally is seen in the form of fine nodular shadows with reticulation scattered throughout the parenchyma.

MISCELLANEOUS

NEUROFIBROMA

The condition, neurofibromatosis or von Recklinghausen's disease, has been discussed in Chapter 2. Neurofibroma occurring as a solitary lesion without the other stigmata of von Recklinghausen's disease is a moderately common lesion. As it involves bone, the roentgen

is noteworthy (Fig. 7-38). Rarely, a small fragment of bone may remain in the cavity, resembling a sequestrum. In the long tubular bones eosinophilic granuloma causes a somewhat different picture. An area of bone destruction is present but the lesion also may cause local expansion of the bone and there may be considerable periosteal calcification about it, forming a laminated shadow around the shaft. Thus it may resemble a bone abscess or even a Ewing's tumor (Fig. 7-39). In the mandible the lesions of histiocytosis cause destruction of bone without any sclerotic reaction. The bone may completely disappear around one or more of the teeth, causing them to appear as if they were "floating," the soft tissues that retain them not being visualized readily (Fig. 7-40). This is a highly significant finding. In the ribs the lesions may appear somewhat expansile with a slight periosteal

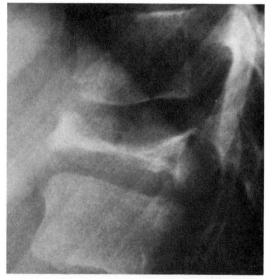

Fig. 7-41. Eosinophilic granuloma involving a vertebral body. The vertebra is undergoing fairly uniform compression which may, in time, become thin and waferlike.

findings are generally similar to those seen in the multiple form of the disease. Neurofibroma of an intercostal nerve causes a soft-tissue mass adjacent to a rib and often with pressure erosion of the cortex of the rib. The rib interspace may be locally widened if the mass is of appreciable size (Fig. 7-42). Tumors arising from a spinal nerve root often are of "dumbbell" type with intra- and extraspinal extensions. Erosion of vertebral pedicles adjacent to the mass is commonly seen and the intraspinal part of the mass may cause a concavity of the posterior surface of the vertebral body. The extraspinal component can be visualized as a rounded, soft-tissue mass adjacent to the spine in the thoracic area. In the lumbar spine the extraspinal mass usually cannot be seen unless very large when it may cause a lateral bulge of the psoas muscle margin. Neurofibroma of a long tubular bone may cause a localized cyst-like translucency in the shaft. Occasionally it is seen as a small excavation in the cortex of the bone, described as a "pit" or "cave" defect. Neurofibromas of the cranial nerves often cause enlargement of the corresponding foramen. The acoustic nerve is the most frequent site of the tumor within the skull.

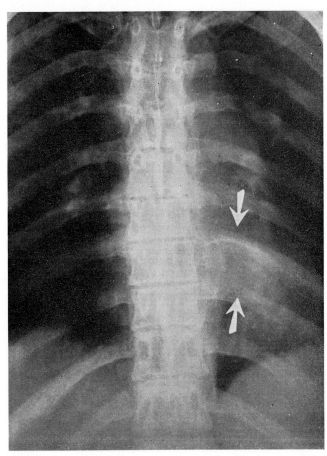

Fig. 7-42. Neurofibroma arising from an intercostal nerve. **Upper arrow** points to erosion of undersurface of a rib, characteristic of pressure erosion. **Lower arrow** indicates inferior margin of the chest-wall mass. The adjacent vertebral pedicle is also eroded indicating intraspinal extension (dumbbell tumor).

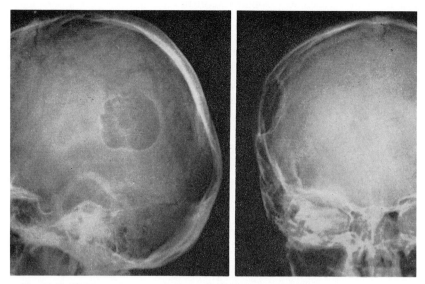

Fig. 7-43. Cholesteatoma of the cranial vault. Anteroposterior (*left*) and lateral (*right*) roentgenograms of the skull. When viewed tangentially in the anteroposterior position the lesion is seen to have caused expansion of the tables, particularly on the inner. In the lateral projection it is visualized as an area of rarefaction with slightly scalloped margins and bounded by a thin zone of sclerotic density. This is a characteristic example of this lesion.

FIBROSARCOMA

Fibrosarcoma of the soft tissues has a great tendency to invade the bone by direct extension. This tumor may arise from the outer layer of the periosteum, which does not have osteogenic properties, or it may arise from tendon sheaths or other fibrous tissue. At first only the roentgen density of the soft-tissue mass is present. Occasionally flecks or larger deposits of calcium are noted within the mass. Later, evidence of invasion of the adjacent bone is seen. This is characterized by local erosion of the outer surface of the cortex at first, and later, by extension of the destruction into the medullary canal. This may become severe enough to cause pathologic fracture. When the destruction of bone is this far advanced it may be impossible to determine whether the lesion originated within the bone or extrinsic to it. Rarely, a fibrosarcoma arises within a bone, causing a local destructive lesion that cannot be distinguished from other malignant tumors, particularly metastatic carcinoma.

CHOLESTEATOMA (EPIDERMOID CYST)

A sharply marginated, cystic-appearing tumor is occasionally encountered in the cranial bones, usually in children or young adults, which, pathologically, shows a lining of squamous epithelium and with the cyst filled with a mushy, pearly colored material consisting of cholesterol and cellular debris. These are known as cholesteatomas or epidermoidomas. When the cyst is lined only by squamous epithelium, the term, epidermoid cyst, is used. When dermal structures (hair, teeth, etc.) also are included the lesion is known as a dermoid cyst.

In the skull epidermoid cysts usually are of congenital origin arising from epidermoid inclusions at the time of closure of the neural groove or of other epithelial fusion lines. A similar lesion is found in the hands, usually in a terminal phalanx; these are believed to be acquired owing to trauma with implantation of epidermoid cells at the time of injury. Epidermoid cysts also may follow a surgical proce-

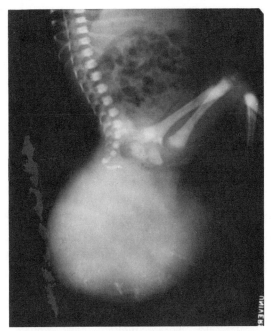

Fig. 7-44. Sacrococcygeal teratoma. Lateral roentgenogram of the pelvis of a newborn infant. The large mass contains scattered areas of calcification and bone formation. The lower parts of the sacrum and the coccyx are deformed.

dure or a spinal puncture and thus have been found in episiotomy scars, in the cecum following appendectomy and in the spinal canal.[27] In the skull the lesion arises in the diploic space and expands the tables and thins them (Fig. 7-43). Viewed *en face* it appears as a sharply outlined, rounded or ovoid area of bone deficit with a thin surrounding zone of sclerosis. The edge of the defect is often slightly scalloped in places, a rather characteristic finding. Viewed tangentially it will be seen that the tables have been expanded symmetrically. The tumor grows very slowly and at first may be asymptomatic except for the deformity caused by the mass. When large it may cause the signs and symptoms of brain tumor because of the intracranial portion of the mass. Those that develop in or near the base of the skull may cause symptoms of pressure on the contiguous cranial nerves plus the evidence of increased intracranial pressure.

TERATOMA

A teratoma is, fundamentally, an attempt at formation of a new individual within the tissues of another. A malignant tumor, either carcinoma or sarcoma, may develop within a teratoma and the lesion then is commonly referred to as a malignant teratoma. There are two sites where external teratomatous malformations are most frequently encountered, the upper jaw and the sacrococcygeal area. In either location a mass of tissue, usually composed of all germinal layers, projects from the body. Because practically all teratomas contain bone or calcified cartilage, the nature of the mass can be recognized by roentgen examination. The characteristic locations, the presence of the mass at birth, and the finding of bone or calcification within it are reliable diagnostic signs (Fig. 7-44). The normal structure, jaw or sacrum, to which the teratoma is attached, often shows abnormal ossification and may be grossly distorted.

CHORDOMA

Chordoma is an infrequent tumor that arises from remnants of the fetal notochord. This is discussed in Chapter 3. The two common sites for chordoma are at the cervico-occipital junction and in the sacral or sacrococcygeal area. It is in these locations where notochordal remnants most frequently occur. The tumor is a rather slowly growing one of a low degree of malignancy that spreads by infiltration, metastasizing only in the late stages of growth. Roentgenologically, chordoma causes localized destruction of bone and evidence of a soft tissue mass. In the cervico-occipital lesions, destruction of the clivus, the margins of the foramen magnum, or portions of the upper cervical vertebrae may be found. The mass may project into the retropharyngeal space and cause a demonstrable thickening of the soft tissues. In the sacral region, the lesion usually causes a sharply marginated area of destruction, often involving a large part of the sacrum. The mass displaces the rectum forward and may compress it. There is usually very little in the appearance of the lesion to establish the diagnosis from roentgen findings alone but whenever localized bone destruction is found in either of these two characteristic regions, one should consider the possibility of a chordoma.

REFERENCES AND SELECTED READINGS

1. AAKUS, T., EID, O., and STOKKE, T.: Parosteal osteogenic sarcoma. *Acta Radiol. 54:* 29, 1960.

2. AEGERTER, E.: Diagnostic radiology and the pathology of bone disease. *Radiol. Clin. North Am. 8:* 215, 1970.

3. AEGERTER, E., and KIRKPATRICK, J. A., JR.: *Orthopedic Diseases,* 3rd ed. Philadelphia, Saunders, 1968.

4. AMSTUTZ, H. C., and CAREY, E. J.: Skeletal manifestations and treatment of Gaucher's disease. Review of twenty cases. *J. Bone Joint Surg. 48-A:* 670, 1966.

5. BARNES, R., and CATTO, M.: Chondrosarcoma of bone. *J. Bone Joint Surg. 48-B:* 729, 1966.

6. BINET, E. F., KIEFFER, S. A., MARTIN, S. H., and PETERSON, H. O.: Orbital dysplasia in neurofibromatosis. *Radiology 93:* 829, 1969.

7. BYERS, B. D.: Solitary benign osteoblastic lesions of bone: Osteoid osteoma and benign osteoblastoma. *Cancer 21:* 1289, 1968.

8. CAMPBELL, C. J., and HARKESS, J.: Fibrous metaphyseal defect of bone. *Surg. Gynecol. Obstet. 104:* 329, 1957.

9. DAHLIN, D. C., COVENTRY, M. B., and SCANLON, P. W.: Ewing's sarcoma: A critical analysis of 165 cases. *J. Bone Joint Surg. 43-A:* 185, 1961.

10. EVINSON, G., and PRICE, C. H. G.: Subungual exostosis. *Br. J. Radiol. 39:* 451, 1966.

11. FALK, S., and ALPERT, M.: The clinical and roentgen aspects of Ewing's sarcoma. *Am. J. Med. Sci. 250:* 492, 1965.

12. FELDMAN, F., HECHT, H. L., and JOHNSTON, A. D.: Chondromyxoid fibroma of bone. *Radiology 94:* 249, 1970.

13. FREIBERGER, R. H., LOITMAN, B. S., HELPERN, M., and THOMPSON, T. C.: Osteoid osteoma. A report of 80 cases. *Am. J. Roentgenol. Radium Ther. Nucl. Med. 82:* 194, 1959.

14. FUCILLA, I. S., and HAMANN, A.: Hodgkin's disease in bone. *Radiology 77:* 53, 1961.

15. GOLDENBERG, R. R., CAMPBELL, C. J., and BONFILGIO, M.: Giant cell tumor; an analysis of two hundred and eighteen cases. *J. Bone Joint Surg. 52-A:* 619, 1970.

16. GREENFIELD, G. B.: Bone changes in chronic adult Gaucher's disease. *Am. J. Roentgenol. Radium Ther. Nucl. Med. 110:* 800, 1970.

17. GROSSMAN, R. E., and HENSLEY, G. T.: Bone lesions in primary amyloidosis. *Am. J. Roentgenol. Radium Ther. Nucl. Med. 101:* 872, 1967.

18. HUNT, J. C., and PUGH, D. G.: Skeletal lesions in neurofibromatosis. *Radiology 76:* 1, 1961.

19. JAFFE, H. L.: *Tumors and Tumorous Conditions of the Bones and Joints.* Philadelphia, Lea & Febiger, 1958.

20. JAFFE, H. L., and LICHTENSTEIN, L.: Benign chondroblastoma of bone; a reinterpretation of the so-called calcifying or chondromatous giant cell tumor. *Am. J. Path. 18:* 969, 1942.

21. JOHNSON, P. M., and McCLURE, J. G.: Observations on massive osteolysis: A review of the literature and report of a case. *Radiology 71:* 28, 1958.

22. KARLSBERG, R. C., and KITTLESON, A. C.: Osteoid osteoma. *Radiol. Clin. North Am. 2:* 337, 1964.

23. LODWICK, G. S.: A probabilistic approach to the diagnosis of bone tumors. *Radiol. Clin. North Am. 3:* 487, 1965.

24. LODWICK, G. S.: *Atlas of Tumor Radiology: The Bones and Joints,* ed. by P. H. Hodes. Chicago, Year Book, vol. 4, 1971.

25. MASZAROS, W. T., GUZZO, F., and SCHORSCH, H.: Neurofibromatosis. *Am. J. Roentgenol. Radium Ther. Nucl. Med. 98:* 557, 1966.

26. McGAVRAN, M. H., and SPADY, H. A.: Eosinophilic granuloma of bone. *J. Bone Joint Surg. 42-A:* 979, 1960.

27. PEAR, B. L.: Epidermoid and dermoid sequestration cysts. *Am. J. Roentgenol. Radium Ther. Nucl. Med. 110:* 148, 1970.

28. POCHACZEVSKY, R., YEN, Y. M., and SHERMAN, R. S.: The roentgen appearance of benign osteoblastoma. *Radiology 75:* 429, 1960.

29. REYNOLDS, J.: The "fallen fragment sign" in the diagnosis of unicameral bone cysts. *Radiology 92:* 949, 1969.

30. RIDINGS, G. R.: Ewing's tumor. *Radiol. Clin. North Am. 2:* 315, 1964.

31. SAENGER, E. L., and JOHANSMANN, R. F.: Letterer-Siwe's disease: Promise in diagnosis and treatment. *Am. J. Roentgenol. Radium Ther. Nucl. Med. 71:* 472, 1954.

32. SHERMAN, R. S., and SOONG, K. Y.: A roentgen study of osteogenic sarcoma developing in Paget's disease. *Radiology 63:* 48, 1954.

33. SHERMAN, R. S., and WILNER, D.: The roentgen diagnosis of hemangioma of bone. *Am. J. Roentgenol. 86:* 1146, 1961.

34. SLOWICK, F. A., JR., CAMPBELL, C. J., and KETTLKAMP, D. B.: Aneurysmal bone cyst. *J. Bone Joint Surg. 50-A:* 1142, 1968.

35. TILLMAN, B. P., DAHLIN, D. C., LIPSCOMB, P. R., and STEWART, J. R.: Aneurysmal bone cyst: An

analysis of ninety-five cases. *Mayo Clin. Proc. 43:* 415, 1967.

36. TORRANCE, D. J., JR.: "Negative" bone density in a case of multiple myeloma. *Radiology 70:* 864, 1958.

37. TURCOTTE, B., PUGH, D. G., and DAHLIN, D. C.: The roentgenologic aspects of chondromyxoid fibroma of bone. *Am. J. Roentgenol. Radium Ther. Nucl. Med. 87:* 1085, 1962.

38. VAN DER HUEL, R. O., and VON RONNEN, J. R.: Juxtacortical osteosarcoma. *J. Bone Joint Surg. 49-A:* 415, 1967.

39. VOHRA, V. G.: Roentgen manifestations in Ewing's sarcoma, a study of 156 cases. *Cancer 20:* 727, 1967.

40. WEINFELD, A., STERN, M. H., and MARX, L. H.: Amyloid lesions of bone. *Am. J. Roentgenol. Radium Ther. Nucl. Med. 108:* 799, 1970.

41. WILLSON, J. K. V.: The bone lesions in childhood leukemia: A survey of 140 cases. *Radiology 72:* 672, 1959.

42. WILSON, T. W., and PUGH, D. G.: Primary reticulum-cell sarcoma of bone, with emphasis on roentgen aspects. *Radiology 65:* 343, 1955.

8

MISCELLANEOUS CONDITIONS

ISCHEMIC NECROSIS; OSTEOCHONDROSIS

The *osteochondroses* or *ischemic necroses* comprise a group of lesions, usually involving an epiphyseal ossification center or one of the small bones of the hand or foot of a child or adolescent and which were considered to be a form of aseptic necrosis. More recently the term, ischemic necrosis, has come into use to indicate that the lesions are caused by local bone ischemia. It is becoming apparent that the terms osteochondrosis or aseptic necrosis have been used in the past for two essentially different conditions. In the one group, the *ischemic necroses,* occlusion of blood vessels supplying a portion of the bone will lead to death of the bone supplied by the vessels. In the other group, the *osteochondroses,* trauma is being stressed as a causative factor, either as an avulsion injury or as a chronic stress type of fracture.[19] A few of the entities are difficult to classify because the pathogenesis still is uncertain. At one time or another practically every epiphyseal ossification center in the body has been described as the site of osteochondrosis or ischemic necrosis and an eponym has been attached to each. It now is recognized that some of these represent only variations in normal ossification and that others should more properly be classified as a form of injury (Table 8-1). The eponyms have become firmly established in the literature and it is difficult to eliminate them.

EPIPHYSEAL AND SMALL BONE LESIONS IN CHILDREN

CAPITAL FEMORAL EPIPHYSIS

Ischemic necrosis or osteochondrosis of the proximal epiphysis of the femur is more commonly known as *Perthes' disease* or *Legg-Calvé-Perthes' disease.* Other names applied to this lesion include *osteochondritis deformans* and *coxa plana.* The etiology of Perthes' disease has been debatable. Some authors have classified it as the idiopathic type of ischemic necrosis based on study of resected specimens even though occlusion of major arteries often cannot be demonstrated. The pathology is one of degeneration and necrosis. Trauma or repeated microtrauma has often been considered as a cause with injury to the vessels supplying the epiphysis. Recently, Caffey[3] has presented evidence which he believes indicates that the early lesion is a form of chronic stress or fatigue fracture; the ischemic necrosis being a later manifestation and secondary to the fracture. His findings again emphasize the role of trauma in the so-called osteochondroses.

TABLE 8-1. Ischemic Necrosis; Osteochondrosis

I. Epiphyseal and Small Bone Lesions in Children
 A. Capital Femoral Epiphysis
 B. Other Areas
  1. Tarsal scaphoid
  2. Tibial tuberosity
  3. Vertebral epiphyses
  4. Second metatarsal head
  5. Apophysis of os calcis
  6. Osteochondritis dissecans
  7. Epiphyseolysis
  8. Others
II. Epiphyseal Ischemic Necrosis Secondary to Other Diseases
III. Ischemic Necrosis of the Ends of the Bones in Adults
 A. The head of the femur
 B. Other areas
IV. Bone Infarction of the Diaphyses

Perthes' disease is a benign condition that runs a self-limited course with eventual healing. Because this takes several years or longer, the epiphyseal ossification center and femoral neck undergo change in shape, permanent deformity usually follows and often leads to the early development of degenerative joint disease. It is a disease of childhood and is more frequent in males than in females. It is bilateral in about 10 per cent of patients.

The relationship of skeletal maturation and the development of Perthes' disease has been evaluated by Girdany and Osman.[7] They found that among boys, skeletal age was below normal in most and that in none of the patients was the value for skeletal maturation above the mean for the age. This observation did not hold true for girls.

The early roentgen findings in Perthes' disease are largely in the soft tissues of the joint. The joint capsule is distended with fluid and the joint space may be widened slightly. Also, a slight lateral displacement of the head of the femur is commonly present owing to hyperemia of the synovium and subsynovial tissues (Fig. 8-1). These changes often are subtle and require careful observation for detection. According to Kemp and Boldero,[12] if the hip is put at rest at this stage, the signs and symptoms will disappear and the joint will return to normal. Others, however, consider changes of this nature with disappearance after a period of rest leaving little or no residuals, as indicative of the entity known as *transient synovitis of the hip*. In a review of cases by Nachemson and Scheller,[20] 6 per cent of those initially thought

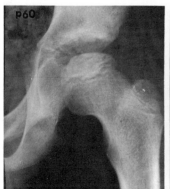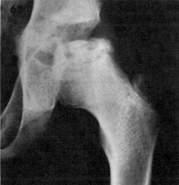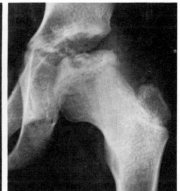

Fig. 8-1. Perthe's disease. *Left,* Early film in the series showing slight, uniform increase in density of the femoral head, several thin and irregular fissures within it, and widening of the joint space (compared with opposite, normal hip). *Center,* Ten months later there is further flattening of the head, increased density of it, and areas of absorption surrounding a small, dense fragment near the center of the articular surface. *Right,* Five months later the central fragment appears to lie within a cavity in the head and it has become fragmented. The remainder of the epiphysis shows more normal density and reformation of trabecular bone. The flattening of the epiphysis will remain after healing is complete.

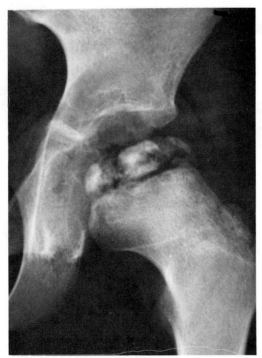

Fig. 8-2. Perthes' disease. Advanced disease showing marked flattening of the femoral epiphysis, several dense, white fragments and areas of absorption. The joint space is wide and the epiphyseal plate is wider than normal. There is broadening of the neck of the femur.

to be transient synovitis of the hip, later developed Perthes' disease. The remainder cleared with only minor residual changes in a small percentage (slight increase in size of the femoral head on the affected side, a few cortical cysts and dense spots in the femoral neck).

The first change in the femoral head usually is a thin arclike translucent zone which develops in the subchondral bone close to the bony articular surface along the anterosuperior aspect of the epiphyseal ossification center. This has been considered to represent a stress fracture occurring through the necrotic bone. Caffey[3] has described the occurrence in some cases of a thin, dark line adjacent to the fracture which he believes is a fissure in the bone filled with gas from the blood or tissue fluids. (Also Martel and Poznanski[17] have demonstrated an increased lucency of the radiolucent crescent line in avascular necrosis of the

femoral head in adults when traction was applied to the leg and which they believe is caused by release of gas secondary to the vacuum caused by the traction). In other cases there is a slight flattening of the center and irregularity of its superior articular surface (see Fig. 8-1). At times during this early stage the entire center will show a slight uniform increase in density. This probably is more apparent than real owing to disuse osteoporosis in the viable bone immediately adjacent (e.g., the acetabulum and femoral neck). The head, having lost its blood supply maintains the density of normal bone and it keeps this density until revascularization takes place.

The next well-defined stage is represented by crushing and fragmentation of the epiphysis or a portion of it (Figs. 8-1 to 8-3). The extent of involvement of the epiphysis varies among patients. In some the entire center is affected; in others the changes are limited to an area of subchondral bone along the superior aspect of the head. Once revascularization has taken place, dead bone can be removed. In some patients this happens before much new bone has been formed and large areas of the epiphysis will be absorbed (Fig. 8-4). In other patients reossification occurs before dead bone has been removed, the new bone being laid down on the scaffolding formed by the dead trabeculae. The increased thickness of the trabeculae causes increased density of the epiphysis and this is probably the major cause of the increased density of the head or its fragments at this stage of the disease. Compression of the bone causes impaction of trabeculae and this may add to the increased radiopacity. At this stage the revascularization process is well advanced and reossification is taking place. Eventually the dead trabeculae are removed and the center returns to a normal density. However, in some cases, the old trabeculae may never be removed and the increased radiopacity of the head persists after healing is complete.[4] Reossification begins adjacent to the epiphyseal plate and the subchondral bone next to the articular surface is the last to ossify. Healing is a slow process and may require several years or longer.

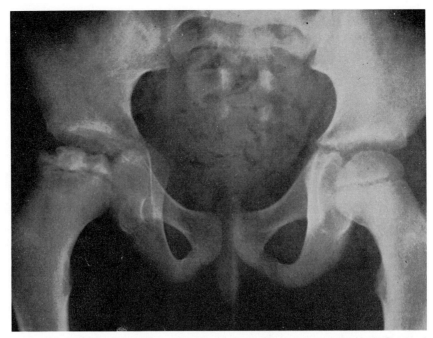

Fig. 8-3. Legg-Perthes' disease of the right hip. The capital epiphysis is flattened and irregular in density, the central portion is uniformly opaque, the articular surface is roughened, and there are areas of absorption. The joint space is widened. Compare with the opposite normal hip.

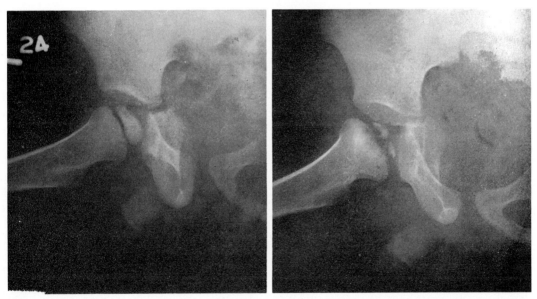

Fig. 8-4. Legg-Perthes' disease. *Left,* Lateral roentgenogram of the hip shows a general flattening of the capital epiphysis of the femur. It is increased in density as compared to the adjacent neck and shaft and the articular surface is irregular and has the appearance of being fragmented. *Right,* Same hip 8 months later. There has been progressive absorption of bone, leaving only small fragments of ossification. In this patient removal of bone occurred much faster than reossification and it will require a considerable period of time, probably several years at least, before restitution of the head has occurred. Note the broadened femoral neck and irregularity of the metaphysis.

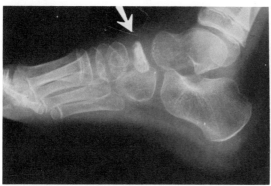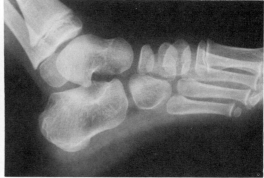

Fig. 8-5. Osteochondritis of the tarsal scaphoid (Köhler's disease). Lateral roentgenograms of both feet of a child, showing on the *left* the dense tarsal scaphoid characteristic of this lesion (**arrow**). Compare with the normal bone on the *right* side.

During the active stage of the disease there often is a slight widening of the epiphyseal line. (The epiphyseal cartilage derives its blood supply from the same vessels that supply the head). The surface of the metaphysis becomes irregular, sometimes with small cystic areas, and the femoral neck broadened and foreshortened (see Fig. 8-2). The acetabulum is not involved in Perthes' disease but, because of disuse, ossification of it lags behind that of the opposite hip and it develops a wavy contour.

OTHER AREAS

Some of the more common sites where osteochondrosis has been said to occur are given below. As noted before some of these now are recognized as being either avulsion fractures or chronic fatigue fractures instead of primary ischemic necrosis.

THE TARSAL SCAPHOID (KÖHLER'S DISEASE). Infrequently this bone may be involved by a process similar to Perthes' disease (Fig. 8-5). It occurs during childhood and the roentgen findings consist of flattening and crushing, increased density, and a tendency for fragmentation of the bone. In some cases the lesion has been asymptomatic.

THE TIBIAL TUBEROSITY (OSGOOD-SCHLATTER DISEASE). The tibial tuberosity develops as a tonguelike extension on the anterior aspect of the proximal tibial epiphysis. While the major part of this epiphysis begins to ossify at or shortly before birth, the tuberosity remains cartilaginous until late childhood. When it does begin to ossify it frequently does so from one or more centers; these fuse to the major part of the epiphysis within a relatively short time and subsequently the entire epiphysis fuses to the shaft. The tuberosity serves for the attachment of the patellar tendon and thus is readily subjected to injury. Most investigators believe this lesion represents either a fracture of the tuberosity or the sequelae of previous fracture. The lesion also may represent a stress or fatigue type of fracture of the tuberosity rather than an ischemic necrosis. It is more frequent in boys than in girls and is more common during adolescence (i.e., 13 to 15 years). When the lesion develops the ossified portion of the tuberosity becomes ragged in outline, it often fragments, and it may develop irregular increase in density (Fig. 8-6). The inferior portion often is elevated slightly from its normal position. Localized swelling of the soft tissues over the tuberosity can be visualized. The roentgen diagnosis of osteochondrosis of the tibial tuberosity should be made with caution. There is considerable variation in the appearance of the normal tuberosity during the process of ossification. It may ossify from several centers and its inferior portion may be elevated. The

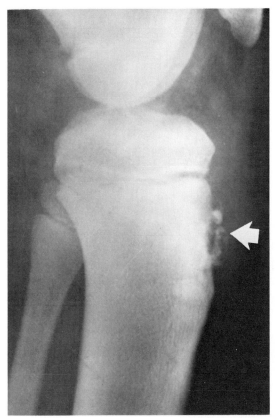

Fig. 8-6. Osgood-Schlatter disease of the tibial tuberosity. The epiphysis for the tuberosity is fragmented (**arrow**) and, in the original roentgenogram, there was localized soft-tissue swelling overlying it.

appearance may resemble rather closely that seen in osteochondrosis. Visualization of soft-tissue swelling over the tuberosity plus the clinical signs of pain and local tenderness should be present before the diagnosis of Osgood-Schlatter disease is made. As a sequela to healing, some of the fragmented portions may not unite but remain as small, round or ovoid bony shadows.

VERTEBRAL EPIPHYSES (SCHEUERMANN'S DISEASE). At about the ages of 13 to 15 there appear narrow ringlike epiphyses along the upper and lower margins of the vertebral bodies. These may be involved by an osteochondrosis particularly those in the midthoracic area. The epiphyseal plates lose their sharp outlines and regular appearances; they often become fragmented and somewhat sclerotic. The adjacent border of the vertebral body becomes irregular. Probably because of disturbance in growth, such vertebrae tend to become wedge-shaped with decrease in height anteriorly and this in turn leads to a dorsal kyphosis (Fig. 8-7). While involvement of several or many vertebral bodies is the rule, occasionally the disease may be confined to only one or two. After the disease has healed, some irregularity of the disc surfaces persists and the anterior wedging and kyphotic deformity continue throughout life. Deficiency of the anterior portions of the epiphyseal plates may cause a notchlike defect along the anterior corners of the bodies. Schmorl's nodes also are common. These are seen as small, concave defects on the disc surfaces of one or more vertebrae. They are said to be caused by the softness of the vertebral body allowing protrusion of disc material into it. However, their presence also suggests that the fault is a defect in ossification of the vertebral end-plate allowing herniation of the nucleus pulposis of the disc into the body and that the process is one of faulty ossification. Some investigators have expressed doubt that the vertebral epiphyses are ever affected by ischemic necrosis; rather, they believe that the irregularities in contour, anterior wedge deformities, and the dorsal kyphosis represent the effects of faulty ossification.

SECOND METATARSAL HEAD (KÖHLER-FREIBERG INFRACTION). This lesion is found in the head of the second metatarsal, less commonly in the third and the first. Although originally considered by Köhler to be a form of aseptic necrosis it now is generally considered to represent an infraction or a stress type of fracture involving the metatarsal head. It is found during late adolescence. The articular end of the bone becomes flattened, sometimes concave, and irregular. With healing the neck of the metatarsal becomes thickened and sclerotic (Fig. 8-8). Tiny fragments of bone may become separated from the articular surface and remain as small ossicles after healing is complete.

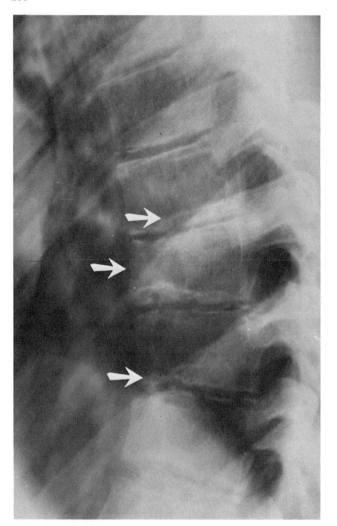

Fig. 8-7. Scheuermann's disease of the thoracic spine. One of the vertebra (**central arrow**) is wedge-shaped and its disc surfaces irregular. This latter change appears to be caused by fragmentation of the ring epiphyses, particularly the inferior. There is minor involvement with Schmorl node defects in several of the other bodies (**upper and lower arrows**).

APOPHYSIS OF OS CALCIS. The apophysis of the os calcis is an epiphyseal plate that develops along the posterior border of the bone. It has been reported as the site of an osteochondrosis with the apophysis becoming dense and sclerotic and undergoing fragmentation. It has been considered to be a frequent cause for painful heels in children. This apophysis normally varies a great deal in density and in many normal children it has a uniform chalky white appearance; it may ossify from several centers. The diagnosis of osteochondrosis involving it should be made with caution and is seldom justified on roentgenologic grounds.

OSTEOCHONDRITIS DISSECANS. This lesion is a form of ischemic necrosis but one that involves only a small portion of bone, usually the articu-

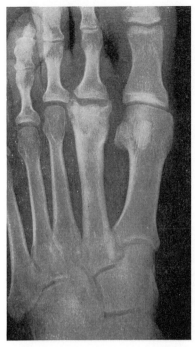

Fig. 8-8. Köhler-Freiberg infraction of the head of the second metatarsal bone. The distal end of the second metatarsal shows an irregular, concave articular surface and the head and neck of the bone are generally thickened. This is a characteristic appearance of this lesion.

lar surface of the medial condyle of the femur. It occurs during adolescence, chiefly in males, and is characterized by the gradual separation of a button-shaped fragment of bone and cartilage from the condylar surface (Fig. 8-9). It is bilateral in about 20 per cent of cases. The disease shows an unusual tendency for involving this particular site for reasons that are not clear. The fragment may separate completely from its bed and become a loose body within the joint cavity, leaving a shallow defect in the articular surface of the femur. If it does not become completely separated the button of bone may remain within its cavity either becoming absorbed or eventually developing a new blood supply and becoming revitalized. Infrequently, this lesion is found in other areas, particularly in the articular surface of the head of the femur, the articular margin of the astrag-

alus, and the internal surface of the patella (Fig. 8-9).

EPIPHYSEOLYSIS (SLIPPING OF THE CAPITAL FEMORAL EPIPHYSIS). This lesion has been classified by some as an ischemic necrosis affecting the epiphyseal plate of the proximal end of the femur; the head of the femur does not become avascular. Other writers, however, believe the lesion is most likely caused by trauma or else that the etiology remains unknown. It is placed here for convenience and because it enters into the differential diagnosis of Perthes' disease. The lesion develops during adolescence and is most frequent in overweight boys of the Froelich type. There is an increased incidence of epiphyseolysis in renal osteodystrophy. The lesion is a gradual slipping of the femoral head on the neck or, more correctly, of the neck on the head as the head remains in the acetabulum. There is upward displacement, external rotation and adduction of the neck on the head. The early deformity is seen to best advantage in a lateral or "frog" view of the hip (Fig. 8-10). In straight anteroposterior views the displacement may not be apparent. There is widening of the epiphyseal line and irregularity of the surface of the metaphysis. The lesion progresses slowly over a period of several years. Since growth is proceeding during this time the neck of the femur is remodeled to some extent. It develops a convex superior surface instead of the normal concavity and the appearance becomes more characteristic in straight anteroposterior views (Fig. 8-11). When the epiphysis fuses the lesion stops progressing but any deformity that has occurred will be permanent. As with Perthes' disease, the early development of degenerative joint disease in the hip is a frequent complication.

In addition to the above, many other epiphyseal centers have been reported as sites of osteochondrosis. Thus the disease has been described as occurring in the epiphyseal plates along the lateral margins of the sacrum, in the carpal scaphoid and in other locations. An example of one of the rare lesions is *Calvé's vertebra plana*. In this lesion a single vertebral

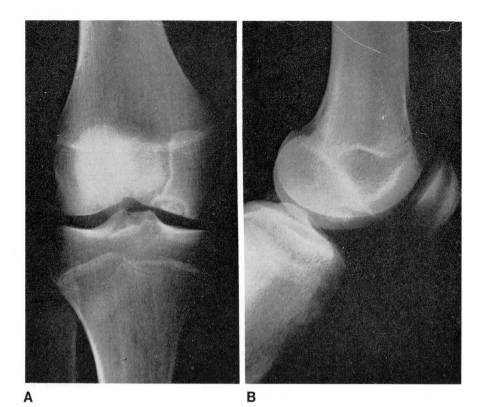

A   **B**

Fig. 8-9. Osteochondritis dissecans of the medial condyle of the femur. *A*, Antero-posterior roentgenogram of the knee showing a buttonlike fragment of bone lying within a cavity in the articular surface of the medial femoral condyle. *B*, Lateral roent-genogram of the same knee. The buttonlike fragment of bone can be visualized clearly. In this case the fragment apparently is still attached and has not become free in the joint. *C*, Osteochondritis dissecans involving the patella. Lateral roentgenogram of the knee shows separation of a small fragment of bone from the inferior articular surface of the patella.

C

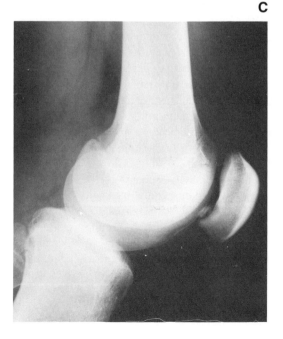

body undergoes a uniform compression and flattening until it comes to resemble a thin disc. A number of cases have been reported in which this configuration has been found to result from involvement of the vertebral body by an *eosinophilic granuloma*. It has also been seen in Hand-Schüller-Christian disease. When this type of lesion is encountered in a child, the diagnosis of histiocytosis usually is justified. These observations again emphasize the need for caution whenever the diagnosis of osteo-chondrosis is a consideration in the growing skeleton.

EPIPHYSEAL ISCHEMIC NECROSIS SECONDARY TO OTHER DISEASE

There are several generalized diseases and toxic agents that can cause ischemic necrosis of an epiphysis, particularly that for the head of

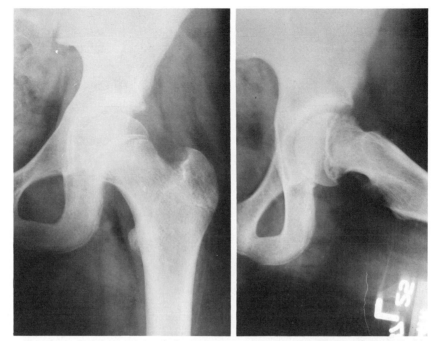

Fig. 8-10. Epiphyseolysis. *Left,* Anteroposterior roentgenogram of the left hip shows very little in the way of abnormality. The epiphyseal plate may be a little wider than normal and the metaphysis slightly irregular in density. *Right,* Lateral roentgenogram of the same hip taken at same time as the anteroposterior view. This projection shows much more clearly the beginning displacement of the neck on the head and the irregularity of the metaphysis. In early cases of epiphyseolysis a lateral roentgenogram is invaluable.

the femur, by occlusion of the vessels supplying the epiphysis. The causes of ischemic necrosis in adults are listed in the section on "Ischemic Necrosis of the Ends of Bones in the Adult" and some of these will also be found in children. In sickle-cell anemia, thrombosis is considered to be the cause of the occlusion. In Gaucher's disease the medullary spaces are filled with Gaucher's cells and the vessels are occluded by pressure. A similar situation may exist in the histiocytoses. In still other entities the mechanism of vascular compromise has not been entirely clarified. Repeated trauma or microtrauma may be responsible in some where the bone and joint structures may have been rendered less sensitive or insensitive to pain.

When the capital femoral epiphysis is the site of the lesion, the roentgen appearance resembles Perthes' disease. However, the metaph-ysis may not be involved as it is in Perthes' disease and the lesion often develops at a later age period. Also, other areas of ischemic necrosis may be found not only in epiphyses but as infarcts involving the shafts of the long and short tubular bones or the vertebrae and the causative disease may have been identified previously.

ISCHEMIC NECROSIS OF THE ENDS OF BONES IN THE ADULT

Changes in the articular ends of the bones in adults and suggesting ischemic necrosis are relatively common. The head of the femur is most frequently involved but other bones may be the sites of the disease. As in the child, these changes appear to have two major causes, (*1*) trauma and, (*2*) vascular occlusion. Posttrau-

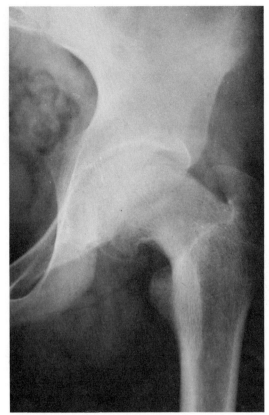

Fig. 8-11. Epiphyseolysis. Anteroposterior roentgenogram of the hip shows more advanced disease than illustrated in Fig. 8-10. There has been a gradual upward displacement of the neck on the head. This has occurred slowly enough so that remodeling of the neck has occurred to some extent. Characteristically there is a convexity of the upper border of the junction of the head and neck instead of the normal concavity.

6. Histiocytosis

7. Sickle-cell anemia

8. Radiation therapy

9. Pain relieving drugs other than steroids

10. Chronic alcoholism

11. Chronic pancreatitis

12. Arteriosclerosis

13. Gout

14. Systemic lupus erythematosis

15. Idiopathic disease

THE HEAD OF THE FEMUR

Following acute injury, either a fracture of the femoral neck or a dislocation of the femoral head, there may be sufficient disruption of the blood supply to the head so that a portion of it undergoes ischemic necrosis.

The area of femoral head involved usually is the superior portion where weight-bearing stress is greatest. The lesion may not develop until some time after healing of the fracture, particularly if operative procedures on the hip have been done, or it may begin immediately after the injury. During the early stage the area of devitalized bone usually appears denser than the adjacent viable bone and may be separated from it by a thin lucent zone. The increased density in this early stage is most likely owing to osteoporosis in the adjacent viable bone. The dead bone, having no blood supply, cannot change density and thus maintains the appearance of normal bone until revascularization has taken place. The dead fragment often has a triangular shape with the apex pointing toward the neck. Later, the fragment undergoes compression causing flattening of the articular surface of the head and it may separate into several pieces. The lucent zone becomes more distinct and a dense sclerotic reaction develops in the viable bone adjacent to the dead fragment (Figs. 8-12 and 8-13). Healing is a slow process with revascularization followed by removal of dead bone and the deposition of new bone.

A similar lesion may develop from a variety of other causes as listed in the section "Is-

matic changes may follow a single, acute injury or be the result of repeated episodes of trauma or microtrauma. A list of the diseases or toxic agents that may cause ischemic necrosis and that have been mentioned in the literature includes the following:

1. Acute trauma—fracture or dislocation

2. Caisson disease

3. Steroid therapy

4. Cushing's disease

5. Gaucher's disease

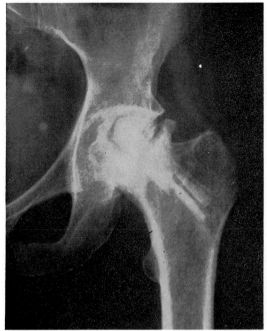

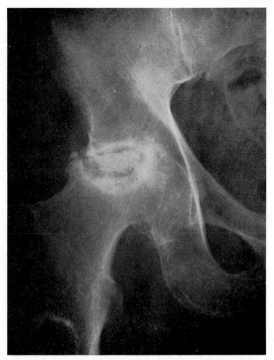

Fig. 8-12. Ischemic necrosis of the head of the femur in an adult. The patient had a previous subcapital fracture of the femur which was openly reduced and a nail inserted. The fracture did not heal, the nail was removed and replaced by split bone grafts. The fracture then healed but a short time later evidence of ischemic necrosis became apparent. There is separation of a rounded fragment of the head superiorly which has lost its blood supply. It is bounded by a lucent zone and a dense, sclerotic border in the adjacent bone.

Fig. 8-13. Ischemic necrosis of the head of the femur, idiopathic type. Note resemblance to the lesion shown in Figure 8-12.

chemic Necrosis of the Ends of Bones in Adults." In many of these the early appearance resembles Perthes' disease with the presence of a thin, curved or arclike translucent zone separating a narrow fragment of subchondral bone from the articular surface. Fragmentation and crushing of the subchondral bone develops and further progress is similar to that seen in Perthes' disease. This appearance is frequent when ischemic necrosis develops after steroid therapy (Fig. 8-14) or in Cushing's disease. In caisson disease and in sickle-cell anemia there often are associated shaft infarctions which are visible roentgenologically. In some patients no causative lesion is apparent and this is known as the idiopathic form of the disease. Many of

these hips also show evidence of well-marked degenerative joint disease.

The pathogenesis of ischemic necrosis developing in chronic alcoholism and in chronic pancreatitis is uncertain although several theories have been proposed including fat embolism. However the high incidence of trauma, often unremembered, in chronic alcoholics is well known. The frequency of chronic subdural hematoma in these individuals is noteworthy. The same factors may be operative in the causation of ischemic necrosis of bone.[19] Many patients with chronic pancreatitis also suffer from chronic alcoholism and the relationship may be significant.

OTHER AREAS

Either as a result of a single injury or following repeated minor traumas, the carpal lunate may develop changes suggesting ischemic

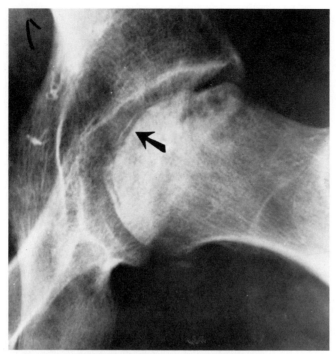

Fig. 8-14. Ischemic necrosis of the head of the femur after steroid therapy. Note the thin, lucent crescent separating a narrow fragment of subchondral bone (**arrow**). The head is moderately flattened and generally selerotic except for areas of absorption superiorly. The joint space and acetabulum are not involved.

necrosis. This lesion has been known as *Kienbock's malacia*. The bone becomes flattened in contour, increased in density and may fragment (Fig. 8-15). The proximal fragment of a fractured carpal navicular may develop a similar type of change. Normally, the blood supply to this part of the bone is poor. A fracture through the neck of the astragalus very often is followed by ischemic necrosis of the articular portion of the bone. *Kümmel's disease* has been considered to be an avascular necrosis of a vertebral body which develops after an injury, with no roentgen evidence of fracture immediately after the injury. The lesion, however, may very well be an unrecognized fracture with compression of the vertebral body occurring later because of continued weight bearing. The lesion is very infrequent and some authors have doubted its existence.

BONE INFARCTION OF THE DIAPHYSIS

In addition to infarcts in the subchondral areas of bone, infarction may involve an area in the shaft and with a different roentgen appearance. In some diseases, such as sickle-cell anemia and caisson disease, infarction may occur in both areas. Also in sickle-cell anemia, infarction of one or more of the short tubular bones may occur (i.e., the "hand-foot syndrome"). At other times only shaft infarction is seen. Not infrequently the roentgen changes characteristic of infarction are completely asymptomatic and are found by chance on examination for some other reason. The role of arteriosclerosis in causation of the infarction in these cases is difficult to assess.

During the acute stage of an infarct of the diaphysis there are no roentgen changes. In-

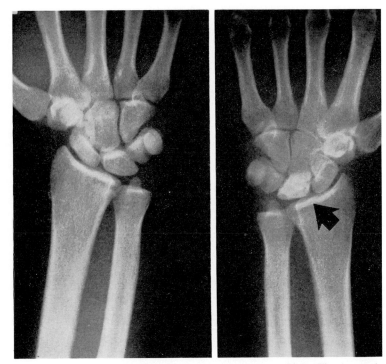

Fig. 8-15. Kienböck's malacia of the carpal lunate. *Right,* The lunate is of increased density as compared to the adjacent carpal bones and is somewhat flattened (**arrow**). Compare with the normal bones in the wrist on the *left.*

farcted bone does not undergo change in density because there are no vessels to carry minerals away or bring new minerals in. Not until revascularization takes place does the density of the infarcted area change. Then the dead bone is gradually removed and the area becomes irregularly calcified. Usually there is a thin rim of sclerosis bounding the lesion (Fig. 8-16). The "scar" of the infarct apparently remains throughout the rest of the life of the individual. Infarction of the shafts of the short tubular bones in the hands and feet in sickle-cell anemia has a different appearance and resembles osteomyelitis very closely. Both infarction and infection may be present in the same patient.

Irregular calcification of cartilage islands that have failed to ossify during the course of bone growth may lead to a rather similar appearance in the long bones. These have been termed *calcified chondromas* or *calcified medullary defects* (Fig. 8-17). Differentiation from a healed bone infarct may be difficult and probably is unnecessary in most instances. Calcified enchondromas are likely to be more mottled in appearance and without a rim of density marking off the boundary as is noted in infarction.

CHEMICAL POISONING

LEAD POISONING

While lead is deposited in the bones of adults, it produces no recognizable alteration in the roentgen shadows of the osseous system and roentgen examination cannot be expected to yield any important information. If lead poisoning occurs before endochondral bone

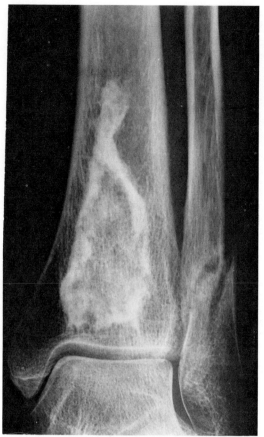

Fig. 8-16. Shaft infarct. The "scar" of the infarct remains as a triangular area of sclerosis bounded by a sclerotic rim. The examination was done because of a fracture of the lateral malleolus.

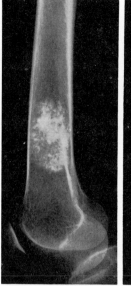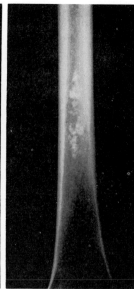

Fig. 8-17. Calcified enchondromas. Two cases showing the characteristic mottled calcification within the medullary canal. Note the lack of a boundary rim of sclerosis as seen in Figure 8-16.

growth is completed, however, changes do occur that may be of considerable value in arriving at the correct diagnosis. The significant alteration is the appearance of dense transverse bands extending across the metaphyses of the long bones and along the margins of the flat bones, such as the pelvis (Fig. 8-18). The width of the "lead line" varies and depends upon the amount of lead ingested and the length of time it has been taken. It has been shown that the increased density is not caused by lead alone but also by increased calcium content. This results from a failure of proper absorption of calcium from the zones of provisional calcification. Except for the development of these transverse zones of density, the bones and epiphyses remain normal. After the intake of lead has been discontinued normal bone forms on the epiphyseal side of the metaphysis and the lead line appears to migrate into the shaft. It usually becomes wider and less dense for a time and then gradually disappears. In normal active infants the metaphyses of the long bones often show an unusual whiteness and appear wider than one might expect. This should not be confused with lead poisoning. The incidence of lead poisoning in infants is low except in children living in "inner-core" areas of large cities.

PHOSPHORUS POISONING

At one time phosphorus poisoning was a serious health hazard during infancy but this is no longer the case. The possibilities for obtaining yellow phosphorus are negligible at the present time. The ingestion of this substance in sufficient amounts produces changes that are indistinguishable from those resulting from the ingestion of lead.

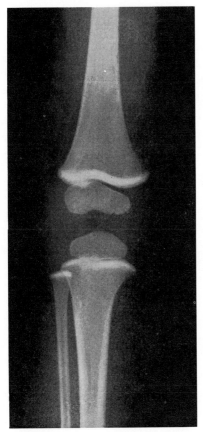

Fig. 8-18. Lead poisoning. Anteroposterior roentgenogram of the knee showing zones of increased density involving the metaphyses. This is characteristic of heavy metal poisoning.

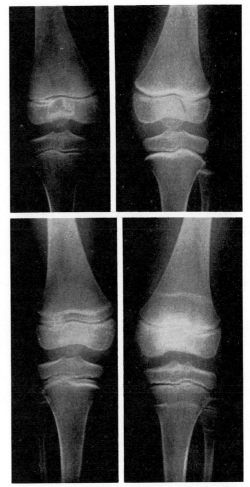

Fig. 8-19. Bismuth lines. The child was treated for congenital syphilis with bismuth preparations. *Upper left,* Appearance of the knee joint before the administration of bismuth. *Upper right,* Appearance shortly after completion of a course of bismuth therapy. *Lower left,* Appearance several months later after discontinuation of the bismuth. The bismuth lines appear to have migrated into the shaft. This appearance is caused by the formation of normal bone during the process of growth. *Lower right,* Appearance approximately 1 year later. The lines have migrated farther into the shafts, indicating the amount of growth that has taken place after the medication was discontinued.

BISMUTH POISONING

Poisoning from bismuth usually has followed the administration of large doses of this substance for the treatment of congenital syphilis. Bismuth produces changes exactly like those caused by lead and as with phosphorus cannot be differentiated from lead poisoning on the basis of roentgen examination (Fig. 8-19).

FLUORINE INTOXICATION

Fluorine poisoning is a rare cause of abnormal bones and is found mainly in adults, either as a result of exposure to high concentrations of fluorides as an occupational hazard or from drinking water containing a high concentration of these substances. There are only a few areas in the United States where such concentrations occur in the drinking water and these are chiefly in certain parts of Texas. In industry the mining and conversion of phosphate rock into fertilizer and the use of fluorides in the smelting of metals offer possible sources for poisoning. The major alteration in the skeleton is a diffuse increase in density. The bones appear abnormally white. The trabecular architecture is, if anything, accentuated. The cortices become thickened. Calcific spurs may form at the sites of ligament attachments. In spite of rather marked alteration in the bones, there usually are few symptoms referable to the condition and the patients may be surprisingly healthy. Fluoride poisoning must be considered as an unusual cause of generalized increase in density of the bones in this country.

HYPERVITAMINOSIS D

Excessive intake of vitamin D may lead to demonstrable changes on roentgen examination. This condition in adults has been seen most frequently in patients with rheumatoid arthritis who were treated with large doses of this vitamin. It has also been found in children where excessive doses or errors in dosage have occurred. The serum calcium is elevated and the urine calcium is high. On roentgen examination of adults there may be found: (1) Deposition of calcium in the soft tissues, particularly around the joints. These deposits have an amorphous puttylike appearance. Calcification of the arteries may be noted even in the young. Renal calcification often occurs. (2) Chronic decalcification of the skeleton is frequent. Since many of these patients have rheumatoid arthritis and this disease usually is accompanied by skeletal decalcification, this finding may be difficult to evaluate.

In infancy hypervitaminosis D usually follows errors in dosage. It results in metastatic calcification in the media of the blood vessels, kidneys, heart, gastric wall, falx cerebri, tentorium, and adrenals. In the tubular bones there is widening of the zones of provisional calcification, causing dense bands extending across the metaphyses similar to lead poisoning. Later, there may be cortical thickening. Also, in the later stages there may be alternating bands of increased and decreased density crossing the ends of the shafts and an overall osteoporosis.

IDIOPATHIC HYPERCALCEMIA

In this rare disorder there is an abnormally high level of calcium in the blood, causing an osteosclerosis similar to that seen in some cases of osteopetrosis (marble bone disease) and in hypervitaminosis D in infants. The cause is obscure, but it has been suggested that the disease may represent an unusual sensitivity to vitamin D. According to Aegerter and Kirkpatrick, the disease has been more prevalent in England than in the United States and in the past the amounts of vitamin D supplement in foods was not well regulated in Britain. It has been suggested that some infants may have ingested excessive amounts of vitamin in food and as a result developed vitamin D poisoning. More recently stricter controls and limits have been put into effect and the incidence of the disease has decreased considerably. The clinical observations mirror the effects of the hypercalcemia and include muscular weakness and hypotonia, anorexia, vomiting, and failure of the infant to thrive and to develop properly. There is mental as well as physical retardation. The roentgen findings are essentially the same as those found in hypervitaminosis D (Fig. 8-20). The most specific sign in both is the demonstration of calcium in the falx, tentorium, and gastric wall during infancy.

HYPERVITAMINOSIS A

Vitamin A poisoning from excessive administration is seen most frequently in the young infant as a result of errors in dosage. Clinically there are anorexia, failure to gain weight, pruritus, pain and swelling over the long bones, and hepato- and splenomegaly. The serum alkaline phosphatase may be increased and the serum proteins lowered. The level of vitamin A in the blood serum is high. On roentgen examination one may find the following:

Periosteal calcification, mainly around the central shafts of some of the long bones. The bones most frequently affected are the ulna and

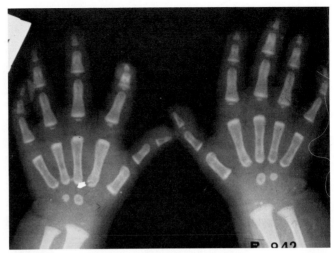

Fig. 8-20. Idiopathic hypercalcemia. There are dense bands crossing the metaphyses, best seen at the proximal metaphysis of the first metacarpal and the distal ends of the second to fifth metacarpals and the adjacent proximal phalanges. The changes resemble heavy metal poisoning and are similar to those of hypervitaminosis D.

clavicle; next in frequency are the femur and tibia. The periosteal calcification is the greatest near the center of the shaft and tapers toward the ends.

This disease must be distinguished chiefly from infantile cortical hyperostosis (see under section "Infantile Cortical Hyperostosis"). In this latter disease the mandible is almost always affected and is usually the first bone to be involved. The disease is accompanied by fever and the other signs of infection. It develops early in life within the first few weeks or months; vitamin A poisoning usually occurs somewhat later, rarely before the age of 1 year. The final diagnosis rests upon the history of the administration of excessive amounts of the vitamin and the determination of the level of vitamin A in the serum.

INFANTILE CORTICAL HYPEROSTOSIS (CAFFEY'S DISEASE)

This is an uncommon disease of infancy, the cause of which is unknown. In many respects the disease behaves like an infection, but there is no proof of this and biopsy of affected bone has failed to show the usual findings of an infection. It is a disease of early infancy, having its onset within the first few weeks of life in most cases. Occasionally the disease has been encountered in older infants up to the age of 2 years. The familial nature of the disease has been reported. Clinically, there is swelling of the soft tissues overlying the affected bone. The skin, however, is neither hot nor red. There are fever, irritability, and other signs suggesting an infection. The disease tends to show remissions and exacerbations but eventually recovery takes place, after a period of weeks or months. The favorite sites for the development of the lesions are the mandible and the clavicles. Less frequently the ulna, radius, ribs, tibia, and fibula are affected. Apparently the mandible is nearly always involved, regardless of what other bones are affected, and this seems to be one of the characteristics of the disease. On roentgen examination there is noted a laminated subperiosteal calcification surrounding the bone. This may involve only a short segment at first but eventually may extend throughout the entire shaft of a long bone (Fig. 8-21). In the jaw the major portion of the mandible may be affected. At first the subperiosteal new bone formation is less dense than the cortex beneath it but eventually the density increases and the two shadows merge (Figs. 8-21 and 8-22). The outer margin may be rather irregular and wavy or it may be smooth. As healing takes place, there is a gradual resorption of the subperiosteal bone formation and the bone gradually returns to a normal or nearly normal appearance. The lesions bear a close resemblance to those found in hypervitaminosis A.

EFFECTS OF RADIATION ON BONE

Damage to bone can result from heavy doses of roentgen radiation. It seems probable that

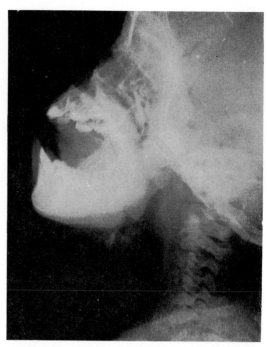

Fig. 8-22. Infantile cortical hyperostosis. Lateral roentgenogram of the jaw showing the characteristic changes in a well-developed case. The patient was a 5-month-old male infant in whom symptoms had been present for approximately 3 months. These consisted of fever, irritability, and the development of swelling of the lower jaw. The mandible is thickened and of increased density. There is a thin shell of periosteal calcification visible along the inferior surface.

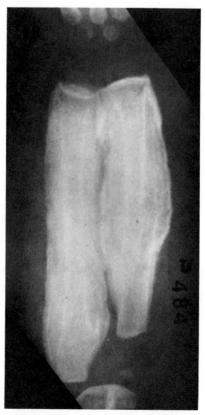

Fig. 8-21. Infantile cortical hyperostosis of the radius and ulna. There is extensive periosteal calcification surrounding the shafts which can be faintly seen through the dense calcification.

the effects of the radiation are largely upon the blood vessels supplying the bone. Initially there may be hyperemia, leading to osteoporosis. In a later stage disintegration of the bone with ischemic necrosis and pathologic fracture may result. The effects can be seen in any bone that has received a sufficient amount of radiation. Fracture of the femoral neck following pelvic irradiation for carcinoma in the female is an occasional complication of the treatment. The bone may appear surprisingly normal to roentgen examination except for the fracture. Fractures of the ribs with focal areas of absorption have been seen after repeated treatment given to the chest wall following mastectomy for carcinoma of the breast.[23] These have been asymptomatic as a rule (Fig. 8-23).

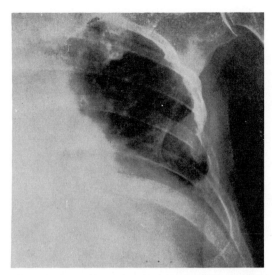

Fig. 8-23. Radiation osteitis of the ribs. The patient had received intensive radiation therapy to the chest as a postoperative treatment for carcinoma of the breast. After an interval of several years areas of absorption developed in the lateral segments of several of the ribs. This progressed to pathologic fractures.

Injury to the growing skeleton can be produced by heavy doses of radiation given either for the treatment of a malignant lesion or at repeated sittings for a benign condition such as a hemangioma. Damage to the active centers of bone growth will lead to retardation or cessation of growth and consequent skeletal deformity.

PAGET'S DISEASE (OSTEITIS DEFORMANS)

The cause of Paget's disease is unknown. Pathologically it is characterized by destruction of bone, followed eventually by attempts at repair. The destructive phase may predominate but most frequently there is a combination of destruction and repair. In the pelvis and the weight-bearing bones of the lower extremities, the reparative process may begin early and be a prominent feature. When widely disseminated, elevation of the serum alkaline phosphatase is present and the values may be very high. Renal

calculi (or nephrocalcinosis) may develop from the hypercalciuria.

The average age of onset is between 50 and 55 years. It is increasingly rare below the age of 50 and its occurrence in young persons is disputed. These latter cases may be instances of fibrous dysplasia rather than Paget's disease. Males predominate over females in the ratio of 2:1. There are a number of reports of Paget's disease occurring in multiple members of the same family. Rosenbaum and Hanson[25] have commented on the marked difference in incidence of the disease in different geographic areas.

Paget's disease may involve any bone in the body. It may affect a single bone and never extend to others. It may begin in one bone with others becoming involved at a later date. At times it is widely distributed throughout the skeleton when first discovered. Its slow spread over a period of years has been observed frequently but this does not always happen. In the order of frequency the following bones are affected: pelvis, femur, skull, tibia, vertebrae, clavicle, humerus, and ribs.

ROENTGEN FEATURES

The roentgen appearance depends upon the extent of the reparative process that has developed. If repair (recalcification) is limited, the destructive phase predominates. This is common in the skull and is known as *osteoporosis circumscripta,* but it is also seen in other bones (Fig. 8-24). It is represented by a sharply demarcated area of decalcification within which the architecture of the bone is poorly made out. The bone also may be thickened. Characteristically, the junction between the rarefied bone and normal bone is very sharp. This lesion may enlarge slowly and later, when repair begins, islands of sclerosis develop, giving the lesion a mottled appearance. In the skull the bone becomes thickened, usually only outward, and this may be very great so that the bone measures 3 cm or more in thickness (Fig. 8-25).

In the weight-bearing bones of the lower extremities a combined destructive and reparative

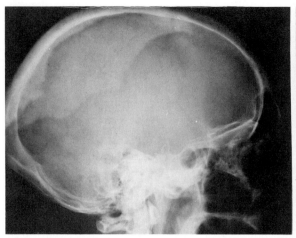 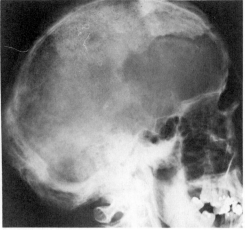

Fig. 8-24. Osteoporosis circumscripta of the skull. *Left,* Lateral roentgenogram of the skull showing the characteristic appearance of a large area of osteoporosis circumscripta. The demineralized bone is sharply demarcated from the normal bone above. *Right,* Lateral roentgenogram of another patient showing osteoporosis circumscripta involving the anterior and inferior portions of the skull with normal bone superiorly. In the occipital area the bone has begun to take on the more characteristic changes of Paget's disease. It has become thickened and rather coarsely trabeculated. The basal angle is flattened.

type of the disease is the most frequent. The bones become bowed because of their softness, the femur outward and the tibia anteriorly. The cortex is thickened but of lessened density and may be mottled as is seen in the skull. The trabeculae that remain are coarse and thickened and extend in the direction required to strengthen the bone for its weight-bearing purposes. Between the coarsened trabeculae, cystlike spaces may be present. Pseudofractures (see Chapter 5) are common along the convex side of the bowed bone. These begin as incomplete transverse fissures and they often are multiple; they may extend completely through the bone and with minor trauma a complete fracture with displacement of fragments may result (Fig. 8-26). Fractures in bones involved by Paget's disease are, characteristically, transverse rather than spiral as they are in ordinary traumatic fracture.

In the pelvis a combination of destruction and repair is most frequent. Coarsening of the trabeculae is present and is best seen, early, along the iliac margins. The sacrum may be the first or the only bone involved and the coarse trabeculation causes a distinctive cross-hatched appearance. Areas of decalcification are common in the central portions of the iliac bones, similar to those found in the skull. The reparative process occasionally predominates so that the affected bone is very dense and somewhat enlarged. The resemblance to osteoblastic metastasis is striking, but careful observation will usually show areas with the typical coarse trabeculation, which is never encountered in metastasis (Fig. 8-29). Because of softening there may be intrapelvic protrusion of the acetabular cavities.

In the vertebrae the disease usually affects multiple bodies but rarely all of them. Coarse trabeculation is prominent along the edges so that the margin of the body is emphasized. The general texture is coarse. The vertebra may be enlarged. Compression fractures are frequent because of the softness of the bones.

In the ribs it is common to find only one or a few affected. The bone is thickened, the general density is increased, but the trabecular structure is typically coarse. The same pattern occurs in the clavicle. Osteogenic sarcoma may develop in an area of Paget's disease and is reported to occur in about 10 per cent of the cases. This figure is based on old statistics and probably is much too high, since isolated bone

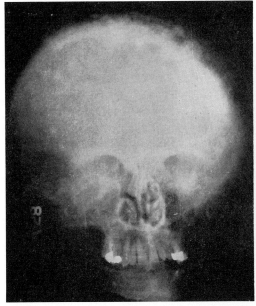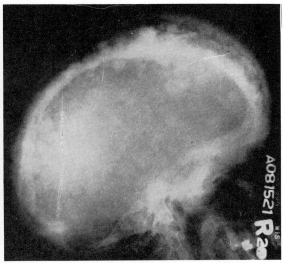

Fig. 8-25. Paget's disease of the skull. Anteroposterior and lateral roentgenograms showing character-istic changes of Paget's disease in an advanced form. There is a pronounced thickening of the bones of the skull. There are many islands of increased density scattered within osteoporotic bone, giving the skull a mottled appearance. The flattening of the basal angle is noteworthy and in the anteroposterior view the widened base of the skull is apparent. This is a characteristic configuration of the skull in advanced Paget's disease.

lesions are being found with considerable fre-quency during routine studies that include the bones of the lower spine and pelvis (such as gastrointestinal and urinary tract roentgenog-raphy). Nevertheless, Paget's disease accounts for many of the cases of osteogenic sarcoma that develop in persons beyond the age of 50 years (see Fig. 7-16).

CHRONIC ANEMIAS

There are a number of congenital anemias, most of them uncommon, that can cause changes in the skeletal system. The three that are best known, roentgenologically, are (1) Cooley's anemia, (2) sickle-cell anemia, and (3) hereditary spherocytosis (familial hemo-lytic anemia). In addition, variants of the above and other rare hemolytic anemias can cause similar changes, although usually much milder. Also, changes in the skull similar to those of the

congenital anemias have been found in chronic iron deficiency anemia, cyanotic congenital heart disease and polycythemia vera in child-hood.

The skeletal alterations are caused by ery-throid hyperplasia of the bone marrow which fills and expands the cancellous bone and dis-turbs the trabecular architecture.

COOLEY'S ANEMIA

This disease also is known as thalassemia major and Mediterranean anemia. It occurs predominately in persons belonging to races living along the Mediterranean Sea (i.e., Greek and Italian). The disease occurs occasionally in persons of other nationalities. In the periph-eral parts of the skeleton roentgen changes consist in widening of the shafts so that bones such as the metacarpals, metatarsals, and phalanges have a rectangular appearance, the normal concavity of the shafts being lost.

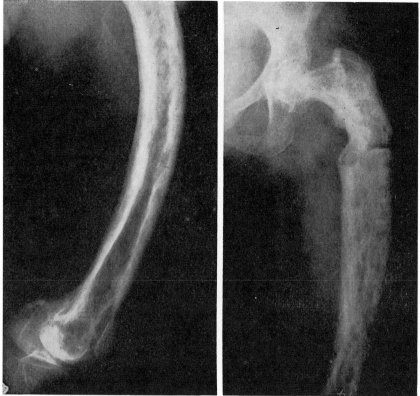

Fig. 8-26. Paget's disease of the femur. *Left,* Lateral roentgenogram of the femur showing characteristic changes of Paget's disease as it involves this bone. There is anterior bowing, the cortex is irregularly thickened, and there is a general coarsening of the trabecular architecture. Pseudofractures in the anterior cortex represented by fine hairline fissures. *Right,* Anteroposterior roentgenogram of another case, showing advanced Paget's disease involving the femur. In this patient there has been a complete fracture through the upper third of the shaft with resulting offset of fragments. The fracture has healed with callus on the medial side but a cleftlike fissure remains on the outer side.

The cortices are thinned. The medullary cavities have a spongy, mottled appearance. The trabecular pattern of the bone is coarsened (Fig. 8-27A). At times thin transverse bands of increased density, the so-called growth lines, can be seen crossing the shafts. In the skull, characteristically, there is a widening of the diploic space, particularly in the frontal and parietal regions (Fig. 8-27B). The occipital squamosa usually is not affected. The outer table is thinned and may become deficient in areas so that marrow can protrude into the subperiosteal space. Frequently there are radiating trabeculae of bone extending at right angles to the inner and outer tables giving a "hair on end" appearance.

In severe cases there is retardation of skeletal growth. In older patients the changes in the small bones of the hands and feet become less striking and may disappear completely by the time puberty is reached. Changes in the skull, spine, and pelvis, where red marrow persists, may become more pronounced after puberty. The paranasal sinuses may be poorly developed, particularly the maxillary sinuses. Encroachment on the sinus air spaces is caused by thickening of the bony walls owing to marrow hyperplasia; it does not affect the ethmoid cells

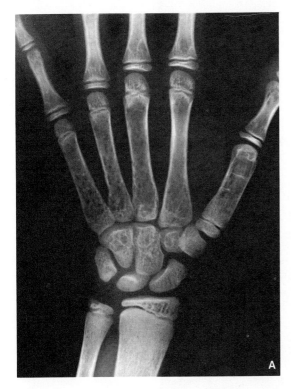

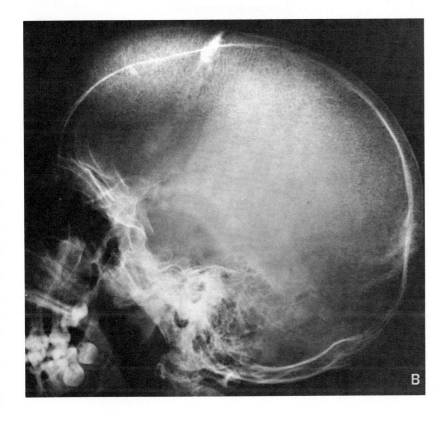

Fig. 8-27. Cooley's anemia (thalassemia major). *A,* The phalanges are less involved than the metacarpals. The cortices are thinned, the mid shafts show decrease in or lack of normal constriction and there is decreased trabeculation. The medullary cavities have a mottled appearance. The carpal bones and radial epiphysis show similar changes. Note transverse "growth arrest" lines in first metacarpal. *B,* Lateral view of the skull illustrates the marked thickening of the bone in the frontal area. The base also is sclerotic. (Courtesy Dr. M. P. Neal, Jr., and Dr. T. R. Howell, Department of Radiology, Medical College of Virginia, Richmond.)

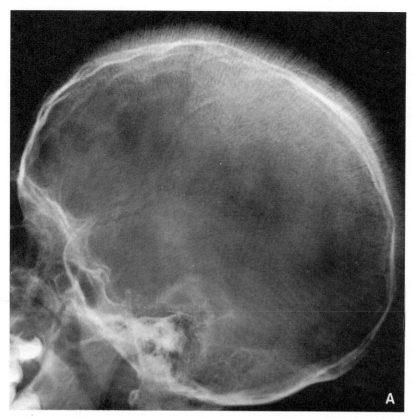

Fig. 8-28. Sickle cell anemia. *A,* Lateral view of skull illustrating thickening of the bones of the vault, particularly in the frontoparietal area with characteristic perpendicular striations ("hair-on-end" appearance). The outer table is indistinct and completely absent in areas. (There also is premature fusion of the vault sutures.) *B,* The "scar" of a shaft infarct is seen in the distal shaft of the femur as an irregularly calcified area (**arrows**). Similar lesion in opposite femur. (Courtesy Dr. M. P. Neal, Jr., and Dr. T. R. Howell, Department of Radiology, Medical College of Virginia, Richmond).

because of a lack of red marrow here. Enlargement of the maxilla may lead to malocclusion and overbite on the mandible. Pathologic fracture may occur through weakened bone, although it is not common. Gallstones occur as a complication of Cooley's anemia.

SICKLE-CELL ANEMIA

This disease occurs in Negroes as a result of an abnormal hemoglobin (hemoglobin S); it is transmitted by heredity as a dominant gene. Those who are heterozygous for the hemoglobin S gene have what is referred to as the *sickle-cell trait*. Those who are homozygous for the gene, inheriting one such gene from each parent, develop sickle-cell anemia.

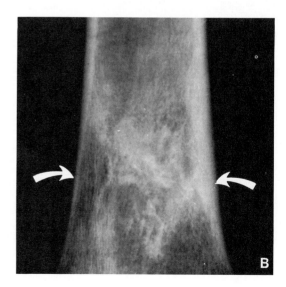

In general the roentgen findings are similar to those found in Cooley's anemia (Fig. 8-28A). In addition, bone infarction is common (Fig. 8-28B). During infancy these tend to involve the small bones of the hands and feet producing a dactylitis (the "hand-foot syndrome"). This appears as an irregular area of destruction with overlying periosteal calcification resembling an inflammatory process. Since both infarction and infection may be present in the same bone differentiation is hardly possible. In older children bone infarction is more common in the epiphyses. This may cause an appearance quite similar to Perthes' disease. There is local rarefaction of bone followed by impaction of the weight-bearing surface. Increase in subchondral bone density especially in the heads of the femur and humerus, appar-

ently owing to previous multiple small infarctions, may be seen. The appearance of a "bone within a bone" also has been described, again probably the result of previous infarction. Osteomyelitis also is a complication of sickle-cell anemia and may develop in any bone. Infection with *Salmonella* is frequent.

In the vertebrae, osteoporosis may be quite severe, leading to compression deformities. The disc surfaces become concave as the discs expand into the softened vertebrae. Reynolds[24] believes the vertebral contour in sickle-cell anemia is characteristic, consisting of localized central depressions of the disc surfaces owing to a disturbance in growth from local ischemia rather than the biconcave contours seen in other causes of vertebral collapse. In adults with long-standing sickle-cell anemia a diffuse

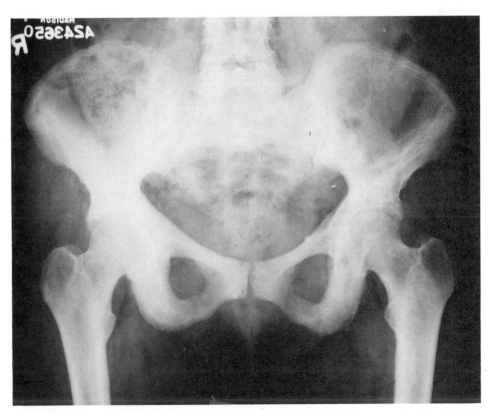

Fig. 8-29. Paget's disease involving the pelvis. All the pelvic bones are involved by the disease. There is a general increase in density but the characteristic coarse trabecular pattern of Paget's disease is predominant. The intensification of trabeculae is noteworthy along the margins of the iliac bones and it is here in early cases that the first changes are often observed.

sclerosis of the bones may be seen, resembling that found in myelofibrosis. The vertebrae, in spite of a sclerotic appearance, are softer than normal and develop biconcave disc surfaces (Fig. 8-30). This, combined with the sclerotic appearance is distinctive for sickle-cell anemia in the older child or adult. In addition there frequently is considerable cardiac enlargement and hepato- and splenomegaly. Cholelithiasis is fairly frequent and may even be found in young individuals.

OTHER ANEMIAS

HEREDITARY SPHEROCYTOSIS

In this disease the bones frequently are entirely normal. When changes are present they resemble those seen in Cooley's anemia, except that they are of a lesser degree and may be limited to the skull.

CHRONIC IRON-DEFICIENCY ANEMIA

Recently, cases have been reported in which skull changes occur which are quite similar to those of Cooley's anemia;[13] we have had similar experience. There is widening of the diplöe and perpendicular trabeculation in the frontal and parietal areas. Changes in other bones, however, are less striking and they may be essentially normal even when well-marked skull changes are present. When long and short tubular bone changes are present they resemble the findings in Cooley's anemia.

SYSTEMIC MASTOCYTOSIS

While this disorder was originally thought to be a disease only of the skin, and known as *urticaria pigmentosa,* it is now recognized that there may be involvement of multiple systems,

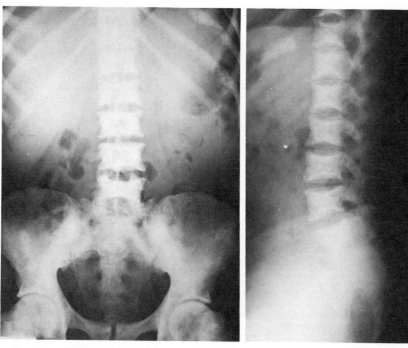

Fig. 8-30. Sickle cell anemia in an adult. Anteroposterior and lateral roentgenograms of the lower spine and pelvis of an adult Negro suffering from sickle cell anemia. The bones are increased in density, having a mottled appearance. There have been expansions of the intervertebral discs causing the disc surfaces of the vertebrae to have biconcave silhouettes. (*Courtesy Dr. J. E. Miller, Dallas, Texas.*)

including the skin, lymph nodes, spleen, liver, and other organs, and the bone marrow. It is characterized by an increased number of connective-tissue mast cells in the involved tissue. The disease is of interest roentgenologically because it can cause an osteosclerosis of the skeleton. In the cases that we have seen this was in the form of generalized increase in density of the bones of the thorax, spine, and pelvis. The appearance closely resembles that seen in cases of myelofibrosis. Others have reported cases where the changes consisted in scattered, well-defined foci of sclerosis. In still other cases radiolucent zones have been found. It is a rare cause of osteosclerosis.

THE RUBELLA SYNDROME

During a virulent epidemic of rubella that occurred in a number of large cities in the United States in 1964, infants born of mothers who had had the disease during the first trimester of pregnancy were found to have a syndrome of anomalies affecting chiefly the cardiovascular system (congenital heart disease), the abdomen (hepatosplenomegaly) and the skeletal system.[26,28] The last is of importance to the present discussion.

In the skull, the anterior fontanelle was unusually large, often extending into the metopic suture. The sutures were not spread but there was deficient mineralization of the margins of the cranial bones. In the long bones changes occurred in the metaphyses, best demonstrated at the knees. The zones of provisional calcification were poorly defined and irregular. The most striking characteristic was the presence of alternating lucent and sclerotic striations extending perpendicular to the epiphyseal plate and parallel to the long axis of the bone (Fig. 8-31). These faded into normal appearing bone in the shafts. Transverse lucent metaphyseal bands were also seen. The bone changes improved rapidly in those infants who thrived and the zones of provisional calcification regained normal smoothness and density. In those infants who did not do well clinically the abnormal trabecular pattern persisted but the zones

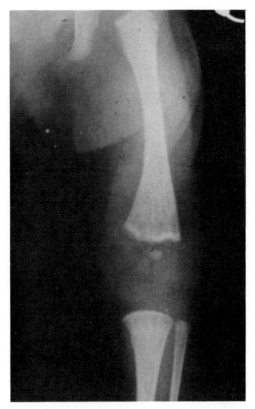

Fig. 8-31. Rubella syndrome. Anteroposterior view of left knee area of a newborn illustrating the alternating longitudinal opaque and lucent striations extending into the shaft from the metaphyses, best seen in the lower femur.

of provisional calcification showed increased density. The most frequent cardiac lesion was a patent ductus arteriosus followed by pulmonary artery branch stenosis. Additional abnormalities included growth retardation, thrombocytopenic purpura, eye defects and deafness. Similar skeletal changes have been reported in a case of cytomegalic inclusion disease so that they may represent a nonspecific response to intrauterine viral infections.[18]

REFERENCES AND SELECTED READINGS

1. Bishop, P. A.: Bone changes in chronic fluorine intoxication. A roentgenographic study. *Am. J. Roentgenol. Radium Ther. Nucl. Med.* 35: 577, 1936.

2. Caffey, J.: Chronic poisoning due to excess of vitamin A. Description of the clinical and roent-

gen manifestations in seven infants and young children. *Am. J. Roentgenol. Radium Ther. Nucl. Med. 65:* 12, 1951.

3. CAFFEY, J.: The early roentgenographic changes in essential coxa plana; their significance in pathogenesis. *Am. J. Roentgenol. Radium Ther. Nucl. Med. 103:* 620, 1968.

4. EDEIKEN, J., HODES, P. J., LIBSHITZ, H. I., and WELLER, M. H.: Bone ischemia. *Radiol. Clin. North Am. 5:* 515, 1967.

5. EHRENPREIS, B., and SCHWINGER, H. N.: Sickle cell anemia. *Am. J. Roentgenol. Radium Ther. Nucl. Med. 68:* 28, 1952.

6. GERLE, R. D., WALKER, L. A., ACHORD, J. L., and WEENS, H. S.: Osseous changes in chronic pancreatitis. *Radiology 85:* 330, 1965.

7. GIRDANY, B. R., and OSMAN, M. Z.: Longitudinal growth and skeletal maturation in Perthes' disease. *Radiol. Clin. North Am. 6:* 245, 1968.

8. HOLMAN, C. B.: Roentgenologic manifestations of vitamin D intoxication. *Radiology 59:* 805, 1952.

9. HOWLAND, W. J., JR., PUGH, D. G., and SPRAGUE, R. G.: Roentgenologic changes of the skeletal system in Cushing's syndrome. *Radiology 71:* 69, 1958.

10. JACOBS, P.: Intra-epiphyseal gas in osteochondritis. *Clin. Radiol. 21:* 318, 1970.

11. JEREMY, R.: Nontraumatic aseptic necrosis of the femoral head. *Med. J. Aust. 1:* 323, 1967.

12. KEMP, H. S., and BOLDERO, J. L.: Radiological changes in Perthes' disease. *Br. J. Radiol. 39:* 744, 1966.

13. LANZKOWSKY, P.: Radiological features of iron deficiency anemia. *Am. J. Dis. Child. 116:* 16, 1968.

14. LEONE, A. J., JR.: On lead lines. *Am. J. Roentgenol. Radium Ther. Nucl. Med. 103:* 165, 1968.

15. LEONE, N.C., STEVENSON, C. A., HILBISH, T. F., and SOSMAN, M. C.: Study of a human population exposed to high-fluoride domestic water; A ten-year study. *Am. J. Roentgenol. Radium Ther. Nucl. Med. 74:* 874, 1955.

16. MALKA, S.: Idiopathic aseptic necrosis of the head of the femur in adults. *Surg. Gynecol. Obstet. 123:* 1057, 1966.

17. MARTEL, W., and POZNANSKI, A. K.: The effect of

traction on the hip in osteonecrosis. *Radiology 94:* 505, 1970.

18. MERTON, D. F., and GOODING, C. A.: Skeletal manifestations of cytomegalic inclusion disease. *Radiology 94:* 333, 1970.

19. MURRAY, R. O.: "Some Current Concepts in Skeletal Radiology," in *Modern Trends in Diagnostic Radiology-4*, ed. by J. W. McLaren. New York, Appleton-Century-Crofts, 1970.

20. NACHEMSON, A., and SCHELLER, S.: A clinical and radiological follow-up study of transient synovitis of the hip. *Acta Orthop. Scand. 40:* 479, 1969.

21. NEUHAUSER, E. B. D., REYERSBACH, G. C., and SOBEL, E. H.: Hypophosphatasia. *Am. J. Roentgenol. Radium Ther. Nucl. Med. 78:* 392, 1957.

22. PAJERSKI, M., and VURE, E.: Late manifestations of infantile cortical hyperostosis (Caffey's disease). *Br. J. Radiol. 40:* 90, 1967.

23. PAUL, L. W., and POHLE, E. A.: Radiation osteitis of the ribs. *Radiology 38:* 543, 1942.

24. REYNOLDS, J.: A re-evaluation of the "fish vertebra" sign in sickle cell hemoglobinopathy. *Am. J. Roentgenol. Radium Ther. Nucl. Med. 97:* 693, 1966.

25. ROSENBAUM, H. D., and HANSON, D. J.: Geographic variation in the prevalence of Paget's disease of bone. *Radiology 92:* 959, 1969.

26. RUDOLPH, A. J., SINGLETON, B., ROSENBERG, H. S., SINGER, D. B., and PHILLIPS, A.: Osseous manifestations of the congenital rubella syndrome. *Am. J. Dis. Child. 110:* 428, 1965.

27. SEAMAN, W. B.: The roentgen appearance of early Paget's disease. *Am. J. Roentgenol. Radium Ther. Nucl. Med. 66:* 587, 1951.

28. SINGLETON, E. B., RUDOLPH, A. J., ROSENBERG, H. S., and SINGER, D. B.: The roentgenographic manifestations of the rubella syndrome in newborn infants. *Am. J. Roentgenol. Radium Ther. Nucl. Med. 97:* 82, 1966.

29. STAHELI, L. T., CHURCH, C. C., and WARD, B. H.: Infantile cortical hyperostosis (Caffey's disease). *JAMA 203:* 384, 1968.

30. VOGT, E. C.: Roentgen signs of plumbism: The lead line in growing bone. *Am. J. Roentgenol. Radium Ther. Nucl. Med. 24:* 550, 1930.

9

DISEASES OF THE JOINTS

In a roentgenogram of a normal joint the ends of the bones are separated by an apparent space; this is occupied by the articular cartilage and the small amount of synovial fluid normally present. For roentgen descriptive purposes this apparent space is commonly referred to as the joint space. Cartilage and synovial fluid are of approximately the same degree of radiopacity and resemble the soft tissues in this respect. The opposing ends of the articular cartilages capping the bones forming a joint cannot ordinarily be identified (see section on "The Vacuum Phenomenon; Gas in the Joints"). Hyaline cartilage, once destroyed, does not regenerate to any degree and loss of articular cartilage is characterized in the roentgenogram as a diminution in the joint space. The synovial membrane cannot be visualized as a structure in roentgenograms. When the joint capsule is distended by fluid, its outer limits often can be seen if there is any fat in the periarticular tissues to offer contrast, but in the normal joint the capsule is an indistinct structure in the roentgenogram. The perichondrium, a fibrous tissue structure that serves to attach the synovial membrane to the bone at the junction of bone and articular cartilage, is an important component of the joint capsule. It is affected in certain inflammatory diseases such as rheumatoid arthritis and in pyogenic and tuberculous lesions of the joints.

CLASSIFICATION OF JOINT DISEASE

I. Infectious Arthritis
   A. Acute infectious arthritis (pyogenic arthritis; septic arthritis)
   B. Chronic infectious arthritis
      1. Chronic pyogenic arthritis
      2. Tuberculous arthritis
      3. Others
II. Rheumatoid Arthritis
   A. Rheumatoid arthritis of the peripheral joints
   B. Rheumatoid arthritis of the spine
   C. Arthritis associated with scleroderma and psoriasis
   D. Still's disease and Felty's syndrome
III. Degenerative Joint Disease (osteoarthritis; osteoarthrosis, etc.)
IV. Gouty Arthritis
V. Neurotrophic Arthropathy
VI. Periarticular Disease (bursitis; tendinitis; fibrositis)
VII. Miscellaneous
   A. Hemophiliac arthropathy
   B. Pigmented villo-nodular synovitis
   C. Xanthomatous tumors of tendons and joints
   D. Synovioma
   E. Chondromatous tumors
      1. Osteochondromatosis
   F. Loose bodies
   G. Other conditions

INFECTIOUS ARTHRITIS

ACUTE AND CHRONIC PYOGENIC ARTHRITIS

Involvement of a joint by pyogenic organisms may be caused by a blood-stream infection, by direct extension into a joint from a focus of osteomyelitis adjacent to it, from surgical procedures on the joint, or may follow compound injuries. The clinical pattern of the disease may vary considerably. In some cases the lesion represents a relatively mild synovial inflammation that subsides and heals; it may become a purulent infection causing a pyarthrosis with rapid destruction of joint cartilages; it may follow a comparatively chronic course from the outset.

Roentgen Observations

SOFT-TISSUE SWELLING. For the first few days and perhaps for a week the only changes to be observed roentgenologically are those of soft tissue swelling and distention of the joint capsule by fluid. This causes a uniform increase in soft tissue density about the joint, the margins of which are usually sharply limited if fluid is present within the joint capsule. Soft tissue changes of this type are of course not specific for any one lesion and at this stage of the disease it usually requires a correlation of the clinical and the roentgen findings for correct interpretation.

JOINT SPACE NARROWING. If the inflammation progresses into a purulent type with pyarthrosis there soon develops destruction of the articular cartilages and this in turn causes a diminution in the roentgen joint space (Fig. 9-1). In this more virulent type of infection the evidence of joint space narrowing usually becomes apparent after a week or 10 days following the onset of the disease. If the disease is untreated or inadequately treated, this narrowing progresses rapidly and the joint space may have disappeared to a large extent within several weeks.

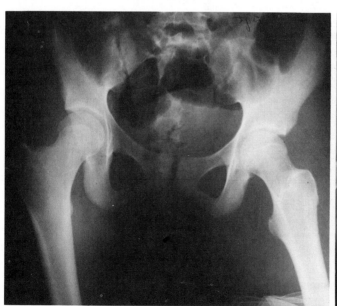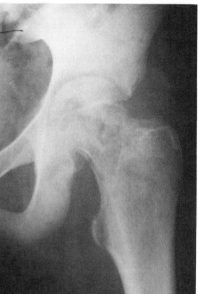

Fig. 9-1. Acute infectious arthritis of the left hip secondary to osteomyelitis. *Left,* Anteroposterior roentgenogram of the pelvis several days after the onset of symptoms. The left thigh is held in abduction and external rotation, the usual position when the hip is involved by acute inflammation. The soft tissues of the hip area are swollen. *Right,* Same hip 2½ months later. There is irregular destruction of bone in the head and neck of the femur, thinning of the joint space, and poor definition of bony articular margins.

Since these changes occur within a short period, there is not sufficient time for osteoporosis to develop and the bones maintain a normal density. This is an important roentgen observation in determining the acuteness of the lesion and, combined with serial examinations, clearly indicates the rapidly progressive nature of the infection.

ANKYLOSIS. If the articular cartilages are completely destroyed, bony ankylosis usually follows. Eventually, bony trabeculae form across the ends of the bones and in time all evidence of the joint disappears.

VARIATIONS. The above description refers mainly to an untreated or inadequately treated infection of high virulence. With present-day therapeutic measures, most cases of acute pyogenic joint infection can be brought under control before appreciable damage to the joint structures occurs. In other cases the acute infection may be transformed into a chronic indolent one with a slowly progressive course extending over a period of months. In a case of this type there is a gradual decrease in the joint space interval, the articular ends of the bones become roughened, and sequestra may separate from them. In time, as the infection subsides, reactive spurs form along the joint edges, the bones gradually regain density, there may be bony ankylosis, and if not, fibrous ankylosis is likely with little or no joint motion possible (Fig. 9-2).

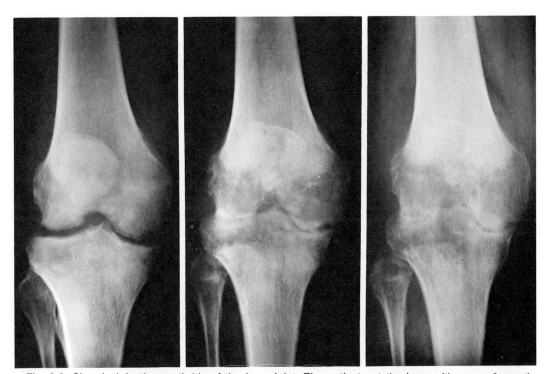

Fig. 9-2. Chronic infectious arthritis of the knee joint. The patient cut the knee with an ax 3 months prior to admission. The wound continued to drain in spite of antibiotic therapy. *Left,* Anteroposterior roentgenogram at the time of admission. There is some erosion of bony articular surfaces, particularly along the inner margins, and a slight thinning of the joint space. *Center,* Four months later. There has been further destruction of articular cartilage. Osteoporosis is prominent in the ends of the bones. *Right,* Five months later. The infection has subsided and bony ankylosis is commencing.

TUBERCULOUS ARTHRITIS

TUBERCULOSIS OF THE PERIPHERAL JOINTS

Tuberculosis of the joints is a chronic, indolent infection having an insidious onset and a slowly progressive course. It usually affects a single joint or at the most only a few joints in an individual case. The joint disease may result from a hematogenous dissemination to the synovial membrane or be secondary to a tuberculous abscess in neighboring bone. The latter is rather common in childhood tuberculosis of joints. Pathologically, tuberculosis usually begins as a synovitis. Proliferation of inflammatory granulation tissue, known as pannus, begins at the perichondrium and spreads over the joint surfaces. It interferes with nutrition of the cartilage, resulting in degeneration and destruction. In weight-bearing joints and, to a lesser degree in the nonweight-bearing joints, there is a tendency for preservation of the joint cartilages at the sites of maximum weight bearing stresses. This is in contrast to pyogenic infections where the joint exudate contains proteolytic enzymes which destroy cartilage rapidly throughout the joint surfaces. Thus, a fairly normal joint space may persist for a considerable period of time.

Roentgen Observations

JOINT EFFUSION (Fig. 9-3). The earliest evidence of tuberculous arthritis of a peripheral joint is that of joint effusion secondary to the synovitis. This can be detected without much difficulty in roentgenograms of the knee, ankle, wrist, and elbow joints but may be more diffi-

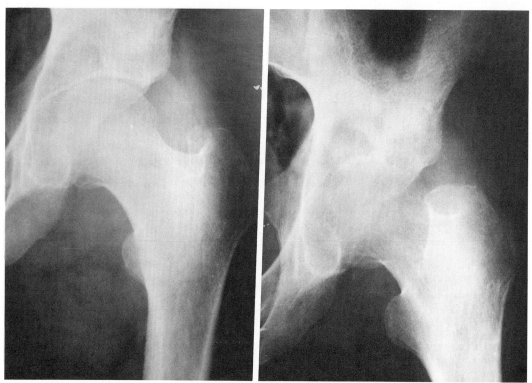

Fig. 9-3. Tuberculous arthritis of the hip joint of an adult. *Left,* The joint capsule is distended with fluid; the joint space is thinned and the bones adjacent to the joint have a "washed out" appearance. *Right,* Three months later the cartilage destruction has progressed to a complete loss of joint space in the roentgenogram.

cult to visualize in the shoulder and hip. Since fluid within a joint may result from a number of causes, this single roentgen observation does not establish the diagnosis.

DECALCIFICATION OF THE BONES. With the passage of time, often a matter of several months, the bones adjacent to the joint undergo a gradual demineralization representing an osteoporosis. The bony trabeculae disappear uniformly causing a washed-out appearance. The degree of osteoporosis often is severe and probably is caused by hyperemia plus disuse of the part.

CARTILAGE AND BONE DESTRUCTION. The disease may remain in the stage noted above for some time but more often there develops gradually the evidence of destruction of articular cartilages and of bone. In the weight-bearing joints, particularly in the knee, there is a tendency for preservation of cartilage at the points of maximum weight-bearing pressure (Fig. 9-4). Thus narrowing of the roentgen joint space may be delayed for a long time, even for several years.

The earliest evidence of bone destruction usually is seen at the margins of the articular ends of the bones. Here marginal erosion becomes apparent. The defects may be punched out and sharply circumscribed and thus resemble very closely those seen in rheumatoid arthritis. In addition to marginal erosion, the infection often burrows beneath the articular cartilage or extends through it to involve the articular ends of the bones. Thus they become ragged in outline and frank abscess cavities may appear (Fig. 9-4, *left*).

DISORGANIZATION OF THE JOINT. With further progression of the disease, gross disorganization of joint structures may result. The articular cartilage disappears, ragged destruction of the articular ends of the bones is noted, and

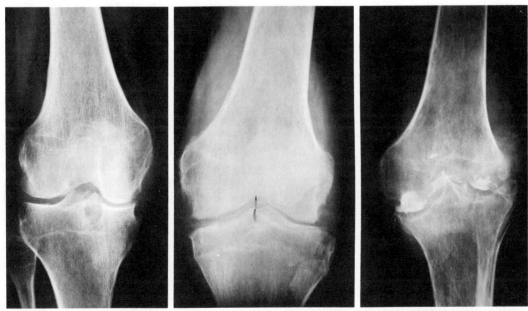

Fig. 9-4. Tuberculosis of the knee joint. Appearance of the knee joint in three different patients shows different degrees of involvement. *Left,* The joint space is intact but there are marginal erosions along the inner margins of the tibia and femur and an abscess cavity in the upper end of the tibia below the tibial spine. *Center,* The disease is more advanced and there is some erosion of articular surfaces of the bones in addition to the marginal erosions. *Right,* Advanced disease with multiple sequestra (**dense, white fragments**), and general disorganization of the joint structures.

separation of dead fragments (sequestra) is common (Fig. 9-4, *right*).

CARIES SICCA. Caries sicca is a relatively uncommon form of tuberculosis characterized by a very chronic and indolent course with an absence of joint effusion. Except for the lack of fluid and the associated swelling of soft tissues, there is little difference in the roentgen findings in this type of the disease from those described above. This lesion occurs most frequently in the shoulder.

Differential Diagnosis

ACUTE PYOGENIC ARTHRITIS. This disease has an acute onset and if untreated or inadequately treated destroys articular cartilage rapidly. With a tuberculous joint, on the other hand, by the time the joint space has decreased as a result of cartilage destruction, chronic osteoporosis, soft-tissue atrophy, and the other signs of chronic disease are clearly apparent.

CHRONIC PYOGENIC ARTHRITIS. Chronic pyogenic infection may subside into a slowly progressive course, particularly if not treated properly; then it may rather closely resemble tuberculosis. In other instances the disease is chronic from the beginning. There are several differences. The loss of articular cartilage is more severe for the duration of the disease and there is no tendency for preservation of cartilage at the points of maximum weight-bearing in the joints of the lower extremities as is noted in tuberculosis. With chronicity, reactive spurs may form along the edges of the bones and sclerotic changes are frequent. Marginal erosion is slight or absent in chronic pyogenic arthritis while in tuberculosis this is a common observation. Bony ankylosis frequently develops after destruction of articular cartilages in chronic pyogenic infection. In tuberculosis there is little tendency for spontaneous healing and bony ankylosis seldom develops without surgical aid.

RHEUMATOID ARTHRITIS. This disease is characterized by multiplicity of joint involvement, characteristically affecting the proximal interphalangeal and metacarpophalangeal joints of the hands. Loss of articular cartilage is uniform, marginal erosion is prominent in the small joints but is usu-

ally minimal when the large joints are involved. Sequestra do not form in rheumatoid arthritis. Serial observations may reveal evidence of spontaneous remissions. When rheumatoid arthritis involves a single joint as it does occasionally, the appearance is very similar to tuberculosis and correlation with the clinical and laboratory findings is important.

TUBERCULOSIS OF THE SPINE

Depending largely upon the location of the initial focus of infection, three main roentgenologic patterns are encountered in tuberculosis of the spine:

Intervertebral Type

In the intervertebral form of the disease the lesion begins in a vertebral body adjacent to the intervertebral disc. There is early extension of the infection into the disc and destruction of cartilage. In turn this results in a thinning of the intervertebral disc space in roentgenograms. The lesion in the bone becomes visualized as a poorly marginated focus of bone destruction. Accumulation of purulent material with abscess formation around the affected area is readily visualized in the dorsal spine as a fusiform soft-tissue shadow surrounding the vertebra (Fig. 9-5). The abscess shadow is present along both sides of the spine but often is larger on one side than on the other. In the lumbar spine, abscess formation is more difficult to demonstrate but its presence is determined by an outward bulging of the psoas muscle shadow (Fig. 9-6).

With further progression of the disease, the intervertebral disc space undergoes further thinning and may disappear. The destruction of the vertebral body also progresses and the infection extends across the disc to involve the adjacent vertebra. Since the arches and articular processes are not affected as a rule, collapse of the vertebral body occurs anteriorly to a large extent. This leads to a sharp angular kyphosis or gibbus. Lateral angulation or scoliotic deformities are infrequent in tuberculosis. Periosteal reaction along the margins of the

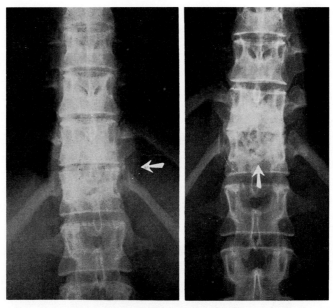

Fig. 9-5. Tuberculosis of the spine. *Left,* There is thinning of the intervertebral disc space (**arrow**) and a fusiform soft-tissue density on either side, representing a paraspinal abscess. *Right,* Same patient showing progression of the disease. The soft-tissue abscess is larger, the disc space is obliterated, and there is more obvious destruction of bone, noted particularly in the upper part of the twelfth thoracic vertebra (**arrow**).

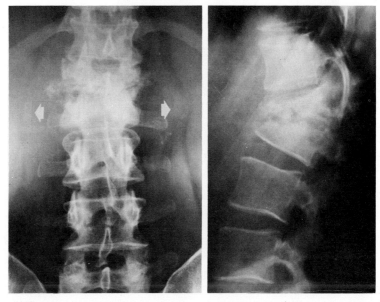

Fig. 9-6. Tuberculosis of the spine. Anteroposterior and lateral roentgenograms of the lumbar spine. There is extensive destruction of the first and second lumbar vertebrae with gibbus formation. The intervertebral disc is completely destroyed. The outward bulging of the psoas muscles (**arrows**) indicates abscess formation.

vertebral body involved by tuberculosis is uncommon and little if any sclerotic response is seen.

Central Type

The primary focus of the infection in the central type occurs within the vertebral body rather than along a margin and it develops as an abscess cavity (Fig. 9-7). The intervertebral discs are not involved as early as in the intervertebral form and some collapse of the vertebra may occur before disc changes are

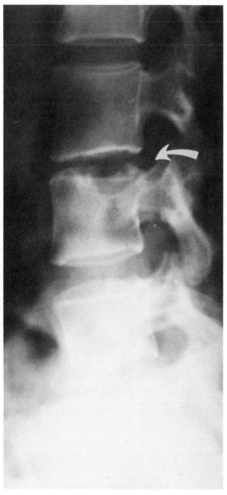

Fig. 9-7. Tuberculosis of the vertebra. Lateral roentgenogram of the lumbar spine. There is thinning of an intervertebral disc (**arrow**) and an abscess cavity in the upper part of the fourth lumbar vertebra.

obvious. Paravertebral abscess formation likewise may be less apparent in the early stages. The central type of the infection is much less common than the intervertebral.

Anterior Type

The anterior type of the disease usually results from extension of the infection from a focus above or below. The infection burrows upward or downward, bathing previously unaffected vertebrae in pus and eventually extending into one or more of the bodies. Roentgenologically, this is seen as an irregular erosion of the anterior border of the vertebral body, or as a smooth saucerized defect. There is little or no vertebral collapse and the disc intervals may be preserved. In long-standing cases of tuberculosis of the spine, very extensive involvement of this type may be present because of the tendency of the disease to extend by sinus formation and by burrowing along fascial planes.

Other Roentgen Observations

1. In very chronic disease calcium may be deposited in the paravertebral abscess, giving it a mottled appearance. Such calcified or partially calcified abscesses will remain throughout life.

2. In very old cases several contiguous vertebrae may have been destroyed to such an extent that their individual outlines are no longer recognizable and all evidence of an intervertebral disc space has disappeared.

3. With quiescence and healing of the disease the bones regain a more normal density and sharpness of outline. Areas of destruction tend partially to recalcify and bony ankylosis may ensue. Paravertebral abscess shadows diminish in size but seldom disappear completely.

Differential Diagnosis

COMPRESSION FRACTURE. There is no destruction of bone, only compression of it. The compressed zone is denser than normal. The intervertebral disc space often is narrowed but not completely absent. The superior surface of the vertebral body usually is concave because of infraction of it and expansion of the disc into the softened bone. Hemorrhage around the injured vertebra may cause a slight thickening of the paravertebral soft tissue shadow but this seldom is a prominent feature. Lateral angulation often is present in addition to a gibbus deformity.

TUMOR. A neoplasm of the vertebra may cause a paravertebral soft-tissue mass that may mimic an abscess shadow very closely. Tumors, however, rarely affect disc cartilage and narrowing of the intervertebral disc space does not develop. Collapse of the vertebral body often is uniform so that the posterior part may be affected as much as the anterior. This is unusual in tuberculosis. Gibbus formation, therefore, may not develop even in the presence of an extensive lesion.

PYOGENIC OSTEOMYELITIS. In pyogenic infections, sclerosis is more pronounced and periosteal calcification usually is a noticeable feature. The disease has an acute onset and is more rapid in its development than tuberculosis.

FUNGAL INFECTIONS. Involvement of the spine is moderately frequent in actinomycosis, blastomycosis, and coccidiodomycosis. The roentgen appearances usually are not distinctive except for the tendency for the development of sinus tracts which may be extensive. Most lesions in the spine resemble tuberculosis and roentgen diagnosis usually is not possible.

SYPHILIS OF THE JOINTS

There is some doubt whether syphilis of the joints ever occurs. A synovitis with joint effusion has been described as being caused by syphilitic infection but not all pathologists agree that this is the case. Roentgenologically, therefore, syphilitic arthritis can be dismissed as a diagnostic possibility since it will rarely enter into the picture.

RHEUMATOID ARTHRITIS

While the clinical pattern of rheumatoid arthritis varies, most cases begin insidiously and run either a protracted and progressive course or undergo remissions of variable length. In many cases the disease eventually leads to more or less crippling deformity of the affected joints. In the typical case the disease begins in the peripheral joints, usually the proximal interphalangeal and metacarpophalangeal of the hand and the ulnocarpal of the wrist. There is a tendency for symmetrical distribution in the two hands. In the feet, metatarsophalangeal joint involvement of one or more toes is common. As the disease progresses it affects the more proximal joints advancing toward the trunk in all extremities, until finally practically every joint in the body may be involved. The disease may become arrested at any stage. If this happens before much structual change has been caused, the joint may return to a normal or almost normal appearance. A curious feature of the disease is the frequent sparing of the terminal joints of the fingers. Females are affected much more frequently than males.

Pathologically, rheumatoid arthritis begins as a synovitis and in the early stages there is edema and inflammation of the synovium and the subsynovial tissues. Joint effusion also is frequent. If the disease advances, the synovium becomes greatly thickened with enlargement of the synovial villi. This is followed by a proliferation of fibrous connective tissue in the region of the perichondrium. This vascular connective tissue is known as pannus; it grows over the surface of the articular cartilage, interfering with its normal nutrition and resulting in cartilage degeneration. In advanced disease the joint becomes filled with pannus, articular cartilages disappear, and a fibrous ankylosis results. Frequently this is followed in time by bony ankylosis. As these changes are occurring in the joint, the bone adjacent undergoes osteoporosis and the muscles atrophy from disuse. Foci of inflammatory cells often accumulate in the bone adjacent to the joint.

Roentgen Observations

SOFT-TISSUE SWELLING. The earliest roentgen evidence of the disease is a diffuse swelling of soft tissues around the joint, leading to a fusiform enlargement (Fig. 9-8). This is easily seen when the proximal interphalangeal joints are affected but can also be observed in some of the other joints, particularly in the knee and ankle. Since the disease tends to attack the proximal interphalangeal and metacarpopha-

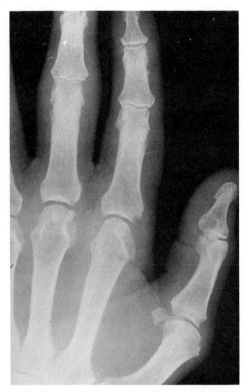

Fig. 9-8. Rheumatoid arthritis. There is fusiform soft-tissue swelling around the proximal joint of the third finger and a slight thinning of the joint space. Small marginal erosions are evident in the heads of the first and second metacarpals and the adjacent proximal phalanges. These are relatively early roentgen changes. Soft-tissue swelling also is present at the second metacarpophalangeal joint.

langeal joints first, these should be observed carefully for such evidence of synovitis. The third area often affected early is the inner aspect of the wrist, where soft-tissue swelling may be observed readily. The swelling observed roentgenologically is caused by joint effusion and also by edema of the subsynovial tissues (Fig. 9-8).

SUBARTICULAR OSTEOPOROSIS; PERIOSTITIS. Another early sign of the disease is local demineralization of bone adjacent to an involved joint. This is seen as a thinning of the cortex in the end of the bone and a decrease in number of trabeculae. It is often seen to good advantage in the metacarpal heads when there is

involvement of one or more metacarpophalangeal joints. Associated with this a thin layer of periosteal calcification around the contiguous portion of the shaft frequently occurs. These early changes, soft-tissue swelling, subarticular demineralization and periostitis, are highly suggestive, if not characteristic, of rheumatoid arthritis particularly when they are found in the joints of the hands and feet commonly affected by this disease.

MARGINAL EROSIONS. After an interval of time, which varies greatly among patients, marginal erosions become apparent. These are seen as small foci of destruction along the margins of the articular ends of the bones. They are caused by the development of granulation tissue at the perichondrium and indicate the early stage of pannus. These erosions may be very minute but they represent one of the significant roentgenologic observations of the disease (Figs. 9-8 through 9-10). The use of a magnifying lens is helpful when searching for the smallest erosions. They commonly involve the joints of the hand and wrist (excluding the distal interphalangeal joints) and the styloid process of the ulna. In the knee area they are seen chiefly along the medial edge of the tibia and the posterior aspects of the tibia and femur. Erosions occasionally occur at the sites of tendinous attachments such as the Achilles and plantar attachments on the os calcis.

THINNING OF THE JOINT SPACE. Narrowing of the joint space results from degeneration of the articular cartilages as pannus spreads across the joint surfaces. Typically, this diminution in space is uniform throughout the joint (Fig. 9-12, *left*). It may progress gradually until the ends of the bones impinge against one another. The articular ends may remain smooth. Often, however, they become roughened. In some joints a deep excavation may form in the base of one bone with the end of the opposing bone projecting into the cavity (Fig. 9-11). This is seen in severe cases and is common in the metacarpophalangeal joints where the rounded or pointed head of the metacarpal lies within an eroded cavity in the adjacent base of the

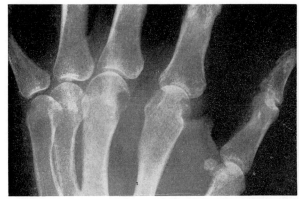

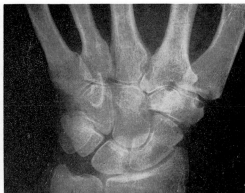

Fig. 9-9. Rheumatoid arthritis. Early changes in some of the joints of the hand and wrist. *Left,* Marginal erosions are apparent in the distal ends of the second, third, and fifth metacarpals and in the proximal phalanx of the index finger. This joint space also is thinned. *Right,* Marginal erosions in the wrist.

phalanx. In advanced cases there may be a striking loss of bone substance at the outer end of the clavicles, with widening of the acromio-clavicular joint space. It resembles the erosion seen in hyperparathyroidism, but the other joint changes are absent in this latter disease. In some patients, again with advanced disease, marked destruction of the articulating ends of the bones may be found. Thus the ends of the metatarsals, metacarpals, and phalanges may be sharpened almost to a point.

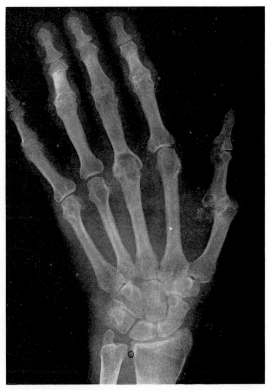

Fig. 9-11. Rheumatoid arthritis of the hand and wrist. Note the concave erosion of the base of the proximal phalanx of the third finger and the subluxation of the metacarpo-phalangeal joint of the thumb. There are small erosions along the margins of some of the carpal bones. These are characteristic changes.

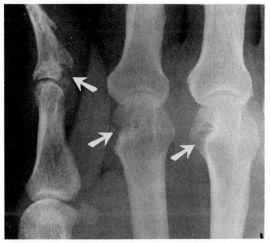

Fig. 9-10. Rheumatoid arthritis illustrating characteristic marginal erosions in the heads of the second and third metacarpals and terminal phalanx of thumb (**arrows**).

When extensive destruction of the articular ends of the bones in the hands, wrists, and feet occurs, the disease has been termed *arthritis mutilans.* Some authors consider this to be a separate entity although its similarity to rheumatoid arthritis in many of its aspects is to be noted.

In the hip, thinning of the central aspect of the joint space causes an inward displacement of the femur (Fig. 9-12). The acetabular cavity becomes deepened and eventually may lead to the characteristic changes of *protrusio acetabuli* (Otto's pelvis) (see section on "Intrapelvic Protrusion of Acetabulum" and Figs. 9-12 and 9-45). Rheumatoid arthritis is one of the common causes of this condition.

GENERALIZED OSTEOPOROSIS. If the disease has become fairly generalized and sufficient to cause limitation of bodily activity, generalized disuse osteoporosis will develop. The bones will become demineralized throughout the skeleton. If the disease remains confined to the peripheral joints, only the bones in these areas will show appreciable demineralization.

CARTILAGE CALCIFICATION. Calcium deposition in the articular cartilages (chondrocalcinosis) is seen occasionally but is more frequent in other entities (see section on "Calcification of Articular Cartilages, this chapter).

SUBLUXATIONS AND CONTRACTURES. In the later stages of the disease soft tissue contractions and subluxations are common. By this time the joint will have been damaged to the point where little or no articular cartilage remains and fibrous ankylosis is present.

BONY ANKYLOSIS. In other joints destruction of articular cartilages leads to the development of bony ankylosis. This is particularly frequent in

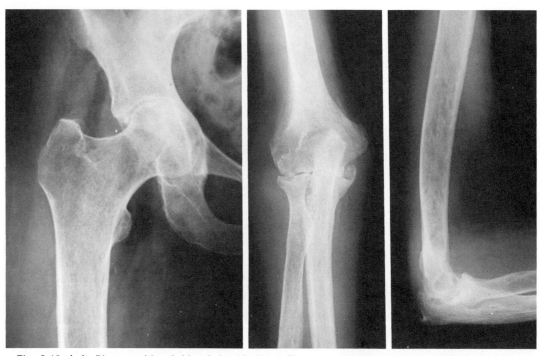

Fig. 9-12. *Left,* Rheumatoid arthritis of the hip joint. There is uniform thinning of the joint space and deepening of the acetabular cavity, causing a moderate degree of protrusio acetabuli (see text). There is chronic osteoporosis of disuse type. *Center* and *right,* Rheumatoid arthritis of the elbow joint. The disease when it involves this joint does not differ appreciably from that of the finger and wrist joints. Note irregular excavations of articular surfaces, decreased joint space interval, and the chronic osteoporosis.

the intercarpal and radiocarpal joints of the wrist. After all cartilage has been destroyed, bony trabeculae form across the previous joint space and the end result is a complete obliteration of the joint cavity and formation of a solid bony ankylosis. Bony ankylosis seldom develops if there has been much destruction of the articular ends of the bones or if there has been any appreciable degree of subluxation.

THE SPINE. Involvement of the spine, particularly the cervical area, may occur especially in long-standing disease. One of the characteristic changes is erosion of the odontoid process of the second cervical vertebra (Fig. 9-13). Erosions and malalignment of the facet joints particularly of the atlantoaxial and atlanto-occipital joints may develop. These changes may lead to forward subluxation of the first cervical on the second (Fig. 9-14). In late stages, ankylosis of these facet joints usually occurs (Fig. 9-15).

REPARATIVE CHANGES. Since, in many cases, remissions and exacerbations of the disease

have occurred, reparative changes may be apparent. Marginal spurs similar to those seen in degenerative disease are frequent along the articulating ends of the bones. There also may be a considerable amount of sclerotic density along the articular surfaces. It may be difficult to determine whether these changes are caused by a combination of rheumatoid arthritis and degenerative joint disease or by rheumatoid disease alone. In weight-bearing joints, such as the hip, knee, and ankle, degenerative changes are common after middle age and combinations of the two diseases may be seen.

RHEUMATOID ARTHRITIS OF THE SPINE (SPONDYLITIS RHIZOMELIQUE; MARIE-STRÜMPEL ARTHRITIS, ANKYLOSING SPONDYLITIS)

While there continues to be some difference of opinion as to the place of this disease in the classification of arthritis, many observers consider it to be a manifestation of rheumatoid arthritis and it is so listed in the classification

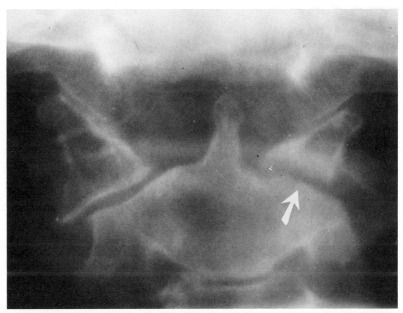

Fig. 9-13. Rheumatoid arthritis. Anteroposterior tomogram showing erosion and thinning of odontoid process, lateral subluxation of C-1 on C-2 and involvement of facet joints, particularly the left one between C-1 and C-2 (**arrow**).

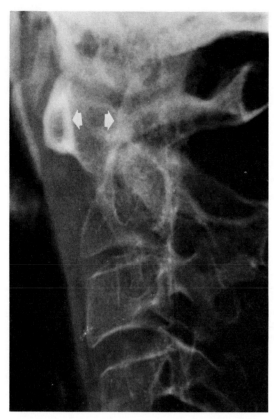

Fig. 9-14. Rheumatoid arthritis. Lateral view of upper part of cervical spine showing anterior subluxation of C-1 on C-2 (**arrows**). The odontoid process is thin and pointed.

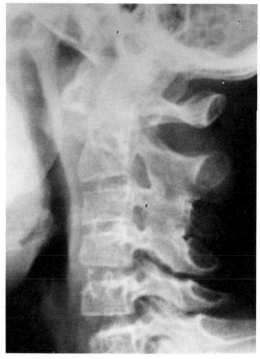

Fig. 9-15. Still's disease. Lateral view of cervical spine illustrating ankylosed facet joints between C-2, 3, and 4 owing to long-standing disease.

of joint disease. It differs in some important respects from rheumatoid arthritis of the peripheral joints in that it affects young adult males predominantly, in the ratio of about 15 to 1, while the disease affecting the peripheral joints is more common in females and the age of onset generally is later in life. It frequently remains confined to the joints of the spine and the sacroiliacs, although occasionally patients with the spinal disease will develop subsequently the manifestations of rheumatoid arthritis in the peripheral joints and vice versa. The lesions are similar pathologically and, allowing for the anatomic differences of the joints involved, the roentgen patterns are the same.

The disease involves the synovial joints of the spine. These include the apophyseal joints between the articulating facets of the vertebrae, the costovertebral joints, and the sacroiliac joints. While the disease may begin in any of these areas, roentgen visualization of the small joints is difficult and thus the sacroiliacs often show the earliest signs of the disease. Special projections have been devised for showing the costovertebral joints and if symptoms point toward this area of the spine they can be used.

Roentgen Observations

1. The articular surfaces of the affected joints become blurred and the joint spaces are irregular in width. The bony edges frequently show a sclerotic reaction. This is noted particularly in the sacroiliac joints (Fig. 9-16). Usually this involves both the iliac and the sacral side of the joint, although it may be more

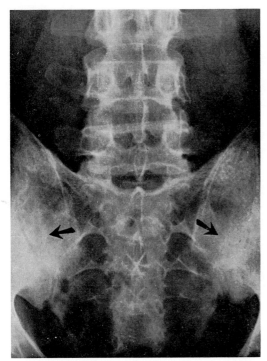

Fig. 9-16. Rheumatoid arthritis of the sacroiliac joints (spondylitis rhizomelique) (**arrows**). The joint spaces are blurred and margins very poorly defined. Where they can be seen the bony surfaces are irregular. There is sclerosis on both sides of the joint.

body appear unusually square and sharp instead of smoothly rounded as is seen in the normal. Later, a shell-like calcification of the ligaments surrounding and between the vertebrae develops and the end result is a shell of calcification forming a sheath around and between the vertebrae and resulting in a fixed, ankylosed spine (bamboo spine; poker spine) (Fig. 9-17).

4. Generalized skeletal osteoporosis is a frequently associated finding in this disease with the decalcification generally more intense in the vertebrae. It is produced, to a large extent, by the inactivity or limited activity caused by the disease.

5. Infrequently, the disease causes a localized destruction of a single intervertebral disc and margins of the adjacent vertebral bodies. The vertebral destruction is more apparent along the anterior margins, but may affect the entire disc surface. The lesion tends to undergo slow repair, with the development of sclerosis. The disc space may or may not be narrowed. This lesion is usually found in patients showing rheumatoid disease of long duration, with extensive ankylosis of the spine, but has been reported as a relatively early finding.

6. Erosion and periosteal calcification may be noted in areas such as the ischial tuberosities, femoral trochanters, and at other sites of ligamentous or muscular attachments. Erosive changes also may occur at the symphysis pubis and the manubriosternal joint in patients with advanced rheumatoid spondylitis.

severe on one side or the other. In the apophyseal joints it is infrequent to find uniform involvement of all the joints at the same time. More often one or several joints are more severely affected than others, and some may appear fairly normal during the early stages. The same is true of the costovertebral joints.

2. One of the characteristic features of rheumatoid arthritis of the spine is the tendency for bony ankylosis to develop in the affected joints. This is seen in the sacroiliac, the apophyseal or facet joints, and the costovertebral joints and represents the end stage of the disease.

3. Calcification of the spinal ligaments is one of the characteristic features of the disease in its later stages. This is first seen as a squaring of the vertebral bodies. In the lateral view the superior and inferior edges of the vertebral

STILL'S DISEASE

Still's disease is rheumatoid arthritis that begins during infancy or childhood. It resembles rheumatoid arthritis in adults in most respects (Fig. 9-18). Roentgenologically it differs somewhat, depending upon the fact that there is a larger amount of unossified cartilage in the epiphyses of the child and as a result early narrowing of the joint space is not as easily detected. For a similar reason marginal erosions commonly seen in the adult joint involved by rheumatoid arthritis are not as frequent

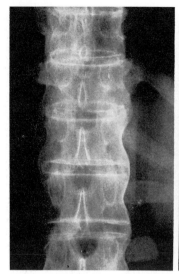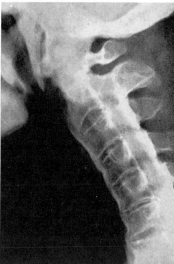

Fig. 9-17. Rheumatoid arthritis of the spine (spondylitis rhizomelique). *Left,* Anteroposterior roentgenogram showing advanced disease with ankylosis of the facet joints and a shell of calcified ligaments forming bridges between the vertebrae. When the disease has reached this stage the condition often is referred to as "bamboo spine" or "poker spine." *Right,* Lateral roentgenogram of the cervical spine of a patient with long-standing rheumatoid arthritis. There is a solid ankylosis of the facet joints and extensive calcification of the ligaments, preventing motion.

in the child. Articular cartilage destruction is a later manifestation. The joints most frequently affected include the wrists, knees, and ankles. Periosteal calcification in the bones contiguous to involved joints is more common than in the adult form of the disease. Subluxations are not infrequent. Spondylitis, especially in the upper cervical spine, occurs and may lead to bony ankylosis. As a complication atlantoaxial subluxation has been noted. Also in the spine, compression fractures have been observed, evidently secondary to the demineralization that is a feature of the disease. In some cases this may have been aggravated by steroid therapy. Transverse bands of diminished density extending across the metaphyses, similar to the change seen in acute leukemia, have been noted. In addition to the deformities caused by these changes there frequently is interference with growth of the affected extremities, which adds to the general skeletal deformity. Clinically there may be enlargement of the spleen and lymph nodes. A rather similar condition in adults has sometimes been called *Felty's syndrome* but the tendency is to discon-

tinue the use of this term and consider the disease as rheumatoid arthritis.

ARTHRITIS ASSOCIATED WITH SCLERODERMA AND PSORIASIS

Occasionally a patient with psoriasis will develop an arthritis that resembles rheumatoid arthritis closely. There is some difference of opinion as to whether the joint disease is related to the psoriasis or whether it occurs as an independent process merely by chance. Roentgen changes in the joints may be indistinguishable from rheumatoid disease. Avila et al.,[1] however, have pointed out that the disease tends to involve the terminal interphalangeal joints, which are seldom involved in rheumatoid arthritis (Fig. 9-19). They list five signs that are of importance in the differential diagnosis: (1) a destructive arthritis involving predominantly the distal interphalangeal joints of the hands and toes; (2) a tendency for bony ankylosis of some of the interphalangeal joints (in rheumatoid arthritis, ankylosis is more com-

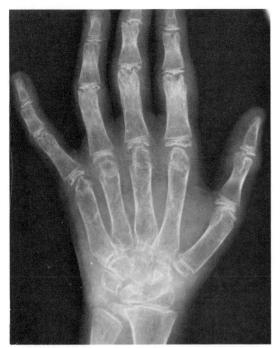

Fig. 9-18. Still's disease of the joints of the hand and wrist. There is erosion of articular surfaces in most of the joints including the terminal. There is severe osteoporosis. The intercarpal joints are involved.

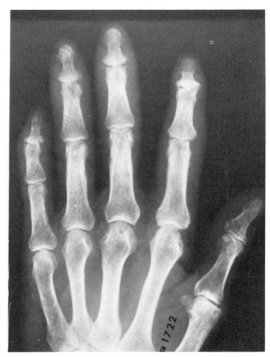

Fig. 9-19. Psoriatic arthritis. The terminal interphalangeal joints are involved.

mon in the intercarpal joints); (3) abnormally wide joint spaces with sharply demarcated bony surfaces; (4) destructive arthritis of the interphalangeal joint of the great toe; and (5) resorption of the terminal tufts of the terminal phalanges.

Some patients with scleroderma likewise develop a rheumatoidlike disease in the joints of the hands. In addition to the arthritic changes certain other findings caused by the scleroderma may be observed in roentgenograms (see Fig. 10-13):

1. Atrophy of the soft tissues in the tips of the fingers, giving them a tapered appearance.

2. Loss of bone substance in the terminal tufts of the distal phalanges, resulting in a pointed or rounded end.

3. Small punctate calcific deposits in the soft tissues, especially in the ends of the fingers (interstitial calcinosis, also see Chapter 10 under heading "Interstitial Calcinosis"). When these changes are observed in association with the joint findings of rheumatoid arthritis the diagnosis of

scleroderma can be made with considerable certainty.

Other collagen diseases may have an associated joint disease similar to rheumatoid arthritis except for a tendency toward a milder course in most cases. In *dermatomyositis* and *disseminated lupus erythematosis* a rheumatoidlike arthritis is frequent. Similar joint changes may be found in *ulcerative colitis* and in *Whipple's disease*.

DEGENERATIVE JOINT DISEASE

The term "degenerative joint disease" has come into use for the condition previously known as osteoarthritis, osteoarthrosis, hypertrophic arthritis, and the like. Its use is preferred since the condition is characterized pathologically by degeneration of the articular cartilages and of the other tissues comprising the joint. It is not an inflammatory lesion and the term "arthritis" is not satisfactory. It is a disease mainly of older individuals affecting the weight-bearing joints (spine, hip, knee, ankle) and the interphalangeal joints of the fingers. It is convenient to think of degenerative joint disease as occurring in two major forms, primary and secondary. The primary form may be a generalized disease affecting the weight-bearing joints, the spine and the terminal interphalangeal joints of the fingers, the cause of which is unknown. The disease often appears to be only the result of the aging process, representing the effects of wear and tear, to which may be added the factor of abnormal weight-bearing stresses and strains. Aging and trauma in one form or another, therefore, are common predisposing factors. The secondary form of the disease develops in a joint that has been subjected to abnormal stresses and strains over a period of time or one that has been traumatized repeatedly. In the hip it often follows congenital abnormalities in the shape and form of the acetabulum or of the femoral head, Legg-Perthes' disease, epiphysiolysis, etc., or it may develop as a result of abnormal weight-bearing such as follows a shortening of one leg or a scoliotic deformity of the spine. The roentgen signs and pathologic changes are similar in the two forms and the dividing line between them often is not distinct. Degenerative joint disease of the fingers (Heberden's nodes) represents a separate clinical entity. It seems to have little relationship to trauma, it may develop in fairly young individuals, is not necessarily associated with disease in other joints, and appears to have a distinct hereditary tendency.

Roentgen Observations

SPURRING. One of the earliest changes is the development of small bony spurs or osteophytes along the articular edges of the bones. This is sometimes referred to as lipping. The osteophytes may become large, particularly in the spine, but rarely form ossified bridges between the bones along the joint edges (Fig. 9-20).

EBURNATION. Increased density of the articular ends of the bones is another relatively early finding. This is noted particularly on the joint

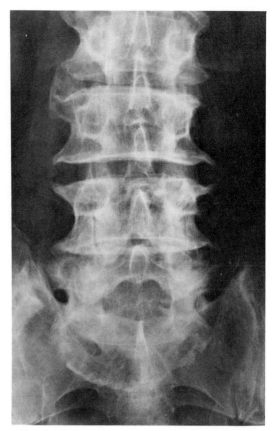

Fig. 9-20. Degenerative joint disease. Anteroposterior roentgenogram of the lumbar spine illustrating osteophyte formation on the margins of the vertebrae.

edges where the maximum weight-bearing stresses and strains occur.

THINNING OF THE JOINT SPACE. Sometimes as an early manifestation and at other times occurring later in the course of the disease, thinning of the joint space develops. In contrast to rheumatoid arthritis, thinning of the roentgen joint space in this condition is almost invariably uneven. It is more pronounced in the part of the joint where weight-bearing strains are greatest and is caused by degeneration of the articular cartilages. In extreme cases the cartilage may be completely destroyed in areas and the articular ends of the bones then form the apposing joint surfaces. The greater the thinning of the joint space, the more severe the sclerosis of the articular ends and the more intensive the spurring is likely to be. These findings, however, do not always follow one another in severity and at times considerable thinning of the joint space may be seen with relatively little marginal osteophyte formation.

CYSTS. In certain joints, notably the hip, cyst-like rarefactions frequently develop along the articular borders. Occasionally these are an early manifestation of the disease in the hip joint (Fig. 9-21). More often they are seen only after the other findings enumerated above have become definite. Cystic cavities vary in size but in the hip may reach a diameter of several centimeters. They are bounded by a dense wall of sclerosis. They extend to the bony articular surface and sometimes are more prominent on one side of the joint than on the other. They may communicate with the joint cavity.

SUBLUXATION. As a manifestation of late disease subluxation is frequent. Relaxation of the joint capsule and the other ligament structures

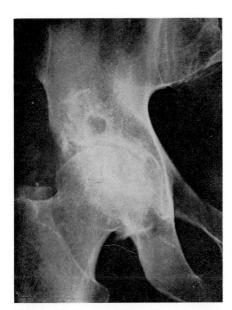

Fig. 9-21. Degenerative joint disease of the hip. There is eburnation of articular surfaces and spurring along the margins of the femoral head. A cyst is seen above the acetabulum.

around the area may allow a certain amount of displacement of one bone upon the other. When this happens the joint becomes even more unstable and thus more subject to trauma and aggravation of the existing disease.

INTRA-ARTICULAR AND PERIARTICULAR OSSIFICATION. In some joints, particularly the knee, formation of calcific or ossified loose bodies is common. These may represent osteophytes that were broken off and became loose bodies but more often they represent fragments of cartilage that have been detached and have undergone calcification. In other instances the loose body may be formed by the synovium. Not infrequently dense masses that have the characteristics of bone are noted along the joint margins, usually in the tendons and not free within the joint. Again, these are particularly common in the knee.

SPECIAL AREAS

JOINTS OF THE FINGERS

The disease affects primarily the terminal interphalangeal joints but need not be limited to these areas. The early findings consist of tiny marginal spurs or small calcific flakes along the bases of the distal phalanges. These spurs enlarge gradually to form well-defined bony protuberances that cause an irregular knobby thickening, palpable and visible, representing the well-known *Heberden's nodes,* one of the significant clinical diagnostic features of the disease. The largest spurs form on the dorsal edges of the articular ends of the bones and thus are best demonstrated in lateral roentgenograms. In more severely affected joints, narrowing of the joint space is present and the bony articular surfaces become irregular. The appearance is somewhat similar to that seen in rheumatoid arthritis. There are, however, no areas of marginal erosion and decalcification of the articular ends of the bones is not present. The bony trabeculae remain sharp and the cortical margin is apparent. The terminal phalanx becomes flexed on the middle and the finger cannot be completely straightened. Lateral angulation of the distal on the middle phalanx is common. Partial subluxations may occur but bony ankylosis does not develop. In some cases small cystic cavities form in the ends of the bones but eburnation of the articulating ends of the bones seldom is striking (Fig. 9-22).

HIP JOINT

In the hip the early signs of this disease are variable. In some, the first evidence consists of increased density along the superior acetabular rim. In others, marginal spurring is the earliest feature, but in most cases narrowing of the joint space is the most significant finding (Fig. 9-21). In contrast to rheumatoid arthritis, decrease in joint space in degenerative disease is characterized by its asymmetry and is related closely to the distribution of weight-bearing in the joint. In the hip this affects the superior portion almost exclusively, since this is the area that receives the thrust of the femoral head in weight-bearing. The joint space narrowing progresses to complete loss of the joint space but without bony ankylosis. This asymmetrical narrowing of the space leads to varying degrees of subluxation or lateral wandering

of the femoral head and, if accompanied by a wearing away of the superior portion of the acetabular fossa, may result in notable deformity. Marginal osteophytes of large size may be present. As the head moves upward and laterally in the enlarged acetabular cavity, considerable amounts of calcium may be laid down along the undersurface as if to fill more completely the enlarged cavity. The joint surfaces, particularly the acetabular, show increased density or eburnation (Fig. 9-23). Cystic-appearing cavities develop as sharply outlined rarefactions surrounded by dense sclerotic walls. In some cases the cysts appear early. The cysts may communicate with the joint cavity. Infrequently degenerative disease in the hip may lead to a general deepening and inward bulging of the acetabular cavity and at least some cases of so-called intrapelvic protrusion of the acetabulum seem to result from this disease.

KNEE JOINT

Degenerative joint disease is the most common chronic joint affection encountered in the knee. Usually the early changes consist in the development of small spurs along the joint margins, on the tibial spine, along the borders of the intercondylar fossa of the femur, and on the edges of the patella. Hypertrophic excres-

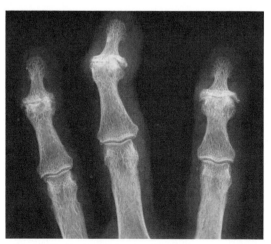

Fig. 9-22. Degenerative joint disease of the terminal joints of the fingers. Note the large spurs (Heberden nodes) and angular deformity of terminal on middle phalanx of the third finger.

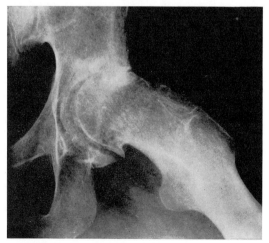

Fig. 9-23. Degenerative joint disease of the hip. Semilateral projection illustrating characteristic changes of the disease.

cences may develop on the joint surface of the tibia, particularly at the attachments of the cruciate ligaments. As in the hip, narrowing of the joint space usually appears early and may be the first sign. It is almost always asymmetrical with the medial aspect undergoing the most severe change (Fig. 9-24). Occasionally the outer side of the joint narrows first. Increased density of the bony articular surfaces also is most pronounced along the site of greatest joint space narrowing. Because of the uneven narrowing of the space and the consequent disturbance of weight-bearing alignment, some degree of lateral subluxation of the tibia on the femur is common in advanced lesions and a varus deformity is frequent. In contrast to the hip, formation of cystic cavities in the articular ends of the bones is infrequent. However, a common feature of the disease in this joint is the development of calcific or bony loose bodies within the joint pouch. The fabella, if present, may be enlarged and roughened. Joint effusion is not infrequently seen in roentgenograms and usually results from either the mechanical irritation of intraarticular loose bodies or because of trauma to a joint rendered unstable by the disease.

JOINTS OF THE SPINE

The same process that involves the peripheral joints may also affect the spine but because of anatomical structures peculiar to this region it requires separate discussion. The most common finding almost universally present in patients above middle age is hypertrophic spurring along the anterior and lateral margins of the vertebral bodies (Fig. 9-25). These marginal osteophytes are particularly prone to develop in the lower cervical, lower dorsal, and lower lumbar areas. When the process begins in younger persons below the age of 50 the lower cervical vertebrae often are affected primarily. In addition to the spurs, small calcific or bony deposits may form in the spinal ligaments, especially the anterior, without any attachment to the adjacent bodies. Bony proliferation along the margins of the spinous

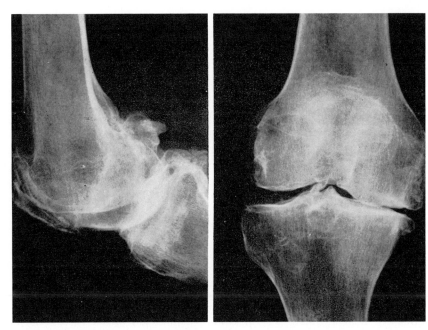

Fig. 9-24. Degenerative joint disease of the knee. Anteroposterior (*right*) and lateral (*left*) roentgenograms. There is thinning of the joint space on the medial side, lateral subluxation of the tibia on the femur, extensive spur formation on the articular margins of the bones, and eburnation of bony surfaces.

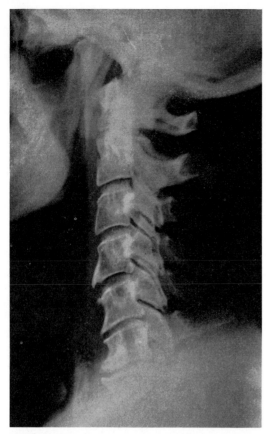

Fig. 9-25. Degenerative joint disease of the spine. Lateral roentgenogram of the cervical spine shows characteristic changes. There are marginal osteophytes and thinning of intervertebral discs between C-5, 6, and 7.

processes often is present, as is marginal spurring of the costovertebral joints. In more severe forms of the disease some degree of thinning of the intervertebral discs is found. This is particularly likely to occur in the lower cervical region and at the lumbosacral joint but other disc spaces may be affected (Fig. 9-25). Narrowing of the disc space usually is uniform except in the dorsal region, where it is more pronounced along the anterior borders (Fig. 9-26). In the presence of scoliosis these changes are more severe along the concave side of the curvature. Because this disease is found chiefly in the older age period, senile decalcification of bone usually is present although the cortical margins of the vertebrae remain distinct and

actually may show increased density. Involvement of the small apophyseal joints may or may not be present. When it is, the roentgen findings are no different from those seen in other weight-bearing joints, allowing for differences in size of the joints. These changes consist in thinning of the joint space, marginal spurring, increased density of bony articular surfaces, and some degree of subluxation, the uppermost facets slipping forward on the ones below. This combined with the thinning of the adjacent intervertebral disc may result in a distinct narrowing of the corresponding spinal foramina and lead to the production of clinical symptoms. The forward displacement of one vertebra on the one below is called spondylolisthesis and a minor degree of this is common in degenerative joint disease (also see p. 83). Marginal spurs are not infrequent on the posterior margins of the vertebrae in the lower cervical and lower lumbar areas. These are more significant from a clinical standpoint than spurs on the other surfaces because of the close association with spinal nerve roots. Occasionally a thin, waferlike, translucent space is visualized within one or more of the discs severely involved by degenerative disease. This is called a *phantom disc* (see p. 300) and is seen mainly in the lower lumbar area (Fig. 9-27).

As a form of degenerative joint disease of the spine there may occur relatively massive ossification of the anterior spinal ligaments, tending to be localized to the lower cervical and upper thoracic areas and causing an accentuation of the thoracic kyphosis. It is found in elderly people as a part of the aging process and is generally asymptomatic. It can be confused with rheumatoid spondylitis, but the absence of change in the lumbosacral spine and sacroiliac joints is significant. The term *Forestier's disease* has sometimes been applied to this condition.

TRAUMATIC ARTHRITIS

The term "traumatic arthritis" should be reserved for that form of degenerative joint disease in which the process is initiated by acute trauma,

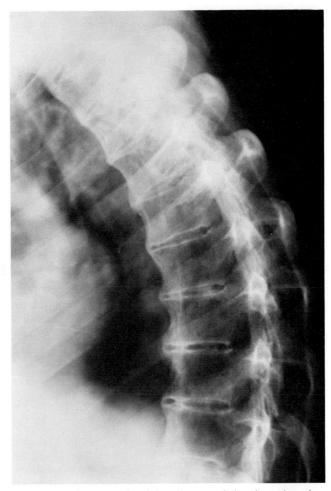

Fig. 9-26. Degenerative joint disease of the thoracic spine, lateral view. Note thinned intervertebral disc spaces, anterior spurs, and ligament calcification.

either as a single episode or as the result of repeated injuries. Thus, traumatic arthritis may develop in a joint following a fracture that extended into the joint; after a hemorrhagic effusion following trauma; as a result of a severe sprain or recurrent injuries to the supporting structures of the joint. Because the diagnosis of traumatic arthritis may have medicolegal implications and because it may be a compensable disease, it is not wise to use this term unless it can be established with reasonable certainty that the joint was normal prior to the trauma and that following the injury the arthritic changes became evident. In general the roentgen findings are similar to those of degenerative joint disease (see section entitled "Degenerative Joint Disease," this chapter) and the pathologic alterations are similar.

GOUTY ARTHRITIS

Gout is a metabolic disturbance of unknown cause. It is characterized by the occurrence of acute attacks of arthritis in certain joints with freedom of symptoms between the attacks; by elevation of the uric acid in the blood serum and the body fluids; by the deposition of sodium urate in various body tissues (joints, bones, periarticular tissues); and by the devel-

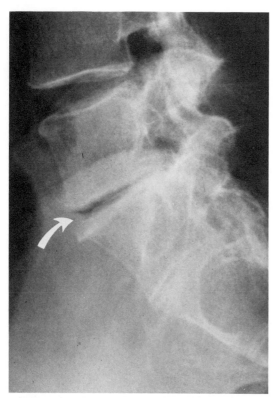

Fig. 9-27. "Phantom disc." There is severe thinning of the lumbosacral disc and a dark, translucent space within the disc (**arrow**).

the attack and the amount of disuse associated with it.

LATER CHANGES. After several attacks of the disease, localized soft tissue swellings appear. These are irregular and lumpy in appearance, representing accumulations of sodium urate, and are known as tophi. Similar deposits occur in the articular cartilages and in the bones adjacent to the joint. As they enlarge, these deposits result in localized punched-out defects in the ends of the bones. These not infrequently have the appearance of cysts with a fairly well-defined cavity surrounded by a thin sclerotic wall (Figs. 9-28 and 9-29). The cyst may lie completely within the bone or be marginal and cause some destruction of cortex. When marginal, the partially eroded cortex may form a characteristic spurlike projection. Involvement of bursae, particularly the olecranon bursa, is common.

opment of degenerative changes, particularly in the blood vessels of the kidneys. The most common joint to be affected is the first metatarsophalangeal, where the disease is clinically known as *podagra*. Other joints commonly involved are the ankle, knee, and the joints of the hands and wrists and the elbow. Roentgen changes are not likely to be present unless the disease has existed for some time and after several attacks of the disease. Thus, a negative roentgenogram does not necessarily exclude gout. The disease affects males predominantly.

Roentgen Features

EARLY CHANGES. The joint may appear entirely normal or there may be soft-tissue swelling during the acute exacerbation of the disease. A variable amount of disuse osteoporosis may be present, depending upon the length of

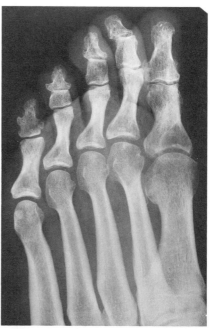

Fig. 9-28. Gouty arthritis of the first metatarsophalangeal joint. Oblique view showing a cystlike rarefaction or cavity in the proximal end of the proximal phalanx of the first toe. There is moderate disuse osteoporosis. This represents a gouty tophus, the cavity being filled with sodium urate.

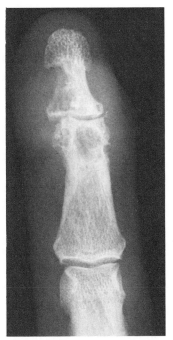

Fig. 9-29. Gouty arthritis. Finger of a patient with gout shows cystlike defect in the distal end of the middle phalanx and cortical erosion of the distal with associated lumpy, soft-tissue swellings.

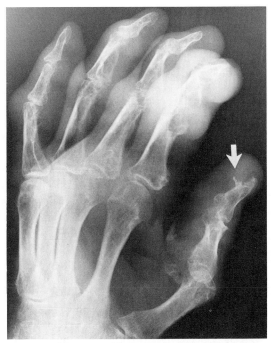

Fig. 9-30. Gouty arthritis with multiple areas of destruction and characteristic lumpy swellings owing to gouty tophi. Note the erosion at the tip of the thumb with a characteristic spurlike projection (**arrow**).

ADVANCED CHANGES. After the disease has existed for many years the roentgen findings usually become typical. There are large marginal erosions and cavities in and along the ends of the bones. There are, in association with these, large, lumpy, soft-tissue swellings representing gouty tophi (Fig. 9-30). The joint spaces may be somewhat thinned as a result of degeneration of articular cartilages but usually this is not particularly severe. Bony ankylosis does not occur. The bones often maintain a surprisingly good density because disuse osteoporosis does not develop since the patients are relatively free of symptoms between the acute exacerbations. Tophi consisting only of sodium urate are radiolucent. Calcification of gouty tophi occurs occasionally, particularly in more advanced disease.

Differential Diagnosis

The diagnosis of gouty arthritis is largely a clinical one in the early stages of the disease

although it may be suspected roentgenologically because of the typical joint or joints involved and the character of the soft-tissue swelling caused by the tophi. However, confusion with rheumatoid arthritis is entirely possible since both of these diseases cause marginal erosions and soft-tissue swelling. The distribution of the disease is significant. In rheumatoid arthritis, characteristically, the proximal interphalangeal, metacarpophalangeal, and ulnocarpal joints are affected early. It is here that one expects to find the more characteristic changes. In gouty arthritis the first metatarsophalangeal joint is the one most frequently involved. This is not a common joint to be involved by rheumatoid arthritis unless the disease is generalized.

NEUROTROPHIC ARTHROPATHY

Any disease that impairs sensation in the joint structures renders it susceptible to repeated traumas and may lead to severe disorganization of the joint. Included among such diseases are tabes dorsalis, syringomyelia, diabetic neuropathy, leprosy, transection of the spinal cord, and peripheral nerve injury. The most frequent cause is tabes dorsalis. The resulting arthropathy is known as a *Charcot joint*. The weight-bearing joints of the lower extremities are the most frequently affected in tabes dorsalis. Less common is involvement of the spine, usually the lower part of the lumbar. Neurotrophic arthropathy in the joints of the upper extremities is much less common and in these areas syringomyelia is the usual cause (Fig. 9-31, *right*). Diabetic arthropathy predominantly affects the foot (Fig. 9-32).

Roentgen Features

Pathologically the lesion is one of repeated infractions, often of minor degree but, with summation of these injuries, considerable breakdown and fragmentation of the articular cartilages and articulating ends of the bones result. Hemorrhage in the soft tissues may also occur. In the early stages the roentgen findings are usually limited to condensation of bone in the articular ends, producing an eburnated appearance of the articular surfaces and some loss of the joint space. There is a tendency for

subluxation to occur rather early. These changes are followed by breakdown of bone structures and eventually considerable disorganization of the joint results. In the hip the acetabular cavity becomes enlarged, the head of the femur undergoes fragmentation and absorption, often with increase in density of the bone (Fig. 9-31). In the knee similar changes take place. Wearing away of the condylar surfaces occurs, particularly on the medial side. Fragmentation and generalized disorganization develops. Soft-tissue swelling is pronounced; multiple calcified and osseous fragments are found in and around the joint. The changes are similar in other large joints that may be affected. The frequency of subluxation is to be noted and instability of the joint is one of the prominent clinical signs. In the spine the affected vertebral bodies develop increased density; they tend to undergo some degree of compression and fragmentation, and alteration in alignment (Fig. 9-33). Thinning or disappearance of the intervertebral discs accompanies these changes in the vertebral bodies. The rapidity of development of these changes is variable but in some cases relatively advanced disease has been reported as occurring in from 9 days to 6 weeks after roentgenograms had shown a normal joint.

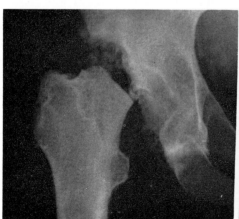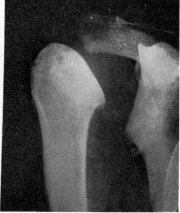

Fig. 9-31. Neurotrophic arthropathy (Charcot joint). *Left,* Anteroposterior roentgenogram of the hip of a patient suffering from tabes dorsalis. There is gross disorganization of the joint with fragmentation of the head of the femur. Because the patient is using the extremity there is no disuse osteoporosis. *Right,* Involvement of the shoulder joint in syringomyelia.

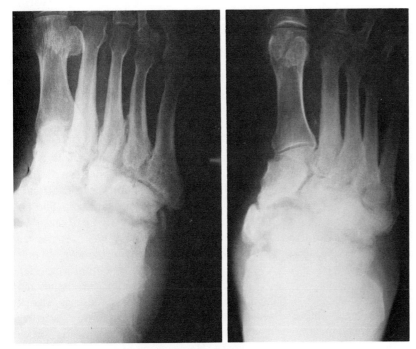

Fig. 9-32. Diabetic arthropathy involving the tarsus.

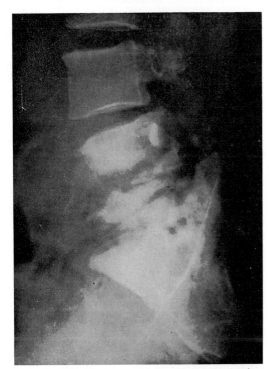

Fig. 9-33. Neurotrophic arthropathy of the lumbar spine. Lateral roentgenogram shows increased density, fragmentation, and malalignment of the vertebrae of a patient with tabes dorsalis.

PERIARTICULAR DISEASE

The various tissues around a joint, such as bursae, tendons, and muscles, may become involved by acute or chronic inflammatory changes. Involvement of the tendons and bursae is common, particularly in the shoulder, and results in limitation of motion and considerable disability. This is referred to variously as periarthritis, periarticular disease, bursitis, fibrositis, tendinitis, and the like. It is the most frequent cause of shoulder disability. Roentgenologically, in addition to disuse osteoporosis, amorphous calcium depositions frequently are seen in the tendons of the shoulder cuff (Fig. 9-34). These usually occur in the tendon of the supraspinatus and are found directly above the greater tuberosity of the humerus. Less common are similar deposits in the tendons of the subscapularis, infraspinatus, and teres minor. Such deposits in the tendons often are associated with inflammation of an overlying bursa, hence the clinical designation of a painful shoulder as bursitis or subacromial

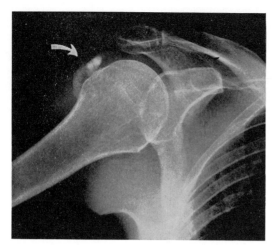

Fig. 9-34. Calcifying tendinitis of the shoulder (**arrows**).

bursitis. Rupture of a mass of calcium into a bursa may occur but as a rule the calcification occurs within the tendon and not in the overlying bursa. Approximately 50 per cent of patients with complaints of pain and disability in the shoulder will show demonstrable calcification on roentgen examination. In the remainder there will be noted only the evidence of disuse osteoporosis if the disability has been present for any appreciable time and the demonstration of limited motion when films are made with the arm in abduction and rotation. It is not at all infrequent to find calcium deposits in the tendinous cuff of the shoulder in patients who have no complaints, or at least none at the time of present examination. Thus the mere presence of demonstrable calcium does not indicate the existence of an active inflammatory process. In addition to the shoulder area similar calcifications sometimes are found in association with the trochanteric bursa that overlies the greater trochanter of the femur. They also are encountered in the periarticular tissues around the elbow, especially on the radial side, at the wrist, along the interphalangeal joints, or in any location where bursae are present with tendons overlying them. Such deposits should be searched for in patients complaining of acute inflammatory changes in any of the joints.

MISCELLANEOUS

HEMOPHILIAC ARTHROPATHY

In hemophilia recurrent hemorrhages into the joints are of frequent occurrence. The knee and elbow are somewhat more vulnerable to repeated injuries than the others but any joint may be involved. As a result of the repeated hemorrhages and the irritating effect of the blood within the joint, a chronic synovitis develops. There is degeneration of articular cartilages and erosion of bony surfaces. The soft tissues become thickened. If there has been recent injury the joint capsule may be distended with fresh blood, and the signs of joint effusion will be present. In chronic cases the deposition of iron pigment in the tissues may lead to areas of cloudy increase in density resembling calcification (Fig. 9-35). Cartilage degeneration is shown by narrowing of the joint space. Hemorrhage into the articular ends of the bones may cause them to appear eroded and irregular. In the knee, enlargement of the intercondylar fossa of the femur may be apparent. Occasionally, hemorrhage may occur within the bone at a distance from the joint and result in a cystlike cavity (Fig. 9-36). The ilium has been reported as an occasional site of this lesion, which may expand and destroy a rather large area of bone.[24] It is well to be acquainted with this fact so that a biopsy will not be done, a very dangerous procedure in patients with hemophilia. The lesion has been called a *pseudotumor of hemophilia*. Acceleration of epiphyseal growth from chronic irritation leads to club-shaped enlargement of the ends of the bones. This is noted in other chronic inflammatory lesions such as Still's disease and tuberculosis. The differential diagnosis of hemophiliac arthropathy may be difficult from roentgen examination alone but it should be considered as a possibility when a destructive arthritis is encountered in a child.

TUMORS AND RELATED LESIONS

Because of the diversity of the tissues entering into the formation of a joint, a wide variety

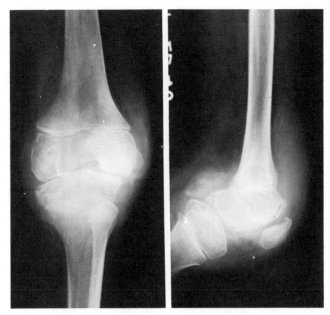

Fig. 9-35. Hemophiliac arthropathy. Anteroposterior and lateral roentgenograms of the knee of a child with hemophilia who had repeated episodes of hemarthrosis. This led to irregular destruction of articular cartilages and of areas in the ends of the bones. The epiphyses are enlarged because of acceleration of growth from the chronic irritation. The joint capsule is distended with fluid (i.e., blood) and the deposition of iron pigment in the synovium from previous hemorrhages causes a diffuse cloudy increase in density noted particularly in the popliteal fossa.

of tumors and tumorlike lesions may develop. Most of these are uncommon but of sufficient importance to warrant some discussion. The ones described below are considered to be the most significant from a roentgenologic point of view.

SYNOVIOMA (SYNOVIAL SARCOMA)

Synovioma (synovial sarcoma) is an uncommon but important tumor. It usually begins in the vicinity of a large joint, starting in the para-articular soft tissues just beyond the confines of the capsule. Occasionally it is found at some distance from a joint. It is most frequent in young adults. The knee area is a favorite site. While there has been some disagreement on the matter, it is generally considered that the tumor must be classed with the malignant neoplasms, although the degree of malignancy may vary from case to case. The lesion is visualized in roentgenograms as a mass of soft-tissue density, adjacent to a joint. Usually the outer margin of the mass is fairly well demarcated from the adjacent soft tissues. Calcification of portions of the tumor occurs rather frequently. This may be in the form of hazy, punctate deposits or linear streaks (Fig. 9-37). During the early development of the tumor the bone beneath it remains normal. Sooner or later the lesion begins to invade the bone and destroy it. At first this is seen as a ragged erosion of the cortex directly beneath the tumor. Subsequently, destruction of the cancellous bone develops (Fig. 9-37). The type of bone destruction is similar to that caused by fibrosarcoma arising in the soft tissues and invading bone. The location of the lesion within

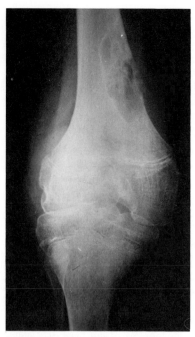

Fig. 9-36. Hemophiliac arthropathy. In addition to changes in the knee joint there is a cystlike cavity in the shaft of the femur, probably resulting from a previous intraosseous hemorrhage.

or close to the joint is presumptive evidence of synovial origin (Fig. 9-38). Calcium deposition also occurs in fibrosarcoma but is less frequent. Before the stage of bone invasion has been reached, and in the absence of calcification within the mass, accurate roentgen diagnosis usually is impossible and recourse must be had to surgical exploration and study of tissue specimens.

PIGMENTED VILLONODULAR SYNOVITIS

The cause of pigmented villonodular synovitis is unknown but most investigators have considered it to be inflammatory rather than neoplastic. In some cases there is a history of trauma but in the majority there is none. Usually the symptoms are mild and of long duration, often extending over a period of years. Two major pathologic types are recognized, the localized and the diffuse. In the former, roentgenograms reveal the outlines of a soft-tissue mass within the joint but not distending the entire joint pouch. The mass may have a nodular outline but more often is smooth. In the diffuse form there is a generalized swelling of soft tissues of the joint indicative of a synovitis. Usually there is very little in the appearance of this swelling to indicate the nature of the lesion. Since the disease does not cause much disability, disuse osteoporosis is not a prominent feature and may be lacking entirely. Narrowing of the joint space also is seen infrequently. If the disease has been present for some time, deposition of iron pigment in the tissues may cause a cloudy increase in density very similar to that found in some cases of hemophiliac arthropathy (see section on "Hemophiliac Arthropathy"). In chronic lesions, local erosions or actual invasion may develop along the margin or within medullary cavity. Accurate diagnosis from roentgen examination alone is difficult and often impossible. Significant features include the presence of a chronic lesion in a young adult characterized by synovitis and causing very little disability, slight or no changes in the roentgen joint space or in the articular ends of the bones and, occasionally, cloudy areas of density in the soft tissues. Surgical exploration and the examination of tissue usually is required to establish the diagnosis with certainty and is indicated in most cases in order to differentiate the lesion from synovial sarcoma.

GIANT CELL AND XANTHOMATOUS TUMORS

There is a group of tumors or tumorlike lesions of the tendon sheaths and joints that have been difficult to classify. Following the investigations of Jaffe, Lichtenstein, and Sutro, many pathologists now consider most of these, if not all, to be closely related to the disease known as pigmented villonodular synovitis (see section on "Pigmented Villonodular Synovitis"). Evidence has been presented to show that these "tumors" are linked rather closely and probably represent only stages in the development of the same disease. Nevertheless agreement on the subject is not completely uniform and there are certain clinical and roentgen features that tend to separate some of

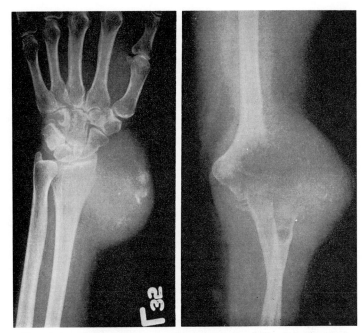

Fig. 9-37. Synovioma (synovial sarcoma). *Left,* Anteroposterior roentgenogram of the wrist. The large soft-tissue mass contains areas of calcification. The adjacent bone is unaffected. *Right,* Synovial sarcoma of the elbow. The lesion had been resected locally but recurred. The large soft-tissue mass is obvious and the tumor has extended to involve the bones on both sides of the joint. A malignant tumor arising within a bone rarely extends across the joint in this manner.

them from pigmented villonodular synovitis, at least from the diffuse form of the disease. The xanthomas and giant cell tumors are prone to develop in the tendon sheaths and are found most frequently in the hands and feet. In roentgenograms they are visualized as discrete masses of soft-tissue density but with no specific features by which their histologic nature can be recognized. In some cases the mass may cause a smooth, pressure type of erosion of the bone beneath it. In an occasional patient the tumor appears to grow directly into the bone, forming an irregular cystlike cavity. A peculiar variant is the disease known as *xanthoma tuberosa.* In this condition multiple nodular masses form along the tendons and synovial membranes in the hands and feet; these cause very little clinical disability. The bones may be perfectly normal and the joint spaces preserved. In some cases, however, erosion and destruction of the bone beneath one or more of the masses may occur. The resulting appearance resembles gout very closely (Fig. 9-39). To avoid confusion it is preferable to consider the single

xanthomas as lesions distinct from xanthoma tuberosa. The former are apparently related closely to the giant cell tumor of the tendon sheaths and to pigmented villonodular synovitis. Xanthoma tuberosa, on the other hand, has no such relationship. Instead, it may be one of the manifestations of hypercholesterolemia.

CARTILAGINOUS TUMORS

Cartilaginous tumors, either benign chondroma or chondrosarcoma, may arise from the articular cartilages, but they are uncommon lesions. Because the tumor forms a hard mass within the joint, symptoms of joint dysfunction may appear early. In other cases the mass has grown chiefly outside the joint cavity and thus has reached a large size before removal became necessary (Fig. 9-40). Cartilaginous tumors are prone to calcify no matter where they may originate and those developing within a joint are no exception to the rule. Typically, the calcium occurs in the form of multiple, very dense, discrete foci, result-

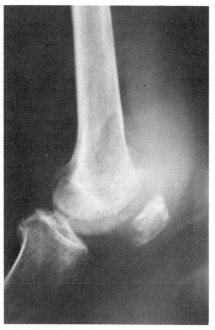

Fig. 9-38. Synovial sarcoma of the knee. Lateral roentgenogram. The soft-tissue mass represents tumor filling and distending the joint capsule. The tumor has invaded the femur anteriorly.

ing in a mottled appearance. If the calcified areas are few in number it may be impossible to distinguish between a chondroma and a synovioma from the roentgen appearances.

OSTEOCHONDROMATOSIS. Probably initiated by trauma, the synovial villi may hypertrophy and, by cellular metaplasia, form cartilaginous masses. These become calcified or even ossified in part and often become detached to lie free within the joint cavity. This condition is known as osteochondromatosis (Fig. 9-41). Usually there are multiple bodies but at times only one or a few are present. Calcification or ossification of the bodies usually is irregular and often has a laminated appearance. The presence of the masses within the joint causes a chronic synovitis with generalized thickening of the synovium and joint effusion. Degenerative changes in the form of joint space narrowing, eburnation of articular surfaces, and marginal osteophytes are common and may be severe. Osteochondromatosis is seen most frequently in the knee, occasionally in the elbow and the hip. Involvement of other joints is rare.

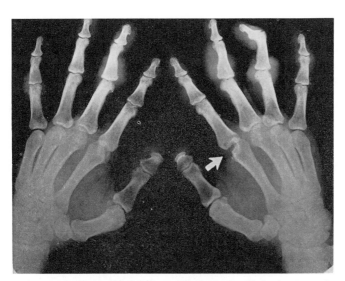

Fig. 9-39. Xanthoma tuberosa. There are multiple, lumpy soft-tissue swellings in the hands, mostly near the joints. Similar lesions are present in the feet. Note erosion of head of metacarpal (**arrow**). Similar bone involvement occurs with solitary xanthoma.

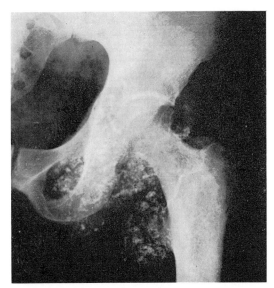

Fig. 9-40. Osteochondromas of the hip joint. There are large masses of partly calcified cartilage in and around the joint.

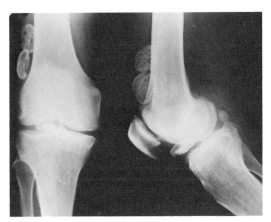

Fig. 9-41. Osteochondromatosis of the knee joint.

HEMANGIOMA

Hemangiomas involving the articular and peri-articular tissues are moderately common lesions. As is true when this tumor develops elsewhere in the body, calcified thrombi may be present, and give a clue concerning the nature of the lesion. A calcified thrombus within a vein appears as a small round or ovoid shadow and is called a phlebolith. Frequently these are ringlike with a dense outer rim and a less dense center, or else the shadow is laminated. Unless such phleboliths are visualized there usually is nothing specific about the appearance of a hemangioma of a joint that will allow its recognition in roentgenograms.

LOOSE BODIES

Intra-articular loose bodies may arise from multiple causes. Among these are (1) intra-articular fracture with separation of a fragment of cartilage, (2) rupture and fragmentation of a meniscus cartilage in the knee, (3) osteochondritis dissecans, (4) osteochondromatosis, (5) degenerative joint disease (see page 279). Injury accounts for the majority of loose bodies and they occur most frequently in the knee. If composed only of cartilage, the fragment cannot be visualized in roentgenograms. Many cartilaginous bodies calcify, becoming radiopaque and thus easily demonstrable in roentgenograms. Such calcified cartilage masses may arise from the synovial membrane as a result of metaplasia and are seen in the condition known as osteochondromatosis (see p. 292). Similar calcified bodies may be formed in degenerative joint disease as a result of fragmentation of articular cartilage or as a sequela to chronic synovial irritation in a joint rendered unstable by the disease.

OTHER CONDITIONS

OCHRONOSIS

This is a rare disorder of metabolism in which there is an abnormal accumulation of homogentisic acid in the blood and urine. The urine is either very dark on voiding or becomes black after standing or after it is alkalinized. The deposition of homogentisic acid (alkapton) in the articular cartilages results in degeneration of them. The significant roentgen observation is the extensive deposit of calcium that occurs in the articular cartilages. This is seen most frequently in the spine. In addition to calcification of the disc cartilages, the intervertebral disc spaces become thinned as a result of degeneration. Because many patients are in the older age group, senile osteoporosis and marginal spurring also may be present. Calcification of the articular cartilages of the peripheral joints is rather frequent as a simple degenerative process; in the spine, however, extensive calcification of the discs should arouse the suspicion of ochronosis. The cartilages in the ears may be extensively calcified.

In the peripheral joints a severe degenerative type of arthritis may develop, with thinning of the articular cartilages and even destructive changes in the bony articular surfaces. Calcifications may form in the synovium and periarticular tissues, such as ligaments and tendons.

REITER'S DISEASE

This is a syndrome characterized by urethritis, conjunctivitis, and arthritis. It occurs almost exclusively in males. The disease shows a tendency for asymmetrical involvement of the sacroiliac joints and asymmetry also is common when other joints are involved. This is a helpful differential feature particularly when rheumatoid arthritis is a consideration. Metatarsophalangeal and interphalangeal involvement, particularly of the first toe are other favorite sites of the disease (Fig. 9-42A and B) and the joints of the lower extremity are more often involved than the upper.[23] However, metacarpophalangeal and interphalangeal involvement of the fingers may be seen in some patients and other joints in the upper extremity infrequently are the sites of the disease. In any individual joint the roentgen findings may resemble those of other chronic inflammatory or infectious diseases. Soft-tissue swelling, joint effusion, local osteoporosis, marginal erosions, and joint-space thinning all may be present. Involvement of the plantar fascia often leads to an osteoperiostitis at its attachment to the os calcis. This is seen as a "wooly" appearing, calcified spur on the inferior surface of the bone but similar findings may occur at the attachment of the Achilles tendon, or, there may be cortical erosions, periostitis, and sclerosis along the entire posterior surface of the heel (Fig. 9-41C). Similar changes may occur at other sites of tendon insertions. Periosteal calcification around the shafts of bones adjacent to involved joints, such as the metatarsals, is common.

CALCIFICATION OF ARTICULAR CARTILAGES; THE PSEUDOGOUT SYNDROME

Calcium deposition in the articular cartilages or *chondrocalcinosis* occurs in a number of diseases including: (*1*) hyperparathyroidism, (*2*) rheuma-toid arthritis, (*3*) gout, (*4*) idiopathic hemochromatosis, and (*5*) the pseudogout syndrome. In addition it is a relatively common finding in elderly individuals whose joints are asymptomatic. When it is found in younger individuals the possibility of hyperparathyroidism should be kept in mind.

In the *pseudogout syndrome* the patients are apt to have intermittent attacks of acute pain and swelling in one or more joints and suggesting true gouty arthritis. Roentgenograms demonstrate chondrocalcinosis; the calcium may be deposited in hyaline or fibrocartilage or both. It often is widespread in multiple joints and there usually is associated degenerative disease. According to Martel and associates[14] the arthritic changes show a predilection for the metacarpophalangeal joints, elbows, wrists, ankles, and knees and are characterized by subchondral rarefactions, probably "degenerative cysts," thinning of articular cartilages with subchondral sclerosis and marginal spurs, and the frequent accompaniment of paraarticular, tendon and bursal calcifications. Examination of joint fluid aspirate usually reveals crystals of calcium pyrophosphate, said to be characteristic of the disease and the acute arthritis that develops is thought to be a crystal-induced synovitis. Calcium deposition in the hyaline articular cartilages is seen as a thin line of increased density paralleling the bony articular surface. In the knee-joint menisci and other fibrocartilages it is seen as a more granular deposit having more or less the shape of the cartilage.

Some investigators have found calcification of the knee-joint menisci in as high as one-third of the patients with *gout*.[8] Other causes of articular cartilage calcification that have been cited include trauma, infection, necrosis, malnutrition, senility, impaired vascularity, anoxia, and hypercalcemia. Calcification of the triangular cartilage of the wrist was found in five of 202 elderly patients (2.5 percent) by Dodds and Steinbach.[9] They also note its frequency in *primary hyperparathyroidism* and point out the necessity for excluding this disease when cartilage calcification is found. In our material, cartilage calcification has been found most frequently in elderly patients and often was asymptomatic or associated with degenerative joint disease. It is apparent, however, that there are multiple causes for it and correlation with the clinical and laboratory findings is important in establishing a cause.

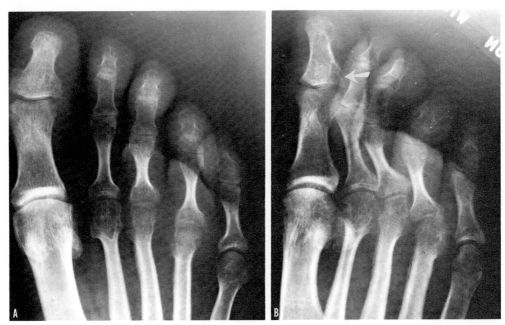

Fig. 9-42. Reiter's syndrome. *A*, Anteroposterior and *B*, oblique views of forefoot. There is involvement of the interphalangeal joint of the first toe with marginal erosions (**arrow**). Of the metatarsophalangeal joints, the fourth shows the most severe changes with local osteoporosis, joint space thinning and roughening of articular surfaces. *C*, Lateral view of the heel. There is cortical erosion (**arrow**), sclerosis along the posterior surface of the os calcis, and beginning spur formation inferiorly at the attachment of the plantar fascia.

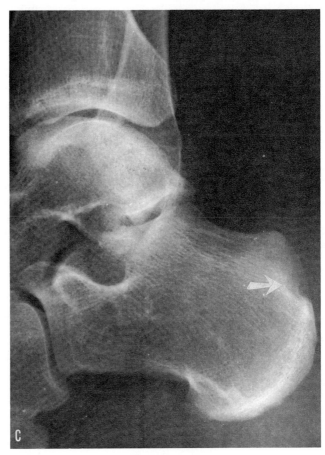

CYSTS CONNECTED WITH THE JOINTS

DISTENDED BURSAE. Any bursa adjacent to a joint may become distended with fluid and present as a cystic mass. Common examples are the prepatellar and olecranon bursae. Trauma is the most common cause for distention of these bursae. Some of the bursae around the major joints may communicate with the joint and become distended whenever joint effusion develops. Bursitis may be a complication of gout, particularly the olecranon bursa. Extensive distention of bursae associated with the hip joint has been found in rheumatoid arthritis of the hip by Melamed, Bauer, and Johnson.[16] The distended bursae bulged into the pelvis and caused pressure on the rectum and bladder suggesting a tumor mass. Similar large, fluid-distended bursae may be found near other large joints involved by rheumatoid arthritis.

BAKER'S CYST. Baker's cyst or popliteal cyst is caused by a herniation of synovial membrane through an opening in the posterior part of the joint capsule of the knee. The cause is not definitely known but it has been considered to be a congenital lesion, at least as far as predisposing factors are concerned. There is nothing characteristic about the roentgen appearance of the cyst and it cannot be differentiated from other soft-tissue masses that may occur in the popliteal space (synovioma, aneurysm of the popliteal artery, fibrosarcoma, etc.).

CYST OF THE SEMILUNAR CARTILAGE OF THE KNEE. These are not very common lesions. There often is a history of antecedent trauma but some investigators have considered the cyst to be of developmental nature. The external semilunar cartilage is involved most frequently and the lesion is seen in roentgenograms of the knee as a small soft-tissue bulge along the outer side of the joint.

OSTEITIS CONDENSANS ILII

This condition is found almost exclusively in females during the childbearing period and it almost always follows one or more pregnancies. It consists in a zone of dense sclerosis that develops along the iliac side of the sacroiliac joint. It is usually bilateral and symmetri-

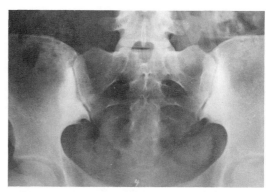

Fig. 9-43. Osteitis condensans ilii. The areas of sclerosis are, typically, on the iliac sides of the sacroiliac joints and the joint spaces are intact.

cal although some variation in intensity sometimes is observed between the two sides. The joint space is not affected and the sacrum is normal (Fig. 9-43). The area of sclerosis may be slight and fade off into normal bone or it may be several centimeters in width and be rather sharply demarcated from adjacent normal bone. The cause of this condition is unknown but because it does seem to be related to pregnancy it may represent the reaction to the abnormal stresses and strains to which this area is subjected during pregnancy and delivery. In many cases the lesion is discovered by accident during roentgenography of the pelvis for some other condition. In other cases the patient complains of pain in the lower part of the back and in the sacroiliac region. The lesion probably disappears spontaneously in most cases. This is borne out by observations of some of these patients carried out over a period of years and by the fact that sclerotic changes of this type are found very infrequently in older women. A similar type of sclerotic reaction is observed in the pubic bones adjacent to the symphysis (Fig. 9-44). This too is seen almost exclusively in women who have borne children and both the pubic and the iliac sclerosis have been seen in the same individual. This lesion is termed *osteitis condensans pubii*. Osteitis condensans ilii must be differentiated from rheumatoid arthritis of the sacroiliac joints. This latter disease affects the joint space and the articular surfaces of the

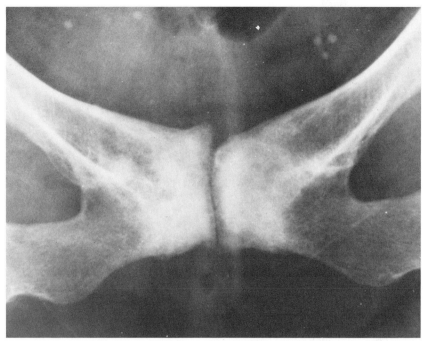

Fig. 9-44. Osteitis condensans pubii. The symphysis pubis is thinned with considerable sclerosis in the pubic bones.

bones on both sides of the joint although the iliac changes may be more noticeable than the sacral. Characteristically, the joint margins become blurred and eventually ankylosed. The disease affects young males predominantly and is relatively uncommon in females (approximate ratio of males to females is 15:1).

INTRAPELVIC PROTRUSION OF ACETABULUM (OTTO'S PELVIS; PROTRUSIO ACETABULI)

In this condition there is a deepening of the acetabular cavity, the head of the femur is deeply seated in the acetabulum, and the floor may bulge into the pelvis (Fig. 9-45). Protrusio acetabuli may arise from a number of causes. In a unilateral lesion, deepening of the acetabulum may have resulted from a destructive arthritis, particularly tuberculosis. Trauma with fracture of the acetabulum and with the head of the femur driven into the acetabular cavity is another cause. Bilateral lesions occur rather frequently as a result of rheumatoid

arthritis. When the pelvic bones are involved by severe osteomalacia, Paget's disease, or any other condition that causes the bones to be abnormally soft, the weight-bearing thrust of the femur may, over a period of time, cause a deepening of the acetabula and the development of a form of intrapelvic protrusion. Severe osteomalacia, in particular, often causes a general inward bending of the pelvic sidewalls which resembles protrusio acetabuli. In some cases the cause is obscure but it seems probable that, barring the presence of a joint disease such as rheumatoid arthritis, bilateral intrapelvic protrusion of the acetabula depends upon softening of the bones.

CALCIFICATION OF INTERVERTEBRAL DISCS IN CHILDHOOD

Calcification of one or more intervertebral discs in childhood is a rare disorder.[10, 17] The patients are usually in the 2- to 11-year age range, with a predominance of males. The patients usually complain of pain, with limitation of motion, muscle

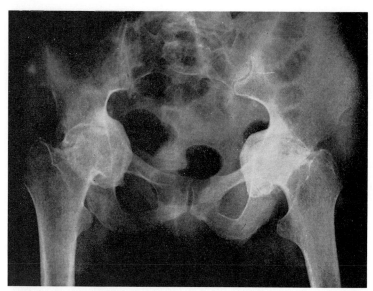

Fig. 9-45. Intrapelvic protrusion of the acetabulum. Anteroposterior roentgenogram of the pelvis demonstrates bilateral involvement in a patient, age 50, with rheumatoid arthritis.

spasm, tenderness, and torticollis. Roentgenograms show calcification in one or more intervertebral discs, mostly in the cervical area. The disease tends to be self-limited and the calcifications gradually disappear over a period of several months. The cause is not understood. Calcification within the discs of adult patients, usually in the thoracic area, is common and appears to be a different entity and related to the aging process, with degenerative changes responsible.

HYPERTROPHIC OSTEOARTHROPATHY

As a result of certain diseases, usually intrathoracic, subperiosteal calcification develops in the bones of the hands and feet and, in many cases, in the other long tubular bones. This condition is known as *hypertrophic osteoarthropathy*. In the past the term "hypertrophic pulmonary osteoarthropathy" was used. However it now is known that diseases involving systems other than the lungs or cardiovascular system can cause similar changes so that it is preferable to delete the "pulmonary" part of the term. In association with the periosteal changes there may be synovial thickening and arthralgia. A related condition is even more

common clinically and is referred to as clubbing of the digits. Clubbing consists of thickening of the soft tissues of the ends of the fingers. Clubbing may exist without the periosteal changes of osteoarthropathy or the two may be found together. Likewise periosteal calcification may be seen occasionally without soft-tissue clubbing. Current opinion indicates that clubbing and hypertrophic osteoarthropathy are closely related; that clubbing follows chronic pulmonary disease, particularly suppurative lesions such as bronchiectasis and lung abscess, and congenital cardiovascular disease; that osteoarthropathy, on the other hand, occurs more often as a result of intrathoracic neoplasms, especially mesothelioma of the pleura and bronchogenic carcinoma, is more rapid in its onset and development, and may recede promptly after removal of the tumor.[31]

In soft-tissue clubbing roentgenograms of the hands and feet reveal the enlarged soft tissues but the bones may be entirely normal. When hypertrophic osteoarthropathy is present the changes are those of subperiosteal calcification (Fig. 9-46). During the early stages this is

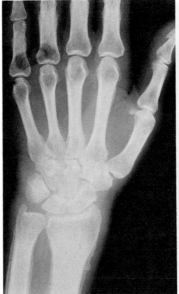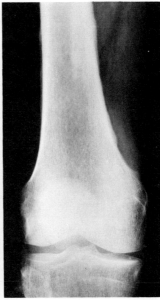

Fig. 9-46. Hypertrophic pulmonary osteoarthropathy. *Left,* Antero-posterior roentgenogram of the hand and wrist showing periosteal calcification around the shafts of the radius and ulna and, to a lesser degree, in the other bones. *Right,* Anteroposterior view of the knee of the same patient. Areas of periosteal calcification are visible along the cortical borders of the femur.

seen as thin pencil-line stripes of increased density along the outer surfaces of the bones. Multiple bones are involved although some may be unaffected or show only slight changes. The radius and ulna and the tibia and fibula are the bones most frequently affected. In the hands and feet the metacarpals and metatarsals are more often involved than the phalanges and the terminal phalanges may escape altogether. Later, the periosteal calcification becomes thicker and denser and may become nearly as dense as normal cortical bone. The outer surface also becomes wavy. In the adult there usually is little difficulty in diagnosis if multiple areas, such as both hands and feet, are examined. No other condition is as likely to cause this type of periosteal calcification involving multiple bones of the hands and feet with the underlying bone structure perfectly normal. In the legs a very similar type of periosteal calcification is seen in association with chronic venous stasis but the involvement is limited to the tibia and fibula and does not affect the upper extremities. During childhood there are a number of causes for periosteal calcification that may be a source of difficulty in diagnosis. These are considered in Chapter 10.

Rarely, an idiopathic type of hypertrophic osteoarthropathy is encountered in which no cause for the periosteal changes is apparent. In some patients there is an associated thickening of the skin of the forehead and face with prominent creases and folds (*pachydermoperiostosis*). This idiopathic form shows essentially the same roentgen features as described above.

CAISSON DISEASE

Caisson disease affects those who have worked under increased atmospheric pressure and is caused by too rapid decompression. It is more familiarly known as "the bends." It is the result of liberation of bubbles of nitrogen from the blood after the body has absorbed an excess of the gas while in compressed air. The bone and joint changes that may develop are the result of infarction. When infarcts have involved the articu-

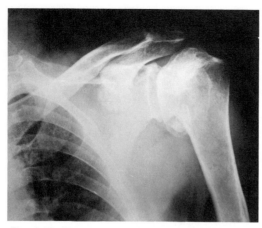

Fig. 9-47. Caisson disease. Anteroposterior roentgenogram of the left shoulder. The patient, age 51, had suffered an episode of "the bends" while working as a "sand-hog" building a river bridge 17 years ago. He has had difficulty with his hip and shoulder joints for 15 years. The changes are essentially degenerative in character owing to multiple small subchondral infarcts.

lar ends of the bones, ischemic necrosis results and the bones become softened. Eventually joint changes develop that resemble those of degenerative joint disease. The joints most frequently affected are those of the lower extremities and the shoulder (Fig. 9-47). In the hip the head of the femur becomes flattened, the superior portion often undergoes fragmentation or compression, and reactive spurring and sclerosis ensue. While the bone and joint changes are not particularly specific, the presence of areas of irregular calcification in the medullary cavities of the bones adjacent to the joints should raise the suspicion of caisson disease since these calcified areas may represent healed bone infarcts. In aviators a rapid ascent to high altitudes may cause aero-embolism similar to that found in caisson disease. In this instance the condition is caused by a rapid reduction in atmospheric pressure. Bone and joint changes similar to those found in caisson disease also have been described in these individuals.

THE VACUUM PHENOMENON; GAS IN THE JOINTS

The normal joint space is only a potential one and ordinarily cannot be identified in roentgenograms. What is often called the "joint space" in the description of roentgenograms refers to the relatively clear or translucent space between the ends of the bones that is occupied by the articular cartilages and what little synovial fluid is present. Under certain circumstances an actual space can be visualized in roentgenograms as a thin, translucent, dark line or space between the articular cartilages. In certain joints, notably the shoulder and the knee, the potential joint space can be made into a real one by proper traction exerted during the exposure. For example, this procedure has been utilized to visualize the semilunar cartilages in the knee. It is not entirely clear whether this space represents a vacuum or whether it becomes filled with gas liberated from the blood. Some authors writing on the subject consider it to be filled with gas and that the term "vacuum phenomenon," is a misnomer.

In other areas more persistent "spaces" will occasionally be demonstrated. For example, in the lumbar spine in association with severe degenerative disease of one or more of the discs, there may be seen a waferlike dark space within the disc. This has been called a "phantom disc." (See Fig. 9-27) A similar appearance has been noted with considerable frequency in the symphysis pubis of women during pregnancy. In these cases it is assumed that the space becomes filled with gas derived from the blood or tissue fluids rather than being a persisting vacuum (Fig. 9-48).

ARTHROGRAPHY

Arthrography consists of the injection of a contrast substance into a joint and the making of a series of roentgenograms to visualize the internal structures of the joint. While the procedure has been practiced for a number of years it has become a commonly done procedure only in recent years. While any of the peripheral joints can be examined by this means, the knee is the joint most often studied because of the frequency of injuries to this joint and its supporting structures. Either a radiolucent substance such as room air or, more frequently, a water-soluble radiopaque material can be used as the contrast agent. Some writers have expressed a preference for double-contrast arthrography, that is, combining a gas with an opaque substance. Our own preference is for a water-soluble, radiopaque contrast agent such as Renografin 60.

After suitable preparation of the skin and the injection of a local anesthetic, from 10.0 to 15.0

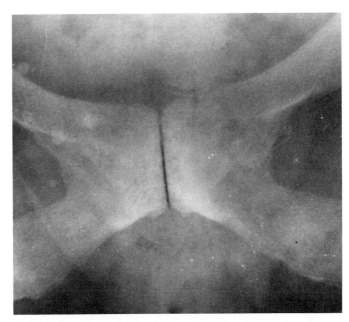

Fig. 9-48. "Vacuum phenomenon" in the symphysis pubis. In addition to being greatly thinned, there is a vertical translucency involving the remaining space. This translucent stripe probably is not a vacuum but rather is filled with gas. It indicates severe degeneration of the cartilage of the symphysis.

ml of Renografin 60 are injected using a 20-gauge needle and with the puncture made on the lateral side of the patella. If fluid is present in the joint it is aspirated before the contrast material is injected. The technique should be done meticulously to prevent infection. The leg is flexed and extended a number of times to distribute the contrast agent throughout the joint. If the examination is being done for possible injury to the internal structures of the joint, an Ace bandage is wrapped tightly around the lower thigh to the level of the joint space to obliterate the suprapatellar pouch and prevent dissemination of the material away from the joint space. Multiple roentgenograms are exposed (usually "spot-films" under fluoroscopic guidance) promptly after injection as the material is absorbed rather rapidly.

By this method tears of the menisci can be visualized. Also ruptures of the collateral ligaments can be recognized by the extravasation of contrast material beyond the confines of the joint cavity. Ruptures of the cruciate ligaments and visualization of nonopaque, cartilaginous loose bodies are other lesions that often can be identified. If the entire joint pouch is examined, synovial abnormalities such as villonodular synovitis often can be recognized. With experience on the part of the examiner the accuracy of the method is very good and it has proved extremely useful in detailing the anatomy of the knee joint structures in cases of acute injury when the results of clinical examination may be equivocal. For details of the technique and its interpretation, references are appended.[12, 19, 29] Among other uses arthrography has been recommended for the study of injuries to the supporting structures of the shoulder joint and in congenital dislocation of the hip in infants.

REFERENCES AND SELECTED READINGS

1. AVILA, R., PUGH, D. G., SLOCUMB, C. H., and WINKELMANN, R. K.: Psoriatic arthritis. A roentgenologic study. *Radiology 75:* 691, 1960.

2. BERENS, D. L., LOCKIE, L. M., LIN, R., and NORCROSS, L. M.: Roentgen changes in early rheumatoid arthritis. *Radiology 82:* 645, 1964.

3. BOCHER, J., MANKIN, H. J., BERK, R. N., and RODNAN, G. P.: Prevalence of calcified meniscal cartilages in elderly persons. *N. Engl. J. Med. 272:* 1093, 1965.

4. CAMIEL, M. R., and AARON, J. B.: The gas or vacuum phenomenon in the symphysis during pregnancy. *Radiology 66:* 548, 1956.

5. CORRIGAN, A. B.: Radiological changes in rheumatoid cervical spines. *Australas. Radiol. 13:* 370, 1969.

6. CRAIG, R. M., PUGH, D. G., and SOULE, E. H.: The roentgenologic manifestations of synovial sarcoma. *Radiology 65:* 837, 1955.

7. DETENBECK, L. C., YOUNG, H. H., and UNDERDAHL, L. O.: Ochronotic arthropathy. *Arch. Surg. 100:* 215, 1970.

8. DODDS, W. J., and STEINBACH, H. L.: Gout associated with calcification of cartilage. *N. Engl. J. Med. 275:* 745, 1966.

9. DODDS, W. J., and STEINBACH, H. L.: Triangular cartilage calcification in the wrist: Its incidence in elderly persons. *Am. J. Roentgenol. Radium Ther. Nucl. Med. 105:* 850, 1969.

10. HENRY, M. J., GRIMES, H. A., and LANE, J. W.: Intervertebral disc calcification in childhood. *Radiology 89:* 81, 1969.

11. JACKMAN, R. J., and PUGH, D. G.: The positive elbow fat pad sign in rheumatoid arthritis. *Am. J. Roentgenol. Radium Ther. Nucl. Med. 108:* 812, 1970.

12. LINDBLOOM, K.: Arthrography of the knee: A roentgenographic and anatomical study. *Acta Radiol. (Suppl. 74):* 1–112, 1948.

13. MARTEL, W.: The pattern of rheumatoid arthritis of the hand and wrist. *Radiol. Clin. North Am. 2:* 221, 1964.

14. MARTEL, W., CHAMPION, C. K., THOMPSON, G. R., and CARTER, T. L.: A roentgenologically distinctive arthropathy in some patients with the pseudogout syndrome. *Am. J. Roentgenol. Radium Ther. Nucl. Med. 109:* 587, 1970.

15. MARTEL, W., HOLT, J. F., and CASSIDY, J. T.: Roentgenologic manifestations of juvenile rheumatoid arthritis. *Am. J. Roentgenol. Radium Ther. Nucl. Med. 88:* 400, 1962.

16. MELAMED, A., BAUER, C. A., and JOHNSON, J. H.: Iliopsoas bursal extension of arthritic disease of the hip. *Radiology 89:* 54, 1967.

17. MELNICK, J. C., and SILVERMAN, F. N.: Intervertebral disc calcification in childhood. *Radiology 80:* 399, 1963.

18. MOSKOWITZ, R. W., and KATZ, D.: Chrondrocalcinosis and chondrocalsynovitis (pseudogout syndrome). Analysis of twenty-four cases. *Am. J. Med. 43:* 322, 1967.

19. NICHOLAS, J. A., FREIBERGER, R. H., and KILLORAN, P. J.: Double-contrast arthrography of the knee: Its value in the management of two hundred and twenty-five knee derangements. *J. Bone Joint Surg. 52-A:* 203, 1970.

20. PAUL, L. W.: Rheumatoid arthritis. *Postgrad. Med. 31:* A-61, 1962.

21. POGONOWSKA, M. J.:, COLLINS, L. C., and DOBSON, H. L.: Diabetic osteopathy. *Radiology 89:* 265, 1967.

22. RAGAN, C.: Primer on the rheumatic diseases. *JAMA 152:* 323, 1953.

23. SHOLKOFF, S. D., GLICKMAN, M. G., and STEINBACH, H. L.: Roentgenology of Reiter's syndrome. *Radiology 97:* 497, 1970.

24. SCHWARZ, E.: Hemophilic tumor of the ilium. *Radiology 75:* 795, 1960.

25. SEAMAN, W. B., and WELLS, J.: Destructive lesions of the vertebral bodies in rheumatoid disease. *Am. J. Roentgenol. Radium Ther. Nucl. Med. 86:* 241, 1961.

26. SEGAL, G., and KELLOGG, D. S.: Osteitis condensans ilii. *Am. J. Roentgenol. Radium Ther. Nucl. Med. 71:* 643, 1954.

27. SMITH, J. H., and PUGH, D. G.: Roentgenographic aspects of articular pigmented villonodular synovitis. *Am. J. Roetgenol. Radium Ther. Nucl. Med. 87:* 1146, 1962.

28. SPENCER, H., and WHIMSTER, I. W.: The development of giant-celled tumours and related conditions (chronic villo-nodular synovitis and cutaneous histiocytoma). *J. Pathol. 62:* 411, 1950.

29. TURNER, A. F., and BUDIN, E.: Arthrography of the knee. A simplified technique. *Radiology 97:* 505, 1970.

30. WHOLEY, M. H., PUGH, D. G., and BICKEL, W. H.: Localized destructive lesions in rheumatoid spondylitis. *Radiology 74:* 54, 1960.

31. WIERMAN, W. H., CLAGGETT, O. T., and McDONALD, J. R.: Articular manifestations in pulmonary diseases. An analysis of their occurrence in 1024 cases in which pulmonary resection was performed. *JAMA 155:* 1459, 1959.

32. WRIGHT, V.: Psoriasis and arthritis. A study of the radiographic appearances. *Br. J. Radiol. 30:* 113, 1957.

10

THE SUPERFICIAL SOFT TISSUES

Because the soft parts are much less radiopaque than the bones they may be overlooked when an average roentgenogram, made primarily to bring out bone detail, is being examined. Nevertheless the soft tissues, even in a heavily exposed film, exert a distinct influence on the appearance of the bones they cover. One has only to observe the difference in density of a part of a bone over which there is a loss of soft-tissue covering because of ulceration, traumatic avulsion, or surgical removal, with that of the adjacent uninvolved part to appreciate how much radiation is absorbed by the soft tissues and thus prevented from exerting a blackening effect on the photographic emulsion of the roentgen-ray film. Conversely, a small, localized, soft-tissue enlargement such as a wart or a mole in close contact with the film cassette or Bucky table can cause a sharply marginated increase in density that may be mistaken for a pathologic process within the tissues. For example, a mole on the surface of the chest wall may produce a round density that can be mistaken for a nodule within the lung and a similar lesion of the soft tissues of the lower back may suggest a renal or gallbladder calculus (see Fig. 10-21). The nipples are a common source of difficulty in the interpretation of chest roentgenograms. If one breast is pressed more firmly against the film

cassette than the other the nipple on one side may form a sharply outlined round density while the other may be invisible. Absence of one breast following a radical mastectomy causes one lung field to be more translucent than the other. After amputation of one upper extremity and the consequent unilateral disuse atrophy of the pectoral muscles in the male, similar increased translucency in the lung field often is observed. These are but a few examples of the influence of the peripheral soft tissues on the radiographic density of the deeper structures.

The soft tissues can be visualized in practically every roentgenogram, even those that have been heavily exposed, by viewing the film with a strong beam of light. Some type of spotlight should always be available in addition to the usual illuminators for the scrutiny of overexposed roentgenograms and particularly for the study of the soft-tissue coverings.

When specifically indicated, a suitable selection of exposure factors (usually a low kilovoltage and a high milliamperage) will produce a roentgenogram of high contrast in which the soft-tissue outlines are preserved and with a good differentiation of the soft-tissue densities. This type of roentgenogram is useful when the examination is made primarily for soft tissue visualization. Such a film will be of very little value for demonstrating bone detail because there will not be sufficient penetration of the dense bone structure; it will appear almost uniformly opaque. The use of high kilovoltages (80 to 125 kV) in diagnostic roentgenology tends to produce a roentgenogram with considerable latitude in density so that the soft-tissue outlines are preserved even though good penetration of the bone is obtained. Such an "all purpose" roentgenogram can be used as a routine type of exposure with considerable satisfaction and it will eliminate the need for special soft-tissue studies except in particular circumstances (Fig. 10-1).

While the specific gravity of the soft tissues as a whole is close to that of water, there is enough difference between fat and other tissues to make the subcutaneous fat zone distinctly visible in roentgenograms as a more translucent area beneath the skin. The fat zone also makes the outer surface of the muscles stand out clearly. Localized accumulations of fat near the joints aid in recognizing joint effusion because of their displacement when the joint capsule is distended. When there has been wasting from disease with consequent loss of fat, the soft parts have a very homogeneous density. Fat, therefore, is very important in giving texture to the soft tissues. The importance of the perirenal fat in enabling visualization of the kidneys has been commented on elsewhere and the value of intra-abdominal fat for soft-tissue differentiation is considerable.

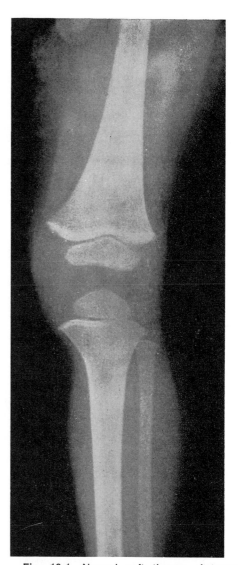

Fig. 10-1. Normal soft tissues. Anteroposterior roentgenogram of the lower extremity of a child illustrates the difference in density of muscles and fat. The more transparent subcutaneous fat causes the muscles to stand out clearly.

THE MUSCULAR DYSTROPHIES

The replacement of muscle by fat in the muscular dystrophies results in a fairly characteristic appearance in roentgenograms of the extremities. The muscles do not shrink appreciably in size but the extensive accumulations of fat within the remaining muscle bundles gives them a fine striated or striped appearance. In later stages most of the muscle tissue is replaced by fat, the fascial sheath bounding the muscle standing out as a thin shadow of increased density as it is visualized on edge (Fig. 10-2). One of the clinical subgroups is known as *pseudohypertrophic muscular paralysis*. It is characterized by the enlargement of certain muscles groups, usually those of the calves and of the shoulder girdles. The appearance clinically is that of a very muscular individual but actually the strength is extremely weak. In addition to the extensive replacement by fat in this type of dystrophy the muscles are enlarged. This

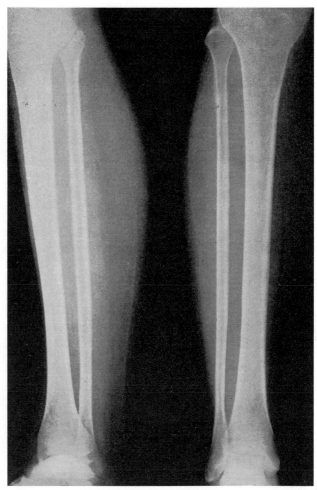

Fig. 10-2. Muscular dystrophy. Anteroposterior (*right*) and lateral (*left*) roentgenograms of the leg. The muscles are not appreciably decreased in size but have been replaced to a large extent by fat. The thin stripes represent the outer fascial boundaries of muscles with subcutaneous fat on the external side and fatty infiltration of the muscle beneath.

is the only condition in which the combination of large muscles interlaced with fat is found (Fig. 10-3). A recently described sign in this disease consists of an unusual widening of the shaft of the fibula in its anteroposterior diameter.[14, 20] This can be seen, for example, in Fig. 10-3, where the midshaft of the fibula is nearly as wide as the narrowest part of the tibial shaft. In patients with long-standing paralysis of one or more extremities from causes other than muscular dystrophy, including such conditions as poliomyelitis, spinal cord injuries, and cerebral vascular accidents,

muscles may contain stripes of fat but the affected muscle groups are decreased in size while the subcutaneous fat layer may be thick. When complete paralysis of an extremity has existed for a long time the muscle bundles may be almost completely absent, with subcutaneous fat making up most of the soft tissues surrounding the bones.

Normal blood vessels are visualized only as they course through the subcutaneous fat and only the larger vessels, chiefly the veins, can be

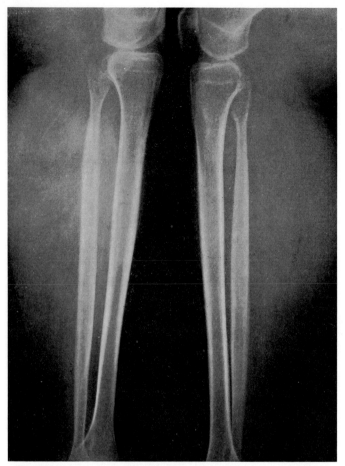

Fig. 10-3. Pseudohypertrophic muscular dystrophy. Lateral roentgenograms of both legs. While the muscles of the calves are very large, the roentgenograms show that they are largely replaced by fat. Note wide fibular shafts.

seen readily. When the superficial veins in the legs become varicose they are easily identified as tortuous linear shadows. Varicosities of the deep veins are not visible as a rule because they have a density similar to the muscles that surround them.

EDEMA AND HEMORRHAGE

Subcutaneous edema or hemorrhage causes a diffuse increase in density that as a rule is not sharply demarcated. The fluid obliterates the normal distinct boundary between the muscles and overlying fat. The subcutaneous space develops a fine striated or occasionally a slightly mottled appearance. The margins fade off gradually into normal density. When the accumulation of fluid is within the muscles or beneath them it causes only a uniform swelling of the part; if small it may go entirely unnoticed. Hemorrhage under the periosteum is invisible until the periosteum reacts to the irritation by depositing calcium. This requires a week or more before sufficient calcium is present to be visible in roentgenograms. Calcification develops more rapidly in the very young than it does in older individuals. In general the type of fluid within the tissues cannot be determined from the roentgen appearances and there is not enough difference in specific gravity of the various fluids to cause an appreciable variation in radiographic density.

CALCIFICATION IN THE SOFT TISSUES

ARTERIAL CALCIFICATION

Calcification in the walls of the larger arteries of the abdomen and of the extremities is a frequent observation in roentgenograms of individuals of middle age or over. Of the three pathologic types of arteriosclerosis, diffuse arteriolar sclerosis is not included in the present discussion; the small size of the vessels involved precludes roentgen visualization even if they should be calcified. The other two types have certain roentgen characteristics by means of which they often can be identified.

MÖNCKEBERG'S MEDIAL ARTERIOSCLEROSIS

This type of arteriosclerosis is characterized by the formation of calcific plaques in the medial layer of the blood vessel wall. These plaques do not narrow the vessel lumen and they cause no interference with the circulation. Mönckeberg's arteriosclerosis is an almost constant finding in elderly individuals and it is not at all infrequent in persons of the 35 to 50 age group, particularly in diabetics. The vessels most often affected are the femoral, popliteal, and radial arteries. This type of arteriosclerosis has the following roentgenologic features:

1. The calcification occurs in the form of closely spaced, fine concentric rings. These may be complete or incomplete but the process generally is diffuse, involving long segments of a vessel and multiple vessels (Fig. 10-4, below).

2. The characteristic changes are seen to best advantage in the femoral, popliteal, and tibial arteries but often can be identified in other moderate-sized vessels, such as the radial, dorsalis pedis, and the like.

INTIMAL ARTERIOSCLEROSIS

This type of arteriosclerosis is characterized pathologically by the formation of atheromatous plaques in the thickened intima of the arteries. The lumen of the vessel is narrowed, thrombosis may develop, and complete occlusion may result. This is the type of arteriosclerosis that leads to the clinical signs and symptoms of arterial insufficiency. The atheromatous plaques may not be calcified. When they are, the calcification is seen as irregular plaque-like areas of variable size and shape, from small flecks to larger areas a centimeter or more in length. The plaques seldom completely encircle the lumen of the vessel and are distributed irregularly along the course of the vessel without any specific arrangement (Fig. 10-4, left and right). The amount of visible calcification bears no relationship to the severity of the vascular occlusion and complete obstruction may exist with no visible calcification.

MIXED TYPES

Combined medial and intimal arteriosclerosis is common and when much medial calcification is present the intimal plaques may be hidden. In the feet it usually is difficult to determine the type of disease that may be present; the small vessels often are heavily calcified and combined forms are frequent. Calcified plaques are very frequently seen in the abdominal aorta and the iliac vessels. The typical ringlike calcification of medial arteriosclerosis is not seen in a vessel the size of the aorta and the type of arteriosclerosis cannot be determined from the roentgen appearances of the calcification. The most frequent type of aortic arteriosclerosis, however, is a form of medial arteriosclerosis that weakens the vessel wall and predisposes to the development of aneurysm.

CALCIFICATION OF THE VEINS

Calcification associated with the superficial or deep veins occurs in one of the following forms.

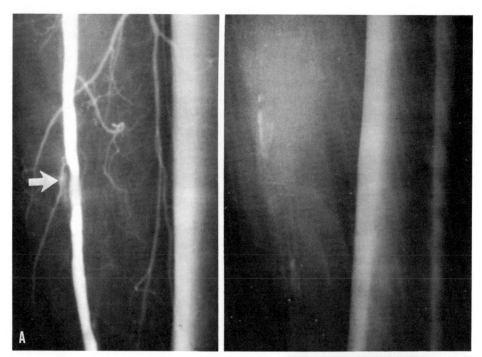

Fig. 10-4. Intimal arteriosclerotic plaques. *Right,* Several irregular plaques are visible in the femoral artery (shaft of femur is on the right). *Left,* Femoral arteriogram, same patient. The uppermost plaque has caused narrowing of the arterial lumen (**arrow**) with lesser encroachment at sites of other plaques. *Below,* Medial arteriosclerosis, femoral artery.

PHLEBOLITHS

A phlebolith is a calcified thrombus within a vein. They are found very frequently in the pelvic veins (see Chapter 13) and most adults will have a few of them. They occur in the form of small round or slightly ovoid calcified shadows of variable size from very tiny ones up to those that measure on the order of 0.5 cm in diameter. The phlebolith may be of homogeneous density, be laminated, or have a ring-like appearance. Phleboliths are common in varicose veins of the lower extremities. They frequently form in the dilated venous spaces of a cavernous hemangioma and result in one of the characteristic roentgen signs of this lesion. When a number of small, rounded calcifications are visualized in a localized area of the superficial soft tissues one should think of the

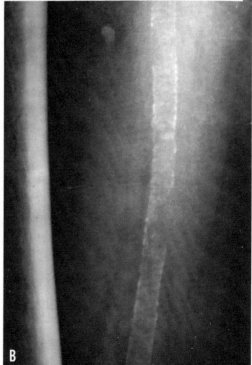

possibility of a cavernous hemangioma (Fig. 10-5). The phleboliths in a hemangioma very often have a ringlike appearance.

CALCIFICATION OF LARGER THROMBI

Occasionally a long thrombus within a vein will calcify and be visible as an elongated, somewhat irregular, calcification following the course of one of the larger veins.

CALCIFICATION ASSOCIATED WITH VENOUS STASIS

In the presence of venous stasis of long duration, usually secondary to varicosities and thrombosis, thin stripelike shadows of calcification may be seen in the subcutaneous tissues. They usually are visualized as double parallel stripes or with distinctly tubular and branching characteristics. Additionally there often are plaquelike calcifications in the subcutaneous tissues throughout the legs (Fig. 10-6) or as a

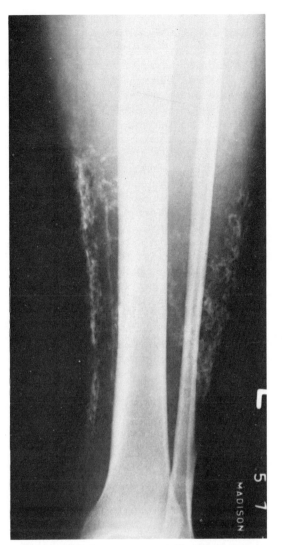

Fig. 10-6. Subcutaneous calcification in venous stasis.

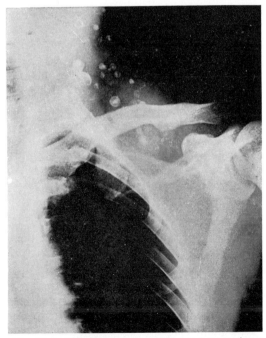

Fig. 10-5. Phleboliths in a cavernous hemangioma of the neck and shoulder. Multiple, round, ringlike and laminated calcareous densities characteristic of phleboliths are seen.

more localized process in the neighborhood of a varicose ulcer. The calcification in some of these cases resembles very closely that seen in diffuse scleroderma or dermatomyositis except that it is localized to the leg. Recent investigations suggest that the calcification is not in the walls of the vessels but rather in the perivascular tissues.[22] Phleboliths are often seen in association with the plaques. Periosteal calcification along the tibial and fibular shafts also is common (Fig. 10-15).

PARASITIC CALCIFICATION

The encysted larvae of the pork tapeworm (*Taenia solium*), known as cysticerus cellulosae, occasionally form in the brain, meninges, muscles, and other structures. Normally the pig is the intermediary host and human infestation occurs from eating improperly cooked pork. The eggs may be swallowed as a result of self-infection, with the larvae subsequently entering the tissues and becoming encysted, man thus acting as the intermediate host. The parasites may become calcified, making them visible roentgenologically. When calcified, the larvae from small round or slightly elongated masses from 1 to several millimeters in diameter or length, which may be widely disseminated throughout the muscles (Fig. 10-7) or the brain and its coverings. The small size of the calcifications and the wide dissemination of them should suggest the proper diagnosis.

The encysted embryos of *Trichina spiralis* are said to undergo calcification very frequently but the parasite is so small that it cannot be visualized readily in roentgenograms and the diagnosis of trichiniasis usually cannot be made from roentgen examination.

CALCIFICATION AFTER TRAUMA

Calcification or ossification often follows trauma to the deep tissues of the extremities. So-called calcified hematomas involving the muscles of the thigh are observed frequently in athletes, particularly football players, but may follow any local injury sufficient to cause bruising of the muscle or a frank hemorrhage within it. An injury of this nature severe enough to cause a deep muscle bruise often traumatizes the periosteum too and there may be hemorrhage beneath it; this also frequently undergoes calcification. Calcification within a muscle that follows trauma is called *traumatic myositis ossificans* because the condition progresses to actual bone formation in most cases. This form of myositis ossificans should not be confused with the disease known as *progressive myositis ossificans,* which begins in the very young, is not associated with trauma, and progresses until the entire body may become fixed

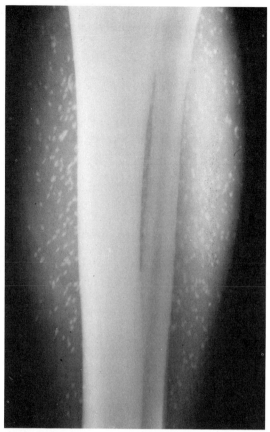

Fig. 10-7. Cysticercosis. Innumerable tiny round and ovoid calcifications in the muscles of the leg. The patient had been a prisoner of war of the Japanease during World War II and had eaten a considerable amount of raw pork. (Courtesy Margaret Winston, M.D., Madison, Wisconsin).

and immobile. This disease is discussed later in this chapter.

The calcified hematoma may become visible as a hazy shadow of increased density within a few weeks after the initiating trauma (Fig. 10-8). Over a period of several weeks this gradually becomes denser and finally it develops the appearance of actual bone. The mass has a laminated character caused by the hemorrhage dissecting along the muscle and fascial planes (Fig. 10-9). Usually after a period of time the ossification gradually decreases in size; smaller masses may disappear completely. Cases have been reported in which osteogenic sarcoma has developed in an area of traumatic myositis

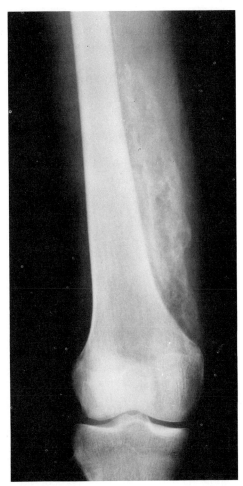

Fig. 10-8. Traumatic myositis ossificans. Calcification in a large hematoma in the inner aspect of the thigh.

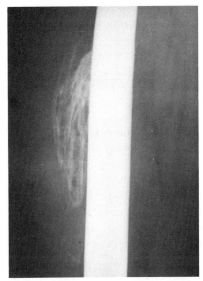

Fig. 10-9. Posttraumatic myositis ossificans. Lateral roentgenogram of the midpart of the thigh. The hematoma followed a deep bruise. The typical laminated calcification of an intramuscular hemorrhage is demonstrated.

ossificans but this appears to be a rare lesion. Calcification or bone formation within a laparotomy scar is occasionally seen and this represents a form of traumatic myositis ossificans.

THE EHLERS-DANLOS SYNDROME

The Ehlers-Danlos syndrome is a rare cause of disseminated subcutaneous calcifications. It is characterized by an unusual hyperelasticity and fragility of the skin and blood vessels, hypermobility of the joints, pseudotumors over the bony prominences, and disseminated movable subcutaneous nodules. In addition, other congenital de-

fects have been noted frequently and the disease is considered to be a congenital dystrophy with hereditary and familial influences. The syndrome is of interest roentgenologically because the subcutaneous nodules may calcify. Holt[16] has described the appearance of these as found in two sisters. The nodules appeared as round, discrete densities, usually ringlike with a central zone of translucency. The calcifications resembled very closely the shadows of venous phleboliths as seen in cavernous hemangiomas, except for the wide dissemination. The nodules had a predilection for the medial and lateral surfaces of the extremities and were more numerous in the legs.

CALCIFICATION IN TUMORS

Calcification is not a specific finding for any single type of tumor of the soft tissues and it results usually because of a deficient blood supply with subsequent necrosis within a solid, slowly growing neoplasm. Deposits of calcium occur in lipomas, liposarcomas, fibrosarcomas, and synovial sarcomas to mention the most common. There is nothing characteristic about the appearance of the calcification to aid in identifying the type of tumor. Rarely, *osteogenic sarcoma* has been found arising in the soft tissues, apparently as a result of cellular metaplasia.

CALCIFICATION AFTER SPINAL CORD INJURY

The development of masses of calcium or bone in the extremities of paraplegics or quadriplegics is one of the interesting and rather poorly understood complications of spinal cord injury. In some patients the calcification appears to follow decubitus ulcers and chronic infection of the deep tissues overlying the bony prominences, particularly the greater trochanters and the ischial tuberosities. In others, extensive calcification or ossification develops along the shafts of the bones and within the muscles of the paralyzed extremities. This may represent a traumatic myositis ossificans (*q.v.*) since the lack of pain sensation predisposes to repeated injuries with intramuscular and subperiosteal hemorrhages and subsequent calcification. However, in some cases this explanation does not seem correct and the exact mechanism at times remains obscure (Fig. 10-10).

Because of the severe disuse osteoporosis in these patients the bones fracture easily and the injury may go undetected for a time. Exuberant callus is common around such a fracture because of the lack of proper immobilization. Dislocation may also occur and not be recognized for some time.

INTERSTITIAL CALCINOSIS

Interstitial calcinosis is an uncommon although not a rare disease in which there is either a localized or a widely disseminated deposition of calcium in the skin, subcutaneous tissues, muscles, and tendons. Calcinosis often is associated with and apparently a part of the collagen diseases, scleroderma, and dermatomyositis. However, it can exist in a relatively asymptomatic form with no signs of any associated disorder. The cause of interstitial calci-

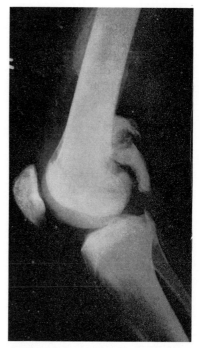

Fig. 10-10. Periosteal and soft-tissue calcification in a paraplegic patient. Large masses of calcium have formed in the popliteal area. Subperiosteal calcification is present along the shaft of the femur.

nosis, therefore, is unknown but the process is generally considered to represent tissue calcification secondary to some type of injury and thus to fall in the general group of dystrophic calcifications. The following types of calcinosis can be recognized.

CALCINOSIS UNIVERSALIS (DIFFUSE CALCINOSIS)

Calcinosis universalis is characterized by the wide dissemination of thin calcific plaques of various sizes throughout the soft tissues, chiefly in the subcutaneous layer, occasionally within the muscles and tendons. From a clinical point of view there are three types of diffuse calcinosis:

1. Asymptomatic. This has been reported but in our experience is a rare lesion.

2. Diffuse calcinosis associated with generalized scleroderma.

3. Diffuse calcinosis associated with dermatomyositis (Fig. 10-11).

The diseases, scleroderma and dermatomyositis, are closely related, both being considered to belong to the group of "collagen diseases." The calcification occurs in the form of thin plaques. In scleroderma these are limited to the skin and immediate subcutaneous tissues; in dermatomyositis calcification also occurs in the muscles. In addition to the plaques there is a general loss of soft-tissue differentiation with the subcutaneous fat layer becoming very scanty or disappearing altogether.

Among the unusual variants of calcinosis associated with scleroderma is the hereditary condition known as *Werner's syndrome*. In addition to the scleroderma and diffuse calcinosis there are other stigmata of congenital origin. Thus there may be premature graying of the hair, juvenile cataracts, and widespread arterial calcification of the Mönckeberg type. These changes may be extensive in a relatively young individual (20 to 30 years of age). The interstitial calcinosis may involve not only the subcutaneous tissues but the tendons, ligaments, and bursae.

CALCINOSIS CIRCUMSCRIPTA

In the localized type of calcinosis the calcifications occur in the form of small rounded foci having an amorphous appearance. These foci are found chiefly in the tips of the fingers and along the margins of the joints in the hands and feet. The changes are found more frequently in the hands than in the feet and when present in both areas are usually more intense in the hands. As is true with the diffuse form of calcinosis, the localized type occurs in several different clinical manifestations:

WITHOUT ASSOCIATED SKIN OR VASOSPASTIC PHENOMENA. The lesions appear most frequently in elderly persons and are more common in women than in men. There may be some aching in the joints of the affected areas or the calcifications may be found by chance. The foci may be numerous and some may be sufficiently large to cause visible swellings (Fig. 10-12). In some cases ulceration of the skin occurs over the larger lumps, followed by extrusion of cheesy, whitish material and subsequent healing. Because of the physical similarity to gout, the condition has been termed

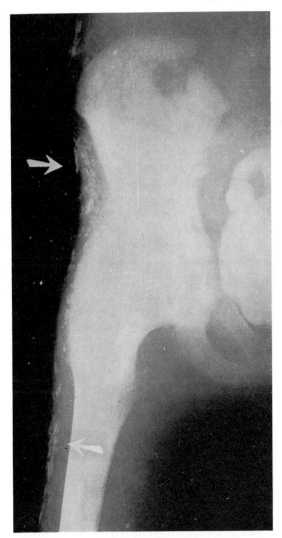

Fig. 10-11. Diffuse interstitial calcinosis in a patient with dermatomyositis. Anteroposterior roentgenogram of the hip area shows extensive plaque formation in the subcutaneous tissues along the outer side (**arrow**). There is complete loss of normal soft-tissue differentiation and the margins of muscles and boundaries of the subcutaneous fat layer cannot be identified. (Barium residue in rectum is from gastrointestinal study.)

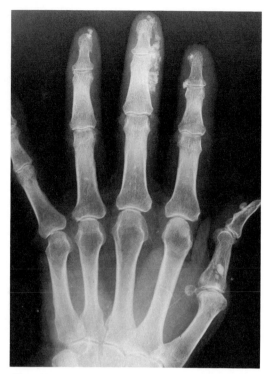

Fig. 10-12. Localized interstitial calcinosis. Deposits of calcareous material are noted in many areas.

chalk gout. This is not good usage and should be discontinued because the disease has no relationship to gout. Gouty tophi, being composed of urates, are radiolucent and of a density comparable to the soft tissues. However, gouty tophi may calcify occasionally but the other bone and joint changes of gout are usually present to aid in diagnosis.

ASSOCIATED WITH SCLERODERMA. Calcinosis is of frequent occurrence when scleroderma affects the fingers and hands. The calcification may be in the form of a few tiny rounded subcutaneous nodules or occur as larger masses. These are found commonly in the terminal phalanges or along the margins of the joints. Other roentgen signs of scleroderma often are present, including (*1*) diminution in the amount of soft tissues in the tips of the fingers so that they develop a tapered or almost pointed appearance, (*2*) uniform density of the subcutaneous tissues with loss of normal soft-

tissue architecture, and (*3*) absorption of bone. This begins in the terminal tufts of the distal phalanges of the affected fingers so that these tufts disappear and the shaft of the phalanx becomes pointed. The absorption may extend to involve the shaft and can be sufficiently severe so that most of the bone disappears or fragments (Fig. 10-13).

ASSOCIATED WITH RAYNAUD'S PHENOMENON AND SECONDARY SCLERODERMA. Clinically these patients usually are women; the disease may begin during adolescence or later. The early symptoms are those of intermittent arteriolar spasm with the scleroderma appearing either contemporaneously or at a variable time afterward. The scleroderma may progress and involve extensive areas of the body. In other cases it is limited to the face and neck, the fingers and hands, with progressive decrease to the elbows; less marked changes may be present in the feet and toes. This more limited disease goes by the name of *acrosclerosis*. The roentgen findings are no different from those described for scleroderma alone.

CRST syndrome.

PERIOSTEAL CALCIFICATION

The periosteum, although intimately related to bone and bone formation, has the same "water-density" as other soft tissues. Regardless of cause, irritation of it usually is followed by reactive calcification. The appearance of this often gives a valuable clue to the nature of the underlying bone disease. The following list of types of periosteal calcification indicates how this information can be used in diagnosis:

I. Continuous layer (mostly benign lesions)
  A. Uniform density [hazy (early); dense (older)]
    1. Parallel surface (infections; hemorrhage; callus)
    2. Wavy surface (osteoarthropathy; venous stasis; tuberous sclerosis)
    3. Convex surface (hemorrhage; benign tumors; callus)
  B. Laminated (some active infections)
  C. Spiculated (anemias; acropachy; hemangioma)

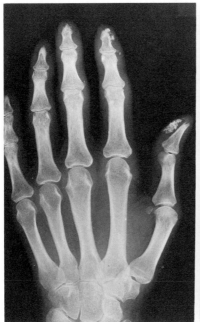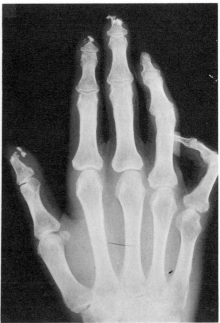

Fig. 10-13. Insterstitial calcinosis associated with scleroderma. *Left,* In addition to the amorphous calcareous deposits in the tips of fingers there is absorption of the terminal tufts, giving the phalanges a pointed shape. The soft tissues of the tips of the fingers are decreased. *Right,* Another case of scleroderma showing more extensive absorption of the terminal tufts of the dstal phalanges of the thumb and second and third fingers.

II. Interrupted layer (many are malignant)
   A. Uniform density
   B. Laminated (multiple layers) (Ewing's)
      1. Codman triangles (usually primary malignancy)
   C. Spiculated (malignant tumors)

The most frequent causes include: (1) fracture (callus), (2) infection, (3) metabolic, (4) tumors, (5) melorheostosis, (6) infantile cortical hyperostosis, (7) vitamin A poisoning, (8) hypertrophic osteoarthropathy, (9) subperiosteal hemorrhage, (10) tuberous sclerosis, (11) others (see following).

CHRONIC VASCULAR STASIS. In the presence of chronic venous stasis in the legs occurring as a result of long-standing varicosities and venous thrombosis, chronic periosteal calcification along the tibial and fibular shafts is frequent (Fig. 10-14). The appearance resembles closely that found in hypertrophic osteoarthropathy. In this latter condition, periosteal calcification also will be present in the hands and possibly other long bones in the upper extremities, and there almost always is evidence of chronic pulmonary disease, usually neoplastic, responsible for the periosteal changes.

PERIOSTEAL STRIPES IN INFANTS. In young, healthy infants thin, stripelike shadows are visible occasionally, paralleling the outer cortical margins of the long bones. The cause of the periosteal stripes is debatable since the infant may be perfectly normal and healthy, but apparently they represent incompletely calcified new bone that is being formed by the inner layer of periosteum. Similar periosteal stripes are seen at times when there has been a chronic illness and where osteoporosis may be the causative factor (Fig. 10-15). In many premature infants fairly pronounced subperiosteal calcification may be found around the shafts of the tubular bones very similar in appearance to

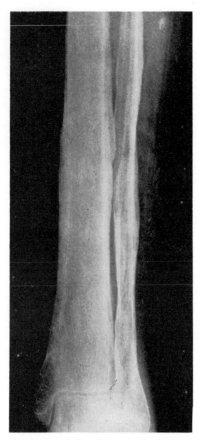

Fig. 10-14. Periosteal calcification associated with chronic venous stasis. There is wavy calcification extending along the tibial and fibular shafts. A few phleboliths (i.e., calcified thrombi) also are visible, indicating the presence of varicose veins.

along the concave side of a bowed, weight-bearing bone, or in any area where strain has existed for any length of time.

THYROID ACROPACHY. This is a rare manifestation of thyroid disease. It usually occurs some years after partial thyroidectomy with resulting hypothyroid or euthyroid state. The cause is unknown. Clinically, there are swelling of the fingers and toes, exophthalmos and pretibial myxedema. Roentgen examination shows periosteal calcification involving the metacarpals and phalanges. The calcification has a somewhat spiculated appearance and tends to be most intense beneath the areas of greatest soft-tissue swelling. The dense, spiculated calcification is

the periostitis found in congenital syphilis. There is, however, no evidence of syphilis in these patients. Caffey has expressed the opinion that the periostitis in these cases may represent the effects of unrecognized trauma to susceptible tissues such as the periosteum which is very vascular and loosely attached to the cortex at this age period.

CHRONIC BONE STRAIN. Abnormal stresses affecting a bone over a long period of time will lead to a thickening of the cortex at the site of maximum stress. This is a buttressing effect. It is seen along the outer sides of the metatarsals in such deformities as congenital clubfoot and in other types of varus deformity of the foot,

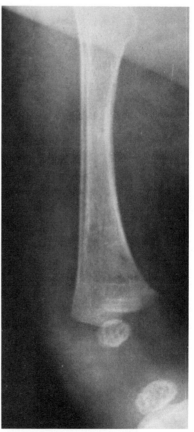

Fig. 10-15. Periosteal stripes in an infant with generalized edema. Note the stripelike density paralleling the outer cortex of the femur. Similar "stripes" may be seen in normal infants.

characteristic. In differential diagnosis hypertrophic osteoarthropathy often involves bones other than those of the hands and feet, and the periosteal calcification has a smoother, wavy outer surface.

NORMAL OSSEOUS RIDGES. In the interpretation of roentgenograms of bone, care must be used not to mistake a normal osseous ridge for periostitis. Such ridges are constantly present for the attachment of the interosseous membranes between the radius and ulna and the tibia and fibula. In some persons these are more prominent than usual without being in any way abnormal. The position of the extremity in its relation to the roentgen film will affect the visualization of the interosseous ridges since they are seen only when along the margin of the bone tangential to the direction of the roentgen-ray beam. The *linea aspera* of the femur, when brought into profile by a lateral view of the thigh, often appears as a rough thickening of the cortex that must be recognized as a perfectly normal anatomical structure. Older persons, particularly males who have worked as laborers, often show increased prominence of the tuberosities and bony ridges where ligaments and muscles are attached.

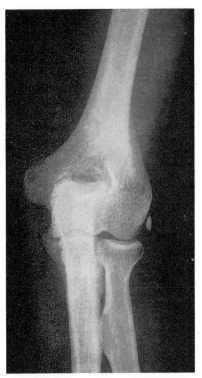

Fig. 10-16. Calcifying tendinitis of the elbow. Calcareous deposit adjacent to the external epicondyle of the humerus.

MISCELLANEOUS FORMS OF SOFT-TISSUE CALCIFICATION

ARTICULAR AND PERIARTICULAR CALCIFICATION

Calcification occurring as a result of inflammation of the tendons and bursae around the joints has been considered in Chapter 9, under the heading of "Periarticular Disease" (see Fig. 10-16).

Periarticular calcification also occurs as a part of vitamin D poisoning following the administration of excessive amounts of this vitamin. In this condition large deposits of calcium have been noted in the soft tissues around various joints. An associated finding has been the presence of widespread chronic osteoporosis. Because many of the patients showing evidence of vitamin-D poisoning have received the vitamin as a part of the treatment for rheumatoid arthritis, it is difficult to evaluate the osteoporosis in terms of vitamin-D poisoning. Chronic osteoporosis is an almost constant accompaniment of chronic rheumatoid arthritis when it has existed for any length of time.

Large deposits of calcium in the subcutaneous tissues in the region of the joints may follow the prolonged ingestion of large quantities of milk, usually by patients suffering from peptic ulcer. This is known as *milk drinker's syndrome* (milk-alkali syndrome). Other components include extensive calcification of the kidneys and of the blood vessels. Poppel and Zeitel[27] believe that a primary requirement is the excess intake of milk. The increase of phosphorus and calcium in the blood leads to calcification of the renal tubules. If there also is an alkalosis because of the excess intake of alkali over a long period of time, the kidneys will excrete an abnormally large amount of acid and this will increase the precipitation of calcium salts in the kidneys. Eventually renal insufficiency supervenes, the levels of calcium and phosphorus remain constantly high, and calcification of various tissues will follow. The subcutaneous calcification occurs either in the form of amorphous masses, often large, or as a more mottled deposit of calcium. These are found in the region of the larger joints. Calcification of the renal tubules, nephrocalcinosis, causes a fine, granular type of renal calcification sometimes limited to the renal papillae, but in other cases more widely disseminated in the kidney parenchyma. In some cases calcium is clearly demonstrated in histologic sections but roentgenograms do not show it well.

Calcification of the articular cartilages of various joints is not uncommon in elderly individuals. The condition, articular calcification, is discussed in Chapter 9.

Periarticular calcification also occurs in pseudohypoparathyroidism and in hyperparathyroidism. The skeletal changes usually present in these diseases are significant in diagnosis.

Juxta-articular and soft-tissue calcification has recently been described in the disease called *pseudoxanthoma elasticum*.[17] This is a rare hereditary disorder characterized by degeneration of elastic tissue and involves many organ systems. The most common clinical findings are reported to be xanthomalike skin lesions, upper gastrointestinal tract hemorrhage, and loss of visual acuity. Arterial calcification, both intimal and medial, is commonly present. Resorption of the terminal tufts of the phalanges may follow narrowing of arteries with diminished blood flow to the fingers.

PROGRESSIVE MYOSITIS OSSIFICANS

This is a rare disorder of unknown cause that appears to belong to the congenital dysplasias. It commences during early childhood with the development of doughy and often painful swellings, chiefly in the muscles of the neck and back. As these subside there is left a diffuse fibrosis and this in turn is followed by the development of platelike masses of bone (Fig. 10-17). There is a slow progression of the disease with periods of remission and exacerbation but eventually there develops a widespread fixation of the muscles until the

body becomes immobile and death ensues. The patient may have considerable limitation of motion in the affected areas before much bone has been formed and the amount of bone demonstrated roentgenographically does not give a true indication of the extensiveness of the process. The first places where roentgenograms often reveal the abnormal ossifications are the muscles of the back and the neck. The ossified lesions at first are relatively hazy and difficult to identify but within a period of time irregular elongated bony plates are observed extending along the long axis of the muscle. In the later stages numerous muscles will be found extensively ossified and the joints practically immobile. This disease should not be confused with traumatic myositis ossificans, which has been described earlier in this chapter. There is no relationship between the two conditions. Anomalies of the skeleton are present almost invariably. Among these are microdactyly of the first toe with ankylosis of the interphalangeal joint and ankylosis of the metatarsophalangeal joint, hallux valgus, hypoplasia of the first metacarpals and of some of the phalanges, and occasional examples of hypoplasia of the middle phalanges of the fifth digits of the hands. Changes in the feet have been encountered more frequently than those in the hands.

CALCIFICATION OF LYMPH NODES

After being involved by infection, usually tuberculosis, the peripheral lymph nodes may calcify. The most frequent site is the cervical chain with the axillary nodes second in frequency. Calcification of other peripheral nodes is very infrequent. The calcifications are visualized as mottled areas of calcific density, often multiple, and distributed along the course of the cervical lymph node chains or in the axilla.

PELLEGRINI-STIEDA CALCIFICATION

A small, flat or slightly curved area of calcification or ossification occasionally is found along the upper border of the medial condyle of the femur that goes by the name of Pellegrini-Stieda calci-

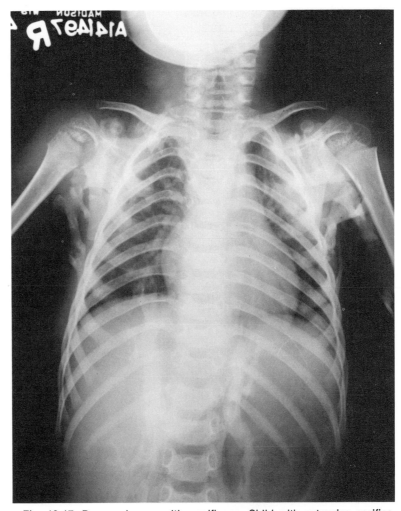

Fig. 10-17. Progressive myositis ossificans. Child with extensive ossification of muscles of back and shoulders. Irregular bony plaques can be seen alongside the lower thoracic spine and throughout the axillas.

fication. While this at first was thought to be an avulsion fracture of the femoral cortex, subsequent studies have demonstrated that it represents a post-traumatic calcification in the tibial collateral ligament at or near its attachment to the femur. The lesion is caused by trauma and represents in effect a small area of traumatic myositis ossificans. The evidence of calcification usually appears within several weeks to a month after the initiating trauma. It gradually increases in density and in time may develop the appearance of actual bone. In some cases followed over a period of months the lesion has gradually diminished in size and disappeared.

CALCIFICATION IN THE FEMALE BREAST

Calcified deposits occasionally are found within the breast and in some instances are large enough to cause confusing shadows in chest roentgenograms and to suggest abnormal changes within the lung parenchyma. Special soft-tissue roentgenograms of the breast show these to best advantage (see section on "Mammography"). Leborgne[19] has called attention to the fact that calcification is frequent in scirrhous carcinomas of the breast. The calcifications occur in the form of a cluster of fine, stippled or sandlike densities and he found this

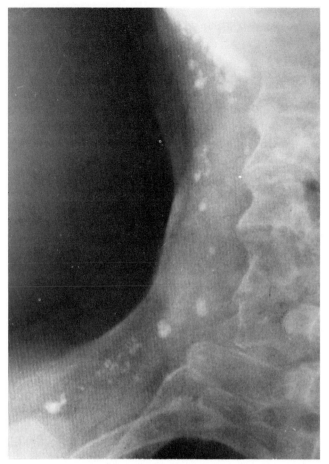

Fig. 10-18. Calcified cervical lymph nodes. Multiple, small, irregular calcified deposits are seen along the cervical chain of lymph nodes.

particular type of calcification to be fairly significant for the diagnosis of scirrhous carcinoma. Benign forms of calcification also are encountered. One of the commonest is that of multiple calcifications within the lactiferous ducts. These are sharply outlined, rounded, or ovoid calcified densites that frequently have a ringlike character, the periphery being denser than the center. Calcification in the blood vessels of the breast is occasionally encountered and usually can be recognized by the tubular nature of the shadows and their branching characteristics. Calcification in benign tumors, particularly in fibroadenomas, may occur and these differ from the calcifications of carcinoma in being larger, fewer in number, and often disposed around the periphery of the tumor capsule.

TUMORAL CALCINOSIS

This is a rare entity characterized by the occurrence of a large calcified mass usually near one of the larger joints, particularly the hip and elbow.[26] In the elbow the lesion may cause flattening of the lower posterior surface of the humerus. Generally, however, the adjacent bone is not involved. Multiple areas may be affected and the lesion also has been reported adjacent to the spine, wrists, lower ribs, and sacrum. Clinically there is pain and localized swelling. The lesion is benign but may recur if surgical removal has been incomplete. The etiology is unknown, but some have considered it to be related to calcinosis circumscripta or universalis. In differential diagnosis, similar calcified masses may be found in hypervitaminosis D, milk drinker's syndrome (milk-alkali syndrome), and hyperparathyroidism, among others. The tumors are found in young, otherwise healthy persons and the blood chemistry findings are normal. These features are of considerable aid in differential diagnosis from other causes of juxta-articular calcification.

GAS IN THE SOFT TISSUES

Accumulations of gas in the soft tissues can be easily recognized in roentgenograms because of the extreme translucency of gas compared to the surrounding soft tissues. Occasionally a localized deposition of fat, such as in a lipoma, may appear sufficiently translucent in roentgenograms with very high contrast so that it suggests a local pocket of gas. An accumulation of air or other gas, of similar size, however, would appear considerably darker and it usually requires little experience to differentiate between the two. There are two major types of gas that can be found in the soft tissues. One is air that may have gained entrance through a traumatic wound or following a surgical procedure or may have been introduced deliberately as a contrast substance. The other is gas that has been formed as a result of anaerobic bacterial action. When there is any appreciable amount of subcutaneous air it is often described as subcutaneous emphysema.

SUBCUTANEOUS EMPHYSEMA

Small bubbles or streaks of air are frequently seen in the region of soft-tissue wounds of penetrating nature. The air shadows may persist for several hours or longer but usually have disappeared after a day or two. Subcutaneous emphysema may follow injuries to the thorax, usually rib fracture. There may or may not be an associated pneumothorax. Occasionally after such an injury the subcutaneous

emphysema becomes very extensive and the air extends widely through the fascial spaces of the body. As a rule such an extensive subcutaneous emphysema develops as a result of a tension pneumothorax. After surgical procedures on the thorax fairly large amounts of subcutaneous emphysema are constantly found for several days after the operation. Traumatic rupture of the trachea or larynx may also result in subcutaneous emphysema (Fig. 10-19). Because of the free communication of the fascial spaces of the body, air may extend far from its point of origin. The recognition of subcutaneous emphysema is not difficult unless the amount of gas is small. Air associated with penetrating wounds often is found in the form of small bubbles, probably because it is associated with hemorrhage. Otherwise any appreciable amount of air tends to accumulate in the form of linear streaks along the fascial planes.

GAS BACILLUS INFECTION

Infection with gas-forming organisms may result in the visualization of bubbles or streaks of gas in the subcutaneous or deeper tissues. This may follow penetrating or crushing injuries or surgical procedures. The organisms most frequently found are *Bacillus welchii, Vibrion septique,* and *Bacillus oedematiens.* It is not possible to distinguish gas formed by anaerobic bacteria from air that has been introduced from without and, therefore, the diagnosis of gas gangrene cannot be made from roentgen evidence during its very early stage. If the gas shadows extend for a considerable distance from the known site of the soft-tissue wound, one can suspect the possibility of gas infection. If serial examinations over a period of hours or several days show definite evidence of increasing amounts of gas and spread of the gas shadows, the evidence for gas bacillus infection is more conclusive (Fig. 10-20).

In diabetic gangrene involving the foot it is common to find small bubbles of gas in the region of the gangrenous tissue and occasionally even more extensively throughout the soft

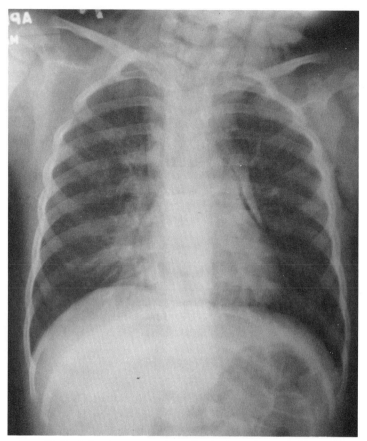

Fig. 10-19. Subcutaneous and mediastinal emphysema. There is air in the soft tissues of the neck, the left axilla, and the left side of the mediastinum. It followed injury to the trachea as a result of foreign-body aspiration.

tissues of the foot or in the distal part of the leg. The occurrence of gas in the gallbladder wall (*emphysematous cholecystitis*) and in the wall of the urinary bladder in the presence of infection of these structures particularly in diabetics has been commented upon in other sections dealing with these organs.

TUMORS OF SOFT TISSUES

Many tumors that involve the peripheral soft tissues of the body cause no roentgen signs other than a diffuse increase in density. Mention has been made earlier of the shadow that may be caused by a circumscribed mass projecting from the skin surface such as a wart or a mole and how it may be confused with a pathologic process within the lung or abdomen (Fig. 10-21).

NEUROFIBROMATOSIS

In von Recklinghausen's neurofibromatosis there are, characteristically, widely disseminated cutaneous nodules over the body and these often cause rounded shadows of increased density. In roentgenograms of the chest these tumor nodules may cause round shadows overlying the lung fields that may, on casual inspection, be considered to be nodules within the lung. If the examination consists of more than one view, the superficial location of the

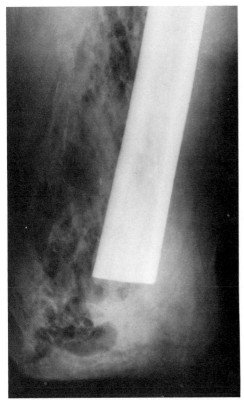

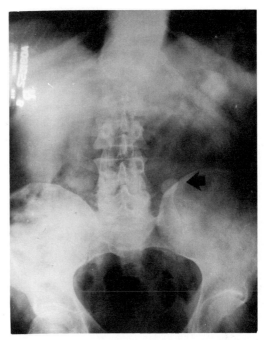

Fig. 10-21. Mole on the skin of the back causing a round density in a roentgenogram of the abdomen (**arrow**).

Fig. 10-20. Gas gangrene of the thigh following amputation. The gas forms irregular streaks and rounded translucent areas in the deep tissues of the thigh.

soft-tissue nodules may be apparent. Nodular shadows along the margins of the chest wall may clearly indicate the nature of the disease and that the lesions are extrapulmonary.

LIPOMAS

A subcutaneous lipoma usually can be identified without difficulty because of the translucency of fat as compared to that of the muscles. Only when the lipoma is small and located superficially is there an absence of this finding. The margin of the tumor is usually sharply defined. Occasionally fibrous tissue septa are seen within the lipoma and these cause a certain amount of striation of the fat shadow (Fig. 10-22). Calcium deposits are found occasionally within a lipoma, although

they are seen somewhat more frequently in other tumors such as fibrosarcomas and synoviomas. Calcification follows necrosis within the central part of the tumor mass as a result of its poor blood supply. Liposarcoma causes roentgen findings similar to its benign counterpart except for the fact that the boundary of the mass may be poorly defined and there may be irregular extensions of fat into the adjacent muscles. It may also erode the adjacent bone.

FIBROSARCOMA

There are no characteristic roentgen findings in fibrosarcoma of the soft tissues but there are some highly suggestive signs that are useful in diagnosis. The mass of the tumor usually is fairly well defined unless it is completely within the major muscle bundles of the extremity. The density of a fibrosarcoma is no different from that of muscle. If the tumor lies largely in the subcutaneous tissues, the normal fat may allow the margin of the tumor to be visualized clearly

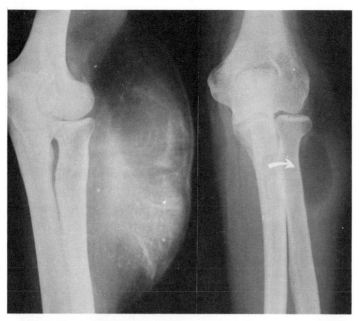

Fig. 10-22. Lipoma of the subcutaneous tissues. *Left,* Large lipoma of the forearm. The darker areas are caused by fat and the striations by fibrous tissue septa and blood vessels. There are a few small areas of calcification in the distal part of the tumor. *Right,* Small lipoma of the forearm (**arrow**). The mass of fat is clearly outlined because it is surrounded by muscle tissue.

so that a fairly good estimate of its size and shape can be obtained. Deep tumors result only in a diffuse enlargement of the part. Calcification is fairly common in fibrosarcomas, occurring as mottled shadows, usually near the center of the mass. Deep-seated fibrosarcomas show a definite tendency to invade contiguous bone. This is seen as a ragged loss of the external cortical surface of the bone. Periosteal reaction at the limits of the erosion is not present very often. The tendency for fibrosarcoma to recur after local excision is noteworthy and soft-tissue roentgenograms may be useful in demonstrating the recurrent tumor mass. Of greater importance, perhaps, is the use of roentgenograms to determine if a recurrent tumor has begun to invade bone; this finding may influence the method of treatment to a considerable degree.

Fibrosarcomas metastasize to the regional nodes and also to the lungs. Roentgenograms of the chest should be obtained in all cases and whenever the patient returns for periodic checkup examinations.

OTHER TUMORS

Tumors of the joints have been considered in Chapter 9 and will not be discussed further in this section. A variety of other tumors of soft-tissue nature may develop in the extremities but with nothing characteristic in their roentgen appearances. Mention has been made earlier, in the section dealing with subcutaneous calcification, of the roentgen findings in *cavernous hemangiomas.* In addition to the visualization of calcified thrombi, the tortuous shadows of dilated vessels may be visible in such a tumor if it extends to involve the subcutaneous fatty layer. The tumor may cause either cortical thickening or erosion of the bone immediately adjacent if it is deeply situated. Otherwise the lesion causes only a diffuse increase in density.

MAMMOGRAPHY

Radiography of the female breast for the demonstration of tumors and other masses is a useful method of investigation. Attention has been called in a previous paragraph to the occurrence of calcification in tumors of the breast and the differential diagnosis of such calcification. In carcinoma of the breast, the lesion appears as a fairly dense nodule (water density) surrounded by the fatty elements of the breast. Characteristically the nodule is irregular in shape with spiculated borders (Fig. 10-23). The center of the tumor tends to be denser than the periphery, especially in the larger lesions. Calcification is frequent and occurs in the form of fine, sandlike granules, or small punctate deposits. This form of calcification is said to be quite characteristic of carcinoma and in one series was found in 118 of 245 patients with the disease. Associated findings are helpful in diagnosis and include localized or diffuse thickening of the skin over the tumor, retraction of the nipple, engorgement of the veins, and evidence of metastatic masses in the axillary nodes. In the presence of fibrocystic disease, mammography may aid in recognizing the dominant nodule and its nature. The more fatty the breast, the easier it is to recognize an abnormal mass. This is in contrast to physical examination where palpation may be unsatisfactory in a large, pendu-

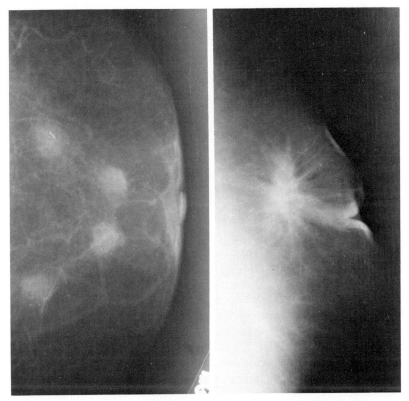

Fig. 10-23. Carcinoma of the breast in two patients. *Left,* Four nodules connected by dense strands. Note thickening of skin around nipple. Several tiny calcifications are seen in uppermost nodule. *Right,* Dense nodular mass with spiculated borders; note dense strand extending to a retracted nipple.

lous breast. Mammography also is useful in confirming palpatory findings and in following the progress of small masses when surgery is deferred for one reason or another.

Benign masses in the breast are homogeneously dense, with rounded or smoothly lobulated contours, sometimes with a surrounding layer of translucent fat. There are no associated changes in the skin. Calcification, when it occurs, is of a coarser and denser type than is seen in carcinomas. Such calcification may be seen in benign conditions such as fibroadenoma, localized areas of mastitis, or even in arteriosclerosis of the blood vessels. Intraductal calcifications are relatively common occurring as small, round ring-contoured densities and are usually multiple. Calcifications associated with benign disease also are often bilateral in contrast to the unilateral calcifications of carcinoma. For satisfactory mammography the technique must be meticulous (the literature should be consulted for details).

VENOGRAPHY

Venography consists in the injection of an aqueous radiopaque substance into one of the peripheral veins of an extremity and the making of one or several roentgenograms. Venography has its greatest use in the examination of the veins of the lower extremities for the detection of thrombosis of the deep veins. In the upper extremity the method can be used for the study of obstructions of the axillary and subclavian veins or of the superior vena cava. The value of venography for the determination of deep venous thrombosis in the lower extremities has been disputed. While many reports have indicated enthusiasm for the method, others have raised doubt about its value. In our experience it is difficult to fill all the veins in the normal extremity. The interpretation of venograms necessarily is difficult and at times the decision cannot be made whether a given vein is pathologically obstructed or did not fill merely as a normal variant. Contrast material injected into one of the small tributaries in the foot, which is the usual site of injection, finds

its way into the larger veins of the thigh by the most direct route as a rule and it is unusual to be able to fill all of the medium-sized or larger veins.

TECHNIQUE

Many technical variations have been introduced to improve the value of venography but, essentially, all of them depend upon the rather slow injection of an aqueous contrast substance such as Hypaque (50%) into one of the small veins on the dorsum of the foot or in the region of the ankle.* In general, we have followed the method outlined by DeBakey, Schroeder, and Ochsner.[6] A tourniquet is placed on the thigh as high as possible and tightened sufficiently so that the superficial veins are occluded and the blood is shunted into the deeper veins. If desired, a blood pressure cuff can be inflated to no more than 25 to 30 mmHg and used in place of the rubber tourniquet but this is not essential. Any vein on the dorsum of the foot can be used for the venipuncture. If none can be found easily, the lesser saphenous vein can be used. This is constantly present directly behind the external malleolus and if necessary a cutdown on this vessel can be done to locate it. If only the veins of the leg are to be examined, a 14 × 17-inch cassette is placed beneath the leg and 20 cc of the contrast solution are injected at the rate of about 1 cc per second. The film is exposed 20 seconds after the injection is completed. If both the leg and the thigh are to be examined, 25 cc of the contrast solution are used. A film of the leg is exposed 20 seconds after the injection is completed, another film is placed beneath the thigh and it is exposed as soon as possible, usually within another 20 to 30 seconds.

Injection of contrast material directly into bone, i.e., intraosseous venography, has been recommended when a superficial vein cannot

---

* See Chapter 20 for a discussion of the contrast substances available for intravenous and intra-arterial injections, with particular reference to the possible dangers, the use of sensitivity tests, and the treatment of drug reactions when they occur.

be cannulated because of edema, infection, obesity, or other cause.[35]

ROENTGEN OBSERVATIONS

The anatomy of the veins of the lower extremity is shown in Figure 10-24. As mentioned previously, failure to visualize any given vein does not necessarily indicate that it is obstructed by a thrombus. If there are no signs of collateral vessels around the nonvisualized vein and if the filled veins have a normal caliber and follow a normal direction, the likelihood of deep venous obstruction is remote. On the other hand, visualization of one of the deep veins up to a certain point with failure of

contrast material to outline it any higher, the presence of dilated and tortuous vessels in the region, and filling of other deep or superficial veins at a higher level in the extremity are valuable observations. In some cases of partial obstruction the thrombus may be outlined. Often it will be found necessary to repeat the examination to determine if a given finding is constant. At other times the evidence of obstruction and its exact site will be reasonably definite.

Most venographic examinations in the upper extremity are done for obstruction of the axillary or subclavian veins. The contrast material can be injected into a branch of the basilic vein at the elbow. One exposure is made at the completion of the injection and another 20 to

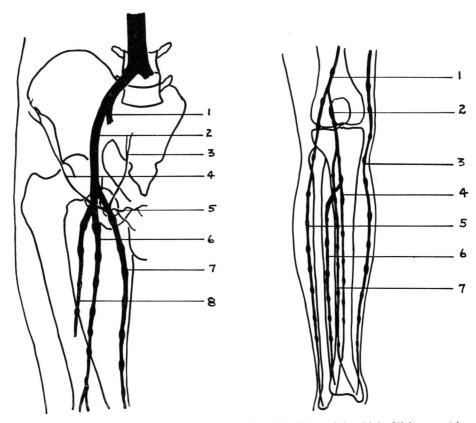

Fig. 10-24. Diagram of veins of lower extremity. *Left,* Veins of the thigh: **(1)** hypogastric; **(2)** external iliac; **(3)** superficial epigastric; **(4)** superficial circumflex iliac; **(5)** superficial external pudendal; **(6)** femoral; **(7)** greater saphenous; **(8)** Deep femoral. *Right,* Veins of the leg: **(1)** femoral; **(2)** popliteal; **(3)** greater saphenous; **(4)** posterior tibial; **(5)** lesser saphenous; **(6)** peroneal; **(7)** anterior tibial.

30 seconds later. If the clinical evidence of obstruction is definite a third exposure can be made as rapidly as film cassettes can be changed. These serial roentgenograms serve to demonstrate the site of obstruction and the collateral circulation around it. It is preferable to use a large sized film so that the entire shoulder area and the upper mediastinum can be included in one view.

ARTERIOGRAPHY

Visualization of the arteries of the lower extremities can be done by injecting the contrast material into the femoral artery in the upper thigh or after puncture of the abdominal aorta. The latter procedure, known as abdominal aortography, has been discussed in Chapter 20.† Direct aortic puncture has been replaced to a great extent by the Seldinger catheter technique or a modification of it. If the aorta or femoral artery is obstructed the catheter can be introduced into the axillary artery or other major vessel and passed to the upper abdominal aorta and the contrast material injected to outline the site of obstruction. Injection of the contrast material into the abdominal aorta has

† See Chapter 20 for discussion of this examination.

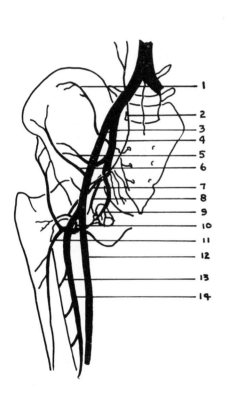
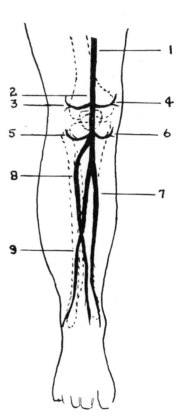

Fig. 10-25. Diagram of the arteries of the pelvis, thigh, and leg. *Left,* Arteries of the pelvis and thigh: **(1)** iliolumbar; **(2)** inferior epigastric; **(3)** external iliac; **(4)** hypogastric; **(5)** superior gluteal; **(6)** deep circumflex iliac; **(7)** inferior gluteal; **(8)** internal pudendal; **(9)** obturator; **(10)** medial femoral circumflex; **(11)** lateral femoral circumflex; **(12)** femoral; **(13)** perforating branch; **(14)** deep femoral (profunda). *Right,* Arteries of lower thigh and leg; **(1)** femoral; **(2)** popliteal; **(3)** lateral superior genicular; **(4)** medial superior genicular; **(5)** lateral inferior genicular; **(6)** medial inferior genicular; **(7)** posterior tibial; **(8)** anterior tibial; **(9)** peroneal. (Based on Morton, S., and Byrne, R., *Radiology 69:* 63, 1957.)

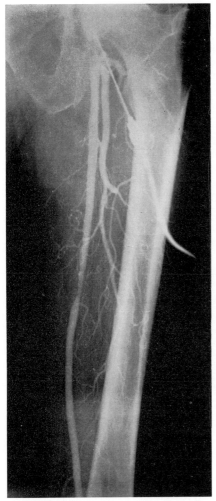

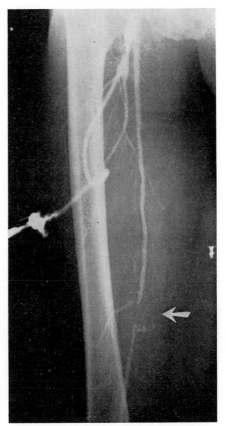

Fig. 10-27. Segmental occlusion of the femoral artery (**arrow**). Refilling below the site of occlusion via collaterals.

Fig. 10-26. Femoral arteriogram. An arteriosclerotic plaque narrows the lumen in the middle third of the thigh.

the advantage that both extremities can be visualized with one injection and information may be obtained concerning the lower part of the aorta and iliac vessels (Fig. 10-25). For localized disease, such as aneurysm, arteriovenous fistula, occlusive disease, and for study of the vascularity of neoplasms, it is advisable to do the injection into the femoral artery. This can be done after surgical exposure of the vessel but most frequently is performed by percutaneous puncture. The contrast material used is similar to that for venography except

that there is an advantage in the use of more concentrated solutions. The blood flow is so much faster in the arteries than in the veins that the medium becomes diluted even when injected rapidly. The contrast solution is injected as quickly as possible. For the examination of a lesion such as an aneurysm where its site is known, the film cassette is placed beneath the region and the exposure made immediately at the completion of injection. When the vessels in both the thigh and the leg are to be examined by means of abdominal aortic injection the technical difficulties increase. Usually it is possible by utilizing multiple films and suitable cones and shielding to expose two roentgenograms in rapid succession so that the pelvis, thighs, and upper parts of

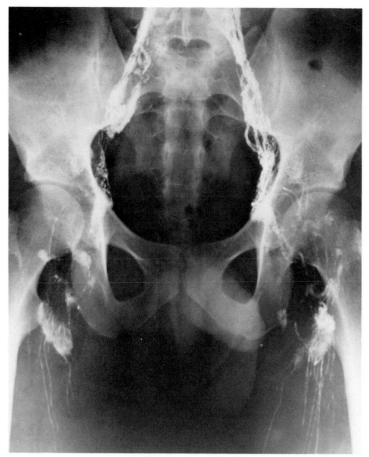

Fig. 10-28. Normal lymphangiogram. Vascular phase showing filling of lymphatic vessels in the upper thighs and pelvis. A few nodes are opacified.

the legs can be visualized. For descriptions of special radiographic techniques the current literature should be consulted.

ROENTGEN OBSERVATIONS

The visualization of an aneurysm usually is made without difficulty and the appearances are characteristic. Occasionally the aneurysm will be partially filled with an old thrombus that may have become canalized and the channel as visualized by the contrast material may give an entirely erroneous impression of the actual size of the vessel. In some cases it may appear fairly normal. One should not rely too

greatly, therefore, upon the size of the aneurysmal sac as visualized by contrast filling as an indication of the actual size of the aneurysm. Arteriovenous fistulae, usually caused by penetrating wounds, give unequivocal signs when examined by means of arteriography. The extension of the contrast material through the fistula into the communicating veins can be clearly demonstrated. The abnormal veins are greatly dilated and tortuous and there is extensive filling of them in the region of the fistula.

The most frequent use of arteriography of the peripheral vessels is in the study of occlusive disease. Intimal arteriosclerotic plaques cause areas of irregular narrowing of the vessel (Fig. 10-26) or, if severe, complete occlusion

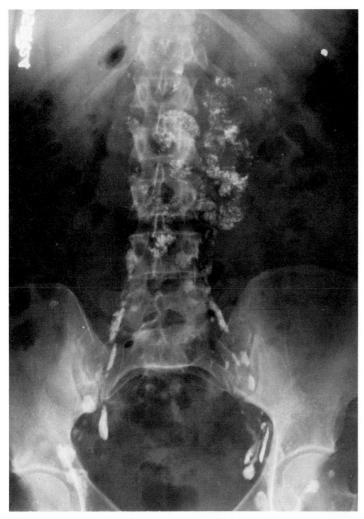

Fig. 10-29. Lymphangiogram of a patient with Hodgkin's disease. This 24-hour film shows a number of midabdominal para-aortic nodes which are enlarged and appear "foamy." Pelvic and iliac nodes are normal.

of it. The lumen may be slightly dilated between areas of constriction. When complete occlusion has taken place as a result of thrombosis the contrast ends with a sharp cutoff. One or more collateral vessels usually can be visualized arising just above the level of obstruction. Frequently these can be followed down to the point where they join the vessel again below the level of the occlusion (Fig. 10-27). If a satisfactory set of roentgenograms can be obtained, arteriography offers a valuable means of identifying the presence and location of arterial occlusion and the extent of disease that may be present in the vessels.

LYMPHANGIOGRAPHY

Lymphangiography has come into use as a method for opacifying the lymphatic channels and lymph nodes.

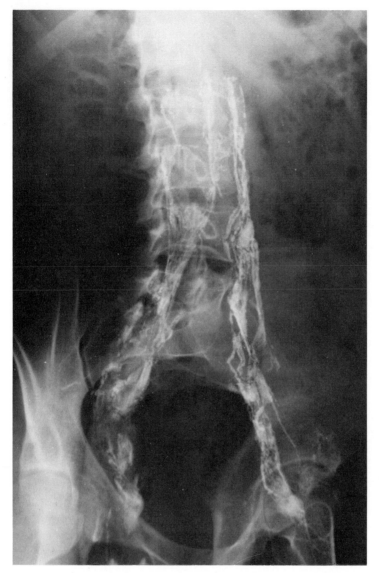

Fig. 10-30. Lymphangiogram. Vascular phase shows displacement of channels by large nodes which are not opacified.

TECHNIQUE

Staining of lymphatic channels in the feet is done by intradermal injection of a mixture of 1% xylocaine (1 cc) and 4% direct sky blue (3 to 4 cc) between the first three toes of each foot. In 15 to 30 minutes the subcutaneous lymphatic vessels are stained. A 1-inch skin incision is then made under local anesthesia over a selected channel in the dorsum of each foot. The vessel is freed from its fibrous sheath for 1½ to 2 cm on each side. The vessel is then stabilized with a small hairclip. A 30-gauge cannula especially designed for the purpose is then inserted with the aid of magnifying lens or glasses. Once the cannula is fixed, 6 to 8 cc of ethiodol are injected in each foot. We use a gravity injector designed by Arts. Scout films of the upper thighs and abdomen are obtained and when the contrast material reaches the level of L 3 or L 4, the injection is discontinued. Films of the abdomen, pelvis, and upper femurs demonstrate the vascular phase. A second set of films is obtained in 24 hours to demonstrate nodal filling.

Indications for lymphography include: (*1*) edema of an extremity of unknown cause; (*2*) evaluation of the extent of adenopathy and staging of lymphomas; (*3*) localization of nodes for treatment planning, either surgical or radiotherapeutic; (*4*) evaluation of the nature of intra-abdominal masses when biopsy material is not readily available; (*5*) a search for metastasis in patients with suspected intra-abdominal nodal disease; and (*6*) localization of lymph fistulas in chylothorax, etc.

Contraindications include known iodine hypersensitivity, severe pulmonary insufficiency, cardiac disease, and advanced renal or hepatic disease.

Complications in the main are related to embolization of the contrast material into the lungs which diminishes pulmonary function temporarily and in some patients may produce a lipid pneumonia. Extravasation is a complication which usually does not cause any clinically significant changes.

Normally the initial films show filling of the lymphatic channels in the thigh, pelvis, and abdomen. Some of the nodes are filled at this time (Fig. 10-28). In the 24-hour film, the lymph channels are no longer visible in the normal and the lymph nodes are filled (Fig. 10-29). Interpretation of lymphangiograms is difficult and there are limitations in that nodes completely replaced by neoplasm may not take up contrast material while nodes involved by inflammatory disease may sometimes show a pattern similar to that observed in lymphoma (Fig. 10-30). Detailed lymphangiographic interpretation is beyond the scope of this book.

REFERENCES AND SELECTED READINGS

1. ARTS, V.: An injection apparatus for lymphangiography. *Am. J. Roentgenol. Radium Ther. Nucl. Med. 100:* 466, 1967.

2. BARNUM, E. N.: The roentgenographic differentiation of peripheral arteriosclerosis. *Am. J. Roentgenol Radium Ther. Nucl. Med. 68:* 619, 1952.

3. BEIGHTON, P., and THOMAS, M. L.: The radiology of the Ehlers-Danlos syndrome. *Clin. Radiol. 20:* 354, 1969.

4. CARLIN, R. A., and AMPLATZ, K.: Downstream aortography. *Am. J. Roentgenol. Radium -Ther. Nucl. Med. 109:* 536, 1970.

5. CRISPEN, J. F., and JEFFRIES, P. F.: Lymphangiography. A simple method of dye infusion. *JAMA 182:* 872, 1962.

6. DEBAKEY, M. E., SCHROEDER, G. F., and OCHSNER, A.: Significance of phlebography in phlebothrombosis. *JAMA 123:* 738, 1943.

7. DEWEESE, J. A., and ROGOFF, S. M.: Functional ascending phlebography of the lower extremity by serial long film technique. *Am. J. Roentgenol. Radium Ther. Nucl. Med. 81:* 841, 1959.

8. DICHIRO, G., and NELSON, K. B.: Soft tissue radiography of extremities in neuromuscular disease with histologic correlations. *Acta Radiol. (Diag.) 3:* 65, 1965.

9. FISHER, H. W., and ZIMMERMAN, G. R.: Roentgenographic visualization of lymph nodes and lymphatic channels. *Am. J. Roentgenol. Radium Ther. Nucl. Med. 81:* 517, 1961.

10. GERSHON-COHEN, J., and BERGER, S. M.: Breast cancer with microcalcifications: Diagnostic difficulties. *Radiology 87:* 612, 1966.

11. GERSHON-COHEN, J., and INGLEBY, H.: Carcinoma of the breast. Roentgenographic technique and diagnostic criteria. *Radiology 60:* 68, 1953.

12. GERSHON-COHEN, J., and SCHORR, S.: The diagnostic problems of isolated, circumscribed breast tumors. *Am. J. Roentgenol. Radium Ther. Nucl. Med. 106:* 863, 1969.

13. HAMOVICI, H., SHAPIRO, J. H., and JACOBSON, H. G.: Serial femoral arteriography in occlusive disease. Clinical-roentgenologic considerations with a new classification of occlusive patterns. *Am. J. Roentgenol. Radium Ther. Nucl. Med. 83:* 1042, 1960.

14. HARRIS, V. J., and HARRIS, W. S.: Increased thickness of the fibula in Duchenne muscular dystrophy. *Am. J. Roentgenol. Radium Ther. Nucl. Med. 98:* 744, 1966.

15. HASSOCK, D. W., and KING, A.: Neurogenic heterotopic ossification. *Med. J. Aust. 1:* 326, 1967.

16. HOLT, J. F.: The Ehlers-Danlos syndrome. *Am. J. Roentgenol. Radium Ther. Nucl. Med. 55:* 420, 1946.

17. JAMES, A. E., JR., EATON, S. B., BLAZEK, J. V., DONNER, M. W., and REEVES, R J.: Roentgen findings in pseudoxanthoma elasticum. *Radiology 106:* 642, 1969.

18. JAMES, W. B., and IRVINE, R. W.: Mammography

in management of breast lesions. *Br. Med. J. 4:* 655, 1969.

19. LEBORGNE, R.: Diagnosis of tumors of the breast by simple roentgenography. Calcifications in carcinomas. *Am. J. Roentgenol. Radium Ther. Nucl. Med. 65:* 1, 1951.

20. LEWITAN, A., and NATHANSON, L.: The roentgen features of muscular dystrophy. *Am. J. Roentgenol. Radium Ther. Nucl. Med. 73:* 226, 1955.

21. LIBERSON, M.: Soft tissue calcifications in cord lesions. *JAMA 152:* 1010, 1953.

22. LIPPMANN, H. I., and GOLDIN, R. R.: Subcutaneous ossification of the legs in chronic venous insufficiency. *Radiology 74:* 279, 1960.

23. MEZAROS, W. T.: The regional manifestations of scleroderma. *Radiology 70:* 313, 1958.

24. MOULE, B., GRANT, M. C., BOYLE, I. T., and MAY, H.: Thyroid acropachy. *Clin. Radiol. 21:* 329, 1970.

25. PACK, G. T., and BRAUND, R. R.: The development of sarcoma in myositis ossificans. *JAMA 119:* 776, 1942.

26. PALMER, P. E. S.: Tumoural calcinosis. *Br. J. Radiol. 39:* 518, 1966.

27. POPPEL, M. H., and ZEITEL, B. E.: Roentgen manifestations of milk drinker's syndrome. *Radiology 67:* 195, 1956.

28. ROY, P.: Peripheral angiography in ischemic arterial diseases of the limbs. *Radiol. Clin. North Am. 5:* 456, 1967.

29. SCHOBINGER, R. A., and RUCZICKA, F. F., JR.: *Vascular Roentgenology.* New York, MacMillan, 1964.

30. SHOPFNER, C. E.: Periosteal bone growth in normal infants: Preliminary report. *Am. J. Roentgenol. Radium Ther. Nucl. Med. 97:* 154, 1966.

31. SIEBERT, S., LIPPMANN, H. L., and GORDON, E.: Mönckeberg's arteriosclerosis. *JAMA 151:* 1176, 1953.

32. SINGLETON, E. B., and HOLT, J. F.: Myositis ossificans progressiva. *Radiology 62:* 47, 1954.

33. TORRES-REYES, E., and STAPLE, T. W.: Roentgenographic appearance of thyroid acropachy. *Clin. Radiol. 21:* 95, 1970.

34. WALLACE, S., JACKSON, L., DODD, G. D., and GREENING, R. R.: Lymphangiographic interpretation. *Radiol. Clin. North Am. 3:* 467, 1965.

35. WEGNER, G. P., FLAHERTY, T. T., and CRUMMY, A. B.: Intraosseous lower extremity venography. *Arch. Surg. 98:* 105, 1969.

36. WHEELER, C. E., CURTIS, A. C., CAWLEY, E. P., GREKIN, R. H., and ZHEUTLIN, B.: Soft tissue calcification with special reference to its occurrence in "collagen diseases." *Ann. Intern. Med. 36:* 1050, 1952.

Section II

THE BRAIN AND SPINAL CORD

11

INTRACRANIAL DISEASES

THE NORMAL SKULL

Fractures, infections, congenital dyplasias, and primary tumors involving the cranial bones have been discussed in the appropriate chapters dealing with these conditions as they affect the general skeletal system. In the present chapter attention will be given to changes in the cranial bones caused by intracranial disease and the examination of the skull done primarily for the detection of intracranial abnormalities. Other specialized methods for study of the intracranial structures will be discussed, including pneumoencephalography, ventriculography, and cerebral arteriography.

Roentgen examination of the skull consists in the making of multiple exposures in different positions, preferably with stereoscopic technique. As a minimum, posteroanterior and lateral stereoscopic roentgenograms are obtained. In many cases other projections are needed, since the shape of the skull and the density of the basal structures make it impossible to visualize all parts of the cranial bones if only two positions are used. It is good practice to supplement the standard forehead down and lateral views with additional projections, depending upon the problem at hand. Thus special positions are available to show the basal structures and the important foramina, the pars petrosa of the temporal bones and

internal auditory canals, the sphenoid wings, etc. Figures 11-1 and 11-2 show two of the standard projections and the major anatomic features that can be demonstrated in each.

In the study of skull roentgenograms it is well for the beginner to adopt a plan of observation, since there are many anatomic structures that must be scrutinized. It is easy to have one's attention attracted by some apparently significant alteration only to miss a more important but less readily visualized abnormality. Any method of observation is satisfactory so long as it allows an orderly review of all the structures depicted.

BLOOD VESSEL MARKINGS

The pattern of the blood vessel grooves should be observed closely. The middle meningeal artery, a branch of the external carotid, enters the cranial cavity through the foramen spinosum. It courses upward, branching fairly extensively, and the branches lie on the internal surface of the skull within sharply defined grooves. These grooves usually are visible in roentgenograms as they extend upward to the vertex along and posterior to the coronal suture. The posterior branch of this vessel sometimes is unusually straight and extends directly upward through the temporal squa-

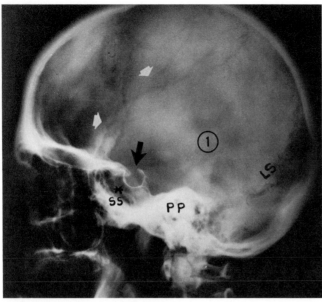

Fig. 11-1. Lateral roentgenogram of normal skull. ①️ indicates position of pineal gland. **Black arrow** points to sella turcica. For details concerning sella, see Figures 11-8 and 11-9. **Short white arrows** indicate branches of middle meningeal artery. **SS**, sphenoid sinus; **PP**, petrous pyramids; **LS**, lambdoidal suture.

mosa, mimicking a linear fracture. Careful observation of stereoscopic views or of right and left lateral roentgenograms will usually show the same line on the opposite side and help to distinguish it from a fracture.

A certain amount of variation in the size of the right and left middle meningeal vessels is found occasionally as a normal variant. If the vessels on one side are appreciably larger than those on the opposite side, the possibility of an underlying meningioma must be considered. This tumor derives most of its blood supply from the middle meningeal artery and it may cause considerable dilatation of the vessels supplying it. When unilateral vascular prominence is encountered, a close scrutiny of the appearance of the bone near the vertex should be made. If a meningioma is responsible for the dilated vessels, the bone may be slightly moth-eaten over the site of the tumor. At other times a localized thickening or hyperostosis may be visible and be a clue to the nature of the lesion. The dilated vessels tend to form an

irregular network at the point of attachment of the tumor to the dura.

Of some significance is the anatomic finding that the branches of the middle meningeal artery lie within accompanying venous channels (middle meningeal veins). Thus the grooves contain both arteries and veins. At their terminations these venous channels enlarge into lakes (lacuna lateralis) within which dangle the cauliflowerlike masses of arachnoid granulations, the pacchionian bodies. These lakes often are large enough to form distinct, sharply outlined areas of rarefaction in roentgenograms. Characteristically, a vessel groove is seen entering and terminating in the lake and this appearance is helpful in distinguishing lakes from foci of destruction caused by disease (Fig. 11-3). Also, if viewed tangentially, a venous lake will be seen to lie within the diploe with intact tables overlying it. The lakes drain into the superior sagittal sinus by means of small venous channels.

The *diploic veins* or *veins of Breschet* lie

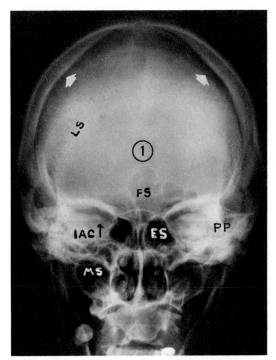

Fig. 11-2. Posteroanterior roentgenogram of normal skull. Figures and lettering the same as for Figure 11-1. In addition, **IAC,** internal auditory canal; **FS,** frontal sinus; **ES,** ethmoid sinuses; **MS,** maxillary sinuses.

of the normal and little attention need be paid to them providing they are equally prominent or nearly so on both sides. The condition has been termed *phlebectasia.* The only significance is when craniotomy is to be done. Then the surgeon may encounter brisk bleeding from the bone and he should be forewarned of this possibility. Unilateral enlargement of the diploic veins has the same significance as unilateral enlargement of the middle meningeal artery (there are no accompanying diploic arteries, the meningeal and pericranial arteries supplying the blood to the diploë).

PHYSIOLOGIC INTRACRANIAL CALCIFICATION

Certain structures within the skull are found to contain calcium deposits with considerable frequency. Such calcification is, as far as is known, without clinical significance. An outline listing the major causes of normal and abnormal intracranial calcification will be found in the tabulation below.

within the diploë of the skull and thus cannot be seen in anatomic specimens unless one of the tables has been removed. Roentgenograms, however, visualize them in most normal skulls. The size and number of these veins is extremely variable (Fig. 11-4). Anatomically the diploic veins tend to form plexuses in the frontal, temporal, and anterior and posterior parietal areas. They are most prominent, as a rule, in the posterior parietal region, where they assume a stellate radiation. The venous channels are more tortuous and irregular than the middle meningeal arterial grooves. They often show localized enlargements or lakes. These venous channels may stand out so prominently in roentgenograms as to suggest strongly that they are abnormal. The bilateral nature of the grooves is always good evidence that such prominent veins are only a variation

CAUSES OF INTRACRANIAL CALCIFICATION

I. Physiologic Causes
   A. Pineal gland
   B. Habenular commissure
   C. Choroid plexus
   D. Dura
   E. Pacchionian bodies
II. Abnormal Findings
   A. Traumatic lesions
      1. Subdural hematoma
      2. Epidural hematoma
      3. Intracerebral hematoma
   B. Parasitic lesions
      1. Cysticercosis
      2. Trichinosis
      3. Toxoplasmosis
      4. Echinococcosis
   C. Vascular lesions
      1. Arteriosclerosis
      2. Aneurysms

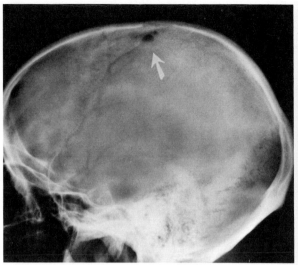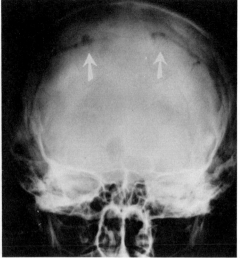

Fig. 11-3. Vascular lakes. Branches of the middle meningeal vessels end in vascular spaces near the vertex **(arrows)**.

3. Arteriovenous malformations
4. Capillary and venous angiomas (Sturge-Weber syndrome)
D. Tuberous sclerosis
E. Inflammatory and other lesions
    1. Tuberculosis
    2. Viral (cytomegalic inclusion disease)
    3. Other infections
        a. Old abscesses
        b. Nontuberculous granulomas
        c. Torulosis
F. Degenerative and atrophic lesions
    1. Congenital atrophy or hypoplasia (lissencephaly)
G. Symmetric calcification of basal ganglia
    1. Hypoparathyroidism
    2. Pseudohypoparathyroidism
    3. Idiopathic disease
H. Neoplasms
    1. Gliomas
    2. Craniopharyngiomas
    3. Dermoids, teratomas, and epidermoids
    4. Meningiomas
    5. Lipomas
    6. Pituitary adenomas
    7. Metastatic tumors

I. Toxicosis
    1. Hypervitaminosis D
    2. Idiopathic hypercalcemia
J. Other causes
    1. Lead poisoning
    2. Fahr's disease

THE PINEAL GLAND

The pineal gland is found to contain sufficient calcium to be visible in roentgenogram in about 60 per cent of adult skulls. Rarely, it is found in the very young, and the frequency of its visualization increases with advancing age. Since it is a midline structure and its position in the lateral view can be plotted with a fair degree of accuracy, displacement of the calcified gland from its normal position may be a valuable clue in indicating the presence of an intracranial lesion (Fig. 11-5). Space-taking lesions such as tumors, hematomas, and abscesses displace the gland away from the mass; atrophic lesions cause displacement toward the side of the abnormality. In general, masses are more apt to cause significant displacement than atrophic processes. Because many skulls are slightly asymmetric when viewed frontally, a slight apparent shift of the pineal from the

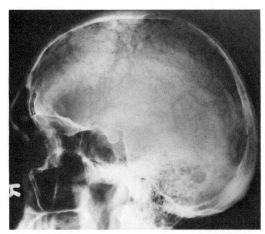

Fig. 11-4. Diploic veins. Lateral roentgenogram of a skull shows a rich network of diploic veins throughout the vault. This is not abnormal but the vascularity is more than is usual.

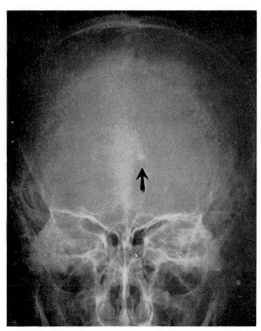

Fig. 11-5. Displacement of calcified pineal toward the left side (**arrow**) by a tumor in the right cerebral hemisphere.

midline may be a normal finding. Ordinarily a variation of from 1 to 2 mm from the midline is allowable as being within the range of normal. Measurement of the position of the pineal in posteroanterior roentgenograms must be made only when the skull has been positioned carefully so that the midsagittal plane is at a right angle with the film. The position of the calcified pineal gland can be determined in the lateral view by measuring its distance from the most distant point on (*1*) the inner table of the frontal bone, (*2*) the inner table of the occiput, (*3*) the inner table of the vault at the vertex, and (*4*) the inner table of the occiput. Using the charts prepared by Vastine and Kinney[29] (Fig. 11-6), measurement 1 is plotted as the abscissa and the sum of measurements 1 and 2 as the ordinate. In like manner measurement 3 is plotted as the ordinate and the sum of measurements 3 and 4 as the abscissa. By this means forward, upward, downward, or posterior displacement of the gland can be identified. These charts are satisfactory only when the skull is reasonably normal in shape. If the skull is of abnormal shape, false results may be obtained and such measurements cannot be relied upon. Some possibility for error also arises from the fact that the habenular commissure, which lies just in front of the

pineal, also calcifies frequently and may be mistaken for the pineal gland. Lack of obvious displacement, of course, does not exclude a space-filling mass since the amount of shift may not be enough to cause the pineal to fall outside the range of normal in the charts; or the lesion may be too small to cause appreciable displacement.

THE CHOROID PLEXUS OF THE LATERAL VENTRICLES

The choroid plexus lies along the floor of the lateral ventricles, its function being to elaborate cerebrospinal fluid. The glomus of the choroid plexus is a localized enlargement found along the posterior part of the floor of the ventricle just in front of the point of origin of the occipital horn. Calcification of the glomus occurs in about 8 per cent of normal adult skulls. Such calcification is seen infrequently in young children. Usually the glomus of each lateral ventricle calcifies and the position of these structures and their relation to the mid-

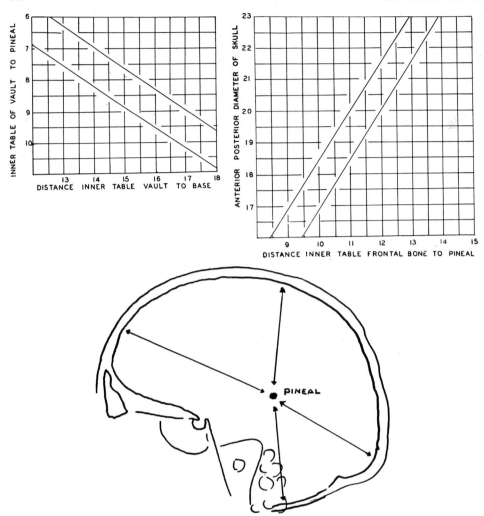

Fig. 11-6. Vastine-Kinney charts for determining displacement of the pineal in the lateral roentgenogram. *Left,* Chart for determining if pineal is displaced up or down from its normal position. The distance in centimeters from the inner table of the vault to the pineal is plotted against the total distance from the inner table of the vault to the base. If normal the position will fall between the two diagonal lines. *Right,* To determine displacement forward or backward the distance in centimeters between the inner tables of the frontal and occipital bones is plotted against the distance from the inner table of the frontal bone to the pineal. The normal range will lie between the two diagonal lines (modified by Dyke, C.). *Below,* Tracing of lateral roentgenogram of skull showing method of measurement.

line of the skull can be determined. Any appreciable shift of one glomus in relation to the other or to the midline suggests the presence of either a space-filling mass on one side or an atrophic lesion on the other side (Fig. 11-7). Displacement of a calcified glomus has less significance than a corresponding amount of displacement of the pineal gland. This is be-

cause the positions of the glomera may vary somewhat on the two sides or different parts may calcify and lead to visible asymmetry of the resulting shadows. When only one glomus is calcified little information can be obtained, since its position cannot be determined too accurately and one must see the opposite one for comparison. Recognition of unilateral cal-

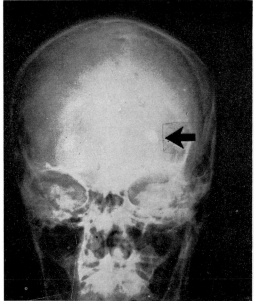 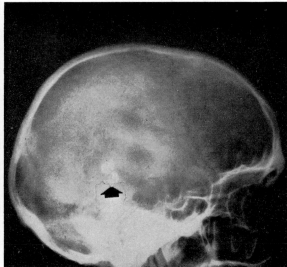

Fig. 11-7. Displacement of calcified glomus of choroid plexus. *Right,* The lateral view shows the two calcified glomera lying above one another (**short arrow**). *Left,* In the posteroanterior view the glomus on the right side is elevated because of an abscess beneath it. **Arrow** points to elevated glomus.

cification is important because the shadow may be mistaken for a displaced pineal gland or for some other serious lesion such as calcification within a tumor.

CALCIFICATION OF THE DURA

Plaquelike areas of calcification are common in the dura, particularly in the falx and along the margins of the superior sagittal sinus. No significance can be attached to the finding of such plaques, so far as is known. Calcification is frequent in the free edges of the tentorium posterior to the sella in the so-called petroclinoid ligaments. These are formed by the margins of the tentorium as it extends from the petrous ridges of the temporal bones to the dorsum sellae. The calcifications are seen as spurlike projections extending posteriorly and downward from the dorsum (see Fig. 11-8c). Calcification in other parts of the tentorium is less common.

CALCIFICATION OF PACCHIONIAN BODIES

The pacchionian granules or bodies are small localized enlargements of the pia arachnoid that lie in pits along the vertex of the skull, mostly along the superior sagittal sinus. Histologically, these granules are said to contain calcium often but they are not observed frequently in roentgenograms. When visible they are seen as small punctate calcified shadows immediately adjacent to the inner table. More often only the small pitlike depressions or the lakes within which the bodies are situated are visualized.

THE SELLA TURCICA

The importance of the sella turcica in the interpretation of skull roentgenograms can hardly be overemphasized. Not only does it harbor an important structure, the pituitary gland, but changes in the thin bony walls and processes of the sella are among the prominent roentgen signs of increased intracranial pressure. This is discussed more fully in the section on "Intracranial Tumors." As visualized in the lateral view of the skull, the normal sella is usually of a flat, oval shape. The normal measurements are given as being 8 to 12 mm in the anteroposterior diameter and 6 to 8 mm in depth (Fig. 11-8) However, many normal sellae exceed these measurements and the upper limits of normal have been given by some authors as 17 mm for the anteroposterior diameter and 13 mm for the depth. The shape of the sella can vary considerably within normal limits from a flattened oval to a rounded or an upright oval contour. The clinical significance of the "small sella" is somewhat doubtful. There is some evidence that a small sella is found in many patients with idiopathic hypopituitary dwarfism, apparently secondary to the small size of the pituitary gland in this condition. In most cases, however, sellar sizes less than those listed above can be disregarded. The sphenoid sinus lies directly below the sella and is separated from the pituitary fossa by only a thin bony wall. The dorsum of the sella is of variable thickness, usually measuring on the order of 2 to 3 mm. At times a large sphenoid sinus will extend into the dorsum. The posterior clinoid processes form the upper limit of the dorsum in the lateral view and often are superimposed upon one another in this projection. They are best demonstrated, individually, in

anteroposterior views. The anterior clinoid processes form the upper anterior boundary of the sella and are seen as pointed bony projections. They, too, tend to be superimposed one upon the other in lateral views, although it usually is possible to visualize them independently in stereoscopic roentgenograms. At times there appears to be a bony bridging between the anterior and posterior clinoid processes as viewed in the lateral projection, either on one or on both sides (Fig. 11-8D). This may be a true bony bridge or only a pseudobridging because long clinoid processes overlap one another. In any event bony bridging is not believed to be of any clinical significance. The extension of the dura that is attached to the clinoid processes and forms a membranous cover over the sella (the diaphragm of the sella) may be partially calcified. The walls of the normal sella are composed of cortical bone and thus appear sharp and dense. Loss of this normal density and sharpness may be an early sign of decalcification from increased intracranial pressure (Fig. 11-9). In elderly individuals and in others showing evidence of skeletal demineralization, the margins

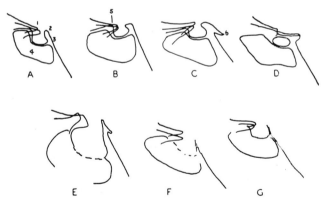

Fig. 11-8. Diagrams of the sella turcica. *A–D,* normal sella and variations. **(1)** Anterior clinoid processes; **(2)** posterior clinoid processes (the two are superimposed in lateral view); **(3)** dorsum sellae; **(4)** sphenoid sinus; **(5)** tuberculum sellae; **(6)** calcific spur along posterior edge of dorsum occurring at attachment of tentorium (petroclinoid ligament). In *D* there is shown bony bridging between the anterior and posterior clinoid processes. *E,* enlarged sella caused by chromophobe adenoma of the pituitary gland (see Fig. 11-34). *F-G,* decalcification of posterior clinoids, dorsum, and floor secondary to increased intracranial pressure.

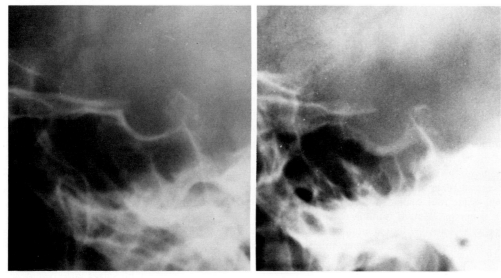

Fig. 11-9. Erosion of sella turcica secondary to increased intracranial pressure. The view on the *right* was made about 6 months after the one on the *left*, illustrating increased demineralization with loss of cortical outlines of the floor and dorsum of the sella.

of the sella may become indistinct as a result of osteoporosis. Some degree of osteoporosis is common in persons over 60 years of age but may be seen in younger individuals. Lateral tomograms are useful in evaluating the sella in the presence of osteoporosis and usually resolve the question as to the presence or absence of pathologic erosion. In addition to senile osteoporosis, demineralization of the sella can occur in any condition that causes generalized skeletal demineralization such as hyperparathyroidism, Cushing's disease, or following steroid therapy.

THE CRANIAL FORAMINA

Most of the important foramina of the skull cannot be seen in the standard lateral and postero-anterior views and require special projections for demonstration. Such views are available and it is possible to visualize clearly the optic and internal auditory canals, the foramen ovale and rotundum, the jugular foramina, the foramen magnum, as well as other smaller openings in the skull base. These projections are utilized when the clinical problem indicates the need for them.

ABNORMAL INTRACRANIAL CALCIFICATION

TRAUMATIC LESIONS

At times, a *subdural hematoma* that has not been recognized and treated surgically may undergo calcification in later life and appear as a dense, plaquelike, calcified mass overlying the cerebral hemisphere. These often are small and thin, occurring as a sheetlike calcification directly beneath the inner table. Occasionally a rather extensive calcified hematoma will be encountered. The usual location is over the superior parietal area but they may be found elsewhere, even in the posterior fossa. In like manner an *intracerebral hematoma* may calcify and be visualized as a dense mass of calcium within the brain. There usually is little in the roentgen appearance of such a calcified mass to determine its nature and a history of previous trauma is important. At times it may be necessary to explore and remove surgically such a mass, either because the diagnosis cannot be made otherwise or because it is felt that the calcified scar is causing significant symptoms.

PARASITIC LESIONS

CALCIFIED CYSTICERUS CYSTS

Cysticercosis is an uncommon disease in this country. The encysted larvae may calcify and be visualized in roentgenograms of the muscles and the brain. These form small calcified masses from 1 to 2 mm in length, either rounded or of an elongated shape, somewhat resembling a small grain of rice. When disseminated small calcifications of this type are found within the brain, the diagnosis of cysticercosis can be suggested. Small, ring-contoured calcifications also have been noted in some patients. If similar calcified lesions are found widely distributed in the skeletal muscles, the roentgen diagnosis becomes more certain (see Fig. 10-7).

TRICHINOSIS

Calcified encysted larvae in the brain and muscles are frequent, pathologically, in this disease but this is an uncommon roentgen observation. The small size of the lesions makes them difficult to detect and probably explains the lack of positive roentgen evidence.

TOXOPLASMOSIS

Toxoplasmic encephalitis is an infection caused by a protozoan parasite. The infection may develop in the fetus and be manifest at birth or shortly thereafter. In the congenital or infantile form of toxoplasmic encephalitis dense nodules of calcification may form (Fig. 11-10). Often these are widely distributed throughout the brain. The foci are variable in size in the individual case and some of the nodules may measure a centimeter or more in diameter. When the basal ganglia are involved the calcification may be more linear or curvilinear in shape. Calcified deposits also have been found in the meninges, choroid plexuses, and the ependyma of the ventricles. The incidence of associated hydrocephalus during infancy is high (reported to occur in 80 percent of patients). Microcephaly also has been noted as a sequela of the infantile form of the disease and is a later manifestation representing the effects of scarring and shrinkage in volume of brain tissue. Toxoplasmosis should be considered as a diagnostic possibility when widely disseminated calcified nodules of variable sizes are found within the brain. If there is evidence of either hydrocephalus or microcephaly, this diagnostic possibility is enhanced. Clinically, these patients show the signs of brain injury with convulsions, and mental retardation. The incidence of chorioretinitis is high. Neutralizing antibodies will be found in the blood serum of these infants and in a high percentage of the mothers. Roentgen differential diagnosis includes tuberous sclerosis and cytomegalic inclusion disease. Skin lesions are usually present in tuberous sclerosis and there is a tendency for lesions to form along the ventricular walls. The patients are usually older when the lesions are first discovered. In cytomegalic inclusion disease, in

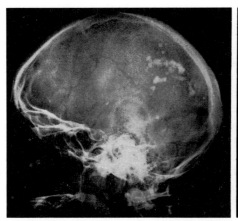 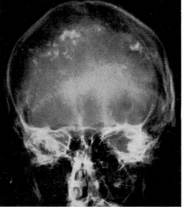

Fig. 11-10. Toxoplasmosis. Calcified areas in the brain following the infantile form of toxoplasmosis. *Left,* Lateral roentgenogram; *Right,* Posteroanterior roentgenogram of the same patient.

addition to disseminated nodules, the calcification often occurs as a thin sheetlike deposition in the walls of the ventricles and forms a cast of them.

VASCULAR LESIONS

CALCIFIED ARTERIOSCLEROTIC PLAQUES

Calcifications in the walls of the intracranial portions of the internal carotid arteries are common in elderly individuals and are occasionally seen in younger persons suffering from vascular disease. In lateral roentgenograms the calcifications are seen as thin, curved calcific shadows alongside the sella (see Fig. 11-11). At times the entire circumference of the vessel will be calcified and it will appear as a ring-contoured shadow when viewed end-on in posteroanterior views. This type of calcification indicates a medial or Mönckeberg form of arteriosclerosis. Intimal plaques tend to be smaller and irregular and usually do not completely encircle the lumen. Because intimal plaques may encroach upon the lumen of the vessel and interfere with bloodflow through it, it is of some importance to be able to determine from the roentgen appearance whether

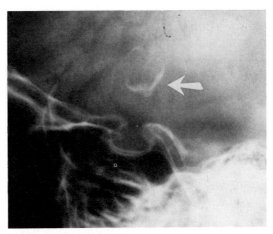

Fig. 11-12. Calcification in the wall of an aneurysm above the sella (**arrow**). (See Fig. 11-24 for arteriogram.)

medial or intimal calcification is present. This is not always possible but in many cases the differentiation can be made. Usually the calcifications lie below the level of the clinoid processes. Calcification above this level may be in the wall of an aneurysm, if plaquelike or circular in nature, or indicate the presence of a tumor or other significant lesion.

CALCIFICATION OF ANEURYSMS

Aneurysms of the internal carotids or of the other components of the circle of Willis and the larger branches arising from the circle are common lesions. In most cases roentgenograms of the skull will be negative. Occasionally calcification in the wall of the aneurysmal sac will be seen (Fig. 11-12). While it is unusual for the entire sac to be calcified, even small plaques may give a valuable clue as to the presence of the lesion. In contrast to simple arteriosclerotic plaques that seldom extend above the upper border of the sella, those in the wall of an aneurysm usually lie above the level of the clinoid processes. The shape of the curve also may indicate the approximate diameter of the sac even though the entire wall is not visualized. Of importance in the diagnosis of these lesions is the occasional finding of unilateral erosion of the sella from pressure.

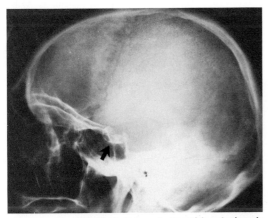

Fig. 11-11. Calcified internal carotid arteries in the circle of Willis. Lateral roentgenogram of the skull. The calcified infraclinoidal portion of at least one internal carotid artery is visualized as a tubular calcified shadow lying alongside the sella turcica (**arrow**).

The combination of unilateral sellar destruction and curvilinear shadows of calcification in the immediate parasellar area forms a highly reliable diagnostic sign complex for this lesion. In the absence of these findings, internal carotid arteriography (see section on "Arteriography") is the method of choice for the roentgen demonstration of these lesions.

ARTERIOVENOUS MALFORMATIONS

Calcified plaques may form in the walls of the dilated vessels making up a congenital vascular malformation with an arteriovenous fistula. There may be only a few small linear shadows or a fairly extensive calcification. The calcific shadows are linear and curved when viewed from the side and circular or tubular when viewed end-on, corresponding to the lumen of the vessel. Usually the nature of the calcification is such that one can recognize its vascular nature without too much difficulty. As with the true neoplasms, the extent of calcification rarely indicates the actual size of the lesion and, as a rule, the malformation will be found to be much more extensive than the calcified areas would suggest. Arteriography is the roentgen method of choice for the diagnosis and study of these lesions.

CAPILLARY AND VENOUS ANGIOMAS

In association with cutaneous angiomas or nevi, often showing a distribution corresponding to that of the trigeminal nerve, an area of abnormal calcification may be found within the cerebral cortex on the ipsilateral side. The lesion is most frequent in the posterior parietal area. It appears as a collection of wavy, curved plaques simulating the convolutions of the brain but lying 1 or 2 cm beneath the inner table (Fig. 11-13). Histologically, the calcium is found in the second and third layers of the cortex, occasionally in the basal ganglia. It is deposited in the perivascular tissues in the cortex rather than in the walls of blood vessels. This combination of cerebral and cutaneous angiomatosis is known as the *Sturge-Weber syndrome;* there may be associated visual defects, contralateral hemiplegia, migraine, epilepsy, and, often, mental deficiency. The cerebral lesion may exist without the facial nevus.

TUBEROUS SCLEROSIS

Tuberous sclerosis is one of the developmental neurocutaneous syndromes (others include von Recklinghausen's neurofibromatosis and the Sturge-Weber syndrome). Clinically this syndrome is characterized by sebaceous, warty adenomas distributed in a butterfly fashion over the nose and cheeks, mental deficiency, and epilepsy. Other malformations may be present including spina bifida, cleft palate, nodulation of the skin and retina, and polydactyly. A characteristic skin lesion, the shagreen patch, is usually found on the trunk as a slightly elevated area of variable size and having an "orange-peel" appearance. Other abnormalities that may be present include premature graying of the hair, *café au lait* spots, and hemangiomas. In the central nervous system, hard,

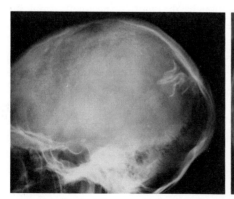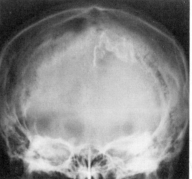

Fig. 11-13. Capillary angioma, parieto-occipital area. *Left,* Lateral view. *Right,* Posteroanterior view.

tumorlike nodules are found scattered widely in the hemispheres. Of significance to the roentgenologist is the fact that these nodules are prone to calcify and thus become visible in skull roentgenograms. The calcified nodules vary greatly in size from very tiny ones up to those measuring a centimeter or more in diameter. There is a distinct tendency for them to develop along the ventricular margins. Thus, even when uncalcified, they may be visualized in pneumoencephalograms or ventriculograms as nodules projecting into the ventricular cavities. The large lesions may obstruct the ventricular foramina or the aqueduct of Sylvius and lead to an obstructive hydrocephalus and the roentgen signs of increased intracranial pressure (Fig. 11-14).

A second roentgen sign of tuberous sclerosis is the occurrence of dense sclerotic islands in the bones of the cranial vault. A combination of such sclerotic foci and scattered areas of intracranial calcification is highly reliable evidence of the disease. Similar sclerotic islands have been found in the spine and pelvis in many cases and probably can occur in any bone. Localization of the sclerosis to the posterior portions of the vertebrae has been reported.

An additional roentgen finding is the occurrence of cystlike defects in the phalanges, especially of the hands, and a wavy periosteal calcification along the shafts of the metatarsals and metacarpals. As with other syndromes, not all these findings need be present in the individual patient. Central nervous system lesions may occur without the typical skin lesions and other parts of the syndrome may be lacking at times.

Tuberous sclerosis of the brain is accompanied by a high incidence of renal masses. The renal tumors are of various connective tissue types, or hamartomas. One of the lesions, known as an angiomyolipoma, may contain enough fat to be visualized in plain roentgenograms. Similar tumors also may be found less frequently in the heart, spleen, lungs, and gastrointestinal tract.

INFLAMMATORY AND OTHER LESIONS

Mention has been made previously of the occurrence of disseminated calcified foci within the brain after *toxoplasmic encephalitis*. Rarely, after other types of encephalitis, scattered, small calcified areas may develop. There is nothing specific in the appearance of such foci and a history of previous inflammatory disease would be necessary to diagnose the lesion correctly. *Tuberculomas* of the brain have been reported as showing the presence of calcification in a relatively small percentage of cases (6 per cent). Multiple lesions are the rule, pathologically, and they are equally common in the cerebral and cerebellar hemispheres. Characteristically, the calcified tuberculoma has an irregular outline with a crenated margin caused by shrinkage of the lesion as it undergoes healing. Calcification in tuberculous meningitis has been reported as occurring in the meninges at the base of the brain, usually immediately above the sella or behind the posterior clinoid processes, and in the form of small, punctate deposits or as calcified plaques.

Calcified plaques along the walls of the lateral ventricles have been reported in *cytomegalic inclusion disease*. At times these form a nearly complete cast of the ventricles. A similar type of calcification has been noted in some cases of toxoplasmosis so that, although highly suggestive, it apparently is not completely pathognomonic of cytomegalic inclusion disease. Calcific deposits have also been found in the cerebral cortex and subcortical white matter in this disease. Also reported have been instances of diffuse bony sclerosis.

Calcification in an old abscess occasionally is

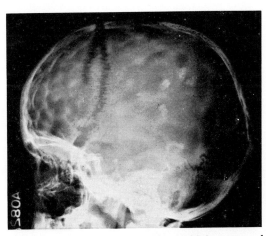

Fig. 11-14. Tuberous sclerosis. Multiple areas of mottled calcification in the brain. The sutures are spread, indicating increased intracranial pressure. Pneumoencephalography revealed a large mass beneath the right lateral ventricle that was occluding the third ventricle and foramen of Monro, leading to obstructive hydrocephalus. The patient was operated on and the diagnosis of tuberous sclerosis confirmed.

found but there is little in the roentgen appearance to aid in recognizing the nature of the original lesion. It is probable that other isolated (or generalized) lesions may heal spontaneously and calcify. It is not uncommon to find one or several small calcified foci within the brain on roentgen study. It usually is impossible to determine the nature of such small lesions from their roentgen appearances. Even when removed surgically or when examined at the time of autopsy an etiologic diagnosis may not be possible; the lesion may be completely "burned out" and healed, leaving only the calcified remains.

DEGENERATIVE LESIONS

Occasionally there is seen a fairly extensive area of calcification of wavy, tortuous form, resembling closely the more restricted calcification seen in the Sturge-Weber syndrome but without the other stigmata of this disease. The calcification may involve much of one hemisphere and tends to form an outline of the cortical convolutions although separated somewhat from the inner table. Histologically, the calcium is found to be deposited in the perivascular spaces, similar to that in the Sturge-Weber lesion. There may be a more stippled calcification in the basal ganglia. In most cases the lesion probably is one of congenital atrophy or hypoplasia of the brain (lissencephaly) and the skull may be smaller in size and the calvarium thickened on the side of the lesion to compensate for the atrophic cortex. Bilateral lesions have been observed.

Fahr's disease, or *idiopathic familial cerebrovascular ferrocalcinosis,* is a rare cause of intracranial calcification.[3] The disease has a familial occurrence and shows the clinical manifestations of severe growth disorder and progressive mental deterioration. The intracranial deposition of iron and calcium causes widespread, irregular, punctate and dustlike densities in the brain. Its cause is not definitely known but it has been thought to be a genetically determined metabolic or vascular disorder.

SYMMETRIC CALCIFICATION OF THE BASAL GANGLIA

In the presence of parathyroid insufficiency, usually the result of surgical removal or injury to the parathyroid glands, fine granular calcifica-

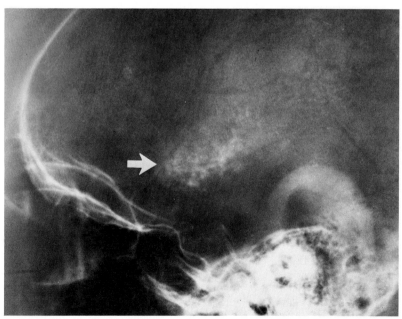

Fig. 11-15. Calcification in the basal ganglia (**arrow**) in a patient with hypoparathyroidism. The ganglia are superimposed in this lateral view.

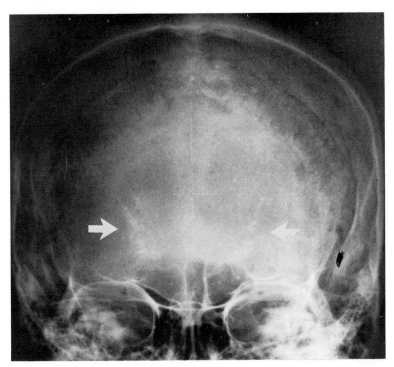

Fig. 11-16. Posteroanterior view of same patient as Figure 11-15 shows the bilateral, symmetric calcifications (**arrows**).

tions have been noted in the regions of the basal ganglia on either side of the midline. Occasionally such calcification is more extensive and wavy calcification in the deeper layers of the cerebral cortex may be found (Figs. 11-15 and 11-16). Cerebellar calcification of similar type can occur. The calcified shadows resemble those seen in other conditions as enumerated above and the pathologic observations are similar. The calcium is found chiefly in the perivascular spaces of the finer cerebral vessels. The fact that the calcification is bilateral and symmetric is helpful in distinguishing this lesion from the cerebral angiomas of the Sturge-Weber syndrome and from the atrophic degenerations described in the previous paragraph. The same type of calcification has been found in cases of *pseudohypoparathyroidism*. Not all these patients, however, show evidence of parathyroid insufficiency and the cause of the abnormal calcification at times remains obscure. A few cases of unilateral calcification of the basal ganglia have been reported, some with no signs referable to the central nervous system and others showing contralateral extrapyramidal symptoms.

CALCIFICATION IN NEOPLASMS

Calcification within a tumor offers one of the certain roentgen signs of the presence of a lesion. As a rule the character of the calcium deposits offers little in the way of information concerning the histologic nature of the tumor. In general, the more slowly growing and benign a lesion may be, the more likely it will calcify. Thus, among the gliomas, the slowly growing oligodendrogliomas usually show extensive calcification when first recognized. Astrocytomas are more likely to show calcification than the more malignant and rapidly growing glioblastoma multiforme. Other tumors that are prone to calcify include the craniopharyngiomas (about 80 per cent), ependymomas, dermoids, teratomas, and meningiomas. For further discussion see the section dealing with "Intracranial Tumors."

HYPEROSTOSIS FRONTALIS INTERNA

Hyperostosis frontalis interna is a peculiar overgrowth of bone developing on the inner table of the frontal bone. The hyperostosis usually is bilateral and symmetric and is found chiefly in females over the age of 35. The abnormal bony proliferation is confined to the internal surface of the inner table; the diploë and external table are not affected. It forms a shaggy, irregular thickening that surrounds the venous sinuses but does not obliterate them. As a result they stand out as prominent translucent zones, the superior sagittal sinus and the veins draining into it forming a recognizable pattern (Fig. 11-17). The extent of the thickening varies considerably among patients but the hyperostosis may measure 1 cm or more in thickness. The process spreads upward and laterally from the midline of the frontal area for a variable distance. The external limits may be abrupt, or the process may fade gradually into normal bone at the periphery. While usually limited to the frontal area, occasionally it extends into the parietal bones and over the orbital roofs. As a variant of hyperostosis frontalis interna there may be a more diffuse thickening of the vault involving both tables with a poorly defined or absent diploë; the term, *hyperostosis calvariae diffusa,* has been applied to this condition.

The significance of hyperostosis frontalis interna from a clinical standpoint has been disputed. By some it has been considered to be a part of a syndrome indicative of endocrine dysfunction and variously called *metabolic craniopathy,* the *Morgagni syndrome,* and the *Stewart-Morel syndrome.* The symptoms and signs included in this syndrome have been numerous and include frequent headaches, obesity, muscular weakness, fatigue, nervousness, menstrual disturbances, and dizziness.

Minor degrees of hyperostosis frontalis are seen frequently by the roentgenologist and it is difficult to ascribe much importance to the finding in most cases.

HYPERVITAMINOSIS D AND IDIOPATHIC HYPERCALCEMIA

During infancy calcification of the falx and tentorium has been observed in *hypervitaminosis D* and also in *idiopathic hypercalcemia.* The occurrence of such calcification during the first year or two of life is almost certain evidence for either of these diseases (see Chapter 8,

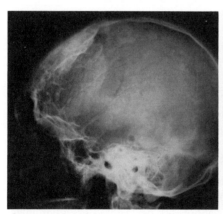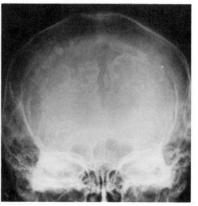

Fig. 11-17. Hyperostosis frontalis interna. Lateral (*left*) and posteroanterior (*right*) roentgenograms showing a heavy calcification on the inner table of the frontal bone. The hyperostosis does not form over the superior sagittal sinus and its major tributaries, leaving a midline translucent area as seen in the frontal view.

under "Hypervitaminosis D" and "Idiopathic Hypercalcemia"). This finding has no significance during adult life since calcified plaques are common, especially in the falx, without clinical signs or symptoms.

INTRACRANIAL TUMORS

The roentgenology of intracranial tumors can be considered under three main divisions: (1) changes produced in the cranial bones and demonstrable in plain roentgenograms of the skull; (2) changes in the fluid pathways and the ventricular system and demonstrated only after injection of air or oxygen into the subarachnoid space (encephalography) or directly into the ventricles (ventriculography); (3) opacification of the intracranial blood vessels (arteriography) is another specialized procedure that may be utilized to give information concerning the presence or absence of a tumor. From 40 to 50 per cent of all tumors will give some evidence of their presence in ordinary roentgen study of the skull. By means of encephalography, ventriculography, and arteriography it is possible to localize accurately almost all intracranial tumors and in many the histologic type can be predicted with considerable accuracy.

CHANGES IN THE CRANIAL BONES

SIGNS OF INCREASED INTRACRANIAL PRESSURE

The roentgen signs of increased intracranial pressure are, of course, not specific for tumors. Other conditions can cause obstructive hydrocephalus by interfering with the free flow of cerebrospinal fluid from within the ventricles where it is formed to the arachnoid granulations over the superior aspects of the cerebral hemispheres where it is absorbed. Inflammatory adhesions and congenital defects are examples of such nonneoplastic obstructive processes. Other mass lesions such as abscesses or

hematomas may take up sufficient space within the skull to cause the signs and symptoms of increased intracranial pressure. The changes described below, therefore, indicate only that a space-taking mass is present within the cranial cavity or that something is obstructing the flow or interfering with the absorption of cerebrospinal fluid.

WIDENING OF THE CRANIAL SUTURES. In children and occasionally in young adults increase in intracranial pressure will cause a spreading of the vault sutures. This widening may amount to as much as several centimeters and it is a very reliable sign of increased pressure (see Figs. 11-14 and 11-30). This sign is not found in adults because the bones are held tightly together and in older persons above the age of 35 the sutures often are completely fused. Widening of the sutures is prevalent in the presence of tumors within the posterior fossa of the skull since these lesions are prone to obstruct the aqueduct of Sylvius or the fourth ventricle and thus cause an obstructive hydrocephalus. In the infant, sutural spread can develop rapidly if there is a sudden increase in intracranial pressure. In the older child or adolescent the sutures are not as likely to spread unless the pressure rises considerably or unless it has existed for some time. It follows that the younger the child the more valuable the sign becomes. In patients with slowly developing increased intracranial pressure, and particularly in older children, the sutures may not be spread to any appreciable degree but the digitations along the suture edges become lengthened.

ENLARGEMENT OF OCCIPITAL EMISSARY FORAMEN. The occipital foramen is a small opening in or near the midline of the occipital bone serving for the passage of an emissary vein. Normally it does not measure more than 2.0 mm in diameter. In increased intracranial pressure it has been reported to enlarge to a diameter of 8 to 10 mm. Some recent observations, however, suggest that this finding is not as significant as previously thought with large foramina being seen in patients without other signs of increased pressure and lack of enlargement in some who do have chronic intra-cranial hypertension.[33] Our own experience has been similar.

DECALCIFICATION AND EROSION OF THE SELLA TURCICA. Loss of density and sharpness of outline of the walls and processes of the sella turcica can develop as a result of chronic increase in intracranial pressure. The time lag between the onset of increased pressure and the detection of changes in the sellar walls in roentgenograms will vary depending upon the degree of increased pressure and its constancy. However, in most cases it is probable that several months must elapse before roentgen evidence becomes distinct. When the ventricular system has been obstructed by a lesion in the posterior fossa there is a resulting dilatation of the lateral and third ventricles; the latter ventricle then projects downward over the sella and may actually bulge into it. Constant pressure from a greatly dilated third ventricle may cause erosion of the posterior clinoid processes and the dorsum of the sella, leaving the rest of the sellar walls intact. The early change is one of loss of the normal sharp cortical margin of the anterior surface of the dorsum and floor. In other patients the margins of the sella undergo a general loss of density. The sharp cortical bone that normally forms the borders of the cavity becomes lost and the edges become ill defined (see Fig. 11-9). This type of change is noticeable particularly in the floor of the sella when the sphenoid sinus is well developed. In such a case the sinus is separated from the intracranial cavity only by the thin floor of the sella and this may undergo decalcification or even actual loss of bony substance. The anterior clinoid processes and the tuberculum of the sella are the last to show effects from increased intracranial pressure. Enlargement of the sellar cavity may or may not occur. It is particularly likely to develop if the dilated third ventricle is responsible for pressure erosion. This ventricle may, as indicated before, actually bulge into the cavity of the sella and thus enlarge it. Such enlargement may be in all directions and resemble very closely that produced by a pituitary

adenoma. At times it may be very difficult to be certain from the contour of the sella whether it has been enlarged as a result of a distant lesion or by an expanding tumor within the confines of the sella. Because pituitary adenomas rarely produce other signs of increased intracranial pressure, the presence or absence of these other findings is of considerable value in differentiation. Thus the presence of widened sutures in the child or prominent convolutional impressions on the inner table in the adult is valuable evidence that the lesion responsible for the sellar enlargement is actually at a distance from the sella. Likewise displacement of the calcified pineal or evidence of calcification within the tumor mass itself may be important signs of the nature of the lesion. In determining whether or not a given sella turcica is abnormal, attention must be paid to the density of the bony walls since the early signs of pressure often are manifested in this way. Enlargement of the sella is a later sign and a less valuable one from the standpoint of extrasellar tumors.

INCREASED CONVOLUTIONAL IMPRESSIONS. Pressure from the developing gyri of the brain causes a variable amount of waviness of the inner table of the skull and in roentgenograms the variation in thickness of the bones produced by these impressions can be visualized as alternating areas of lessened and increased density (while the visualized impressions may not actually correspond to the convolutions of the brain anatomically, the term has received wide usage). In general the infant skull does not show evidence of these convolutional impressions. They are more prominent during late childhood and early adolescence. The adult skull frequently shows little evidence of them. In the presence of increased intracranial pressure an increase in prominence of these convolutional impressions may develop. If this becomes at all marked the appearance of the skull is striking and has been likened to that of beaten silver. If in the infant or child the sutures are not fused prematurely, increase in pressure will cause a spreading of them before it will produce much change in the convolutional impressions. Thus this sign is seldom encountered in the child unless there is abnormal fusion of the cranial sutures (see Fig. 3-6). Even in the adult it is not too reliable a sign of increased intracranial pressure. It requires the existence of increased pressure over a considerable period of time to produce these changes, at least of a degree sufficient that they can be recognized from the normal variation. Occasionally, in an adult who has had a low-grade increase in intracranial pressure dating back to childhood and caused by some type of benign lesion such as inflammatory adhesions or congenital stenosis of the aqueduct, this beaten-silver appearance will be a striking manifestation of the chronic increase in intracranial pressure. The pressure in these patients may have existed for such a length of time and have been of relatively mild degree that sutural spread is not apparent. In practically all patients, however, the sella turcica will be abnormal if the convolutional impressions are increased as a result of pressure. The same pressure is more likely to affect the thin walls and processes of the sella and produce decalcification or erosion. Thus in borderline cases where there is some question as to the presence or absence of abnormal convolutional impressions the appearance of the sella may be helpful in deciding whether abnormality exists or not.

LOCALIZING EVIDENCE OF TUMOR

DISPLACEMENT OF CALCIFIED PINEAL GLAND. In previous paragraphs the importance of displacement of the calcified pineal gland and methods for determining its position have been given. The significance of this finding is emphasized by the fact that Vastine and Kinney found pineal displacement occurring in 39 per cent of all cases of tumor of the brain. Frequently the shift of the pineal only indicates the existence of a mass in the contralateral hemisphere and does not localize the lesion more closely (see Fig. 11-5). Occasionally the pineal will be shifted in two planes, laterally from the midline and in one other direction. Such a shift is of value in localizing the site of the mass lesion responsible for it. In general, tumors of the frontal lobe displace the pineal backward and toward the contralateral side. Lesions of the temporal lobe produce a shift away from the side of the lesion with little or no other displacement. Parietal lobe tumors are likely to cause a downward displacement of the pineal and some degree of lateral shift. Occipital lobe tumors displace it forward and in some subtentorial tumors an upward displacement will be noted. Other space-taking masses such as subdural hematomas and intracerebral abscesses may also cause pineal displacement. Unilateral atrophic lesions may cause a shift toward the side of the lesion but the amount is seldom very large. As has been noted before, a variation of 1 to 2 mm from the midline as viewed in the frontal position should be allowed as a normal variation before a diagnosis of lateral shift of the pineal is made. In the lateral view, as the charts of Vastine and Kinney[29] indicate, there is a range of normal variation in the position of the pineal and small degrees of shift may not be apparent when the position of the pineal is plotted on these charts. In general, mimimal degrees of pineal shift are more accurately recognized in the frontal view than they are in the lateral projection.

DISPLACEMENT OF CALCIFIED CHOROID PLEXUS. This has been discussed in the section on "The Choroid Plexus of the Lateral Ventricles." Displacement of the calcified glomus of a choroid plexus is a less significant finding than a corresponding degree of pineal displacement. These structures may be asymmetric in position in a normal skull since the glomus may not be at similar levels in the two lateral ventricles or different parts of it may calcify on the two sides. Thus minor asymmetry in position of the glomera can be a normal finding. If asymmetry of the glomera is encountered, careful observation of the appearance of the sella, the determination of the position of the calcified pineal, and special observation for other possible signs of intracranial disease as enumerated in previous paragraphs should be done.

CALCIFICATION OF THE TUMOR. Calcification within an intracranial tumor forms one of the significant roentgen signs of intracranial disease. Roentgen evidence of calcification is found in about 15 per cent of all intracranial tumors. Certain tumors show a very high incidence of calcification while others rarely if ever calcify. Thus, in individual lesions the incidence of calcification may be high. Among the tumors that frequently show calcification are the oligodendrogliomas, astrocytomas, meningiomas, craniopharyngiomas, and ependymomas. Mention will be made of these lesions in more detail in the summaries of brain tumors in the following sections.

LOCAL CHANGES IN THE CRANIAL BONES. Change in the bone overlying a meningioma is a common finding but is rare in other types of tumor. Infrequently, local thinning and outward bulging of the bone directly overlying a tumor is seen. This is more common in the temporal area in children and the lesion usually is a slowly growing or expanding process. The meningioma shows a tendency to invade the overlying bone and may actually extend through it to form a visible and palpable soft-tissue mass on the outer side of the calvarium. The changes described below, therefore, refer largely to meningiomas.

Increased Vascularity. The blood supply to a meningioma comes largely from the middle meningeal artery. Dilatation of this artery and its branches and of the accompanying veins causes a widening and tortuosity of the bony vascular grooves when the meningioma arises from the vertex of the skull (Figs. 11-18 and 11-19). When the tumor is situated close to the coronal suture and near the midline, a network of dilated vascular grooves may develop in and around the area of attachment of the tumor to the dura. The bone may have a fine moth-eaten appearance because of the numerous small vascular channels. Since there normally can be some variation in the prominence of the middle meningeal grooves, this finding must be interpreted with caution and with correlation of other roentgen and clinical findings. It is not unusual to find one or more branches of a middle meningeal on one side ending in a well-defined vascular lake with no similar change on the opposite side. This is usually a normal variation. Pathologic dilatation of these vessels is likely to form a much more irregular network of vascular spaces. When the tumor lies more posteriorly or lower down over the con-

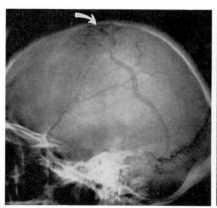 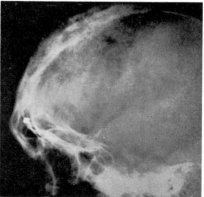

Fig. 11-18. *Left,* Convexity meningioma with increased vascularity of the bone. Note the dilated tortuous vessel groove extending to the vertex. There is loss of outline of the floor and dorsum of the sella indicative of increased intracranial pressure. **Arrow** indicates site of attachment of the tumor at the time of craniotomy. *Right,* Meningioma of the frontal area that has caused an extensive change in the bone overlying it. There is a mixture of destruction and proliferation with the latter predominating. The result is a thickened bone. There is fine spiculation extending at right angles to the bone on the external surface. Middle meningeal vessel channels are prominent behind the area of hyperostosis.

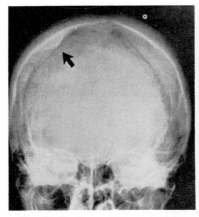
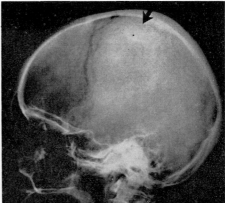

Fig. 11-19. Convexity meningioma causing a localized hyperostosis on the inner table at the site of its attachment to the dura (**arrows**). *Right*, The lateral view also reveals a dilated channel for the middle meningeal artery leading to the region of the tumor. The hyperostosis is seen clearly only in the posteroanterior view (*left*).

vexity, only one or several dilated vessels may be visualized extending to the region of the tumor (Fig. 11-18, *left*).

Localized Erosion of Bone. The bone directly overlying a meningioma may be invaded by the tumor with resulting dissolution of bone structure (Fig. 11-18, *right*). This varies widely from a fine moth-eaten appearance to an occasional case where the bone is completely destroyed over the tumor and the mass protrudes into the soft tissues of the scalp.

Proliferative Response. Meningiomas also tend to envoke a hyperostotic response in the bone directly overlying them. In some cases this is manifested by a local hyperostosis producing an elevated area of cortical bony density on the inner table (see Fig. 11-19). At other times the tumor may extend through the bone and cause a dense hyperostotic reaction on the outer table, with resulting external swelling. In other instances there is a mixture of bone destruction and proliferation (see Fig. 11-18, *right*). Variations in meningiomas and the effects on the overlying bone are remarkable and one must allow a wide range of roentgen changes in the bone to cover all possible variations that can be produced by this tumor.

PNEUMOENCEPHALOGRAPHY AND VENTRICULOGRAPHY

Ventriculography is a surgical procedure in which a needle is inserted through a trephine opening or drill hole directly into one of the lateral ventricles, the fluid is withdrawn and substituted for by air or oxygen, and roentgenograms are made. The ventricular system thus is made visible because of the contrast between the density of the gas and the surrounding brain tissue. In pneumoencephalography the gas is introduced into the lumbar subarachnoid space after lumbar puncture. The cerebrospinal fluid is removed in small increments and replaced by gas, and this can be continued until the major portion of the fluid has been drained from the system. However, attempted complete drainage is seldom necessary and usually unwise. Small amounts of gas, e.g., 20 to 30 cc, generally will allow satisfactory visualization if multiple projections are used. In pneumoencephalograms, in addition to visualization of the ventricles, the subarachnoid fluid pathways over the hemispheres and the basal cisterns can be demonstrated (Figs. 11-20 and 11-21). If there is increase in intracranial pressure, herniation of the cerebellar tonsils through the foramen magnum may

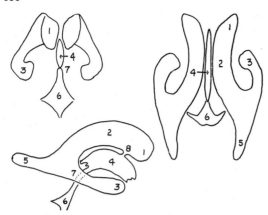

Fig. 11-20. The normal ventricular system. Diagrams show the appearances of the ventricles as viewed from different directions. *Upper left,* Anteroposterior view. *Upper right,* Appearance as viewed from above. *Lower,* Side view. **(1)** Anterior horn, **(2)** body, **(3)** temporal horn, and **(5)** occipital horn of lateral ventricle, **(4)** third ventricle, **(6)** fourth ventricle, **(7)** aqueduct of Sylvius, **(8)** foramen of Monro.

occur so that pneumoencephalography carries some risk in this situation. It should be done only when neurosurgical personnel and facilities are available to tap the ventricles and relieve the pressure. The neurosurgeons with whom we are associated prefer doing a ventricular tap in these circumstances through drill holes through the posterior parietal areas. With this method reduction of intraventricular pressure can be accomplished in a matter of minutes if the situation is critical. With proper precautions pneumoencephalography is particularly useful in showing small masses that may encroach upon the basal cisterns or the ventricular cavities and in many posterior fossa lesions it may be preferable to arteriography. Ventriculography has a limited field of usefulness because the subarachnoid spaces and cisterns are not demonstrated and it often is impossible to fill the third and fourth ventricles even though the ventricular system is patent.

The complicated pneumographic diagnosis of brain tumors is briefly summarized here. Generally speaking, cerebral neoplasms show evidence of their presence by deformities in the outline of the adjacent ventricle and displacement of the ventricular system away from the tumor. Tumors of the third ventricle reveal absence of filling of this cavity or a portion of it and a bilateral and symmetrical dilatation of the lateral ventricles if the lesion is large enough to obstruct the foramina of Monro. Tumors of the cerebellum and adjacent structures are likely to obstruct the ventricular system, resulting in dilatation of the third ventricle and a symmetrical enlargement of the lateral ventricles. When in the midline, deformity or absence of filling of the fourth ventricle is the rule. When the tumor is in a cerebellar hemisphere, the fourth ventricle will be shifted away from the side of the lesion. Many of these tumors, however, are large enough to prevent filling of the fourth ventricle. In these cases the aqueduct usually fills, and a sharp forward angulation of the lower on the proximal portion can be identified in lateral views (see Figs. 11-37 and 11-38). Tumors arising within a lateral ventricle or very close to it cause a localized filling defect in the ventricular cavity in addition to the evidence of displacement of the system away from the mass. The effect of a neoplastic mass on the ventricular system, therefore, will depend to a considerable extent upon its position, its size, and to some degree on its cellular characteristics. The most pronounced shift and deformity of the ventricular system often is encountered in glioblastoma multiforme because of the invasive characteristics of this tumor and the associated edema that may be present. In contrast, a small globular-shaped meningioma along the surface of a hemisphere may cause only a slight displacement of the ventricular system and very focal indentation of the roof of the lateral ventricle directly beneath the mass (see Fig. 11-32). Lesions in the posterior fossa are prone to cause obstructive hydrocephalus, and even a small tumor mass situated in or close to the fourth ventricle may readily obstruct the aqueduct of Sylvius and produce a high-grade dilatation of the ventricular system above the level of the aqueduct (see Fig. 11-38). Pneumoencephalography may be useful in the study of tumors of the pituitary gland and those arising in the immediate parasellar region because of the ability to visualize the basal

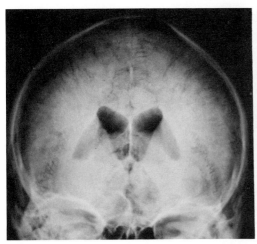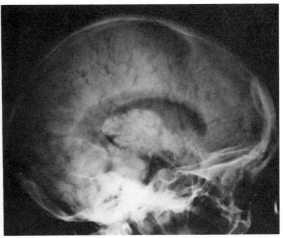

Fig. 11-21. Normal encephalogram. *Left,* Upright posteroanterior view. *Right,* Upright lateral view. Compare with diagrams of normal ventricular system shown in Figure 11-20. Because it is practically impossible to drain all the cerebrospinal fluid from the ventricles and replace it with gas, the entire ventricular system cannot be completely visualized unless multiple projections both in upright and recumbent positions are used. By shifting the fluid and gas with change in position of the head, all parts can be seen in the various films. In addition to the ventricles, the basal cisterns around the sella are visualized and there are subarachnoid channels over the surfaces of the cerebral hemispheres seen as dark streaks.

cisterns by this procedure. These tumors tend to encroach into the cavities of the basal cisterns and the outline of the tumor often is clearly seen when it is surrounded by gas (see Fig. 11-36).

ANGIOGRAPHY

Intracranial angiography consists in the rapid injection of an iodine-containing substance such as 40 to 50% Hypaque into the carotid artery in the neck or in the vertebral artery and the making of a series of roentgenograms in rapid sequence while the material is passing through the cerebral or cerebellar circulations. Angiography has received wide acceptance and in many cases is preferred to pneumography. Not only can space-taking masses be identified, but at times a good idea of their nature can be obtained. For vascular lesions such as aneurysms, arteriovenous malformation, and occlusive disease it is the method of choice. In some examinations the puncture of the vessel is done percutaneously. In some circumstances, particularly in the study of occlusive disease, it may be preferable to insert a catheter into the aortic arch via either the brachial artery or the femoral artery. By this means multiple vessels can be outlined with one injection or individual vessels may be catheterized selectively allowing better opacification of the vessel and its smaller branches. By means of arteriography it is possible to visualize clearly the cerebral vessels and as the contrast material is followed in the series of roentgenograms, sequential filling of the arteries, capillaries, and veins is obtained. Usually it is advisable to obtain roentgenograms in both lateral and frontal positions so that the vessels can be studied in two different planes (Figs. 11-22 and 11-23). With special equipment this can be done with one injection of contrast substance. In the absence of such equipment, two separate injections must be made. The amount of contrast material injected should be kept as small as possible and from 10 to 15 cc or less usually is sufficient for each injection.

The angiographic findings in brain tumors depend upon (*1*) stretching or displacement of vessels by the mass, (*2*) the demonstration of

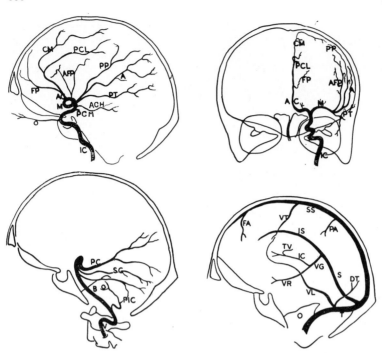

Fig. 11-22. The normal arterial and venous systems. Diagrammatic anatomy of intracranial vessels as visualized by means of arteriography. *Upper left,* Lateral internal carotid arteriogram: **IC,** internal carotid artery; **M,** middle cerebral artery; **AC,** anterior cerebral artery; **FP,** frontopolar artery; **CM,** calloso-marginal artery; **PCL,** pericallosal artery; **AFP,** ascending frontoparietal artery; **PP,** posterior parietal artery; **A,** angular artery; **PT,** posterior temporal artery; **ACH,** anterior choroidal artery; **PCM,** posterior communicating; **O,** ophthalmic artery. *Upper right,* Anteroposterior internal carotid arteriogram (same lettering as above). *Lower left,* Lateral vertebral arteriogram. **PC,** posterior cerebral artery; **SC,** superior cerebellar artery; **B,** basilar artery; **V,** vertebral artery; **PIC,** posterior inferior cerebellar artery. *Lower right,* Lateral view of venous drainage. **FA,** frontal ascending vein; **SS,** superior sagittal sinus; **IS,** inferior sagittal sinus; **VT,** anastomotic vein of Trolard; **PA,** parietal ascending vein; **IC,** internal cerebral vein; **VG,** vein of Galen; **S,** straight sinus; **VR,** basal vein of Rosenthal; **VL,** anastomotic vein of Labbe; **T,** transverse sinus. The site of the foramen of Monro (interventricular foramen) is indicated by the location of a small angular vein (**TV,** thalamostriate vein) entering the internal cerebral vein.

tumor vessels or a diffuse "blush" or "stain" within the lesion, (*3*) early or delayed filling of veins draining the lesion, and (*4*) the visualization of an avascular area if the mass is cystic, necrotic, or otherwise has little circulation within it. In glioblastoma multiforme, for example, multiple small, tortuous vessels may be identified. In some tumors, particularly the more vascular meningiomas, a deep tumor stain develops during the phase of late arterial or capillary filling (see Figs. 11-27 and 11-33). This tends to persist after visualization of the major arteries and veins has disappeared. In some cases of metastatic carcinoma, "tumor vessels" may become opacified clearly outlining the mass; in others a dense blush or tumor stain develops; in still others there is only displacement of vessels away from the lesion. Intracranial angiography is particularly useful when, for one reason or another,

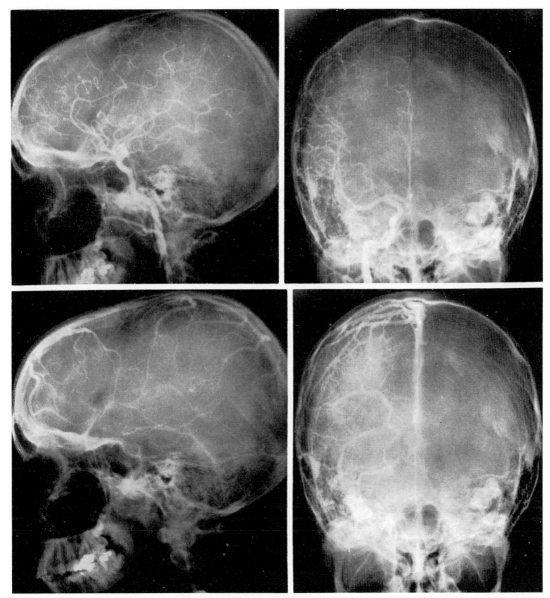

Fig. 11-23. Normal internal carotid arteriograms and venograms. *Top,* Anteroposterior (*right*) and lateral (*left*) roentgenograms during the phase of arterial filling. Compare with Figure 11-22. *Bottom,* Anteroposterior (*right*) and lateral (*left*) roentgenograms during phase of venous filling.

pneumographic examination has been unsatisfactory or cannot be performed. It also is useful in giving some indication of the histologic nature of the tumor in some cases, as noted above. It is valuable in the study of vascular malformations and aneurysms. Arteriography also is a worthwhile procedure in the diagnosis of subdural hematomas. This will be discussed in the section on "Subdural Hematoma and Hygroma."

In occlusive disease, arteriography is the method of choice for the study of the intracranial vessels, as well as for the examination of the arteries in the neck. Arteriosclerotic plaques are visualized as areas of narrowing of the vessel lumen. With complete obstruction there is a sharp cutoff of the column of contrast material. The accompanying illustrations demonstrate some of the more characteristic changes that may be found in the presence of intracranial neoplasms and vascular lesions by means of angiography (Figs. 11-24 through 11-26).

OBSERVATION IN SPECIFIC TUMORS

A brief résumé of the findings in specific tumors will be given in the following section. Special emphasis will be paid to the roentgen findings on plain-film examination and with reference to the pneumographic and arteriographic changes that may be expected. From a clinical point of view it is customary to consider brain tumors, according to location in relation to the tentorium, as being either supratentorial or infratentorial. The location of the lesion is important not only from the aspects of symptomatology and clinical signs but also because of differences in surgical approach. Roentgen findings are also best considered in

the same way because the location of a tumor in its relation to the tentorium may alter the roentgen findings considerably. Only the pertinent roentgen observations will be given here, chiefly to indicate to the student the ways in which roentgen diagnosis can be used in the study of intracranial neoplasms and to illustrate the more frequently encountered signs of various lesions. The incidence of various intracranial tumors as listed by Potts[22] is as follows: Gliomas, 43 per cent; meningiomas, 15 per cent; pituitary adenomas, 13 per cent; acoustic neuromas, 6.5 per cent; metastatic tumors, 6.5 per cent; congenital tumors, 4 per cent; blood vessel tumors, 3 per cent; and miscellaneous, 9 per cent.

SUPRATENTORIAL TUMORS

GLIOMAS

GLIOBLASTOMA MULTIFORME

This is an invasive, locally malignant tumor and is the most common of the gliomas occurring above the tentorium, forming about 40 per

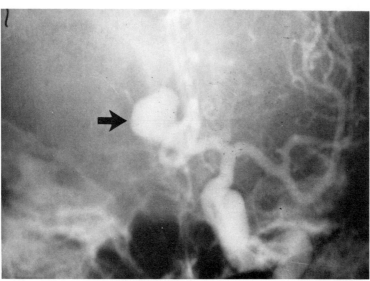

Fig. 11-24. Aneurysm of anterior communicating artery fills from a left-sided carotid injection but projects to the right. (Same patient as seen in Fig. 11-12).

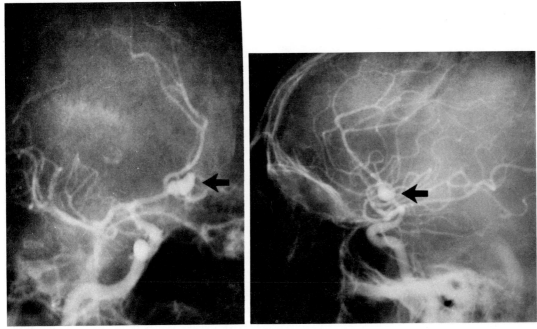

Figure. 11-25. Aneurysm of the anterior cerebral artery (**arrows**). The location of the aneurysm is best demonstrated in the oblique view on the *left*.

cent of all such tumors.[2] The tumor is most frequent between the ages of 40 and 60 years. The duration of symptoms usually is short and averages about 6 months prior to the initial examination. However, in many cases the symptoms are of very short duration, sometimes only a matter of days. The tumor may occur anywhere in the brain; it is characterized by its infiltrating nature and its ability to spread rapidly.

Roentgenograms of the skull frequently reveal nothing abnormal because of the short duration of the tumor. This is true in spite of the clinical signs of severe increase in intracranial pressure. Calcification sufficient to be visible in roentgenograms occurs infrequently because of the rapid growth of the lesion. Some decalcification of the sella, especially of the dorsum, may be seen if the tumor has been present for several months or longer. If calcified, the pineal will usually be found to be displaced from its normal position and a pronounced lateral shift is frequent. Occasionally the tumor destroys brain tissue as it grows, so

that the mass effect of the tumor is not apparent and the pineal may remain in the normal location. Absence of pineal displacement, therefore, does not completely rule out an infiltrating glioblastoma.

On pneumoencephalography or ventriculography significant displacement of the ventricular system away from the lesion is usual (see Fig. 11-27). Temporal lobe tumors displace the temporal horn of the lateral ventricle or prevent its filling with gas. Often there is gross distortion of the ventricle on the side of the lesion and it may be difficult to fill it with gas because of compression by the tumor. When the tumor involves a frontal lobe, it is prone to extend across the midline beneath the falx or by way of involvement of the corpus callosum so that some deformity of the opposite ventricle may be visualized. Following internal carotid angiography, displacement of the vessels away from the area of the lesion with stretching and straightening of their branches is a common observation. Frequently vessels within the tumor will become opacified and

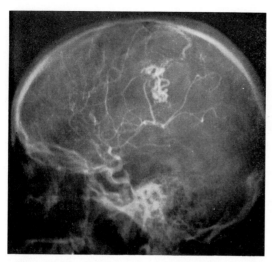

Fig. 11-26. Arteriovenous malformation in the right parietal area. The lesion originates from a branch of the middle cerebral artery and consists of a tangled mass of dilated vessels.

characteristically will show the presence of multiple irregular dilatations. Early filling of veins draining the area is usual. In some cases a stain or blush develops during the late arterial or capillary phase (Figs. 11-28 and 11-29). During the venous phase, displacement of veins may be seen. These findings in the presence of a space-occupying lesion are characteristic for this tumor. Angiography is the preferable method for demonstrating this tumor and has supplanted ventriculography to a considerable extent.

ASTROCYTOMA

Astrocytoma is the second most common glioma occurring above the tentorium, representing approximately 32 per cent of gliomas in this area. The duration of symptoms averages 3 years. The tumor may involve any part of the brain. Large cysts commonly form in astrocytomas and the cystic element may predominate in the pathologic appearance of the lesion.

Roentgenograms of the skull may reveal calcification and this finding is reported to occur in 13 per cent of astrocytomas (Fig. 11-

30).[2] The calcium frequently is seen in the form of coarse, strandlike densities with intermixed small punctate shadows. At times, in a predominantly cystic lesion, a nodule of tumor tissue along the wall of the cyst will calcify and appear as a more or less rounded calcific density (see Fig. 11-30). The amount of calcium often is small and by no means indicates the extent of the tumor. Only occasionally when a lesion is cystic and calcium is deposited in the wall of the cyst does the calcium shadow indicate reasonably well the extent of the lesion. Because of the duration of this lesion prior to its recognition, roentgen signs of increased intracranial pressure often are noted. Decalcification and erosion of the sella are frequently observed. Displacement of the calcified pineal is frequent in this tumor.

Pneumograms demonstrate the characteristic findings of a space-filling mass with local deformity of the ventricle adjacent to the lesion and a general shift of the ventricular system away from the side of the tumor.

On angiography the findings are similar to

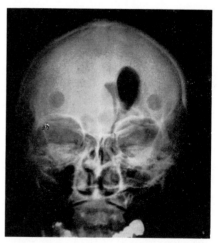

Fig 11-27. Right temporal lobe tumor. Anteroposterior ventriculogram. The lateral ventricle is displaced beneath the falx, the roof of the right being flattened by the rigid falx. The third ventricle also is displaced and lies obliquely, a characteristic position for this ventricle in the presence of a temporal lobe mass. Burr holes for ventricular puncture are visible as round translucent areas on either side.

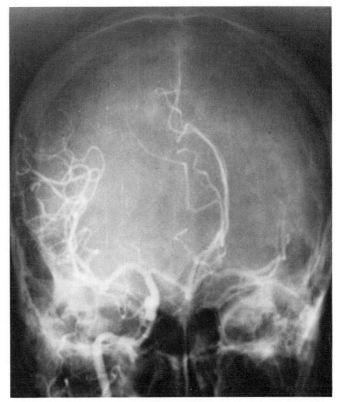

Fig. 11-28. Frontal lobe glioblastoma multiforme. Anteroposterior internal carotid arteriogram shows displacement of the anterior cerebral to opposite side.

those of glioblastoma multiforme except that there tends to be fewer and shorter tumor vessels. If the mass is largely cystic, an avascular area will be seen together with stretching and displacement of vessels adjacent to the mass. Contralateral shift of the anterior cerebral artery will be present, the amount of shift depending upon the size of the mass. A tumor blush may be present at times in the nodular component of the lesion or if the entire mass is solid but the blush is not very intense.

OLIGODENDROGLIOMA

This tumor comprises about 7 per cent of the supratentorial gliomas. The average age of the patients is 35 years. The duration of symptoms is long and it is the most slowly growing and benign of the supratentorial gliomas; the average duration of symptoms is given as 11 years.[2] This tumor is predominantly one of the cerebral hemispheres.

Because of its slow growth, calcification within the tumor occurs very frequently. The calcium usually is distributed in the form of coarse, irregular strands (Fig. 11-31). As with the other gliomas, the extent of calcification rarely indicates the actual extent of the tumor. Roentgen signs of increased intracranial pressure are frequent, with evidence of sellar erosion and decalcification, and displacement of the pineal if it is calcified.

Pneumograms show only the evidence of space-filling mass displacing the ventricular system. Because these tumors often have attained a large size by the time they are dis-

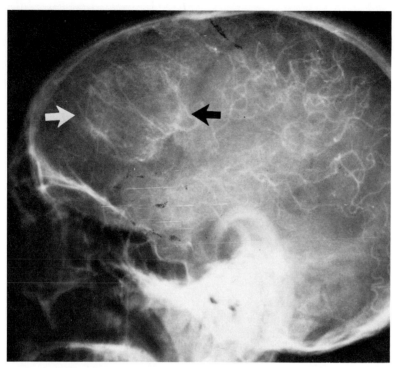

Fig. 11-29. Lateral view of same patient seen in Figure 11-28. During the late arterial and capillary phase the lesion shows a tumor blush (**arrows**).

covered, rather marked ventricular displacement may be seen.

Arteriography will show displacement of vessels away from the mass, with stretching of smaller vessels and occlusion of some. The interior of the tumor usually does not develop a tumor stain during the capillary phase.

EPENDYMOMA

This tumor comprises about 5 per cent of the supratentorial gliomas. The average age of appearance is reported to be 30 years. The duration of symptoms is relatively short and usually less than 1 year. Most of these tumors which develop above the tentorium, arise from and lie within a lateral ventricle.

The tumor frequently contains small, scattered, punctate, calcified deposits. Otherwise it shows only the roentgen findings of increased intracranial pressure which are not specific. Pneumograms reveal the mass of the lesion usually projecting into one of the lateral ventricles, which may be sufficiently large to occlude the major portion of one ventricle. There also will be a shift of the ventricular system away from the side of the mass. If the tumor blocks the foramen of Monro it may cause a pronounced dilatation of the ipsilateral ventricle.

MENINGIOMAS

Meningiomas constitute between 13 and 15 per cent of all intracranial tumors and the majority are situated above the tentorium. The age period is from 30 to 60 years and the tumor becomes more frequent with advancing age. It is rare below the age of 30. The duration of symptoms usually is long and may cover a period of many years. Meningiomas commonly develop at the sites of attachment of the dura and in the areas where arachnoid villi

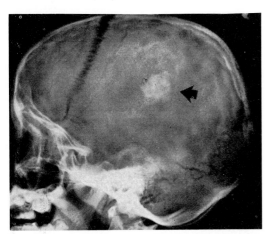

Fig. 11-30. Astrocytoma of the parietal lobe. Lateral roentgenogram of the skull of a child demonstrates a mottled calcified area (**arrow**) situated deeply in the brain (depth also established by an anteroposterior view). There is spreading of the vault sutures, particularly the coronal, characteristic of increased intracranial pressure.

are frequent. Thus the common locations of meningiomas include sites alongside the superior sagittal sinus in the posterior frontal and parietal areas and along the convexities of the cerebral hemispheres a short distance away from the midline. Other favorite sites for development of these tumors are in the region of the tuberculum sellae or just anterior to the tuberculum along the olfactory groove, along the edges of the sphenoidal ridge, and somewhat less frequently along the falx cerebri and the tentorium. Grossly, meningiomas vary from a globular shape to a flat type of growth that spreads over the surface of the cerebral hemisphere, the *meningioma en plaque.*

Roentgen Findings

Positive evidence of the presence of a tumor is frequently demonstrated. This is because of the long duration of the lesion and the frequent findings of sellar erosion or decalcification plus the evidence of pineal displacement. The latter finding is less common, however, than is seen in the gliomas. Of greater importance is the fact that meningiomas tend to evoke a response in the bone overlying the point of attachment and to cause hypervascularity of the overlying bone. Convexity meningiomas usually receive a major portion of their blood supply from the middle meningeal artery, a branch of the external carotid. Enlargement of the grooves of the middle meningeal branch of the external carotid and its accompanying veins is frequently seen in convexity and parasagittal meningiomas (see Fig. 11-18). The vessels may end in a network of dilated tortuous grooves overlying the region of the tumor. In addition a localized hyperostosis may be formed on the surface of the inner table (see Fig. 11-19). Occasionally the tumor invades the bone and extends through it to form a similar hyperostotic density along the external table. In other cases extensive bone destruction is apparent and, rarely, the bone overlying the tumor will be completely destroyed with a soft-tissue mass bulging externally.

Calcification within the tumor is found in 15 to 20 per cent of cases. The calcium deposits typically are in the form of small punctate densities rather uniformly distributed throughout the tumor mass and known as psammoma bodies.

Pneumographic studies reveal the evidence

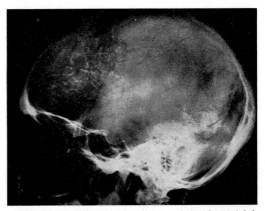

Fig. 11-31. Oligodendroglioma of the frontal lobe. There is extensive calcification within the tumor that involves practically all one frontal lobe. The floor of the sella is decalcified and the dorsum and posterior clinoid processes are almost completely destroyed by the increased intracranial pressure. The calcified pineal is displaced backward from its normal position.

of a space-filling mass with displacement of the ventricular system. The displacement is usually less marked than with gliomas since the latter tumors, particularly glioblastoma multiforme, tend to incite an edematous reaction in the surrounding brain that adds to the space-filling characteristics. Meningiomas do not invade the underlying brain, they only displace it (Fig. 11-32).

If following carotid arteriography, contrast material has opacified the branches of the external carotid, the vascularity of the tumor may become apparent. This is best demonstrated in the capillary or venous phase of filling (Fig. 11-33). Then the tumor may become uniformly opaque and the entire mass of it will be clearly outlined as a dense stain. Such a tumor stain is fairly characteristic of a meningioma; if it arises as a result of external carotid opacification, it is almost certainly indicative of this lesion. If the vessels supplying the tumor do not fill with contrast substance and only branches of the internal carotid opacify, then the positive finding may be limited to displacement of the vessels away from the site of the mass. Meningiomas arising from the falx or tentorium, and occasionally at other sites, however, receive blood from the internal carotid; some tumors derive their blood supply from both internal and external carotid arteries. Selective catheterization of each of these vessels will demonstrate this. Also, some are supplied largely from branches of the internal carotid so that, generally, it is good practice to opacify both vessels. Angiography is probably the method of choice, at least as the initial method of investigation, because the findings not only locate the lesion but frequently give changes indicating the nature of the tumor.

TUMORS IN AND NEAR THE SELLA

PITUITARY ADENOMAS

CHROMOPHOBE ADENOMA. This is a nonsecretory tumor of the pituitary gland. The age period for its occurrence is given as between 30 and 50 years. Clinically it produces the picture of hypopituitarism.

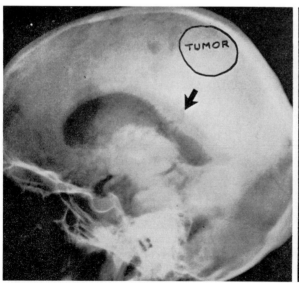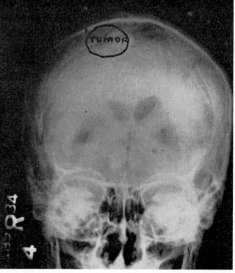

Fig. 11-32. Parasagittal meningioma in the posterior parietal area causing localized depression of the lateral ventricle beneath it as seen in the lateral pneumoencephalogram on the *left*. The depression of the ventricle and the slight shift of both ventricles to the opposite side is shown in the posteroanterior view on the *right*.

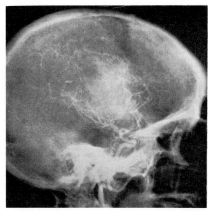
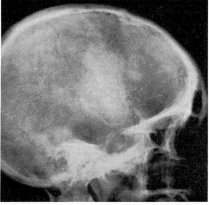

Fig. 11-33. Meningioma in the frontoparietal region visualized by means of arteriography. *Left,* During late arterial filling the tumor has become diffusely opaque (Tumor stain). There also is a network of larger vessels that have filled via the middle meningeal artery (both internal and external carotid arteries have been opacified). *Right,* Several seconds later. There continues to be a dense tumor stain as the fine vessels and capillaries of the tumor retain the contrast substance.

Characteristically, a chromophobe adenoma of the pituitary causes a generalized enlargement of the sella turcica that has been described as "ballooning." The growth of the tumor is slow and as a result the sella becomes enlarged without the walls actually being destroyed. In very large tumors, however, the wall may become so thin that it is practically nonexistent along the posterior and inferior portions. As the floor is expanded the tumor tends to bulge into the sphenoid sinus and with destruction of the bony floor the lesion may actually decompress itself by growing into the sphenoid sinus. Calcification in chromophobe adenomas is uncommon. There are no other changes in the cranial bones. There is no displacement of the calcified pineal (Fig. 11-34).

EOSINOPHILIC ADENOMA. This is a secretory tumor of the pituitary and clinically results in the picture of acromegaly in the adult. If the tumor develops before bone growth has ceased it will cause gigantism. Enlargement of the sella by this tumor is sometimes less than is usually seen in association with a chromophobe adenoma. In some patients the sella may be of normal size.

Mixed types also occur and with considerable enlargement of the sella. In some patients at the time of surgery or autopsy only the chromophobe adenoma remains. In other patients degeneration of the tumor leads to the formation of a cyst. In either event the acromegaly ceases progression although signs of hypopituitarism may increase.

The roentgen diagnostic findings in acro-

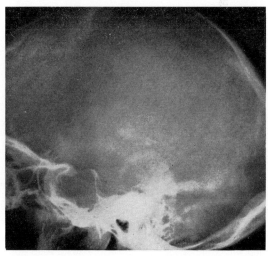

Fig. 11-34. Chromophobe adenoma of the pituitary enlarging the sella in all dimensions.

megaly have been discussed in Chapter 1 under the heading "Hyperfunction of the Pituitary Gland."

BASOPHILIC ADENOMA. Basophilic adenomas usually are microscopic lesions and it is hardly to be expected that enlargement of the sella or any change in its bony walls will be demonstrated. Basophilic adenomas often are found in association with Cushing's syndrome and thus there may be demonstrated a generalized skeletal decalcification with collapse of the vertebrae, multiple fractures, and a granular osteoporosis of the flat bones, including the skull. This granular appearance often is striking. It is not specific for Cushing's syndrome since a similar type of osteoporosis is seen in hyperparathyroidism.

CRANIOPHARYNGIOMA. This is a congenital tumor arising from remnants of Rathke's pouch. It is a tumor of childhood and adolescence, although an occasional case is found later in life. The clinical picture is one of hypopituitarism with infantilism.

Calcification is very frequent in cranio-pharyngiomas and has been reported in as high as 80 per cent of cases (see Fig. 11-35). The calcium is found in the form of a cloudy density or as punctate deposits in and above the sella turcica. In addition, abnormality in the appearance of the sella is present almost constantly. Erosion of the dorsum sellae is the most frequent finding. Occasionally the sella is enlarged and at times considerable destruction of its bony walls may be seen. In some cases the signs of generalized increase in intracranial pressure will be apparent and because this tumor occurs mainly in childhood, spreading of the cranial sutures may be present. This is usually caused by a large suprasellar mass that either displaces the brain stem and occludes the aqueduct, producing an obstructive hydrocephalus, or else the tumor encroaches upon the third ventricle and interferes with flow of fluid out of the lateral ventricles. Pneumoencephalography is helpful in identifying the lesion in those cases where calcification is not present. The mass of the tumor projecting above the sella into the basal cisterns is the major finding.

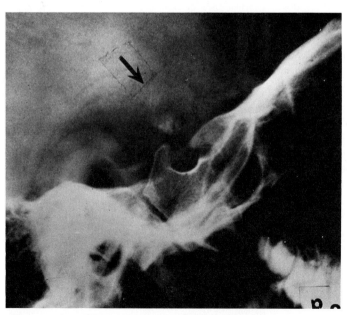

Fig. 11-35. Craniopharyngioma. **Arrow** points to the calcification within the lesion just above the sella. Also note the depression between the anterior clinoid processes giving a J-shaped sella or a duplicated floor.

OTHER SUPRATENTORIAL TUMORS

TUMORS OF THE PINEAL GLAND

Pineal tumors are uncommon; not infrequently the tumor calcifies. Calcification in the region of the pineal gland in a child below the age of 10 years is strongly suggestive of a pinealoma since the normal pineal gland usually does not calcify at this age. If in older patients calcium in the region of the pineal extends over a distance of more than a centimeter, the possibility of a pinealoma should be considered. Teratomas of the pineal body may exhibit a combination of calcium and fat. The density of the fat is less than that of the brain tissue surrounding it and the fatty portion of the tumor may appear as an area of translucency within the brain, while the calcified portion of the tumor appears very dense. This combination occurring in the region of the pineal is characteristic of a teratoma of this structure. In the absence of calcification, pinealoma can be diagnosed roentgenologically only on pneumographic study. The mass of the tumor projects into the posterior part of the third ventricle. If very large it may obstruct the inferior outlet of the third ventricle, occluding the aqueduct of Sylvius and causing a pronounced dilatation of the lateral ventricles.

BENIGN CYST OF THE THIRD VENTRICLE

This lesion develops in the anterior portion of the third ventricle, usually arising from the roof. Because of its situation it blocks the foramina of Monro and causes a bilateral dilatation of the lateral ventricles. If gas is injected into one ventricle during ventriculography the tumor may prevent the gas from extending across into the opposite ventricle. Failure to displace gas from one ventricle to the other during ventriculography is presumptive evidence of obstruction of the foramina of Monro. If gas enters the third ventricle the margin of the cyst may be outlined as a smooth, convex soft-tissue shadow encroaching into the air space of the ventricle. Because this is a benign lesion it is important to recognize it if possible so that curative surgery may be attempted.

OPTIC NERVE TUMORS

Glioma of the optic nerve is a congenital tumor. It causes enlargement of the optic foramen. Be-

cause the tumor is developmental in origin the tuberculum of the sella usually fails to develop properly and there may be a concave depression between the anterior clinoid processes. When viewed in the lateral position, the floor of the sella may appear duplicated in the region of the tuberculum. Neurofibroma also causes enlargement of the optic foramen. The other clinical stigmata of neurofibromatosis may be present, including subcutaneous tumors and *café au lait* pigmentation. Encephalography is an excellent method for studying tumors of the optic nerves or chiasm because filling of the cisterns above the sella may outline the tumor mass very clearly even though it is of small size (Fig. 11-36).

ANGIOMAS

The roentgen findings in vascular tumors have been discussed in the section on "Capillary and Venous Angiomas."

EPIDERMOID AND DERMOID CYSTS; LIPOMAS

Epidermoid Cyst. (Cholesteatoma). This tumor is more frequent in the cranial bones than it is as an intracranial lesion. In the brain it is found most frequently in a lateral ventricle, the

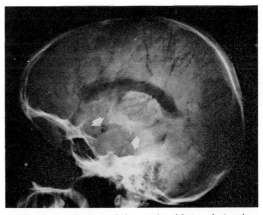

Fig. 11-36. Tumor of the optic chiasm. Lateral upright pneumoencephalogram. There is a small mass in the suprasellar area outlined by gas in the narrowed cisterns above and behind it (**arrows**). The anterior floor of the third ventricle is elevated. The tuberculum of the sella is flattened (J-shaped sella). Compare with normal gas-filled basal cisterns shown in Figure 11-21.

fourth ventricle, or at the cerebellopontine angle. On pneumography, gas may outline all or a portion of the mass. Characteristically, the surface is rough, nodular, or cauliflowerlike with gas extending into deep clefts on the surface of the tumor.[28] Otherwise the findings are only those of a space-filling mass.

INTRACRANIAL DERMOIDS. These are rare lesions. They differ from epidermoids in that the lesion also may contain hair or dermal elements other than squamous epithelium. Because of their high fat content a portion of the mass may be sufficiently translucent so that it can be recognized in plain skull roentgenograms. Calcification may be found in the lesion. Dermoids are found most frequently in the region of the pineal, in the cerebellum, or in the fourth ventricle.

INTRACRANIAL LIPOMAS. These also are infrequent lesions. Rarely a lipoma may develop in the region of the corpus callosum and is sometimes found in association with agenesis of the corpus callosum. As with dermoids the fat content of the lesion may allow it to be visualized in plain skull films as an area of translucency. The lateral limits of the lesion often contain calcified plaques visible in posteroanterior views of the skull on either side of the midline.

SUBTENTORIAL TUMORS

GLIOMAS

Astrocytoma is one of the most frequent tumors involving a cerebellar hemisphere. Occasionally it may extend to the midline or even to the opposite side. Like its counterpart above the tentorium it often becomes cystic with a mural nodule of tumor tissue and the cyst may predominate in the gross specimen. It behaves like any other space-occupying mass and because of its nearness to the fourth ventricle, displacement, encroachment, or obstruction of the ventricle or its outlets is commonly seen (Fig. 11-37). Displacement of the fourth ventricle usually is to the opposite side but in some cases the ventricle is displaced only for-

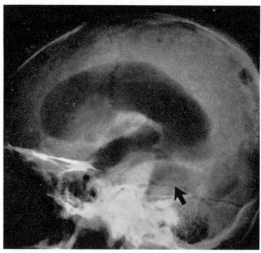

Fig. 11-37. Astroblastoma of cerebellum. Lateral recumbent ventriculogram with the left side uppermost. The dilated fourth ventricle (**arrow**) is displaced forward and upward by a mass directly behind and below it.

ward. The differentiation by pneumography from other hemispherical masses, particularly hemangioblastoma, is difficult or impossible. Calcification in the tumor is less frequent than in supratentorial lesions and the plain-film findings, if present, are usually those referable to increased intracranial pressure. On angiography, stretching and displacement of vessels may be seen. A tumor stain also is encountered in some cases which may resemble that seen in hemangioblastoma so that the differential diagnosis may be difficult regardless of the roentgen method of examination.

HEMANGIOBLASTOMA

This lesion, also known as *Lindau's disease,* develops in a cerebellar hemisphere. It is a highly vascular lesion and causes a deep stain or blush during the capillary phase of arteriography. The tumor displaces the fourth ventricle toward the opposite side during pneumoencephalography and may obstruct it. Calcified deposits usually are not seen. This tumor sometimes is associated with a retinal hemangioma-tosis known as *von Hippel's disease,* or the combination as *von Hippel-Lindau disease.* Cysts of the kidneys, pancreas, and other abdominal organs may be present.

The angiographic appearances that have been noted have been of several types:[32]

A. Dense nodule
   1. Homogenous
   2. With central translucency
B. Tangle of vessels
   1. Homogenous
   2. With central translucency

Also enlarged feeding arteries and draining veins may be seen with either type. Cysts often are associated and cause more vascular displacement than would be expected from the size of the dense nodule.

MEDULLOBLASTOMA

This tumor is encountered chiefly during childhood. It is a malignant tumor and tends to spread to various parts of the subarachnoid space by seeding. The tumor arises in or near the roof of the fourth ventricle and thus may cause obstructive hydrocephalus while it is still very small.

Because this tumor is most frequent during childhood and is very prone to obstruct the outlets of the fourth ventricle or the aqueduct of Sylvius, the signs of increased intracranial pressure are often noted. Spreading of the cranial sutures is a common observation. Decalcification or erosion of the sella turcica may or may not be present, depending upon how readily the sutures give and how long the increased pressure has existed. The tumor seldom calcifies.

Pneumoencephalography or ventriculography reveals evidence of obstructive hydrocephalus with dilatation of the lateral and third ventricles. Gas may or may not extend into the fourth ventricle, depending upon the size of the tumor and the amount of its encroachment on the ventricular space (Fig. 11-38). Often the

ventricle is not identified and a sharp cutoff of the gas shadow in the aqueduct is noted. The inferior part of the aqueduct often is angled forward on the proximal to form nearly a right angle. When viewed in the frontal position the aqueduct is not displaced from the midline. Vertebral arteriography shows displacement of vessels away from the mass or occlusion of some of the major branches of the basilar artery.

Metastasis to the osseous system occurs infrequently in medulloblastoma. Characteristically, the lesions are of sclerotic type and may involve the skull, pelvis, and long bones.

EPENDYMOMA

This tumor is similar to its counterpart occurring above the tentorium and it arises in or adjacent to the floor of the fourth ventricle. Small, punctate, calcified deposits are relatively common in this tumor and it is a frequent cause of subtentorial calcification during childhood. The roentgen findings otherwise are those of increased intracranial pressure and pneumographic evidence of a mass that usually obstructs the fourth ventricle and prevents filling of it by the gas.

POLAR SPONGIOBLASTOMA

This is the most common tumor involving the pons and immediately contiguous structures. Its rate of growth is moderately slow. It is mainly a tumor of childhood or adolescence. The tumor causes a diffuse swelling of the pons and this results in a smooth backward displacement of the fourth ventricle with elongation of the aqueduct as it is stretched over the mass. The pontine cistern, which is the subarachnoid space between the pons and the clivus and dorsum sellae, is narrowed. The distance between the floor of the fourth ventricle and the dorsum sellae is increased. Normally this measurement varies from 3.5 to 3.75 cm. As a rule there is little or no dilatation of the third

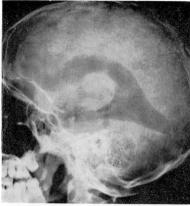

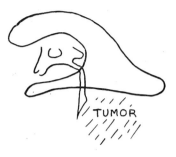

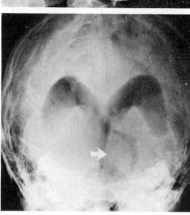

Fig. 11-38. Medulloblastoma. *Left*, Lateral recumbent ventriculogram with the left side of the head uppermost. The left lateral ventricle is filled with gas and the third ventricle, aqueduct of Sylvius, and the upper part of the fourth ventricle are visible. The fourth ventricle is displaced forward and its inferior portion obliterated. *Right*, Tracing of roentgenogram. *Below*, Posteroanterior ventriculogram of medulloblastoma involving the fourth ventricle. The mass of the tumor encroaches upon the ventricular cavity and is bounded by a small amount of gas along the margin of the ventricle (**arrow** indicates tumor).

and lateral ventricles in spite of the fact that the mass displaces the aqueduct and fourth ventricle. Apparently the growth of the lesion is slow enough so that the structures tend to accommodate and little interference with the flow of the cerebrospinal fluid results. Pneumoencephalography is an excellent method for the study of these lesions, since by this procedure the cisterns around the base of the brain can be visualized in addition to the ventricular system and the enlargement of the pons becomes obvious as it is outlined by gas anteriorly and posteriorly.

PERINEURAL FIBROBLASTOMA (ACOUSTIC NEUROMA; CEREBELLOPONTINE ANGLE TUMOR; SCHWANNOMA)

This tumor arises from the nerve sheath of the acoustic nerve. It is found chiefly in the age period between 30 and 50 years. The duration of symptoms is moderately long and may be several years or even longer.

The tumor most frequently develops within the internal auditory canal and causes enlargement of the canal and the internal acoustic meatus. This is a smooth pressure type of erosion resulting in a generalized enlargement of the canal or, occasionally, only of its meatus (Fig. 11-39). The latter lesions produce a funnel-shaped canal and the mass of the tumor develops largely outside of the canal. It is helpful to compare the abnormal with the normal side. As a rule the internal auditory canals are of similar appearance on the two sides of the skull. Slight degrees of variation in size do occur and occasionally different degrees of pneumatization of the petrous pyramids are noted. A variation in height of the meatus on the two sides of 1.0 mm is considered within normal limits. A variation of 2.0 mm or more is highly suggestive of pathologic enlargement.[13] Tomography, or body-section roentgenography, is of considerable value in visualization of the canals and meati and should be done in most cases when this tumor is a diagnostic consideration. In most cases, however, careful study of both petrous pyramids will enable the observer to recognize pathologic enlargement. In borderline cases it is usually necessary to correlate the roentgen findings with the clinical observations. The latter often are so typical that the diagnosis can be made from the clinical findings alone. In some cases the tumor causes no change in the bony structure of the pyramid. This is because of its development within the cranial cavity rather than in the meatus or canal. However, proper roentgen study will show changes in most cases.

On pneumography evidence of internal hydrocephalus is commonly seen with the larger lesions. The fourth ventricle frequently fills and is seen to be flattened on the side of the lesion and often displaced away from the midline toward the contralateral side and somewhat posteriorly. Less frequently the ventricle is displaced anteriorly rather than posteriorly.

Positive-contrast visualization of the cerebellopontine cisterns has come into use in recent years for the demonstration of this tumor. The contrast material used is Pantopaque, the same as used for myelography. The procedure is carried out the same as myelography except that the contrast medium is allowed to flow into the posterior fossa. By proper positioning of the patient's head it can be displaced into one or both cerebellopontine cisterns and thus outline the tumor as a filling defect. If other methods of examination do not demonstrate the tumor, positive-contrast visualization should be done in most cases.

OTHER TUMORS

CHORDOMA

This tumor arises from remnants of the fetal notochord and its common locations are at the cervico-occipital junction and in the sacrococcygeal area of the spine. It is a slowly growing tumor that results in bone destruction. The cervico-occipital lesion, therefore, leads to destruction in the base of the occiput or the clivus together with evidence of a soft-tissue mass in the retropharyngeal soft tissues and occasionally some destruction of the first or second cervical vertebral body. Extensive destruction of the coccyx and lower part of the sacrum is found in lesions of the lower end of the spine.

METASTATIC TUMORS

Metastasis to the brain from distant primary tumor is common. Carcinomas of the lung, breast,

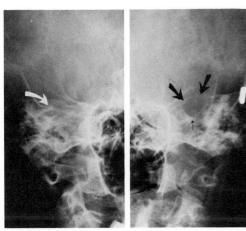

Fig. 11-39. Acoustic neuroma. Oblique projections (Stenver's views) of right and left temporal bones show a normal internal auditory canal on the right (**white arrow**) and an enlarged canal and internal meatus on the left (**black arrows**).

and kidney frequently metastasize to the brain. While multiple metastatic foci may be present, usually the clinical and roentgen signs point toward the presence of a solitary lesion. The roentgen findings of intracranial metastasis do not differ significantly from those described for other brain tumors, particularly the gliomas. The mass of the tumor causes displacement of normal structures away from it. Displacement of a calcified pineal gland is frequent. Ventriculography and encephalography show the signs of ventricular displacement and deformity. Occasionally multiple areas of deformity will be apparent and suggest the nature of the disease. On arteriography the vessels will be displaced away from the lesion and those in proximity appear stretched. With the more vascular lesions, increased vascularity may be seen and a distinct tumor stain may occur during the capillary phase of filling. Evidence of increased intracranial pressure in plain roentgenograms of the skull is usually absent since the duration of the disease is relatively short. *Every patient suspected of harboring a brain tumor should have routine roentgen examination of the chest;* this may demonstrate an otherwise silent bronchogenic tumor or perhaps evidence of pulmonary metastasis from some other primary site.

OTHER CONDITIONS

BRAIN ATROPHY

The causes of atrophy of the brain are numerous and include arteriosclerosis and hypertensive disease leading to encephalomalacia, certain degenerative diseases such as Pick's disease and Alzheimer's disease, multiple sclerosis, trauma, and local vascular occlusion and rupture. Roentgen evidence of brain atrophy is elicited only by specialized procedures such as encephalography. The amount of cerebrospinal fluid that can be drained varies among patients and depends to a considerable extent upon the degree of atrophy that may be present. In the average normal adult from 100 to 150 cc can be removed. This does not necessarily represent a complete drainage of the subarachnoid space and ventricles of the brain; this is usually impossible via lumbar puncture. Usually it is preferable to use less gas than this as the diagnosis of brain atrophy can be made without complete drainage. However, enough gas must be present to determine the degree of ventricular dilatation and enlargement of subarachnoid spaces and to exclude space-occupying masses. The interpretation of pneumoencephalograms is complex and beyond the scope of this text. However, an idea of the structures that can be visualized intracranially by this procedure can be gained from the illustrations of a normal encephalogram shown in Figure 11-21. The ventricles are clearly outlined as they are filled with the radiolucent gas. The subarachnoid cisterns around the base of the brain are identified. The sulci and fissures over the surfaces of the cerebral hemispheres also become visible to a certain extent when drainage of the cerebrospinal fluid has been reasonably complete. These are seen as dark linear markings. These channels do not correspond completely with the anatomic sulci and fissures because septa and blood vessels interfere with the continuity of the flow of gas through them. It is preferable to speak of these air-filled spaces as the subarachnoid channels rather than as sulci.

When brain atrophy is generalized it is practically impossible to state the cause from roentgen examination alone because there is nothing specific in the findings. As a matter of fact, it is usually impossible to distinguish between a congenital hypoplasia of the brain and an acquired atrophy. When the atrophy is localized or focal the causes are few in number. Focal atrophy most often is caused either by truama or by occlusion or rupture of a blood vessel.

The pneumoencephalographic signs of brain atrophy are essentially those of increased size of the subarachnoid cisterns, the surface subarachnoid pathways or channels, and the ventricles. In some cases there is a dilatation of all these spaces or cavities (Fig. 11-40); the diagnosis of atrophy then is obvious. In others, the dilatation is limited either to the ventricular system or the superficial subarachnoid spaces. The term "cortical atrophy" often is used when the dilatation is limited to the superficial channels, with the ventricular system reasonably normal. This term may not be anatomically correct even under these circumstances, and it

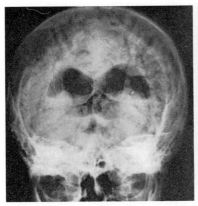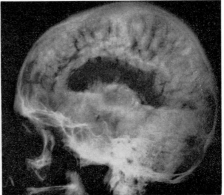

Fig. 11-40. Generalized cerebral atrophy. Upright posteroanterior (*left*) and lateral (*right*) encephalograms. The ventricles are dilated and the subarachnoid channels over the surfaces of the cerebral hemispheres are enlarged. Clinical diagnosis, Alzheimer's disease.

is preferable to speak of cerebral atrophy rather than cortical atrophy (Fig. 11-41). Occasionally the atrophy is limited to or is more severe in the cerebellum than in the cerebrum. This is shown by an enlarged fourth ventricle, increased accumulations of gas over the surface of the cerebellar hemispheres, and enlargement of the cisterns, especially the cisterna magna.

Focal atrophy or cicatrix formation is recognized by a localized dilatation of one ventricle or a portion of a ventricle nearest the site of

scarring, a retraction of structures toward the side of the atrophy, and by a local enlargement of the subarachnoid pathways over the site of the lesion (Fig. 11-42).

SUBDURAL HEMATOMA AND HYGROMA

Bleeding into the subdural space is a frequent complication of head injuries and results in the formation of a subdural hematoma. The most common location is over the superior

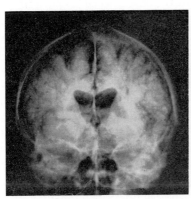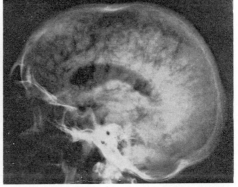

Fig. 11-41. Generalized cerebral atrophy. Upright posteroanterior (*left*) and lateral (*right*) encephalograms. The lateral and third ventricles are moderately dilated but there is a greater degree of enlargement of the subarachnoid channels. Note the large amount of gas outlining deep sulci over the surfaces, particularly on the right.

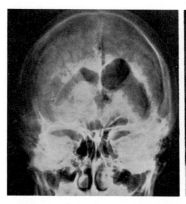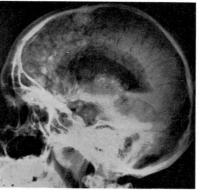

Fig. 11-42. Unilateral cerebral atrophy following birth injury. Upright lateral (*right*) and posteroanterior (*left*) encephalograms. There is a decrease in volume of the left cerebral hemisphere with a shift of midline structures to this side and dilatation of the homolateral ventricle.

parietal area but occasionally the lesion develops at some other site; we have observed it infrequently in the posterior fossa. The roentgen findings are essentially those of an intracranial mass. A fracture may or may not be present; most frequently a fracture is not demonstrated. There is some difference in the roentgen findings, depending upon whether the hematoma is an acute or a chronic one. Acute subdural hematomas give the clinical and roentgen signs of an intracranial mass with increase in intracranial pressure. Hematomas of more than 4 weeks' duration are usually designated as chronic. Shift of the calcified pineal is frequent in these cases. In very chronic cases, where the hematoma has been present for months or longer, there often is associated atrophy of the brain beneath the hematoma and there may be little evidence of a mass, the atrophy compensating for the space occupied by the hematoma. With acute unilateral hematomas, displacement of the pineal, if it is calcified, is demonstrable. Bilateral hematomas are not uncommon (approximately 20 per cent of patients) and absence of pineal shift is not reliable in excluding hematoma.

ENCEPHALOGRAPHY AND VENTRICULOGRAPHY

When the ventricular system is outlined with gas in the presence of an acute subdural hema-

toma a shift of the ventricular system away from the lesion is invariably present. The shift is a general one but the roof of the homolateral ventricle becomes flattened as it is displaced beneath the rigid falx. From the type of ventricular displacement it is usually possible to postulate the presence of a rather diffuse and superficial lesion; however, differentiation between a diffusely infiltrating tumor such as a glioblastoma and a subdural hematoma may be impossible. When bilateral hematomas are present there may be no ventricular displacement and little if any recognizable contour deformity. If the superficial subarachnoid channels are visualized adequately and extend to the inner table it is possible to exclude a hematoma with considerable certainty. If they do not fill, no statement as to the condition of the spaces can be made. Failure of filling or scattered, incomplete filling of these channels happens so frequently in otherwise normal cases as an artifact of filling or because of inadequate drainage of cerebrospinal fluid that it is not safe to attach diagnostic significance to the finding as an isolated observation. In certain cases, usually where the hematoma is chronic, gas may enter the space between the limiting membrane of the hematoma and the arachnoid. When this happens a typical configuration results. Posteroanterior roentgenograms show the gas as a sickle-shaped shadow displaced away from the inner table and clearly marking the inner boundary of the hematoma. In other patients enough gas may enter the subarachnoid space beneath the hematoma so that the subarachnoid channels can be seen to be displaced away from the inner table of the skull (Fig. 11-43). As noted above, a large chronic hematoma may constrict the hemisphere and result in atrophy so that the ventricle on the side of the hematoma is enlarged. Because of the cerebral atrophy there may be no displacement of the ventricular system away from the hematoma; in fact, in very long-standing cases there can actually be some retraction toward the side of the lesion. The presence of calcification in an old subdural hematoma has been commented on in the section dealing with intracranial calcification.

ARTERIOGRAPHY

Arteriography is a very useful procedure in the diagnosis of subdural hematoma. When the internal carotid and its branches have been opacified by the injection of contrast substance, a subdural hematoma will cause an inward displacement of the branches of the middle cerebral artery easily seen in anteroposterior arteriograms (Fig. 11-44). On the other hand, if the vessels are seen to be closely apposed to the inner table, a convexity hematoma can be excluded with assurance. In acute hematomas the vessels may be displaced over a relatively wide area. Chronic hematomas tend to be more localized and to cause a convex inward displacement of the vessels because the hematoma is limited by a membrane. Chronic subdural hematoma may, therefore, resemble an acute epidural hematoma in its arteriographic appearances (see section on "Epidural Hematoma") and the clinical history is important in differential diagnosis (see Fig. 11-44).

With a unilateral hematoma the anterior cerebral artery is displaced toward the contralateral side. Absence of displacement of this vessel or minor degrees of shift in the presence of characteristic shift of the middle cerebral vessels is highly suggestive of the presence of a hematoma on the contralateral side and warrants carotid arteriography on the opposite side. Displacement of the deep veins (internal cerebral vein) has the same significance as shift of the anterior cerebral artery, and in the absence of filling of this latter vessel, the position of the internal cerebral vein may be the deciding factor as to the presence or absence of a contralateral hematoma. If the hematoma is small there may be little or no shift of the anterior cerebral artery and in the presence of such a small lesion it may be necessary to perform arteriography on the opposite side to rule out a hematoma there.

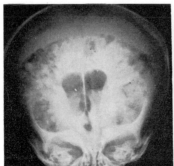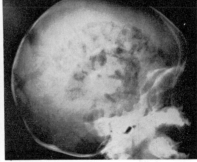

Fig. 11-43. Subdural hematoma, bilateral. Posteroanterior and lateral pneumoencephalograms demonstrate a pronounced displacement of the subarachnoid channels away from the inner table of the vault by large subdural hematomas. These occurred in association with extensive fractures in the parieto-occipital area that can be seen in the lateral view. The fracture surfaces are separated because of the increased intracranial pressure (diastatic fracture).

SUBDURAL HYGROMA (SUBDURAL EFFUSION; EXTERNAL HYDROCEPHALUS)

In a subdural hygroma there is an accumulation of fluid in the subdural space; the fluid may be either loculated or freely movable. A limiting membrane as in subdural hematoma may or may not be demonstrable and the fluid is either clear or slightly xanthochromic. Some subdural hygromas, particularly those that are limited by adhesions, undoubtedly represent the effects of trauma and some appear to be the residues of previous subdural hematomas. In other cases, however, the cause is obscure.

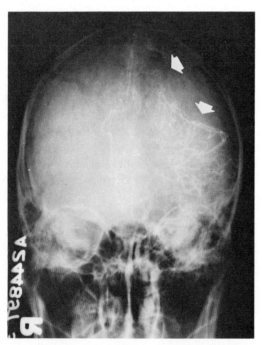

Fig. 11-44. Subdural hematoma demonstrated by means of internal carotid arteriography. Anteroposterior arteriogram shows opacification of the anterior and middle cerebral branches of the internal carotid on the left side. **White arrows** point to inward displacement of the vascular structures by a large subdural hematoma. This is an example of a chronic subdural hematoma characterized by the convex displacement of the vessels. Note the displacement of the anterior cerebral artery toward the contralateral side, which would tend to exclude a hematoma on this side.

Roentgenologically an encapsulated subdural hygroma gives findings identical with those of a subdural hematoma. Free effusions behave somewhat differently. The fluid accumulations usually are bilateral because there is, normally, free communication between the subdural spaces over both hemispheres. Thus little or no ventricular shift is apparent. Occasionally enough gas will enter the subdural space to demonstrate clearly the presence of a gas-fluid level and establish the diagnosis. In some cases delayed roentgenograms made from 6 to 24 hours after pneumoencephalography will show gas and a fluid level in the subdural space when none was present in the immediate encephalograms. This is a useful supplemental procedure when either a subdural hematoma or hygroma is a diagnostic consideration.

EPIDURAL HEMATOMA

An epidural hematoma results from laceration of a branch of the middle meningeal artery, these vessels coursing in grooves on the inner table of the skull. Less frequently the bleeding is caused by rupture of a vein. The tear often occurs secondary to a fracture and the fracture can be identified in skull roentgenograms. The diagnosis of an epidural hematoma is often made from the clinical examination. The history is that of an individual who suffers a head injury that is followed after a period of time, usually several hours, by progressive stupor and other signs of increased intracranial pressure. At times the clinical course is not characteristic and the diagnosis may be in doubt. The roentgen demonstration of a fracture extending across a meningeal arterial vascular groove is important; otherwise pneumography or arteriography may be resorted to for information. The roentgen signs are those of a mass lesion, usually in the frontoparietal or temporal area. The maximum diagnostic information is obtained by means of internal carotid arteriography. The inward displacement of the branches of the middle cerebral artery away from the inner table of the skull as seen in anteroposterior arteriograms is diagnostic of either a subdural or an epidural hematoma. The latter are more localized than subdural hematomas because of the normal adherence of the dura to the skull. The subdural space, on the other hand, is potentially a free one and hemorrhage within it can spread over a wide area. However, in chronic subdural hematomas, as noted above, the mass of the hematoma tends to be more localized and thus may mimic an epidural hematoma in its arteriographic appearances. In some epidural hematomas, extravasation outlines the site of bleeding.

BRAIN ABSCESS

The roentgen signs of brain abscess are usually nonspecific and consist only of the evidence of a mass lesion. In most patients, plain roentgenograms of the skull will be essentially normal. If the pineal is calcified it may be displaced from its normal position; displacement of a calcified choroid plexus is observed occasionally. During childhood, spreading of the cranial sutures may be demonstrable. These findings only indicate the existence of a mass lesion or the presence of increased intracranial pressure. Pneumoencephalography, ventriculography, and cerebral arteriography, if these specialized procedures are done, will also reveal the signs of a mass lesion. In a few patients we have observed gas within an abscess cavity when the lesion followed a fracture through the frontal or ethmoid sinuses. In these cases it is impossible to state, from roentgen findings alone, whether one is dealing with an abscess caused by anaerobic gas-forming organisms or whether the gas represents air introduced through the fracture (traumatic pneumocephalus). For all practical purposes, therefore, the roentgen signs of brain abscess are only those of a space-occupying mass. When the clinical findings point to the possibility of a brain abscess, roentgen examination of the nasal accessory sinuses and mastoids may reveal evidence of infection and thus indicate that a potential source for intracranial abscess exists.

HYDROCEPHALUS

Hydrocephalus means an increased amount of cerebrospinal fluid within the cranial cavity, usually associated with dilatation of the ventricles. It may be either congenital or acquired. Hydrocephalus may be further subdivided into the following:

I. Internal hydrocephalus. This type indicates a dilated ventricular system.
  A. Obstructive
    1. Communicating: The ventricular system is patent but there is obstruction to the flow of CSF either in the basal cisterns, the subarachnoid pathways over the surface of the brain, or in the arachnoidal villi.
    2. Noncommunicating: The obstruction is in the ventricular system or at the outlets of the fourth ventricle.
  B. Nonobstructive
    1. Communicating: This is also known as *hydrocephalus ex vacuo*. The ventricles are dilated because of a decrease in volume of brain tissue. This may be either a congenital or an acquired brain atrophy.
    2. Excess secretion of CSF. This is uncommon and usually results from a choroid plexus tumor (papilloma).
II. External hydrocephalus. There is increased fluid in the subdural space surrounding the brain; also known as subdural effusion. The ventricles may or may not be enlarged.

It is generally accepted that the cerebrospinal fluid is formed by the choroid plexuses within the ventricles. From the ventricles the fluid passes through the outlets of the fourth ventricle, the foramina of Luschka and Magendie, into the subarachnoid cisterns around the base of the brain. It then flows upward over the convexities of the cerebral hemispheres to the arachnoid villi where it is absorbed.

ACQUIRED HYDROCEPHALUS

It is possible to have an obstruction develop anywhere along the cerebrospinal fluid pathway from the foramina of Monro, the openings between the lateral ventricles and the third ventricle, to the points of absorption along the superior surface of the brain. Tumors and adhesive processes may block the flow of fluid at any of these sites and the roentgen findings are those of the causative lesion as described in previous sections of this chapter.

CONGENITAL HYDROCEPHALUS

The cause of congenital hydrocephalus is not completely understood but it is the belief of many investigators that the fault often lies in some defect in the absorbing mechanism so that the cerebrospinal fluid, which continues to be elaborated by the choroid plexuses, cannot be removed properly from the subarachnoid space. Many cases of congenital hydrocephalus are of the communicating type.

The clinical diagnosis of congenital hydrocephalus is usually made without difficulty but roentgen examination, particularly encephalography, is utilized frequently to confirm the diagnosis, to determine the type, to establish the severity of ventricular dilatation, and to follow the progress of treatment. Plain roentgenograms of the skull reveal the large size of the head and demonstrate spreading of the sutures. In the infant, the cranial bones often are poorly ossified and their margins are indistinct. The anterior fontanelle is large. If the condition becomes arrested the bones ossify and, with growth, fill in the defects caused by the previous spreading of the sutures.

Pneumoencephalography is used to determine whether the hydrocephalus is of the communicating or noncommunicating type. In the former, the gas will ascend and enter the dilated ventricles. If the ventricular system is obstructed, only the subarachnoid space will fill and direct ventricular puncture and introduction of gas into the ventricles will be necessary if information concerning them is wanted (Fig. 11-45). During encephalography it usually is not necessary and actually is not wise to drain all the fluid that can be obtained. Even in the infant this may amount to several hundred cubic centimeters. The removal of 50 cc or less of fluid and replacement with gas will give sufficient information in most of these patients.

ADHESIVE ARACHNOIDITIS

Adhesions involving the arachnoid may arise from a number of causes, including inflammatory disease, subarachnoid hemorrhage following rupture of an aneurysm or other vascular malformation, and trauma. Roentgen diagnosis is difficult. The ability to fill the normal subarachnoid space with gas during pneumoencephalography is variable and lack of complete visualization is usual. When filling of the subarachnoid pathways is poor,

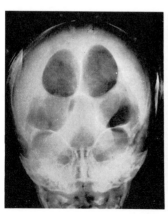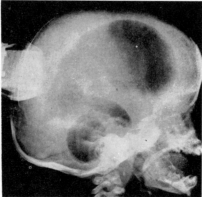

Fig. 11-45. Obstructive internal hydrocephalus following meningitis. Lateral (*right*) and posteroanterior (*left*) roentgenograms after ventricular puncture (ventriculogram). All the ventricles are greatly dilated. The fourth ventricle forms a large rounded cavity in the posterior fossa. The obstruction was caused by adhesions blocking the outlets of the fourth ventricle (foramina of Luschka and Magendie).

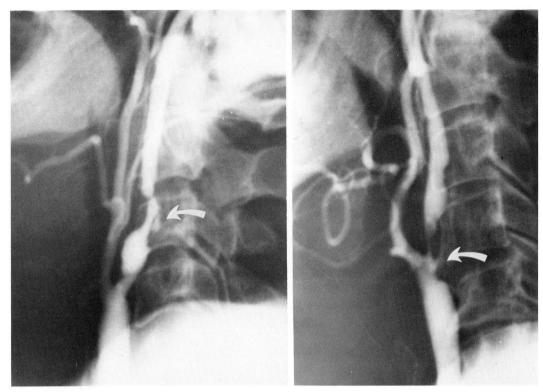

Fig. 11-46. Arteriosclerotic plaques in the internal carotid artery at and above the carotid bifurcation in the neck (**arrows**). These are two different patients and ulceration has occurred in both (operative proof).

not too much emphasis can be placed upon the finding providing the rest of the examination is normal. Presumably any extensive obliteration of the subarachnoid space by adhesions will obstruct the flow of cerebrospinal fluid and result in ventricular dilatation. Scattered adhesions or the involvement of relatively localized areas may exist, however, with a perfectly normal ventricular system. Because drainage of cerebrospinal fluid from the subarachnoid space and its replacement with gas is variable and difficult to control, the diagnosis of adhesive arachnoiditis should be made with caution in these cases.

Arachnoidal adhesions around the base of the brain, particularly if the process involves the region of the cisterna magna, give more definite signs than when the condition exists over the surfaces of the cerebral hemispheres. This is because of the greater likelihood of the flow of fluid being obstructed with resulting internal hydrocephalus. Posterior fossa adhesions of rather limited extent may obstruct the outlets of the fourth ventricle completely and lead to severe signs of increased intracranial pressure (see Fig. 11-45).

OCCLUSIVE (ATHEROMATOUS) DISEASE

As mentioned earlier in this chapter, arteriography is the method of choice for the identification and study of occlusive disease of the vessels supplying the brain. The site of injection depends on the problem at hand. Puncture may be done of the internal carotid or the vertebral artery in the neck. When multiple vessels are to be investigated, retrograde catheterization of the aortic arch via either the brachial artery or the femoral artery may be preferable. These methods also allow study of the subclavian and innominate vessels. Vascular occlusions occur most frequently at the origin of a vessel or at the site of branching. Thus one finds the most frequent location of internal carotid occlusion is at or directly adjacent to the bifurcation of the common carotid in the neck. In the case of the vertebral artery, the most frequent site of occlusion is at its point of origin.

Incomplete occlusion is manifested in the arteriogram as a localized area of narrowing of the vessel. This may be in the form of a plaquelike encroachment on the vessel lumen or by a more or less annular or fusiform narrowing (Fig. 11-46). In complete occlusion there is a sharp cutoff of the column of contrast material, with nonvisualization distally. In some cases, the anterior cerebral artery may fail to fill during injection, without an actual occlusion of the vessel. This may be the result of spasm or a malformation of the circle of Willis. Both anterior cerebral arteries may arise from one side. Bilateral angiograms aid in identifying this malformation. Sometimes the vessel will fill after one injection, but not after another. In equivocal cases, correlation with the clinical history and physical findings is extremely helpful.

An interesting manifestation of occlusive disease recently described is known as the "subclavian steal syndrome." In this condition there is obstruction of the proximal portion of the subclavian, usually on the left, with refilling of the vessel distal to the obstruction by reverse flow through the vertebral artery by way of the basilar artery. Roentgen visualization is obtained after retrograde catheterization of the aortic arch via the right brachial artery or after retrograde femoral artery catheterization. The lesion may lead to the signs and symptoms of cerebrovascular insufficiency. Retrograde brachial or femoral arteriography are useful methods for the study of the vessels arising from the aortic arch and for simultaneous visualization of the carotid and vertebral components of the circle of Willis.

Ulceration of carotid artery atheromata can occur and give rise to emboli.[16] The appearance has been likened to that seen in ulcer craters of the stomach and duodenum with a craterlike pocket filled with contrast material (Fig. 11-46). Other evidence of atheromatous

disease usually is present with variable degrees of stricture formation.

REFERENCES AND SELECTED READINGS

1. ALLEN, J. H., and RILEY, H. D., JR.: Generalized cytomegalic inclusion disease, with emphasis on roentgen diagnosis. *Radiology 71:* 257, 1958.

2. BOLDREY, E.: The pathology of brain tumors and its relationship to roentgenologic diagnosis. *Radiology 41:* 107, 1943.

3. BABBITT, D. P., TANG, T., DOBBS, J., and BERK, R.: Idiopathic familial cerebral vascular ferrocalcinosis (Fahr's disease) and review of differential diagnosis of intracranial calcification in children. *Radiology 105:* 352, 1969.

4. CAMP, J. D.: Pathologic non-neoplastic intracranial calcification. *JAMA 137:* 1023, 1948.

5. CRONQVIST, S.: Total angiography in evaluation of cerebrovascular disease: Correlative study of aortocervical and selective cerebral angiography. *Br. J. Radiol. 39:* 805, 1966.

6. FELSON, B., ed.: A primer on cerebral angiography. *Semin. Radiol. 6:* 1–33, 1971.

7. GOLD, L. H. A., KIEFFER, S. A., and PETERSON, H. O.: Intracranial meningiomas. A retrospective analysis of the diagnostic value of plain skull films. *Neurology 19:* 873, 1969.

8. HINCK, V. C., and DOTTER, C. T.: Appraisal of current techniques for cerebral angiography. *Am. J. Roentgenol. Radium Ther. Nucl. Med. 107:* 626, 1969.

9. HOLT, J. F., and DICKERSON, W. W.: The osseous lesions of tuberous sclerosis. *Radiology 58:* 1, 1952.

10. KALAN, C., and BURROWS, E. H.: Calcification in intracranial gliomata. *Br. J. Radiol. 35:* 589, 1962.

11. KOMAR, N. N., GABRIELSEN, T. O., and HOLT, J. F.: Roentgenographic appearance of lumbosacral spine and pelvis in tuberous sclerosis. *Radiology 89:* 701, 1967.

12. LAGOS, J. C., HOLMAN, C. B., and GOMEZ, M. R.: Tuberous sclerosis. Neuroroentgenologic observations. *Am. J. Roentgenol. Radium Ther. Nucl. Med. 104:* 171, 1968.

13. LAPAYOWKER, M. S., and CLIFF, M. N.: Bone changes in acoustic neuromas. *Am. J. Roentgenol. Radium Ther. Nucl. Med. 107:* 652, 1969.

14. LEMAY, M.: The radiologic diagnosis of pituitary disease. *Radiol. Clin. North Am. 5:* 303, 1967.

15. LOFSTROM, J. E., WEBSTER, J. E., and GURDJIAN, E. S.: Angiography in the evaluation of intracranial trauma. *Radiology 65:* 847, 1955.

16. MADDISON, F. E., and MOORE, W. S.: Ulcerated atheromata of the carotid artery: Arteriographic

appearance. *Am. J. Roentgenol. Radium Ther. Nucl. Med. 107:* 530, 1969.

17. MUENTER, M. D., and WHISNANT, J. P.: Basal ganglia calcification, hypoparathyroidism and extrapyramidal manifestations. *Neurology 18:* 1075, 1968.

18. MUSSBICHLER, H.: Radiologic study of intracranial calcification in congenital toxoplasmosis. *Acta Radiol. (Diag.) 7:* 369, 1968.

19. NATHAN, M. H., COLLINS, V. P., and COLLINS, L. C.: Premature unilateral synostosis of the coronal suture. *Am. J. Roentgenol. Radium Ther. Nucl. Med. 86:* 433, 1961.

20. NEW, P. F. J., and WEINER, M. A.: The radiological investigation of hydrocephalus. *Radiol. Clin. North Am. 9:* 117, 1971.

21. PEAR, B. L.: Epidermoid and dermoid sequestration cysts. *Am. J. Roentgenol. Radium Ther. Nucl. Med. 110:* 148, 1970.

22. POTTS, D. G.: Brain tumors: Radiologic localization and diagnosis. *Radiol. Clin. North Am. 3:* 511, 1965.

23. SALMI, A., VOUTILAINEN, A., HOLSTI, L. R., and UNNERUS, C-E.: Hyperostosis cranii in a normal population. *Am. J. Roentgenol. Radium Ther. Nucl. Med. 87:* 1032, 1962.

24. SANTIN, G., and VARGAS, J.: Roentgen study of cysticercosis of the central nervous system. *Radiology 86:* 520, 1966.

25. SCOTT, W. G., SIMRIL, W. A., and SEAMAN, W. B.: Intracerebral arteriovenous malformations; their diagnosis and angiographic demonstration. *Am. J. Roentgenol. Radium Ther. Nucl. Med. 71:* 762, 1954.

26. SOTER, C. S., and GILMORE, J. H.: Roentgenologic study of the vascular markings of the skull. *Am. J. Roentgenol. Radium Ther. Nucl. Med. 82:* 823, 1959.

27. STEINBERG, I., and HALPERN, M.: Roentgen manifestations of the subclavian steal syndrome. *Am. J. Roentgenol. Radium Ther. Nucl. Med. 90:* 528, 1963.

28. TAVERAS, J. M., and WOOD, E. H.: *Diagnostic Neuroradiology.* Baltimore, Md., Williams & Wilkins, 1964.

29. VASTINE, J. H., and KINNEY, K. K.: The pineal shadow as an aid in the localization of brain tumors. *Am. J. Roentgenol. Radium Ther. Nucl. Med. 17:* 320, 1927.

30. WESCOTT, J. L., CHYNN, K. Y., and STEINBERG, I.: Percutaneous transfemoral selective arteriography of the brachiocephalic vessels. *Am. J. Roentgenol. Radium Ther. Nucl. Med. 90:* 554, 1963.

31. WILSON, M.: Angiography in cerebrovascular occlusive disease. *Am. J. Med. Sci. 250:* 554, 1965.

32. WOLPERT, S. M.: The neuroradiology of hemangioblastomas of the cerebellum. *Am. J. Roentgenol. Radium Ther. Nucl. Med. 110:* 56, 1970.

33. YUHL, E. T., and SCHMITZ, A. L.: The occipital emissary foramen and increased intracranial pressure. *Acta Radiol. (Diag.) 9:* 124, 1969.

12

THE SPINAL CORD AND RELATED STRUCTURES

The present chapter will consider the roentgen diagnosis of tumors of the spinal cord and its coverings, herniation of intervertebral discs, and brief reference to the findings in certain inflammatory lesions and vascular malformations. Roentgen examination for the detection of these conditions will be discussed under two main headings, plain roentgenograms of the spine without the use of contrast media and myelography, or contrast examination, of the spinal canal.

METHODS OF EXAMINATION

PLAIN ROENTGENOGRAMS

Roentgenograms of the spinal column should always be obtained as the first step whenever a lesion of the cord or of the intervertebral discs is suspected. Not only will these roentgenograms reveal positive evidence of considerable value in many cord tumors, they are useful in excluding or in demonstrating infections, tumors, degenerative changes, and injuries involving the vertebrae. In many cases the examination can be limited to a single anteroposterior and a lateral view. In others it may be necessary to use multiple projections, including oblique views or roentgenograms

made with the patient flexing or extending the spine.

As is true with other anatomic parts, when observing roentgenograms of the vertebral column the student should develop an orderly system of viewing the structures so that small changes from the normal will not be overlooked. It makes little difference how one proceeds as long as all parts are observed carefully.

MYELOGRAPHY

Myelography consists in the introduction of a contrast substance into the spinal subarachnoid space to render it visible in roentgenograms. Either a gas such as air or oxygen, which is less opaque than the cerebrospinal fluid, or a material such as an iodized oil, which is more radiopaque than the fluid, can be introduced. The main advantage from the use of air or oxygen is that the gas is absorbed rapidly from the subarachnoid space and leaves no residues. Disadvantages include (*1*) the contrast between the gas and the soft tissues is not very high and visualization often is poor; (*2*) it is difficult to control the gas once it has been introduced and it will ascend rapidly into the cerebral ventricles and other intracranial spaces if the head and thorax are elevated unless the head is in full extension; (3) unless there is a complete block full drainage may be required in the examination of the thoracic and cervical parts of the canal. In the cervical region, air in the trachea interferes with visualization in the anteroposterior position. If gas is used, tomography is essential to improve visualization and help eliminate objectionable shadows. In our experience, gas myelography has a limited field of usefulness.

Water-soluble contrast materials have been used more extensively in the Scandinavian and a few other countries than in the United States. These materials are more irritating than oily media and adverse side effects have prevented their wide acceptance in this country. We prefer an oily medium such as iodophenylundecylic acid (Pantopaque). It should be noted that water-soluble materials can only be used for lumbar myelography which further limits their field of usefulness.

OIL MYELOGRAPHY

Oil myelography consists in the injection of a small quantity of radiopaque oil into the spinal subarachnoid space, usually via lumbar puncture. Early investigations of the spinal canal by this method were done using an iodized poppyseed oil known as Lipiodol. During the past 25 years this material has been supplanted to a large extent by iodophenyl-undecylic acid (Pantopaque). This is an oily substance that depends upon its iodine content for radiopacity. It produces a very opaque shadow in roentgenograms, is visualized easily during fluoroscopy, and can be removed after the examination is completed. Being an oil, Pantopaque is not miscible with the cerebrospinal fluid. It is heavier than the fluid and can be displaced up or down the spinal canal by means of gravity. For this reason the examination is done on a tilting fluoroscopic table that can be changed from vertical to at least a 45° Trendelenberg position.

Pantopaque is slightly irritating and if allowed to remain in the subarachnoid space will cause a temporary pleocytosis. There has been some difference of opinion concerning the long-term effects of the oil on the arachnoid membrane when it is left in contact over a period of time. However, experience with Pantopaque now extends over many years and a great many thousands of examinations and from published reports the chance for reactions from its use appears very remote. While in some departments the oil is left in place after the examination is completed we prefer to remove it if possible.

TECHNIQUE. The injection usually is made in the lumbar area. The preferred site of lumbar puncture varies and depends to a large extent upon the clinical findings. If the examination is being done for a suspected herniation of a lumbar intervertebral disc the puncture should be made at the second or third lumbar interspace. The majority of herniated lumbar discs are found at the fourth and fifth interspaces and it is better to do the puncture at a site other than at the level of the lesion. If the clinical signs and symptoms indicate that the lesion may be at a higher level, the puncture should be made in one of the lower lumbar interspaces. It is important, particularly when investigating for a possible disc herniation, to do the needle puncture with the patient in a prone position, being careful to see that the needle enters directly in the midline. This can be checked by fluoroscopy and by spot roentgenograms if necessary. A direct midline puncture lessens the chance for injection of the material into the subdural or epidural spaces, and makes it much easier to aspirate the oil when the examination has been finished. Should the point of the needle enter the subarachnoid space to one side of the midline, the bevel of the needle may only partially penetrate the arachnoid and part of the oil may be injected directly into the subdural space. A satisfactory study cannot be done if much of the oil is extra-arachnoidal. An offset needle also makes it difficult to aspirate the oil.

The amount of oil to be injected varies from 6 to as much as 12 or 15 cc. For the average examination 9 cc is used. In an occasional patient a larger amount will be needed. In some patients the lumbar spinal canal is unusually wide. In searching for small defects, an oil column long enough to bridge two interspaces and the intervening vertebral body is essential and 6 cc will not do this if the canal is wide. In examining the thoracic part of the canal, amounts larger than 9 cc are an advantage. It often is difficult to keep the oil in a solid column while passing it over the dorsal curvature. With a larger amount of oil this difficulty is lessened. For cervical myelography from 6 to 9 cc is adequate.

After the oil has been injected into the subarachnoid space, the needle is left in place while fluoroscopy is carried out and the oil displaced throughout the region of interest. The examiner watches for defects in the oil column and obstructions to its free flow. Spot roentgenograms are made during fluoroscopy of the various parts of the canal and particularly of any defects or suspicious areas. For cervical myelography the head of the table is lowered gradually and the oil moved over the dorsal curvature. By keeping the patient's head in extreme extension it is usually

possible to prevent the oil from entering the cranial cavity. As soon as the oil has accumulated in the upper cervical region the table is brought to the horizontal position and the oil then will remain in the dependent part of the cervical curve so that by slight changes in the level of the table the entire cervical canal can be inspected without much chance of the oil escaping into the intracranial cisterns. Oil that has entered the cranial cavity is difficult to dislodge and most of it will remain. At times it is necessary to examine the upper part of the cervical canal, including the cisterna magna. By proper tilting and positioning of the head it is usually possible to carry the oil into the cranial cavity overlying the clivus almost to the level of the dorsum sellae. In these cases some of the oil may spill into the cisterns and cannot be removed. In fact, Pantopaque is being used for positive-contrast ventriculography, the oil being injected directly into one of the lateral ventricles. Pantopaque also is being used for visualization of structures in the posterior fossa of the skull, particularly for the investigation of acoustic nerve tumors, as an extension of cervical myelography.

When the examination has been completed, the

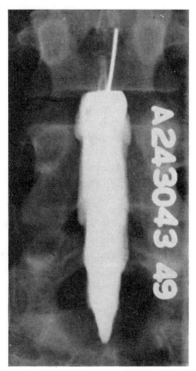

Fig. 12-1. Normal lumbar myelogram. Posteroanterior view with patient upright. The lumbar-puncture needle is visible, the hub overlies the upper end of the oil column. The typical cone-shaped configuration of the sacral cul-de-sac is shown. The axillary root pouches vary slightly on the two sides but this is not abnormal.

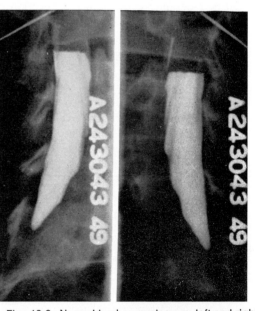

Fig. 12-2. Normal lumbar myelogram, left and right oblique views with patient upright. The linear translucent stripes of the nerve roots are visible. The upper end of the oil column is flat, indicating that the patient is in a vertical position.

oil column is brought under the point of the needle by fluoroscopic control and it then is aspirated. If a satisfactory placement of the spinal puncture needle was accomplished, complete removal of the oil usually is possible with the exception of a few small drops or streaks that may be caught around the nerve roots. If a poorly placed needle is responsible for difficulty, sometimes it is advisable to remove it and attempt another puncture at a different level.

The rate of absorption of Pantopaque that may have been left in the subarachnoid space is extremely slow and has been estimated to be about 1 cc per year or less. The oil tends to remain freely movable and can be displaced by gravity for a long time after the injection. It is common to find small droplets of oil in the basal cisterns of the skull in patients who have had an oil myelogram without complete removal. Should an individual with oil in the spinal canal stoop over or assume a position where the head and trunk are lower than the buttocks the oil can move rapidly into the cranial cavity and once there, may become lodged. The chance for harm from oil lodged in the intracranial subarachnoid space is

remote. Myelography should be performed only when there are sufficient clinical indications for it and it should not be looked upon as a screening procedure.

NORMAL RESULTS. The appearance of normal myelograms is shown in the accompanying illustrations (Figs. 12-1 through 12-4). In the lumbar region there usually are small triangular projections on either side of the oil column at each vertebral level. These are known as axillary pouches or root pouches and they represent extensions of the arachnoid along the inferior edges of the nerve roots. Except for these projections, the normal canal is smooth along its lateral borders. The distal end of the

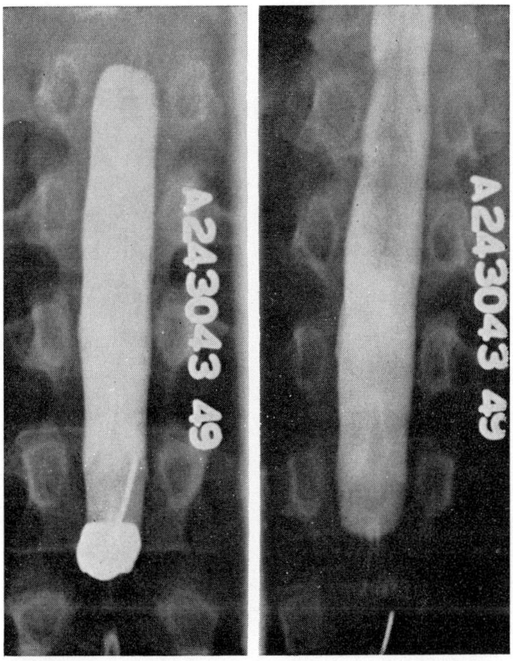

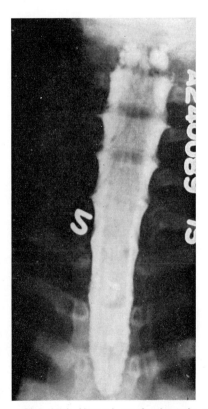

Fig. 12-4. Normal cervicothoracic myelogram. In the upper thoracic region there are only slight projections at the sites of exit of nerve roots. In the cervical canal the axillary pouches again appear. The nerve roots are clearly visible as they extend through the pouches. The cord forms a distinct translucent central area as it is surrounded by the radiopaque oil.

Fig. 12-3. Normal myelogram of the lower thoracic and upper lumbar region. The axillary pouches representing the sites of exit of nerves are not apparent in this part of the canal.

thecal sac generally extends below the level of the lumbosacral joint, sometimes as far as the second sacral segment. As an anatomic variant, occasionally a shortened lumbosacral cul-de-sac is present that does not extend below the lumbosacral joint level. This anomaly prevents adequate myelography of the lumbosacral disc.

When viewed from the side there occasionally is seen a smooth anterior bulging of the oil column at the level of each vertebral body, apparently caused by an anatomic variation in the shape of the vertebrae, which have more concave indentations of their posterior surfaces than is usual. This particular configuration may be sufficient to cause the oil to pool at each vertebral body level when the patient is placed in the prone position. It is difficult to examine the discs adequately in these cases and a larger amount of oil than usual may be necessary to form a continuous column. In the thoracic region axillary pouches are not present except for the upper two or three roots; they are found in the cervical part of the canal and form distinct notchlike shadows at each nerve exit.

In general, examination of the midthoracic part of the canal is unsatisfactory unless there is an obstruction present. It is difficult to keep the oil in a solid column when the head of the table is tilted so that the oil will flow over the dorsal curvature. To detect small lesions it may be necessary to turn the patient onto his side or to remove the spinal puncture needle and place him in a supine position so that the contrast material will pool in the midthoracic region.

ARTIFACTS

Needle Defects. A traumatic spinal puncture with laceration of a blood vessel may lead to the formation of a hematoma at the site of puncture. This is more likely to happen when difficulty has been encountered in attempting to enter the subarachnoid space or when the needle is laterally situated and does not enter the dural sac in or close to the midline. A needle defect interferes with interpretation because it resembles a herniated disc. As a rule it can be recognized as an artifact because the needle will be centrally situated within the area of the filling defect and the upper and lower

borders taper smoothly and gradually (Fig. 12-5). It is possible, of course, to have a herniated disc and a needle defect at the same location; if the clinical signs point to a lesion at the same level and on the same side, it is almost impossible to determine the true state of affairs. For this reason, as recommended in the paragraphs dealing with technique, when a herniated lumbar intervertebral disc is suspected clinically, the needle puncture should be done at a level other than where clinical localization indicates the hernia to be. The preferred sites are at the second and third lumbar interspaces. When a needle defect causes difficulty in interpretation it is advisable to discontinue the examination, aspirate as much of the oil as possible, and repeat the study at a later date, preferably after an interval of a week or ten days.

Globule Formation. At times the oil breaks up into multiple drops or globules during injection or globule formation occurs while the examination is in progress (Fig. 12-6). Slow or intermittent injection of the oil favors globule formation. The contrast substance should be injected in a steady stream so that it flows from

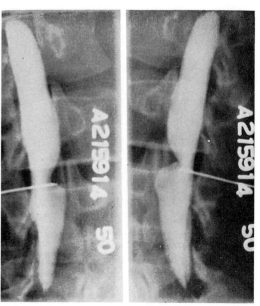

Fig. 12-5. Needle defect. Left and right oblique lumbar myelograms. The defect occurs directly beneath the point of the needle.

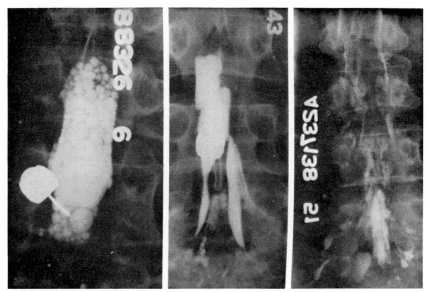

Fig. 12-6. *Left,* Globule formation in a lumbar myelogram. *Center,* Extra-arachnoidal, subdural oil injection. The oil separates into masses of irregular shape but characteristically with tapered ends. *Right,* Epidural oil injection.

the needle in a solid column rather than in drops. In displacing the oil into the cervical region it sometimes breaks up into globules as it passes over the thoracic curvature. Proper tilting of the table helps to prevent this but in some cases it cannot be avoided. Fortunately, globule formation often disappears during the examination, so that by the time roentgenograms are to be made the oil has become a solid mass.

Subdural Oil. Improper placement of the needle so that the bevel is only part way through the arachnoid membrane may lead to a partial injection of the oil into the subdural rather than into the subarachnoid space. Difficulty in doing the spinal puncture with repeated attempts to enter the subarachnoid space may result in a laceration of the filmy arachnoid and allow escape of the oil. If the myelography is done within a week or 10 days after a spinal puncture, there is some chance for leakage of oil. It is preferable not to precede oil myelography by another spinal puncture or, if a puncture has been done, to wait a week or longer before doing the myelography. Oil in the subdural space can be recognized by the sluggish way that it moves

when the table is tilted and by the characteristic tapered ends of the oil accumulations. An example of subdural oil is shown in Figure 12-6, *center.* It is very important to recognize that the oil is in the subdural space because the contours of such oil masses simulate filling defects when none actually exist. The subdural space rarely fills completely and the spaces that remain suggest the presence of tumor or disc herniation. Typically these defects do not remain constant during tilting of the table. Inconstancy of a filling defect during fluoroscopy should alert the examiner to the possibility that the oil is subdural rather than subarachnoid in location. When oil has entered the subdural space an attempt should be made to aspirate it. If this is not possible, it may be necessary to discontinue the examination and wait until the oil has become more widely dispersed. This may require several weeks or even longer.

Epidural Injection. Oil that has been injected or that extravasates extradurally accumulates in the form of streaky shadows along the spinal canal and extends for some distance along the nerve roots. A characteristic example of epi-

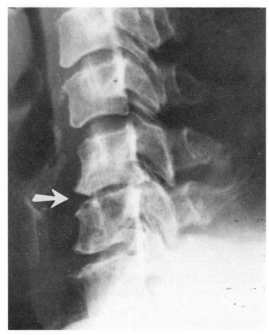

Fig. 12-7. Posterior bony ridging at the C-5 and C-6 levels. There is thinning of the disc between these vertebrae (**arrow**), slight backward offset of C-5 on C-6, and posterior spurs. (Patient also has a metastatic lesion in C-6 from a carcinoma of the breast but the degenerative changes are independent of the tumor deposit).

dural oil is shown in Figure 12-6, *right*. The presence of extradural oil interferes greatly with the examination and it usually is necessary to defer further study for several weeks, until the material has become dispersed or partially absorbed.

DISCOGRAPHY

Discography consists in the direct injection of a contrast material such as 50% Hypaque into the intervertebral disc and the making of suitable roentgenograms. The contrast material is injected through a needle that has been inserted via lumbar puncture through the posterior annulus fibrosis into the disc substance. First introduced by Lindblom of Sweden in 1950, the method has received some acceptance in this country. It has been recommended for use particularly in those patients complaining of low back pain with sciatic radi-

ation, in whom standard contrast myelography has yielded negative results. Degenerative changes in the disc, anterior ruptures, and rupture into the vertebral body can be visualized. Discography does not replace oil myelography for the detection of herniated disc and, in our experience, has a limited field of usefulness.

POSTERIOR HERNIATION OF INTERVERTEBRAL DISC

Rupture of an intervertebral disc with extrusion of disc material into a vertebral body has been considered in Chapter 3. When the rupture occurs along the posterior or posterolateral surface of the disc, the mass of herniated disc material projects into the spinal canal or an intervertebral foramen. It may impinge upon a nerve root and is a frequent cause of low back pain with sciatic radiation. The clinical aspects of herniated intervertebral disc have been treated extensively in the literature and pertinent references are given at the end of this chapter. The diagnosis of a herniated intervertebral disc often can be made with considerable assurance from the clinical history and physical findings. However, many clinicians believe that the diagnosis should be confirmed by myelography in most cases. Clinical localization may not always be possible or completely reliable, the diagnosis may be in doubt, and other lesions can give rise to clinical findings resembling those of a herniated disc. The indications for the procedure must be definite, however; the possible dangers have been mentioned previously.

The majority of herniated discs occur in the lumbar spine and most of these affect either the fourth or fifth disc. Only a small percentage of lumbar disc herniations are found above the fourth interspace level. The lesion is uncommon in the thoracic area except for an occasional case encountered in the lower thoracic disc interspaces. Posterior disc herniation in the cervical area is not infrequent, although less common than in the lumbar spine.

The varied terminology used in discussions concerning herniated discs is somewhat confus-

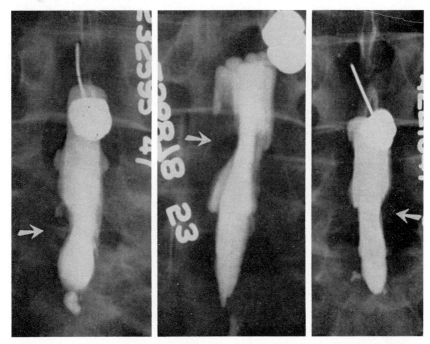

Fig. 12-8. Lumbar intervertebral disc herniation. *Left,* Large herniated disc on the right at the fourth interspace level. The notchlike filling defect is characteristic. Note the distortion of the nerve root adjacent to the hernia. *Center,* Herniated disc on the right side of the lumbosacral interspace. *Right,* Small defect on the left caused by herniated disc at the lumbosacral interspace.

ing; in order to avoid misunderstanding, in the present discussion the following usage is implied:

1. *Posterior disc herniation* and *ruptured intervertebral disc* are terms used synonymously to denote a rupture of the posterior part of the annulus fibrosus with extrusion of a mass of disc substance that projects into the spinal canal.

2. *Posterior disc protrusion* or *ridging* is a condition in which the annulus fibrosus is intact but there is a smooth, ridgelike bulging of the disc posteriorly. This condition is usually associated with and a part of degenerative disease affecting the spine. In association with a weakened annulus and a posterior bulging of the disc there frequently is hypertrophic bony spurring or osteophyte formation along the posterior or posterolateral edges of the adjacent vertebral bodies, resulting in a bony ledge projecting into the canal.

PLAIN ROENTGENOGRAMS OF THE SPINE

Roentgenograms of the spine may be entirely normal in the presence of a herniated intervertebral disc. More often there are one or more abnormal findings which, in the main, while suggestive of the presence of a disc hernia, are not specific for this condition. A combination of these signs is more significant than any one alone. These include:

STRAIGHTENING OR REVERSAL OF THE LUMBAR LORDOTIC CURVE. This abnormality is usually the result of muscle spasm. Because there are many causes for spasm of the low-back muscles, it is of limited value as an isolated observation.

LISTING OF THE LUMBAR SPINE TO ONE SIDE. This finding also is the result of muscle spasm. The list may be toward the side of the hernia or away from it.

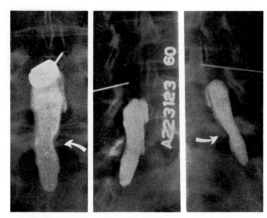

Fig. 12-9. Lumbar intervertebral disc hernia. *Left,* Posteroanterior roentgenogram of the lower lumbar canal. *Right,* Left and right oblique views. Note the filling defect on the left anterolateral aspect of the canal (**arrow**) and compare with the opposite normal oblique view (**center**).

NARROWING OF THE DISC INTERSPACE. The amount of disc material that has been extruded is seldom enough to cause a discernible thinning of the intervertebral disc space as seen in roentgenograms. When thinning of the interspace is present in association with a disc hernia it is an indication of degenerative disease of the disc. This may have preceded the herniation or it may have followed it. Because

localized thinning of an intervertebral disc, usually the fourth or the fifth lumbar, is a very frequent observation in this area without an associated hernia, thinning cannot be relied upon as a good diagnostic sign. It is not at all infrequent to find a thinned disc at one lumbar interspace and to demonstrate by myelography and at subsequent surgery a hernia at a different level where the height of the disc space was normal.

POSTERIOR OFFSET OF THE FIFTH LUMBAR VERTEBRA ON THE SACRUM. Associated with a reversal of the lumbar lordotic curvature, the posterior surface of the fifth lumbar vertebra may appear to lie slightly behind the corresponding surface of the upper sacrum (reverse spondylolisthesis). This finding too is not specific for a herniated disc but when combined with some of the other observations as noted above it becomes of greater significance.

CALCIFICATION OF THE EXTRUDED DISC MATERIAL. This is a very reliable sign but is not observed very often.

POSTERIOR OSTEOPHYTES ON THE VERTEBRAL BODIES. Spurs or osteophytes may be found along the posterior or posterolateral edges of the vertebrae contiguous to a disc hernia. The

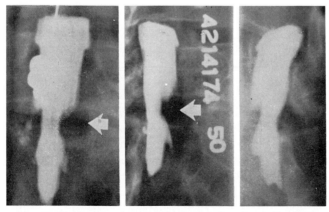

Fig. 12-10. Lumbar intervertebral disc hernia. *Left,* Anteroposterior and *right,* left and right oblique views. There is a bilateral defect but it is much larger on the right side (**arrows**).

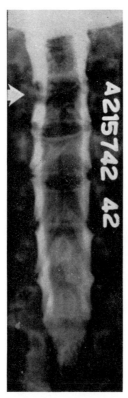

Fig. 12-11. Cervical intervertebral disc hernia. The defect is small (**arrow**) but there is lack of filling of the axillary pouch and a local indenting of the oil column. Note the clarity with which the spinal cord is seen. This is usual when enough radiopaque oil is used to extend along the lateral aspects of the cord.

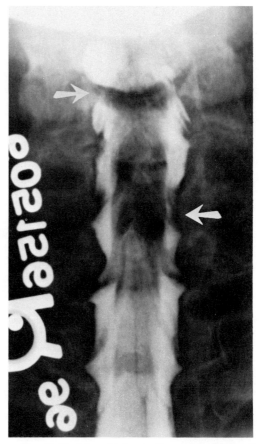

Fig. 12-12. Disc ridging in the cervical area. Posteroanterior myelogram demonstrates a transverse, translucent defect (**upper arrow**) indicative of a transverse ridge and a unilateral deformity on the left (**lower arrow**) owing to posterolateral spurring.

presence of such spurs is positive evidence that at least a posterior bulging or protrusion of the disc is present but they do not indicate whether there has been an actual rupture of the annulus fibrosus with extrusion of disc material. These osteophytes are a manifestation of degenerative disease (Fig. 12-7).

OIL MYELOGRAPHY

Because a herniated disc is a space-taking mass that encroaches upon the subarachnoid space it will cause a filling defect when radiopaque oil is injected into the space. Characteristically the defect is seen as a sharply outlined, smooth, unilateral indentation or notch in the oil shadow along the anterolateral aspect of the spinal canal. The axillary root pouch is either obliterated at the site of the defect or else it is displaced or distorted. Oblique views often bring out the defect to best advantage because they show it tangentially. Some typical examples of lumbar disc hernias are shown in Figures 12-8 through 12-10. Herniation at the fourth lumbar interspace usually causes a clearcut and characteristic defect because the meninges are closely approximated to the anterior and lateral bony walls of the spinal canal and encroachment upon the space by the

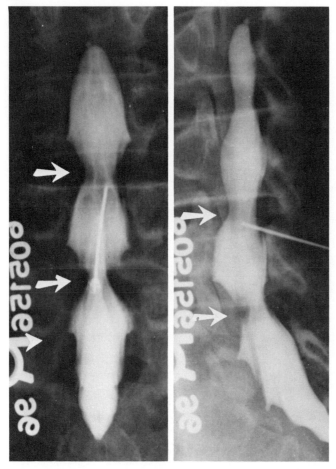

Fig. 12-13. Disc ridgings in the lumbar area. *Left,* In the posteroanterior view the deformities assume an hour-glass configuration (**arrows**). *Right,* the oblique view shows anterior indentations
on the oil column (**arrows**).

hernia readily deforms the oil column. Because
the lumbosacral cul-de-sac narrows gradually
to a smooth rounded or pointed termination,
there may be considerable space in the canal
outside the dural sac at the level of the lumbosacral disc. The defect of a hernia often is less
obvious at this interspace than when a mass of
similar size has herniated at the fourth disc
level. At times a lumbosacral defect is quite
inconspicuous, being limited to a slight anterolateral indentation on the oil column with slight
elevation of the axillary root pouch. Even a
minor defect of this nature at this interspace
must be viewed with considerable suspicion. In
itself a unilateral failure of filling of an axillary

root pouch is not sufficient to indicate the existence of a hernia since this is not infrequent as
a normal variation. There must be some evidence of encroachment upon the canal proper
even though this be very slight. It is in these
cases that oblique views are particularly helpful. If the cul-de-sac is unusually short and
terminates at or above the level of the lumbosacral disc, it is possible to have a rather large
hernia without myelographic evidence of its
presence.

Occasionally a very large hernia will completely or almost completely obstruct the canal
and mimic a tumor very closely. In fact a
herniated disc, being an extradural mass, can

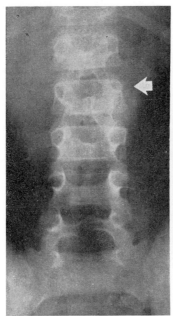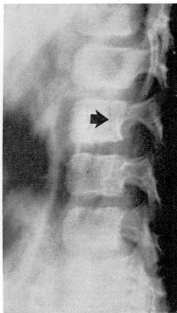

Fig. 12-14. Neurofibroma of the lumbar area. The tumor was of dumbbell type, protruding through an intervertebral foramen. *Left,* Anteroposterior roentgenogram. The tumor has eroded the inner and inferior surface of the left pedicle of the second lumbar vertebra (**arrow**) and widened the space between this pedicle and the one below where they bound the intervertebral foramen. The pedicles are visualized as ringlike shadows because they are seen end-on, the cortical margin forming the ring. *Right,* Lateral roentgenogram, same patient. The intraspinal part of the tumor has eroded the posterior surface of the vertebral body (**arrow**). Note how it has enlarged the intervertebral foramen.

cause myelographic evidence hardly different from that of a tumor such as a small neurofibroma. It is chiefly the characteristic location of the lesion that is significant in diagnosis. At other times the extruded cartilage will become separated completely from the disc and come to lie free in the subarachnoid space. It may be displaced from its site of origin. In these cases the defect may be found behind a vertebral body rather than at a disc interspace and in rare instances it will be found along the posterior aspect of the canal rather than the anterior. It may be impossible to exclude a neoplasm as a cause for such a defect.

In the cervical region disc hernias are found most frequently at the fifth and sixth interspaces. The defect of the hernia may be large and notchlike and resemble that of a lumbar hernia. In other patients the hernia is small and laterally placed. The myelogram defect is correspondingly small and inconspicuous. The chief manifestation is a deformity of the axillary root pouch (Fig. 12-11). Because the hernia projects into a spinal foramen, the clinical signs of nerve root impingement may be severe; the small size of a myelographic defect does not necessarily indicate a clinically insignificant lesion.

FURTHER OBSERVATIONS

TRANSVERSE DISC RIDGING

Posterior bulging of a disc without actual herniation of disc material is known as "posterior disc protrusion" or "ridging." The lesion is a frequent accompaniment of degenerative joint disease of the spine. Also, hypertrophy of the ligamenta flava is frequently associated. As a result of these changes pressure on a spinal nerve root may cause signs and symptoms suggestive of a herniated disc. The lesion may be found in any part of the spine but is infrequent in the thoracic area. In the cervical and lumbar areas, multiple disc ridging often is present. Neurosurgeons frequently speak of ridging as a "hard disc" in contrast to the "soft disc" of a true hernia. The bony marginal osteophytes are particularly prone to encroach upon the contiguous spinal foramen.

Roentgen Findings

Disc-space thinning and posterior or posterolateral spurs may be noted on plain roentgenograms (Fig. 12-7). However, disc ridging can occur without significant plain-film findings although this is unusual. Often one can postulate the presence of the lesion from these plain-film findings. On myelography, disc ridging causes a transverse lucent defect in the oil column. If lateral cross-table views are obtained with the patient prone, a smooth, anterior indentation on the oil column will be seen at the affected disc level. In posteroanterior views the ridge may cause a transverse band-like lucency (Fig. 12-12). Also bilateral indentations may be seen causing an hourglass type of deformity. If there is associated hypertrophy of the ligamenta flava these defects are accentuated (Fig. 12-13). Herniated disc may be present at the same level as the ridge but more often it exists alone. It accentuates the filling defect on the side of the herniation, and elevates and compresses the corresponding nerve root more than is seen with ridging alone. At times it is difficult to determine if both conditions are present or not.

THE POSTOPERATIVE MYELOGRAM

The interpretation of myelograms performed after laminectomy and surgical removal of a herniated disc is difficult and often unsatisfactory. In many patients there is irregularity and deformity of the oil column at the level of the previous surgery, which are only the result of adhesions in the subarachnoid space. In some cases a filling defect resembling a herniated disc is found but at reoperation there is no evidence of recurrent hernia. In patients with the most severe deformity there may be a complete obstruction to the flow of oil at the level of the previous hernia and laminectomy. In general, slight to moderate irregularities in filling that do not show the characteristic notch defect of a herniated disc are most likely the result of adhesions. If a defect that fulfills the criteria for a herniated disc is found, one is justified in interpreting it as evidence for recurrent disc herniation.

SPINAL CORD TUMORS

Primary tumors of the spinal cord and its coverings can be classified as intramedullary, and extramedullary intradural, or extradural. Such a breakdown is important, not only from the standpoint of operability but because of differences in roentgen findings in the three groups. The histologic types of tumors in the order of frequency are as follows: neurofibroma, meningioma, ependymoma, astrocytoma, glioblastoma, and a miscellaneous group including infrequent and rare lesions such as dermoid and epidermoid cysts, epidural cysts, lipomas, and hemangiomas. In addition to the group of primary tumors, metastatic neoplasms involve the cord very frequently. This may be from extension of a focus in a vertebral body or its arch; less frequently the metastasis is directly to the cord or the meninges. Any malignant tumor can metastasize in this way.

NEUROFIBROMA

Neurofibroma is an extramedullary tumor that can be either intradural or extradural in location, with the majority lying beneath the dura. Neurofibromas arise from the spinal nerve roots. In the lumbar area the tumor often is completely within the dural sac. In the thoracic and cervical regions the lesion tends to be of dumbbell type with an intraspinal portion and an extraspinal extension through an intervertebral foramen. In the thoracic area the extraspinal portion of the tumor often is visible because of the contrast afforded by the air-filled lungs. In the cervical region a mass is rarely demonstrated. In the lumbar spine the extraspinal part of the tumor may, if very large, cause an outward bulge of the psoas muscle margin. The intraspinal part of the tumor leads to erosion of the pedicle on one or both sides. Normally the pedicles are seen end-on in anteroposterior roentgenograms as vertical ovoid ringlike shadows (see Fig. 12-14). The inner surface usually is convex but may vary from a flattened surface to one slightly concave. Pressure erosion from a neurofibroma causes a thinning of the pedicle with or without a loss of its inner cortical margin. Because of the variations in the contour of normal pedicles, Elsberg and Dyke[6] measured the difference between the inner surfaces of the two pedicles of each vertebra, called the inter-

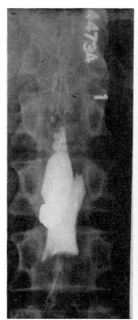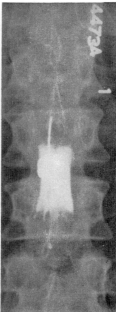

Fig. 12-16. Neurofibroma of a lumbar nerve root. Two views of oil myelogram with patient partially upright (*left*) and upright (*right*). The oil was injected at the first interspace level and has descended to cap the superior surface of the tumor, which is almost completely obstructive.

pedicular distance, and published the results in the form of a chart. Erosion from a neurofibroma usually is limited to one or two vertebrae and comparison of the pedicle shadows above and below the lesion will clearly indicate the presence of abnormality without the need for measurement in most cases. If very large, an intraspinal neurofibroma will cause a smooth, pressure type of erosion of the posterior surface of the vertebral body so that it will have a concave contour as seen in the lateral roentgenogram (Fig. 12-15). A dumbbell tumor will erode the upper and lower surfaces of the pedicles bounding an intervertebral foramen (Fig. 12-14). Bone changes occur in about 20 per cent of neurofibromas.

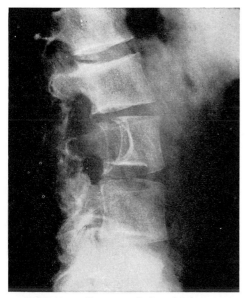

Fig. 12-15. Neurofibroma of the lumbar area. Lateral roentgenogram showing erosion of the posterior surface of the third lumbar vertebra with a smooth, concave pressure type of defect. One pedicle is completely destroyed, better visualized in an anteroposterior view.

MYELOGRAPHY

An intradural neurofibroma causes a sharply outlined, round or oval-shaped filling defect. Because the tumor often is large enough to

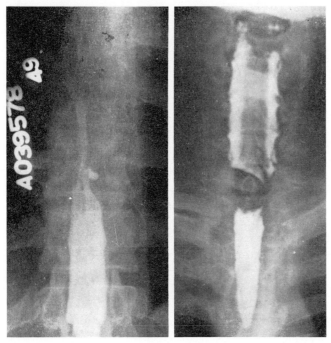

Fig. 12-17. Meningioma. *Left,* Meningioma at the tenth thoracic level that has obstructed the flow of radiopaque oil during myelography. Roentgenogram made with the patient's head lowered, showing the oil column narrowed and obstructed by a mass that is extramedullary in type. *Right,* Meningioma at the cervicothoracic junction. The oil was injected in the lumbar subarachnoid space and displaced by gravity. It flowed slowly around the tumor, which was thus outlined almost in its entirety. Usually a tumor of this size will cause high-grade obstruction to oil flow.

block the canal completely, obstruction to the flow of oil is easily demonstrated and the end of the oil column has a sharp concave margin as it caps the end of the tumor (Fig. 12-16). Although this type of defect is not specific for a neurofibroma, it is always most suggestive of this tumor and if erosive changes in the pedicles also are present the diagnosis is more certain. Sometimes it is important to know the upper limits of a neurofibroma that is above the level of lumbar oil injection. This can be obtained by injecting a small amount of the oil into the cervical cisterna magna and allowing it to drop down to the level of the lesion by gravity. Then it will cap the superior surface and the entire extent of the lesion can be established.

MENINGIOMA

Meningiomas are second only to neurofibromas in frequency and are the most common tumor encountered in the thoracic region. Being extramedullary in type, the main mass of the tumor usually lies subdurally. Meningiomas of the cord resemble their counterparts within the cranial cavity in being slowly growing tumors and symptoms usually extend over a period of several years or even longer before the diagnosis is established. The plain roentgen findings in meningiomas are few. While calcification in the tumor is common in pathologic specimens it is an infrequent finding in roentgenograms. This is caused in part by the rather small amount of calcification and in part to the

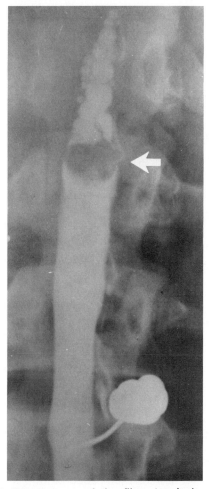

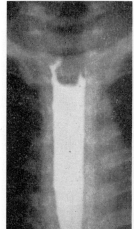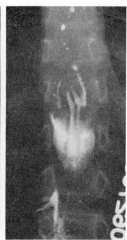

Fig. 12-19. *Left*, Intramedullary tumor (ependymoma) at the level of the first thoracic vertebra. The oil has extended part way around the tumor but the obstruction was nearly complete. *Right*, Intramedullary tumor at the thoracolumbar level (intramedullary teratoma). The myelogram was made with the patient inverted about 45° from the horizontal. Streaks of oil extend around the fusiform enlargement of the conus caused by the tumor. Obstruction is not complete.

Fig. 12-18. Ependymoma of the filum terminale. The lesion presents as a round, centrally situated filling defect at the level of L-1 (**arrow**). It was movable over a distance of several centimeters during fluoroscopy.

difficulty of visualizing small hazy calcific shadows within the thoracic part of the spinal canal. Meningiomas do not erode pedicles or vertebral bodies very often and this sign, of great help in detecting neurofibromas, is not available. The roentgen diagnosis depends to a large extent upon myelography.

MYELOGRAPHY

The tumor causes either partial or complete obstruction to the flow of oil. When the block is partial the oil column often narrows slightly just below the lesion and then ends with a fairly sharp cut off (Fig. 12-17). In other cases the oil column is effaced more gradually. If the block is incomplete, the oil that passes by the defect does so along one side of the canal only and the column has the appearance of being squeezed off rather than sharply cut off as with a neurofibroma. The myelographic signs alone seldom are sufficiently characteristic to make a diagnosis of meningioma; when taken in conjunction with the clinical history and the thoracic location of the lesion the diagnosis is frequently possible.

INTRAMEDULLARY TUMORS

As a group, the intramedullary tumors are uncommon lesions that resemble one another rather closely in their roentgen findings. Ependymomas are the most frequent. In the lumbar region they arise from the filum termi-

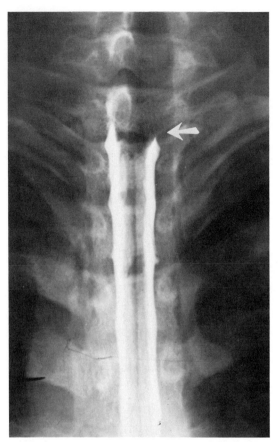

Fig. 12-20. Intramedullary lesion at the level of T-1. Note apparent widening of the central translucency which is the spinal cord (**arrow**), and then a complete obstruction to the flow of oil cephalad. The lesion was a hematoma (hematomyelia).

nale. An ependymoma is more likely to erode the vertebral pedicles than the other lesions in this group and thus may cause roentgen findings similar to a neurofibroma. Even on myelography it may be impossible to distinguish between the lesions because an ependymoma of the filum terminale is usually a well-circumscribed mass and the myelographic defect may resemble that of an intradural neurofibroma (Fig. 12-18). When the spinal cord is involved by any of the tumors of this group, the myelogram often is clearly indicative of the intramedullary location of the lesion (Figs. 12-19 and 12-20). Obstruction of the flow of oil

may be either partial or complete. When partial, the oil column will be seen to widen out at the level of the tumor with thin streaks of it passing alongside the enlargement of the cord (Fig. 12-21). When the obstruction is complete, the oil shadow widens slightly and is effaced gradually without the sharp cut-off characteristic of an extramedullary intradural mass.

METASTATIC NEOPLASMS

Metastatic tumors, usually metastatic carcinomas, are frequent lesions often involving the cord by extension from a focus in a vertebra. Roentgenograms of the spine may reveal the lesion as an area of destruction. Metastatic lesions that cause clinical signs of cord or nerve root compression often have developed in the vertebral arch and the roentgen findings may be minimal and difficult to visualize. A loss of outline of one pedicle sometimes is the only clue to the presence of the lesion.

MYELOGRAPHY

A metastatic lesion large enough to cause clinical signs and symptoms of cord compression will produce some degree of obstruction to the flow of radiopaque oil and in many cases this is complete. If the tumor is extradural, the oil column narrows slightly where the dura is being compressed by the mass. The end of the column tapers gradually (Fig. 12-22). If the block is only partial, droplets of oil may break off the main mass and flow upward on one side of the canal when the patient's head is lowered. Occasionally a metastatic nodule is intradural and extramedullary; rarely it is intramedullary in location. Unless there are associated signs in the vertebrae that clearly indicate the nature of the tumor, it usually is impossible from myelographic evidence to determine whether a given defect is caused by a metastatic tumor or a primary one.

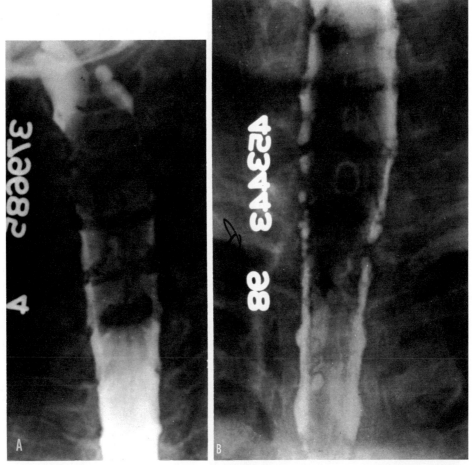

Fig. 12-21. *Left,* Intramedullary tumor (astrocytoma) involving the cervical cord. The lesion has caused expansion of the cord but is not completely obstructive. *Right,* Syringomyelia. A large intramedullary cyst has caused fusiform expansion of the cord in the cervicothoracic area simulating a solid intramedullary tumor.

FURTHER OBSERVATIONS

ADHESIVE ARACHNOIDITIS

Arachnoidal adhesions arise from a number of causes, including inflammatory processes and chemical irritation. In some patients the cause remains obscure. The adhesive process can be localized or widespread. There are no plain-roentgen findings in adhesive arachnoiditis. If during myelography the adhesive process is localized, an obstruction to the flow of oil is encountered and this may be complete. More often the block is incomplete and the oil passes through the region, outlining a rather tortuous channel with irregular filling defects. When the process is more diffuse it may be impossible to displace the oil to any extent after it has been injected into the subarachnoid space and it may accumulate in numerous linear and irregularly shaped pockets. Less extensive adhesions cause correspondingly less deformity. The diagnosis of adhesive arachnoiditis is a difficult one to make by myelography in some patients. One must be certain that the oil has been injected properly into the subarachnoid space

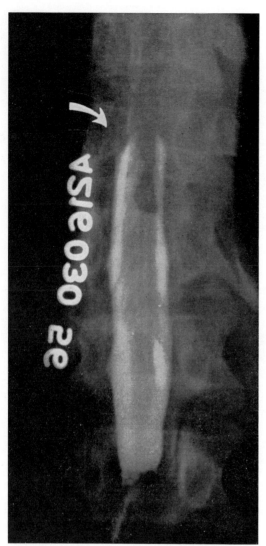

Fig. 12-22. Metastatic tumor (lymphosarcoma) obstructing the canal at the eleventh thoracic level. Roentgenogram made with the head lowered approximately 45° from the horizontal. The tumor is extradural but has surrounded the dura and obstructed the subarachnoid space.

rather than subdurally or epidurally. The latter injections cause artifacts and defects that may resemble those of arachnoid adhesions. One must also be certain that defects suggesting arachnoid adhesions are not merely associated findings secondary to some other lesion such as a herniated disc or a spinal cord tumor.

HEMANGIOMA; ARTERIOVENOUS MALFORMATIONS

Hemangioma is a rather rare lesion involving the cord and meninges. A cavernous hemangioma causes irregular tortuous linear defects in oil filling at the site of the lesion (Fig. 12-23). There may be some interference with oil flow but seldom a complete obstruction. As a complication of a cavernous hemangioma, there may be a sudden rupture of one of the vessels with the development of a subdural or epidural hematoma. This causes the rapidly progressive signs of pressure on the spinal cord. Myelography is useful in demonstrating the site of the hematoma.

In recent years angiography has been utilized to demonstrate hemangiomas and other vascular lesions such as arteriovenous malformations and hemangioblastomas. The initial injection of contrast material can be made into the aorta following catheterization of the femoral, axillary, or subclavian arteries. Once the lesion has been identified and localized, selective catherization of the major feeder vessels can be done to more clearly define the lesion and its nature.

Arteriovenous malformations cause myelographic changes similar to cavernous hemangiomas and differentiation may be impossible (Fig. 12-23). Even on angiography it may be difficult to decide which of these lesions is present.

PERINEURIAL CYSTS

As originally described by Tarlov,[14] perineurial root cysts consist of one or more cystlike spaces surrounding the nerve roots, usually in the sacral area. The cysts may or may not communicate with the subarachnoid space of the spinal canal. If they do not, roentgen diagnosis is hardly possible. With the larger cysts a rounded area of smooth erosion along one or more of the sacral foramina may be demonstrated. When the cysts communicate with the spinal subarachnoid space, they fill with oil during myelography or subsequently and then are visualized as rounded pockets close to the sacral *cul-de-sac* and contiguous to the sacral nerve roots (Fig. 12-24, *left*). It has been our experience that these cysts are demonstrated most frequently when some of the radiopaque oil has

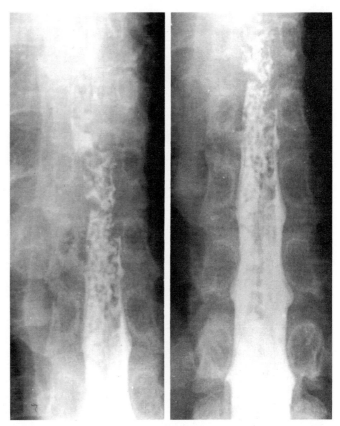

Fig. 12-23. Arteriovenous malformation or cavernous hemangioma in the thoracic area. Two views of oil myelogram outline
numerous tortuous filling defects caused by the dilated vessels
of the lesion. At subsequent angiography it was thought the
lesion was more likely an arteriovenous malformation.

been left in the canal and a reexamination of the
spine is performed some weeks or months after
myelography. Failure to demonstrate a root cyst
during immediate myelographic examination does
not exclude its presence. Similar cystlike extensions of the arachnoid along the nerve roots have
been found, rarely, in the lower cervical and
upper thoracic regions.

EPIDURAL OR MENINGEAL CYSTS

An epidural cyst is a rare lesion found chiefly
in the thoracic region. Here it results in the
gradual development of a progressive spastic paraplegia. The patient usually is an adolescent and
the history usually indicates a gradually progres-

sive lesion. Erosion of the pedicles of multiple
vertebrae is common. In some cases there have
been findings indicative of a *vertebral epiphysitis
of Scheuermann's type* with irregularity of disc
surfaces, anterior wedging of the vertebra, and a
kyphotic deformity in the spine. This has been
thought to be due to disturbance of the blood
supply to the vertebrae as a result of the cyst.
Myelograms reveal obstruction of extradural type
with compression of the oil column (Fig. 12-24,
center). Some epidural cysts communicate with
the subarachnoid space and fill with contrast
medium during myelography. Others do not and
the myelographic signs then are those of an extradural mass. A similar cystlike lesion has been
reported as a rare finding in the lumbosacral area
and we have observed cases in which the cyst had

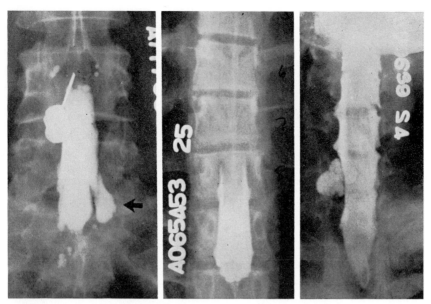

Fig. 12-24. *Left,* Perineurial sacral root cyst that has filled with radiopaque oil during myelography (**arrow**). *Center,* Epidural cyst. The upward flow of oil is obstructed at the lower margin of the cyst and the appearance suggests that the dura and cord are being compressed by an extrinsic mass. The cyst has caused a thinning of pedicles of several vertebrae above the level of oil block. *Right,* Traumatic avulsion of a cervical nerve root allowing an escape of the radiopaque oil. The two axillary pouches above the rupture are enlarged and these roots have been partially avulsed.

eroded the sacral laminae. These are essentially *sacral meningoceles* and are not to be confused with the perineurial cysts described in the preceding section. The sacral cyst occasionally fills with oil and its nature thus becomes apparent (Fig. 12-25).

LIPOMA

Intraspinal lipomas are rare lesions but cause some fairly characteristic roentgen findings. The lesion often is large when first discovered and may extend through several vertebral segments. It is encountered most frequently in the thoracic area. Preliminary roentgenograms may show erosion and thinning of the pedicles of two or more vertebrae with widening of the interpedicular distances. On myelography a variable degree of obstruction is found and this may be complete. The lesion arises extradurally and compromises the spinal cord by compression and the myelographic

appearance is that of an extramedullary mass. Spinal epidural cysts may show similar roentgen findings and cause the major difficulty in differential diagnosis. In some cases the cyst communicates with the spinal subarachnoid space and fills with the radiopaque oil during myelography; this is diagnostic.

AVULSION OF CERVICAL ROOTS

As a part of a severe injury to the neck and shoulder region, one or more of the cervical nerve roots forming the brachial plexus may be avulsed. Myelography often gives unequivocal evidence of the injury by demonstrating an extension of oil beyond the normal limits of a cervical axillary root pouch. The oil forms a rounded pocket or a linear extension for a short distance along the path of the avulsed root (see Fig. 12-24, *right*). The appearance is somewhat similar to that caused by a perineurial cyst as described

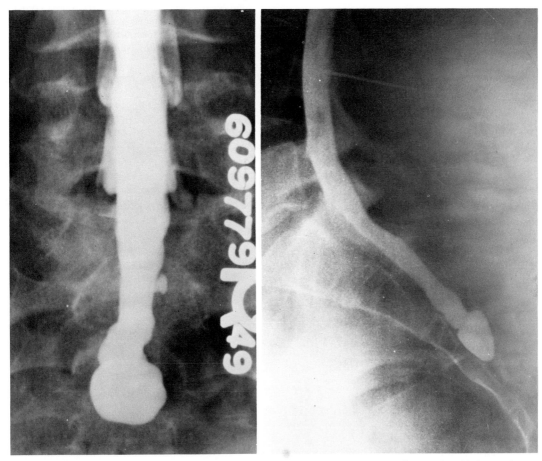

Fig. 12-25. Occult sacral meningocele. The spinal canal is elongated, extending to the third sacral segment and ends in a saclike dilatation representing the small meningocele. (*Courtesy Dr. V. C. Hinck.*)

above. Differentiation depends upon the history of injury with clinical signs of brachial plexus involvement. Root cysts usually are bilateral while brachial plexus injury is almost always unilateral.

EPIDURAL ABSCESS

Epidural abscess may occur with any infection of the vertebrae or intervertebral discs. The most common cause of chronic epidural abscess or granuloma is tuberculosis. In addition to chronic lesions, an acute suppurative infection can develop in the epidural space, either by direct extension from an acute osteomyelitis of a vertebra or as a primary focus of infection in the epidural tissues. Because the lesion is a serious one that

may compromise the blood supply of the cord, early diagnosis is imperative. The plain roentgenograms of the spine often are unrevealing. In the thoracic region one may see a widening of the soft-tissue paraspinal shadow indicative of the paraspinal abscess. If caused by an acute osteomyelitis it will be several weeks after the onset of symptoms before roentgen signs of the disease become evident in the vertebral body or disc. Myelography is an extremely valuable procedure in these cases because the clinical diagnosis may be in doubt. Myelograms reveal evidence of a block to the flow of oil. The nature of the obstruction often cannot be determined from the myelograms but when correlated with the clinical signs a preoperative diagnosis of epidural abscess frequently is possible.

EPIDURAL SARCOMAS

A sarcoma arising in the epidural area is a rather infrequent lesion. Plain roentgenograms often show a paraspinal mass when the lesion is in the thoracic area. Invasion of a vertebral body may lead to the finding of irregular erosion and loss of substance. More often this is a fairly late manifestation. Myelography will demonstrate a partial or complete block of extradural type but will not indicate the nature of the lesion otherwise. The final diagnosis usually rests upon surgical exploration.

REFERENCES AND SELECTED READINGS

1. BRIERRE, J. T., and COLCLOUGH, J. A.: Total myelography. Complete visualization of the spinal subarachnoid space. *Radiology 64:* 81, 1955.

2. CAMP, J. D.: Contrast myelography past and present. *Radiology 54:* 477, 1950.

3. CRONQVIST, S.: The postoperative myelogram. *Acta Radiol. 52:* 45, 1959.

4. DAVIES, E. R., SUTTON, D., and BLIGH, A. S.: Myelography in brachial plexus injury. *Br. J. Radiol. 39:* 362, 1966.

5. DJINDJIAN, R., HOUDART, R., and HURTH, M.: Angiography of the spinal cord. *Acta Radiol. (Diag.) 9:* 707, 1969.

6. ELSBERG, C. A., and DYKE, C. G.: The diagnosis and localization of tumors of the spinal cord by means of measurements made on the x-ray films of vertebrae, and the correlation of clinical and x-ray findings. *Bull. Neurol. Inst. New York 3:* 359, 1934.

7. EPSTEIN, B. S.: Spinal canal mass lesions. *Radiol. Clin. North Am. 4:* 185, 1966.

8. ERICKSON, T. C., and VAN BAAREN, H. J.: Late meningeal reaction to ethyl iodophenylundecylate used in myelography. *JAMA 153:* 636, 1953.

9. HIRSCH, C., ROSENCRANTZ, M., and WICKBOM, I.: Lumbar myelography with water-soluble media with special reference to the appearances of root pockets. *Acta Radiol. (Diag.) 8:* 54, 1969.

10. HOLMAN, C. B.: The roentgenologic diagnosis of herniated intervertebral disc. *Radiol. Clin. North Am. 4:* 171, 1966.

11. JIROUT, J.: Pneumographic examination of lumbar disc lesions. *Acta Radiol. (Diag.) 9:* 727, 1969.

12. KECK, C.: Discography: Technique and interpretation. *Arch. Surg. 80:* 580, 1960.

13. LILIEQUIST, B.: Gas myelography in the cervical region. *Acta Radiol. (Diag.) 4:* 79, 1966.

14. TARLOV, I. M.: Cysts (perineurial) of the sacral roots. *JAMA 138:* 740, 1948.

15. TENG, P., and PAPATHEODOROU, C.: Myelographic findings in adhesive spinal arachnoiditis. *Br. J. Radiol. 40:* 201, 1967.

16. YOUNG, I. S., and BRUWER, A. J.: The occult intrasacral meningocele. *Am. J. Roentgenol. Radium Ther. Nucl. Med. 105:* 390, 1969.

Section III

THE ABDOMEN AND
GASTROINTESTINAL TRACT

13

THE ABDOMEN

METHODS OF EXAMINATION

Roentgenograms of the abdomen made without the use of contrast material serve many purposes. When limited to one or two, these sometimes are referred to as "scout roentgenograms." Such an examination frequently consists of a single roentgenogram made with the patient prone or supine. The addition of a lateral view or a roentgenogram made with the patient standing or sitting is desirable under certain circumstances. Another commonly used projection consists of a lateral decubitus view made with the patient lying on one side, the film cassette placed in front of the abdomen, and the roentgen-ray beam directed through the body in a horizontal plane. For example, in examining for the signs of bowel obstruction, recumbent upright and decubitus views are obtained more or less as a routine. This becomes more than a simple scout examination but rather is a fairly detailed study of the soft tissues of the abdomen without the use of contrast media. As a preliminary step in the examination of the gastrointestinal tract, the gallbladder, or the urinary tract, it is customary to obtain a single scout roentgenogram of the abdomen for visualization of the soft tissues.

INDICATIONS FOR EXAMINATION

In addition to the use of a scout roentgenogram as a routine procedure prior to contrast visualization, roentgen examination of the abdomen without contrast media is useful in the study of the following:

1. Abnormal accumulations of gas within the intestinal tract

2. Calculi or other abnormal intra-abdominal calcifications

3. Size, shape, and position of the liver, spleen, and kidneys

4. Abnormal intra-abdominal masses

5. Free gas within the peritoneal cavity (pneumoperitoneum)

6. Ascites

7. Intra-abdominal abscesses

8. Radiopaque foreign bodies in the gastrointestinal tract or within the peritoneal cavity.

THE NORMAL ABDOMEN

The liver forms a homogeneous shadow in the right upper quadrant of the abdomen. Its upper border is limited by the right leaf of the diaphragm and thus is visualized easily because of the contrast afforded by the air-containing lung above it. The right lateral margin of the liver usually is separated from the density of the abdominal wall by a thin layer of fat. The lower edge of the right lobe of the liver usually is visualized in normal individuals and is seen to best advantage in the obese. It parallels the lower costal margin as a rule. In persons of asthenic habitus, however, the liver is more vertical in shape and the outer inferior edge of the right lobe may extend down almost to the same level as the posterior iliac crest. Gas in the hepatic flexure and the transverse portion of the colon also aids in determining position of the lower margin of the right lobe. When the liver is enlarged the hepatic flexure is displaced downward. The inferior margin of the left lobe is indistinct and seldom seen clearly in the normal individual.

The spleen or a part of it can be visualized in the normal as a rule. The inner surface and the inferior pole often can be outlined. The normal spleen is about 10 to 14 cm in length. The medial surface is seen to best advantage when gas is present in the stomach; also gas in the splenic flexure of the colon aids in outlining the inferior pole. In rare instances the spleen is unusually mobile and it may be found medial to the splenic flexure of the colon, below the body of the stomach, or even above the gastric fundus.

The kidneys are visualized on either side of the lumbar spine and they are more readily seen when there is an increased amount of perirenal fat. In emaciated persons the renal outlines may be completely lost. Fat is an important substance in rendering the margins distinct because of its relative radiolucency as compared to the density of the parenchymatous viscera. The right kidney usually is at a slightly lower level than the left.

The pancreas cannot be visualized in the normal abdomen and even when enlarged the mass is seldom seen distinctly.

The outer margins of the psoas muscles form stripelike shadows on either side of the spine, extending from the level of the first lumbar vertebra down to the pelvis. The border becomes indistinct as the muscle passes over the midportion of the ilium. The integrity of the psoas muscle borders is important in excluding retroperitoneal lesions of inflammatory or neoplastic nature. Retroperitoneal hemorrhage may also obliterate the psoas line. The muscles are normally symmetrical but scoliosis may cause

one to stand out more prominently than the other. If the patient is rotated slightly, one shadow may be less distinct than the other; gas shadows in the bowel may blur the outline of one psoas margin while the other remains distinct. At times it may be necessary to reexamine in order to be certain of the condition of these muscle shadows and allowance must be made for the fact that in the normal, visualization of the muscle margins may be asymmetric, one standing out more clearly than the other. The outer margins of the quadratus lumborum also can be visualized in many individuals. This muscle lies lateral to the psoas and its lower border angles slightly more toward the lateral aspect of the ilium.

The lateral margins of the peritoneum often are bounded externally by thin layers of fat sufficient to cause a radiolucent stripe along the flanks. This is known as the extraperitoneal or properitoneal fat line (Fig. 13-1). Obliteration of this line occurs in the presence of peritonitis when the infection involves the lateral aspect of the peritoneal cavity.

The urinary bladder usually is visible if it contains urine and its density may be increased considerably over that of adjacent structures if the specific gravity of the urine is high. Usually there is little difficulty in recognizing it as urinary bladder because of its contour and its position behind and extending directly above the symphysis pubis. In adult females the shadow of the uterus often can be seen and especially so if there is much intra-abdominal fat.

In roentgenograms of the abdomen made in the supine position, the fluid-filled gastric fundus may appear as a rounded mass in the left upper quadrant and which may be mistaken for a tumor. The patients usually are obese. In the prone position the duodenal bulb likewise may appear as a round or ovoid mass below the liver or overlying the kidney.

The appearance and distribution of gas in the intestinal tract and the types of intra-abdominal calcification often seen in the normal individual are discussed separately in the sections that follow.

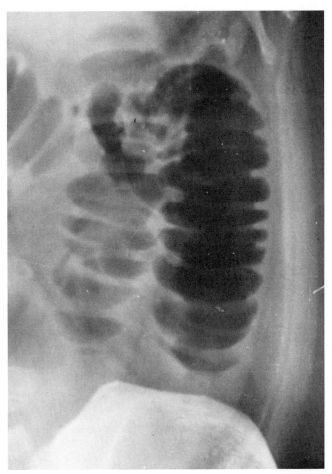

Fig. 13-1. Left flank stripe. Note the translucent properitoneal fat line lateral to the loop of gas-filled small intestine. (Patient had obstruction secondary to carcinoma of the cecum). The peritoneum parallels the outer wall of the intestine and the narrow distance of the bowel gas from the properitoneal fat excludes fluid in this flank. There also is a thin layer of fat separating the lateral abdominal muscles.

ABNORMAL ACCUMULATIONS OF GAS WITHIN THE INTESTINAL TRACT

Gas is present normally in the stomach and in the colon. Small accumulations of gas may be found in the duodenum and the upper part of the jejunum. In bedridden patients and in those who swallow large amounts of air habitually, scattered bubbles of gas may be present throughout much of the small intestine (Fig. 13-2). These are seen as more or less individual bubbles or gas accumulations of rounded or ovoid shape. If a single loop of intestine can be recognized because of gas filling, the shadow is seldom more than 5 to 8 cm in length and the caliber of the lumen is on the order of several centimeters or less. More often, the gas does not form any specific loop pattern. When individual segments of small intestine can be recognized as such, are dilated in width, and of greater length than 8 to 10 cm,

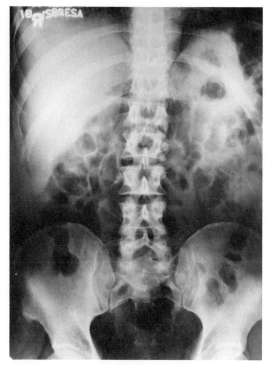

Fig. 13-2. Normal abdomen. Excess gas is noted in the small intestine because of air swallowing (aerophagia). The gas is seen in the form of multiple small accumulations of irregular size and shape. There are no long segments of bowel and the caliber of the visible portions is normal.

one should consider the possibility that the gas is abnormal.

The intestinal gas pattern during infancy differs from that of the adult. Swallowed air can be visualized in the stomach immediately after birth. Within a few hours it will be found distributed throughout the intestinal tract, including the colon. The small intestine of the infant normally contains considerable amounts of swallowed air. Between the ages of 6 months and a year, as the infant gradually receives an adult diet and assumes an ambulatory existence, the pattern of intestinal gas resembles more and more that of an adult. In feeble or premature infants or in those in whom there is severe respiratory distress, appearance of intestinal gas after birth may be delayed. Care should be taken not to interpret

this as evidence of high intestinal obstruction in the newborn.

ACUTE OBSTRUCTION OF THE SMALL INTESTINE

METHOD OF EXAMINATION

In examining for acute obstruction, roentgenograms of the abdomen without contrast media in the intestinal tract usually are sufficient. Barium sulfate should never be given orally if bowel obstruction is a possibility until the colon can be eliminated as the site of the obstructing lesion. Should the obstruction be in the colon, the barium sulfate may become impacted above the lesion, absorption of water from the mixture follows, and the barium becomes a hard mass. Masses of impacted barium sulfate also may cause difficulty for the surgeon when operating for the relief of an obstruction. Barium sulfate by mouth is not likely to cause harm if the obstruction is in the small intestine since the accumulation of fluid above the lesion keeps the barium from becoming inspissated.

If the obstruction is high in the small intestine, induced vomiting or the use of a negative suction apparatus may remove most of the gas and fluid that ordinarily would accumulate. Thus the typical findings described below may not be apparent. In these cases a barium-water meal examination may be required to establish the diagnosis (Fig. 13-3). When the obstruction is in the lower part of the small intestine, the motility of the bowel usually is so impaired that it requires considerable time for the head of the opaque column to reach the site of block and reveal significant information about it. In these cases plain roentgenograms can usually be depended upon to furnish adequate information.

If a double-lumen tube of the Miller-Abbott type has been introduced, it is often possible to obtain valuable information concerning the level of the obstruction and nature of the lesion causing it by injecting an opaque mixture

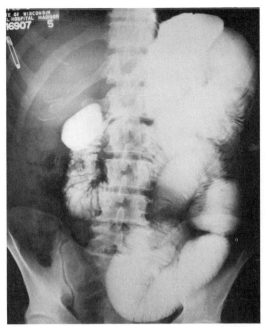

Fig. 13-3. Obstruction of the jejunum caused by an adhesive band. Roentgenogram of the abdomen after barium meal. The duodenal and jejunal loops are considerably dilated down to the level of obstruction. Even though greatly distended the transverse mucosal folds of the jejunum have not been obliterated and the appearance resembles a stack of coins.

through the tube under fluoroscopic control. After completion of the examination the barium mixture can be aspirated if desired.

The type and number of roentgenograms required in the study of bowel obstruction will vary with the nature of the case. As a rule, a recumbent and an upright roentgenogram should be obtained as the minimum. If the patient is too ill to sit or stand, lateral decubitus views, as described in previous paragraphs, are useful to show the distribution of gas within the bowel and to demonstrate fluid levels.

SIMPLE OBSTRUCTION

In a simple obstruction the intestinal lumen is occluded at a single point without any significant interference with its blood supply. An example, and one of the common causes, of simple obstruction is a band of adhesions; another is the obstruction caused by an intraluminal tumor.

Roentgen Observations

Within a few hours after the onset of an acute obstruction, gas and fluid begin to accumulate above the lesion. The gas is swallowed air. The gas is visualized readily in recumbent roentgenograms but the presence of the fluid can be confirmed only in upright or lateral decubitus views. In these positions the gas rises to the top, overlying the fluid, and the interface between gas and fluid forms a straight horizontal margin. A fluid level is generally to be considered as abnormal in the small intestine. (A fluid level is observed normally in the stomach because swallowed air is present almost invariably. A fluid level is frequent in the superior portion of the duodenum where air may be trapped temporarily when the patient assumes an upright position.)

The gas-filled loop or loops are increased in caliber over the normal. In an early stage of obstruction only one or two such gas-distended segments are visualized. The loop tends to form part of a circle, and in the upright roentgenogram each end of the segment is limited by a fluid level. The fluid level in one limb of the loop may be at different height from the level in the other end. With increasing distention more loops become visible; they tend to lie transversely one above the other forming a ladderlike arrangement (Figs. 13-4 and 13-5). The time lag between the onset of an acute obstruction and distinct roentgen visualization of gas-distended loops and fluid levels varies but usually is from 4 to 6 hours. After this interval positive roentgen signs should be present in most cases.

The gas-filled loops are recognized as small intestine rather than colon by:

1. Location of the loops in the central part of the abdomen rather than around the periphery.

2. Fine serrations along the margins caused

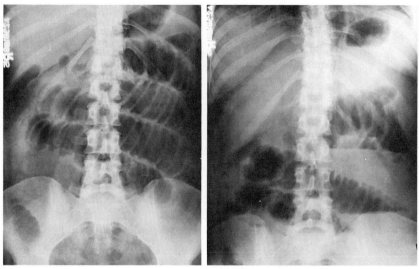

Fig. 13-4. Small intestinal obstruction. Supine (*left*) and upright (*right*) roentgenograms. Note the ladderlike arrangement of distended segments showing the
pattern of jejunum in the supine roentgenogram. In the upright roentgenogram gas-
fluid levels are present. There are a few small areas of gas in the right side of the
colon and some is present in the stomach. There is, however, no gas distention
of the large intestine and the abnormal pattern is confined to the jejunum.

by the mucosal folds, the volvulae conniventes
(Fig. 13-6). These are finer and closer together than the colonic haustra. In the jejunum,
simple distention, no matter how severe, will
not efface the folds completely and in the obstructed segment they frequently show an appearance that has been likened to a stack of
coins (it should be noted that edema and inflammatory changes may cause a diminution or
absence of the folds). In the ileum the folds
are fewer in number and the internal surface is
much smoother. When the ileum is distended
the folds disappear and the gas-filled loop has a
smooth surface. This is an aid in distinguishing
ileum from jejunum.

Where two gas-filled loops of bowel approximate one another the soft-tissue shadow between the gas represents a double thickness of
bowel wall. Thus, information concerning the
thickness of the intestinal wall is available. In
simple obstruction such a double thickness seldom amounts to more than a few millimeters
since the walls are thinned considerably by the
distention. Inflammatory changes in the wall,
exudate on the external surface, or fluid in the

peritoneal cavity results in a thickening of this
soft-tissue shadow. Abnormal thickening of the
bowel wall is an important sign that the obstruction is no longer a simple one (see
below).

If the obstruction of the small intestine is
complete little or no gas will be found in the
colon, a valuable differential point between
mechanical obstruction and adynamic ileus.
Small amounts of gas or fecal accumulations
may be present in the colon if the examination
is done within the first hours after the onset of
symptoms. In late obstruction the colon usually
contains very little gas. When gas is found in
the colon in the late stages of a completely
obstructed small bowel it may be the result of
putrefaction or it may be air introduced during
the administration of an enema. If the small
bowel obstruction is incomplete, some gas may
pass through it and thus be visualized in the
colon. There will be a discrepancy, however, in
the caliber of the distended small bowel and
the colon, the latter being of normal or decreased width. This finding is useful in differentiating between a partial small bowel

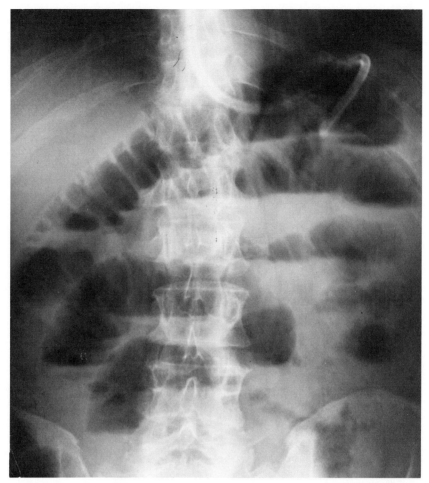

Fig. 13-5. Small-intestine obstruction. Upright roentgenogram demonstrates air-fluid levels in gas-distended loops of small bowel.

obstruction and one in the lower colon. In low colonic obstruction, the major distention affects the large intestine.

Early in the course of an obstruction it may not be possible to determine if abnormal gas accumulations are present or not. In such cases the value of serial observations is considerable. If the gas-visualized loops are the result of obstruction, the amount of gas will increase rapidly and often within a few hours the findings become more definite (Figs. 13-7 and 13-8). Conversely, if the gas shadows are insignificant they may be gone at the second examination or at least not increased. Constancy in position of gas-filled loops and increasing dis-

tention in serial roentgenograms are valuable signs of a significant obstructive process.

GALLSTONE OBSTRUCTION. Occasionally a large calculus in the gallbladder will ulcerate through the wall into an adherent duodenum and, because of its size, become impacted somewhere in the small intestine. In addition to the signs of simple bowel obstruction the stone may be partially calcified and thus be visible. More often it is non-opaque. A very significant finding in these cases is the frequent observation of gas outlining the common and hepatic ducts and forming a Y-shaped translucent gas shadow in the right upper quadrant. The demonstration of gas in the biliary duct system plus the signs of a simple obstruction is

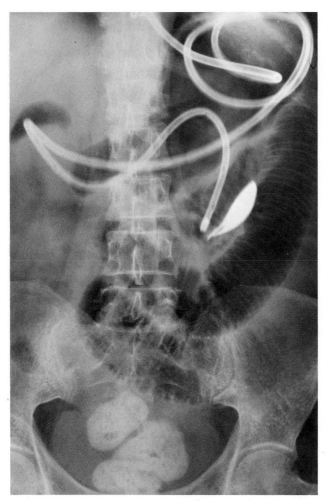

Fig. 13-6. Small-intestine obstruction. Recumbent view showing gas-distended loops of small intestine. A decompression tube has been passed into the jejunum. The colon contains very little gas (barium residue in the rectum from previous barium enema). Note the "stacked coin" appearance of the jejunum.

good evidence of gallstone obstruction with a fistulous communication between the gall bladder and the duodenum.

OBSTRUCTION WITHOUT GAS DISTENTION. Rarely, in the presence of obstruction, the bowel above the lesion is filled with fluid but there is an absence of gas. The fluid-filled loops may form recognizable shadows in the abdomen but at other times they do not and the lack of gas may make it impossible to establish the diagnosis without the use of a barium-water meal (Fig. 13-9).

MECONIUM ILEUS. The absence of normal pancreatic and intestinal gland secretions during fetal life, the result of cystic fibrosis, leads to the formation of a thick, sticky, almost mucilagenous meconium which may cause bowel obstruction during the immediate postnatal period. The obstruction occurs in the distal ileum where the meconium may form into hard pellets (Fig. 3-10). If a barium enema examination is done the colon will be found to have a very small caliber since it has never been used during fetal life (*microcolon*). The caliber may be so narrow that

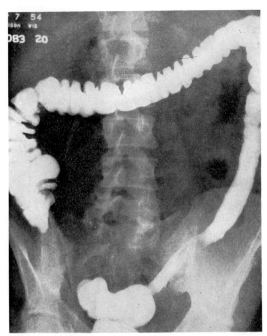

Fig. 13-7. Early partial obstruction of the small intestine. Barium enema roentgenogram done at 9:30 A.M., shows a normal colon. There are a few accumulations of gas in the small intestine but these are no more than is commonly seen and represent swallowed air. Compare with Figure 13-8.

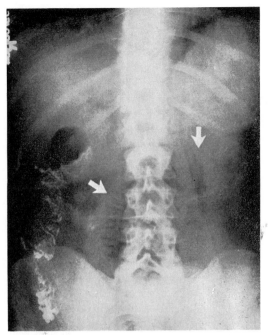

Fig. 13-8. Same patient as shown in Figure 13-7. Anteroposterior roentgenogram of the abdomen made at 1:00 P.M. of the same day. Patient began having cramping abdominal pain about 1½ hours prior to this examination. There is a small barium residue in the colon from the barium enema. Note the finely serrated gas shadow representing a dilated segment of jejunum (**arrows**) indicative of obstruction. Several days later a malignant polyp of the jejunum was removed. It was causing intermittent obstruction because of intussusception.

an erroneous diagnosis of rectal obstruction may be made on the basis of a rectal examination or after attempts to pass a tube through the rectum.

On plain-film examination loops of gas-distended bowel will be seen. Often it is impossible at this age to distinguish small intestine from colon based on the gas pattern and a barium enema may be required. In addition to showing a microcolon, the barium mixture may reflux through the ileocecal valve and partially surround the masses of meconium thus giving a valuable diagnostic clue.

Two signs have been described as highly suggestive of meconium ileus on plain roentgenograms: (*1*) Bubbles of gas mixed with the hard or sticky meconium causes a finely mottled or granular appearance, usually in the right lower quadrant (Fig. 3-11).[26] This finding is not entirely specific as similar changes have been noted with other causes of postnatal obstruction such as Hirschsprung's disease and imperforate anus. However, the diagnosis of the latter condition can be made by inspection; in the former, the barium

enema findings are different. (*2*) Paucity or absence of air-fluid levels in upright roentgenograms.

One of the most frequent complications of meconium ileus both pre- and postnatally is volvulus (Fig. 3-12). In prenatal volvulus, if the twist is of sufficient degree, the blood supply to the closed loop is compromised and it undergoes necrosis. It eventually may be absorbed leaving an atresia of the bowel. In other patients the closed devitalized loop may lose its continuity with the bowel, become adherent, and form a "pseudocyst," again with resulting atresia of the intestine.[21] Single or multiple areas may be affected in this way. Rupture of the bowel may occur *in utero* and result in meconium peritonitis which may be recognized on plain roentgenograms made shortly after birth by the presence of scattered calcified deposits on the peritoneal surfaces (see under

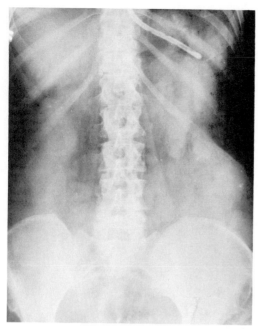

Fig. 13-9. Obstruction of the small intestine without gas distention. Recumbent roentgenogram of the abdomen shows irregular soft-tissue masses. These are caused by fluid-filled loops of bowel. The obstruction was caused by a carcinoma of the cecum. This patient emphasizes the fact that complete obstruction of the small intestine can be present without significant gas accumulation; fluid-filled loops of bowel may simulate tumor masses.

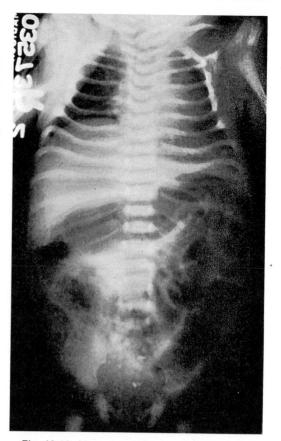

Fig. 13-10. Meconium ileus in newborn infant with clinical signs of bowel obstruction. There is a mottled shadow in the right lateral abdomen representing gas mixed with solid material. At operation this was found to be a mass of inspissated meconium.

"meconium peritonitis," this chapter). Prenatal rupture of the bowel from any cause will result in the same roentgen finding so that it is not specific for meconium ileus. In postnatal volvulus, a closed-loop obstruction is formed and gangrene and peritonitis may result. The closed loop may be visualized as a mass (*the pseudotumor sign*) but roentgen diagnosis generally is difficult. The demonstration of a mottled or granular collection of gas bubbles, the absence or paucity of air-fluid levels, the presence of calcified deposits on the peritoneal surfaces and the barium enema finding of a microcolon are signs to be looked for when meconium ileus is a diagnostic consideration.[21]

In some infants without signs of cystic fibrosis there is difficulty in passing the first meconium stool and signs of intestinal obstruction develop. As soon as the meconium is passed the obstructive symptoms disappear. This entity has been called the *meconium plug syndrome*. It has been stressed that this diagnosis should not be made without

first excluding cystic fibrosis and Hirschsprung's disease, both of which may present initially as the meconium plug syndrome.

Intestinal obstruction in cystic fibrosis occurring after the newborn period, particularly in older children, and caused by inspissated contents in the small intestine has been called *meconium ileus equivalent*. Inspissated material also may cause intussusception in the older child.

CLOSED-LOOP OBSTRUCTION

Closed-loop obstruction refers to a closure of the lumen at two points, leaving a loop of bowel obstructed at both ends. Among the common causes are volvulus and incarcerated

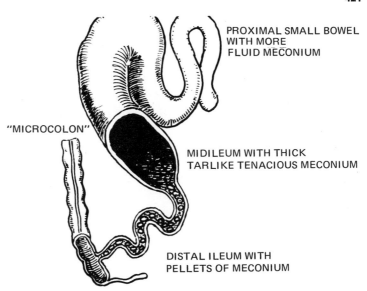

Fig. 13-11. Meconium ileus. The diagram illustrates the pathologic findings. (From Leonidas, J. C., Berdon, W. E., Baker, D. H. and Santulli, T. V. *Am J Roentgenol Radium Ther Nucl Med* 108:598, 1970. Reproduced by permission of the authors, Editor, and Publisher. Modified from an illustration by Santulli, T. V. in Benson, C. D., Mustard, W. T., Ravitch, M. M., Snyder, W. H., Jr., and Welch, K. J. (eds.), "Pediatric Surgery" Chicago, Yearbook, 1962.)

hernia. The significance of the lesion lies in the fact that the blood supply may be compromised. Serious interference with the blood supply may develop even though the loop of bowel is incompletely obstructed. Because the venous pressure is lower than the arterial, the veins are obstructed first and there often is extravasation of blood into the loop. If the lumen is not blocked completely, gas may enter it from above. In the colon gas may accumulate within a completely obstructed loop as a result of putrefaction. It is imperative to distinguish a closed-loop obstruction from a simple one as soon as possible, so that measures may be undertaken for its relief. The roentgen diagnosis is difficult and often impossible. Signs to be watched for are listed below but it always is important that these findings be considered in conjunction with the clinical observations.

Roentgen Observations

GAS WITHIN THE LOOP. During the early stage of a closed-loop obstruction the roentgen signs may be indistinguishable from a simple obstruction. In some patients, however, gas will be trapped within the obstructed loop, which may assume the form of two short segments of distended bowel lying parallel to one another and separated by the soft-tissue space of the thickened intestinal walls ("coffee bean" sign of Mellins and Rigler). When gas-distended bowel is also present above the obstructed loop this sign is difficult to recognize. In other patients the loop has the form of a U, usually inverted. This is a frequent observation in volvulus of the sigmoid colon (q.v.). Gas is almost always present in a closed-loop obstruction of the colon, probably the result of putrefaction. In the small intestine there may be nearly complete absence of gas above the obstruction.

FLUID WITHIN THE LOOP. The closed loop may contain only fluid and result in a mass shadow similar to that of a solid tumor (pseudotumor of Frimann-Dahl).[15] The outline of a pseudotumor shadow is easier to detect if

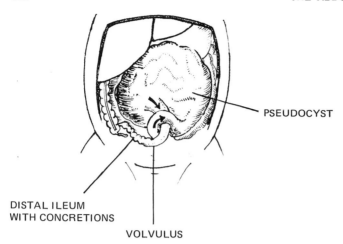

PSEUDOCYST

DISTAL ILEUM
WITH CONCRETIONS

VOLVULUS

Fig. 13-12. Meconium ileus. Diagram illustrates the formation of a pseudocyst secondary to volvulus in meconium ileus (see also Fig. 13-11 and credit citation).

there is gas distention of bowel above the obstruction (Fig. 13-13). It is more difficult to demonstrate when there are no gas-distended loops.

FIXATION OF LOOP. Lack of movement of the closed obstructed loop may be demonstrable in roentgenograms made in recumbent, upright, and lateral decubitus positions.

LOSS OF MUCOSAL MARKINGS. In simple obstruction the valvulae conniventes of the jejunum are never completely obliterated, even when the distention is severe and these cause the margins of the gas shadows to be serrated. When the blood supply of a closed-loop obstruction has been compromised, the folds tend to disappear and the margins of the gas shadow become smooth. This sign is of value only if one can recognize the loop as being jejunum rather than ileum, since the folds disappear readily in the ileum under the effects of simple distention.

SIGNS OF PERITONITIS AND FLUID IN PERITONEAL CAVITY. In the later stages of a closed-loop obstruction the signs of exudate and free fluid in the peritoneal cavity appear. The soft-tissue spaces separating two adjacent loops of intestine become widened. Shifting fluid density

may be demonstrable when roentgenograms are made in multiple positions. These are serious signs although they do not necessarily indicate that the bowel has perforated. Bacteria may pass through the wall of an intact gut if the blood supply has been damaged and peritonitis may develop without frank rupture. If actual perforation does occur, free gas may be demonstrated in the peritoneal cavity in upright or lateral decubitus views.

INTRAMURAL GAS. If necrosis develops, gas may be found within the wall of the involved bowel and seen as linear, lucent stripes paralleling the lumen.

OBSTRUCTION OF THE COLON

Roentgenograms of the abdomen may be sufficient for the diagnosis of colonic obstruction. The same type of film examination is used as described above for small bowel obstruction. Because gas is present in the normal colon, the diagnosis of obstruction can be made only when the colon is found to be dilated from the cecum to the level of the lesion (Fig. 13-14). Usually the abnormal distention ends abruptly at the level of the lesion, with the colon distal to it being free of gas. In case of doubt it is

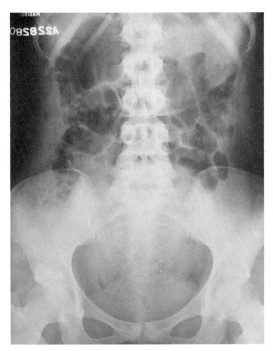

Fig. 13-13. Strangulated obstruction of the small intestine. There is a mass density in the lower central part of the abdomen extending to the upper border of the fifth lumbar vertebra. There are segments of gas-distended small intestine in the upper abdomen. At operation the mass was found to be a fluid-filled and distended loop of ileum that had been obstructed because of herniation through a rent in the mesentery apparently following a previous intra-abdominal surgical procedure. This is an illustration of the "pseudotumor sign" of strangulated obstruction.

advisable to proceed with a barium enema. This will establish either the presence of a lesion or the patency of the colonic lumen. Because the tissues at the site of an obstruction may be friable, care should be used to prevent undue pressure within the colon during the administration of the enema; palpation of the abdomen also should be done carefully.

As noted in the preceding section, colonic loops usually can be distinguished from the small intestine by the haustral sacculations and by the position of the loops, situated around the periphery of the abdomen. The haustra are deeper than the mucosal folds of the small intestine and the sacculations are considerably wider. When solid fecal matter is also present

in the colon the gas shadows often have a finely mottled appearance. This appearance is not seen in the small intestine except in some cases of meconium ileus in newborn infants.

If the ileocecal valve is incompetent, gas may back up into the small intestine and some degree of small bowel distention may be present. If the ileocecal valve is competent, small-bowel gas distention is slight or absent; instead the colon becomes increasingly dilated. Because of its thinner walls the cecum undergoes the greatest distention and perforation is most likely to occur here even when the obstruction is in the distal part of the colon (Fig. 13-15). When gas can back up into the ileum and jejunum there is less likelihood of perforation. If the cecum distends to more than 9 or

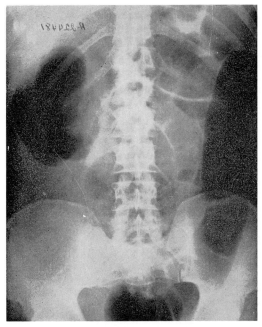

Fig. 13-14. Obstruction of the colon caused by a carcinoma of the rectum (recumbent anteroposterior roentgenogram). There is gas distention of the colon from the hepatic flexure to the rectum. The ascending colon is filled with fluid. There are some moderately gas-distended loops of small intestine in the central part of the abdomen, which indicate that the ileocecal valve is patent. The pattern of gas distention is not unlike that seen in adynamic ileus and in some cases of obstruction of this type it may be necessary to do a barium enema to determine if there is a lesion in the distal colon or rectum.

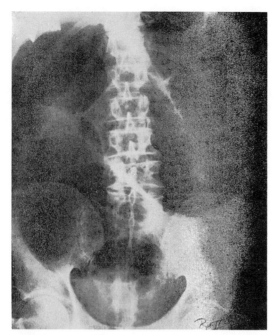

Fig. 13-15. Obstruction of the sigmoid colon caused by incarceration of the bowel in a left femoral hernia. While the obstruction is in the sigmoid, the gas distention ends in the upper descending colon. The end of the gas column in a single roentgenogram of this type does not always indicate the site of obstruction. The cecum is greatly distended and did rupture shortly after this roentgenogram was made. In this patient the ileocecal valve prevented back-up of gas into the ileum to aid in decompression of the distended colon.

10 cm, perforation becomes a very likely possibility.

Fluid levels are of less significance in the diagnosis of colonic obstruction than they are in the small bowel. Patients frequently have had enemas prior to roentgen examination and residual fluid from the enema will lead to the formation of fluid levels. If enemas have not been administered and fluid levels are demonstrable in the colon they have the same significance as they do in the small intestine.

VOLVULUS OF THE SIGMOID COLON

A long redundant loop of sigmoid colon may undergo a twist on its mesenteric axis and thus form a closed-loop obstruction. Usually the loop of sigmoid becomes distended with gas forming an inverted U-shaped shadow rising out of the pelvis and with the limbs of the loop extending into or pointing toward the pelvis (Fig. 13-16). Fluid levels may be revealed in the loop if an upright or a lateral decubitus view is obtained. Because of the obstruction the colon proximal to the sigmoid also becomes abnormally distended with gas. A barium enema sometimes is needed if the diagnosis remains in doubt. As the barium column reaches the sigmoid the end assumes a pointed or tapered form; the twisted appearance of the mucosal folds may be apparent. The obstruction may be incomplete and enough of the barium mixture may pass through to outline clearly the twist and establish its nature (Fig. 13-17).

VOLVULUS OF THE CECUM

The ascending colon and cecum may have a long mesentery as a fault of rotation and fixa-

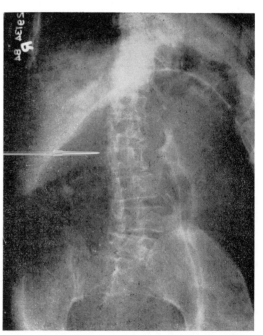

Fig. 13-16. Volvulus of the sigmoid colon. Anteroposterior supine view of the abdomen showing a gas-distended loop of colon filling the major part of the abdomen. This has the configuration of an inverted U with the limbs extending into the pelvis.

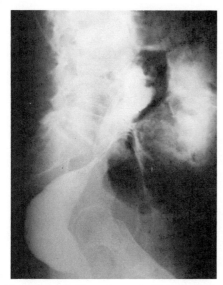

Fig. 13-17. Same patient as shown in Figure 13-16. This is a lateral view of the rectum and lower sigmoid after barium filling by means of barium enema demonstrating the twisted appearance characteristic of volvulus. The obstruction is not complete and some of the barium has extended into the dilated sigmoid.

tion during development of the gut; this condition predisposes to volvulus, with the cecum undergoing a twist on its long axis. The cecum becomes greatly distended with gas and some degree of distention of the ileum and jejunum usually is present as well (Fig. 13-18). The colon distal to the volvulus will contain little or no gas. Because of its mobility, the cecum may be found in almost any part of the abdominal cavity. Thus the gas shadow of the distended cecum not infrequently is found in the left upper quadrant of the abdomen, or even in the left lower quadrant. When a rounded or ovoid, gas-distended structure is visualized in such a location the possibility of a volvulus of the cecum should be entertained. When the cecum is displaced in this manner the long axis of the distended loop will point toward the right side of the abdomen. Also there will be an absence of normal colonic gas shadows in the right lower quadrant; instead one may see loops of gas filled–small bowel where normally the cecum should be. If the ileocecal valve can be identified by the visualization of its lips, it will be found on the undersurface or on the right side of the cecum.

ADYNAMIC (PARALYTIC) ILEUS

In adynamic ileus the lumen of the bowel remains patent but loss of propulsive power and tone lead to local or general distention with accumulation of gas and fluid within the paralyzed loops. Local ileus may be associated with localized inflammations within the abdomen, such as acute appendicitis, cholecystitis, or pancreatitis. Generalized ileus has many causes. It may follow intra-abdominal operations or develop as a result of trauma to the abdomen, spine, or thorax. Ileus constantly accompanies peritonitis but it also may develop in the presence of any severe infection such as pneumonia.

ADYNAMIC ILEUS WITHOUT PERITONITIS

In the absence of peritoneal inflammation, adynamic ileus usually results in generalized gas and fluid distention of the entire gastrointestinal tract. The colon often shows a relatively greater degree of distention than the small intestine. The loops of small bowel usually are shorter than those seen in mechanical obstruction; also they are not as likely to form smoothly arched curves or appear to be under as much tension. Fluid levels will be seen but they are not as prominent a feature as in mechanical obstruction (Fig. 13-19). In early cases differentiation between the two conditions may be difficult, or impossible, on roentgen examination. Progressive examinations are helpful in such patients. In adynamic ileus the gas pattern does not change remarkably over a period of hours or even days, as it does in mechanical obstruction. Because the colon may be distended the question of an obstructive lesion in the distal part of the large bowel may arise. A barium enema examination is indicated in such a case and usually will make the differential diagnosis.

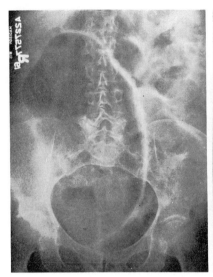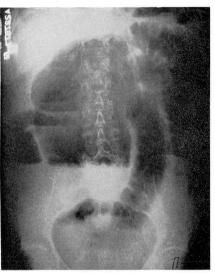

Fig. 13-18. Volvulus of the cecum. *Left,* Recumbent view. *Right,* Upright view. The distended cecum forms an oval-shaped translucency, the tip pointing upward and to the right. There is gas distention of the small intestine in the left lateral abdomen. In the upright roentgenogram there is a gas-fluid level in the cecum and smaller levels in the loops of small intestine.

ADYNAMIC ILEUS SECONDARY TO PERITONITIS

When peritonitis is present, in addition to the generalized distention as noted above, the signs of exudate or of free fluid in the peritoneal cavity will be seen. There is a widening of the soft-tissue spaces between contiguous gas-filled loops of bowel. In addition there may be shifting density demonstrated when upright or lateral decubitus views are obtained, to indicate the presence of free fluid. Evidence of apparent thickening of the bowel wall in the presence of distended bowel is a fairly reliable sign of an inflammatory process; simple distention causes a thinning of the wall.

COMBINED DYNAMIC AND ADYNAMIC ILEUS

Because certain lesions may cause both a mechanical block and a paralytic ileus (e.g., some cases of appendiceal abscess), both conditions may be present at one time. It may be impossible to make an accurate estimate of the changes purely from roentgen examination. In general, it is important to remember that if the colon is gas-distended, a barium enema can be given to distinguish between a mechanical obstruction and a paralytic bowel. In small-bowel obstruction the colon will be free or almost free of gas. Adynamic ileus may occasionally be limited to the small bowel. When it is, serial observations are important and, of course, correlation with the clinical findings may be the deciding factor.

ACUTE INTERMITTENT PORPHYRIA

This is a familial metabolic disease characterized by attacks of severe colicky abdominal pain in association with obstipation. The character of the clinical symptoms and signs often leads to the erroneous diagnosis of bowel obstruction and many patients are operated upon for this reason. In some patients signs of central nervous system involvement are present, including an ascending Landry's type of paralysis, parasthesias, delirium and hallucinations, and coma. The diagnosis usually is made from the chance observation that the urine becomes dark on exposure to light or by the development of neurologic symptoms that may suggest the disease and lead to investigations for the presence of abnormal porphyrins in the urine and feces. The disease is of interest roentgeno-

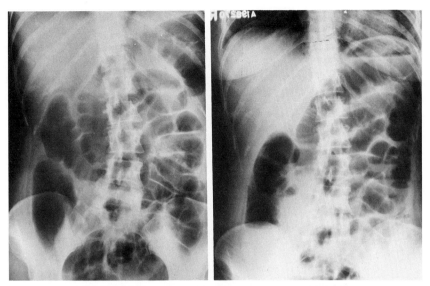

Fig. 13-19. Adynamic ileus. Recumbent (*left*) and upright (*right*) roentgenograms. There is gas in the colon and in the small intestine. While dilated, the small bowel loops are relatively short and do not appear to be under very great tension. Fluid levels are inconspicuous in the upright view except in the cecum. This is a case of acute appendicitis.

logically because of the signs and symptoms pointing toward bowel obstruction. Abnormal amounts of gas are present in the intestinal tract and the pattern is that of adynamic ileus rather than mechanical obstruction. Gas usually is present in both the small intestine and colon but the distention may be more pronounced in the small bowel.

The distended segments are short, fluid levels are not particularly prominent in upright roentgenograms, and the gas pattern shifts from day to day in serial studies.

"SENTINEL" LOOP

In certain localized acute inflammatory processes within the abdomen a loop of bowel adjacent to the lesion may become distended with gas representing, in effect, a localized paralytic ileus (Fig. 13-20). This has been called a sentinel loop and it may offer a clue to the presence of the lesion. In acute pancreatitis the duodenum, the transverse colon, or a loop of jejunum may be visualized in this manner. In the presence of acute appendicitis, localized gas accumulation in loops of bowel in the ileocecal area is frequent. Acute cholecystitis may have an associated localized ileus in the right upper quadrant. While a sentinel

loop is a valuable sign for such disease, it must be interpreted in relation to other findings and particularly to the clinical signs and symptoms in any given case, for the visualization of gas limited to a single segment of intestine often is a chance observation without significance.

ACUTE MESENTERIC VASCULAR OCCLUSION

Acute mesenteric arterial occlusion may result from thrombosis in arteriosclerotic disease or from lodgement of an embolus from the left side of the heart. The superior mesenteric artery is more frequently involved than the inferior and the arteries more frequently than the veins. Venous occlusion usually is secondary to some disease that impairs venous flow. Unless there is an adequate collateral circulation acute occlusion of a major vessel results in a severe, acute illness with infarction of the bowel, necrosis, peritonitis, and death. In plain roentgenograms a characteristic gas pattern has been described consisting of adynamic ileus limited to the ileum and proximal part of the

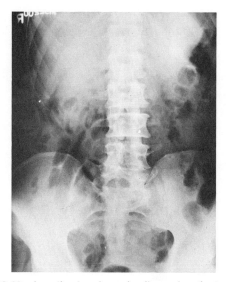

Fig. 13-20. Localized adynamic ileus (sentinel loops) in a patient wtih acute appendicitis. There are several segments of ileum in the right lateral abdomen that are moderately distended. The gas pattern elsewhere is normal.

colon as far as the splenic flexure corresponding to the distribution of the branches of the superior mesenteric artery. In most cases, however, the distribution of gas is not as specific. The ileus may be limited to the small intestine simulating obstruction (pseudo-obstruction) or may involve both small intestine and colon. The appearance in some may suggest a low colonic obstruction although this is unusual. When there is gas distention of the small bowel and ascending and transverse portions of the colon, the cecum may be of smaller diameter than the transverse colon.[34] When necrosis develops, gas may be found within the wall of the intestine or even in the portal venous system within the liver. This is a significant sign of intestinal necrosis. Other causes for intramural gas must be excluded (see pages 435 and 442). Occasionally the bowel is filled with fluid with little or no gas present. The roentgen signs in such cases are too nonspecific to allow a diagnosis to be made. In late stages the mucosal folds may disappear and the luminal surface becomes quite smooth. Most patients with acute mesenteric thrombosis are too ill to undergo barium studies.

In recent years selective mesenteric angiography has been used to demonstrate the obstruction if the diagnosis is in doubt. Serial roentgenograms demonstrate the site of occlusion and the collateral blood supply, if present. The severity of any associated arteriosclerotic disease can be defined.

INTRA-ABDOMINAL CALCIFICATION

For a discussion of calculi in the biliary and urinary tracts and in the pancreas the appropriate sections dealing with these structures should be consulted. In addition to such calculi there are a number of other causes of intra-abdominal calcification including those listed in the following sections (see also Index).

CALCIFIED LYMPH NODES

Calcification of the mesenteric lymph nodes is observed most frequently in the right lower quadrant or in the lower central part of the abdomen and occasionally to the left of the midline. Calcification of these nodes represents the effects of previous infection, usually tuberculosis. The roentgen appearance of a calcified node is that of a mottled density seldom more than 1 to 1.5 cm in diameter (Fig. 13-21). Occasionally the shadow is more uniform in density. Often two or more nodes will be found clustered together or within a relatively small area. In serial films or in those made with the patient in different positions such as recumbent and upright, the shadows of the calcified mesenteric nodes will move over a fairly wide area. Such an observation is a useful one in differential diagnosis if there is doubt concerning the nature of the lesions. Calcification in other abdominal nodes occurs infrequently.

VASCULAR CALCIFICATION

Plaquelike areas of calcification in the aorta are common in persons beyond middle age. Such plaques may be seen occasionally in

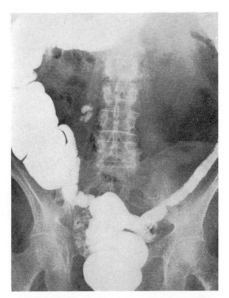

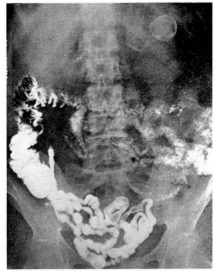

Fig. 13-21. Calcified mesenteric lymph nodes. Roentgenogram of the colon after a barium enema demonstrates the calcified nodes as mottled areas of density along the right margin of the fourth lumbar vertebra.

Fig. 13-22. Calcified arteriosclerotic aneurysms of the splenic artery found during a gastrointestinal examination. The aneurysms are visualized in the left upper quadrant as circular areas of calcific density occurring along the course of the splenic artery. (*Courtesy Dr. Wayne Rounds, Madison, Wisconsin.*)

younger individuals, particularly in those suffering from diabetes. The plaques overlie the lumbar vertebrae in anteroposterior roentgenograms and they are seen to best advantage in oblique or lateral projections. In some cases practically all the abdominal aorta will be visualized. Calcification of the arterial wall allows an estimation to be made of the diameter of the vessel. If aneurysmal dilatation is present, it can be recognized if there is sufficient calcification to delineate all or a part of the dilated segment.

In addition to the aorta, calcification occurs frequently in the iliac and splenic arteries. The splenic artery usually becomes tortuous and the calcification appears as one or more segments of tubular shape in the left upper quadrant. If the vessel turns so that it is seen end-on, the calcification appears as a thin-walled ring. Arteriosclerotic aneurysms of this artery can be demonstrated occasionally when the wall is calcified (Fig. 13-22). Calcification in other branches of the celiac axis is less frequent and the same is true of the renal arteries. Visualization of crescentic or ringlike calcified shadows

in the region of the kidney hilus should suggest the possibility of an aneurysm of a renal artery.

Calcification of the veins occurs mainly in thrombi and such calcified thrombi are called "phleboliths." These are observed very frequently in the pelvic veins and most adults have a few of them. Phleboliths are round or slightly oval in shape and vary in size from very tiny ones up to those that measure 0.5 cm or more in diameter. The small ones usually are evenly dense throughout; the larger ones tend to be ring-contoured or even laminated. They are found throughout the pelvis but are more frequent along the lateral aspects. It is easy to confuse a phlebolith with a calculus in the lower part of the ureter. A calculus often is irregular in shape and its long axis will lie parallel to the long axis of the ureter. Ureteral calculi seldom are found below the level of the ischial spine; phleboliths often occupy this position. At times it is impossible to determine the nature of the shadow until the ureter has been opacified by means of intravenous or retrograde pyelography. In a patient having the symptoms of ureteral colic, a calcific density in the plane of the ureter must be looked upon as evidence of a ureteral calculus. Occasionally a long thrombus within a vein will calcify and be visualized as an elongated and somewhat irregular linear shadow of calcification. The location in the region of the larger pelvic veins helps to identify the nature of the shadow. Rarely, a calcified thrombus in the portal vein has been identified.

CALCIFIED FOCI IN THE SPLEEN AND LIVER

Small, round, dense foci of calcification are observed frequently in the spleen, occasionally in the liver. They may be extremely numerous and evenly distributed throughout these viscera. Usually they are considered to be the healed foci of previous widely disseminated infection, either tuberculosis or one of the fungi, such as histoplasmosis (Fig. 13-23). Recent observations suggest that histoplasmosis is responsible in most cases. Similar foci of calcification may be found in the lungs of some of these patients, distributed widely throughout the pulmonary parenchyma.

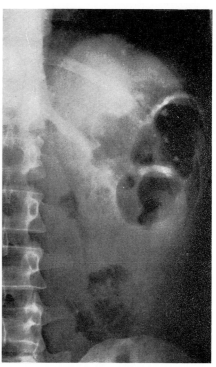

Fig. 13-23. Calcified foci in the spleen. There are multiple, small, nodular calcifications throughout the spleen, some of them visualized through gas in the splenic flexure of the colon.

ENTEROLITHS AND APPENDICEAL FECALITHS

Enteroliths are uncommon causes for radiopaque objects in the abdomen, usually occurring in the colon. The enterolith may be primary or secondary. In the latter instance it forms usually after ingestion of foreign material such as a fruit pit, the pit serving as a nidus for the calcium salt deposition. In the primary type there is no predisposing foreign object to serve as a nidus. An enterolith may form within a Meckel's diverticulum or above a stenosing lesion of the small intestine such as regional enteritis. A large radiopaque gallstone may become lodged in the intestine after ulcerating through the duodenal wall.

Concretions within the lumen of the appendix may calcify (see Fig. 19-37). These are known as appendiceal fecaliths or coproliths. They are rounded or ovoid in shape and the

calcium often is deposited in concentric laminations so that the shadow is not uniformly dense. Since they are located in or near the tip of the appendix, they may be found distributed over a fairly wide area in the right lower quadrant of the abdomen or even below the brim of the pelvis. When inflammation of the appendix develops in the presence of a coprolith, gangrene and rupture are prone to follow. When examining roentgenograms of the abdomen in a patient in whom an acute appendicitis or appendiceal abscess is a diagnostic possibility, search for evidence of a coprolith should be made. Because the shadow often overlies the ilium, it may be difficult to visualize unless this area is inspected with care.

CALCIFICATION IN THE ADRENAL GLANDS

Mottled shadows of calcification may be found in one or both adrenal glands when involved by tuberculosis and such an observation forms one of the positive roentgen signs of *Addison's disease* (Fig. 13-24). The calcification is seen in the form of irregular mottling located directly over the superior pole of the kidney and sometimes forming almost a complete outline of the adrenal. Observation of the adrenal glands is facilitated if roentgenograms are made with the patient rotated slightly to the right and to the left of a supine position. Ordinarily a rotation of 15° is sufficient. This degree of rotation will tend to displace any confusing calcified areas in the costal cartilages away from the adrenal region.

Occasionally calcification is demonstrated in one or both adrenals of a patient who has none of the clinical signs of Addison's disease. Such calcifications have been observed in young infants and in children. In some cases, at least in infants, the calcification appears to have followed hemorrhage into the gland but in others its cause remains obscure. In these patients the calcification often is an incidental finding and does not seem to have any relationship to the patient's present complaints.

Calcification in the adrenal glands occurs in the lipidosis known as *Wolman's disease*.[23]

The adrenals are enlarged bilaterally and this, combined with the diffuse calcification, allows the diagnosis to be made. This is the only condition in which diffuse calcification in enlarged adrenal glands is found.

CALCIFIED CYSTS

Calcification in the wall of an intra-abdominal cyst is seen occasionally and the cystic nature of the lesion can be surmised by the crescentic or ring-shaped form of the calcification. Such cysts may be found in the mesentery, spleen, kidney, or in the liver and rarely in the adrenal (Figs. 13-25 and 13-26). Usually they are simple cysts of congenital origin. Calcification is frequent in the wall of an appendiceal mucocele and cystlike calcification in the right lower quadrant may indicate this lesion to be present (see Chapter 19).

Another type of intra-abdominal cyst that frequently calcifies is an echinococcus cyst. This disease is rare in this country and particularly so in persons who have never lived outside the United States. Echinococcus cysts in the abdomen may be found in the spleen or

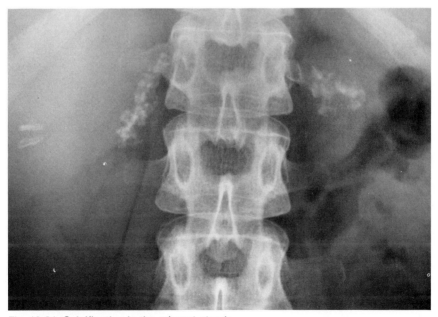

Fig. 13-24. Calcification in the adrenal glands.

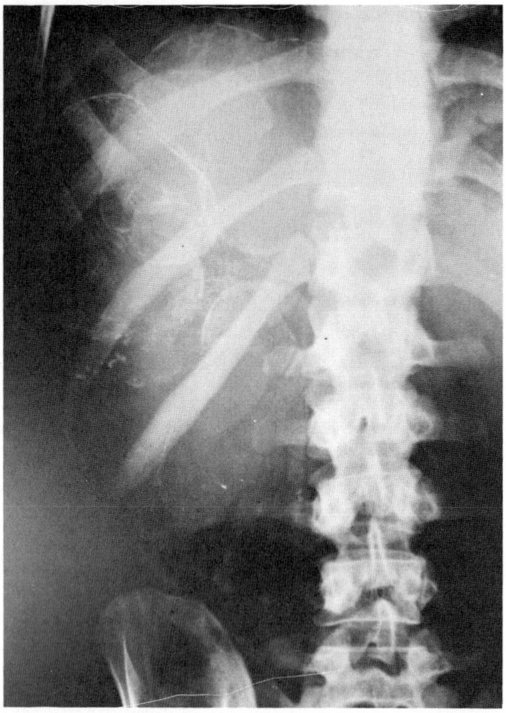

Fig. 13-25. Multiple calcified cysts in the liver. There are numerous thin-walled, rounded and ovoid calcified masses distributed throughout the liver, which is enlarged. They were believed to be congenital cysts although histologic confirmation was not possible.

liver, occasionally elsewhere within the peritoneal cavity. Calcified echinococcus cysts usually have thicker walls than simple cysts and there is somewhat less tendency for the entire wall of the cyst to be calcified.

Dermoid cysts constitute about 10 per cent of all ovarian cysts. The cyst may contain partially calcified or incompletely formed teeth, a characteristic feature of the lesion. Less frequently the wall of the cyst may be partially calcified. In addition to the presence of teeth the interior of a dermoid cyst, being filled with a fatty material, is more translucent than the surrounding tissues and thus appears as a sharply circumscribed area of lessened density within the pelvis (fat is the most transparent of all the tissues). Even when the wall is not calcified, it may stand out as a thin ring sur-

rounding the more radiolucent interior of the cyst (Fig. 13-27).

CALCIFICATION IN OTHER TUMORS

UTERINE LEIOMYOMA

In females of middle age or over, roentgenograms of the lower abdomen frequntly show the shadows of calcified uterine fibroids. The calcification forms a mottled "mulberry type" of shadow in the midpelvis or close to the midline (Fig. 13-28). The size of the lesion of course may vary considerably and occasionally a very large calcified fibroid will be found that will occupy the entire pelvis or even extend out of the pelvis.

CYSTADENOCARCINOMA OF THE OVARY

The papillary growths characteristic of this tumor frequently contain calcified deposits or psammoma bodies. These may be found not only in the primary tumor but in its peritoneal implants and even in its more distant metastases. The calcification is seen as scattered fine amorphous shadows, hardly denser than the normal soft tissues, and therefore easily missed unless they are extensive. The hazy calcifications may be confused with semiopaque material in the gastrointestinal tract, such as a small residue of barium mixed with other fecal material. This type of calcification is almost characteristic of this tumor and when distributed in various parts of the abdominal cavity indicates the presence of peritoneal implants. In benign cystadenoma of the ovary, similar psammoma bodies may form but there are, of course, no implants and the calcification is limited to the ovarian mass.

NEUROBLASTOMA

Neuroblastoma, usually arising in the adrenal gland, is a rather uncommon tumor of childhood that very frequently shows the pres-

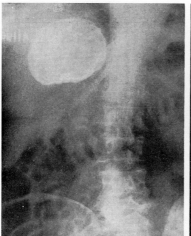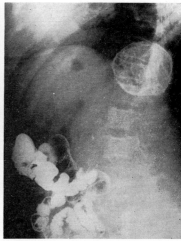

Fig. 13-26. Calcified cyst of the adrenal. *Left,* Anteroposterior and *Right,* lateral roentgenograms of the abdomen reveal a large cyst with densely calcified wall directly above the right kidney. At the time of operation the lesion was found to be an adrenal cyst, probably of congenital origin.

ence of calcification in the form of hazy granular deposits. Such calcification in a mass lying above the kidney in a young child is almost certain evidence of this tumor. Other malignant tumors of childhood occurring within the abdomen, such as Wilms' tumor of the kidney, infrequently calcify.

RENAL CARCINOMA

Calcification in a renal carcinoma is not unusual and is found in about 25 per cent of these tumors. The calcification must be distinguished from renal calculi and other causes of renal calcification (see Chapter 20).

GASTROINTESTINAL CARCINOMA

As a rare finding in gastrointestinal carcinoma there may be small mottled or punctuate deposits of calcium. The tumors have invariably been of the mucinous type and the lesions have been found in the stomach or colon. The patients have generally been in the younger or middle-aged groups. Calcification in metastases to the liver from mucinous carcinomas of gastrointestinal tract origin have also been reported, and we have observed one from a primary in the breast.

OTHERS

Calcified deposits occasionally are seen in carcinoma of the urinary bladder and in adrenal carcinoma. Calcification of the vas deferens is seen occasionally in older male patients. Calcification of the uterine arteries is an occasional finding in females, particularly in diabetics. The calcification forms a tubular, slightly tortuous density extending laterally from the uterus on both sides of the midline.

CALCIFICATION IN FETAL MECONIUM PERITONITIS

Fetal meconium peritonitis has been defined as a chemical inflammation of the peritoneum caused by the escape of sterile meconium into the peritoneal cavity. The condition usually results from perforation in utero, secondary to a congenital stenosis or atresia of the bowel and in meconium ileus. The clinical manifestations of obstruction

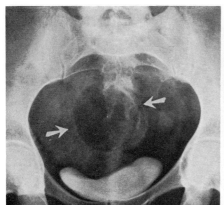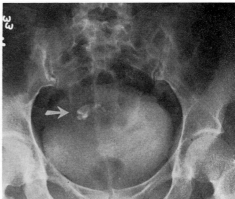

Fig. 13-27. Dermoid cyst of the ovary. Two patients with small dermoid cysts. *Left,* The cyst has a translucent center because of fatty content, but the wall is seen as a thin, ringlike density (**arrows**). The bladder contains contrast material from a previous intravenous urogram. *Right,* The cyst indents the dome of the contrast-filled urinary bladder. **Arrow** points to a cluster of well-formed teeth.

usually are recognizable at birth or shortly thereafter. Calcification of the cornified epithelial cells of the meconium occurs and may be visualized as small irregular calcifications widely distributed throughout the peritoneal cavity (Fig. 13-29). This is a very reliable sign of meconium peritonitis in the newborn when the calcification can be identified as being in the peritoneal cavity. Another finding which is seen occasionally in newborn males is the presence of calcified deposits in the scrotum. In one series this occurred in 20 per cent of the infants. Cases of intestinal atresia have been reported in which the calcified deposits were located within the intestinal lumen only, without perforation having developed. If the amount of calcified material is small it may be impossible to determine whether or not it has escaped from the intestinal tract. In patients with intramural calcification there often is an associated duplication of the bowel at the site of calcification. Wolfson and Engel[36] have described the occurrence of dense bands across the metaphyses of newborn infants as a significant finding in neonatal meconium peritonitis. They did not find similar bands in infants with intestinal obstruction without complicating meconium peritonitis.

PNEUMOPERITONEUM

The roentgen demonstration of free gas within the peritoneal cavity is a valuable sign in the diagnosis of perforation of the gastrointestinal tract. There are, however, other causes for pneumoperitoneum and the possible sources for such free gas in the peritoneal cavity are discussed below.

RUPTURE OF A GAS-CONTAINING VISCUS (STOMACH OR INTESTINE)

The most frequent cause of spontaneous pneumoperitoneum is rupture of a peptic ulcer, either gastric or duodenal. Other causes include perforation of a carcinoma of the stomach or colon, rupture of a colonic diverticulum, and traumatic rupture of the intestine or of the stomach. It is not observed very often following rupture of the small intestine other than the duodenum because of the usual absence of gas in this part of the intestinal tract. The time interval following rupture and the appearance of sufficient gas to be visualized roentgenologically obviously will vary, depending upon the size of the rupture, the location of the lesion, and the amount of gas present within the lumen of the segment. It has been noted within an hour after rupture.

Pneumoperitoneum does not always follow rupture of a peptic ulcer and approximately 25

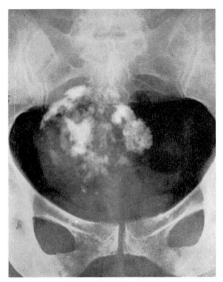

Fig. 13-28. Calcified uterine leiomyoma.

per cent of patients will not reveal free gas on roentgen examination. Failure to demonstrate such gas therefore is of no value in excluding a perforated ulcer.

PERITONITIS

Septic infection of the peritoneal cavity from gas-forming organisms may result in the production of a considerable amount of gas and the roentgen demonstration of pneumoperitoneum. There is nothing characteristic in the appearance of this gas to identify its source except that other signs of peritonitis will be present, including the evidence of ileus and of fluid in the spaces between the loops of gas-distended bowel.

PNEUMATOSIS CYSTOIDES INTESTINALIS

Gas "cysts" in the intestinal wall are found in the condition known as *pneumatosis cystoides intestinalis*. The intramural gas may be found in the small intestine or colon or in both. Gas in the wall of the stomach also has been reported. The entity is usually asymptomatic but rupture of a gas cyst may cause pneumoperitoneum. The gas is visualized roentgenologically as small bubbles, or less

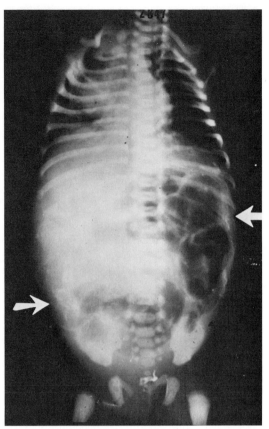

Fig. 13-29. Meconium peritonitis in a newborn. There are scattered, small irregular calcifications along the peritoneal surfaces (**arrows**).

frequently, as linear streaks within the intestinal wall. The cause is unknown but the condition usually clears spontaneously. Some investigators have expressed the opinion that the gas arises as a result of interstitial emphysema of the lungs brought about by forceful vomiting. The gas extends to the mediastinum and then along fascial planes to the retroperitoneal space and from there to the subserosa of the bowel. In other cases the intramural gas has been found above an obstructing lesion such as a carcinoma of the colon. In these it is assumed that the increased intraluminal pressure above the obstruction combined with the friable, ulcerated tissue sometimes seen above a carcinoma, is responsible for the entrance of gas into the wall (Fig. 13-30). Pneumatosis intestinalis also has been found in the small intestine when it is involved by scleroderma. The mechanism whereby gas enters the wall in these cases is unknown.

In addition to this form of intramural gas, it

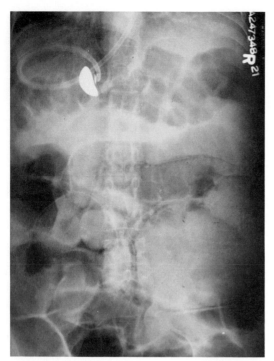

Fig. 13-30. Pneumatosis cystoides intestinalis. In addition to the signs of bowel obstruction, linear stripes of gas can be seen in the walls of intestinal loops.

also may be found in association with certain diseases, particularly where intestinal necrosis has occurred, such as mesenteric vascular thrombosis and strangulated obstruction. This is discussed in the section entitled "Intramural Gas."

INJECTION OF FALLOPIAN TUBES

Gas injected into the fallopian tubes as a part of the Rubin test for tubal patency may escape into the peritoneal cavity and be present in sufficient amounts to be visualized roentgenologically. Following vaginal lavage it has been reported that gas may enter the peritoneal cavity through the fallopian tubes in sufficient amounts to be demonstrable.

POSTLAPAROTOMY AIR

Some air is almost always present within the abdominal cavity following laparotomy. Under ordinary circumstances sufficient air remains to be visualized roentgenologically for several days; occasionally it will persist for a week to 10 days and has been reported to remain visible at times for as long as 4 weeks after the laparotomy. Demonstration of pneumoperitoneum during the postoperative period is of no significance unless (1) the amount of gas is large, or (2) increasing gas is shown in serial roentgenograms. The latter observation is good evidence that the gas is abnormal and may indicate breakdown of a surgical anastomosis or other rupture of the intestinal tract. Occasionally a large amount of air is seen in the peritoneal cavity as a normal observation during the first day or two following laparotomy; however, such large accumulations should be viewed with suspicion and they warrant close observation for progress and a careful correlation with the clinical signs and symptoms.

Air frequently is introduced into the peritoneal cavity at the time of paracentesis for removal of fluid or during peritoneoscopy. The amount usually is small. Following peritoneal dialysis for chronic renal failure, a small amount of pneumoperitoneum is common.

DIAGNOSTIC AND THERAPEUTIC PNEUMOPERITONEUM

In these instances the source of the gas should be obvious. In diagnostic pneumoperitoneum the gas is introduced to aid in delineating the abdominal viscera, particularly the liver and spleen, to outline abdominal masses, and to demonstrate the undersurface of the diaphragm, etc. In therapeutic pneumoperitoneum the gas usually is introduced as part of the therapy for pulmonary tuberculosis.

IDIOPATHIC SPONTANEOUS PNEUMOPERITONEUM

In very rare instances spontaneous pneumoperitoneum of unknown etiology is encountered. It is generally considered that most if not all of these cases result from rupture of emphysematous gas cysts occurring as part of an otherwise un-recognized instance of pneumatosis cystoides. Pneumoperitoneum may result from air arising in the mediastinum, a mediastinal emphysema. This, in turn, may follow an interstitial emphysema of the lung. We have observed it as a complication of pneumothorax.

ROENTGEN OBSERVATIONS

Free gas within the peritoneal cavity is best demonstrated in roentgenograms made with the patient upright, either sitting or standing. The gas ascends and accumulates beneath the summit of the diaphragm. It then can be visualized as a translucent zone limited by the thin, curved shadow of the diaphragm above and the density of the abdominal tissues beneath (Fig. 13-31). If the amount of gas is very small it forms a thin, curved, dark streak or a semilunar-shaped shadow, having a smoothly curved superior surface where the gas is bounded by the diaphragm and a horizontal flat inferior margin if there is fluid also present. The gas may be found under one or both diaphragmatic domes. It is easier to recognize on the right side because of the homogeneous density of the liver. On the left the normal gas and fluid shadows present in the fundus of the stomach may be confusing (Fig. 13-32). Close observation, however, will usually show the presence of two shadows, one representing the normal gas-fluid level of the stomach and the other the abnormal gas in the subdiaphragmatic space.

If the patient is too ill to sit or stand, lateral decubitus views as explained in previous paragraphs may be obtained. The gas will rise to the highest point in the flank and be visible as a horizontal translucent area. It is somewhat easier to recognize a small amount of gas when the patient is examined in a left lateral decubitus position because the right side of the abdomen is uppermost and the small gas accumulation sometimes will be found between the lateral surface of the liver and the abdominal wall; the homogeneous density of the liver again makes it more readily apparent.

If a relatively large amount of gas is present or if the gas is localized it can be recognized at times in roentgenograms made with the patient supine. The gas accumulated between the loops of bowel outlines their external surfaces. Visualization of the outer surfaces of loops of intestine is good evidence of the existence of

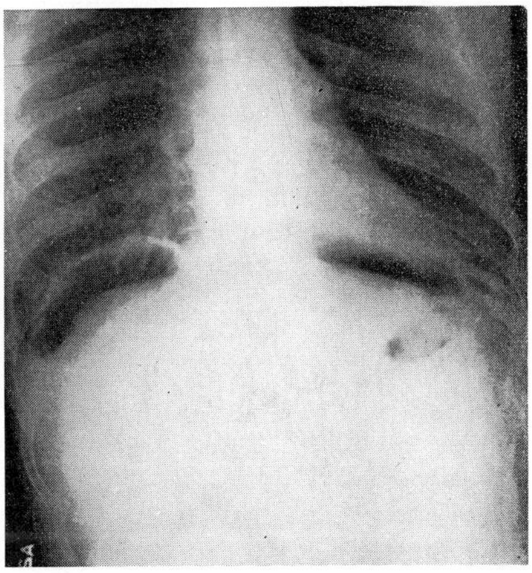

Fig. 13-31. Pneumoperitoneum following rupture of a peptic ulcer. Upright roentgenogram of the abdomen. There is air beneath both leaves of the diaphragm. Air in the gastric fundus can be seen beneath the pneumoperitoneum on the left.

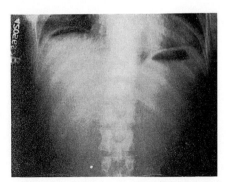

Fig. 13-32. Pneumoperitoneum secondary to rupture of a gastric ulcer. The amount of gas is small and is seen mainly beneath the right leaf of the diaphragm. On the left side the gas with fluid level is in the fundus of the stomach. Directly along the upper outer margin of the fundus there is a small amount of pneumoperitoneum. The fact that the major gas accumulation is in the stomach and not free in the peritoneal cavity is determined by the shape of the summit of the gas shadow, which does not follow the curve of the diaphragm laterally.

gas since, normally, these cannot be demonstrated. If gas is also present within the lumen, the thickness of the wall may be clearly visualized because both surfaces are demonstrated. When there is ample intra-abdominal fat the outlines of intestinal loops sometimes are visible, particularly if they are filled with fluid (Fig. 13-33). However, they are never seen with as much clarity as when pneumoperitoneum is present. In infants with intestinal perforation very large amounts of gas may escape into the peritoneal cavity. This can be recognized, even in supine roentgenograms, by the demonstration of a large oval translucency, with sharp margins overlying the central part of the abdomen ("football sign"). It may be divided cephalad along its central axis by a

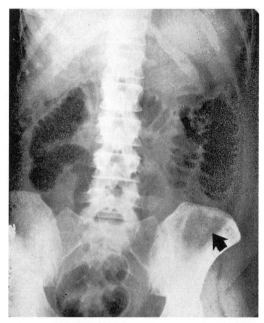

Fig. 13-33. Obstruction of the small intestine caused by a carcinoma of the cecum. Anteroposterior roentgenogram with the patient supine, illustrates the "stacked coin" appearance of gas-distended segments of jejunum in the left side of the abdomen and the smoother margins of ileum in the right side. The presence of intra-abdominal fat allows the outer surface of some of the segments of bowel to be visualized (**arrow**). Note also the properitoneal fat forming a thin translucent stripe along the lateral margin of the abdominal cavity.

narrow streak representing the falciform ligament. Free gas also tends to accumulate along the inferior surface of the liver when the patient is prone or supine. This region should be observed carefully when searching for the signs of pneumoperitoneum.

ASCITES

When roentgenograms are made with the patient supine, free fluid in the peritoneal cavity causes a generalized increase in density of the abdomen. The margins of the liver, spleen, and kidneys become indistinct and the psoas muscle margins also become poorly visualized. Normally the lower lateral margin of the liver can be identified. If fluid is present in the area the liver edge becomes indistinct or disappears altogether. It should be noted that in emaciated individuals the margins of the abdominal viscera are seen very poorly because of a lack of fat around the viscera, which normally offers contrast because of its more radiolucent nature. If gas is present within loops of small bowel they are spread apart and the soft-tissue space between contiguous gas shadows is increased over the normal. Fluid in the flanks causes increase in the soft-tissue space between the radiolucent flank stripe (properitoneal fat line) and the adjacent gas-filled colon. It also causes an outward bulging and increased definition of the properitoneal fat line. In upright roentgenograms the fluid sinks to the most dependent part of the abdominal cavity and forms a homogeneous increase in density. This is limited to the pelvis if the amount of fluid is small or it may extend higher if a large effusion is present. The upper boundary of the fluid is not sharp but the density gradually diminishes superiorly. It is limited inferiorly by a convex margin and frequently delineated from the urinary bladder by a narrow translucent zone. If gas is present in the small intestine, the loops float above the fluid and thus are not found within the pelvis as they normally would be. Similar findings are to be noted in lateral decubitus roentgenograms with the fluid sinking to the dependent side and the gas-filled loops of bowel rising. If fluid for one reason or another should be loculated, it will not shift in position but remain in the same position regardless of the position of the patient. Such loculations may simulate the appearance caused by solid tumors or abscesses and usually the differentiation is not possible from roentgen observation. For the identification of small to moderate-sized accumulations of fluid it is recommended, therefore, that roentgenograms be obtained with the patient recumbent and in upright or lateral decubitus positions.

INTRA-ABDOMINAL ABSCESSES

The shadow of the abscess may be visualized as an area of increased density, particularly if it is surrounded by gas-filled loops of bowel. Frequently, however, it is too indistinct in outline to be recognized clearly except as a zone of ill-defined density. The signs of generalized peritonitis may be present, including separation of the gas-filled loops, because of exudate on the surface of the bowel wall or fluid in the peritoneal cavity. A paralytic ileus is likely to be found in association with the infection so that distention of loops of small intestine and of colon is very often present. The shadow of an abscess may be confused with that of a tumor or even with a fluid-filled strangulated loop of bowel (the pseudotumor sign of Frimann-Dahl, *q.v.*) (see Fig. 13-13). Correlation of the roentgen observations with the clinical findings is essential in many of these cases in order more clearly to evaluate the roentgen findings.

If the abscess has developed as a result of perforation of the stomach or bowel, gas may enter it; or gas may form as a result of infection by gas-forming organisms (Fig. 13-34). When this happens, the interior of the abscess may have a mottled radiolucent appearance

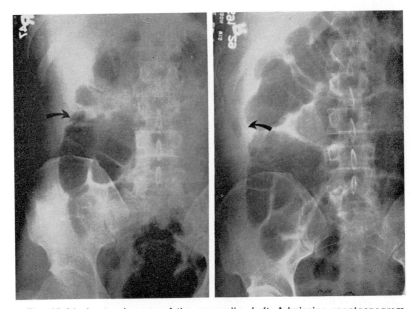

Fig. 13-34. Acute abscess of the appendix. *Left*, Admission roentgenogram. There is gas distention of the cecum. There are small irregular gas shadows along the upper outer margin of the cecum (**arrow**). *Right*, Several days later. The gas distention (ileus) of the bowel has increased. The extraluminal gas is more definite and there is a soft-tissue mass along the lateral abdominal wall (**arrow**). Findings indicate a ruptured retrocecal appendix with abscess formation.

caused by gas bubbles intermixed with necrotic material or pus (Fig. 13-35). In upright or lateral decubitus roentgenograms a gas-fluid level may be demonstrated if the cavity contains pus. This may be confused with gas accumulations within the bowel. Distinguishing features include the constancy in position of the gas shadows regardless of the position of the patient when multiple roentgenograms are obtained and constancy of the shadows in serial roentgenograms; at times the location of the shadows clearly indicates them to be outside the lumen of the bowel. Barium enema or barium-meal studies may show the lesion responsible and reveal the sinus tract leading from the lumen to the abscess (e.g., a ruptured colonic diverticulum).

SUBDIAPHRAGMATIC ABSCESS

Infection in the subphrenic space is more common on the right side than on the left. The earliest roentgen findings are those of elevation of the hemidiaphragm and restriction of its motion (Fig. 13-36). These changes are not characteristic of a subdiaphragmatic abscess, since other causes may be responsible for them. It is necessary at this stage, therefore, that the roentgen findings be considered in conjunction with the clinical signs and only when there is evidence to indicate the likelihood of a subphrenic abscess are these observations to be considered significant. During the immediate period after upper abdominal surgery, it is not at all uncommon to find the

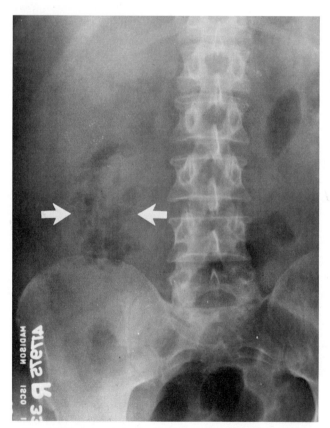

Fig. 13-35. Intra-abdominal abscess secondary to perforation of a carcinoma of the colon. The accumulation of mottled gas shadows (**arrows**) is extraluminal as shown by constancy in serial roentgenograms and confirmed by barium enema, and, later, by surgery.

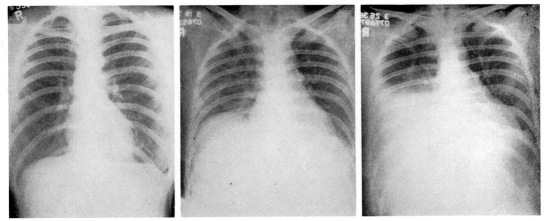

Fig. 13-36. Acute subdiaphragmatic abscess. *Left,* Normal appearance of the chest prior to the onset of subphrenic infection. *Center,* Roentgenogram of chest at the bedside several days after the onset of symptoms referable to developing subphrenic infection, following a laparotomy. The right leaf of the diaphragm is elevated but this finding is not specific and may be from a number of causes. *Right,* Seven days later. There is pleural effusion on the right side that obscures the diaphragm. The progressive changes as observed in serial roentgenograms and considered with the clinical findings led to the diagnosis of subdiaphragmatic abscess. This was evacuated surgically. The pleural effusion was not purulent (sympathetic effusion).

diaphragm elevated, especially the right leaf, and its motion restricted because of abdominal distention or pain or a combination of both. This sign must be interpreted with particular caution during the postoperative period.

The next change to be observed is an inflammatory pleural reaction at the base of the lung and the development of pleural effusion. The fluid usually is not purulent and is sometimes referred to as a "sympathetic effusion." Once an appreciable amount of fluid has formed, the diaphragm becomes obscured and it may be difficult to determine its position. Examination of the chest with the patient recumbent and in right and left lateral decubitus positions may cause enough shifting of the fluid to allow at least a partial visualization of the diaphragm.

Gas formation within the abscess cavity is rather frequent and can be demonstrated in upright or lateral decubitus roentgenograms. These should always be obtained as a part of the study of a suspected or known subdiaphragmatic abscess. The gas surmounting the fluid leads to the formation of a fluid level and this gives one of the most significant roentgen findings for the diagnosis (Fig. 13-37).

The signs of a left-sided subphrenic abscess are similar to those described above. In addition, displacement of the stomach downward, medially, and often anteriorly may be seen. In some cases the displacement can be recognized by the position of the gastric air bubble; at other times the introduction of a small amount of barium-water mixture may be needed to more clearly outline the entire stomach and demonstrate the evidence of the extragastric mass.

The roentgen findings in perirenal abscess are discussed in Chapter 20.

FOREIGN BODIES

A scout roentgenogram is useful for determining the presence or absence of opaque foreign bodies in the gastrointestinal tract or within the peritoneal cavity. In order to be sufficiently radiopaque to be visualized, metallic objects must be made of or contain one of the heavier metals such as iron, gold, or silver. Objects composed entirely of aluminum are of almost the same density as the soft tissues and

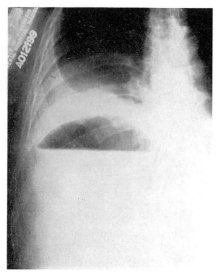

Fig. 13-37. Subdiaphragmatic abscess. Upright roentgenogram reveals gas and fluid in the abscess cavity. The dome-shaped upper boundary of the gas represents the diaphragm. There is fluid in the pleural cavity, accounting for the increased density above the diaphragm.

therefore not readily visualized. During infancy and early childhood the swallowing of coins, pins, and nails is very common. Psychiatric patients in mental hospitals often swallow objects such as pins, paper clips, and the like. Roentgenograms are useful to confirm the presence of the foreign body and to follow its course through the gastrointestinal tract.

Attention has been called to the occurrence of radiopaque shadows in the gastrointestinal tract following the eating of dirt. This condition is known as *geophagia*. The practice of dirt-eating apparently is widespread among female Negroes in parts of the South. According to Clayton and Goodman[10] the diagnosis is suggested by "the finding of unusually radiopaque contents in a patient who has not had any roentgenographic contrast studies and who is not taking any medicine containing radiopaque ingredients."

The presence of retained surgical sponges can be established if a radiopaque type of sponge has been used. There are several varieties of these sponges and they depend for radiopacity upon an insert of barium or other metallic impregnated string or cloth. This type of sponge should be used routinely in surgical procedures within the body cavities. Because sponge counts occasionally indicate a missing sponge a roentgenogram of the abdomen made in the operating room before closing the incision will give the operating surgeon peace of mind if no radiopaque shadows are seen or allow him to search for and remove the object before closure.

INTRAMURAL GAS

In addition to the entity known as pneumatosis cystoides intestinalis (see page 435) gas may be found within the wall of one or more loops of bowel in certain other diseases. These include: (1) necrotizing gastroenterocolitis, usually in infants; (2) mesenteric vascular thrombosis; (3) necrosis secondary to strangulated obstruction; (4) toxic ulcerative colitis; and (5) in ulcerative disease developing above an obstructing carcinoma of the colon. Some authors prefer to use the term, pneumatosis cystoides intestinalis, to include all entities in which intramural gas is found. Others limit it to the idiopathic, usually asymptomatic form. The pathogenesis may vary but in most cases there is necrosis of a segment of intestine and the gas probably enters through a break or breaks in the mucosa. In patients with obstruction the increase in intraluminal pressure above the lesion also may play a part (Fig. 13-38). Infection with gas-forming organisms has been noted less frequently but can be a cause of intramural gas.

In patients with necrosis or impending necrosis there may be a solitary abnormal segment of bowel or, at the most, several segments adjacent to one another. The segments contain an excessive amount of fluid, the mucosal folds are widened owing to edema and there is thickening of the wall of the bowel. These changes can be determined if there also is gas within the lumen to outline the folds and two adjacent abnormal segments are found so that wall thickness can be estimated.

The intramural gas is seen as linear, stripe-like translucencies paralleling the lumen of the

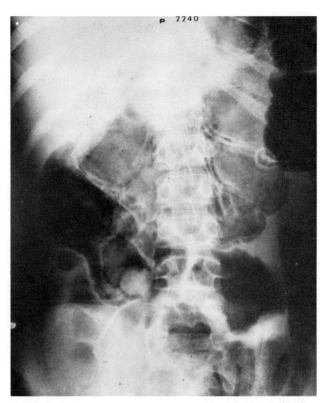

Fig. 13-38. Pneumatosis intestinalis in a patient with low colonic obstruction. The intramural gas is seen as thin radiolucent stripes along the margins of the gas-distended bowel.

intestine (see Fig. 13-30). If the segment is seen end-on, a ring-contoured translucency is formed as the intramural gas surrounds the gas-filled lumen of the bowel. Later as frank necrosis develops the mucosal folds tend to disappear and the internal surface becomes relatively smooth.

In association with the intramural gas there may be gas filling of the portal veins which are seen as linear branching translucencies in the peripheral parts of the liver (Fig. 13-39); these two findings form a highly significant roentgen complex for the diagnosis of intestinal necrosis.

THE PANCREAS

ROENTGEN ANATOMY

The pancreas is situated along the posterior abdominal wall in the upper abdomen in intimate relationship to the stomach and duodenum. The head of the gland usually lies directly in front of the lumbar spine and is surrounded by the duodenal loop. The third portion of the duodenum crosses obliquely in front of the pancreas to its junction with the jejunum, where it forms the angle of Treitz. The central portion or body of the pancreas usually lies directly posterior to the body and antrum of the stomach, separated from it by the omental bursa, which in turn is bounded posteriorly by the pancreas and anteriorly by the posterior wall of the stomach. The tail of the pancreas is in contact with the medial surface of the spleen. The pancreas cannot be identified in roentgenograms of the abdomen. Its borders are indistinct and it blends with the soft tissues of the posterior wall of the abdomen. In recent years considerable investigative work has been done on arteriography of the celiac axis and superior mesenteric arteries in diseases of the pancreas, particularly carcinoma. This is discussed on page 453. Otherwise the roentgen diagnosis of pancre-

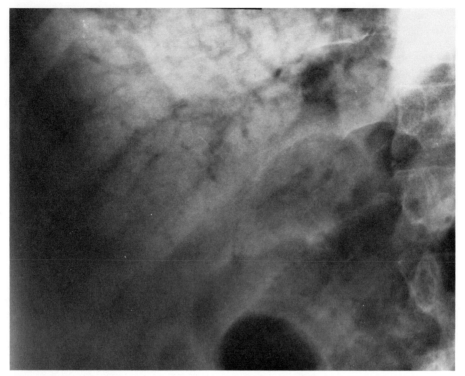

Fig. 13-39. Gas within the portal veins secondary to intestinal necrosis. The gas is seen as branching, translucent shadows extending to the peripheral parts of the liver.

atic disease depends to a large extent upon the changes produced in adjacent structures, particularly the stomach, duodenum, and transverse colon. Only when calcifications are found within the pancreas is there characteristic and direct roentgen evidence of disease. In spite of these drawbacks there are a number of findings that occur in various diseases of the pancreas and that offer considerable information, particularly when they are correlated with the clinical signs and symptoms. Scout roentgenograms of the abdomen as well as gastrointestinal studies with barium sulfate and angiography have a place in the study of the pancreas, as will be indicated in succeeding paragraphs.

ACUTE PANCREATITIS

In the presence of acute pancreatitis, roentgen examination may be of considerable value in helping to exclude other causes of acute abdominal pain, such as calculi in the biliary or urinary tracts, ruptured peptic ulcer, and acute bowel obstruction. In addition, in many patients other findings will be present to direct attention to the pancreas as the site of disease. In general the roentgen findings must be interpreted in the light of clinical symptoms and signs since by themselves the changes may be too nonspecific to allow definitive diagnosis.

SCOUT ROENTGENOGRAMS

Preliminary or "scout" roentgenograms should include supine and upright projections as a routine with the addition of lateral decubitus views in cases with equivocal findings. Among the changes that may be observed are the following:

REGIONAL OR LOCALIZED ILEUS ("SENTINEL LOOPS"). Localized gas distention of one or more loops of bowel immediately adjacent to the pancreas may be found. The duodenum may be filled with gas or a loop of jejunum may be visualized in this manner (Fig. 13-40). In some cases a segment of the transverse colon is distended. The more localized the distention and the closer the relationship of the loops to the pancreas, the more significant is the observation. Fluid levels usually are present in the loops when upright or lateral decubitus views are obtained. When both the stomach and the transverse colon are distended with gas there may be an unusually wide soft-tissue space between them; normally they are in close relationship and separated by a thin space equivalent to the thickness of their walls.

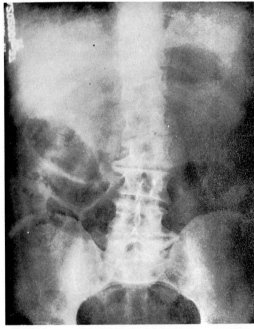

Fig. 13-40. Acute pancreatitis. Anteroposterior roentgenogram of the abdomen shows gas-distended loops of small intestine, probably ileum, in the right upper quadrant and extending across the midline (sentinel loops). This represents localized adynamic ileus and while it is not characteristic of acute pancreatitis, it is highly suggestive of the presence of an acute inflammation in the vicinity. Similar findings are observed in acute appendicitis (Fig. 13-20), acute cholecystitis, and other localized inflammations.

Because of its close relationship to the pancreas, gas distention of the duodenum is more suggestive of acute pancreatitis than is distention of a jejunal loop. The finding of localized gas distention of the midtransverse colon also is significant.

GENERALIZED ILEUS. Not infrequently by the time the patient is examined roentgenologically the signs have become those of a more or less generalized adynamic ileus. If there has been a spread of inflammation beyond the confines of the pancreas so that fairly extensive peritoneal inflammation is present, there may be evidence of exudate separating the gas-filled loops. In the later or more advanced stages of the inflammation such generalized signs are frequent and by themselves are of little value in establishing the exact cause of the difficulty.

LOCALIZED ACCUMULATIONS OF FLUID. With extension of the inflammation beyond the confines of the pancreas localized accumulations of fluid may form either in the immediate area of the pancreas or occasionally at some distance from it. These are known as pseudocysts. Such a mass may be visible as a soft-tissue shadow with ill-defined borders. When a collection of fluid forms adjacent to the pancreas or in the lesser peritoneal sac, displacement of the stomach, colon, and duodenum may indicate the presence of the lesion. The inflammation may spread to the subphrenic space and form a subphrenic abscess on either side although this complication is more frequent on the left. Spread to the subphrenic space results in elevation of the hemidiaphragm, restriction of its motion, and within a short time the development of pleural effusion. Rarely the infection may burrow through the diaphragm and cause an empyema or it may extend into the mediastinum with formation of a mediastinal abscess.

CHANGES IN THE LUNGS. As indicated in the preceding paragraph, extension of inflammation to the subphrenic space will cause elevation and fixation of the diaphragm. Linear streaks of density frequently can be visualized crossing the lung field in its basal portion in these patients. These linear shadows represent foci of platelike atelectasis and are the result of restriction of diaphragmatic motion. They are, of course, not specific for acute pancreatitis.

PANCREATIC CALCULI. If the attack represents an acute exacerbation of a chronic pancreatitis, calculi may be visualized in some cases (see discussion of pancreatic lithiasis to follow).

BARIUM MEAL EXAMINATION

Many patients with acute pancreatitis are too ill to be subjected to gastrointestinal examinations but, according to Poppel,[29] important information can be obtained by this method. Some of the changes that may be observed in acute pancreatitis or during an acute exacerbation of chronic disease are the following:

ENLARGEMENT OF THE PAPILLA OF VATER. The normal papilla is sometimes seen as a smoothly rounded, filling defect along the medial aspect of the descending duodenum approximately 1 cm in diameter and 0.5 cm in height. During the acute stage of pancreatitis the papillary defect enlarges. The mucosal folds of the duodenum adjacent to it become thickened. With a greater degree of swelling the pancreas may bulge into the duodenum and surround the ampulla, causing a defect that resembles a figure 3 in reverse. This sign, originally described by Frostberg,[16] is not specific for pancreatitis; it also occurs when the pancreas is enlarged as a result of neoplasm of the periampullary region.

FUNCTIONAL DISTURBANCES OF THE DUODENUM. The duodenal motility may be altered, often being increased over the normal. Peristalsis is hyperactive and reverse peristalsis may be seen. The duodenum often undergoes spasmlike contraction and is unduly irritable. The mucosal folds may be altered, being coarsened or thickened.

OTHER SIGNS OF ACUTE PANCREATITIS. The left psoas muscle margin and the left renal outline may be blurred in the presence of acute pancreatitis. The left kidney at times is displaced slightly downward and outward. The stomach may be displaced forward if the pancreas is enlarged.

Intravenous urography may reveal impairment of the left renal function if there has been sufficient pressure on the renal artery or vein to interfere with its circulation. Localized tenderness directly over the region of the pancreas may be elicited during fluoroscopic observation. With recurrent attacks of acute pancreatitis (relapsing pancreatitis), calculi may be demonstrable within the gland (see section on "Pancreatic Lithiasis").

ENLARGEMENT OF THE PANCREAS

Enlargement of the pancreas may be caused either by inflammation or neoplasm and in many cases it is impossible on the basis of roentgen examination to determine which condition exists. In some cases the invasive nature of a carcinoma may be apparent as it extends into the duodenum or the stomach. In others the roentgen signs are minimal or completely absent. The chief roentgen findings that may be observed when the pancreas enlarges include the following:

ENLARGEMENT OF THE DUODENAL LOOP

Because the duodenum surrounds the head of the pancreas and is in intimate relationship to it, any appreciable enlargement of the pancreatic head causes widening of the duodenal loop. The duodenal curve becomes rounded (Fig. 13-41). This sign has long been described as one of the important roentgen features of pancreatic enlargement. It is of considerable diagnostic value when present but minor to moderate degrees of enlargement are difficult to recognize. The range of normal variation in the appearance of the duodenal curve is considerable and must be taken into account when considering the possibility of pancreatic enlargement. In obese individuals it is always more rounded and smooth than in persons of average habitus, and in some of these, it may appear actually enlarged. This is caused by the high transverse position of the stomach and the accumulations of fat in the pancreatic area.

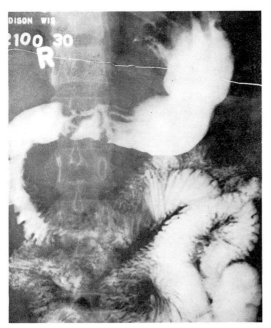

Fig. 13-41. Chronic pancreatitis. The enlargement of the head of the pancreas has widened the duodenal loop. There is flattening of the mucosal folds on the inner side of the descending duodenum.

FORWARD DISPLACEMENT OF THE STOMACH

This is another sign difficult to evaluate unless the displacement is of considerable degree. The normal distance between the posterior surface of the stomach and the anterior border of the spine varies considerably in different persons and is much influenced by the habitus of the individual. A distended colon, the presence of ascites, or a large mass such as an ovarian cyst may elevate the stomach and cause the retrogastric space to appear unusually wide. The most accurate determination of the width of the retrogastric space is obtained by examining the patient in a supine position with a horizontally directed roentgen-ray beam passing transversely through the abdomen, the film cassette being placed along one side. This gives a lateral view of the abdomen with the stomach riding over the anterior surface of the pancreas. The stomach can be filled either with air introduced through a tube placed within it or with orally administered barium meal. The latter is generally preferred because of its simplicity. For standard examination the ordinary right lateral view of the stomach is adequate and this is obtained as a routine during examination of the upper gastrointestinal tract.

CHANGES IN THE MUCOSAL PATTERN OF THE DUODENUM; HYPOTONIC DUODENOGRAPHY

The effect of pancreatic enlargement upon the mucosal pattern of the duodenum often is a significant roentgen observation and is a more obvious sign of early enlargement than is rounding of the duodenal curve or forward displacement of the stomach. These folds may appear unusually thick and rigid. They may be flattened along the inner side of the duodenum and relatively normal on the outer (Figs. 13-42 and 13-43). When carcinoma of the head of the pancreas is present there may be actual invasion of the duodenal wall shown by a loss

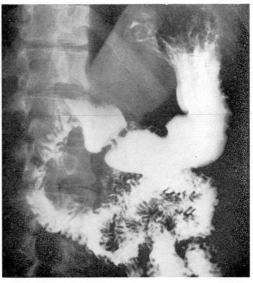

Fig. 13-42. Carcinoma of the head of the pancreas. Barium filling of the stomach and duodenum. There is a pressure defect on the inner side of the descending duodenum and the mucosal folds are flattened and distorted. The mass lies adjacent to the ampulla of Vater. The sharp junction between the first and second portions of the duodenum is caused by the dilated common duct, which is obstructed by the tumor.

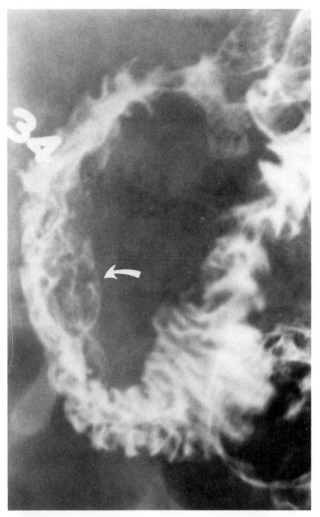

Fig. 13-43. Carcinoma of the head of the pancreas. The duodenal curve is shown with the mass indenting the wall and distorting the mucosa on the inner side of the descending duodenum (**arrow**). Chronic pancreatitis might cause similar changes.

of mucosal pattern, with irregular nodular protrusions into the duodenal lumen; or constricted stenotic areas may be produced leading to duodenal obstruction. When the body of the pancreas is enlarged there may be evidence of compression of the transverse portion of the duodenum where it passes over the pancreas, the folds being flattened and the lumen of the duodenum narrowed in an anteroposterior direction.

HYPOTONIC DUODENOGRAPHY. This is a method for giving a more detailed study of the effects of pancreatic and other disease upon the mucosa of the duodenum. In brief, the technique consists in the intramuscular injection of 30 to 60 mg of Pro-Banthine after the duodenum has been intubated. Within about 5 minutes after injection of the drug, the duodenum becomes dilated and hypotonic with absence of peristalsis. About 50 to 75 ml of barium sulfate mixture is then introduced through the tube and spot films are made. The barium is aspirated and from 100 to 150 ml of air are injected and further spot films are obtained. The finer detail of the duodenal mucosa is brought out to good advantage and the effects of pressure or invasion from a contiguous mass can be identified more easily than with a routine barium meal. The procedure is, in effect, an extension of the usual barium sulfate meal. A similar procedure but without intubation has been advocated by some. The normal amount of swallowed air is used for double contrast, being manipulated into the duodenum by positioning of the patient and the barium sulfate being given orally.

THE REVERSE FIGURE 3 SIGN

Frostberg[16] originally called attention to a distinct alteration in the appearance of the inner wall of the descending duodenum in cases of pancreatic enlargement, which he described as a reverse figure 3. This is caused by swelling of the pancreas either from inflammation or neoplasm, with bulging of the gland into the duodenal lumen surrounding the papilla of Vater. This causes a smooth filling defect above and below the papilla that resembles a figure 3 in reverse (Fig. 13-44). It is a valuable sign of pancreatic disease but in itself does not distinguish between swelling caused by inflammation and that resulting from tumor.

EVIDENCE OF A DILATED COMMON BILE DUCT

The common bile duct lies in close relationship to the duodenum, usually crossing just posterior to the junction of the first and second portions. Because of this close relationship, dilatation of the common duct may cause a pressure defect on the duodenum. This may be in the form of a bandlike compression or flattening of the duodenum, or a sharp angulation of the apex of the duodenal bulb and its continuation into the descending portion (see Fig. 13-42). The right lateral position is of value in showing this deformity but it also can be demonstrated frequently in the standard right

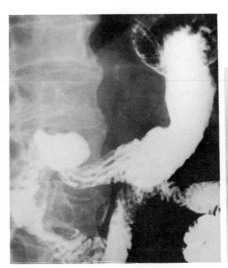
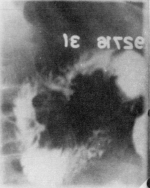

Fig. 13-44. Two patients having changes in the duodenum secondary to carcinoma of the head of the pancreas illustrate the reversed figure 3 sign of Frostberg. The inner margin of the descending duodenum resembles a figure 3 in reverse. The illustration on the right is a spot roentgenogram made at the time of fluoroscopy, showing the duodenal loop and the nodular encroachment on the lumen by the tumor mass that surrounds the ampulla.

anterior oblique position. This sign only indicates obstruction of the distal portion of the common duct but its significance in relation to pancreatic disease is obvious. Tumors of the periampullary region are prone to cause dilatation of the common duct and this may be the only roentgen abnormality that can be demonstrated.

THE "PAD" SIGN

The pad sign is a localized, smooth, pressure type of deformity, usually on the inferior surface of the gastric antrum or duodenal bulb, resembling closely that which can be produced by applying pressure over the anterior abdominal wall by a pressure pad or by manual palpation (Fig. 13-45). Occasionally the pad defect is observed along the superior surface of the duodenal bulb or gastric antrum since the relationships of the stomach and pancreas need not be constant. This sign originally described by Case[11] and reemphasized by Hodes and others[17] is best brought out by having the patient face the top of an upright fluoroscopic table and then tilting the table slowly toward the horizontal position under fluoroscopic observation. Pressure of the spine on the gastric antrum can simulate the pad sign when the patient is prone on the fluoroscopic table, but the effect of pressure from an enlarged pancreas will appear before the table has reached a horizontal position. Careful palpation of the abdominal wall with the patient upright also may demonstrate this defect.

VISUALIZATION OF THE COMMON BILE DUCT (CHOLANGIOGRAPHY)

Using one of the newer cholecystographic media, such as iopanoic acid (Telepaque), it is usual to be able to visualize the common duct when good gallbladder function is present. Even when the gallbladder is diseased, the common duct often is visualized if a double dose of iopanoic acid is administered. Demonstration of the duct occurs most frequently during the phase of gallbladder contraction following a fat meal. Another method for visualization of the common duct, of value particularly when gallbladder dis-

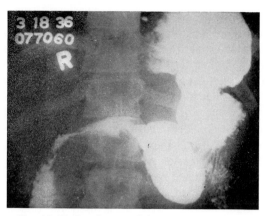

Fig. 13-45. Carcinoma of the head of the pancreas illustrating the "pad sign." Smooth-pressure defect on the inferior surface of the duodenal bulb and gastric antrum, indicates a mass in the region of the head of the pancreas.

ease interferes with its function or in patients in whom the gallbladder has been removed, consists in the intravenous injection of a contrast substance known as Cholografin. This material is excreted by the liver in a sufficiently high concentration so that the bile is radiopaque as it leaves the liver and thus the common duct may be outlined. These methods of examination are discussed in more detail in Chapter 14. If the common duct can be identified by rendering its bile content radiopaque, obstruction in the distal portion may be demonstrated because of the dilatation of the duct above the level of obstruction. These methods require reasonably good liver function and if there has been very much liver damage results often are unsatisfactory. The method does offer some chance for detection of early obstructions caused by tumors involving the ampulla.

More recently the method of direct puncture of the common duct or of a hepatic radicle through the abdominal wall and liver (percutaneous transhepatic cholangiography) has been used to demonstrate the presence of common duct obstruction and, often, the nature of the lesion responsible. This is discussed in Chapter 14 under the section entitled "Percutaneous Transhepatic Cholangiography."

PANCREATIC LITHIASIS

The formation of calculi within the ducts or possibly in the parenchyma of the pancreas gives one of the most striking and direct roentgen signs of pancreatic disease. In most cases the calcifications occur in association with chronic pancreatitis and the roentgen demonstration of them usually indicates the existence of this disease. Occasionally, however, pancreatic lithiasis is found in an individual who shows none of the clinical signs or symptoms of pancreatitis. Some investigators believe that all pancreatic calcifications form within the ducts; others consider that the concretions may form either in the ducts or in the gland parenchyma.

Pancreatic calculi are usually multiple and are seen in the roentgenogram as dense, small calcified areas throughout a portion or the entire gland. The effect is usually one of calcific stippling, since most of the stones are likely to be small (Fig. 13-46). The calculi are found most frequently in the head of the pancreas but it is not uncommon to have them widely distributed throughout the gland. When relatively few in number and limited to the region of the head, the stones may be overlooked in routine supine or prone roentgenograms of the abdomen because the head of the pancreas usually lies directly over the upper lumbar vertebrae. They are seen to best advantage when the roentgenograms are made with the patient turned to a slightly oblique position that projects the pancreatic head to one side of the spine. If there is doubt concerning the nature of the shadows, a barium meal can be given and the relationship of the calcifications to the duodenal loop determined. In most cases the small dense and discrete calcifications clustered in the region of the pancreas make the diagnosis of pancreatic lithiasis not too difficult. Renal and gallbladder calculi seldom cause difficulty in differential diagnosis because of the location and character of the shadows. Gallstones often are laminated while pancreatic calculi rarely are. In doubtful cases cholecystography or intravenous urography may be used to localize the calculi in relation to these structures. Calcified lymph nodes cause the greatest difficulty. When the pancreatic calcifications are few in number they may resemble the appearance of calcified nodes rather closely. Roentgenograms of the barium-filled

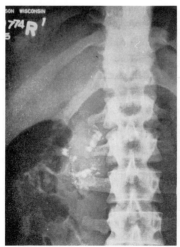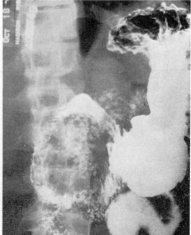

Fig. 13-46. Pancreatic lithiasis. *Left,* Anteroposterior roentgenogram of the right upper abdomen showing a cluster of small irregular calcifications in the head of the pancreas. *Right,* Extensive calcifications throughout the pancreas. Roentgenogram of the stomach and duodenum shows the numerous granular calculi in the pancreas. Note the enlargement and rounding of the duodenal curve, indicating that the head of the pancreas is enlarged. The duodenal mucosa also is flattened from pressure.

stomach and duodenum will help to localize the calculi and establish their position in relation to the pancreas. In most cases the small discrete calcifications distributed over a fairly wide area differ from the larger mulberry type of calcifications found in lymph nodes. Calcified plaques in the aorta or in branches of the celiac axis or other branches of the aorta also must be considered. Usually the linear nature of such plaques when they are viewed on edge or their curvilinear or circular shape when seen on end are sufficiently characteristic for proper identification.

CHRONIC PANCREATITIS

The roentgen signs of chronic pancreatitis include the evidence of pancreatic enlargement, the presence of pancreatic calcifications, and changes secondary to pancreatic steatorrhea. The changes caused by enlargement of the pancreas have been enumerated and discussed above and, as indicated in the previous section, the roentgen demonstration of an enlarged pancreas frequently does not allow a differential diagnosis to be made between inflammation and tumor. The presence of pancreatic lithiasis is reasonably good evidence of the coexistence of chronic pancreatitis. This has been discussed in the section entitled "Pancreatic Lithiasis." Steatorrhea may be caused by disease of the pancreas, particularly by chronic pancreatitis. The clinical features of pancreatogenic steatorrhea resemble those of idiopathic sprue and the roentgen findings in the gastrointestinal tract may be similar. These conditions have been discussed in Chapter 18 under the heading, "Malabsorption Syndromes." Some recent observations indicate that the small-intestinal changes are less severe in pancreatogenic steatorrhea than they are in the idiopathic form of the disease (nontropical sprue) and in some cases the small-bowel pattern may be normal or nearly so. Rather infrequently chronic pancreatitis may cause an osteomalacic picture in the skeletal system characterized by generalized demineralization of the skeleton and the occurrence of pseudofractures in some of the

bones. These are highly characteristic of osteomalacia and are visualized as fissure-like defects or clefts extending transversely part way or completely through a bone. They represent fracture fissures filled with uncalcified osteoid. They are seen most frequently along the axillary borders of the scapulas, the inner margins of the femoral necks, and in the ribs. In severe cases, however, they may be rather widely distributed in the skeleton.

CARCINOMA OF THE PANCREAS

The roentgen findings in carcinoma of the pancreas have been covered, to a large extent, in the section dealing with enlargement of the pancreas. Some observations concerning tumors of the periampullary region also have been made in this chapter. As indicated earlier, it often is impossible to distinguish between inflammatory and neoplastic enlargements of the gland. In some cases direct invasion of the duodenum or the gastric antrum may have occurred and the infiltrative and destructive nature of the lesion may be readily apparent. For example, a carcinoma arising in the head of the pancreas may extend into the duodenum, causing an irregular nodular filling defect, loss of mucosal folds, abnormal fixation, stiffening of the duodenal wall, and ulceration. Partial or complete obstruction of the duodenum may be caused by carcinoma of the pancreas; this is an unusual complication of pancreatitis. The demonstration of pancreatic lithiasis in association with the signs of pancreatic enlargement is good evidence of the presence of chronic pancreatitis, although the possibility of coexisting carcinoma cannot be excluded entirely even in these cases.

The frequency of positive roentgen evidence in cases of pancreatic carcinoma depends upon the location of the tumor within the gland and to some extent upon its duration. Those lesions arising in the head of the pancreas, particularly in the periampullary region, will give positive roentgen findings more often and earlier than those that develop in the body or tail of the gland. In general about 50 per cent of all pancreatic carcinomas will show some evidence of their presence on roentgen examination if careful attention is paid to the early signs of pressure and invasion as noted above. It is emphasized again that even when findings are present it may not be possible to state the nature of the lesion from roentgen examination alone and the diagnosis may have to be limited to that of a mass in or near the pancreas.

PANCREATIC CYSTS

True cysts of the pancreas are infrequent lesions from a roentgen point of view because they seldom become large enough to cause the signs of a pancreatic mass. They arise as a result of ductal obstruction, usually from a chronic pancreatitis. A more common lesion is the pancreatic pseudocyst. This represents an encapsulation of fluid caused by escape of pancreatic juice beyond the confines of the pancreas. It may follow an acute pancreatitis, a surgically produced injury to the gland, or trauma to the abdomen with rupture of the pancreas. The history often is that of a rapidly enlarging mass in the upper abdomen that follows one of the episodes listed above. When the stomach and duodenum are outlined with barium, the mass of the cyst causes a smooth rounded pressure enlargement of the duodenal curve. The stomach is pushed forward and it may be displaced upward or downward, often being freely movable over the mass so that the pressure defect varies upon change in position of the patient (Fig. 13-47). The cyst may present itself at a distance from the pancreas although it usually is in close relationship. It may burrow in any direction and it is possible to have the mass lie below the transverse colon, displacing the colon upwards.

Differentiation of a pancreatic cyst from other retroperitoneal masses may be difficult and often is impossible. To be considered in this connection are carcinoma of the pancreas, primary and metastatic neoplasms of the retroperitoneal lymph nodes, aneurysm of the abdominal aorta, and mesenteric cysts. Carcinoma of the pancreas usually does not reach the size that cysts commonly

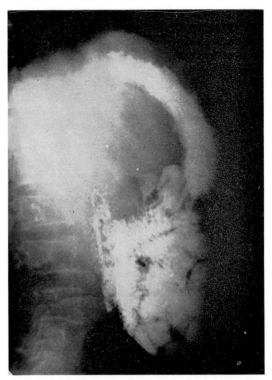

Fig. 13-47. Pseudocyst of the pancreas. Lateral roentgenogram of the barium-filled stomach, shows it displaced anteriorly by a large retrogastric mass. The cyst was secondary to a chronic pancreatitis.

do and the invasive nature of the tumor may be evident. Fixation of the stomach to the tumor is frequent while this is less common with cysts, the stomach moving freely over the mass. Primary or metastatic tumors of the lymph nodes resemble carcinoma of the pancreas more than they do cysts. Mesenteric cysts usually are freely movable over a fairly wide area; pancreatic cysts are fixed.

ANGIOGRAPHY OF THE PANCREAS

Visualization of the vessels supplying the pancreas is obtained following catheterization of the celiac axis and superior mesenteric arteries using the Seldinger method of percutaneous puncture of the femoral artery. There is some difference of opinion as to the value of the procedure in pancreatic disease, particularly in the diagnosis of carcinoma of the pancreas. The arteriographic findings include (*1*) irregular encasement of arteries by the tumor, (*2*) occlusion of larger arterial branches, (*3*) compression of veins, and, (*4*) abnormal tumor vessels and tumor stain. Unfortunately in most patients the latter findings are not often observed and diagnosis depends upon the findings of irregular constriction, displacement and occlusion of vessels, signs which are often difficult to interpret (Fig. 13-48). Nebesar and Pollard[25] in a retrospective study found that approximately 10 per cent were falsely positive, i.e., cases where carcinoma was diagnosed on the basis of angiographic findings but with tumor not found. Also, in 17 cases of proved malignant tumor there were eight false negatives. Others have commented on the fact that practically all patients with positive signs on arteriography were found to be inoperable at the time of surgery even though the clinical history was short, indicating its limited value in the detection of early lesions, particularly of

the body and tail of the pancreas. The diagnosis of pancreatitis could rarely be made in the series reported by Nebesar and Pollard.[25] Others, however, have reported better results and consider arteriography as the best method presently available for roentgen investigation of the pancreas.[7]

THE LIVER

The homogeneous density of the liver in the right uppper quadrant makes it rather easy to identify in roentgenograms of the abdomen. If not obscured by fluid or other pathologic changes within the thorax, the upper surface of the liver is outlined by the contour of the diaphragm. Part of the lower border of the right lobe usually is visible unless there is very little intra-abdominal fat to offer contrast or unless there is fluid in the peritoneal cavity. In these patients the liver blends imperceptibly with the general soft-tissue density of the abdomen. When the lower margin is not visualized, some information concerning the size of the liver can be obtained by noting the position of the gas-filled hepatic flexure of the colon. The lower margin of the left lobe of the liver cannot be identified.

The liver is transverse in position in persons of sthenic habitus; in the thin asthenic individual it assumes a much more vertical position and not infrequently the inferior edge of the right lobe extends to the plane of the posterior iliac crest. In certain of these individuals, notably in thin-waisted females, the medial surface of the vertically placed liver may present a V-shaped indentation so that the lower part of the lobe has a tonguelike downward extension. This is known as *Riedel's lobe* (Fig. 13-49). This formation causes the liver to project below the costal margin; it can be palpated and may lead to the erroneous impression of a tumor mass. An anomalous lobe along the superior surface of the liver has been described, causing a dome-shaped localized elevation of the anteromedial portion of the right diaphragm. It is more likely that this is actually a molding of the liver secondary to a

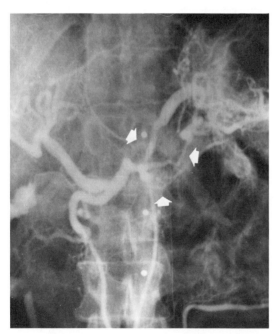

Fig. 13-48. Carcinoma of the pancreas. Celiac axis arteriogram shows obstruction, straightening, and narrowing of a group of vessels, i.e., tumor encasement (**left and right arrows**). There also is a small area of neovascularity (**lower arrow**).

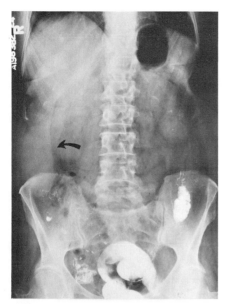

Fig. 13-49. Riedel's lobe of the liver. There is a tongue-like downward extension of the right lobe of the liver (**arrow**). Roentgenogram made after evacuation of a barium enema.

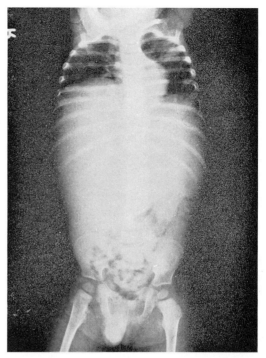

Fig. 13-50. Enlargement of the liver in a child with an undifferentiated carcinoma. The lower border of the greatly enlarged liver is demarcated by the gas in the displaced bowel.

localized developmental weakness or eventration of the diaphragm. Contrast visualization of the liver is discussed under the heading "Splenoportography."

LIVER SIZE

The determination of slight to moderate degrees of hepatomegaly by roentgen examination of the abdomen is difficult; this is more accurately done by clinical examination. The inferior costal margin is a good clinical landmark but it often is poorly localized in roentgenograms. When a moderate or more severe enlargement is present, downward displacement of the hepatic flexure of the colon can be demonstrated (Fig. 13-50). The stomach is displaced toward the left and backward. Posterior displacement of the stomach occurs with enlargement of the left lobe of the liver. A localized mass projecting from the surface of the liver may result in a more localized pressure deformity upon the stomach. In the presence of hepatic enlargement the right kid-

ney often is displaced downward. Generalized enlargement of the liver tends to cause an elevation of the diaphragm, the right side more than the left.

TUMORS OF THE LIVER

In many cases it is impossible to determine the nature of a tumor involving the liver from plain abdominal roentgenograms alone. Primary and metastatic neoplasms often cause only the signs of local or general enlargement. Calcification within the tumor is occasionally present. Hepatoma, the most common primary tumor of the liver, will show areas of mottled calcification in about one-third of all patients. Otherwise hepatoma causes only general or local enlargement of the liver. In some patients the liver becomes very large. Cavernous hemangioma may calcify, and, characteristically, the calcifications are in the form of trabeculae radiating from a densely calcified center. Metastatic deposits from mucinous adenocarcinoma of the gastrointestinal tract may show areas of hazy calcification. Intrahepatic cysts may show calcification in the wall thus outlining the mass (also see the section on "Calcification within the Liver"). The use of angiography in the detection of tumors of the liver is discussed under the section entitled "Angiography of the Liver."

LIVER ABSCESS

The roentgen signs of liver abscess usually are too indefinite to permit a diagnosis from plain roentgenograms. The size of the liver may be increased. If the abscess is near the superior surface there may be some restriction of motion of the right side of the diaphragm on fluoroscopic examination. Linear strandlike densities may be seen in the basal lung owing to atelectasis. If the abscess extends into the subphrenic space the roentgen signs become those of subphrenic infection (see discussion). Infection may extend to the pleura or even to the lung with the development of a lung abscess. Amebic abscesses cause changes similar to those of abscess from other causes. Radioisotope scanning of the liver may demonstrate the abscess as a "filling defect." On hepatic arteriography the abscess is seen as an avascular area within the liver. These two procedures are complementary and taken in conjunction with the clinical signs and symptoms often allow a correct diagnosis to be made.

CALCIFICATION WITHIN THE LIVER

Small, discrete, calcified areas, usually multiple, are occasionally seen within the liver. Often there are similar shadows within the spleen. These lesions probably are old, healed foci of tuberculosis or histoplasmosis. Current opinion leans toward the belief that widely disseminated calcified lesions of this nature are most often the result of a previous infection with *Histoplasma capsulatum*. Occasionally one or several larger areas of mottled calcification are visualized within the liver substance; these usually are the calcified residues of previous abscesses. *Echinococcus cysts* frequently involve the liver but this disease is

rare in this country. The cysts often are multiple and calcification in the wall is of common occurence (also see the section entitled "Tumors of the Liver"). Congenital cysts of the liver may be associated with polycystic disease of the kidneys. The calcified wall, if present, is usually thinner than is seen with hydatid disease and the cysts tend to be of uniform size (see Fig. 13-25).

INCREASED DENSITY OF THE LIVER

A homogeneous increase in density of the liver is found in some cases of hemochromatosis (bronze diabetes), presumably because of the heavy deposition of iron that occurs in this disease. The spleen is affected in the same manner. When diffuse increase in density of these organs is seen in abdominal roentgenograms, particularly when they are found to be enlarged, the diagnosis of hemochromatosis should be given consideration.

Another cause of increased density of the liver and spleen is the presence of retained thorium dioxide. This substance may have been used as a contrast agent for cerebral arteriography at some previous time. Thorium dioxide (Thorotrast) is picked up by the cells of the reticuloendothelial system and retained by them almost indefinitely. It is a very radiopaque substance and even the amount ordinarily used for cerebral arteriography (15 to 30 cc) may be sufficient to cause a relatively permanent increase in density of the liver and spleen. About 35 years ago this substance had a rather wide usage for contrast visualization of these structures but it is not employed at the present time.

Thorium possesses a low degree of radioactivity and its fixation in the tissues may lead to harmful effects over a period of years; there is evidence that it is carcinogenic.

GAS WITHIN THE PORTAL VEINS

This is a rare condition which may develop as a complication of mesenteric thrombosis or other cause of intestinal gangrene. The gas is found in the form of linear and branching shadows (see Fig. 13-39). Characteristically the gas is found in the more peripheral parts of the liver. This aids in distinguishing portal vein gas from gas in the biliary tract (see Chapter 14, the section entitled

"Gas in the Gallbladder or Biliary Ducts"). The condition carries a grave prognosis, since it usually indicates intestinal gangrene. In addition to mesenteric thrombosis, other forms of intestinal obstruction may be responsible.

ANGIOGRAPHY OF THE LIVER

The liver has two blood supplies, one arterial via the hepatic artery and the other venous via the portal vein. Blood leaves the liver through the hepatic veins which drain into the inferior vena cava. Methods for opacifying the portal venous system have been described under the section on "Splenoportography." Opacification of the hepatic artery and its branches is usually done after catheterization of the celiac axis or the hepatic artery selectively, the catheter being inserted percutaneously into the femoral artery using the Seldinger technique. Catheterization of the superior mesenteric artery should also be done as the liver may obtain part of its blood supply from this vessel. After the hepatic arteries have been

opacified the normal liver develops a uniform blush during the arterial hepatogram phase, as the small vessels and capillaries fill. This is followed by opacification of the hepatic veins. If the contrast material is injected into the celiac axis and the splenic artery is filled the splenoportal venous system will be visualized later (Fig. 13-51). After the portal veins empty, another blush of the liver occurs representing the venous hepatogram phase.

The method is particularly useful for the study of neoplasms, both primary and metastatic. The determination of the presence or absence of metastatic deposits in the liver is particularly important when assessment for operability is being done. Radioisotopic scanning methods also are useful in determining the presence of metastases and in some patients are preferred because of their simplicity and absence of complications. However most agree that the two procedures are complementary and both have a place in the investigation of the liver.

The roentgen findings during the arterial phase depend upon (*1*) stretching or displacement of ves-

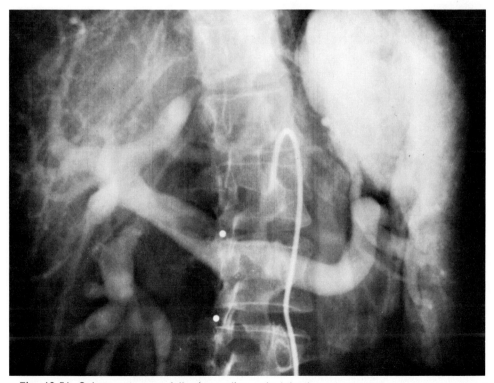

Fig. 13-51. Splenoportogram following celiac axis injection of contrast material. The tip of catheter is in celiac axis (note pyelogram from a previous injection). The splenic and portal veins are patent.

sels, (2) an area or areas of avascularity, and (3) neovascularity (the visualization of tumor vessels).[28] The first two signs are relatively nonspecific and are seen in some tumors, abscesses, cysts, and in necrotic tumors. The most significant findings are the visualization of abnormal vessels within the tumor or a tumor stain or blush in the hepatogram phase (Figs. 13-52 and 13-53). Of the metastatic lesions, the most vascular according to Pollard, Fleischli, and Nebesar[28] are those arising from malignant carcinoids, malignant islet cell tumor, leiomyosarcoma, and renal cell carcinoma. The first two demonstrate an intense tumor stain; the last two show large vessels within the tumor. Lesser degrees of neovascularity occur with metastatic adenocarcinoma of the breast, endometrium, and colon, carcinoma of the adrenal gland, seminoma, and some types of pancreatic carcinoma (other than adenocarcinoma). Avascular metastatic deposits are seen with adenocarcinoma of the pancreas, gallbladder, and bile ducts, and squamous cell carcinoma of the lung

and esophagus. If there are multiple avascular metastases the arterial hepatogram phase shows a diffusely mottled appearance which is relatively nonspecific.

Among the primary malignant tumors, hepatoma is the most common. It is a very vascular lesion with many tumor vessels and a dense stain in the hepatogram phase. Other malignant neoplasms show less specific angiographic changes. Of the benign tumors, hemangioma is one of the most common and shows characteristic changes in the arteriogram consisting of multiple, dilated vascular channels similar to cavernous hemangiomas elsewhere.

THE SPLEEN

The spleen lies in the posterior part of the abdomen in the left upper quadrant directly below the left leaf of the diaphragm and lateral to the fundus of the stomach. Its medial surface

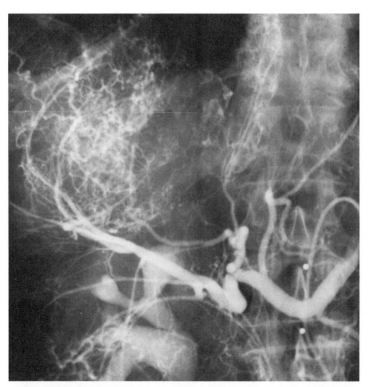

Fig. 13-52. Arteriogram in a patient with metastatic leiomyosarcoma of the liver. In addition to downward and lateral displacement of hepatic artery branches there is extensive filling of tumor vessels in the right lobe of the liver.

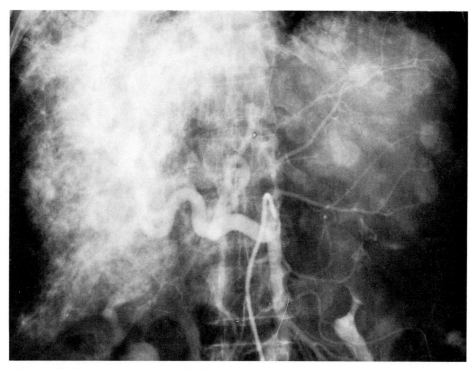

Fig. 13-53. Same patient as seen in Figure 13-52, during the capillary phase of angiogram. Note mottled blush throughout the right lobe of the liver and the more discrete, rounded areas of tumor blush on the left.

is in relationship to the stomach and the tail of the pancreas. Visualization of the spleen in routine roentgenograms of the abdomen is variable. The lower pole often is outlined by gas in the splenic flexure of the colon and the medial surface by the gastric air bubble or by the colon, which may lie medial to the spleen. Rarely, a tonguelike extension of the spleen projects into the space between the fundus of the stomach and the diaphragm, causing a filling defect that resembles closely that of an intramural tumor of the fundus. Infrequently the spleen is located below its usual position or it may be movable and descend when the patient is examined in an upright position. Such an abnormal location may cause it to be mistaken for a tumor mass.

Congenital absence of the spleen is a rarity. It has been reported along with associated anomalies. These include partial situs inversus and multiple congenital cardiovascular anomalies. The liver may show a symmetric lobulation, the left lobe being as large as the right.

Symmetric lobulation of the lungs may also be present, with three lobes on the left, the same as the right.

Increased density of the spleen is found in hemochromatosis and after the intravenous injection of thorium dioxide (see discussion above dealing with increased density of the liver).

ENLARGEMENT OF THE SPLEEN

Splenomegaly usually is demonstrated more readily and with greater accuracy in roentgenograms than is a comparable enlargement of the liver. Even slight to moderate degrees of enlargement often make the splenic shadow easily visible as it presses against the stomach and colon and is outlined by the gas in these structures (Fig. 13-54). When the stomach is filled with barium, pressure of the enlarged spleen on the greater curvature usually is obvious. When

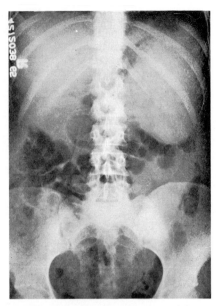

Fig. 13-54. Splenomegaly. The spleen displaces the stomach toward the midline and the splenic flexure of the colon downward, and forms a well-defined mass in the left upper quadrant.

very large, the spleen may displace the entire stomach toward or even beyond the midline. The splenic flexure of the colon is displaced downward. The left kidney also is pushed downward as the spleen increases in size. When significant enlargement occurs, the left side of the diaphragm becomes elevated (normally the left half of the diaphragm lies at a slightly lower level than the right).

CALCIFICATION IN THE SPLEEN

It is very common to find multiple, small round or ovoid calcified foci distributed throughout the spleen (see Fig. 13-23). These may be phleboliths within the splenic veins or the healed lesions of some widely disseminated infection. In the past, tuberculosis has been thought to be responsible for these lesions but current opinion favors the belief that they represent the healed foci of histoplasmosis. There often are similar foci distributed extensively in the lungs and occasionally in the liver.

Calcified splenic cysts are infrequent. In this country they are usually simple cysts, often of congenital origin. Occasionally a posttraumatic hematoma may become cystic with a calcified wall. A calcified cyst forms a rounded ringlike shadow, easily recognized because of the calcification outlining the wall of the cyst. According to published reports, echinococcal disease is a frequent cause of calcified intraabdominal cysts in many foreign countries. It is a rare disease in persons who have spent their entire lives in the United States. The calcified wall of an echinococcal (hydatid) cyst often is thicker and coarser than a simple cyst. Multiple cysts are the rule.

Splenic infarcts are infrequent causes of calcified areas within the spleen. The calcification may appear in the form of a wedge if the infarct is seen in profile or as a more rounded or oval-shaped area if seen *en face*. Unless calcified, splenic infarcts are not demonstrable in roentgenograms.

RUPTURE OF THE SPLEEN

In many individuals suffering a traumatic rupture of the spleen, the severity of the clinical symptoms and rapid loss of blood into the abdominal cavity lead to operative intervention without roentgen investigation. Only in those cases where the leakage of blood ceases temporarily or where there is a slow leakage over a period of days is roentgen examination requested. A number of signs have been described in rupture of the spleen including (*1*) prominent mucosal folds on the greater curvature of the stomach, (*2*) gastric dilatation, (*3*) displacement of the stomach to the right or downward, (*4*) separation of intestinal loops by intraperitoneal fluid, and (*5*) pleural reaction at the left base. However, the most significant observation is that of a progressively increasing mass in the splenic area in serial roentgenograms covering a period of several hours or days after an episode of trauma. A left lateral decubitus view with barium in the stomach also has been recommended. Normally the greater curvature of the stomach is closely adjacent to the abdominal wall and has a convex outline. If the spleen is enlarged or if there is a perisplenic hematoma the greater curvature will be concave and separated from the wall by a soft-tissue space up to 8 cm in width. The escape of blood into the peritoneal cavity causes the development of adynamic ileus. Definite visualization of a normal splenic outline is good evidence that splenic rupture does not exist. The observation of one or more fractures in the lower left ribs should call attention to the possibility of splenic injury when the other signs are equivocal.

Splenic arteriography is a useful procedure when rupture of the spleen is suspected.[4, 22] Among the significant findings are (1) extravasation of the contrast material into the splenic parenchyma, and (2) simultaneous visualization of the splenic artery and vein. Other findings that have been described include (1) stretching of splenic arterial branches, (2) distortion and irregular opacification of the splenogram, and (3) splenic enlargement. It has been recommended that this procedure be done in all patients where doubt exists and other examinations have proved inconclusive.

Cases of so-called spontaneous rupture of the spleen have been described in which rupture occurs without obvious trauma; a diseased spleen is probably a prerequisite. The initiating trauma in these cases may be so slight as to be considered insignificant. The roentgen findings are the same as those occurring after acute traumatic ruptures.

SPLENOPORTOGRAPHY

Splenoportography consists in the visualization of the splenoportal venous system, and the liver parenchyma to some extent, by the injection of a radiopaque contrast substance. This may be done in one of several ways. The first method introduced consisted in injection of the material into the splenic pulp by direct splenic puncture. The contrast substance passes rapidly into the splenic vein, then into the portal vein and the liver (Fig. 13-55). Normally tributaries to these veins do not fill by reflux. However, if there is obstruction anywhere from the splenic to the hepatic veins there will be

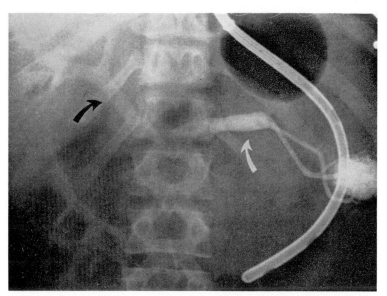

Fig. 13-55. Normal splenoportogram. The contrast material was injected directly into the spleen and a small amount remains in the splenic pulp. There has been rapid passage of the material into the splenic (**white arrow**) and portal (**black arrow**) veins. There has been no filling of collaterals and thus no signs of obstruction at any point along the pathway (including the intrahepatic branches).

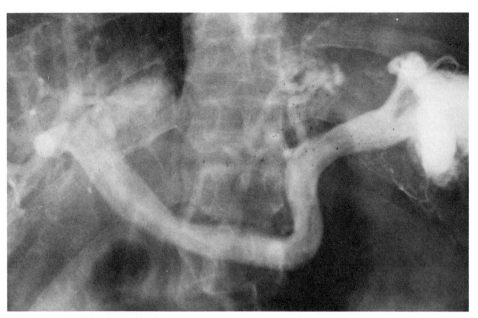

Fig. 13-56. Splenoportogram demonstrates varices in gastric fundus and lower esophagus. The injection was made directly into the spleen.

reflux into the mesenteric and gastric veins and if varices are present they will be opacified. Obstruction of the splenic or portal veins can be demonstrated, usually owing to thrombosis or to occlusion by pressure or invasion from a malignant tumor or inflammatory process in the vicinity. If the splenic and portal veins are patent but collaterals are demonstrated, portal hypertension is present usually owing to intrahepatic block, most commonly cirrhosis (Figs. 13-56 and 13-57). In cirrhosis the intrahepatic branches of the portal vein fill but are thin and attenuated and during the phase of small vein and capillary filling (i.e., the hepatogram phase) the liver may show a mottled appearance. The procedure has its greatest usefulness in the study of portal hypertension particularly when surgical measures for relief are being considered. It is the best method for the radiographic demonstration of the presence and extent of varices. If the obstruction is in the hepatic veins, usually owing to thrombosis (the *Budd-Chiari syndrome*), the intrahepatic portal branches tend to be dilated.

Portography also may be done using the umbilical vein. The lumen of this vein does not become occluded after its function ceases. It is exposed and cannulated through a supraumbilical, extraperitoneal "cut-down." The method has the advantage of eliminating the possibility of hemorrhage which is present when direct splenic puncture is done.

Direct portography has been done using general anesthesia and a small, paraumbilical incision. A tributary of the portal vein, usually a branch of a mesenteric vein is cannulated and the contrast material injected.

Adequate visualization of the splenoportal system usually can be obtained during the venous phase of splenic or celiac axis angiography (see Fig. 13-51). Direct splenic artery catheterization is preferred if the main reason for doing the study is to visualize the venous system. This method has become popular in recent years as a replacement for direct splenic puncture.

MISCELLANEOUS CONDITIONS
PSEUDOMYXOMA PERITONAEI

This rare but interesting condition is caused in most patients by the rupture of a malignant

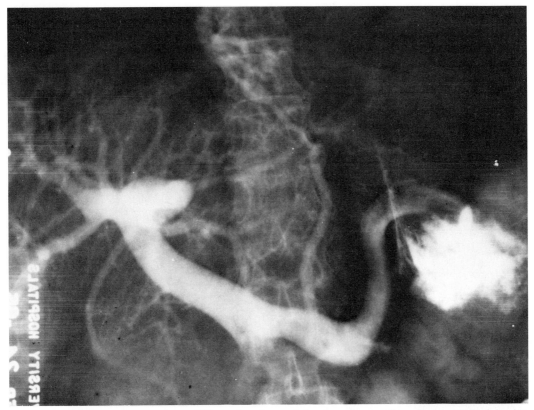

Fig. 13-57. Splenoportogram shows filling of varices of the esophagus after direct splenic injection.

mucocele of the appendix or of a pseudomucinous cystadenoma or cystadenocarcinoma of the ovary leading to the formation of masses of gelatinous material over the surface of the peritoneum. For practical purposes, in the male, the condition is caused only by rupture of a malignant mucocele of the appendix. The release of a large quantity of mucinous material causes a foreign-body type of peritonitis with thickening and fibrosis. The implantation of tumor cells on the surface of the peritoneum results in the formation of daughter tumors and cysts. These cysts also may rupture. Pugh[30] described two cases in which the walls of the cysts became calcified, giving numerous ring-like calcifications widely distributed throughout the peritoneal cavity. Apparently this does not happen very often. (A similar type of cystic or ringlike calcification, sometimes widely distributed throughout the abdominal cavity, is seen rarely as a result of a previous instillation of mineral oil into the peritoneal cavity at the time of laparotomy in the belief that it might prevent the formation of postoperative adhesions. One of the com-

plications of the oil instillation is the development of oil granulomas and it is the calcification of these that gives the roentgen findings. This is a rare cause of intra-abdominal calcification at the present time.) There are no other roentgen diagnostic signs of the disease and there is nothing characteristic about the appearance of the masses; usually individual mass shadows cannot be identified. In later stages bowel obstruction may supervene and the roentgen findings then become those of obstruction.

MESENTERIC CYSTS

Mesenteric cysts are infrequent lesions but when present often have fairly characteristic roentgen findings. The cystic mass can be visualized as a sharply outlined, round shadow of soft-tissue density. Characteristically, the mass is freely movable and is displaced readily by altering the position of the patient or by palpation. Multiple position roentgenograms are useful in demonstrating this mobility. When the intestinal tract is outlined with barium sulfate, particularly during a small intestinal study, the mass is sharply delineated as it is surrounded by the barium-filled loops of bowel. Unless very large no obstructive signs are present and the bowel is displaced but not invaded or compressed. Calcification of the wall of the cyst is seen occasionally.

LIPOMAS

Lipomas or liposarcomas occasionally develop in the retroperitoneal tissues and they have been reported as occurring in the mesentery. It is sometimes difficult to determine if one is dealing with an actual fatty tumor or simply with a localized accumulation of fat ("depot fat"). Because fat is more translucent than other soft tissues, a lipoma

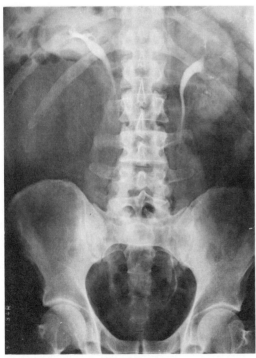

Fig. 13-58. Retroperitoneal lipoma. Intravenous urogram shows a mass in the right lateral abdomen that is more translucent than the normal abdominal structures and indicates that it is a fatty tumor. It is displacing the kidney upward and the ureter toward the midline, which locates it in the retroperitoneal tissues. (*Courtesy Dr. Wayne Rounds, Madison, Wisconsin*)

of any appreciable size may be visualized as an area of lessened density (Fig. 13-58). The translucency of fat is clearly shown when such a tumor develops in an extremity where it can be easily seen. In the abdomen, soft-tissue differentiation is not as good so that the lipoma must be fairly large for this sign to be obvious. Even when not clearly translucent, a disparity in the size of the mass and its radiographic density may be a lead to the correct diagnosis in some cases.

REFERENCES AND SELECTED READINGS

1. BARON, M. G., and WOLF, B. S.: Splenoportography. *JAMA 206:* 629, 1968.
2. BARRY, W. F., JR.: Roentgen examination of the abdomen in acute pancreatitis. *Am. J. Roentgenol. Radium Ther. Nucl. Med. 74:* 220, 1955.
3. BAUM, S., and NUSBAUM, M.: The control of gastrointestinal hemorrhage by selective mesenteric arterial infusion of vasopressin. *Radiology 98:* 497, 1971.
4. BERK, R. N., and WHOLEY, M. H.: The application of splenic arteriography in the diagnosis of rupture of the spleen. *Am. J. Roentgenol. Radium Ther. Nucl. Med. 104:* 662, 1968.
5. BOIJSEN, E., and ABRAMS, H. L.: Roentgenologic diagnosis of primary carcinoma of the liver. *Acta Radiol. (Diag.) 3:* 257, 1965.
6. BONTE, F. J., WEISBERGER, A. S., and PIAVELLO, C.: An evaluation of portal venography performed by intrasplenic injection of contrast material (splenography). *Radiology 66:* 17, 1956.
7. BOOKSTEIN, J. J., REUTER, S. R., and MARTEL, W.: Angiographic evaluation of pancreatic carcinoma. *Radiology 93:* 757, 1969.
8. BUDIN, E., and JACOBSON, G.: Roentgenographic diagnosis of small amounts of intraperitoneal fluid. *Am. J. Roentgenol. Radium Ther. Nucl. Med. 99:* 62, 1967.
9. CALVY, G. L., and DUNDON, C. C.: Roentgen manifestations of acute intermittent porphyria. *Radiology 58:* 204, 1952.
10. CLAYTON, R. S., and GOODMAN, P. H.: The roentgenographic diagnosis of geophagia (dirt eating). *Am. J. Roentgenol. Radium Ther. Nucl. Med. 73:* 203, 1955.
11. CASE, J. T.: Roentgenology of pancreatic disease. *Am. J. Roentgenol. Radium Ther. Nucl. Med. 44:* 485, 1940.
12. EATON, S. B., BENEDICT, K. T., JR., FERRUCCI, J. T., and FLEISCHLI, D. J.: Hypotonic duodenography. *Radiol. Clin. North Am. 8:* 125, 1970.
13. ELKIN, M., and COHEN, G.: Diagnostic value of the psoas shadow. *Clin. Radiol. 13:* 210, 1962.

14. FREY, C. F., REUTER, S. R., and BOOKSTEIN, J. J.: Localization of gastrointestinal hemorrhage by selective angiography. *Surgery 67:* 548, 1970.

15. FRIMANN-DAHL, J.: *Roentgen Examinations in Acute Abdominal Diseases.* Springfield, Ill., Thomas, 1951.

16. FROSTBERG, N.: Characteristic duodenal deformity in cases of different kinds of perivaterial enlargement of the pancreas. *Acta Radiol. 19:* 164, 1938.

17. HODES, P. J., PENDERGRASS, E. P., and WINSTON, N. J.: Pancreatic, ductal and vaterian neoplasms: Their roentgen manifestations. *Radiology 62:* 1, 1954.

18. JARVIS, J. L., and SEAMAN, W. B.: Idiopathic adrenal calcification in infants and children. *Am. J. Roentgenol. Radium Ther. Nucl. Med. 82:* 510, 1959.

19. KANTER, I. E., SCHWARTZ, A. J., and FLEMING, R. J.: Localization of bleeding point in chronic and acute gastrointestinal hemorrhage by means of selective visceral arteriography. *Am. J. Roentgenol. Radium Ther. Nucl. Med. 103:* 386, 1968.

20. KEEFE, E. J., GAGLIARDI, A., and PFISTER, R. C.: The roentgenographic evaluation of ascites. *Am. J. Roentgenol. Radium Ther. Nucl. Med. 101:* 388, 1967.

21. LEONIDAS, J. C., BERDON, W. E., BAKER, D. H., and SANTULLI, T. V.: Meconium ileus and its complications. *Am. J. Roentgenol. Radium Ther. Nucl. Med. 108:* 598, 1970.

22. LUNDSTRÖM, B.: Angiographic demonstration of rupture of the spleen. *Acta Radiol. (Diag.) 10:* 1451, 1970.

23. MARSHALL, W. C., OCKENDEN, B. G., FOSBROOKE, A. S., and CUMINGS, J. N.: Wolman's disease. A rare lipidosis with adrenal calcification. *Arch. Dis. Child. 44:* 331, 1969.

24. NEBESAR, R. A., and POLLARD, J. J.: Portal venography by selective arterial catheterization. *Am. J. Roentgenol. Radium Ther. Nucl. Med. 97:* 477, 1966.

25. NEBESAR, R. A., and POLLARD, J. J.: A critical evaluation of selective celiac and superior mesenteric angiography in the diagnosis of pancreatic diseases, particularly malignant tumors: Facts and "artefacts." *Radiology 89:* 1017, 1967.

26. NEUHAUSER, E. B. D.: The roentgen diagnosis of fetal meconium peritonitis. *Am. J. Roentgenol. Radium Ther. Nucl. Med. 51:* 421, 1944.

27. POCHACZESKY, R., CALEM, W. S., and RICHTER, R. M.: Umbilical vein portography. *Radiology 89:* 868, 1967.

28. POLLARD, J. J., FLEISCHLI, D. J., and NEBESAR, R. A.: Angiography of hepatic neoplasms. *Radiol. Clin. North Am. 8:* 31, 1970.

29. POPPEL, M. H.: The roentgen manifestations of relapsing pancreatitis. *Radiology 62:* 514, 1954.

30. PUGH, D. G.: A roentgenologic aspect of pseudomyxoma peritonaei. *Radiology 39:* 320, 1942.

31. RIAN, R. L., and EYLER, W. R.: Aortic, iliac and visceral arterial lesions. *Radiol. Clin. North Am. 5:* 409, 1967.

32. RIGLER, L. G.: Roentgen signs of intestinal necrosis. *Am. J. Roentgenol. Radium Ther. Nucl. Med. 94:* 402, 1965.

33. SANDS, W. W.: Extraluminal localized gas vesicles. An aid in the diagnosis of abdominal abscesses from the plain roentgenograms. *Am. J. Roentgenol. Radium Ther. Nucl. Med. 74:* 195, 1955.

34. TOMCHIK, F. S., WITTENBERG, J., and OTTINGER, L. W.: The roentgenographic spectrum of bowel infarction. *Radiology 96:* 249, 1970.

35. WIOT, J. F., and FELSON, B.: Gas in the portal venous system. *Am. J. Roentgenol. Radium Ther. Nucl. Med. 86:* 920, 1961.

36. WOLFSON, J. J., and ENGEL, R. R.: Anticipating meconium peritonitis from metaphyseal bands. *Radiology 92:* 1055, 1969.

14

THE GALLBLADDER

SCOUT ROENTGENOGRAMS

As the first step in the radiologic investigation of the gallbladder a preliminary or scout roentgenogram of the abdomen can be useful. The position of the gallbladder may vary widely in different persons. It may be situated high in the right upper quadrant in the obese individual or overlie the lower lumbar spine or even the right ilium in those of asthenic habitus. As pointed out by Stevenson, its relation to the inferior edge of the liver and the hepatic flexure of the colon remains fairly constant regardless of the habitus. The liver edge usually can be visualized in roentgenograms of the upper part of the abdomen and the hepatic flexure of the colon often is seen because of its gas and fecal content. Location of these structures aids in identifying the approximate site of the gallbladder. The descending duodenum and the gallbladder also are related closely in their anatomic locations and if the duodenum can be visualized, either because it contains air or because it has been rendered opaque as part of a barium meal examination, the position of the gallbladder becomes more certain. Rarely, the gallbladder will be found to the left of the midline.

VISUALIZATION OF THE GALLBLADDER IN SCOUT ROENTGENOGRAMS

The normal gallbladder is visualized rarely in scout roentgenograms. If it is enlarged, as in hydrops, it may be seen as a mass along the undersurface of the liver. An excess amount of gas in the hepatic flexure of the colon or gas distention of the small intestine aid in outlining the mass. Visualization of a normal-sized but pathologic gallbladder with thickened walls happens occasionally, but it always is difficult to be certain that the shadow in question actually represents the gallbladder and not some other structure such as the first portion of the duodenum filled with fluid, or another loop of fluid-filled bowel seen on end. In general, the diagnosis of a pathologic gallbladder is seldom justified on the basis of an apparent visualization in a scout roentgenogram unless it is enlarged or unless some of the other findings described below are present.

CALCIFICATION OF THE GALLBLADDER WALL

Extensive calcification of the gallbladder wall is an infrequent finding but is an obvious sign of a diseased organ. The calcified wall forms an oval-shaped density corresponding to the size and shape of the gallbladder (*porcelain gallbladder*) (Fig. 14-1). A single large calculus may fill the gallbladder and if only its outer layer is calcified it may resemble closely calcification of the wall; at times it is impossible to distinguish between the two conditions.

GALLSTONES

A scout roentgenogram of the gallbladder area will demonstrate gallstones if they contain sufficient calcium to be radiopaque (only about 15 per cent of gallstones fall within this category). The chief constituent of most gallstones is cholesterol. Other constituents include

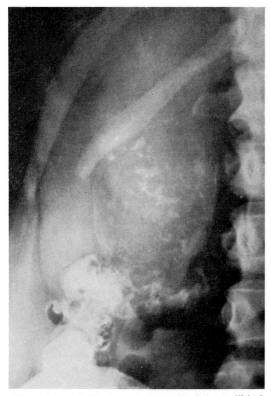

Fig. 14-1. Calcification of the wall of the gallbladder. There is an incomplete calcific shell formed by irregular plaques of calcium in the wall of the gallbladder (there is barium in the hepatic flexure of the colon).

bile pigments and calcium salts, usually calcium carbonate or calcium bilirubinate. Stones composed of pure cholesterol or a mixture of cholesterol and bile pigments are nonopaque to roentgen rays. In fact, cholesterol has a density somewhat less than that of the soft tissues of the body and occasionally a large cholesterol stone may be demonstrated as a negative shadow because of the decreased radiopacity of the stone in comparison to the density of the liver and other abdominal structures immediately around it. In order for a stone to be radiopaque it must contain calcium, usually in the form of calcium carbonate. Opaque gallstones vary greatly in their roentgen appearances but in general they have a denser outer rim and a more transparent center (Fig. 14-2). The dense portion consists of calcium carbonate while the transparent center is composed of cholesterol or bile pigment or both. Sometimes gallstones are laminated, consisting of alternating opaque and transparent rings. If multiple, gallstones usually are faceted. Occasionally a calculus is seen that has a dense opaque center surrounded by a transparent outer zone. Some of the larger stones, particularly those of cholesterol type, may show a stellate fissuring of the center with gas-filled fissures present. The fissures are even more transparent than the surrounding cholesterol and aid in visualization of the calculus as a negative density rather than an opaque one. Opaque stones must be differentiated from a variety of other causes of localized increased density in the right upper quadrant, including calcification of the costal cartilages, calcified foci in the liver, calcified lymph nodes, renal stones, warts and moles on the skin surface, film artifacts, and foreign material in the gastrointestinal tract. As a rule, the position of the shadow or shadows in relation to the liver edge and the hepatic flexure, the ringlike or laminated character, and the faceted contour make correct recognition possible. Differentiation from renal stones usually is made without difficulty if roentgenograms are obtained with the patient rotated to an oblique position. A gallstone that may overlie the renal shadow in the anteroposterior roent-

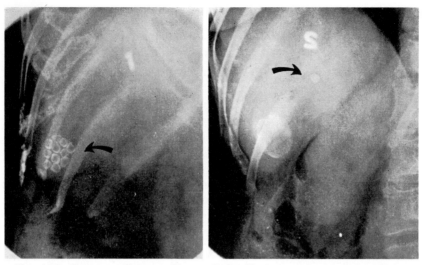

Fig. 14-2. Opaque gallstones. Two patients illustrate opaque stones that are visualized because of the amount of calcium salts they contain. *Left,* The gallbladder contains a number of ring-contoured and faceted calculi (**arrow**). The centers of the calculi are more translucent than the periphery because of cholesterol content. This is a common type of calculus in the gallbladder. Not infrequently the stones are somewhat laminated because of alternating layers of calcium salts and cholesterol. *Right,* There is a single large ring-contoured calculus with a more transparent center. There is a smaller calculus (**arrow**) situated above the larger stone and impacted in the cystic duct.

genogram will be displaced away from the kidney in the oblique projection. Multiple exposures aid in distinguishing gallstones from other calcareous shadows or similar densities for the same reason, i.e., they either reveal the shadow remaining in the gallbladder area regardless of the relation of the patient to the roentgen film or they show displacement away from the gallbladder region, indicating clearly that the shadow cannot be a gallstone.

GAS IN THE GALLBLADDER OR BILIARY DUCTS

Gas within the gallbladder or the biliary ducts always is abnormal. Gas may enter the gallbladder from the intestinal tract because of a fistula between the two, as a result of a surgical anastomosis, or because of a patulous sphincter of Oddi. Spontaneous biliary fistulas usually develop between the gallbladder and the duodenum, less frequently between the transverse colon and the gallbladder. A common cause is ulceration of a large gallstone through the wall into the adherent duodenum. The stone, because of its size, may become impacted in the small intestine and cause a gallstone ileus (see page 417). Cholecystoduodenal fistula also may be caused by perforation of a duodenal ulcer. Any malignant tumor arising in the vicinity may cause a fistulous communication between the intestinal tract and some part of the biliary duct system or the gallbladder. Gas in the biliary duct is recognized without difficulty (Fig. 14-3). It forms a Y-shaped translucent shadow in the right upper quadrant corresponding in position to the common and right and left hepatic ducts. At times there is extensive filling of the smaller hepatic radicles. If the gallbladder is present and the cystic duct patent or if the fistula is between it and the intestine, it too becomes visible as a gas-filled structure.

Rarely gas may enter the biliary tract be-

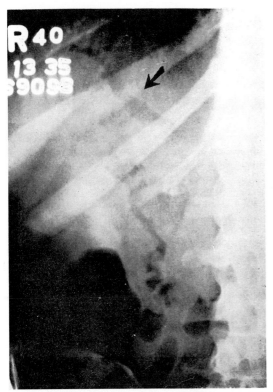

Fig. 14-3. Gas in the biliary ducts. The **arrow** points to the common duct, which is visualized as a translucent bandlike shadow because of the gas within it. In this case there was a fistulous communication between the common duct and the duodenum caused by a carcinoma of the head of the pancreas.

cause of a patulous sphincter of Oddi, a finding that may be confirmed by noting during a gastrointestinal barium study that the barium mixture refluxes into the common duct through the ampulla of Vater.

Infection with gas-forming organisms may be a cause of gas formation within the gallbladder, within its walls, or in both places. *Emphysematous cholecystitis* is a rare entity characterized by an acute infection of the gallbladder. It is found mainly in patients with poorly controlled diabetes but has been observed in others. The organisms involved are usually *Clostridium welchii* or *Escherichia coli*. Roentgenograms reveal gas within the gallbladder lumen, in the wall of the gallbladder, or in the pericholecystic tissues. It may be distributed throughout all these areas. It is probable that gas distention of the gallbladder lumen occurs first and that subsequently there is extension of the gas into the wall and later into the pericholecystic tissues. In the early stages a fluid level may be present if upright roentgenograms are obtained. In other instances the gallbladder contains only gas and is distended. In the early stages gas is absent in the biliary ducts since there is almost universally obstruction of the cystic duct. Later the infection may spread into the ducts and gas then will be visualized within them. When gas is present in the wall of the gallbladder it forms a rim of translucent bubbles or streaks outside of the gallbladder lumen and roughly paralleling it. The roentgen appearance at this stage is diagnostic. When only the gallbladder lumen contains gas it may be mistaken for a normal gas accumulation in the stomach or intestine. It may also be necessary to exclude an internal biliary fistula as a cause for the gas. The lack of gas in the biliary ducts is against the diagnosis of a fistula. Barium studies may be required at times for differential diagnosis. Later, when gas bubbles form in the wall of the gallbladder, the diagnosis can be made from scout roentgenograms.

GAS IN THE PORTAL VEINS

Accumulation of gas in the portal veins is an unusual finding sometimes seen in association with distention of the small bowel secondary to mesenteric thrombosis or other cause for devitalization of the bowel wall. The gas appears roentgenologically in the form of fine linear translucent streaks, usually in the periphery of the liver (see Fig. 13-37). It resembles to some extent the changes seen in cholecystoduodenal or cholecystocolic fistula. However, in this latter condition the abnormal gas shadows are found in the common duct and central hepatic radicles and have a characteristic branching pattern. Gas in the portal veins is found in the peripheral parts of the liver. It carries a grave prognosis and most patients succumb to the primary disease, most frequently mesenteric thrombosis. In addition to the portal veins, gas may be found within the walls of the gangrenous segments of bowel in the form of linear streaks or bubbles (pneumatosis cystoides).

CHANGES IN THE STOMACH AND DUODENUM

Alterations in the stomach or the duodenum may be caused by gallbladder disease but the signs are difficult to interpret in many cases and are not too reliable. An enlarged gallbladder may cause a smooth, pressure defect on the superior surface of the duodenal bulb when the latter has been filled with barium mixture during a gastrointestinal examination. Adhesions between the gallbladder and the duodenum may cause irregularity in contour of the duodenal bulb that may at times be difficult to distinguish from duodenal ulcer. Adhesions also may cause a sharp angulation between the first and second portions of the duodenum or between the stomach and duodenum. They rarely cause obstruction of the pylorus or the duodenum.

CHOLECYSTOGRAPHY

Cholecystography is the roentgen method of choice for study of the gallbladder. It consists in making the bile sufficiently radiopaque to give a dense shadow and thus to outline the gallbladder. Cholecystography is primarily a test of gallbladder function since it depends upon the ability of the gallbladder mucosa to concentrate the bile stored within by removing water.

TECHNIQUE OF THE EXAMINATION

After a light, fat-free supper the patient is given 3 gm of iopanoic acid (Telepaque). The drug is supplied in tablet form, each containing 0.5 gm. Another drug which has been introduced recently

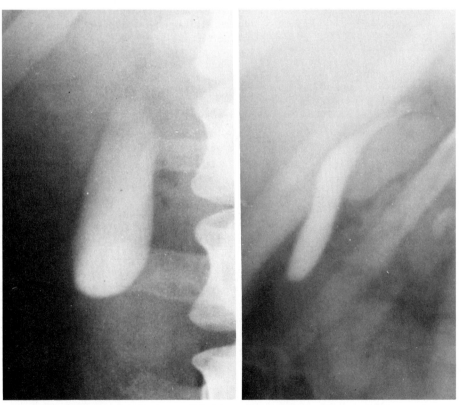

Fig. 14-4. Normally functioning gallbladder without stones. The post-fatty meal roentgenogram is on the *right*.

and which has been found satisfactory is Oragrafin (sodium ipodate) and it now is the drug we prefer. Food is withheld thereafter until the roentgen examination is completed the following morning. Water and coffee or tea without cream may be taken. At 8 A.M. the following day a series of roentgenograms of the gallbladder region is made. At least three exposures are made, one with the patient lying on the abdomen, another with the right side of the body elevated away from the table approximately 30°, and a third with the patient lying on the abdomen but the roentgen-ray tube angled toward the head approximately 15°. In addition a roentgenogram with the patient sitting or standing upright or placed in a right lateral decubitus position, as described on page 411, is usually obtained. Fluoroscopy with upright spot films is a useful adjunct and we do this routinely on our patients. The patient then is given a fatty meal consisting of an eggnog made with cream and a final roentgenogram is obtained 1 hour later. This completes the examination in most cases. Occasionally, because of indeterminate results, the examination is repeated and usually with a double dose of the drug (i.e., 6 gm). The remainder of the procedure is carried out as before.

Various other methods have been used to reinforce the density of the gallbladder when it is not visualized or poorly seen at the first examination. One method consists in giving the patient a 3-gm dose of calcium ipodate immediately after the initial examination and repeating the filming procedure 5 hours later. Crummy[3] found it to be a rapid, accurate method for obtaining additional information in about 25 per cent of the patients in whom gallbladder opacification was initially unsatisfactory. It should be pointed out that oral cholecystography is essentially a test of gallbladder function. Using large doses of present-day cholecystographic media it is possible to render the bile radiopaque as it is excreted by the liver and the gallbladder may be opacified even though its mucosa is diseased. Because of this some investigators prefer not to use reinforcement techniques. The ability to render the gallbladder visible, however, does increase the chance for the detection of nonopaque calculi even though it does make the examination less sensitive as a test of function.

The drugs mentioned have few side reactions when given in the dosages listed. Occasionally, nausea will be complained of or mild diarrhea will develop. Sensitivity to iodine is a

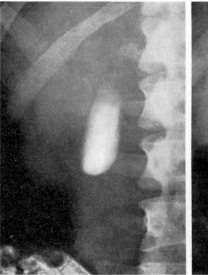 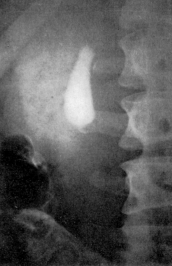

Fig. 14-5. Normally functioning gallbladder. *Left,* Appearance of the gallbladder when fully distended. *Right,* Appearance 1 hour after a fatty meal shows moderate contraction. The density of the gallbladder is homogeneous and there is no evidence of stones. The degree of contraction after a fatty meal is variable, but this is a fair response.

definite contraindication to administration of any cholecystographic medium since all drugs now employed for this purpose depend upon iodine for their radiopacity. Other contraindications to the use of Telepaque or related compounds include obstructive jaundice, vomiting, diarrhea, and severe liver or renal disease.

PHYSIOLOGY OF THE PROCEDURE

The drugs used for cholecystography contain a high percentage of iodine. Iopanoic acid has an iodine concentration of 66.68 per cent. The drug is absorbed from the gastrointestinal tract and secreted by the liver. The bile as it comes from the liver ordinarily does not contain enough of the drug to be radiopaque. The gallbladder receiving the bile concentrates it by

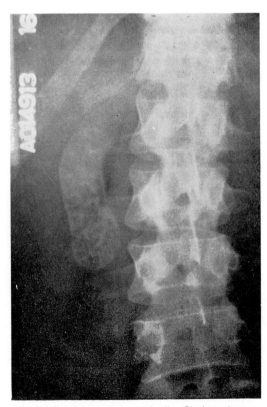

Fig. 14-6. Nonopaque calculi. Cholecystogram shows the gallbladder to be functioning; it has concentrated material sufficiently to render it opaque. There is extensive mottling of the shadow, caused by numerous small, irregular, cholesterol type of stones.

removing water. The amount of iodine in the bile then becomes sufficient to make it radiopaque and a dense shadow of the gallbladder, or more accurately, of its contents, results. In order for this to happen the mucosa of the gallbladder must be intact and functioning normally. If the gallbladder wall is diseased, usually as a result of chronic cholecystitis, the concentrating ability of the mucosa is lost and there is a failure of gallbladder visualization. The following possibilities must be taken into account whenever nonvisualization occurs:

1. The patient did not take the drug or did not retain it.

2. Obstruction at the cardia or the pylorus may have prevented the material from entering the small intestine. Roentgenograms may show the medium remaining in the esophagus or stomach in these cases.

3. There may be faulty absorption in the small intestine. Severe diarrhea may influence the result.

4. The liver function may be impaired to the point where an insufficient amount of the material is secreted. The examination should not be done if liver function is impaired seriously. Results are unsatisfactory in the presence of obstructive jaundice.

5. Obstruction of the cystic duct may prevent entrance of the bile into the gallbladder.

6. The gallbladder may have been removed at some previous time.

7. Disease of the gallbladder may have damaged the concentrating ability of the mucosa to the point where no shadow results.

8. The gallbladder may be in an unusual location and not be visualized on the film.

RESULTS

The results of the examination can be expressed in one of the following ways:

NORMALLY FUNCTIONING GALLBLADDER WITHOUT STONES. The gallbladder has become opaque so that its shadow is clearly visualized and the density of the shadow is uniform with no filling defects indicative of stones (Fig. 14-4). Usually it will have undergone some decrease in size after the fatty meal and occasionally will have emptied itself completely of the radiopaque bile. Contraction of the gallbladder in response to a fatty meal is the result of the production of a hormone by the mucous membrane of the small intestine; this hormone is called cholecystokinin. There is considerable variation in the response of the gallbladder to a fatty meal (Fig. 14-5) and evidence of contraction is not required for the results to be considered normal.

Using contrast substances such as sodium ipodate (Oragrafin), visualization of the cystic and common bile ducts is possible in many of the patients who have normally concentrating gallbladders. The best filling is obtained in the postfat-meal roentgenogram, particularly if this is a right lateral decubitus view. The cystic duct has a twisted corkscrew appearance caused by the valves of Heister. The diameter varies between 0.2 and 0.3 cm. The diameter of the normal common bile duct varies from about 0.2 to 0.7 cm. Shehadi[17] has found that the diameter varies from time to time in the individual patient, the smaller measurement being most frequently obtained during the early phase of gallbladder contraction. The ability to visualize the ducts makes it possible to demonstrate partial obstruction, provided that gallbladder function remains reasonably good. Visualization of the bile ducts with Telepaque in the cholecystectomized patient is discussed later in the section on "Cholangiography."

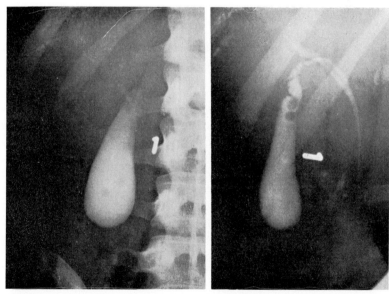

Fig. 14-7. Nonopaque calculi. *Left,* Cholecystogram before a fatty meal. *Right,* Cholecystogram after fatty meal. The gallbladder has concentrated satisfactorily and shows adequate contraction. There are two negative calculi that are seen to better advantage in the post-fat-meal roentgenogram on the *right.* This roentgenogram also was made in a right lateral decubitus position. The patient actually was lying on his right side with the roentgen-ray beam directed horizontally through the body in an anteroposterior direction (Kirklin's position). The calculi have risen to the uppermost part of the gallbladder adjacent to the cystic duct. Note the clarity with which the ducts are visualized, including the major portion of the common duct. The valves of Heister in the cystic duct are clearly visualized. This is a frequent observation in this type of roentgenogram.

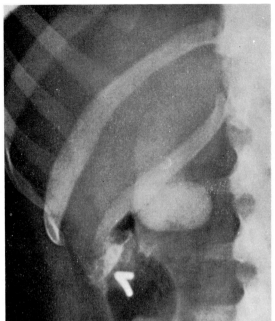 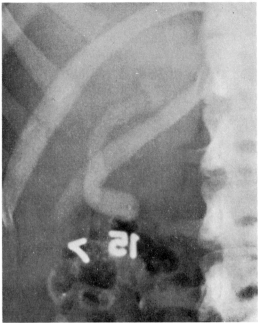

Fig. 14-8. Nonopaque calculi. *Left,* Roentgenogram before fatty meal. *Right,* Roentgenogram after fatty meal. While the gallbladder has concentrated well and contracted in a satisfactory manner, there is a fine granular mottling caused by a large number of cholesterol stones. These are seen to better advantage in the post-fat-meal film because of the contraction of the gallbladder and its decreased volume.

NORMALLY FUNCTIONING GALLBLADDER WITH STONES. The gallbladder has concentrated normally and a good shadow is present but stones are visualized as filling defects in the shadow (Fig. 14-6). Thus, nonopaque calculi can be demonstrated where otherwise they could not be seen. Because about 85 per cent of all gallstones are of the nonopaque variety (chiefly cholesterol stones), the method is a very useful one providing the concentrating ability of the organ has not been lost. For the demonstration of very tiny calculi the postfat-meal roentgenogram often gives the best results, since the decreased size of the gallbladder makes it possible to see the small defects more clearly (Figs. 14-7 and 14-8). The "layering phenomenon" also is used to demonstrate small calculi. If a roentgenogram is made with the patient upright or in a lateral decubitus position the stones, being of similar composition and having the same specific gravity in each individual case, tend to form a transverse layer in the bile (Fig. 14-9). Sometimes the stones gravitate to the dependent part of the gallbladder, particularly if they contain any calcium salts; at other times they float in the bile but invariably at the same level (Fig. 14-9). Thus it becomes possible by bringing a number of small calculi into the same plane with reference to the beam of roentgen rays to visualize them more easily than if they were spread out indiscriminately as they would be with the patient in the recumbent position. The explanation for floating of gallstones within the bile is based on the fact that bile tends to stratify in different layers with different specific gravities. The stones seek the level corresponding to the specific gravity of the calculi. The right lateral decubitus roentgenogram (Kirklin's position) also is useful in displacing the gallbladder away from gas shadows in the bowel and is a part of the routine series of roentgenograms made during cholecystography. Gas bubbles in the duodenum may overlie the gallbladder in some positions and closely resemble stones. Larger accumulations of gas in the colon may interfere with clear visualization of the gallbladder. By the use of multiple positions and tube angulations it is possible as a rule to obtain one or more roentgenograms free of overlying gas shadows and thus allow correct interpretation. Gas in the duodenum does not remain constant in position for very long and may be completely gone in some of the later roentgenograms.

Theoretically a calculus might contain enough calcium evenly distributed through it to make it of exactly the same density as the bile around it and thus be obscured during cholecystography. This chance for error is eliminated if a scout roentgenogram is obtained prior to the cholecystographic procedure, since the calculus will be radiopaque. Actually a calculus seldom is of homogeneous density and the chance for error is minimal.

NONFUNCTIONING GALLBLADDER WITH STONES. In this instance a shadow of the gallbladder does not appear but opaque stones are present. Such calculi of course can be demonstrated in scout roentgenograms but the failure of visualization during cholecystography gives the added information that damage to the gallbladder wall has occurred; usually this indicates cholecystitis.

NONFUNCTIONING GALLBLADDER. The gallbladder is not visualized and no opaque calculi can be seen. Provided that the extraneous factors, as listed above, that may influence the examination can be eliminated, this finding indicates gallbladder disease in a very high percentage of patients. If there is doubt concerning the accuracy of the test, a repetition of the examination using a double dose of the contrast material can be done. Or, the intravenous administration of Cholografin as performed for cholangiography can be used. This

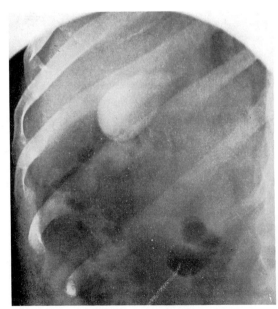 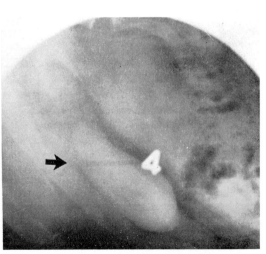

Fig. 14-9. Layering of gallstones. *Left,* Roentgenogram with patient in posteroanterior position. The calculi are not identified clearly. There are some gas shadows in the colon overlying the tip of the fundus. *Right,* Lateral decubitus roentgenogram. The patient is lying with the right side down, the left side uppermost, and the roentgen-ray beam is directed horizontally through the body. In this position numerous stones have accumulated in a layer in the upper part of the body of the gallbladder and are visualized as a translucent line parallel to the table top (**arrow**). The calculi are very tiny and are too small to be visualized as individual defects but when accumulated in a layer in the bile they are sufficiently translucent to be clearly identified.

is discussed more fully under the heading "Intravenous and Oral Cholangiography." The most common cause for a nonfunctioning gallbladder is chronic cholecystitis with stones. Salzman[16] and others have reported on the use of multiple doses of Telepaque for the opacification of gallstones which are otherwise nonopaque in a nonfunctioning gallbladder. The method consists in giving 3-gm doses of the drug each day for 3 or 4 days (1 gm after each meal), with subsequent roentgenography of the gallbladder. At times the margins of a stone may become opaque after this procedure, allowing its recognition. The method has been

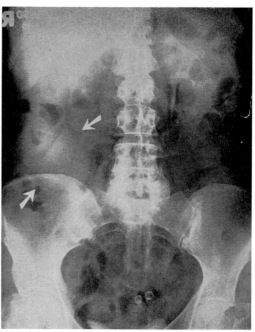

Fig. 14-11. Hydrops of the gallbladder. Roentgenogram of the abdomen made during an intravenous urographic study and contrast material can be visualized in the renal pelves and urinary bladder. The **arrows** point to the enlarged gallbladder, which projects downward from the lower margin of the liver, and its outline is clearly visualized.

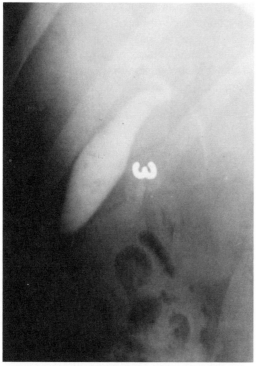

Fig. 14-10. Cholesterolosis of the gallbladder. The gallbladder has concentrated normally and the contrast medium is present in the cystic and common bile ducts. Within the gallbladder are a number of small, irregular translucent defects. These persisted in various roentgenograms with the patient in different positions, including a lateral decubitus view. The defects did not change in position and remained constant in a post-fat-meal roentgenogram. They represent small accumulations of cholesterol below the mucosa of the gallbladder and projecting into the lumen.

successful even in patients with jaundice who have one or more stones impacted in the common duct.

SUBNORMALLY FUNCTIONING GALLBLADDER. A shadow of the gallbladder is visible but it is faint and below the expected normal in density. The density may be so low that the presence or absence of stones cannot be determined. Usually it is advisable to repeat the examination, using a double dose of the contrast material or, preferably, the immediate administration of 3.0 gm of calcium ipodate as previously described with reexamination 5 hours later. Frequently on reexamination much better visualization is obtained and a better idea of the function and the presence or absence of stones results. If the repeat examination again shows only a faint shadow a diagnosis of subnormal function can be made. With present-day contrast material it is unusual to find a faint gallbladder shadow and the diagnosis of subnormally functioning gallbladder is not made very often. If more information is wanted, a study with intravenous Cholografin should be done. As mentioned above, lack of contraction alone, occurring after the fatty meal, is not sufficient to warrant a diagnosis of poor function or of gallbladder disease but if the gallbladder shows definite decrease in size it is probably normal even though its density is less than is usually considered normal. Persisting faint shadows sufficient to indicate subnormal function and with failure of contraction after the fat meal are usually the result of chronic cholecystitis.

OTHER ASPECTS OF GALLBLADDER ROENTGENOGRAPHY

Fixed Defects in the Gallbladder; Cholesterolosis. Not infrequently one encoun-

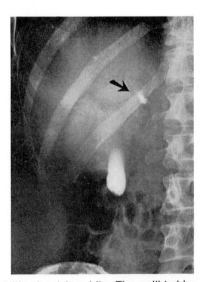

Fig. 14-12. Milk of calcium bile. The gallbladder is seen as a dense shadow below the right twelfth rib, simulating the appearance of a gallbladder that has concentrated material during cholecystography. However, this patient had no contrast material given and the opacity of the gallbladder is caused by the so-called "milk of calcium bile." The **arrow** points to an opaque calculus impacted in the cystic duct and obstructing it.

ters one or more small, round, translucent defects which are attached to the gallbladder wall. These vary in size from 1 to 2 mm to 6 to 8 mm. Their attachment to the wall is determined by lack of movement and failure to layer when roentgenograms are made with the patient in upright and lateral decubitus projections as well as in a recumbent position and by noting that the defect, when viewed tangentially, is not separated from the gallbladder wall by a layer of contrast material. A large number of polypoid lesions have been reported showing these findings including (*1*) inflammatory polyps, (*2*) neurinoma, (*3*) fibroadenoma, (*4*) metastatic tumors, and other rare lesions.[13] However, the most frequent are cholesterol polyps (Fig. 14-10), adenomas, and adenomyomas. In one series of 17 proved cases, 11 lesions were found to be cholesterol polyps.

Fixed defects also may be classified as follows:[6]

I. Epithelial Tumors
  A. Papilloma
  B. Adenoma
  C. Carcinoma
II. Mesenchymal Tumors
III. Pseudotumors
  A. Cholesterol polyps
  B. Inflammatory polyps
  C. Adenomyoma
  D. Congenital malformations

A *cholesterol polyp* is not a tumor but consists of a small collection of cholesterol crystals beneath or on the epithelial surface. It may form a sessile mass or be attached to the wall by a thin, delicate stalk. The lesion may be single or multiple, most frequently the latter. The designation of *cholesterolosis of the gallbladder* has been used for this entity (see Fig. 14-10). It also has been called lipid gallbladder and "strawberry gallbladder" because of the gross appearance of multiple tiny collections of cholesterol on the surface of reddened mucosa resembling strawberry seeds. The gallbladder with cholesterolosis tends to concentrate the contrast material unusually well and to show increased contraction after the fat meal.

According to Jutras and associates,[8,9] cholesterolosis is one of the noninflammatory conditions which they have termed the *hyperplastic cholecystoses,* which also includes the entity known as adenomyomatosis.

Adenoma is a true benign tumor resembling adenomas found in other parts of the gastrointestinal tract. It too may be sessile or pedunculated. The term *papilloma* has been used when the surface has a papillary or villous appearance. Most are very small, measuring a few millimeters in diameter and best seen in the postfat-meal roentgenogram.

Adenomyoma usually is found at the fundus of the gallbladder as a smoothly elevated or sessile mass, often with a central dimple, when viewed in tangent. Rokitansky-Aschoff sinuses (see below) are frequently associated findings. Jutras and Levesque[9] consider adenomyoma to be a localized form of *adenomyomatosis,* one of the entities they have called the hyperplastic cholecystoses.

As far as roentgen diagnosis is concerned it usually is impossible to distinguish one of these lesions from the others which present as small, fixed defects and roentgenologists often report them as "polypoid lesions." On chance alone, cholesterol polyp is the most likely diagnosis in a given case.

The diagnosis of *carcinoma of the gallbladder* has been reported rarely on cholecystographic study. Some of these tumors have reached a size by the time of the initial examination that opacification of the gallbladder is impossible. In others, the lesion develops in a gallbladder which has been chronically inflamed, with or without stones, and concentration of the bile does not occur. Also, the cystic duct may be occluded by the tumor so that bile cannot enter it.

In general, many observers agree that, in the absence of significant symptoms, it is advisable to refrain from doing cholecystectomy when single or multiple, small, fixed defects are found in a normally functioning gallbladder. Repeat cholecystograms can be done at intervals and if no change in size of the lesion or in function occurs, only interval reexaminations are necessary.

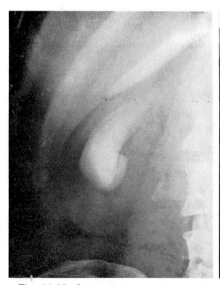 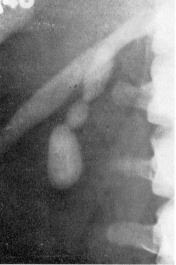

Fig. 14-13. Congenital anomalies of the gallbladder. *Left,* Phrygian cap gallbladder. The fundus appears to be folded over on the body. *Right,* Trilocular gallbladder. The gallbladder is divided into three locules by partial septa. There are several tiny negative stones in the fundic portion.

Occasionally on repeat study the defects will have disappeared. This happens because the thin pedicle attaching the lesion to the gallbladder wall may break allowing the polyp to float free. It may remain in the gallbladder simulating a small stone or pass through the ductal system into the duodenum.

Because they believe that carcinoma cannot be excluded when a fixed defect is found, some investigators have recommended cholecystectomy in all patients showing this type of defect. We favor the more conservative approach as outlined above.

ROKITANSKY-ASCHOFF SINUSES: ADENOMYOMATOSIS. These sinuses consist of tiny projections of the gallbladder mucosa into or through the muscularis resulting in small diverticulumlike outpouchings when they become filled with the contrast-containing bile. The appearance is one of multiple, tiny, beadlike densities paralleling the gallbladder lumen and separated from it by a thin translucent space. When the diverticula are particularly tiny and numerous, the appearance may be that of a fine, almost linear, band of density paralleling the lumen. In many cases there is a stricturelike narrowing in the body of the gallbladder dividing it into two loculi. Jutras[8] and Jutras and Levesque[9] consider this process as part of the entity called *adenomyomatosis* of the gallbladder, also known as *cholecystitis glandularis proliferans*. This, in turn, is one of the noninflammatory conditions they have called the *hyperplastic cholecystoses*. These entities are characterized by a noninflammatory hyperplasia of one of more elements of the gallbladder wall. In adenomyomatosis there is thickening of epithelium and muscularis. They consider adenomyoma to be the localized form of the disease (see above).

HYDROPS OF THE GALLBLADDER. Hydrops results in nonvisualization during cholecystography because the cystic duct is obstructed. The gallbladder is enlarged and this often is sufficient so that it can be seen as a mass along the inferior edge of the liver (Fig. 14-11).

ADHESIONS. Adhesions may distort the outline of the opacified gallbladder. However, considerable variation in the shape and position of the normal gallbladder exists and the diagnosis of pericholecystic adhesions should be made with considerable reservation in most patients.

MILK-OF-CALCIUM GALLBLADDER. Milk-of-calcium bile is a condition in which the gallbladder becomes filled with an accumulation of bile containing a high percentage of calcium carbonate. It follows obstruction of the cystic duct. Because the high concentration of calcium carbonate in the bile makes the entire gallbladder opaque the shadow resembles very closely that of a normally functioning gallbladder during cholecystography. Usually the obstruction of the cystic duct is caused by a calculus and this also is of the opaque calcium carbonate variety so that it is clearly visualized (Fig. 14-12). It gives an important clue to the

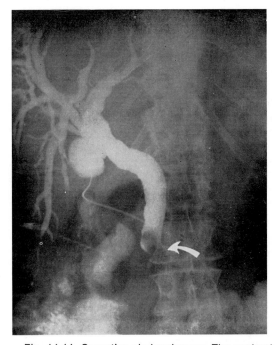

Fig. 14-14. Operative cholangiogram. The contrast material was injected into the gallbladder during laparotomy. There is a stone impacted in the distal end of the common duct (**arrow**).

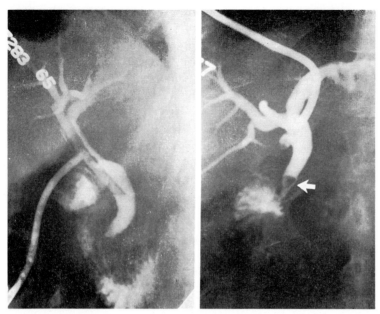

Fig. 14-15. Postoperative T-tube cholangiography. *Left,* Normal post-operative cholangiogram. Contrast material has been injected into the T-tube, outlining the common duct, and has extended through the ampulla into the duodenum. The duct is somewhat dilated over the average normal but this patient had a stone impacted in the lower end of the duct, which was removed, and the dilatation is residual from that which was present preoperatively. *Right,* Postoperative T-tube cholangiogram showing a residual stone in the lower end of the common duct. The calculus is visualized as a triangular translucent defect (**arrow**). It has not completely obstructed the duct and contrast material has entered the duodenum.

diagnosis. The shadow of a milk-of-calcium gallbladder does not change in size after a fat meal; if a scout roentgenogram was made prior to cholecystography the shadow, of course, would be present before the administration of the contrast material. In addition to the amorphous calcium carbonate material the gallbladder may contain one or more larger calculi.

CONGENITAL ANOMALIES

Phrygian Cap Gallbladder. In this developmental anomaly an incomplete septum extends across the fundus separating it partially from the body. The fundus appears to be folded over the body, resulting in a caplike appearance (Phrygian cap, a conical cap represented in Greek art as that worn by orientals and identified in modern art with the so-called liberty cap). The deformity has no clinical significance (Fig. 14-13).

Hourglass Gallbladder. In this anomaly the gallbladder is divided into two locules by a partial septum in its midportion. Occasionally a trilocular gallbladder is found (Fig. 14-13).

Double Gallbladder. The gallbladder may be bifurcated with both sacs emptying into a common cystic duct or with individual cystic ducts. This is a rare anomaly. A rather common finding, possibly related to double gallbladder, is a diverticulumlike projection from the gallbladder; this usually involves the fundus.

Left-Sided Gallbladder. Rarely, the gallbladder is found to the left of the midline while the position of the liver is normal. If small-sized roentgen-

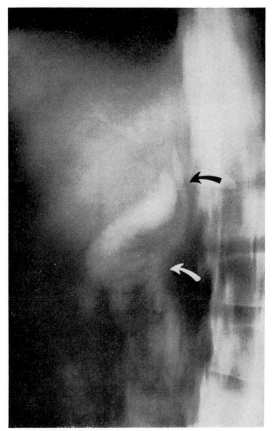

Fig. 14-16. Intravenous cholangiogram. The common duct has become opacified during intravenous cholangiography. This is a body-section roentgenogram in which structures anterior and posterior to the level of the common duct have been blurred during the exposure so that the duct stands out more clearly. Contrast has entered the duodenum through the ampulla. The **white arrow** points to the region of the ampulla. **Black arrow** indicates the upper part of the common duct.

ograms are used that include only the area usually occupied by the gallbladder, this condition may be missed and an erroneous diagnosis of a nonfunctioning gallbladder be made.

Intrahepatic Gallbladder. In this anomaly a part of or the entire gallbladder lies within liver substance. The condition can be recognized or at least suspected if the relationship of the gallbladder to the liver edge is studied carefully. Multiple roentgenograms with the patient in different posi-

tions and with different angulations of the roentgen-ray tube usually are necessary in order to be certain that the position of gallbladder shadow over the liver is not just an artifact of projection.

Absence of the Gallbladder. Congenital absence of the gallbladder has been reported but is a very rare anomaly. It is an extremely remote possibility to explain failure of function during cholecystography.

Choledochal Cyst. A cystlike dilatation of the common duct is met with infrequently, usually in children, and more so in females than males. The clinical diagnostic triad of abdominal pain, jaundice, and a palpable mass of the right upper quadrant in a child is said to be highly significant. The condition is generally considered to be of congenital origin and in some cases the duct has been dilated without any evidence of obstruction to account for it; in others obstruction has been present. The roentgen signs are essentially those of a mass in the gallbladder area that may become very large and as it does so it displaces the duodenum anteriorly and to the left. Visualization of the gallbladder and the dilated common duct is usually not to be expected during cholecystography and has been reported only infrequently. Direct percutaneous injection of contrast material into the cyst is a useful procedure in some cases.

SCLEROSING CHOLANGITIS

This is a rare inflammatory disease of the biliary ductal system characterized by fibrosis and stricture formation leading to biliary obstruction and cirrhosis.[10] On cholangiography strictures of variable lengths are seen both in the extra- and intrahepatic ducts. Obliteration of some of the smaller radicles within the liver gives a "pruned tree" appearance. Other ducts have an irregular or beaded contour. Recently the association of this disease with chronic ulcerative colitis has been reported. In other patients no causative factors are apparent.

CHOLANGIOGRAPHY

Cholangiography is a procedure whereby the biliary ducts are filled with an opaque material so that roentgen demonstration of the ductal system may be obtained.

OPERATIVE CHOLANGIOGRAPHY

This procedure consists in the injection of a contrast material, such as Renografin 60 or Renografin 76, directly into the ductal system or into the gallbladder at the time of surgical exploration. If the material is injected directly into the gallbladder the contents are aspirated and from 40 to 50 cc of the contrast substance are injected. If injected directly into the common duct, from 10 to 15 cc are ample unless the duct is dilated. A portable roentgen-ray generator is brought into the operating room to obtain the roentgenograms. Usually the surgeon punctures the common duct with a 20-gauge needle and injects the solution directly

into it. The roentgenograms are processed immediately for inspection in order to allow evaluation of the condition of the ducts before closure of the abdomen. The method is particularly useful to determine if any calculi are present within the common or hepatic ducts that cannot be palpated by the surgeon. Visualization of the ducts without filling defects and with evidence of free extension of contrast material into the duodenum enables the surgeon to be certain that no calculi remain and that there is no obstruction in the distal part of the duct. Calculi are visualized as negative filling defects within the denser shadow of the contrast material (Fig. 14-14). Air bubbles may be confused with calculi. Care in injection is important in eliminating the chance for bubbles to enter the duct. At times a repeat injection is required.

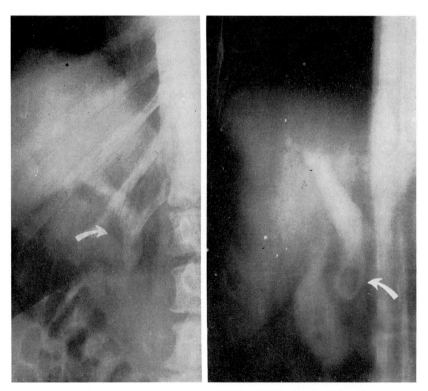

Fig. 14-17. Intravenous cholangiography demonstrating calculi in the common duct. *Left,* The common duct is opacified. It is dilated and in the lower end are two faceted negative stones (**arrow**). *Right,* Body-section roentgenogram of another patient demonstrated a dilated common duct with a large calculus impacted in the lower end (**arrow**). Contrast medium, however, has passed around the stone and can be visualized in the duodenum adjacent to the ampulla.

POSTOPERATIVE T-TUBE CHOLANGIOGRAPHY

After T-tube drainage of the common duct the contrast material can be injected directly into the duct through the drainage tube to determine if the duct is patent and functioning satisfactorily before the tube is removed. The injection should be done under fluoroscopic control and films exposed as necessary during the procedure. Normally a free flow of contrast material into the duodenum is observed and the ducts can be seen to be free from defects indicative of residual stones. If calculi are present they are seen as negative defects within the contrast medium (Fig. 14-15). Obstruction due to strictures and neoplasm can be recognized by failure of entrance of material into the duodenum and the dilatation of the ductal system above the site of obstruction. Cholangiography should be done in all cases of common duct drainage before removal of the T-tube.

INTRAVENOUS AND ORAL CHOLANGIOGRAPHY

With the use of a substance called iodipamide methylglucamine (marketed under the trade name of Cholografin methylglucamine) it is possible to demonstrate the common and hepatic ducts in cholecystectomized patients or in those in whom the gallbladder is nonfunctioning by oral cholecystography. Cholografin depends on a high concentration of iodine for its radiopacity. It is administered intravenously in doses of 20 to 30 cc for the average adult patient and with the injection given slowly over a 10-minute period. The slow, drip-infusion technique using larger doses of contrast material given over a longer period of time has been recommended for better visualization of the ductal system.[2] The material is secreted rapidly by the liver and appears in relatively high concentrations in the bile in from 10 to 15 minutes after injection. The concentration is sufficient to make the ducts opaque to roentgen rays (Fig. 14-16). Ordinarily a series of roentgenograms of the gallbladder region is obtained, beginning at 20 to 30 minutes after injection and spaced at intervals of 20 to 30 minutes. While the timing of the exposures will depend upon the results noted in the first roentgenogram, the usual spacing is 20, 30, 45, and 60 minutes. The technique is varied from patient to patient as the roentgenograms are processed immediately. Tomograms are obtained routinely when optimal opacification is noted. If the gallbladder is present and the cystic duct is patent the gallbladder will be visualized from 1 to 2 hours after injection.

In many patients a sufficient amount of the Cholografin is excreted by the kidneys so that a pyelogram is obtained. If liver function is diminished, renal excretion of the substance is increased and in the presence of serious liver damage roentgenograms reveal only opacification of the renal pelves and calyces and no visualization of the biliary ducts.

According to Shehadi and others the caliber of the normal common bile duct postoperatively is on the order of 5 to 6 mm, the same as in normal ducts visualized by intravenous or oral cholangiography. In our experience the common duct may be somewhat larger than this and we have allowed an upper limit of normal to be 10 mm. When the greatest diameter of the duct exceeds this figure the finding should be considered as evidence of some type of obstruction.

Caution must be exercised in the interpretation of these observations, however, and correlation with the clinical history and the physical findings is needed in borderline cases. The finding of an enlarged duct may indicate spasm of the sphincter of Oddi, stricture formation, tumor infiltration, or impaction of a calculus. Calculi may be demonstrated within ducts that are of normal caliber. They are recognized as negative or filling defects in the shadow (Fig. 14-17). Difficulty in interpretation caused by gas shadows in the intestinal tract is considerable. Special procedures such as planigraphy or body section roentgenography are useful to bring out the shadow of the duct clearly in some patients. It is possible to have partial obstruction of a duct which is not found to be dilated on cholangiography. If the causative

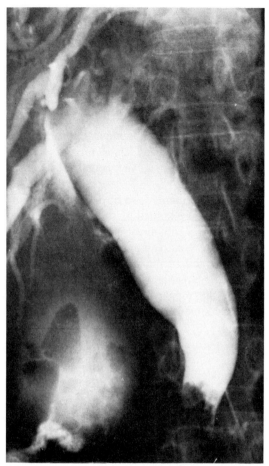

Fig. 14-18. Carcinoma of the ampulla. Transhepatic cholangiogram showing obstruction near the distal end of the duct which is greatly dilated. The contour at the site of obstruction is ragged, characteristic of a malignant tumor. There are numerous translucent stones in the gallbladder.

lesion cannot be identified (stone, stricture, etc.) Wise and O'Brien[21] use what they have called the time-density-retention concept. Briefly, their concept states that if the density of the common duct is greater at 120 minutes than at 60 minutes postinjection, partial obstruction is present. By using this criterion they found considerable improvement in the diagnostic accuracy of the procedure.

If the gallbladder has not been removed but has failed to visualize after oral cholecystography, the intravenous injection of Cholografin may show it or may, by failure of visualization,

indicate that the cystic duct is occluded and that the radiopaque bile cannot enter. If the cystic duct is patent the gallbladder will become opaque even though its wall is seriously diseased because concentration of the bile by the gallbladder mucosa is not required.

In the cholecystectomized patient the cystic duct may dilate to the point where it simulates

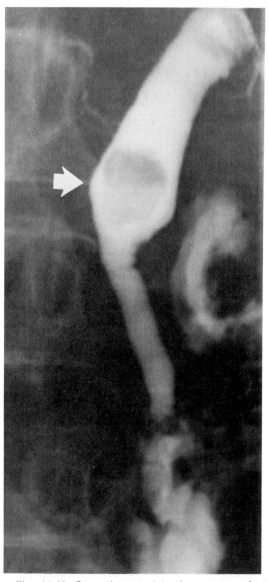

Fig. 14-19. Stone impacted in the common duct without complete obstruction (**arrow**). Transhepatic cholangiogram. There is contrast material in the duodenum.

a "reformed" gallbladder. The clinical significance of the so-called "reformed" gallbladder has been in dispute. In most cases where a remnant of the cystic duct or even the neck of the gallbladder is visualized it is doubtful that clinical significance can be attached to the finding. The gallbladder, itself, does not reform.

Contraindications to the procedure include sensitivity to iodine, severe liver damage, or concomitant impairment of liver and renal functions. A test for iodine sensitivity by the slow intravenous injection of a test dose of 1 cc of solution about 30 minutes before the procedure can be done. However, sensitivity tests have not been found particularly reliable and most investigators do not believe that they are very helpful.

It is possible to visualize the urinary and biliary tracts simultaneously by the intravenous administration of a substance known as Duografin. This is a combination of Cholografin methylglucamine (40%) and Renografin (60%). The procedure is useful, if both tracts are to be examined, because of the saving of time. The usual procedures are employed for obtaining the roentgenograms.

In some patients it is possible to visualize the common duct after cholecystectomy by the oral administration of large doses of Telepaque. A dose of 6 gm, or twice the amount used for cholecystography, will show the duct frequently even though the gallbladder is severely diseased or has been removed. The material is secreted by the liver in a high enough concentration so that the concentrating ability of the gallbladder is not needed to make the bile radiopaque. This method has been largely supplanted by intravenous cholangiography.

PERCUTANEOUS TRANSHEPATIC CHOLANGIOGRAPHY

This procedure consists in direct needle puncture of the common duct or one of the hepatic ducts through the abdominal wall and liver. Mujahed and Evans[12] list the following indications for the procedure:

1. To differentiate between obstructive and nonobstructive jaundice

2. To demonstrate the presence and site of carcinoma of the biliary system

3. To demonstrate the site and number of calculi

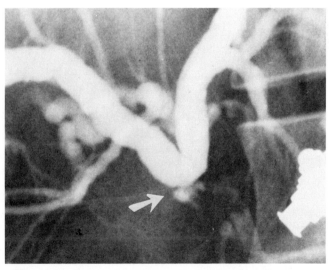

Fig. 14-20. Obstruction of the common hepatic duct just below the junction of the right and left hepatic ducts (**arrow**) caused by a ligature placed around the duct at previous operation. Transhepatic cholangiogram.

4. To determine the status of the biliary tree in cases of congenital biliary atresia

5. To decompress the biliary tree in preparation for surgery.

Major complications are uncommon and are mainly those of peritonitis or hemorrhage. It is generally recommended that operation should follow the examination in jaundiced patients if there is obstruction of the common duct or nonvisualization of the ductal system. In most patients the examination is done to determine the nature and location of biliary ductal obstruction. Involvement of the common duct by carcinoma, particularly of the pancreas, causes a smoothly tapering obstruction in most cases. With carcinoma arising in the periampullary region the contour is ragged and irregular in some (Fig. 14-18); in others the obstructed end of the duct is marked by a smooth concavity. These signs vary between patients, however, and it often is difficult or impossible to determine the site of origin of the tumor particularly in advanced disease. A calculus impacted in the duct (Fig. 14-19) causes a smoothly concave defect as the contrast material partially surrounds it. Calculi may be demonstrated in other ducts as well. Benign stricture is seen as a smooth area of narrowing with a variable amount of dilatation of the ductal system above it (Fig. 14-20).

Recently the transjugular approach to ductal cannulization has been recommended by Weiner and Hanafee[19] in order to minimize the complications of the procedure. Their original article should be consulted for technical details.

REFERENCES AND SELECTED READINGS

1. Arcomano, J. P., Heroy, W. W., and Barnett, J. C.: Fixed filling defects of the gallbladder. *Am. J. Digest. Dis. 8:* 222, 1963.

2. Bornhurst, R. A., Heitzman, E. R., and McAfee, J. G.: Double-dose drip infusion cholangiography: Analysis of 107 consecutive cases. *JAMA 206:* 1489, 1968.

3. Crummy, A. B.: Same day re-enforcement oral cholecystography. *Wis. Med. J. 65:* 84, 1966.

4. Han, S. Y., Collins, L. C., and Wright, R. M.: Choledochal cyst. Report of five cases. *Clin. Radiol. 20:* 332, 1969.

5. Hughes, J., LoCurcio, S. B., Edmunds, R., and Finby, N.: The common duct after cholecystectomy. Initial report of a ten year study. *JAMA 197:* 247, 1966.

6. Jones, H. W., and Walker, J. H.: Correlation of the pathologic and radiologic findings in tumors and pseudotumors of the gallbladder. *Surg. Gynec. Obstet. 105:* 599, 1957.

7. Juhl, J. H., Cooperman, L. R., and Crummy, A. B.: Oragrafin, a new cholecystographic medium. *Radiology 80:* 87, 1963.

8. Jutras, J. A.: Hyperplastic cholecystoses. *Am. J. Roentgenol. Radium Ther. Nucl. Med. 83:* 795, 1960.

9. Jutras, J. A., and Levesque, H. P.: Adenomyoma and adenomyomatosis of the gallbladder: Radiologic and pathologic correlations. *Radiol. Clin. North Am. 4:* 483, 1966.

10. Krieger, J., Seaman, W. B., and Porter, M. R.: The roentgenologic appearance of sclerosing cholangitis. *Radiology 94:* 369, 1970.

11. LeQuesne, L. P., and Ranger, I.: Cholecystitis glandularis proliferans. *Br. J. Surg. 44:* 447, 1957.

12. Mujahed, Z., and Evans, J. A.: Percutaneous transhepatic cholangiography. *Radiol. Clin. North Am. 4:* 535, 1966.

13. Ochsner, S. F.: Solitary polypoid lesions of the gallbladder. *Radiol. Clin. North Am. 4:* 501, 1966.

14. Ross, W. D., Finby, N., and Evans, J. A.: Intramural diverticulosis of the gallbladder (Rokitansky-Aschoff sinuses). *Radiology 64:* 366, 1955.

15. Sachs, M. D.: Routine cholangiography, operative and postoperative. *Radiol. Clin. North Am. 4:* 547, 1966.

16. Salzman, E.: Opacification of bile duct calculi. *Radiol. Clin. North Am. 4:* 525, 1966.

17. Shehadi, W. H.: Radiologic examination of the biliary tract: Plain film of the abdomen: Oral cholecystography. *Radiol. Clin. North Am. 4:* 463, 1966.

18. Turner, F. W., and Costopoulos, L. B.: Percutaneous transhepatic cholangiography. A study of 115 cases. *Can. Med. Assoc. J. 99:* 513, 1968.

19. Weiner, M., and Hanafee, W. N.: A review of transjugular cholangiography. *Radiol. Clin. North Am. 8:* 53, 1970.

20. Wise, R. E.: Current concepts of intravenous cholangiography. *Radiol Clin. North Am. 4:* 521, 1966.

21. Wise, R. E., and O'Brien, R. G.: Interpretation of the intravenous cholangiogram. *JAMA 160:* 819, 1956.

15

THE ESOPHAGUS

THE GASTROINTESTINAL EXAMINATION

In Chapter 13, the roentgen investigation of the gastrointestinal tract without the use of contrast media is discussed, with particular reference to the diagnosis of intestinal obstruction. In this and succeeding chapters, examination of the gastrointestinal tract by means of contrast material introduced into it either orally or given as an enema will be considered.

BARIUM SULFATE

The material most frequently used for contrast visualization of the intestinal tract is barium sulfate. This is obtained as a finely ground powder specially prepared for roentgen purposes. It is important that only chemically pure barium sulfate be used since the commercial product may contain highly poisonous impurities. Various concerns manufacture barium sulfate expressly for roentgen diagnostic purposes and only material in containers bearing such a label should be used. Barium sulfate is completely inert in the gastrointestinal tract and it is very radiopaque. It is insoluble in water and is given, orally and rectally, as an aqueous suspension. Commercial preparations are available that contain suspending agents that help to keep the heavy powder from settling too rapidly. Such mixtures also serve to coat the mucosal surfaces somewhat better than the plain barium-water mixtures.

WATER-SOLUBLE IODINATED COMPOUNDS

Water-soluble iodinated compounds such as Hypaque and Gastrografin have been recommended as contrast agents particularly when obstruction is present or suspected. However, it has been shown that barium sulfate does not become impacted above an obstructing lesion in the small intestine and these compounds have a limited field of usefulness in roentgen studies of the gastrointestinal tract, including the esophagus.

TERMINOLOGY OF EXAMINATIONS

Each part of the gastrointestinal tract will be dealt with separately in the discussions to follow and the techniques of examination will be found under the specific anatomic subdivisions. The colon is examined by means of a barium mixture given as an enema and this is commonly referred to as a barium enema examination. The esophagus, stomach, duodenum, and upper part of the jejunum are examined together by means of a barium mixture given orally; by common usage this is referred to as an upper gastrointestinal series (GI series). The mesenteric small intestine is not included routinely as a part of the upper gastrointestinal study. If it is to be examined this is done as a continuation of the gastrointestinal series by following the oral meal as it passes through the small bowel; this is referred to as a small-intestinal examination or as a "small bowel study."

SPOT FILMS

Modern fluoroscopes are equipped with a device whereby a roentgen-film cassette can be brought in front of the patient being fluoroscoped and an exposure made using the fluoroscopic tube as the source of roentgen rays. Such a device enables the fluoroscopist to obtain a film image of something observed on the fluoroscopic screen within a second or two after it is seen. This makes it possible to record on film, rapidly changing images and transient defects in the barium shadow which otherwise might be difficult to register. These roentgenograms are referred to as "spot films," since they usually cover only a small field and the examiner "aims" the exposure at a definite area. Spot films are very useful in gastrointestinal roentgenography because of the changing contours of the viscera brought about by peristalsis and respiration and by palpation on the part of the examiner.

CINEFLUOROGRAPHY

With modern image amplifiers it is possible to obtain moving pictures of the gastrointestinal tract. This technique has the advantage of recording on film the rapidly changing images seen fluoroscopically and allows a more leisurely viewing and repeated viewings of the various parts of the tract. The quality of reproduction is very good. It is also possible to televise the fluoroscopic image, thus allowing more than one individual to view the procedure, even in a distant room. Devices also are available which allow the examiner to be in an adjacent room, the control of the apparatus being done remotely. Television fluoroscopy has become an important adjunct in the examination of the gastrointestinal tract. It is also possible to register the fluoroscopic image on television tape for later playback.

THE ESOPHAGUS

The esophagus is examined routinely as a part of the study of the upper gastrointestinal tract. In addition it may be investigated because of specific complaints referable to it. The technique of examination will of necessity vary, depending on the presence or absence of a lesion, the amount of obstruction, etc.

METHODS OF EXAMINATION

PRELIMINARY ROENTGENOGRAMS

The contracted esophagus may be visualized as a narrow stripelike shadow in the upper mediastinum in frontal roentgenograms of the chest. Also the external wall of the barium-filled esophagus may occasionally be visualized particularly in the lower third in lateral and oblique roentgenograms as it is outlined by the air-filled lungs adjacent to it. Roentgenograms of the neck and thorax without contrast material in the esophagus are useful for the detection of opaque foreign bodies. Such roentgenograms also may demonstrate the dilated fluid-filled esophagus of achalasia. In congenital esophageal atresia the dilated, air- or fluid-

filled upper esophageal segment may be outlined. It also may cause some forward displacement of the trachea. If perforation of the esophagus is suspected, plain-film roentgenograms may reveal air or fluid in the mediastinal tissues or in the pleural cavities. Occasionally a carcinoma of the esophagus may cause an abnormal shadow and widening of the mediastinum. However, in most lesions affecting the esophagus an adequate examination requires the use of contrast material to outline its lumen.

CONTRAST VISUALIZATION

MATERIALS

A suspension of barium sulfate powder in water is the contrast material used for most esophageal examinations. The same mixture used for the examination of the stomach and small intestine is satisfactory for the preliminary study of the esophagus and consists of 125 gm of the powdered barium sulfate to 180 cc of water. For a more detailed study of the mucosa and to elicit small defects a thicker mixture is needed. Only enough water is added to the barium sulfate to form a creamy paste. This is given in tablespoonful amounts.

Iodized oil sometimes is used in place of barium, usually because there is the possibility of aspiration of the material into the tracheobronchial tree or because a fistula exists between the two. It is often used in examining the esophagus of the newborn when atresia is suspected. However, the danger from aspiration of barium sulfate is not great; in fact it has been recommended as a contrast agent for bronchography. When the possibility of aspiration exists the examiner should use caution regardless of the contrast agent used.

The swallowing of small pledgets of cotton soaked in the barium mixture is useful when examining for the presence of small or sharp foreign bodies such as fish bones. A small piece of bread soaked in the barium mixture is used occasionally to demonstrate the ability of the esophagus to transport solid food. Such a bolus may elicit spasm better than the liquid mixture. To determine the maximum diameter of a stricture, gelatin capsules of various sizes filled with barium powder can be given. By noting the largest size capsule that will pass through the stricture, an idea of its maximum diameter can be obtained.

TECHNIQUE OF EXAMINATION

This will vary among patients, depending on the problem at hand.

FLUOROSCOPY. The examination is begun with the patient standing behind the fluoroscopic screen; after a brief preliminary screening of the heart and lung fields, the patient is asked to take several swallows of the thin barium mixture. This is watched as it passes through the entire esophagus and into the stomach and the patient is rotated into various positions so that the entire circumference of the esophagus is brought into profile. Swallows of the thick paste are then given and again observation is carried out with the patient in various degrees of obliquity in relation to the fluoroscopic screen. Usually the examination is continued with the fluoroscopic table lowered to a horizontal position; with the patient supine the

esophagus again is examined with the several mixtures.

ROENTGENOGRAMS. Spot roentgenograms are made during the fluoroscopic study, the number depending upon what is observed and what it seems desirable to record. As a rule these are the only roentgenograms that are necessary.

CINEFLUOROGRAPHY. The image intensifier has made possible the use of movies in the study of the gastrointestinal tract and these are often of particular value in the investigation of disorders of the esophagus. Television viewing and television tape recording are additional methods that can be incorporated in the study. These devices can be used in conjunction with standard roentgenograms and in some cases can supplant the routine views.

THE NORMAL ESOPHAGUS

ANATOMY

The esophagus begins at the level of the cricoid cartilage in the neck. It passes to the right of the transverse aortic arch, with which it is in close relationship. The arch causes a smooth indentation on the barium-filled esophagus; this becomes more prominent with advancing age (Fig. 15-1). The right branch of the pulmonary artery passes anterior to the esophagus; the left main bronchus crosses it directly below the level of the aortic arch and may cause a slight, smooth indentation in the barium shadow. The distal part of the esophagus lies to the right of and anterior to the descending thoracic aorta. In elderly persons, where the aorta is elongated and tortuous, it may displace the lower part of the esophagus forward. The descending aorta in these patients usually executes a curve to the left and may project beyond the left cardiac margin in posteroanterior roentgenograms. The esophagus remains in close relationship to the right aortic border and will also curve to the left and then back to the midline as it descends through the diaphragm. The distal part of the esophagus lies directly behind the posterior surface of the heart and thus it is in close relationship with the left atrium. The abdominal portion of the esophagus is of variable length and the exact anatomy of this segment is in dispute. In many persons, par-

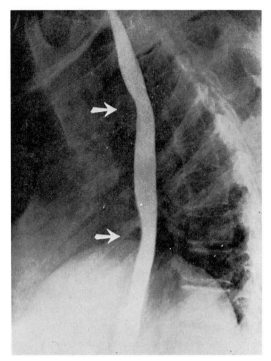

Fig. 15-1. Normal esophagus. Left anterior oblique roentgenogram of the thorax with the esophagus filled with barium mixture. The indentation produced by the transverse aortic arch is shown (**upper arrow**). The **lower arrow** points to a slight impression on the esophagus at the level of the left atrium.

ticularly in those who are obese, there often appears to be a lack of an abdominal portion, the cardia being at the level of the diaphragmatic hiatus. In others, a short segment is seen to lie below the diaphragm. This is discussed more fully in the section entitled "the Lower Esophagus and Cardia."

ROENTGEN OBSERVATIONS

THE ACT OF SWALLOWING

The act of swallowing is a complicated process that has been under recent investigation by means of roentgen cinematography. As an extremely brief description of this complicated act it may be stated that the bolus to be swallowed is pushed backward by the tongue. The uvula and soft palate rise to close off the nasopharynx. The larynx rises, the glottis is closed, and the epiglottis tips backward over the laryngeal vestibule. The bolus passes rapidly through the pharynx, filling the pyriform sinuses momentarily, and is propelled into the esophagus by a powerful contraction of the pharyngeal muscles.

MOVEMENT OF MATERIAL THROUGH THE ESOPHAGUS

In the upright position, once a liquid bolus has reached the esophagus, it passes rapidly through the cervical portion, propelled by a stripping peristaltic wave that is a continuation of the propulsive contraction of the pharynx. Gravity is the major factor in further progress of the material through the remainder of the esophagus. Peristalsis ordinarily is not visible except as a contraction wave behind the advancing bolus, which serves to strip the residue into the stomach. With thick barium paste, and particularly if the swallowing act is performed with the patient in a horizontal position, the material is propelled by a broad contraction that passes rapidly down the esophagus. This is known as the primary wave or contraction. After the esophagus has been emptied of the major portion of the material there is a general relaxation and in the normal resting phase the esophagus remains in a slightly relaxed state. If the initial primary wave has not emptied the esophagus of most of the material a second wave occurs and this may be repeated until no more contrast material remains. These contractions, which are not initiated by swallowing, are called secondary waves.

There is much variation in this process. Ordinarily movement is much slower in older individuals; often the first swallow is arrested at the level of the diaphragm and may remain there until more swallows have been taken. On deep inspiration the diaphragm seems to act as a pinchcock, closing the esophagus until exhalation is performed.

FURTHER ROENTGEN OBSERVATIONS

With rapid swallowing the entire esophagus remains filled except the cervical portion, which contracts rapidly after each swallow. The margins of the distended esophagus are smooth. The pressure indentation by the aortic arch is readily seen. The portion in contact with the left atrium of the heart will pulsate with the atrial pulsations. If, in the contracted state, a thick barium paste has been given, sufficient will cling to the walls to outline the mucosal folds. They become visible as thin, vertical, stripelike shadows paralleling the long axis of the esophagus; the stripes represent barium caught in the valleys between the folds. Normally only three or four folds are present (Fig. 15-2). Frequently a smooth indentation is noted on the posterior wall of the upper end of the esophagus. This is called the "esophageal lip" and is believed to be caused by the

transverse fibers of the cricopharyngeus muscles. It has no clinical significance.

PRESBYESOPHAGUS. With increasing age there often is a change in the motor activity of the esophagus. Peristaltic waves are slowed, shallow, and at times traverse only the upper part of the esophagus or are absent altogether. Tertiary contractions ("curling") are prominent and characteristic (see p. 493). If there is lack of normal relaxation of the lower esophageal sphincter the esophagus becomes dilated. All of these factors lead to poor or incomplete emptying of the esophagus since both primary and secondary peristalsis are not efficient in transporting the contents into the stomach. Most patients do not have symptoms.

THE PHRENIC AMPULLA. Frequently, as the esophagus contracts behind a bolus of barium, the lower end becomes dilated, the primary wave stopping before it reaches the level of the diaphragm. There results a pouchlike dilatation of the esophagus. After a few moments this segment usually contracts, pushing the retained barium mixture into the stomach, and it does not fill again until another swallow has been taken. This dilated segment is known as the phrenic ampulla (Figs. 15-3 and 15-4). It is of importance because of the necessity for distin-

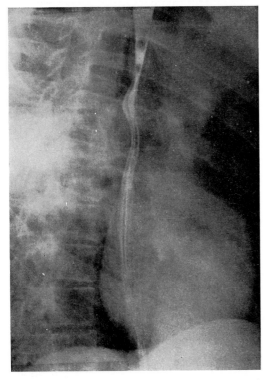

Fig. 15-2. The normal esophagus in a contracted state. Right anterior oblique roentgenogram of the thorax made after patient swallowed a thick barium-water paste. Enough of the material clings to the mucosal surface of the esophagus to outline its folds. These are seen as several fine stripelike, translucent areas separated by stripes of increased density, representing the valleys between the elevated folds.

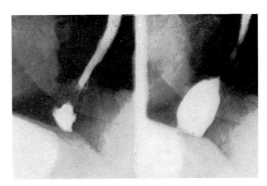

Fig. 15-3. The phrenic ampulla. Two spot roentgenograms made during the fluoroscopic observation of the swallowing act and centered at the level of the cardia. On the *right* the lower end of the esophagus is dilated. The roentgenogram was made shortly after the primary contraction wave had reached the level of the ampulla. On the *left* another wave has caused most of the barium in the ampulla to enter the stomach with a certain amount of reflux into the esophagus proximal to the ampulla.

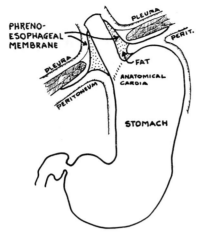

PHRENO-
ESOPHAGEAL
MEMBRANE

PLEURA

PERIT.

PLEURA

FAT

ANATOMICAL
CARDIA

PERITONEUM

STOMACH

Fig. 15-4. Diagram illustrates the anatomy of the cardiac region. The elastic phrenoesophageal membrane serves as a support for the lower end of the esophagus and allows the diaphragm to move up and down without too much disturbance of the cardia. (*Based on Harrington.*)

guishing it from an esophageal hiatal hernia, which it closely resembles. This is discussed more fully in the section entitled "Hiatal Hernia" in Chapter 16.

BARRETT'S ESOPHAGUS, OR THE ALLISON-JOHNSTONE ANOMALY. This anomaly consists of a columnar epithelial lining for a variable portion of the lower esophagus.[14, 22] The mere presence of this type of epithelium in the esophagus cannot be detected roentgenologically. However, in many patients, there is a stricture several centimeters or more above the esophagogastric junction. This may be in the form of a thin ring or be several centimeters long. The lower limit of the stricture marks the squamocolumnar junction. The longer strictures show tapering ends and the lumen through the stricture may vary in some patients from swallow to swallow suggesting that muscle spasm rather than fibrosis is the cause. In others the stricture appears fixed, evidently from fibrosis. Occasionally a deep ulcer niche is encountered. If an ulcer is found it indicates that there is gastric epithelium at this point. Also hiatal hernia or esophageal reflux is frequently present. In these cases differentiation from stricture associated with a short esophagus type of hiatal hernia depends on visualizing peristaltic waves passing through the stricture and through a segment of esophagus be-

low before reaching the esophagogastric junction at the summit of the hernia. The character of the motor activity of this segment below the stricture is that of esophagus and not stomach. In some cases esophagoscopy and biopsy will be necessary. The cause is not definitely known; both congenital and acquired theories have been proposed. In those patients with stricture, dysphagia usually is present. If there is only a thin ring, symptoms may be absent.

THE LOWER ESOPHAGUS AND CARDIA. The anatomic junction between the esophagus and stomach is termed the cardiac orifice or cardia. A considerable amount of investigative work has been done, much of it in recent years, on the anatomy and physiology of the distal end of the esophagus and the mechanisms for closure of the cardia to prevent reflux of stomach contents into the esophagus. There have been differences of opinion regarding the presence of an abdominal portion of the esophagus, the exact site of esophageal closure, and the mechanism whereby competency of the cardia is maintained. It is no longer believed by many that the junction of esophageal and gastric mucosa represents the cardia or the site where closure occurs. The mucosal junction often is irregular with fingerlike projections of one type of mucosa into the other. Gastric mucosa also may continue a considerable distance above the level of the diaphragmatic hiatus (see section on "Barrett's Esophagus or the Allison-Johnstone Anomaly"). Also, it has been shown by Palmer[17] and others, using metal clips attached to the mucosal junction at the time of esophagoscopy, that it is not fixed but that there is a certain amount of up and down migration of the mucosa on the muscularis with swallowing or even during the resting state. Some authors consider the esophagogastric junction to be at the site where esophageal and gastric epithelium meet. It has been pointed out by others that the nature of a given segment, i.e., whether it is functionally esophagus or stomach, is determined not by the type of epithelial lining, but by the character of its motor activity or peristalsis.

Roentgenologically, the junction between esophageal and gastric mucosa may or may not

[handwritten margin note, left:] ie Schatzkis ring? see p 512

[handwritten note, bottom:] in short esoph. due to oesophagitis stricture may be much higher than a Schatzki ring.

be obvious. The transition from three to four vertical parallel folds in the contracted esophagus to the larger, more tortuous, or crinkled folds of the stomach may be distinct but in some individuals the esophageal folds appear to be directly continuous with the gastric folds and pass without interruption into the stomach. Also, when gastric mucosa extends some distance above the diaphragm, as in Barrett's esophagus, the fold appearance is that of esophagus rather than stomach. This difficulty becomes significant when the diagnosis of a small hiatal hernia is being considered (see sections on hiatal hernia, Chapter 16, and "Lower Esophageal Ring," this chapter.)

While a tubular structure considered by some to represent an abdominal portion of the esophagus can be identified at times, other investigators have considered this to be a part of the stomach rather than of the esophagus or else have thought that it represents an intermediate structure to which the name vestibule or abdominal gullet has been given. The latter concept has received considerable support in the recent literature on the subject. According to Wolf and associates[21] the term, "esophago-gastric junction," refers to a segment about 5 cm in length between the body of the esophagus and the stomach. The upper part of this tract, about 3 cm in length, consists of the phrenic ampulla which extends to the diaphragmatic hiatus. Between the ampulla and body of the stomach is another tubular structure which is intra-abdominal in location and designated as the submerged segment or abdominal gullet. This part is lined by squamous epithelium proximally and cylindric epithelium distally. Because the closing mechanism appears to lie at the level of the diaphragm, the opinion has been expressed that this represents the cardia, at least from a functional viewpoint.[6] (Also see page 543.)

The mechanism whereby the lower end of the esophagus is closed, thus preventing reflux from the stomach, is not agreed upon. With but few exceptions investigators have failed to find evidence of a true anatomic sphincter in the lower end of the esophagus, i.e., a localized thickening of the circular muscle. Nevertheless, most observers agree that the muscle must exert a sphincterlike action and this has come to be known as the physiological sphincter. It is also generally agreed that this sphincteric action is relatively weak and that there must be some other mechanism to aid it. For a long time the pinchcock action of the diaphragm has been considered to be one of these factors. The right crus of the diaphragm surrounds the hiatus, encircling the esophagus in a slinglike manner. On deep inspiration, contraction of the diaphragm can be seen fluoroscopically, closing the esophagus and preventing swallowed material from passing through into the stomach. On expiration, as the diaphragm relaxes, the swallowed material passes readily into the stomach.

The obliquity of the insertion of the esophagus into the stomach also has been considered to be important. The direction of the esophagus in relation to the fundus results in a sharp angular sulcus or incisura between the two. This sulcus is deepened when the fundus is distended. Another possible mechanism is the presence of a valvelike action of a lip of mucosa along the left border of the cardia. The final answers to these problems remain unsettled but, as pointed out by Fleischner,[6] roentgenologically, the point of closure, and therefore what may be termed the functional cardia, appears to lie at the level of the diaphragm.

THE "CURLING PHENOMENON." Curling is a peculiar aberration of motility seen rather frequently in elderly individuals and occasionally in younger persons. It is brought out to best advantage when the examination is done with the patient recumbent. As the mass of barium descends into the lower part of the esophagus and distends it, multiple ringlike contractions rapidly appear and disappear, recurring at short intervals until finally a peristaltic wave moves the bolus into the stomach (Fig. 15-5). This condition also is known as *"corkscrew esophagus"* or *"beaded esophagus,"* and as *tertiary contractions* of the esophagus. In most instances it does not seem to be of clinical significance and does not cause symptoms. Occasionally the contractions are particularly deep and lasting and the contraction rings

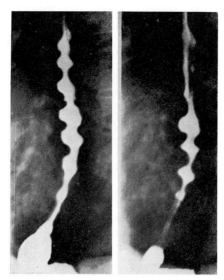

Fig. 15-5. The curling phenomenon. Two roentgenograms made during the fluoroscopic procedure while the patient was swallowing barium mixture, illustrating the characteristic circular contractions that develop in the esophagus and the rapid change in form.

divide the esophagus into multiple dilated segments. Some patients with this more severe form of curling complain of dysphagia. This usually is intermittent and often initiated by the swallowing of poorly chewed food. Also, in this severe form of curling diverticulumlike outpouchings may be seen between two or more of the contractions. These may be only temporary and as the spastic contractions relax the outpouchings disappear. These are known as *pseudodiverticula*. Less frequently, true pulsion diverticula are seen, the pouches remaining filled during the contraction and relaxation phases. It is believed that these arise from the increased pressure within the segments between the contraction rings, the pseudodiverticula being the precursors of the permanent or true diverticula.

GASTROESOPHAGEAL REFLUX. In some individuals under certain circumstances reflux from the stomach into the esophagus may occur frequently. It often accompanies hiatal hernia, especially of the sliding or short esophagus types. The bathing of esophageal epithelium with acidic gastric juice promotes the development of esophagitis, often followed by esophageal stricture and this becomes one of the serious complications of hiatal hernia.

Reflux also may occur in some persons without hernia and also may lead to esophagitis. The most positive way to determine if reflux is present is to observe it fluoroscopically after the stomach has been filled with the barium mixture. It is seen most frequently when the examination is done with the patient supine.

To detect reflux otherwise, the water-siphonage test has been recommended.[5] The patient is placed in a right posterior oblique supine position after barium has been given. In this position the barium mixture will gravitate to the cardia, the most dependent part of the fundus. Several swallows of water then are given. As the lower esophageal sphincter relaxes to allow passage of the water, barium may be seen to reflux into the esophagus. This is considered a positive test and the advocates of the method have found a good correlation between a positive test and the symptoms of esophagitis such as pyrosis. It should be noted, however, that reflux is found only with the patient in a supine position and only after drinking of a liquid in this position so that it is not an entirely physiologic procedure.

CONGENITAL ANOMALIES

ATRESIA OF THE ESOPHAGUS

Complete congenital occlusion of the esophagus is a relatively frequent anomaly, the site of obstruction usually being in the upper third just below the level of the sternal notch. The types of esophageal atresia, according to Vogt's classification,[20] are as follows:

Type   I. Complete absence of the esophagus.

Type II. Atresia of the esophagus with both *[2ᵈ most freq]* upper and lower segments ending in a blind pouch

Type III. Atresia of the esophagus with tracheoesophageal fistula

      a. Fistula between the upper segment and the trachea

      b. Fistula between the lower segment *[Most freq]* and the trachea, the upper ending blindly

      c. Fistula between the trachea and both esophageal segments

In Type II the length of the atretic segment is variable but usually is fairly short. Occasion-

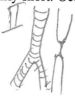

[handwritten: III b]   *[handwritten: II]*

[handwritten: 85—90 %]

ally extensive agenesis of the lower part of the esophagus has been found. The most frequent type is IIIb and this has been reported to constitute from 85 to 90 per cent of all cases. The next most frequent lesion is Type II.

Roentgen Observations

Preliminary roentgenograms of the chest and abdomen in anteroposterior and lateral directions are obtained. If the atresia is of either type IIIb or IIIc, air will be present in the gastrointestinal tract (Fig. 15-6). With the other types of atresia the abdomen will be completely free of air. The presence or absence of intestinal air, therefore, is important in distinguishing between the types of defect. Plain

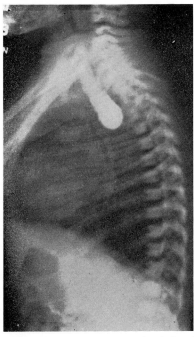

Fig. 15-6. Congenital esophageal atresia. Lateral roentgenogram of the thorax of a newborn infant with esophageal atresia. Contrast material has been instilled into the upper end of the esophagus, demonstrating it to end blindly just above the level of the tracheal bifurcation. This is a Type III-B atresia. Note the gas in the stomach and intestinal tract beneath the diaphragm, indicating that there must be a communication between the tracheobronchial tree and the lower part of the esophagus below the level of the atresia.

roentgenograms may show an aspiration pneumonitis or atelectasis. Occasionally the upper esophageal segment will be outlined by swallowed air. Dilatation of the proximal segment may be sufficient to cause some forward displacement of the trachea.

The next step in the examination is to insert a soft-rubber catheter into the upper end of the esophagus (under fluoroscopic guidance) as far as it will go. A small amount of an iodized oil or barium sulfate, usually not more than 2.0 cc, is injected. This will outline the lower end of the segment and clearly demonstrate the presence of the atresia. If the anomaly is of either Type IIIa or IIIc, the oil will flow into the trachea and be aspirated into the tracheobronchial tree. It is for this reason that iodized oil rather than a barium mixture has been recommended, because aspiration of any appreciable amount of the insoluble barium might cause severe respiratory embarrassment. A large amount of oil also is dangerous because it can fill the small bronchi to the point where respiratory difficulty may develop. Insufflation of oil into the finer bronchioles and pulmonary alveoli may lead to retention of the material and cause difficulty later on (lipid pneumonia). It is wise, therefore, regardless of what medium is used, to inject the material into the esophagus with caution, always under fluoroscopic guidance and with only enough of the contrast material to establish the presence and the type of the defect.

As a rather rare variation of Type IIIc, a small fistulous opening may be present between the esophagus and the trachea but with little or no narrowing of the esophageal lumen. The opening may be very small but be sufficient in size to allow aspiration of swallowed material. In such patients an intractable chronic pneumonitis or atelectasis may result. The infant is noted to have a chronic cough and choking spells develop, particularly during feeding. If the opening is very small and if there is no narrowing of the esophageal lumen it may be difficult to demonstrate the fistula roentgenologically. Leigh et al.[12] recommend examining the infant in an anterior oblique position since the opening is usually in the

[handwritten margin note:] lie baby prone on step of upright X-ray table — underneath then gives horizontal beam films

anterior wall of the esophagus and posterior wall of the trachea. This position facilitates visualization of the tract because it will be dependent to the esophageal lumen. Barium sulfate, or an iodized oil such as Lipiodol, may be used. The contrast material can be instilled through a catheter inserted down to the level of the carina or slightly above it and fluoroscopic observation carried out while several cubic centimeters of the material are injected.

CONGENITAL STRICTURE OF THE ESOPHAGUS

Congenital stricture of the esophagus is an uncommon lesion and represents an incomplete occlusion. The lesion can be diagnosed without much difficulty on roentgen examination. It results in a smooth fusiform narrowing of the esophageal lumen, causing a variable degree of obstruction. In the newborn such a stricture is almost invariably of congenital origin. In the older infant or child it may be impossible to distinguish between a congenital stricture and one of acquired origin caused by the swallowing of caustic material, since the roentgen appearances may be similar. Usually acquired strictures are multiple and involve longer segments of the esophagus.

DUPLICATION OF THE ESOPHAGUS

Duplication of the esophagus is a rare congenital anomaly. A closed duplication results in a cystic mass lined with esophageal epithelium and filled with fluid. It is found, as a rule, in the central or posterior portion of the mediastinum. The cyst may enlarge rapidly during infancy causing symptoms of pressure upon the other mediastinal structures. Most esophageal cysts or duplications, therefore, are discovered during the first few years of life. The lesion is seen as a rounded or oval-shaped mass lying within or along a border of the mediastinum in close relationship to the esophagus. There are few features to distinguish this lesion from a variety of other tumors and mass lesions that may occur in the mediastinum and surgical exploration usually is necessary. Occasionally the cyst is lined with gastric or other type of epithelium.

Open duplication of the esophagus is another extremely rare developmental anomaly in which the lumen of the duplication is patent and communicates with the normal esophagus resulting in a double lumen.[7]

DISEASES OF THE ESOPHAGUS

DIVERTICULA

Diverticula are common lesions in the esophagus as they are in most other portions of the gastrointestinal tract and they may be found in any part of the structure. Diverticula of the esophagus may be either of the pulsion or traction types but almost all are acquired lesions. The most significant from a clinical point of view is the one that develops along the posterior wall of the upper end of the esophagus at its junction with the pharynx (Zenker's diverticulum). This is an acquired pulsion type of diverticulum that forms at a site of anatomical weakness in the pharyngoesophageal wall. The diverticulum may cause symptoms of difficulty in swallowing because of retention of food and consequent pressure upon the cervical portion of the esophagus at the level of the thoracic inlet.

Diverticula of the intrathoracic portion of the esophagus are found mainly in its middle third, in the region of the lung hila, and most of them probably are of traction type, caused by pull from fibrous adhesions following infection of mediastinal lymph nodes. Calcified nodes frequently can be demonstrated adjacent to the diverticulum, the nodes being the end result of previous infection, often primary tuberculosis.

Diverticula in the lower end of the esophagus are most often of pulsion type. They are seen frequently in association with the curling phenomenon as described on page 493, probably developing as a result of increased pressure in the areas between the spastic contraction rings.

Most esophageal diverticula other than the Zenker's type are asymptomatic and are incidental findings during a gastrointestinal roentgen examination. Within the thorax a diverticulum has adequate space to enlarge without causing pressure upon vital structures; they usually do not retain material to any appreciable degree, and secondary complications are infrequent. Exceptionally, a large diverticulum will form in the distal end of the esophagus just above the level of the diaphragm; it may be symptom-producing because of its large size and the retention of food within it (Fig. 15-7) (epiphrenic diverticulum).

Intramural diverticulosis is a rare form of the disease characterized by the formation of small diverticula within the wall of the esophagus.[4] The appearance has been likened to a chain of beads and to the Rokitansky-Aschoff sinuses of the gallbladder. The cause is unknown but the congenital theory has been favored.

Roentgen Observations

The diverticulum is visualized as an outpouching or sac protruding outside of the esophageal lumen and connected to it by a narrow neck (Figs. 15-8 and 15-9). The sac

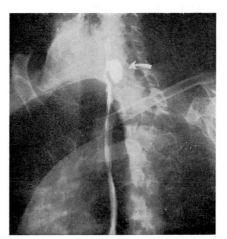

Fig. 15-8. Zenker's type of pharyngoesophageal diverticulum. The **arrow** points to the small diverticulum that arises from the posterior aspect of the esophagus at its junction with the pharynx.

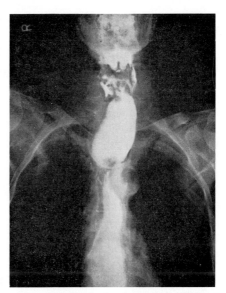

Fig. 15-9. Zenker's pharyngoesophageal diverticulum. There is a large saclike diverticulum projecting backward and downward in the midline behind the upper end of the esophagus as shown in the anteroposterior roentgenogram.

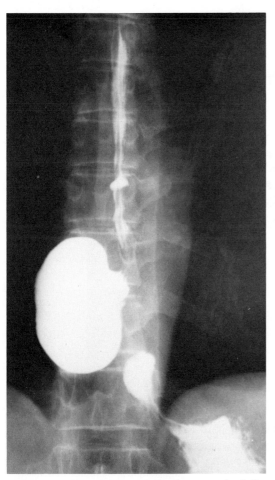

Fig. 15-7. Diverticulum of the lower end of the esophagus. The neck is along the side of the sac.

has a rounded contour in most cases; small traction diverticula may have a more pointed contour. The Zenker's type often reaches a large size (8 to 10 cm or more). This diverticulum as it enlarges extends downward and posteriorly, eventually reaching into the posterior mediastinum. The opening of the sac then is near the upper margin and retention of swallowed material is enhanced. The distended sac pushes the esophagus forward and, confined by the thoracic inlet, pressure obstruction will develop. This type of diverticulum may retain the barium mixture for many hours or even days. Diverticula in the remainder of the esophagus usually have the opening situated along one side of the pouch, retention of barium may be only for short periods, and some of the smaller ones may not be visualized at all unless the examination is conducted with the patient recumbent.

CARCINOMA OF THE ESOPHAGUS

Carcinoma may develop in any part of the esophagus and the tumor often is in an advanced stage when the patient is first examined roentgenologically. Preliminary roentgenograms of the thorax are not informative as a rule since the tumor mass may be small and not detected readily within the mediastinal shadow. Infrequently, the tumor infiltrates rather widely into the mediastinum and produces a visible soft tissue mass; occasionally it may invade the lung. The esophageal origin of such a mass can hardly be determined until contrast visualization of the esophagus is done. Even then, in some of the advanced cases, it may be impossible to determine whether the lesion originated in the esophagus and invaded the lung and mediastinum or whether the reverse is true. The decision may be difficult even at autopsy examination.

Roentgen Examination

The early lesion causes a filling defect in the barium-filled lumen situated along one side of the esophageal wall. The edges of the lesion are sharply demarcated and the defect caused by the mass produces a sharp angle, often an acute one, where it joins the esophageal wall. This is characteristic of polypoid carcinoma throughout the gastrointestinal tract. The surface of the filling defect is irregular or nodular (Fig. 15-10).

More advanced lesions encircle the lumen completely resulting in an annular constricting filling defect, narrowing the lumen, and causing some degree of obstruction. The upper and lower margins of the defect tend to overhang as they do in the unilateral defect described in the previous paragraph. The lumen through the stenotic area is irregular and mucosal folds are absent (Figs. 15-11 and 15-12). The defect is constant and reproducible. The esophagus above the lesion usually is slightly to moder-

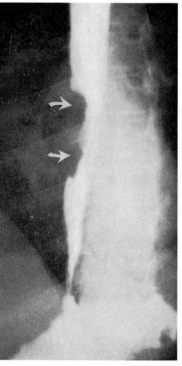

Fig. 15-10. Carcinoma of the esophagus. This is a relatively early lesion and the filling defect is limited to one wall. It is visualized as a filling defect in the barium-filled lumen of the esophagus (**arrows**). The surface of the filling defect is irregular and there is overhanging of edges where the lesion is sharply demarcated from the normal esophageal wall.

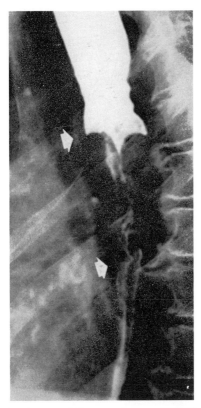

Fig. 15-11. Carcinoma of the esophagus. Lateral roentgenogram of the midportion of the esophagus shows an annular lesion completely encircling the lumen of the esophagus and causing moderate obstruction. The upper and lower ends of the lesion are indicated by the **arrows.** The channel through the lesion is irregular. Note the acute angles formed by the junction of the defect and normal esophageal walls.

ately dilated; the amount of dilatation depends largely upon the amount of obstruction.

High esophageal carcinoma usually causes considerable difficulty in swallowing and there may be aspiration of some of the material into the trachea as the patient attempts to swallow the barium mixture. Carcinoma of the cervical part of the esophagus often causes a forward displacement of the tracheal shadow in lateral roentgenograms of the neck and a corresponding increase in thickness of the prevertebral soft-tissue shadow. When barium outlines the channel through the lesion, it will be seen to lie within the central part of the soft-tissue

thickening. This observation helps to distinguish carcinoma of the esophagus from secondary invasion by an extrinsic malignant tumor. The latter tumor also may result in increase in the soft-tissue space anterior to the cervical spine and the esophagus may be irregular and narrowed by the tumor; but it also will be displaced and not surrounded uniformly by the mass.

Sinus tracts often develop in the late stages of carcinoma of the esophagus and these are outlined by the barium mixture as irregular extensions into the contiguous mediastinal tissues (Fig. 15-13, *left*). Occasionally a fistula will perforate into the trachea if the carcinoma lies adjacent to this structure. As the barium mixture is swallowed, some of it will be seen to

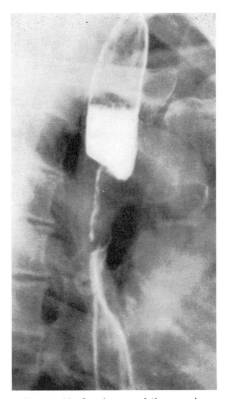

Fig. 15-12. Carcinoma of the esophagus. There is an annular lesion completely encircling the lumen of the esophagus in its middle third. This is an upright roentgenogram and the barium in the esophagus above the level of the lesion is surmounted by swallowed air.

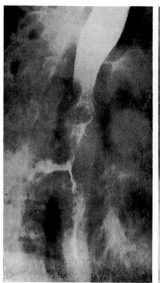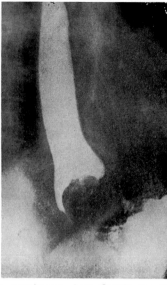

Fig. 15-13. Carcinoma of the esophagus. *Left*, Carcinoma in the midthird of the esophagus, which has developed a fistulous tract extending into the mediastinal tissues. The defect caused by the tumor is long and irregular. *Right*, Polypoid or fungating carcinoma involving the lower end of the esophagus. The tumor forms a bulky mass but is not highly obstructive and barium mixture has entered the stomach.

pass rapidly into the tracheobronchial tree. Usually this initiates a spasm of severe coughing but in some individuals such aspiration causes little distress. The aspiration of the barium sulfate does not appear to cause any acute reaction and is no more harmful than the aspiration of food and water, which happens every time the patient attempts to eat or drink. Aspiration pneumonitis in the lung bases is an accompaniment of tracheobronchial fistula and is present to some extent in all such cases.

In the lower end of the esophagus carcinoma occasionally is of a fungating type, causing a bulky, lobulated, filling defect but with only moderate obstruction. Extension of a carcinoma of the distal esophagus to involve the cardiac end of the stomach and vice versa is common. It may be impossible from roentgen examination to determine where such a tumor originated (Fig. 15-13, *right*).

Infrequently a carcinoma of the esophagus causes a smooth, fusiform type of stricture, resembling closely the appearance of a benign fibrous stricture. The edges do not overhang but taper smoothly. Most benign strictures found in patients within the carcinoma age period occur in the lower end as a result of esophagitis or follow the ingestion of caustic materials and the resulting chemical esophagitis. Any stricture above the level of the distal few inches of the esophagus in a patient in the carcinoma age period with no history of ingestion of caustic material should be considered most likely caused by carcinoma. An exception occurs in Barrett's esophagus where the stricture forms several centimeters or more above the level of the diaphragmatic hiatus. Esophagoscopy and biopsy should be performed if there is any doubt. For the distinguishing features of esophagitis with stricture formation in the cardiac end of the esophagus see discussion to follow.

Rarely, carcinoma of the distal end of the esophagus causes an appearance closely simulating achalasia. The esophagus is greatly dilated and atonic. The lower end tapers gradually. The stricture caused by the tumor usually is at or close to the level of the disphragmatic hiatus. Close observation may show a certain amount of irregularity of the stricture margins and absence of mucosal folds. A slight degree of overhang may be present at either end. These changes are in contrast to the smoothly narrowed segment in achalasia. If one finds an appearance similar to achalasia developing in an older individual without previous symptoms related to the esophagus, carcinoma should be suspected and esophagoscopy and biopsy should be done.

ESOPHAGITIS AND ESOPHAGEAL ULCER

Esophagitis is said to be the most common disease affecting the esophagus. It is probable that mild forms of transient inflammation may occur very frequently but, because of the brief duration of the lesion and the lack of significant symptoms, roentgen and endoscopic examinations are seldom requested. Even excluding these examples of evanescent disease, sufficient cases of esophageal inflammation are encountered in radiologic practice to place this lesion in one of its forms at the head of the list of esophageal diseases.

TERMINAL ESOPHAGITIS

The frequency of esophagitis in autopsy material is surprisingly high, Burke discovering 96 cases of acute and chronic inflammation in a series of 570 autopsies. This high incidence in patients coming to necropsy probably results from multiple factors including debilitation, the lowered resistance of the tissues to trauma and infection during the terminal state, relaxation of the cardia allowing regurgitation of gastric juice, frequent vomiting, and the use of a stomach tube or negative-suction apparatus.

CHEMICAL ESOPHAGITIS

The swallowing of caustic materials such as household lye or an acid such as sulfuric acid will cause a severe erosive inflammation of the esophagus. As the inflammation subsides, fibrosis and scar-tissue formation develop and the end result is usually one or more fibrous strictures. Roentgen examination usually is not done until after the acute inflammation has subsided and then is performed to determine the location and extent of stricture formation. The strictures are most frequent at the sites of anatomic narrowing where the caustic material may have been held up momentarily. Thus they are seen at the level of the thoracic inlet, at the level of the aortic arch, and at or above the level of the diaphragmatic hiatus. The strictures are characterized by tapering edges and the fact that they are relatively long and also multiple (Fig. 15-14). If the injury has been very severe and if proper treatment has not been carried out, complete obstruction may develop.

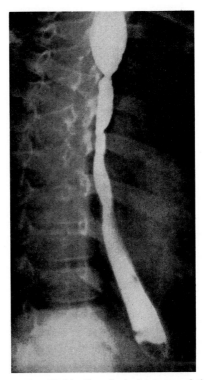

Fig. 15-14. Chemical strictures of the esophagus. Oblique roentgenogram of the barium-filled esophagus showing multiple areas of stricture formation that followed the swallowing of caustic household lye.

ACUTE ULCERATIVE ESOPHAGITIS

In addition to ulcerative or erosive inflammation developing as a result of the ingestion of caustic materials as described in the preceding paragraph, acute ulcerative esophagitis is seen occasionally in patients with peptic ulcer, usually a duodenal ulcer, or following operation for relief of an ulcer. The cause of the disease is undetermined but frequent vomiting, the use of a decompression tube in the esophagus, and the trauma and shock associated with upper abdominal operations seem to be of importance. The same lesion has been observed in patients with persistent vomiting from other causes (e.g., pernicious vomiting of pregnancy). The regurgitation of highly acid gastric juice undoubtedly plays an important role although other factors may enter the picture.

Roentgen Observations

The roentgen findings (Figs. 15-15 and 15-16) in acute ulcerative esophagitis are as follows:

The involvement is limited to the lower third to half of the esophagus.

The first evidence is that of esophageal spasm, which usually is intense. This causes a diffuse narrowing of the affected portion and results in varying degrees of obstruction. The spasm may relax intermittently to allow passage of the barium mixture into the stomach.

After a short period, often only a matter of a few weeks, the deformity becomes fixed because of fibrosis. The lumen narrows gradually from above downward to the cardia. The obstruction may be severe and occasionally becomes complete. There is a complete absence of peristalsis in the involved segment.

The mucosal folds normally seen in the contracted esophagus are absent and the surface appears smooth or occasionally finely granular. In the early stages of the disease a fine roughening of the margin of the lumen may be noted, apparently representing the effects of the fine superficial ulceration that is present; in the late stages after the disease has subsided to a fibrous stricture the margins become smooth.

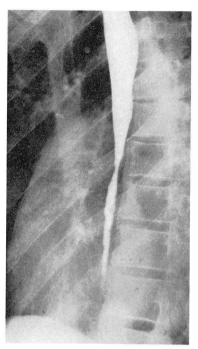

Fig. 15-15. Acute ulcerative esophagitis. Oblique roentgenogram of barium in the esophagus. The patient developed signs and symptoms of esophageal obstruction during the postoperative period, following gastric resection for duodenal ulcer. Examination revealed intense spasm involving the lower half of the esophagus, which relaxed only slightly to allow a minimal amount of material to enter the stomach.

CHRONIC FIBROSING ESOPHAGITIS

Of the pathologic varieties of chronic inflammation of the esophagus, fibrosing esophagitis is the lesion of greatest interest and importance to the roentgenologist. This lesion may be only the fibrous residues of a previous acute inflammation as described above or it may represent an active chronic inflammation without antecedent acute erosive disease.

Roentgen Observations (Fig. 15-17)

The disease involves the distal part of the esophagus almost exclusively. The length of the involved segment varies but usually is on the order of 1 to 5 cm.

The lumen of the esophagus tapers rather rapidly into the area of stenosis but without a

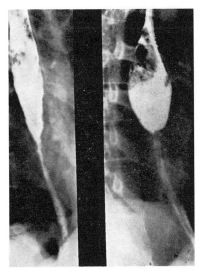

Fig. 15-16. Ulcerative esophagitis. The lesion developed in a patient who was suffering from pernicious vomiting of pregnancy. There is intense spasm in the lower third of the esophagus, which is beginning to progress into fibrous stricture formation. These are two views made during the act of swallowing.

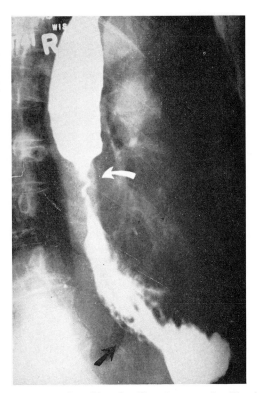

Fig. 15-17. Chronic fibrosing esophagitis. The esophagus is shortened and the fundus of the stomach has been pulled into the thorax. There is an irregular fibrous stricture involving the lower end of the esophagus (**arrow**). The lower **black arrow** indicates the level of the diaphragm.

sharp junction between normal and abnormal.

Herniation of a portion of the stomach through the esophageal hiatus is present in a very high percentage of patients and has led to the belief that the cause of the esophageal inflammation may lie in the incompetency of the cardia often found with hiatal hernia. This would allow free reflux of gastric juice into the esophagus (see Fig. 15-18).

The esophagus almost invariably is shortened so that the cardiac orifice lies on the summit of the herniated part of the stomach.

There is a fairly high incidence of associated peptic ulcer, notably duodenal ulcer. This naturally raises the question as to the effect of the highly acid gastric juice often present with duodenal ulcer and the effect of frequent vomiting on the esophageal mucosa.

In many patients there is an associated ulcer in the distal end of the esophagus or at the esophagogastric junction (see Fig. 15-19 and discussion to follow). The presence of an ulcer is considered by many to indicate that gastric epithelium is present at this point.

Obstruction of some degree is present. Rarely is the obstruction complete to thin barium-water mixture and filling of the stomach usually occurs without too much difficulty. In some patients there will be present a combination of fibrosing esophagitis, peptic ulcer of the stomach or duodenum, hiatal hernia, shortening of the esophagus, and an ulcer of the esophagus. All parts of the syndrome are present in some patients; in others one or more of the lesions may be missing. It is probable that the shortening of the esophagus is acquired rather than developmental and that it results from spasm and fibrosis. There is evidence that esophageal reflux occurs commonly in the presence of a sliding type of hiatal hernia and it is the consensus that it is an important factor in the causation of the inflammation.

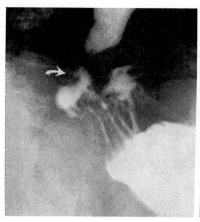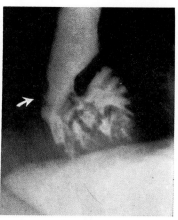

Fig. 15-18. Esophageal ulcer with patulous cardia. There is a small esophageal hiatal hernia. There is a shallow ulcer crater on the posterior wall of the esophagus in its lower end (**arrow**). There is no narrowing of the esophagus. Instead, the cardia is widely patent and a free reflux of the barium mixture from the stomach occurs through it. These are two spot roentgenograms showing different phases as seen fluoroscopically.

PEPTIC ULCER OF THE ESOPHAGUS

As noted above the relation between ulcer of the esophagus, esophagitis, and hiatal hernia is a close one. Esophageal ulcer also is seen in Barrett's columnar-lined esophagus.

Roentgen Observations

The roentgen evidence of esophageal ulcer is similar to that of ulcer in other parts of the gastrointestinal tract and depends upon the visualization of the ulcer crater as an out-pouching or barium-filled pocket. The crater often is shallow and may be difficult to visualize unless seen tangentially (Fig. 15-19).

Mucosal relief studies often show thickened mucosal folds radiating away from the edges of the crater, similar to the configuration seen in gastric or duodenal ulcers.

Spasm often is prominent and may cause a diffuse narrowing of the lumen around the ulcer. Spastic narrowing is characterized by its inconstancy during fluoroscopic observation.

A hiatal hernia is found in a high percentage of patients.

Usually the lumen of the esophagus is narrowed for a short distance above the ulcer and

sufficient fibrosis may have developed to cause high-grade obstruction. The appearances then are those of a fibrosing esophagitis with the addition of the ulcer crater.

Less frequently the esophageal lumen is widely patent, the cardia relaxed, and free reflux from the stomach into the esophagus occurs. This nonstenotic variety has been considered as a possible precursor to the stenotic lesion, representing the phase of the disease whereby the relaxed cardia allows free regurgitation of acid gastric juice into the esophagus. The ulcer crater must be searched for rather carefully in some of these patients because, in the absence of spasm and fibrosis, there is no narrowing or obstruction to draw attention to the lesion (Fig. 15-18).

ACHALASIA (CARDIOSPASM)

Achalasia of the cardia, often referred to as cardiospasm, is a lesion the cause of which has been in some doubt. Most observers now consider it to be a result of a deficiency or lack of the myenteric plexuses of Auerbach with failure of inhibition of contraction rather than a spastic contracture. Because of this the term

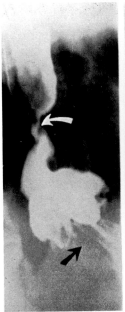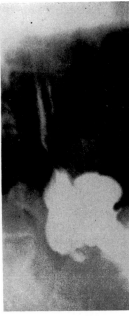

Fig. 15-19. Esophagitis with esophageal ulcer. The esophagus is shortened and the fundus of the stomach has been pulled above the level of the diaphragm. There is a stricturelike narrowing of the esophagus immediately adjacent to the cardia and a small flat ulcer crater is visualized; barium fills the area (**arrow**). These are two spot roentgenograms made at fluoroscopy. On the *right* side the esophagus is almost completely empty and the ulcer crater is not readily identified. The **lower arrow** points to the level of the esophageal hiatus.

"achalasia" or absence of relaxation is favored. Pressure studies have shown that hypertension of the gastroesophageal sphincter with incomplete relaxation on swallowing is present in achalasia. Recent investigations suggest that the hormone, gastrin, may play an important role and that achalasia may be caused by hypersensitivity to endogenous gastrin with resulting increase in tone of the sphincter. Conversely, a decreased effect of the hormone will lead to sphincter incompetence.[23]

Roentgen Observations

The obstruction in achalasia is located at the level of the diaphragm in almost all patients.

Dilatation of the esophagus above the diaphragm is pronounced. Elongation is frequent and the esophagus may be tortuous or angulated. The distal end often curves to the right and then back to the midline just before it passes through the diaphragmatic hiatus (Fig. 15-20). The sharp angulation that results may prevent the ready passage of bougies or dilators and blind instrumentation should be done with caution in these patients.

The dilated esophagus filled with fluid and food may project to the right of the mediastinum and cause a distinct widening of the mediastinal shadow in chest roentgenograms. This may be confused with a mediastinal neoplasm. In many of these patients a fluid level with air above it may be seen in the upper esophagus in properly exposed roentgenograms and be a valuable clue to the correct diagnosis.

There is an absence of normal peristaltic contractions. What waves are seen are ineffective in propelling material into the stomach.

The distal end of the barium-filled esophagus tapers smoothly to a point; this lies even with the diaphragmatic hiatus.

Small amounts of the mixture may pass intermittently into the stomach during the examination but the greater portion of the meal is retained in the dilated esophagus; some of it may be present for hours or even days after ingestion. The esophagus seldom becomes completely empty.

There are sometimes pulmonary complications also. In a fairly high percentage of patients with cardiospasm, inflammatory changes will be found in the lungs on roentgen examination, presumably the result of aspiration. Because the dilated esophagus is rarely empty, nocturnal regurgitation and the aspiration of contents into the tracheobronchial tree must be frequent in this disease. The pulmonary involvement may take the form of one or more episodes of acute pneumonitis with recovery between the attacks, or be a more chronic indurative inflammatory disease that changes very little when observed over long periods of time. It has been considered that a high lipid content in the aspirated material is responsible for these more chronic changes. The pulmonary lesions may be completely asymptomatic or, occasionally, may lead to respiratory symptoms that overshadow those caused by the difficulty in swallowing.

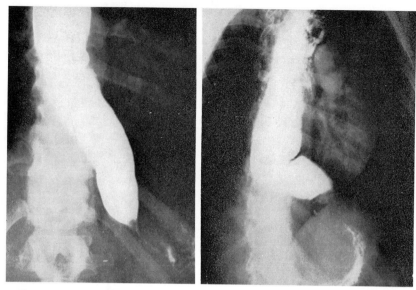

Fig. 15-20. Achalasia of the esophagus (cardiospasm) illustrating two examples of this condition. *Left,* Anteroposterior roentgenogram of the lower half of the esophagus, showing the characteristic dilatation and the tapering lower end of the esophagus at the level of the diaphragm. *Right,* Oblique roentgenogram of another patient with achalasia, showing elongation of the esophagus and the typical angulation of the distal part of the esophagus toward the right.

The lesions seen roentgenologically vary greatly from single or scattered patchy foci of consolidation, or areas of linear fibrosis, to granular, almost miliarylike infiltrations. The lesions may be found in any part of one or both lungs but are more frequent on the right side and tend to involve the midportion of this lung. In some of our patients the roentgen finding has been that of a fairly large area of density resembling pneumonic consolidation or atelectasis. In other cases the changes have been those of closely approximated linear densities involving one or both basal lung fields. The affected segment or segments often appear reduced in volume and frequently show a fine miliary granularity intermixed with the linear fibrosis. These pulmonary lesions are of course not specific for cardiospasm but often are sufficiently suggestive of an aspiration pneumonia to make this the presumptive diagnosis. Other inflammatory lesions that have been reported as occurring with cardiospasm include lung abscess and bronchiectasis.

Carcinoma may develop as a complication of achalasia apparently because of the long-continued chronic inflammation secondary to stasis. The tumor may reach a considerable size before the diagnosis is made because the symptoms are masked by those of the achalasia and the dilated fluid-filled esophagus may obscure the filling defect of the carcinoma.

CHALASIA OF THE ESOPHAGUS (CARDIOESOPHAGEAL RELAXATION)

This condition, the reverse of achalasia or cardiospasm, is found during the immediate postnatal period and is a cause of vomiting in infancy. The esophagus is dilated and flaccid, with diminished peristaltic activity. The cardia is patulous and there is free reflux of stomach contents into the esophagus (Fig. 15-21). The condition is thought to be caused by autonomic imbalance with a lack of proper coordination of muscle function at the cardia and failure of development of the sphincteric action at this point. The difficulty tends to disappear after a short time and treatment consisting of the use of a thickened formula and the keeping of the infant upright during and after feedings has been found satisfactory in controlling symptoms.

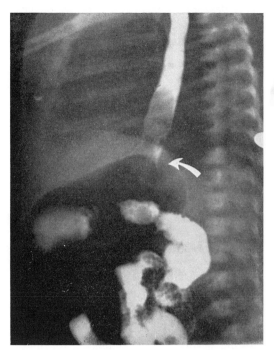

Fig. 15-21. Chalasia of the esophagus in a newborn infant. The **arrow** points to the patulous cardia. The barium in the esophagus has refluxed into it from the stomach.

seen only when the patient is examined in a recumbent position. During fluoroscopic examination the lower third to half of the esophagus undergoes a diffuse, almost tetaniclike spasm when a liquid barium mixture is swallowed (Fig. 15-22). Occasionally the spasm relaxes, allowing the mixture to enter the stomach, but it soon recurs. The appearance under the fluoroscope is one of rapidly changing contour but without the concentric contraction rings characteristic of curling. It has been suggested that diffuse spasm of the esophagus is only a manifestation of peptic esophagitis but it seems more likely that the chronic inflammation usually present in the wall of the esophagus in these cases is the result of the chronic spasm and not the cause of it.

OTHER MANIFESTATIONS OF SPASM

It is probable that acute spasm of the esophagus sufficient to cause substernal pain and difficulty in swallowing occurs not infrequently but unless the spasm can be initiated deliberately, roentgen examination may be entirely negative, the esophagus being perfectly normal between the short episodes of spasm.

ESOPHAGEAL SPASM

CURLING

The severe form of curling as described under the section on "The Curling Phenomenon" may be a cause of difficulty in swallowing and substernal pain and therefore can be considered as one of the manifestations of esophageal spasm.

DIFFUSE SPASM

Diffuse spasm of the esophagus resembles the curling phenomenon to some extent and is considered by many observers to be only a variant of it. There are, however, certain differences. Diffuse spasm is seen most frequently in middle-aged persons, usually those of a nervous type or in those suffering from anxiety tension states; curling is found in both sexes and particularly in the elderly. Diffuse spasm is equally intense in the upright and recumbent positions; curling is exaggerated by recumbency and in its milder forms is

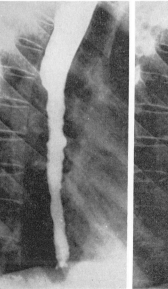
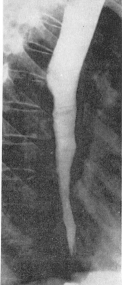

Fig. 15-22. Diffuse spasm of the lower half of the esophagus. Two roentgenograms made at short intervals apart, illustrating the changing contour of the spastic segment.

*best seen when oesophagus is
relaxed, obscured if
full of barium.*

508

THE ABDOMEN AND GASTROINTESTINAL TRACT

VARICES OF THE ESOPHAGUS

Dilatation of the veins of the lower part of the esophagus occurs chiefly as a result of cirrhosis of the liver, the esophageal veins serving as channels to bypass the obstructed portal system. The roentgen demonstration of esophageal varices by gastrointestinal examination is not always successful and the examination may yield negative results in patients who are later proved to have varices. They also may be difficult to demonstrate at autopsy after the veins have collapsed. When varices are suspected, the roentgen examination of the esophagus must be done with particular care in many cases in order to elicit signs of their presence.

Roentgen Observations

The dilated veins project into the lumen of the esophagus and cause tortuous linear defects in the barium shadow (Figs. 15-23 and 15-24). These defects vary from time to time,

being less prominent when the esophagus is distended and becoming more obvious when the patient is examined in the recumbent position or when the intra-abdominal pressure is raised as during a Valsalva maneuver. The defects become obliterated temporarily by a primary contraction wave.

Small varices are best demonstrated by using a thick barium paste that clings to the mucosal surface. After most of the material has passed into the stomach, enough will remain on the surface to form a thin coating on the mucosa. Spot films are particularly valuable to obtain serial roentgenograms of the esophagus in various degrees of filling and contraction because the defects produced by the varices may be seen well in only one or perhaps several of the multiple exposures. When varices are extensive there may be some delay in passage of barium through the lower part of the esophagus. The varices frequently involve the gastric fundus, causing a tortuous thickening of the mucosal folds.

The best radiographic method for the de-

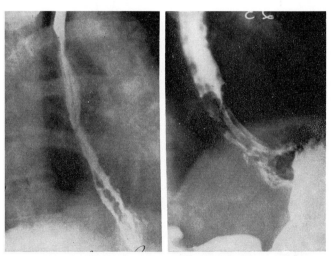

Fig. 15-23. Varices of the esophagus. Two examples illustrating roentgen findings. *Left,* Oblique roentgenogram of the lower end of the esophagus in a partially contracted stage, showing the varicose veins as linear tortuous defects. *Right,* Roentgenogram of the cardioesophageal area showing linear and circular translucencies in the barium filling of the esophagus, representing large varicose veins.

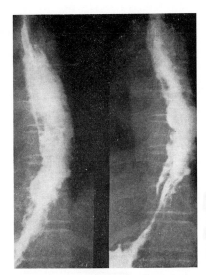

Fig. 15-24. Varices of the esophagus. Two roentgenograms of the same patient made at short intervals apart, illustrating extensive varicosities in the lower half of the esophagus.

tection of varices is the opacification of the dilated veins themselves and the demonstration of the collateral blood flow. This is accomplished by the procedure of splenoportography, described in Chapter 13.

FOREIGN BODIES

METALLIC FOREIGN BODIES

Metallic objects such as pins, coins, small toys, etc. are swallowed frequently by infants and young children. Except for aluminum and some of the lighter alloys, the metals are very radiopaque and easily visualized during fluoroscopy and in roentgenograms. The latter must be made with short exposure times to eliminate motion; otherwise the shadow of even a fairly large object may be blurred to the extent that it cannot be visualized. Objects made of aluminum may be impossible to detect in this manner because the density of this metal is so nearly equal to that of the soft tissues of the body.

NONOPAQUE FOREIGN BODIES

Nonopaque foreign bodies can only be demonstrated after the ingestion of a barium mixture. If the foreign body has caused a complete or nearly complete obstruction, the diagnosis is made without difficulty. Occasionally the swallowing of a large solid bolus such as a piece of poorly chewed meat will result in the object becoming impacted, usually in the lower end of the esophagus just above the level of the diaphragm. The resulting defect when barium is given may resemble that of a completely obstructing carcinoma. The short duration of symptoms and absence of complaints prior to the onset of obstruction point to the benign nature of the lesion. Usually after a few days the bolus becomes sufficiently softened so that it will pass spontaneously into the stomach. Solid objects of wood or other nonopaque material are seen infrequently; the obstruction resulting from such foreign bodies may be complete or incomplete.

IMPACTED BONE

Pieces of chicken bone or other meat bones may be swallowed accidentally and if large enough will become impacted. The favorite site of impaction is in the cervical part of the esophagus at or just above the level of the thoracic inlet. Lateral roentgenograms of the neck will demonstrate most of these foreign bodies since the bones are radiopaque. Care must be taken not to confuse a normal ossification of the laryngeal cartilages for a bony foreign body. Such ossification is invariably present in these cartilages in adults. Small calcified or ossified areas may overlie the upper end of the esophagus in the lateral roentgenogram and are a possible source of error. Familiarity with the appearance of these cartilages is the best insurance against mistakes.

With very small foreign bodies such as fish bones or other small sharp objects that may have penetrated the mucosa and thus become lodged, the defect in barium filling caused by the foreign body may be so small that it cannot be visualized readily and the shadow of the opaque bone may be too small to be detected. Diagnosis then depends upon the following:

1. A temporary delay in the passage of a solid or semisolid barium-containing mass such as a gelatin capsule filled with barium sulfate powder or a lump of bread soaked in barium-water mixture. This is caused by localized spasm at the site of the foreign body.

2. Delay in the passage of a small wisp of cotton that has been soaked in the barium-water mixture. This is particularly useful in detecting the presence and location of objects such as fishbones.

COMPLICATION OF FOREIGN BODIES

Penetration of the esophageal wall may result in a periesophageal abscess or a more diffuse mediastinitis. If the penetration occurs in the cervical area, air shadows may be visible in the soft tissues of the retroesophageal space. The soft-tissue space between the larynx, trachea, and the spine may be widened. Barium mixture may extend into a sinus tract. If the injury occurs within the thorax, mediastinitis may result. The mediastinal shadow becomes broadened at the level of the lesion and streaks of air may be visible in and along the mediastinal borders. Extension of infection can lead to pleural effusion.

MISCELLANEOUS CONDITIONS

POLYPS AND INTRAMURAL TUMORS

Tumors other than carcinoma are uncommon lesions in the esophagus. Polyps apparently are extremely rare and seldom enter into the diagnostic picture. Tumors arising within the wall of the esophagus, such as leiomyomas or leiomyosarcomas, also are uncommon lesions with only an occasional case having been reported. An intramural tumor of this type causes a filling defect in the barium shadow, which resembles that of pressure deformity from a mass lying extrinsic to the esophagus. Because the lesion arises within the wall, intact mucosa usually is present over the surface of the mass. An important point of differentiation is the fact that an intramural tumor causes a filling defect that has sharp angular junctions between the defect and the wall of the esophagus. A pressure defect caused by an extrinsic mass is more likely to have a smooth, concave junction between the defect and the wall. A leiomyoma can grow to large size; a large part of the tumor may project outside the esophageal lumen and, having space to expand in the thorax, it may not cause very much obstruction. The mass may be large enough to be visualized as a dense round shadow in roentgenograms of the thorax. It is usually impossible to differentiate between leiomyomas and other extramucosal tumors of the esophagus.

PLUMMER-VINSON SYNDROME

The Plummer-Vinson syndrome consists essentially of difficulty in swallowing and the presence of a sideropenic anemia in females. There usually is evidence of glossitis. While originally it was believed that the dysphagia was functional, many observers since have demonstrated the presence of webs or bands in the upper part of the esophagus in these cases and it is possible that the nutritional deficiencies are secondary to the difficulty in swallowing rather than being the primary disorder. The web also has been found in patients who have no evidence of anemia.

In a typical patient the web is found just below the pharyngoesophageal junction and when barium mixture is swallowed, the lesion appears as a thin, concentric constriction (Fig. 15-25). The degree of narrowing varies from case to case and in

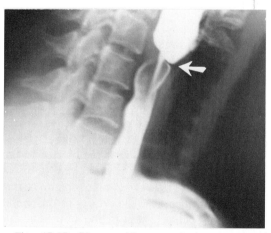

Fig. 15-25. Plummer-Vinson web in upper end of the esophagus (**arrow**).

some it requires careful observation for detection. The weblike constriction is a constant defect and is brought out with every swallow (Fig. 15-26).

SCLERODERMA (PROGRESSIVE SYSTEMIC SCLEROSIS)

Involvement of the esophagus is relatively common in patients suffering from scleroderma. In the early stages the esophagus shows a loss of tone, it is moderately dilated, the cardia is relaxed, and reflux of material from the stomach into the esophagus occurs (Fig. 15-27). The esophagus may empty more slowly than is normal and in recumbency the barium mixture may remain for some time after swallowing, even for several hours. In later stages variable degrees of stricture formation in the lower end of the esophagus are found. This probably results from the esophagitis that follows the relaxation of the cardia and the reflux of gastric juice into the esophagus. The narrowing is smooth and usually is found a short distance above the level of the diaphragm; there may be evidence of some shortening of the esophagus and upward displacement of the cardia. The esophagus above the level of narrowing is dilated and atonic. Peristalsis is much diminished or completely absent. In spite of the

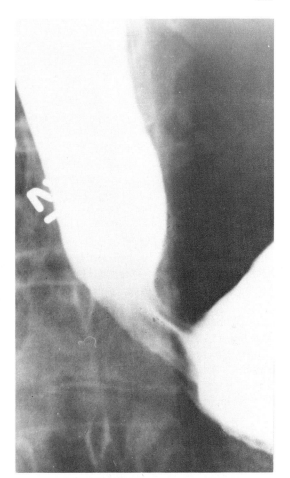

Fig. 15-27. Scleroderma of the esophagus. Enlarged view of lower esophagus and cardia. The esophagus is dilated and atonic. The cardia is relaxed and there was free reflux from the stomach into the esophagus observed during fluoroscopy.

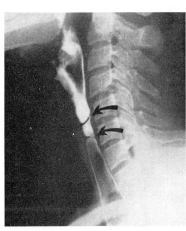

Fig. 15-26. Plummer-Vinson webs. Lateral roentgenogram of the neck made during the swallowing procedure illustrates two thin, weblike, annular strictures in the esophagus just below the level of the cricoid (**arrows**).

narrowing, material passes through the lower end of the esophagus into the stomach without too much difficulty. The appearance may be confused with achalasia but the dilatation is less pronounced than is commonly seen in achalasia and the narrowed segment, if present, is situated some distance above the cardia.

The finding of air in the lower esophagus (air esophagram) in chest films of patients with scleroderma has been reported and may serve to direct attention to the possibility of esophageal involvement in this disease. Sclero-

calcinosis circumscripta
Raynaud's
Scleroderma of esophagus
telangiectasia

} CRST syndrome
see p 514.

derma also may involve other parts of the gastrointestinal tract.

LOWER ESOPHAGEAL RING

Schatzki and Gary,[19] and Ingelfinger and Kramer[9] have reported the occurrence of a symmetric, thin, ringlike contraction in the lower end of the esophagus several centimeters above the diaphragm. The diameter of the lumen at the level of the ring varies from a few to as much as 38 mm (Fig. 15-28). The smaller rings of less than 10 to 12 mm are prone to cause symptoms of intermittent dysphagia, usually present over a period of years. The cause of the ring has been the subject of speculation but it now is recognized as representing the junction between esophageal and gastric epithelium. Because of this some authors consider that the demonstration of a ring indicates some degree of upward displacement of the gastric mucosa, or, a sliding hiatal hernia. As noted before, others consider the type of motor activity of the segment below the ring as determining whether it is, functionally, esophagus or stomach and that, in most cases, the segment will show an esophageal type of peristalsis.[3]

In addition to this mucosal junction ring, Wolf, Heitman, and Cohen[21] have described a functional ring 1 to 2 cm above it. It varies in length and caliber and usually disappears completely with maximum filling. They have called it the "A ring" or "contractile ring." When both rings are present, as in many patients with small, sliding hiatal hernias, the segment of esophagus between the rings shows a variety of configurations during filling and emptying and which distinguishes it from the esophagus proximal to it.

SPONTANEOUS RUPTURE OF THE ESOPHAGUS

Spontaneous rupture of the esophagus is an infrequent lesion that usually follows forceful vomiting. The lesion occurs more frequently in males than in females. Other causes that have been noted include convulsive seizures, straining at stool, and childbirth. The rupture occurs in a normal esophagus. In most cases the tear has been found in the lower end of the esophagus along the left lateral wall. Clinically the symptoms of vomiting followed by low thoracic pain and evidence of subcutaneous emphysema in the neck are considered highly significant for the diagnosis. Roentgenograms may reveal translucent streaks of air in the mediastinal tissues or even in the cervical area. Pneumothorax, usually on the left side, is frequent. Escape of gastric contents through the rent causes a diffuse increase in density of the

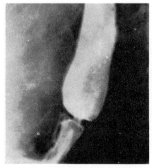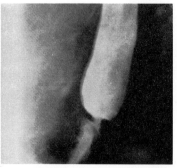

Fig. 15-28. Lower esophageal contraction ring. Two spot roentgenograms of the lower end of the esophagus made during the swallowing act. They demonstrate a thin circular constriction of the esophageal lumen with a slight dilatation above. Note the appearance of the esophagus directly below the constriction. It is somewhat collapsed because of the obstructing nature of the ring. It is probable that this actually represents gastric mucosa extending up to the level of the ring.

lower posterior mediastinum extending to both sides of the midline. Pleural effusion may be present. Infrequently these findings occur on the right side. In most cases the fistula may be demonstrated by the swallowing of barium.

DIFFICULTY IN SWALLOWING CAUSED BY PHARYNGEAL PARALYSIS

Among the less common causes of difficulty in swallowing are conditions that lead to weakness or paralysis of the muscles of deglutition, such as bulbar palsy and myasthenia gravis. The roentgen findings are rather similar in these diseases although they usually are more severe when the bulbar centers are involved. Plain roentgenograms of the neck reveal the dilated air-filled pharynx. When during fluoroscopy the patient is asked to swallow a mouthful of barium it will be noted that there is difficulty in pushing the material into the pharynx by the action of the tongue. Once in the pharynx the barium is held there for a variable time with only weak contrac-

tions or, in advanced cases, with complete absence of motor activity by the pharyngeal muscles. The pharynx is dilated and atonic and the barium collects in the pyriform sinuses and epiglottic vallecula alongside the glottis, remaining there for a time before gradually passing into the esophagus (Fig. 15-29). This retention facilitates aspiration of the material into the trachea and this is almost invariably noted during the attempted swallowing of the barium. There may be sufficient aspiration to cause severe respiratory embarrassment and the examination is not without hazard. There also tends to be reflux of material into the nasal cavities. Except for a thin coating that remains on the mucosa the normal pharynx does not retain barium. In myasthenia gravis there is less atonicity of the pharynx and in general less difficulty in swallowing unless the muscular weakness is pronounced. There is difficulty in propelling the bolus into the pharynx and movements of the tongue are weak and ineffective. Also, rapid fatigue of deglutition is noted; it returns to near normal after a rest or after administration of an anticholinesterase drug.

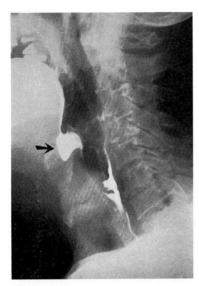

Fig. 15-29. Bulbar palsy. Lateral roentgenogram of the neck made directly after the swallowing act shows barium accumulated in the epiglottic vallecula (**arrow**) and clinging to the posterior surface of the tongue and lower wall of the pharynx. The pharynx is dilated and air-filled because of the paralysis of its musculature. This amount of air is never visualized in the normal pharynx during a resting phase.

REFERENCES AND SELECTED READINGS

1. ADLER, R. H.: What is the cardia? *JAMA 182:* 1045, 1962.
2. ALLISON, P. R.: Reflux esophagitis, sliding hiatus hernia and the anatomy of repair. *Surg. Gynecol. Obstet. 92:* 419, 1951.
3. CAUTHORNE, R. T., VANHOUTTE, J. J., DONNER, M. W., and HENDRIX, T. R.: Study of patients with lower esophageal ring by simultaneous cineradiography and manometry. *Gastroenterology 49:* 632, 1965.
4. CULVER, G. J., and CHAUDHARI, K. R.: Intramural esophageal diverticulosis. *Am. J. Roentgenol. Radium Ther. Nucl. Med. 99:* 210, 1967.
5. CRUMMY, A. B.: The water test in the evaluation of gastroesophageal reflux. *Radiology 87:* 501, 1966.
6. FLEISCHNER, F. G.: Hiatal hernia complex. *JAMA 162:* 183, 1956.
7. FRANK, R. C., and PAUL, L. W.: Congenital reduplication of the esophagus. Report of a case. *Radiology 53:* 417, 1949.
8. HUTTON, C. F.: Plummer-Vinson syndrome. *Br. J. Radiol. 29:* 81, 1956.
9. INGELFINGER, F. J., and KRAMER, P.: Dysphagia produced by contractile ring in lower esophagus. *Gastroenterology 23:* 419, 1953.

10. JOHNSTONE, A. S.: Observations on the radiologic anatomy of the oesophagogastric junction. *Radiology 73:* 501, 1959.

11. JOHNSTONE, A. S.: The diagnosis of early gastric herniation of the oesophageal hiatus. *J. Fac. Radiol. 3:* 52, 1951.

12. LEIGH, T. F., ABBOTT, O. A., and HOPKINS, W. A.: Roentgenologic considerations in tracheo-esophageal fistula without esophageal atresia, with report of two cases. *Radiology 57:* 871, 1951.

13. MCNALLY, E. F., and KATZ, M. I.: The roentgen diagnosis of diffuse esophageal spasm. *Am. J. Roentgenol. Radium Ther. Nucl. Med. 99:* 218, 1967.

14. MISSAKIAN, M. M., CARLSON, H. C., and ANDERSEN, H. A.: The roentgenologic features of the columnar epithelial lined lower esophagus. *Am. J. Roentgenol. Radium Ther. Nucl. Med. 99:* 212, 1967.

15. MURRAY, J. R.: Neuromuscular and functional disorders of the pharynx. *J. Fac. Radiol. 9:* 135, 1958.

16. NEUHAUSER, E. B. D., and BERENBERG, W.: Cardio-esophageal relaxation as a cause of vomiting in infants. *Radiology 48:* 480, 1947.

17. PALMER, E. D.: An attempt to localize the normal esophagogastrie junction. *Radiology 60:* 825, 1953.

18. RAMSEY, G. H., WATSON, J. S., GRAMIAK, R., and WEINBERG, S. A.: Cinefluorographic analysis of the mechanism of swallowing. *Radiology 64:* 498, 1955.

19. SCHATZKI, R., and GARY, J. E.: The lower esophageal ring. *Am. J. Roentgenol. Radium Ther. Nucl. Med. 75:* 246, 1956.

20. VOGT, E. C.: Congenital esophageal atresia. *Am. J. Roentgenol. Radium Ther. Nucl. Med. 22:* 463, 1929.

21. WOLF, B. S., HEITMANN, P., and COHEN, B. R.: The inferior esophageal sphincter, the manometric high pressure zone and hiatal incompetence. *Am. J. Roentgenol. Radium Ther. Nucl. Med. 103:* 251, 1968.

22. WRIGHT, J. T.: Allison's and Johnstone's anomaly. *Am. J. Roentgenol. Radium Ther. Nucl. Med. 94:* 308, 1965.

23. EDITORIAL: Gastrin and the gastroesophageal sphincter. *JAMA 217:* 1098, 1971.

16

THE STOMACH

METHODS OF EXAMINATION

PRELIMINARY ROENTGENOGRAMS

The use of preliminary or scout roentgenograms in the diagnosis of perforation of the stomach is discussed in Chapter 13. Roentgenograms prior to the administration of contrast material are also useful to detect or exclude the presence of metallic foreign bodies. Some swallowed air is almost always present in the normal stomach and when the patient is examined in an upright position an air-fluid level can be visualized in the fundus. Displacement of the gastric air bubble may indicate the existence of an extrinsic mass or the normal contour of it may be deformed by intrinsic tumor. If there is ample intra-abdominal fat the external surface of the stomach occasionally can be seen at least in part. Thickening of the gastric wall caused by scirrhus carcinoma sometimes can be identified in this way. These aspects are discussed more fully under the specific disease categories concerned.

CONTRAST VISUALIZATION

The esophagus, stomach, and duodenum are examined as a unit and what has been said about the conduct of the examination in the discussion dealing with the esophagus is equally true for the stomach and duodenum.

CONTRAST MATERIAL

The thin, barium-water mixture used for examination of the esophagus is the standard opaque meal for study of the stomach and duodenum. This consists of 125 gm of barium sulfate powder to 180 cc of water. This amount is adequate for fluoroscopic examination in most patients. If there is a delay between completion of the fluoroscopic examination and the making of roentgenograms or if gastric emptying is unusually rapid, an additional 40–60 cc of the mixture is given. If the small intestine is to be examined an additional 120 to 180 cc of the mixture should be given routinely after completion of the preliminary fluoroscopic study.

For examination of the fundus the use of a carbonated drink is often of value. After completing the initial study of the stomach and duodenum the carbonated drink is given. Within a few minutes the fundus becomes distended by the carbon dioxide released. Tumors of the fundus often are brought out very clearly as they project into the translucent gas shadow.

Water-soluble iodinated compounds have come into general use, particularly when there is evidence of small intestinal obstruction. Hypaque (50 per cent) or Gastrografin are the substances most commonly used. The latter is similar to Renografin, except for added flavoring to mask the bitter taste. When possible it is preferable to instill these substances through a tube. They are hypertonic and act somewhat like a saline laxative. Also the material becomes considerably diluted in the distal small bowel. It does not cling to the mucosa as does barium and it is not as satisfactory for mucosal relief studies. It has been shown experimentally that barium sulfate does not become impacted in the small intestine in the presence of obstruction, and clinical experience confirms this. Thus if the colon can be ruled out as the site of the obstruction, usually by means of a barium enema, it is safe to give barium orally.

FLUOROSCOPY

Fluoroscopy is an essential part of the examination of the stomach as it is for other parts of the gastrointestinal tract. Fluoroscopy is more than a method for obtaining spot films. The ability to "see" and "feel" at the same time is a valuable part of the procedure. To the trained fluoroscopist, the look and feel of an area of stomach wall infiltrated by carcinoma is unmistakable. With fluoroscopy, peristalsis can be observed rapidly and the effect of a lesion on peristaltic activity easily determined. Spot films can be obtained to record what is seen under the fluoroscope or to show finer detail that cannot be recognized by fluoroscopy. Unfortunately, palpation is more difficult when an image intensifier is used because of the bulkiness of the machine. The use of a television monitor by the examiner instead of the viewing mirror of the intensifier obviates most of this difficulty. Unless the patient is too ill to stand, the examination is begun with the fluoroscopic table in an upright position and the patient standing behind the fluoroscopic screen. Unless there are specific complaints referable to the esophagus, attention is first centered on the cardia and the first few swallows of the barium mixture are watched as they pass through the cardia and then "canalize" the stomach. Pressure by the lead-gloved hand is used to spread the material over the surface of the stomach and into the mucosal folds (see Fig. 16-4). In this way the undistended stomach is examined for filling defects, ulcer craters, pliability of walls, and integrity of mucosal pattern. Some authors have stressed that manual palpation should be avoided during fluoroscopy. Even though the hand is protected with a leaded glove, some radiation may reach the examiner's skin. They prefer using specially constructed pal-

pating spoons and other compression devices. However, we have found that satisfactory palpation can be done in most cases by keeping the protected fingers directly outside of the edge of the coned-down roentgen ray beam. When palpating for deep masses the fluoroscope can be turned off momentarily. When this preliminary survey detects definite or questionable abnormalities, spot films can be made under fluoroscopic guidance with or without compression to bring out the maximum detail of the lesion or the area in question. The remainder of the barium mixture then is given and the esophagus is examined. Frequently the duodenum will begin to fill while the preliminary survey of the stomach is being done. If it does not, pressure applied over the antrum after the stomach is more completely distended usually will cause the duodenal bulb to fill and this is examined for contour deformities, ulcer craters, filling defects, etc. After the duodenum has been studied thoroughly, and the spot films made if desired, attention is returned to the stomach and search is again made for evidence of organic disease in the more distended organ. The examination usually is continued by lowering the table into a horizontal position and with the patient in various positions. In this manner the margins of the stomach can be brought into profile, peristaltic waves can be observed as they pass along the curvatures, filling and emptying of the duodenal bulb can be studied, and posturing can be used to bring out ulcer craters and filling defects to best advantage. For the demonstration of posterior-wall ulcers it is helpful to lower the table to about 45° from the upright and turn the patient slightly toward the right. The ulcer crater then will fill with barium and the air overlying it makes a good "double contrast."

ROENTGENOGRAMS

Reference has been made in the above paragraph to so-called spot roentgenograms made under fluoroscopic guidance (see also page 488). These are of considerable aid in bringing out deformities in relatively inaccessible locations, in showing small ulcer craters, and in giving a permanent record of details observed during fluoroscopy. After completion of the fluoroscopic study the patient is given another 60 to 90 cc of the barium mixture and a series of films (three or four) is obtained with the patient prone in a right anterior oblique position. This is the most useful routine position to show both stomach and duodenum to advantage. As a rule we also obtain at least one roentgenogram with the patient lying on his right side and frequently one with him on the left side. These complete the film study of the stomach and duodenum.

CINEFLUOROGRAPHY

With the use of the image intensifier good movies of the gastrointestinal tract can be obtained and this method is coming into wide use. Also it is possible to store the image on television tape for play-back at any desired time.

ABDOMINAL ARTERIOGRAPHY IN GASTROINTESTINAL BLEEDING

Arteriography of the abdominal vessels has been found useful in the study of acute and chronic gastrointestinal bleeding when other studies have failed to show a causative lesion. The vessels of the celiac axis and the superior and inferior mesenteric arteries can be catheterized by the percutaneous technique of Seldinger, usually using the femoral artery approach. Vascular lesions such as hemangiomas and arteriovenous malformations can be visualized readily. Other tumors may be identified at times owing either to their vascularity or because they displace or occlude normal vessels. The actual bleeding point can be visualized in many cases by the finding of local extravasation of contrast material into the gastrointestinal lumen (Fig. 16-1). Bleeding from gastric or duodenal ulcers, various kinds of tumors and from colonic diverticula have been diagnosed in this way. Most investigators agree that arteriography should be done in all patients where the source of bleeding cannot be found by other methods; this occurred in 22 per cent in one reported series. In acute bleeding it has been recommended that arteriography be done as the initial procedure. If a bleeding site is found, the direct selective injection of vasopressor substances has controlled the hemorrhage in some patients, at least temporarily.

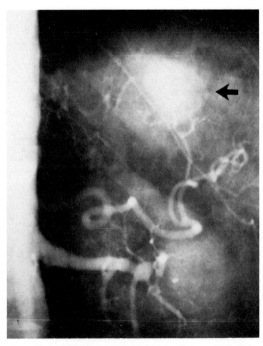

Fig. 16-1. Bleeding gastric ulcer demonstrated by abdominal aortography. There is cloudy density in the gastric fundus (**arrow**) representing contrast material extravasated into the lumen from a bleeding ulcer. (The dense stripe along the left margin of the figure is the opacified abdominal aorta.) Note filling of the left renal artery.

ANTICHOLINERGIC DRUGS

The use of Pro-Banthine (propantheline bromide) to reduce muscle tone and peristalsis in the duodenum when searching for minor defects particularly in pancreatic disease has been discussed in Chapter 13, under the section on "Hypotonic Duodenography." This drug also can be used to reduce or eliminate spasm in the stomach, small intestine, and colon when it interferes with satisfactory filling or to rule out spasm as a cause for a defect which might indicate a serious organic lesion such as carcinoma. The usual dose varies from 30 to 60 mg intramuscularly depending upon body weight. The smaller doses are preferred as they usually produce adequate hypotonicity within five to ten minutes without significant side effects. The effects of the drug usually wear off about fifteen to twenty minutes after onset. The usual contraindications to the use of atropine and similar drugs should be noted; these include glaucoma, prostatism, and serious cardiovascular disease.

ANATOMY AND PHYSIOLOGY

ANATOMIC DIVISIONS AND TERMINOLOGY

1. Cardia: The junction of the esophagus and stomach.

2. Fundus: That part of the stomach above the level of the cardia.

3. Body of the stomach: The central two-thirds from the level of the cardia to the proximal part of the pyloric antrum.

4. Pyloric antrum: The distal one-third of the stomach.

5. Pylorus: The junction of the stomach and duodenum.

6. Pyloric canal: The channel through the pylorus. In the roentgenogram this measures about 7 to 8 mm in width and 5 mm in length.

7. Sulcus angularis. A relatively acute angle formed at or just below the middle of the stomach on the lesser curvature, becoming particularly pronounced when the stomach is of the J or fishhook form. It marks the boundary between the stomach and the pyloric antrum.

FORM AND POSITION OF THE STOMACH

The form and position of the stomach vary greatly in different individuals. In the person of asthenic habitus it tends to lie in a vertical position having the form of a J or fishhook. In the sthenic individual it lies more transversely and in the very obese it assumes the shape of a "steer horn." In between these two extremes are many variations. The average shape of the normal stomach lies part way between the elongated fishhook contour and the more transverse and thus tends to assume the form of a shallow J or a reverse L (Figs. 16-2 and 16-3). An interesting variant is the type of stomach known as a *cascade* or *cup and spill* form. In this condition the fundus of the stomach hangs downward and to the left, lying behind the body of the stomach, and with a sharp angle formed between the two portions. The fundus usually is enlarged and when the

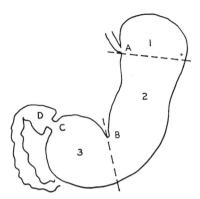

Fig. 16-2. Diagram of normal stomach to show the major anatomic divisions. **(1)** Fundus, **(2)** body, **(3)** antrum, **(A)** anatomic cardia, **(B)** incisura angularis, **(C)** pyloric canal, **(D)** first portion of the duodenum or duodenal bulb.

meal is taken with the patient upright the major portion of it will accumulate in the dilated fundus before spilling over into the distal part of the stomach. It is because of this feature that the term *cup and spill* was coined. The cause of this type of stomach is debatable but in many of these individuals the transverse colon is high in position, usually the result of obesity, and it is probable that this is responsible for the configuration in most cases.

THE FUNDUS AND CARDIA

The fundus of the stomach normally lies close to the left leaf of the diaphragm. The soft-tissue space between the fundic air bubble and the air-containing lung represents, therefore, the combined thickness of the gastric wall and the diaphragm. This measures on the average about 1 cm. Any appreciable increase in width of this soft-tissue space usually indicates a pathologic process involving the gastric wall, the subphrenic space, or the diaphragm. Exceptions occur where this space is unusually thick and yet nothing is found to account for it at the time of surgical exploration. The space is thicker in obese individuals and this must be allowed for in interpretation. Occasionally a tonguelike extension of the spleen may extend into the space between the fundus and the

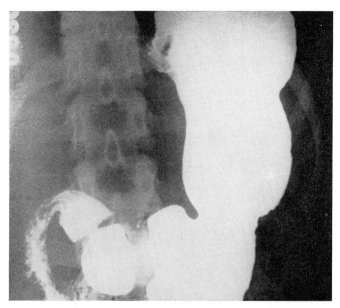

Fig. 16-3. Roentgenogram of normal stomach and duodenum. Compare with diagram shown in Figure 16-2. Note three peristaltic waves, a shallow one near the fundus, a deeper one near the sulcus angularis, and a still deeper wave in the pyloric antrum.

diaphragm and cause a localized indentation of the gastric wall, simulating a neoplasm. An enlarged left ventricle of the heart may cause a downward bulge of the left diaphragm and suggest a filling defect in the fundus of the stomach. In general, minor uniform variations in thickness of this space can be disregarded. Localized thickening is of greater significance but it may be extremely difficult to determine the nature of such a finding prior to laparotomy.

The cardia represents the anatomic junction between esophagus and stomach. It is a relatively fixed part; the pylorus also is a point of fixation but is less stationary in position. The body of the stomach moves freely and can be displaced readily by pressure. The anatomy of the cardia is discussed more fully in Chapter 15.

MUCOSAL FOLDS

The gastric mucosal folds produce distinct, ridgelike, translucent zones when the stomach is partially distended by barium mixture. These translucent ridges are separated by dense stripes representing barium accumulated in the valleys between the folds (Fig. 16-4). Along the lesser curvature the folds run parallel to the curvature; the margin of the curvature is smooth when viewed in profile except for the indentations caused by peristaltic contractions. About 1 or 2 cm proximal to the pylorus, a fairly constant transverse mucosal fold crosses the lesser curvature causing a sharp but smooth indentation in the margin. This is known as the prepyloric fold. It is the only transverse fold normally seen crossing the lesser curvature. Along the gastric walls the folds tend to diverge toward the greater curvature and frequently cross this curvature in a transverse direction. This causes a certain roughness or a serrated appearance of the greater curvature and this is most pronounced, as a rule, in the upper half. In the antrum the folds tend to lie horizontally along the greater curvature as they do along the lesser. The prepyloric fold may extend completely across the antrum and result

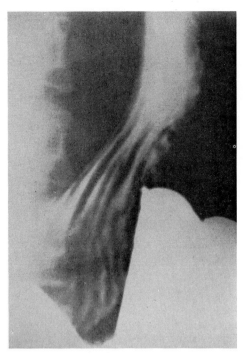

Fig. 16-4. Mucosal folds of the stomach. Spot roentgenogram made during fluoroscopy with the patient upright and with pressure being applied over the body and antrum of the stomach by the lead-gloved hand of the examiner. This expresses barium away from the area but leaves enough to coat the mucosa and show the character of the folds extending down from the fundus along the lesser curvature, branching and curving laterally toward the greater curvature side.

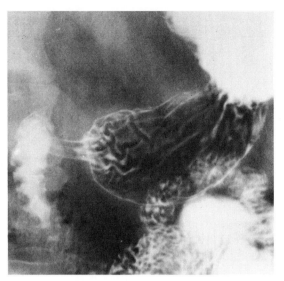

Fig. 16-5. Mucosal pattern of the distal two-thirds of the stomach. Anteroposterior roentgenogram made with the patient supine. The swallowed air in the stomach occupies the lower part while the heavier barium has gravitated into the dependent fundus in this position. A peristaltic wave has reached the pylorus, causing the antrum to be contracted. Note the parallel folds of mucosa in the contracted prepyloric region. The coating of barium on the mucosal surface, combined with the air overlying it, gives a good double contrast and shows the character of mucosal folds in this part of the stomach.

in an indentation on the greater curvature similar to that commonly seen on the lesser. Occasionally more than one such prepyloric fold is present or the fold may branch (Fig. 16-5). These prepyloric folds may appear unusually thick but still be within normal limits and considerable variation must be allowed for in the normal. Rarely, a thin, diaphragmlike septum is found in the gastric antrum near the pylorus which may cause sufficient narrowing to lead to partial outlet obstruction. It is probably of congenital origin. In the fundus the folds generally are larger than those seen elsewhere and course in varying directions without a definite pattern. Surrounding the cardia the folds may show a star-shaped radiation when viewed *en*

face, or appear as a circular fold surrounding the orifice (Fig. 16-6). The mucosal pattern of the normal stomach varies widely and considerable caution must be used in interpreting the significance of apparently prominent folds in terms of disease.

PERISTALSIS

Peristaltic contractions begin in the upper third of the stomach and progress slowly to the pylorus, becoming deeper as they advance. It requires about 20 seconds for a wave to travel from the cardia to the pylorus and usually not more than two or three waves are visible at any one time. Peristaltic activity tends to occur intermittently with periods of relative quies-

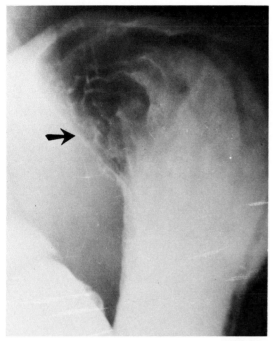

Fig. 16-6. Circular and stellate radiation of mucosal folds at the cardia (**arrow**).

cence in between. As a wave reaches the prepyloric area the distal few centimeters may contract uniformly; this is known as antral systole. Material may or may not be forced through the pylorus by such a contraction. In the normal, roentgenograms of the stomach show the smooth indentation of peristaltic waves to be of uniform depth on both curvatures and the spacing of the indentations is equal. The wave is narrower on the lesser curvature and broader on the greater curvature as it passes through the body of the stomach. Toward the pylorus the wave becomes of similar width on both curvatures (see Fig. 16-3). Peristalsis is an extremely valuable aid in determining the pliability of the gastric walls. Lesions that involve the muscularis will invariably cause an interruption of peristalsis at the site of the disease. Peristalsis is best studied by means of fluoroscopy. Multiple serial films made at frequent intervals (one every 15 or 20 seconds) can be taken if a permanent record is desired.

TONE

The gastric tone varies to a considerable degree. It is related to the habitus of the individual, being increased in the sthenic person and decreased in the asthenic. Gastric tone also is affected by many extraneous factors such as fear, nervousness, nausea, etc.

MOTILITY

Using a barium-water mixture, gastric emptying ordinarily is rapid and the stomach frequently will be empty at the end of 1 or 1½ hours. Longer periods need not be abnormal and small residues in the stomach at the end of 3 hours are not significant. Again, extraneous factors may influence the rate of emptying of the stomach to a considerable extent.

CONGENITAL ANOMALIES

DEXTROPOSITION

The stomach is involved along with the other viscera in *situs inversus totalis*. In this anomaly the thoracic and abdominal viscera are reversed in position so that they form a mirror image of the normal. The anomaly usually is found by chance. Rarely, the thoracic viscera are reversed in position while the situs of the abdominal organs is normal and even less frequent is the finding of reversal of the abdominal structures while the thoracic viscera are normal. A few cases of isolated situs inversus of the stomach and duodenum have been reported.

DUPLICATIONS

Duplications involve the stomach as they do other parts of the gastrointestinal tract. The anomaly is rare. The duplication usually is closed, consisting of a cystic structure having a wall composed of the normal coats of the stomach. This cyst is attached to the gastric wall or develops within the wall of the stomach. Roentgenologically, a closed duplication resembles a solid intramural tumor such as a leiomyoma and correct preoperative diagnosis is hardly possible. Open duplications in which the accessory stomach communicates with the gastric lumen are very rare.

DISEASES OF THE STOMACH

GASTRIC ULCER

The majority of benign gastric ulcers are found on or immediately adjacent to the lesser curvature in the middle third of the stomach. The greater the distance from this area the less the frequency of the lesion. While formerly it was believed that benign gastric ulcer rarely, if ever, occurred directly on the greater curvature, recent reports indicate that such is not the case and that the finding of an ulcer directly on the greater curvature need not indicate that the lesion is malignant. Gastric ulcer is less frequent than ulcer of the duodenum, the frequency ratio being on the order of 1:5 or even less. Benign ulcers can vary greatly in size from tiny ones of a few millimeters in diameter to huge excavations 6 to 8 cm in size or even more (Fig. 16-7). The size of the ulcer is not too significant from the standpoint of malignancy or benignancy. The majority of benign gastric ulcers fall within the range of 1 to 2 cm. Many gastric ulcers are unequivocally benign on roentgen examination. Others are frankly malignant. There also is a borderline group in which some doubt may exist as to the benignancy of the lesion. In general it is good practice to follow all supposedly benign ulcers undergoing medical therapy with repeat examinations at 2- to 4-week intervals. Definite evidence of healing with reduction in size should be present at the first follow-up study with eventual disappearance of the ulcer crater.

Roentgen Observations

THE ULCER NICHE. The ulcer niche represents the crater or cavity of the lesion. When seen in

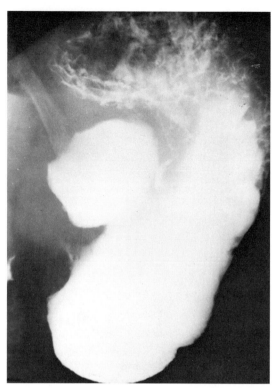

Fig. 16-7. Giant benign ulcer of the lesser curvature illustrates the large size that some ulcers may attain. Large ulcers, and some smaller ones, will have penetrated the gastric wall and the base will be bounded by the adjacent tissue, in this patient, the liver.

profile the niche projects outside of the normal barium-filled lumen because the ulcer is an excavation in the wall of the stomach. Most gastric ulcers are round or slightly oval and the walls tend to run perpendicular to the gastric wall with a relatively flat or slightly rounded base. Sometimes, however, the crater has inward sloping walls and the base is more rounded than flat. Many ulcers tend to show undermining beneath the mucosa apparently because the tissues within the wall are more subject to the digestive action of the acidic gastric juice than is the mucosa. The term "collar-button ulcer" has been used to describe ulcers of this type. If there is little edema or inflammatory reaction around the crater, the overhanging edge of mucosa may be visualized as a thin translucent line (Hampton's line) crossing the orifice of the crater when viewed in profile. This is seldom more than 1 to 2 mm in width and is perfectly smooth (Fig. 16-8). It is a highly significant finding for the diagnosis of benignancy but is not seen very frequently. More often there is considerable edema and inflammatory reaction in the wall surrounding the crater and this results in a much wider translucent line (Figs. 16-9 and 16-10), provided, of course, that there is some undermining and that the crater is in true profile. The width of this line is uniform from one side of the crater to the other. It is known as the "ulcer collar" (Fig. 16-11).

When viewed *en face* a benign gastric ulcer is seen as a sharply marginated, round, dense collection of barium. If there is much edema, the crater will be surrounded by a translucent "halo" when compression is applied over the area. The width of the halo is variable but its inner edge is sharply defined while it fades gradually at the periphery into normal appearing gastric wall. This zone of edema and induration is sometimes known as the "ulcer mound." When viewed in profile, if the ulcer mound is of appreciable size, it will project into the gastric lumen. The ulcer crater will be situated in the center of the mound and it may not project beyond the apparent gastric lumen. Lesions of this type may be difficult to differentiate from ulcerating carcinomas. In the latter the mound often has a nodular or irregular surface, the crater may be situated off-center in relation to the mound and the external limits of the mound are more sharply defined. Also, the crater tends to be more irregular in shape and the floor may appear nodular.

Frequently the mucosal folds radiate away from the crater in a spokelike fashion (Fig. 16-12). This is another highly significant finding in benign ulcers.

In some craters there will be a small, round, filling defect in the center of the crater base. This has been interpreted as a blood clot surrounding a vessel which has recently bled. We have also seen specimens where the tiny defect represented the end of a thrombosed artery projecting slightly above the crater floor. Figure 16-13 *left,* shows a similar defect along the superior wall of a crater.

For posterior or anterior wall ulcers it usu-

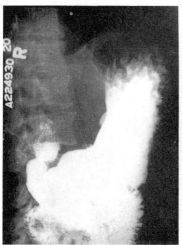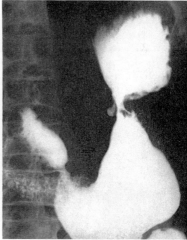

Fig. 16-8. Benign gastric ulcer. *Left,* Shallow ulcer crater on the lesser curvature of the stomach at the junction of the upper and middle thirds. There is a slight undermining of the edges and a narrow band of translucency can be seen surrounding the neck of the crater representing the edge seen in profile. *Right,* Benign ulcer of the lesser curvature with an associated deep incisura on the greater curvature side.

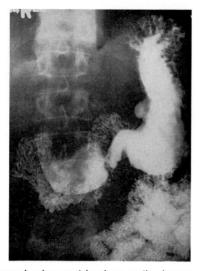

Fig. 16-9. Large benign gastric ulcer on the lesser curvature. The base of the crater is rounded and smooth and there is a smooth halo of induration around the neck. The lesser curvature has been foreshortened as the result of fibrosis so that the antrum has been angled upward moderately.

ally is necessary to displace the barium away from the lesion by suitable compression. Then, the *en face* details noted above will be brought out to best advantage. As noted above posterior-wall ulcers often are seen best by examining the patient in a semierect position and turned somewhat to the right. This allows the crater to fill with barium and to be seen *en face* with air overlying it to give a "double-contrast" effect.

The ulcer crater infrequently is seen as a "ring" rather than a dense fleck or rounded accumulation of barium. This happens when the crater is on the superior wall. The dense barium coats the walls of the crater while the crater itself is filled with air so that its margins are outlined rather than the pocket of the ulcer; the result is a ring-shaped image.

THE INCISURA. Opposite the crater there may be a fingerlike indentation of the greater curvature. This may be caused by spasm and be an inconstant indentation or, in chronic ulcers, it

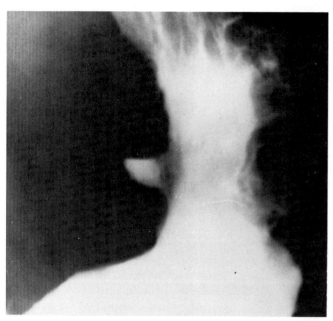

Fig. 16-10. Benign gastric ulcer on the lesser curvature. The base is pointed. There is a fairly wide ulcer collar around the orifice of the crater.

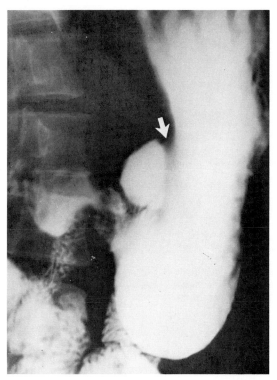

Fig. 16-11. Benign gastric ulcer on the lesser curvature. There is a large crater with a translucent halo or ulcer collar (**arrow**) around the orifice. The lesser curvature of the antrum has been fore-shortened.

may be a fixed, constant defect caused by scar-tissue contraction. In these patients the incisura may be so deep as almost to bisect the stomach and result in an hour glass configuration (see Fig. 16-8, *right*). Even though the ulcer heals, the incisura caused by scar-tissue formation will remain as a fixed persisting defect.

PERISTALSIS. Peristalsis is interrupted at the site of the indurated zone including the ulcer crater within it if the induration involves the muscularis, as it does in most penetrating types of ulcer. The wave will continue, however, on the opposite curvature and, momentarily, it becomes quite deep directly opposite the crater, forming a temporary incisura. As the wave passes beyond the zone of induration it will appear again on the lesser curvature and continue to the pylorus. Thus the width of the zone of induration can be established by observing peristaltic waves as they traverse the area. Small, superficial ulcers do not affect peristalsis appreciably and the crater "rides" the peristaltic wave.

SPASM. In addition to the presence of a spastic incisura gastric ulcers frequently cause spasm in the prepyloric segment of the stomach. If such spasm exists for a long period of time it may cause more or less permanent narrowing of the prepyloric segment as a result of hypertrophy of the pyloric musculature. Spasm results in an inconstant and irregular narrowing of the involved area that can be effaced by palpation and that changes in contour as a result of peristalsis. Hypertrophy of the pyloric muscle results in a more or less fixed narrowing that may involve the immediate prepyloric segment of the stomach for a distance of several centimeters or more (see Fig. 16-28). Under fluoroscopic observation the narrowing usually changes slightly from time to time and is not fixed completely. Mucosal folds can be identified within the narrowed area and this, plus the slightly changing contour, helps to identify the lesion and distinguish it from an infiltrating annular carcinoma.

CHANGES IN THE MUCOSAL FOLDS. The tendency for a spokelike radiation of folds away from the base of the ulcer crater has been noted in a preceding paragraph. The folds often are thickened throughout the stomach when gastric or duodenal ulcer is present, probably a manifestation of gastritis.

PALPABLE MASS. If the ulcer has penetrated and become walled-off by inflammatory tissue a mass may be palpable but in the usual case a palpable mass does not exist.

GASTRIC RETENTION. Retention of material in the stomach for abnormally long periods of time or frank evidence of pyloric obstruction is an extremely variable finding and depends to a large extent upon the location of the gastric ulcer. If the lesion is near the pylorus there

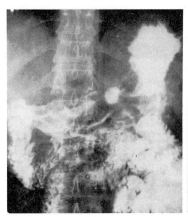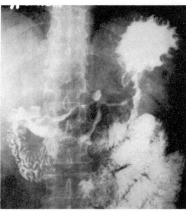

Fig. 16-12. Benign gastric ulcer. The lesion is on the posterior wall in the middle third close to the lesser curvature and these roentgenograms are made with the patient supine so that the crater is seen *en face*. *Left,* The appearance of the crater at the time of initial examination. Note the thickened mucosal folds radiating away from its base. *Right,* The same lesion after medical therapy for 1 month. Note the decrease in size of the crater. The thickened folds persist.

may be enough interference with emptying to cause a significant degree of obstruction. Even ulcers situated higher up on the lesser curvature often cause some retention because they interfere with normal peristaltic activity and because they cause pylorospasm. In other instances even in the presence of a large gastric ulcer the stomach empties promptly.

DIFFERENTIAL DIAGNOSIS OF BENIGN AND MALIGNANT ULCERS. The term "carcinomatous or malignant ulcer" is used for a lesion that initially was a benign ulcer but that subsequently underwent carcinomatous change. There is not complete agreement as to whether a benign ulcer ever becomes malignant, but the pathologists with whom we are associated believe that this happens occasionally. The term "ulcerating carcinoma" is used for a lesion that was carcinomatous from the beginning but with the development of central necrosis and ulceration the gross features are essentially those of an ulcer. To avoid confusion in this discussion the term "ulcerating carcinoma" will be used for both. Ulcerating carcinomas of a type that might be confused with benign gastric ulcer are uncommon. It has been reported that only about 5 per cent of all ulcers are malignant and therefore the chance for any ulcer being a carcinoma is small. Nevertheless, there are cer-

tain roentgen findings that are quite useful in differentiating the two lesions:

1. Benign ulcers usually are sharply marginated and round or slightly ovoid when viewed *en face.* Malignant ulcers often are of irregular shape and uneven in depth.

2. Benign ulcers project beyond the gastric lumen. An exception occurs when there is a mound of edematous and inflamed tissue around the crater as described previously. The malignant lesion usually lies within the outline of the lumen because it develops in a mass of tumor tissue (Fig. 16-14).

3. The edematous halo surrounding a benign ulcer is relatively smooth and fades gradually at the periphery. In carcinomatous ulcers the halo is wider, often nodular, and usually more sharply defined from normal stomach wall at its periphery. The crater may be situated off-center in relation to the halo.

4. When viewed in profile the combination of an intraluminal crater surrounded by a nodular halo resembles the *meniscus sign* or *complex* first defined by Carman and later elaborated by Kirklin. The surface of the barium-filled crater facing the gastric lumen was described originally as being concave, giving the appearance of a meniscus. However, as more commonly seen, the internal surface is convex. The floor of the crater tends to

except in superficial spreading carcinoma

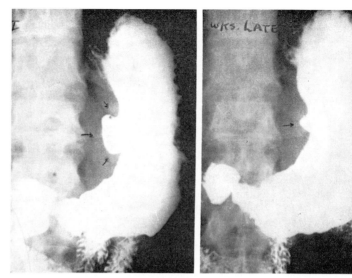

Fig. 16-13. Benign gastric ulcer showing the effect of medical therapy. *Left,* Appearance at the time of initial examination. The crater projects from the lumen and shows the usual features of a benign ulcer. *Right,* Appearance 3 weeks later after patient was under medical therapy. The crater has reduced in size and has become more triangular or pointed in appearance as the base has filled in with granulation tissue.

be flat (Fig. 16-14 *right*), sometimes rounded (externally convex), or irregular and nodular.

5. Spokelike radiation of mucosal folds is characteristic of a benign ulcer and is not seen in carcinoma.

6. The size and location of the ulcer no longer are considered to be important in differential diagnosis. Formerly it was believed that an ulcer crater larger in diameter than 2.5 cm was, in all probability malignant. The same was true of an ulcer on the greater curvature. It is now well established that benign ulcer can occur anywhere in the stomach although greater-curvature ulcers are infrequent. Some benign ulcers reach a very large size and some ulcerating carcinomas are small.

7. Under proper therapy most benign ulcers decrease in size, the halo of edema regresses, and eventually the crater and the induration around it disappear. Some decrease in size should be noted at the first reexamination, usually done within three weeks of the initial study (see Fig. 16-13 *right*). Unfortunately, some benign ulcers heal very slowly or not at all in spite of proper medical management. If the roentgen criteria for benignancy are present, operation can be de-

ferred but in most of these patients, resection eventually must be done to effect a cure.

On the other hand, some ulcerating carcinomas may appear smaller on reexamination. There are several possible reasons for this. The inflammatory element may improve under therapy. Food particles or blood clots may fill the crater so that it cannot be completely outlined by the barium mixture. Also growth of neoplastic tissue may encroach on the crater decreasing its size. It is important, therefore, to determine whether the halo of induration is also decreasing as the ulcer crater appears to diminish in size. If it does not, one should view the lesion with considerable suspicion and close observation.

CARCINOMA OF THE STOMACH

A number of classifications of carcinoma of the stomach have been suggested, based upon pathologic characteristics. From a roentgen point of view it is sufficient to consider the following types: (*1*) polypoid or fungating, (*2*) infiltrating, (*3*) ulcerating, and (*4*) mixed types. Certain roentgen characteristics are

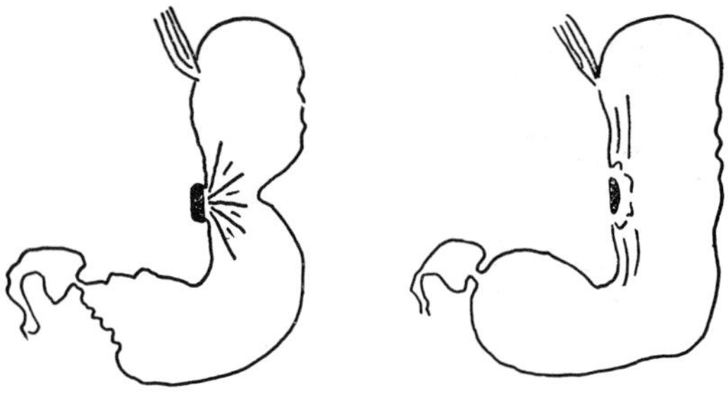

Fig. 16-14. Diagrams illustrating benign (*left*) and malignant (*right*) ulcers on the lesser curvature of the stomach. The ulcer crater of the benign lesion projects outside the normal lumen, the mucosal folds radiate away from its base in spokelike fashion, and the edges of the crater tend to be undermined slightly. There is irregular spasm narrowing the pyloric antrum and an incisura opposite the crater. The malignant meniscus type of ulcer does not project beyond the gastric lumen. It is surrounded by an irregular and rather nodular halo. The mucosal folds do not radiate but rather are obliterated at the edges of the halo.

common to all gastric carcinomas regardless of the pathologic type. The tumor stiffens the gastric wall where it is involved by the neoplasm; the soft, pliable appearance of the normal stomach, as brought out by palpation during fluoroscopy, is lost; peristalsis does not pass through the lesion; the normal mucosal pattern over the surface of the tumor either is destroyed completely or altered markedly in its appearance.

FUNGATING CARCINOMA

In the fungating or polypoid type of gastric carcinoma (Figs. 16-15 to 16-17) the tumor forms a bulky mass that projects into the gastric lumen and causes a filling defect in the barium shadow. The surface of the defect is irregular or nodular. Superficial or deep ulcer pockets may be present but the evidence of ulceration is less obvious than is the mass of the tumor. The mucosal folds are completely absent over the surface of the lesion. The defect is constant, rigid, and reproducible throughout the examination or at repeat examinations. The junction of the filling defect and the gastric wall usually is distinct and

often forms an acute angle, giving an effect of overhanging edges (Figs. 16-15 and 16-16). With small lesions the defect is limited to one wall or one curvature; larger lesions completely encircle the stomach and cause an irregular, fixed narrowing of the gastric lumen.

INFILTRATING CARCINOMA

The infiltrating type of gastric carcinoma does not cause a distinct intraluminal mass but rather infiltrates the gastric wall, spreading in or beneath the mucosa.

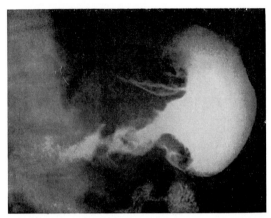

Fig. 6-15. Large fungating or polypoid carcinoma involving the distal half of the stomach.

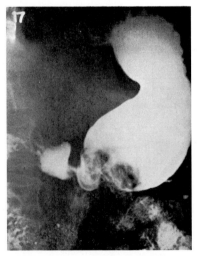

Fig. 6-16. Polypoid carcinoma arising on the greater curvature side of the gastric antrum.

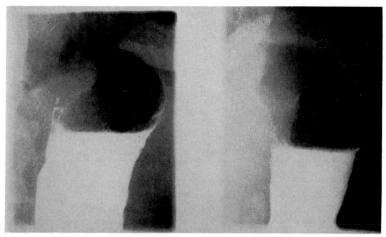

Fig. 16-17. Polypoid carcinoma of the gastric fundus. Two spot roentgenograms made at the time of fluoroscopy with the patient standing. An effervescent beverage has been given to increase the gas content of the fundus. The tumor projects into the fundus from the medial side in the region of the cardia and can be clearly outlined as a soft-tissue mass.

SCIRRHUS CARCINOMA. The scirrhus form of carcinoma is characterized by its infiltrating nature and by the fact that the tumor evokes a pronounced fibrous tissue response in the gastric wall. The wall becomes thickened and rigid at the site of the tumor and peristalsis does not pass through it. The mucosal folds usually are obliterated; instead the surface has a fine granular or occasionally a rough, cobblestone appearance. Scirrhus carcinoma may be local or general. In the latter lesion the limits of the process are poorly defined as a rule and there is a gradual transition from normal to abnormal. Because of this and the absence of a distinct filling defect, the detection of early lesions is extremely difficult, particularly in the fundus or the upper third of the stomach where peristalsis normally is feeble or absent and palpation is difficult (Fig. 16-18). Eventually the infiltration of the tumor may involve practically the entire stomach and it is this extensive lesion that is sometimes called the *leather bottle stomach* or *linitis plastica* (Fig. 16-19). Characteristically this type of carcinoma does not obstruct the orifices until late; in fact the cardia and pylorus often are gaping, held open by the rigid gastric walls, so that the liquid barium mixture literally pours through the stomach into the duodenum and it is difficult to keep sufficient filling for adequate observation. The localized form of scirrhus carcinoma behaves somewhat differently. It tends to encircle the gastric lumen rather early in its development and cause a more or less localized narrowing of the lumen. This lesion is most frequent in the pyloric antrum, where it results in an annular stricturelike narrowing. The limits of the lesion are more sharply defined than in the generalized or linitis plastica form of the disease and obstruction of the pylorus may develop relatively early. Occasionally, the outer wall of the stomach can be visualized and the great thickening caused by the tumor can be confirmed.

SUPERFICIAL SPREADING CARCINOMA. Golden has described the roentgen features of this form of carcinoma. It differs grossly from the scirrhus by the absence of appreciable fibrosis and by the tendency for ulceration. An intraluminal mass is not a prominent feature. The involved area in the wall is stiffened and rigid. Ulceration occurs in a high percentage of patients and the ulcer cavity may be the most obvious roentgen deformity. Because there is no intraluminal mass, the ulcer crater projects outside

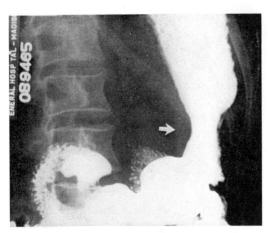

Fig. 16-18. Scirrhus carcinoma of the stomach. The lesion is manifested by a moderate fusiform narrowing of the gastric lumen (**arrow**). During fluoroscopy this was fixed and could not be made to distend at any time. Peristaltic waves were absent through the area although they were present in the distal part of the stomach. The margins of the lesion are very poorly defined.

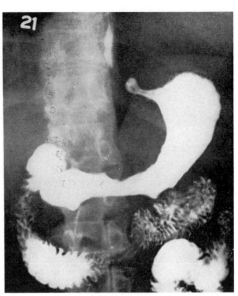

Fig. 16-19. Scirrhus carcinoma of the stomach (linitis plastica). The entire stomach except the distal 1 or 2 cm is involved by the lesion, which has infiltrated and thickened the wall and produced a completely stiff and rigid structure. In spite of the extensive involvement, there is no obstruction at either orifice.

the gastric lumen when viewed in profile. Characteristically the wall around the ulcer is stiffened for some distance and fails to transmit peristalsis. The mucosal pattern is destroyed over the surface of the infiltrated area in most patients. Rarely the tumor has been observed to spread beneath the mucosa, leaving the folds intact, or else causing them to appear unusually thick. This appearance resembles closely that seen in some cases of malignant lymphoma. If the lesion is limited to a moderate-sized area along one curvature, one or several incisuralike indrawings of the opposite curvature may be present. When ulceration develops, the ulcer pocket is more irregular than is seen in a benign ulcer, there is little tendency for the edges to overhang, the area of stiffness and induration around the crater is larger, and the mucosal pattern is obliterated in the vicinity or else is altered.

More recently Mainzer, Amberg, and Margulis[21] have reported their experience with this lesion and note the controversy in the literature concerning the roentgen findings. The roentgen appearances in their patients fell into four main categories, (1) gastric ulcer, (2) polypoid filling defect, (3) contracted lesser curvature or antral rigidity, and (4) normal stomach. The ulcers were interpreted as benign. Those showing antral rigidity or contracted lesser curvature simulated a healed gastric ulcer deformity. The polypoid lesions usually were small and often thought to be benign. Their findings emphasize the need for early diagnosis of this lesion because of the high curability rate, e.g., a 93 per cent 5-year survival rate in one series.

ULCERATING CARCINOMA

Ulceration may develop in any gastric carcinoma. As used here the term is meant to imply a lesion in which necrosis has led to deep ulceration and with the ulcer cavity dominating the gross picture (Fig. 16-20). When a polypoid or fungating carcinoma develops extensive

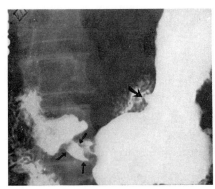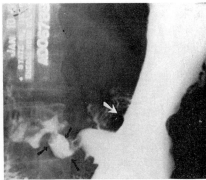

Fig. 16-20. Benign and malignant gastric ulcers. *Left,* Appearance at the time of initial examination. **Upper arrow** points to benign ulcer on the lesser curvature at the sulcus angularis. **Lower arrows** point to another ulcerating lesion on the greater curvature side in the immediate prepyloric area of the stomach. This is a meniscus type of lesion and does not project beyond the lumen; it is bounded by an irregular and rather nodular halo. *Right,* Appearance after several weeks of medical regime. The benign ulcer has decreased in size and only a small pointed projection (**white arrow**) remains. The malignant ulcer in the prepyloric area has increased in size (**lower arrows**).

necrosis to the point where the lesion is predominantly an ulcer, the ulcer is of the meniscus type (described under the heading "Differential Diagnosis of Benign and Malignant Ulcers"). This is because the ulcer forms within a mass that projects into the lumen and thus the cavity of the ulcer will not extend beyond the luminal margin as a rule. When an infiltrating carcinoma ulcerates, the cavity of the ulcer does project outside the lumen when viewed tangentially and resembles a benign ulcer in this respect. Differences between the two are mentioned in the section above. The question as to the frequency with which a benign ulcer may undergo malignant transformation has not been settled but it probably is an infrequent occurrence. The differential diagnosis is given on page 526.

MIXED TYPES

It is to be expected that many gastric carcinomas will show roentgen features of more than one of the above types. A predominantly fungating tumor may undergo extensive ulceration, an infiltrating carcinoma may develop fungating characteristics, or different parts of a single tumor may resemble several of the types described. This is particularly true in advanced lesions, as many of these are when first examined.

CALCIFICATION IN GASTRIC NEOPLASMS

Rarely, calcifications may be found in gastric carcinoma. In the reported cases this has been a mucinous type of adenocarcinoma, as is true when calcification occurs in carcinoma of the colon. Benign tumors may calcify and we have reported an example occurring in a leiomyoma of the gastric fundus.[10]

GASTRIC POLYPS AND INTRAMURAL TUMORS

GASTRIC POLYPS

Adenomatous polyps of the stomach are similar in all respects to polyps of the colon (see page 613). Polyps develop less frequently in the stomach than they do in the colon. Because of the effects of active peristalsis in the stomach, a gastric polyp is likely to develop a fairly long pedicle. When situated near the pylorus the pedunculated polyp is prone to prolapse through the pylorus into the duodenum and thus may be a cause of pyloric obstruction. Otherwise, bleeding is the only symptom to be expected. There may be one or several polyps present in the individual patient; rarely a diffuse polyposis of the gastric wall is encountered. Inflammatory polyps also are found in the stomach and resemble in all respects the roentgen appearances of true adenomatous polyps. The diagnosis cannot be made purely from roentgen examination.

Roentgen Observations

A polyp causes a smoothly rounded, translucent defect in the barium shadow. If the polyp has a pedicle, the defect caused by the polyp may move over a distance of several centimeters under the influence of peristalsis. The pedicle may be visualized as a narrow stalklike defect extending from the head of the polyp to the margin of the stomach. If the polyp is sessile, no motion of it in relation to the gastric wall is seen. A polyp of less than 0.5 cm in

diameter is difficult to detect on roentgen examination unless situated directly on one of the curvatures where it can be visualized easily in profile (Fig. 16-21). The normal tortuosity of gastric mucosal folds offers difficulty in recognition of small lesions because of the similarity to polyps that may be produced when these folds are a little thickened. Occasionally a more or less generalized thickening and tortuosity of the gastric mucosal folds is found, the folds causing polyp-like defects when they are seen on edge. It often is impossible to determine if one is dealing with a multiple polyposis of the stomach or a hypertrophied mucosa. Most frequently it is the latter condition that is, in fact, an inflammatory type of polyposis or polypoid hyperplasia.

A prolapsing polyp may cause the signs of pyloric obstruction with obvious gastric retention and delay in gastric emptying. Peristaltic waves are deep and vigorous and there is some degree of gastric dilatation. During fluoroscopy the defect caused by the polyp may change position, being seen in the pyloric antrum at times and then prolapsing into the duodenal bulb (Fig. 16-22). When situated within the bulb, the head of the polyp causes a circular

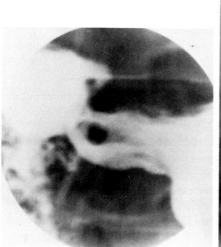 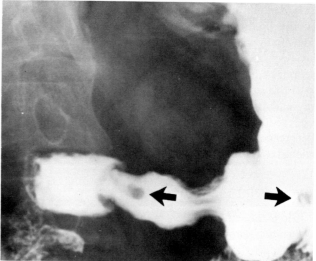

Fig. 16-21. Polyp in the gastric antrum. *Left,* Spot film made during fluoroscopy, and (*right*) recumbent film after fluoroscopy showing constancy of the defect (**left arrow**). Two other small polyps were demonstrated in other roentgenograms (**right arrow** points to one near the greater curvature).

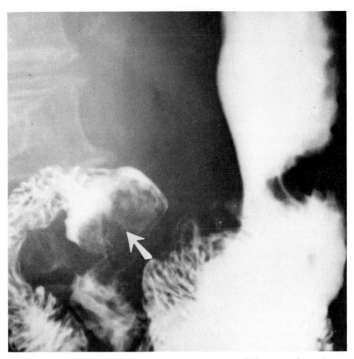

Fig. 16-22. Prolapsed pedunculated polyp of the gastric antrum. In this roentgenogram the head of the polyp is in the duodenal bulb (**arrow**) but other roentgenograms and fluoroscopy showed it to move back into the stomach intermittently.

and centrally placed filling defect. The stalk may be visible, extending through the pylorus and causing a puckering of the wall of the stomach at its point of origin. It may be possible to dislodge the polyp from the duodenal bulb by manual palpation during the fluoroscopic study.

Because adenomatous polyps of the stomach may undergo malignant transformation and because the early stages of carcinomatous degeneration cannot be recognized on roentgen examination, most authorities recommend that such polyps be removed surgically at the time they are discovered.

CRONKHITE-CANADA SYNDROME

Polyposis of the stomach, small intestine and colon occurs in this rare syndrome in association with a malabsorption syndrome and ectodermal changes. The latter include alopecia, atrophy of the nails, and hyperpigmentation. There is severe diarrhea and loss of protein from the intestinal tract. In addition to polyps there may be thickened folds in the stomach and colon and either villous atrophy or thickened folds in the small bowel.[22]

INTRAMURAL GASTRIC TUMORS

A variety of intramural nonmucosal tumors occur in the stomach but as a group these lesions are uncommon. Among these tumors of intramural origin one will find leiomyomas, neurofibromas, lipomas, etc. Since it often is difficult to identify accurately the histologic nature of many of these tumors, some authors prefer to describe them simply as "spindle-cell tumors." The most common tumor in this group is the leiomyoma. Any of these lesions may occur as sarcomas.

Grossly the intramural tumor is usually well circumscribed and encapsulated (Fig. 16-23). The tumor bulges into the gastric lumen but is covered by mucosa. An ulcer often develops on the summit

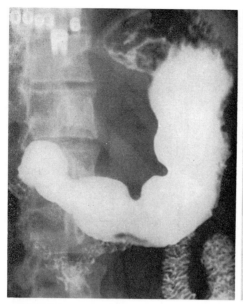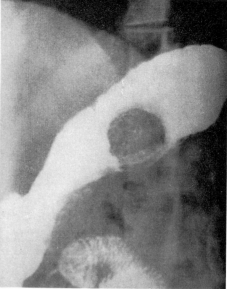

Fig. 16-23. Benign intramural tumor of the posterior wall of the stomach. Posteroanterior roentgenogram on the *left* does not show any evidence of the lesion. *Right*, A lateral view with the defect of the tumor clearly seen as it is brought into profile. The lesion is a neurofibroma.

of the mass and this may be a cause of gastric hemorrhage (Fig. 16-24). Otherwise, these lesions usually are asymptomatic.

With the larger lesions, and particularly those that are frankly malignant, the major portion of the tumor may grow to the outside, causing little intraluminal deformity but with a bulky exogastric mass.

Roentgen Observations

A small intramural tumor nodule resembles a sessile gastric polyp closely, causing a circumscribed, rounded, filling defect (Fig. 16-23) that is best brought out by pressure over the lesion. It may be impossible to distinguish between the two. If an ulcer has formed, it will be visualized as a pocketlike shadow of barium extending into the mass from its inner surface. Gastric peristalsis is interfered with little if any unless the lesion is large or unless it is malignant and has begun to invade the gastric wall. A lipoma, being relatively soft, may change shape under the influence of palpation or peristalsis. Most gastric lipomas are too small for the lucency of fat to stand out clearly from the adjacent gastric wall, a sign that is helpful in diagnosing lipomas of the peripheral soft

tissues. Large lesions, as indicated above, may show very little intragastric protrusion but the large exogastric mass may cause displacement of the stomach, suggesting that the lesion is entirely extrinsic. In some patients it is impossible to be certain if the lesion originated within or outside of the stomach.

ABERRANT PANCREATIC NODULES

Nodules of pancreatic tissue occasionally are found in the wall of the stomach but are somewhat more frequent in the first and second portions of the duodenum. Some of these nodules are almost microscopic in size and cause no roentgen signs. Others may measure up to 1 cm or more in diameter and be large enough to cause a filling defect. The defect of an aberrant pancreatic nodule is identical to that of a small intramural tumor as described above, and there frequently is no certain way to differentiate between them on roentgen examination. One sign that is helpful when present is the demonstration of a thin, hairline radiopaque stripe extending into the center of the defect and which represents a small aberrant duct leading from the nodule. A small central pit on the surface of the nodule may

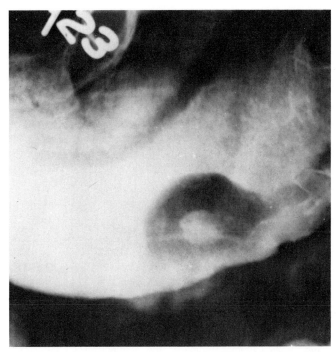

Fig. 16-24. Leiomyoma with central ulcer near the greater curvature of the stomach. The intramural tumor causes a sharply marginated translucent defect as seen *en face* with the central dense spot representing the ulcer. This is an example of a "target" or "bull's eye" deformity.

also be noted in some patients. Because pancreatic nodules are found in the proximal part of the duodenum while other intramural lesions are uncommon in this location, any such duodenal defect is more likely to be a pancreatic nodule than some other type of lesion. Ulceration may develop on the surface of a pancreatic nodule and bleeding may result; usually, however, the lesions are asymptomatic.

EOSINOPHILIC GRANULOMA

This rare granulomatous disease may occur either as a generalized or diffuse involvement of the stomach, small intestine, or both, or as a localized granuloma presenting as an intramural or polypoid mass. In the diffuse form there often is an increase in the eosinophils in the circulating blood. This is not found in the localized type.

In the diffuse form, roentgen findings similar to those of the malabsorption syndrome have been described.[12] These include coarsening of the mucosal folds with segmentation and puddling of the barium. The local form presents as a small intramural mass or as a polypoid lesion, sometimes with a pedicle at or near the pyloric antrum, less commonly in the small bowel. Roentgen findings are not distinctive and histologic examination is necessary for diagnosis. Peroral small bowel biopsy has been used to diagnose the generalized type.

The disease is found usually in adults. The cause is not known but allergy has been considered by some because of the eosinophilia.

OTHER GASTRIC NEOPLASMS

Malignant lymphomas occasionally involve the stomach. Rarely a gastric lesion is the only one demonstrable. The roentgen findings are extremely variable. Some of the lesions resemble carcinoma closely so that roentgen differentiation is impossible. In other instances the roentgen findings are those of an ulcerating

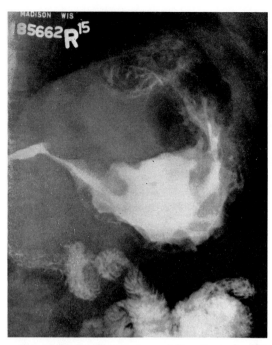

Fig. 16-25 Lymphosarcoma of the stomach. The lesion has infiltrated the gastric wall extensively, producing thickening of the rugae and stiffening of the wall. There is a large extragastric component, causing enlargement of the duodenal curve. The lesion has extended across the pylorus to involve the duodenal bulb.

lesion, even resembling rather closely a benign gastric ulcer. In still others, large portions of the gastric wall may be infiltrated by the tumor, causing gross thickening of the mucosal folds that resembles a hypertrophic gastritis (Fig. 16-25). Localized thickening of the rugae, therefore, must be regarded with suspicion since it may indicate the presence of a malignant lymphoma. Large bulky tumors of lymphomatous origin are less likely to cause obstruction than is carcinoma. Multiple tumors (i.e., a tumor of the stomach and another in the colon or small bowel) always should suggest the strong possibility of malignant lymphoma. *Hodgkin's disease* may involve the stomach. The roentgen findings are variable. The lesion may present as an ulcer simulating a benign lesion. In other cases the lesion causes submucosal infiltration resembling scirrhus carcinoma of the stomach. In a third type, the disease may present as a mass projecting into the gastric lumen. In most cases of Hodgkin's disease, therefore, the disease cannot be distinguished from other, more common lesions.

Villous tumors (villous adenomas) have been reported as occurring in the stomach and duodenum. The lesion resembles the more common villous tumor of the colon clinically and roentgenologically. Malignant changes have been present in most of the tumors. The roentgen appearance is that of a filling defect with a frondlike appearance owing to the numerous villous projections of the lesion, again, similar to that seen in the colon.

GASTRITIS

The problems concerning the significance of gastritis as a clinical entity and the roentgen patterns of the disease have not been completely settled. Gastritis as an accompaniment of other diseases of the stomach (e.g., carcinoma, ulcer) is common. Gastritis of severe degree may result from the ingestion of acids and caustic substances. The major types of chronic gastritis are usually considered to be the atrophic and the hypertrophic.

Roentgen Observations

In *chronic atrophic gastritis* the mucosal folds are thinned and scanty. The normal serrations seen along the greater curvature are lacking. However, many patients showing histologic evidence of the disease have a normal roentgen mucosal pattern and the diagnosis of chronic atrophic gastritis often cannot be made on roentgen findings alone.

In the *chronic hypertrophic type,* similar diagnostic difficulties may be encountered. The following changes may be found:

THICKENING OF THE MUCOSAL FOLDS. Thickening and increased tortuosity of the mucosal folds as a sign of gastritis must be interpreted with considerable caution because of the wide variation in the normal size of these folds. There is no complete agreement as to what the maximum width of a mucosal fold in the stomach should be. As has been observed, a widened fold in the antrum is of more significance than in the fundus because in the latter location the folds normally are thicker and more tortuous than in the distal part of the stomach. It has been suggested that a fold shadow measuring 0.5 cm in width in the antrum is probably abnormal, where the same width in the upper part of the body or in the fundus is probably not abnormal. In general, localized thickening is more significant than a generalized prominence and may indicate a localized hypertrophic gastritis. Occasionally a rather marked thickening of mucous-membrane folds occurs in a localized area of the stomach sufficient to cause a filling defect that may resemble carcinoma rather closely (Fig. 16-26). Surgical exploration and resection may be necessary to settle the problem. This condition is uncommon and is known as *giant hypertrophy of gastric rugae,* or *Menetrier's disease* (Fig. 16-27). In one form of the disease the involvement is predominantly in the middle third involving the greater curvature or both curvatures. However, the lesion may affect any part of the stomach with massive, localized thickening of rugae. At times the tortuous

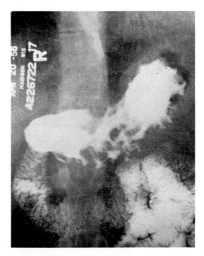

Fig. 16-27. Menetrier's disease. There is marked thickening and tortuosity of folds in the fundus and body of the stomach somewhat suggestive of diffuse polyposis.

thickened folds resemble a mass of polyps. In another type of the lesion the mucosa is stretched over the mass and the surface may be quite smooth. The lesion is uncommon in the pyloric area. In some cases of Menetrier's disease there is a considerable loss of protein, leading to hypoproteinemia and intestinal edema. Excess mucus secretion is common and may add to the mottled effect of the lesion. Eosinophilia and anemia are often present.

STIFFNESS OF THE FOLDS. Of equal and possibly greater importance than thickening of the folds is unusual stiffening of them. Normal gastric folds tend to be completely obliterated or nearly so as the stomach is distended with barium mixture. Folds also are flattened and decreased in width as peristaltic waves pass over them. In the antrum during antral systole, normal folds disappear except for the presence of fine hairline stripes representing thin valleys between the flattened folds as the antrum contracts over them. Normal folds can be obliterated if sufficient pressure is applied over the abdominal wall. This sign is of value only in the lower two-thirds of the stomach where palpation normally can be carried out. Stiffened folds also may be thrown into tortuous eleva-

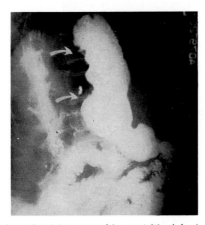

Fig. 16-26. Localized hypertrophic gastritis (giant rugae). Lateral roentgenogram of the stomach shows an irregular filling defect on the posterior wall (**arrow**). At operation and examination of the resected gross specimen the lesion was thought to be a carcinoma. Microscopic examination, however, failed to reveal any evidence of cancer and showed nothing but inflammatory reaction.

tions that resemble polypoid defects and the differentiation from adenomatous polyps may be difficult if not impossible.

ANTRAL GASTRITIS. Probably the most significant form of gastritis from the roentgen standpoint is that which involves the antrum of the stomach. This is a fairly common condition. There may be a localized thickening of the mucosal folds as noted above. The prepyloric area of the stomach is likely to be uniformly narrowed for a distance of several centimeters or even more, proximal to the pylorus; the narrowing is concentric and usually not entirely constant during fluoroscopic observation. Peristalsis through the area is deficient but seldom completely lacking. The antral wall is thickened and relatively stiff but lacks the complete rigidity of an annular carcinoma. These changes possibly are caused by associated pyloric muscle hypertrophy secondary to the chronic spasm and inflammation. Similar findings are seen in the adult form of hypertrophic pyloric stenosis. In some cases the mucosal folds are unusually thin and scanty suggesting an atrophic type of gastritis. Superficial ulcer

craters may be present although frank ulceration is the exception. The lesion must be differentiated chiefly from an annular carcinoma of the antrum (Fig. 16-28). Significant roentgen differential points include:

1. The change from normal gastric wall to involved segment is a smooth one and there are no overhanging edges.

2. The narrowing is even and concentric in antral gastritis; in carcinoma the involvement may be greater on one curvature than on the other.

3. Mucosal folds are present through the contracted area in antral gastritis, they are absent in carcinoma.

4. There almost always is some flexibility of the wall in antral gastritis and if fluoroscopic observation is done carefully or serial roentgenograms are obtained slight relaxation and contraction may be determined. The wall, in annular carcinoma, is completely rigid.

CHEMICAL GASTRITIS. Inflammation of the stomach from the swallowing of caustic substances such as lye or strong acids causes an extensive fibrosis of portions of the gastric wall, leading

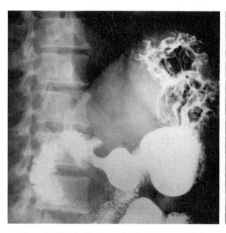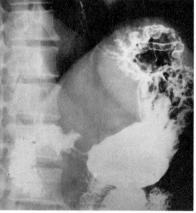

Fig. 16-28. Antral gastritis. Two serial roentgenograms showing the fusiform narrowing of the prepyloric area of the stomach but with a change in contour of the segment in the two roentgenograms. *Right,* There has been increased contraction as a result of peristalsis and a coarse fold of mucosa can be seen extending through the area of narrowing. The lesion never expanded more than shown in the figure on the *left* at any time during fluoroscopy. Note the concavity of the base of the duodenal bulb where the thickened pyloric muscle projects into it.

eventually to irregular constrictions. Involvement of the prepyloric area is frequent and pyloric obstruction may result. In some patients the end result of an extensive chemical gastritis may cause a deformity that resembles a scirrhus carcinoma in many respects. The lumen of the stomach is generally narrowed and the gastric walls show loss of pliability. The history is important in the evaluation of this lesion.

CROHN'S DISEASE OF THE STOMACH. A number of cases of this entity have been reported in the literature but it must be considered as distinctly infrequent. It corresponds, pathologically, to the same disease found in the small intestine (regional enteritis), granulomatous colitis in the colon, and the infrequent similar lesions found in the esophagus and duodenum. The roentgen findings include (1) involvement of the gastric antrum in most patients; (2) associated disease in the duodenum; (3) multiple, tiny or shallow ulcers; (4) thickened mucosal folds and cobblestone mucosal relief in some patients; and (5) lack of antral distensibility. The roentgen diagnosis is difficult unless there are associated changes in the duodenum or elsewhere in the small intestine characteristic of regional enteritis.

THE ZOLLINGER-ELLISON SYNDROME

This syndrome consists of:

1. Fulminating peptic ulceration. The majority of ulcers occur in the duodenal bulb but an atypical location of the ulcer, as in the distal duodenum or proximal jejunem, is found in about 40 per cent of the patients.[8]

2. Marked hypersecretion of hydrochloric acid by the stomach.

3. Nonbeta islet cell tumors of the pancreas. Ectopic locations of the tumors (stomach, duodenum, etc.) occur in about 10 per cent of patients.

4. If only partial gastric resection is done, recurrence of an ulcer occurs in the majority of patients.

In some cases the pancreatic tumor is part of a syndrome with multiple tumors in other endocrine glands including the parathyroid, thyroid, pituitary and adrenal. Severe diarrhea is among the clinical symptoms experienced by many patients. The basic abnormality is the secretion of large amounts of the hormone gastrin by the tumor. This causes the hyperchlorhydria and the resultant symptomatology.

Roentgen Observations

The roentgen findings include:[8,22]

1. Increased gastric fluid content after overnight fasting.

2. Thickened, tortuous, gastric rugae resembling Menetrier's disease.

3. Peptic ulceration. An atypical location of the ulcer (other than the duodenal bulb or stomach) should alert the examiner to the possibility of this syndrome.

4. Dilatation of the duodenum, particularly the descending portion. The mucosal folds are thickened and coarse. In the early stage, spasm and irritability may cause apparent narrowing of the descending duodenum.

5. Changes in the small intestine resembling a malabsorption syndrome. Mucosal fold changes similar to those seen in the duodenum, increased fluid content, hypermotility, and segmentation are commonly encountered. Complete loss of folds may be seen in some segments similar to the "moulage sign" of sprue.

6. Failure of the ulcer to heal under medical therapy. After partial gastric resection, stomal and proximal jejunal ulcers develop in the majority of patients, sometimes within a few weeks after operation.

FOREIGN BODIES

A wide variety of indigestible foreign material may be swallowed and become lodged in the stomach and this is particularly frequent during childhood and among individuals who are psychotic. Most of the swallowed objects are metallic, including pins, coins, etc. Even such objects as spoons and knives may be swallowed, particularly by the mentally deranged. Diagnosis is made without difficulty on plain-film examination because of the extreme density of the metallic foreign bodies.

Certain food substances may result in the formation of indigestible food balls (phytobezoars) in the stomach, the most common of these being persimmons. The continued ingestion of hair, usually by psychotic individuals, may result in the formation of a hair ball (trichobezoar).

Roentgen Observations

1. Metallic objects are readily visualized and the relationship to the stomach identified by the position of the object and its relation to the gastric air bubble. If necessary a small amount of barium-water mixture can be given to localize the object more certainly.

2. Nonmetallic objects can be visualized only after the ingestion of a barium-water meal. They will cause filling defects in the barium shadow. A foreign body is characterized by the fact that the defect can be displaced by manual palpation and by altering the position of the patient. The most common cause for such defects is retained food particles. Reexamination often will clarify the problem if doubt arises concerning the nature of the shadow or shadows.

3. Bezoars are visualized as masses within the gastric lumen, often of large size and sufficient nearly to fill the stomach. The barium mixture will be observed to flow around and completely to surround the mass so that, no matter in what position the patient is placed, a layer of barium can be seen between the defect and the gastric wall. The barium mixture may penetrate into the interstices of the mass and remain after the rest of the stomach is empty; this results in a persistent mottled shadow that is characteristic of a bezoar.

GASTRIC DIVERTICULA

Diverticula of the stomach are uncommon, occurring about once in every 1500 to 2000 gastrointestinal examinations. Diverticula are usually located on the posterior wall of the gastric fundus close to the cardia. It is believed that such diverticula are in all likelihood acquired lesions rather than congenital ones. The fact that practically all gastric diverticula occur in a localized area of the fundus has been explained on the basis of this being a region of anatomic weakness so that diverticulum formation can occur more readily here than elsewhere. Diverticula in the prepyloric area are much less frequent. The sac may contain an island of pancreatic tissue. In the majority of patients it is doubtful if gastric diverticulum is the cause of clinical complaints. A rare case of a tumor, either carcinoma or sarcoma, developing in a gastric diverticulum has been reported. Bleeding from a diverticulum, usually the result of ulceration, also has been reported but is an uncommon occurrence.

Roentgen Observations

The diverticulum when filled with barium is visualized as a smoothly rounded outpouching connected to the stomach by a narrow neck (Fig. 16-29). While they vary in size the majority are small, measuring several centimeters in diameter. Retention of the barium mixture in the pouch for hours after the rest of the stomach is empty is the rule. If follow-up roentgenograms of the abdomen are obtained, the small, round barium shadow will remain in the region of the gastric cardia long after the remainder of the stomach has emptied. A gastric diverticulum can be distinguished from a gastric ulcer without difficulty

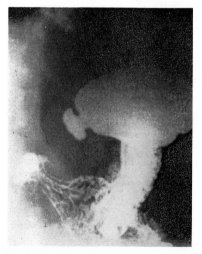

Fig. 16-29. Diverticulum of the gastric fundus.

by its characteristic shape, the typical location, by the absence of spasm, and by the retention of contrast material for hours after the stomach is empty.

HYPERTROPHIC PYLORIC STENOSIS

There are two major forms of hypertrophic pyloric stenosis, the infantile and the adult. The adult type probably is not related to the infantile although the cause is obscure in many patients. In some it appears to develop on the basis of a preexisting antral gastritis as a result of the chronic inflammation and the long-continued spasm. In others it is seen in association with a chronic ulcer and in these it may result from chronic pylorospasm. In still other patients an etiologic factor is not evident and perhaps some of these represent hypertrophy persisting into adult life, following an earlier infantile type of lesion.

In the cases reported by du Plessis[13] atrophic gastritis was present in all those who had biopsy or surgical resection. He believes that the probable cause is a congenital deficiency in the longitudinal muscle over the pyloric canal with hypertrophy of the circular muscle and that the gastritis, gastric ulceration, and mucosal strictures are secondary.

Roentgen Observations

INFANTILE TYPE. The stomach usually is enlarged but pronounced gastric dilatation is not common. Deep peristaltic waves occur intermittently but these force only small quantities of the barium mixture through the pylorus with each wave and the gastric emptying time is delayed. As the barium is forced through the pylorus into the duodenum by peristalsis, the pyloric canal is visualized as a narrow elongated tract from 1 to 2 cm in length (Fig. 16-30). The appearance is one of a thin "string" of barium (Fig. 16-31). The diameter of this segment may vary slightly from time to time but never becomes entirely normal. As the duodenal bulb becomes visualized, its base

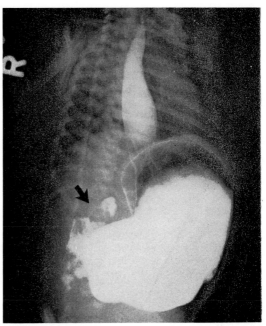

Fig. 16-30. Infantile type of hypertrophic pyloric stenosis. Oblique roentgenogram of the barium-filled stomach shows a thin stringlike shadow of barium extending through the narrowed prepyloric segment of the stomach (**arrow**). Some of the barium has passed through the narrowed area sufficient to outline a small duodenal bulb.

often is seen to be concave because of the thickened pyloric muscle bulging into it.

ADULT TYPE. The roentgen signs are similar to the infantile form except that they are somewhat easier to demonstrate. The narrow elongated pyloric canal may measure 3 to 4 cm in length. The caliber often changes slightly during fluoroscopic observation and mucosal folds can be demonstrated as thin, stripelike shadows paralleling the long axis of the antrum. A concave indentation in the base of the duodenal bulb is often seen owing to the hypertrophied muscle. In the adult, gastric emptying often occurs at a normal rate and the stomach empties within an average length of time. Occasionally gastric retention occurs and in rather uncommon instances a fairly high-grade obstruction may develop at the pylorus.

The lesion must be differentiated from an

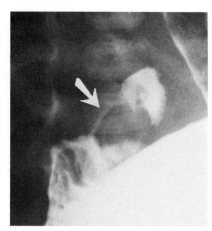

Fig. 16-31. Enlarged view of string sign in infantile hypertrophic pyloric stenosis (**arrow**). Same patient as shown in Figure 16-30. The triangular accumulation of barium above the narrowed pylorus is the duodenal bulb.

annular carcinoma of the gastric antrum. The chief differential points include: (*1*) the presence of mucosal folds in the constricted area; (*2*) concavity of the base of the duodenal bulb. This may also occur in the presence of an annular carcinoma although it is more commonly seen in benign hypertrophy; (*3*) slight changes in contour of the narrowed prepyloric area during fluoroscopic observation and as demonstrated in serial roentgenograms; (*4*) a smooth rather than an abrupt change from normal to abnormal gastric wall; and (*5*) absence of a palpable mass.

None of these signs is absolutely specific for a benign lesion but a combination of them is significant (Fig. 16-32).

EXTRINSIC MASSES

The stomach is displaced easily by masses arising in its vicinity. The nature of the displacement may give some indication of the lesion responsible for it.

LIVER

Enlargement of the liver displaces the stomach to the left and posteriorly. Enlargement of the

left lobe of the liver causes a greater degree of posterior displacement.

SPLEEN

Enlargement of the spleen displaces the stomach toward the midline and anteriorly. Moderate enlargement of the spleen may deform only the fundus and body of the stomach, resulting in a smooth concave indentation of the gastric wall. In rare instances the spleen may project into the space between the fundus and the diaphragm.

LEFT KIDNEY

Enlargement of the left kidney causes a forward displacement of the stomach. A large mass may also displace it to the left and produce a pressure deformity on the lesser curvature.

RIGHT KIDNEY

Enlargement of the right kidney usually has little effect upon the stomach but it does cause displacement of the descending duodenum to the left and anteriorly.

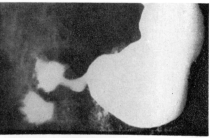

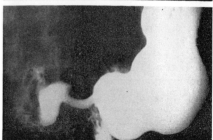

Fig. 16-32. Adult type of benign hypertrophy of the pylorus. This lesion probably developed on the basis of an antral gastritis. Because of impossibility of excluding a localized scirrhus carcinoma of the stomach, the patient was operated upon. The lesion was found to be benign.

PANCREAS

Lesions of the head of the pancreas cause a smooth, pressure defect on the greater curvature side of the gastric antrum (the "pad" sign) displacing it upward and forward. Occasionally the deformity will be on the lesser rather than the greater curvature side and change in position of the patient may alter the effect of pressure to a considerable degree. Lesions of the body of the pancreas displace the stomach forward.

TRANSVERSE COLON

Upward displacement of the stomach may result from a mass in the transverse colon if it is large. Usually no deformity is present from a transverse colon mass.

OTHER MASSES

Any intra-abdominal mass if large enough may cause some displacement of the stomach. Thus a very large ovarian cyst may elevate the stomach considerably. Mesenteric cysts may do likewise. Retroperitoneal sarcomas, metastatic enlargement of lymph nodes, and aneurysm of the abdominal aorta are examples of other mass lesions that may deform and displace the stomach.

ESOPHAGEAL HIATAL HERNIA

Herniation of a part of the stomach through the esophageal hiatus is one of the common lesions of the upper gastrointestinal tract. The frequency of diagnosis of the lesion depends to some extent on whether the small, inconstant protrusions of gastric mucosa, so-called "hiatal insufficiency," are included. Also some have considered the esophagogastric junction to be at the site where squamous esophageal and columnar gastric epithelium meet. Since it is not infrequent to find the epithelial junction above the diaphragmatic hiatus, these cases would be considered as hiatal hernias. Others believe that the motor activity of the distal segment is the determining factor. If esophageal peristaltic waves pass without interruption through the distal segment, it would be considered, functionally, a part of the esophagus

regardless of the type of epithelium present. We subscribe to this opinion which, of course, will lead to fewer diagnoses of small, asymptomatic lesions.

Demonstration of a hiatal hernia is best accomplished when the patient is examined while in a recumbent position. The barium mixture can be fed through a drinking tube and the cardia observed as the patient is rotated into various positions. Usually the hernia will fill readily when the patient is in either a supine or a right lateral position. The Valsalva maneuver is useful to show small hernias and to determine the competency of the cardia. Fixed hernias of any appreciable size often can be recognized in chest roentgenograms, the fundus of the stomach and the gas-fluid level within it forming a recognizable shadow in the lower part of the posterior mediastinum.

TYPES OF HIATAL HERNIA (FIG. 16-33)

SLIDING HERNIA. The most common type of hiatal hernia is the sliding, the herniated portion consisting of the gastric fundus, and with the cardia displaced above the level of the hiatus. The esophagus usually is somewhat kinked or buckled in its lower portion and the cardiac orifice lies along the posteromedial side of the fundus. The hiatus often is very wide, measuring 3 to 4 cm in diameter. In some cases the hernia is inconstant and reducible. In others it is fixed in the thorax. Reflux of material from the stomach into the lower esophagus is frequent in this type of hernia and is generally considered to be an important factor in the subsequent development of esophagitis and esophageal stricture (Figs. 16-34 and 16-35).

PARAESOPHAGEAL HERNIA. The paraesophageal type of hernia (Fig. 16-36) is less frequent than the sliding. It is characterized by the fact that the cardia remains at or below the diaphragm, the fundus herniating through the hiatus to lie alongside the distal part of the esophagus. The esophagus remains of normal length and reflux through the cardia does not usually occur.

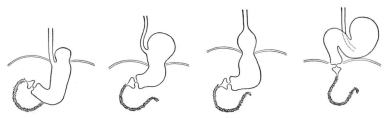

Fig. 16-33. Diagrams illustrating types of hiatal hernia. *Left*, Paraesophageal. *Left center*, Sliding hernia. *Right center*, Short esophagus type of
hernia. *Right*, Intrathoracic stomach.

SHORT ESOPHAGUS TYPE OF HERNIA. The
short esophagus type resembles the sliding except that the esophagus is shortened and the
cardia is situated on the summit of the herniated fundus. While some of these cases undoubtedly are of congenital origin, it is probable that in the majority the lesion began as a
sliding type of acquired hernia, the esophagus
having become shortened as a result of spasm
or inflammation and fibrosis. It is to be noted
that the esophagus almost invariably is somewhat shortened in even the most typical forms
of sliding hernia and that it tends to become as
short as is required, a certain amount of contraction of the longitudinal muscle fibers de-

veloping when the cardia has been displaced
above the diaphragm (see Fig. 16-39).

THORACIC STOMACH. Rather infrequently the
entire stomach or the major portion of it lies
above the diaphragm, representing an advanced form of one of the three types described
above. In most patients the pylorus is below
the diaphragm, the cardia either directly above
or just below the hiatus, and the stomach
rotated upon its long axis so that the body is
inverted.

HIATAL INSUFFICIENCY. While the use of the
term "hiatal insufficiency" to distinguish a type
of hernia is somewhat debatable, there is a
reasonably distinct roentgen pattern that is best
described as insufficiency of the hiatus rather
than as hiatal hernia. It is characterized by an

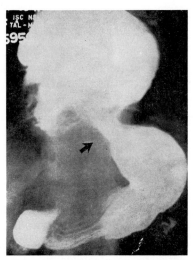

Fig. 16-34. Large sliding type of hiatal hernia. **Arrow** points to the level of the diaphragmatic hiatus
and the large portion of stomach above this represents the hernial sac lying above the diaphragm.

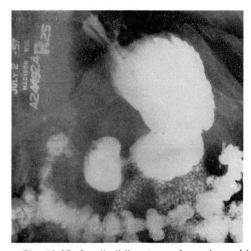

Fig. 16-35. Small sliding type of esophageal hiatal
hernia.

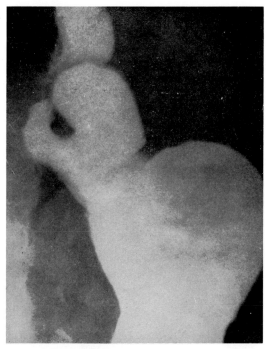

Fig. 16-36. Paraesophageal type of hiatal hernia.

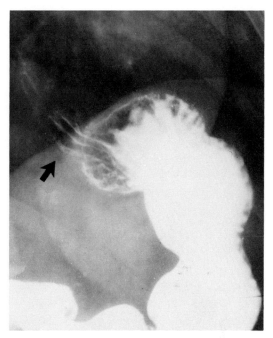

Fig. 16-37. Small protrusion (**arrow**) of gastric mucosa through the hiatus (hiatal insufficiency).

inconstant bulging or protrusion of a small segment of the fundus or of only gastric mucosa through the hiatus. At times during the examination there may be no sign of abnormality at the cardia but under certain circumstances and during some phases of filling or contraction of the distal part of the esophagus, a small knucklelike protrusion of fundus appears (Fig. 16-37). It is recognized as stomach rather than the phrenic ampulla of the lower esophagus by the character of the mucosal folds, which are tortuous or crinkled and sharply distinct from the straight parallel folds of the esophagus. The cardiac orifice usually remains below the diaphragm. A superimposition of straight esophageal folds upon tortuous gastric folds directly above the diaphragm may be observed in some patients and is characteristic of the lesion. Differentiation of this so-called hiatal insufficiency from a phrenic ampulla of the esophagus may be difficult but usually can be made. Usually the ampullary portion of the esophagus when contracted shows straight and parallel folds rather than tortuous ones; the ampulla usually contracts

after a short interval and does not refill from the stomach. At times a distinct line of demarcation between esophageal and gastric folds is not apparent and the exact location of the mucosal junction between the two structures cannot be determined. The clinical significance of hiatal insufficiency is doubtful unless esophageal reflux can be demonstrated.

COMPLICATIONS OF HIATAL HERNIA

BLEEDING. Hiatal hernia may be responsible for bleeding from the upper gastrointestinal tract. This may be caused by an ulcer that has formed within the herniated portion or directly at the constricted zone at the level of the hiatus (Fig. 16-38). Bleeding also may result from hyperemia, gastritis, and superficial mucosal erosions without a frank ulcer crater being present. It may be difficult to visualize an ulcer situated within the hernia because of overlapping of the wall, thickening of the folds, absence of peristaltic contractions in this part of the stomach, and inability to palpate through the abdominal wall.

OBSTRUCTION. Obstruction is infrequent except in the thoracic stomach type of hiatal hernia. In this

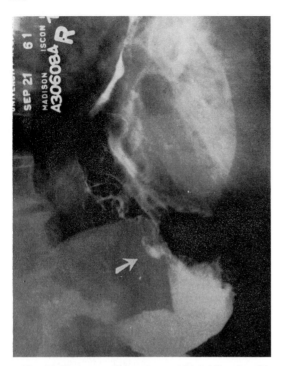

Fig. 16-38. Large sliding type of hiatal hernia with a gastric ulcer at the level of the hiatus (**arrow**).

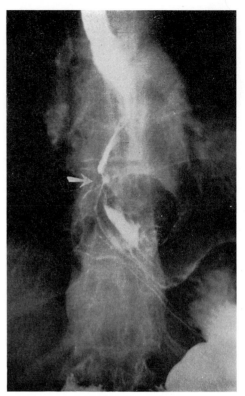

Fig. 16-39. Hiatel hernia with shortening of the esophagus, esophagitis, and peptic ulcer (**arrow**) at the esophagogastric junction. This is a frequently associated combination of lesions. The esophagitis is manifested by a fixed narrowing of the distal part of the esophagus.

lesion torsion of the stomach on its long axis may result in volvulus and this in turn may cause partial or complete obstruction at either the cardia or the pylorus or at both orifices.

ESOPHAGITIS, STRICTURE, AND ULCER (Fig. 16-39). These complications and the relationship between hiatus hernia and inflammation of the distal part of the esophagus have been discussed in Chapter 15 in the section on "Esophagitis and Esophageal Ulcer."

VOLVULUS OF THE STOMACH

Minor degrees of torsion of the stomach are not infrequent and often are asymptomatic. One of the most common is the so-called cup and spill or cascade stomach, mentioned earlier in this chapter. The term "volvulus" probably should be limited to those cases where there is a rotation of the stomach, usually on its long axis, sufficient to obstruct its orifices. This is an infrequent condition. While volvulus may occur in a chronic, intermittent form, the acute type is the most significant and represents an acute surgical emergency. Observers

have pointed out that a torsion of more than 180° is likely to compromise the blood supply; a twist of less than this may not completely obstruct the orifices or seriously disturb the blood supply. Relaxation of the ligaments supporting the stomach must be present for volvulus to develop. This relaxation may be congenital in origin because of abnormal peritoneal attachments or it may be acquired. In the reported cases there has been a high incidence of diaphragmatic hernia and this seems to be the most common predisposing factor. The clinical symptoms include the sudden onset of severe epigastric pain, and retching without vomiting. Because the cardia is obstructed, a gastric tube cannot be passed. A tender mass is present in the upper abdomen.

Roentgen examination will demonstrate a gas-distended viscus in the upper abdomen, representing the stomach, and with one or several fluid levels present in the upright position. In other cases there is very little gas but the distention of the stomach is caused largely by the accumulation of gastric secretions. Even when the distention is predominantly caused by fluid, there is usually enough air in the stomach to show a fluid level. If a hiatal hernia is present there may be a second gas shadow with fluid level in the hernia sac above the diaphragm. On giving barium by mouth, the lower esophagus will be found to be obstructed. If it contains much gas the distended stomach may be mistaken for a segment of volvulated colon, particularly a volvulus of the cecum. If this is a real diagnostic problem, a barium enema can be given to exclude the colon as the site of obstruction. The demonstration of lower esophageal obstruction, however, in the presence of the other findings noted previously, should establish the diagnosis.

INTRAMURAL GAS

Air or other gas within the wall of the stomach is a rare finding.[3] It may be a part of the disease known as pneumatosis cystoides intestinalis and have little or no significance (see page 435). In other cases it is due to infection of the gastric wall by gas-forming organisms or emphysematous gastritis. This is a serious and often fatal malady with the symptoms of a severe, acute infection. In still other cases it represents air that has gained entrance through a break in the mucosa (interstitial emphysema). This may follow intubation or ulceration and usually there is a chronic pyloric obstruction which has caused a rise in the intraluminal pressure. Roentgen findings consist of numerous mottled, cystic, translucencies within the gastric wall or linear translucent streaks of air density. Cystic accumulations are found in pneumatosis cystoides and emphysematous gastritis. Linear streaks of air are seen most frequently in the interstitial emphysema type of the disease. Differentiation can be made on the basis of the clinical symptoms.

THE POSTOPERATIVE STOMACH

A variety of surgical procedures can be done on the stomach and duodenum and the roentgen anatomy often is altered to such an extent that it is difficult to recognize anatomic land-

marks or to determimne the type of operation that has been performed. It is important that the examining roentgenologist be aware of the nature of any surgical procedure that has been done, if it is known, so that he can alter his fluoroscopic technique as needed. Otherwise an anastomosis may be obscured by the first few swallows of the barium mixture and rapid flooding of the loops of small intestine may occur so that the area of maximum interest never can be visualized adequately.

The surgical procedures that are encountered most frequently include (1) posterior gastroenterostomy, (2) subtotal gastric resection, (3) total gastric resection, and (4) esophageal resection with esophagogastric anastomosis. Section of the vagus nerves supplying the stomach is done occasionally but usually in association with one of the other operations or after the development of a marginal or jejunal ulcer following previous gastroenterostomy. Anterior gastroenterostomy is met with infrequently and the same is true of some of the other surgical procedures such as local excisions.

When examining a patient known to have had a gastrointestinal anastomosis, the fluoroscopist centers his attention first on the region of the stoma and watches the first swallow or two of the barium mixture as it reaches this level. If it passes through the stoma, careful palpation and the application of pressure are made to bring out the mucosal relief, to determine the pliability of the walls about the opening, and to demonstrate an ulcer crater if one is present. Rotation of the patient in the various degrees of obliquity aid in bringing the stoma into profile. Spot roentgenograms are obtained and are particularly useful in the study of gastroenterostomy stomas.

POSTERIOR GASTROENTEROSTOMY

Normally the first swallows of the barium mixture will pass through a gastroenterostomy stoma and outline it clearly. If the stoma is located closer to the pylorus or farther away from the greater curvature than is usual, it may take a larger amount of the mixture before stomal emptying is seen. Very often, after the full barium meal has been given, some emptying will occur through the pylorus sufficient to visualize the duodenum. If spontaneous pyloric emptying does not occur, manual pressure may express enough through the pylorus to determine the condition of the duodenum. The gastric mucosal folds usually are thickened in the presence of a gastroenterostomy, especially around the stoma and in the gastric antrum; this is not abnormal. If emptying is prompt through the stoma, peristalsis is apt to be shallow and generally diminished. If a gastroenterostomy opening has been present for a long time, the antrum of the stomach may fill poorly and appear generally contracted with little or no emptying through the pylorus. In some of these cases it is difficult to exclude an organic filling defect such as might be caused by an annular carcinoma because of the poor filling of the antrum and failure to demonstrate the pylorus. Careful attention to the presence of mucosal folds and the absence of a palpable mass or of localized tenderness are helpful in differential diagnosis.

PARTIAL GASTRIC RESECTION

In most cases the type of gastric resection that has been done cannot be determined accurately from roentgen examination, since most of the procedures commonly employed resemble one another rather closely in their roentgen features. In the normal there is immediate emptying through the stoma and the line of anastomosis can be demonstrated easily by proper rotation of the patient, by the application of manual pressure, and by the taking of spot roentgenograms. The abrupt transition from gastric folds to a jejunal fold pattern is distinct. The subsequent rate of gastric emptying is variable but usually it is rapid and it often is difficult to keep the fundic portion distended sufficiently to examine it thoroughly. It is our practice, after the initial observations of the stoma have been completed, to place the patient supine and give the balance of the barium mixture through a drinking tube, completing the examination with the table horizontal. Extremely rapid emptying into dilated loops of jejunum adjacent to the stoma has sometimes been referred to as the "dumping syndrome"; in our experience this has been an infrequent finding. Normally the width of the jejunum adjacent to the stoma is only slightly more than the normal and its mucosal pattern and motility are unaltered.

TOTAL GASTRECTOMY

Following complete removal of the stomach and anastomosis of the jejunum to the lower end of the esophagus, the site of anastomosis often lies at the diaphragmatic level or just above it. The patient is unable to take a large meal but enlargement of the jejunum and the rapid progress of the liquid meal along it serve to compensate partly for loss of the stomach. The esophagus generally does not enlarge to any appreciable degree.

ESOPHAGEAL RESECTION

In recent years resection of large portions of the esophagus has become possible and occasionally the stomach or a part of the colon is brought high up into the thorax, as far as the level of the aortic arch or even above it, where it has been anastomosed to the proximal stump of the esophagus. The intrathoracic portion of the stomach often becomes distended with air and fluid in the immediate postoperative period but is less likely to do so later on. Peristalsis is sluggish or absent in this part of the stomach and its tone is diminished, evidently secondary to the vagotomy that accompanies the resection.

POSTVAGOTOMY STOMACH

Following vagotomy, usually done for the treatment of peptic ulcer, the stomach undergoes pronounced changes. There is a general loss of tone and the stomach dilates. Peristalsis is sluggish and gastric emptying is delayed. Food and fluid residues usually are present even though the patient has been fasting overnight or longer. In spite of the gastric atony, it usually is possible to fill the duodenum during fluoroscopy and thus establish the patency of the pylorus. This is important because otherwise the appearance of the stomach resembles that of pyloric obstruction. Pyloroplasty has come into use to avoid these complications.

MARGINAL OR JEJUNAL ULCER

An ulcer occurring after a gastroenterostomy or subtotal gastric resection is most likely to develop on the jejunal side of the anastomosis and not infrequently it is entirely jejunal in location. The roentgen detection of a marginal or jejunal ulcer is dependent upon the following observations:

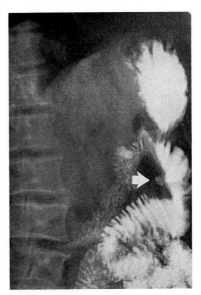

Fig. 16-40. Jejunal ulcer. There has been a subtotal gastric resection. **Arrow** points to the ulcer crater in the efferent loop of the jejunum several centimeters below the stoma.

THE ULCER CRATER. The crater of a marginal ulcer often is broad and shallow and therefore may be difficult to visualize. Otherwise it has the same roentgen characteristics as a gastric ulcer. Upon the application of a suitable amount of compression over it, the crater retains an accumulation of the barium mixture while in the adjacent pliable loops it is expressed out of the lumen, leaving only a coating on the mucosal surface. When situated along an edge so that it can be brought into profile, the crater is seen as a projecting niche (Fig. 16-40).

ALTERATION OF MUCOSAL FOLDS. Obliteration of the mucosal folds around the crater is the usual finding and the surface as coated with barium appears smooth. Radiation of folds in a spokelike fashion away from the edges of the crater, which is common in gastric ulcers, is also seen at times in this lesion.

CHANGES IN CALIBER OF LUMEN. When the ulcer is located in the efferent loop, a smooth constriction of the jejunal lumen adjacent to

the crater often is present. This may or my not be sufficient to cause obstruction. If the ulcer is truly marginal and is situated along the edge of the stoma, stomal narrowing is the rule and in some cases the stoma may become completely nonfunctioning.

TENDERNESS. Local tenderness to palpation directly over the lesion is frequent and may serve to direct the examiner's attention to the presence of the lesion. Otherwise local tenderness has no specific diagnostic value.

GASTROCOLIC FISTULA

Fistulous communication between the stomach, jejunum, and colon, or directly between the stomach and colon usually follows a marginal or a jejunal ulcer and therefore is more frequent as a complication of gastroenterostomy than it is of other surgical procedures. The first evidence of the presence of such a fistula is often obtained during a barium enema examination, the barium mixture being observed to extend directly from the transverse colon into the stomach (Fig. 16-41). It may be easier to visualize the lesion in this manner than by an oral meal. After the oral administration of barium the region of the fistula may be obscured as loops of jejunum and colon fill simultaneously and flood the area. At times the fistula may not fill at all when the meal is given orally. The ulcer responsible for the fistula often is visualized but again rapid filling of the jejunum and colon may prevent its clear visualization and the crater may be completely hidden.

Less frequently, a gastrocolic fistula is caused by carcinomatous invasion and necrosis, the lesion being primary either in the stomach or in the transverse colon. The filling defect of the carcinoma may be quite apparent but, since any fistula is likely to have an associated inflammatory mass, it may be difficult to distinguish between the two. In these patients the history is important and if there has been no previous surgical procedure a diagnosis of carcinoma is justified.

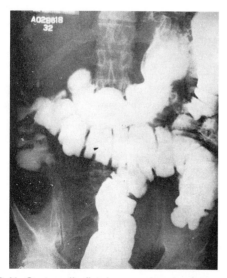

Fig. 16-41. Gastrocolic fistula secondary to a gastro-jejunal ulcer. The patient had had a gastroenterostomy some years previously. On barium enema examination the contrast material was seen to enter the stomach as the transverse colon filled. Roentgenogram of the filled colon shows extensive filling of the stomach and of some of the loops of jejunum, which has occurred through the fistula.

OTHER POSTOPERATIVE COMPLICATIONS

DELAYED EMPTYING. During the immediate postoperative period examination of asymptomatic individuals who have had gastroenterostomy or subtotal gastric resections often will show the presence of retained fluid in the stomach, delayed gastric emptying, poor visualization of efferent and afferent loops, and a narrow stoma. These postoperative changes disappear gradually and after a few weeks the stomach is found to empty promptly. Occasionally a patient will have difficulty in the immediate postoperative period, being unable to retain fluid and food satisfactorily, and examination will show the changes noted above only in an exaggerated form. There is little or no emptying through the stoma, gastric retention is present, and the efferent loop if visualized at all appears small and contracted. In most cases these changes will subside after a few days and symptoms will disappear. At times the symptoms continue or worsen and repeat examinations show no improvement in the roentgen findings. When the patient is explored a mechanical obstruction is found. This may be caused by a torsion of the bowel, by an adhesive band, or by a number of other difficulties of a mechanical nature resulting from the surgical procedure. The exact nature of the obstruction is difficult to determine roentgenologically but it usually is possible to state whether the obstruction is directly at the stoma or involves one of the loops.

STOMAL POUCHES. As a rather infrequent complication of posterior gastroenterostomy a pouch-like dilatation of a segment of jejunum immediately adjacent to the stoma may form. This loop has the outline of a globular sac that fills promptly from the stomach and that comes to resemble stomach rather than small intestine. The pouch fills promptly but may retain the barium for abnormally long periods of time.

JEJUNAL INTUSSUSCEPTION. Another rare complication of gastroenterostomy is the occurrence of retrograde jejunal intussusception when the jejunum herniates through the stoma into the stomach. The intussuscepted segment forms a sausage-shaped mass projecting into the gastric lumen at the site of the stoma and obstructs the stoma. Characteristically the barium is caught in the

crevices formed by the stretched valvulae conniventes of the jejunum resulting in a "coiled-
spring" appearance which is typical of intussusception.[26]

RECURRENT CARCINOMA. Recurrence of carcinoma in the stump of the stomach remaining after
partial gastric resection may be difficult to recognize in its early stages. Frequently the amount of
stomach that remains is small and situated so high
beneath the ribs that it cannot be palpated through
the abdominal wall. There also is, normally, an
absence of peristalsis in this part of the stomach
and thus it is difficult to determine if the stomach
wall has lost its pliability or not. Only when the
lesion becomes large enough to project into the
lumen as a distinct filling defect or encroach upon
the stoma and cause obstruction is it possible to
be certain that recurrence has developed. Careful
attention to the mucosal pattern of the stomal
area is important since the mucosal folds will be
obliterated in the area involved by the carcinoma
even before a distinct filling defect is produced. As
is true with the colon, it is useful to have a base-
line study done 3 or 4 weeks postoperatively for
comparison with later follow-up examinations.

REFERENCES AND SELECTED READINGS

1. ABRAMS, H. L.: Leiomyoma of the stomach. *Am. J. Roentgenol. Radium Ther. Nucl. Med. 72:* 1023, 1954.

2. BAUM, J., NAUSBAUM, M., BLADEMORE, W. S., and FINKELSTEIN, A. K.: The preoperative radio-graphic demonstration of intra-abdominal bleed-ing from undetermined sites by percutaneous selective celiac and superior mesenteric arteri-ography. *Surgery 58:* 797, 1965.

3. BERENS, S. V., MOSKOWITZ, H., and MELLINS, H.: Air within the wall of the stomach. *Am. J. Roent-genol. Radium Ther. Nucl. Med. 103:* 310, 1968.

4. BERLIN, L.: Gastritis: A medical dilemma. *Am. J. Roentgenol. Radium Ther. Nucl. Med. 88:* 627, 1962.

5. BLOCH, C.: Roentgen features of Hodgkin's di-sease of the stomach. *Am. J. Roentgenol. Radium Ther. Nucl. Med. 99:* 175, 1967.

6. BOIJSEN, E., WALLACE, S., and KANTER, I. E.: Angiography in tumors of the stomach. *Acta Radiol. (Diag.) 4:* 306, 1966.

7. BURNS, B., and GAY, B. B., JR.: Menetrier's di-sease of the stomach in children. *Am. J. Roent-genol. Radium Ther. Nucl. Med. 103:* 300, 1968.

8. CHRISTOFORIDIS, A. J., and NELSON, S. W.: Radio-logical manifestations of ulcerogenic tumors of the pancreas. The Zollinger-Ellison syndrome. *JAMA 198:* 511, 1966.

9. CRONKHITE, L. W., and CANADA, W. J.: General-ized gastrointestinal polyposis. An unusual syn-drome of polyposis, pigmentation, alopecia and onychotrophia. *N. Engl. J. Med. 252:* 1011, 1955.

10. CRUMMY, A. B., and JUHL, J. H.: Calcified gas-tric leiomyoma. *Am. J. Roentgenol. Radium Ther. Nucl. Med. 87:* 727, 1962.

11. CULVER, G. J., BEAN, B. C., and BERENS, D. L.: Gastric lymphoma. *Radiology 65:* 518, 1955.

12. CULVER, G. J., PIRSON, H. S., MONTEZ, M., and PALANKER, H. K.: Eosinophilic gastritis. *JAMA 200:* 641, 1967.

13. DU PLESSIS, D. J.: Primary hypertrophic stenosis in the adult. *Br. J. Surg. 53:* 485, 1966.

14. EKLOF, O.: Benign tumors of the stomach and duodenum. *Acta Radiol. 57:* 177, 1962.

15. EVANS, J. A., and WEINTRAUB, S.: Accessory pan-creatic tissue in the stomach wall. *Am. J. Roent-genol. Radium Ther. Nucl. Med. 69:* 22, 1953.

16. FERRUCCI, J. T., JR., and BENEDICT, K. T., JR.: Anticholinergic-aided study of the gastrointestinal tract. *Radiol. Clin. North Am. 9:* 23, 1971.

17. HARPER, R. A. K., and GREEN, B.: Malignant gastric ulcer. *J. Fac. Radiol. 12:* 95, 1961.

18. HOWARTH, F. H., COCKEL, R., ROPER, B. W., and HAWKINS, C. F.: The effect of metoclopramide upon gastric motility. *Clin. Radiol. 20:* 294, 1969.

19. JOHNSTONE, A. S.: Editorial: Reflections on hiatus hernia and related problems. *Radiology 62:* 750, 1954.

20. KOEHLER, P. R., and SALMON, R. B.: Angio-graphic localization of unknown acute gastro-intestinal bleeding sites. *Radiology 89:* 244, 1967.

21. MAINZER, M., AMBERG, J. R., and MARGULIS, A. R.: Superficial carcinoma of the stomach. *Radiology 93:* 109, 1969.

22. MARSHAK, R. H., and LINDNER, A. E.: *Radiology of the Small Intestine.* Philadelphia, Saunders, 1970.

23. NELSON, S. W.: The discovery of gastric ulcers and the differential diagnosis between benignancy and malignancy. *Radiol. Clin. North Am. 7:* 5, 1969.

24. OCHSNER, S.: Benign ulceration on the greater curvature of the stomach: Report of seven proved cases. *Am. J. Roentgenol. Radium Ther. Nucl. Med. 75:* 312, 1956.

25. PALMER, P. E. S.: Giant hypertrophic gastritis. *J. Fac. Radiol. 9:* 175, 1958.

26. PAUL, L. W., and BENKENDORF, C.: Retrograde

jejunogastric intussusception. *Radiology 73:* 234, 1959.

27. REESE, D. F., HODGSON, J. R., and DOCKERTY, M. B.: Giant hypertrophy of the gastric mucosa (Menetrier's disease). A correlation of the roentgenographic, pathologic, and clinical findings.

Am. J. Roentgenol. Radium Ther. Nucl. Med. 88: 619, 1962.

28. SAWYER, K. C., HAMMER, R. W., and FENTON, W. C.: Gastric volvulus as a cause of obstruction. Report of seven cases. *Arch. Surg. 72:* 764, 1956.

17

THE DUODENUM

METHODS OF EXAMINATION

The examination of the duodenum is done as an integral part of a gastrointestinal series during and after the study of the stomach. The same filming technique is used as the duodenum is shown along with the stomach in the routine roentgenograms and with spot films taken as needed in the individual case. The method of *hypotonic duodenography* is discussed in Chapter 13 ("Changes in the Mucosal Pattern of the Duodenum"), and is used for the more detailed study of the mucosal fold pattern. Arteriography of the duodenum can be accomplished by celiac axis catheterization or by selective catheterization of the hepatic artery. A recently introduced drug, metoclopramide, has been found useful in the examination of the duodenum. Given intravenously in a dose of 20 mg, it stimulates gastric peristalsis, relaxes the pylorus, and allows prompt filling of the duodenum (see page 571). The effects of the drug are noted within minutes after administration. Small-intestinal transit also is increased, shortening the time needed for a complete upper gastrointestinal series and small-bowel study.

ROENTGEN ANATOMY AND PHYSIOLOGY

The superior or first portion of the duodenum has a distinct roentgen appearance that differs considerably from the remainder. As viewed in profile, it has a triangular shape with the base at the pylorus and the apex continuous with the descending duodenum. Because of its shape it is known as the duodenal bulb or cap (see Figs. 16-2 and 16-3). The mucosal folds in the bulb are relatively sparse and usually disappear completely when the bulb is distended. Peristaltic contractions resemble those of the stomach and tend to occur in rhythm with gastric peristalsis.

The second or descending portion of the duodenum is retroperitoneal in location and has no mesentery. The change in the roentgen appearance from the first to the second portions is striking (Fig. 17-1). The latter has a rich mucosal pattern, even when distended, with crisscrossing folds of mucosa (the valvulae conniventes or folds of Kerkring) causing a fine serration of the margins when the surface is coated with barium mixture. Peristalsis is relatively rapid with broad waves sweeping the contents forward into the jejunum. Peristaltic waves never empty the lumen completely of barium as long as gastric emptying is in progress and a thin layer will coat the mucosal surface even after passage of a wave. The papilla of Vater is located on the inner side of the descending portion and occasionally is visualized as a small filling defect or localized mucosal irregularity.

The remainder of the duodenum resembles the descending portion in all respects. The duodenum surrounds the head of the pancreas and the ascending portion passes over the body of the pancreas to its junction with the jejunum at the angle of Treitz.

The superior mesenteric artery crosses the third portion of the duodenum just proximal to the

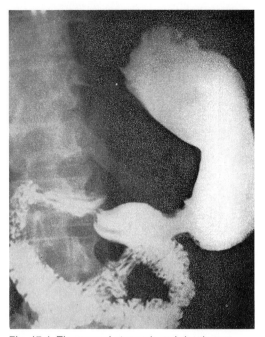

Fig. 17-1. The normal stomach and duodenum.

dence of duodenal obstruction in newborn mongoloids owing to atresia and also to annular pancreas has been reported frequently. If the obstruction is complete, the stomach and the duodenum down to the level of the atresia will be distended with swallowed air; no gas will be visualized in the gastrointestinal tract below this level. The diagnosis can be made from plain-film roentgenograms of the abdomen that will clearly show the gas distention of the stomach and the dilated proximal portion of the duodenum, with complete absence of gas elsewhere in the tract (the "double-bubble" sign). If a contrast substance is given it will stop at the level of the atresia (Fig. 17-2). If there is only a partial obstruction, gas will be visible below the duodenal level but distention of the stomach will be present and the distended segment of duodenum may also be

angle of Treitz. In asthenic persons pressure from this vessel may cause the appearance of mild duodenal obstruction with the duodenum somewhat dilated in its proximal portion and with reverse peristalsis occasionally seen (*the superior mesenteric artery syndrome*). Reverse peristaltic or churning movements occasionally are noted in otherwise normal-appearing individuals without there being any signs of obstruction. The visualization of churning movements in the duodenum, therefore, need not be of significance and it is probable that such movements can be initiated by deep palpation on the part of the examiner.

ANOMALIES OF THE DUODENUM

CONGENITAL OBSTRUCTION

INTRINSIC

Congenital stenosis or atresia may be caused by delay or arrest in development at some stage in the formation of the duodenum. The duodenum is a frequent site of high gastrointestinal obstruction in the newborn. The increased inci-

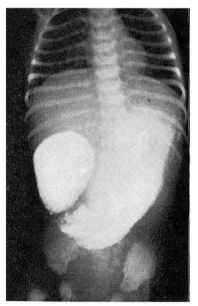

Fig. 17-2. Congenital atresia of the duodenum. Barium filling of the stomach and proximal duodenum of a newborn infant. The stomach is greatly dilated. The oval-shaped accumulation of barium along the right side represents the greatly dilated proximal or first portion of the duodenum. The obstruction is in the second portion of the duodenum. Note the complete absence of gas below this level, indicating that the obstruction is complete.

recognized by gas filling. The diagnosis can be confirmed by giving a small barium-water meal or one of the iodinated compounds such as Hypaque or Gastrografin, but this is seldom necessary. Partial obstruction may be caused by stenosis or incomplete atresia.

EXTRINSIC

CONGENITAL PERITONEAL BANDS OR "VEILS." Cholecystoduodenocolic bands or membranes are of congenital origin and may cause obstruction of the duodenum in the infant. More often they do not, and are found with considerable frequency in the adult. They may cause a certain amount of deformity and distortion of the duodenal outline, particularly of the bulbar portion, and this deformity may be confused with that caused by duodenal ulcer. Persistence of a mesoduodenum may allow the duodenum to twist upon itself, resulting in volvulus and consequent obstruction. Although these bands are of developmental origin, they may remain asymptomatic until adult life is reached, at which time obstructive phenomena may appear (Fig. 17-3). Symptomatic peritoneal bands in the adult, however, must be considered as relatively uncommon lesions.

Congenital peritoneal bands occurring in association with faulty rotation of the gut during its final stages of development may cause obstruction of the duodenum in the infant and occasionally in the adult. The site of obstruction is more frequent in the third portion of the duodenum than elsewhere. If the colon is examined by means of a barium enema, its abnormal position and the failure of complete rotation may be obvious. Otherwise the diagnosis of the type of duodenal obstruction cannot be made with certainty and the roentgen findings will resemble those described for duodenal atresia (see above).

ANNULAR PANCREAS. A ring of pancreatic tissue may encircle the duodenum, causing a smooth, annular constriction of the lumen. This may be sufficient to be the cause of obstructive symptoms or the lesion may be entirely asymptomatic. The obstructive symptoms may develop in the im-

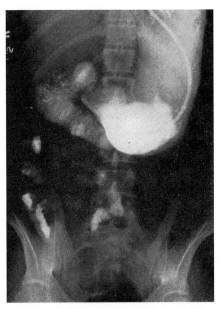

Fig. 17-3. Partial obstruction at the duodenojejunal junction secondary to faulty rotation of the gut. A volvulus developed that caused the obstruction. Barium instilled into the stomach through a decompression tube is diluted by retained fluid. The dilated duodenum can be visualized. There has been some extension of barium beyond the site of obstruction, which lies behind the stomach and is not clearly visualized in this projection; the obstruction is incomplete. Note the presence of small bowel containing barium in the right lateral abdomen where normally the colon should be. In this patient the colon is nonrotated, lying almost entirely to the left of the midline.

mediate neonatal period or be delayed until adult life is reached. The roentgen diagnosis depends upon the demonstration of a smooth annular constriction, usually occurring in the upper part of the descending duodenum. In the adult this lesion must be differentiated from a primary malignant tumor of the duodenum and from an ulcer of the second portion of the duodenum. In the former lesion the constriction is usually more irregular in nature and involves a longer segment of the duodenum. The mucosal pattern is destroyed through the area of constriction. Ulcers of the postbulbar part of the duodenum depend upon the demonstration of an ulcer crater. In the very young infant, annular pancreas must be differentiated from congenital bands and veils. The defect of an annular pancreas is usually longer than that of a veil or band. However, it usually is impossible to determine the exact nature of the lesion prior to operation and the roentgen diagnosis in these cases must be limited to that of an obstructing lesion.

OTHER CAUSES. In addition to the causes of duodenal obstruction listed above there are other rare causes. These include duplication cysts, which may be large enough to cause obstruction, and other rare tumors. The majority of cases however are owing to stenosis or atresia, congenital bands or volvulus, and annular pancreas.

REDUNDANCY OF THE SUPERIOR PORTION

The superior portion of the duodenum may be unusually long and hang downward as a loop between the bulb and the superior duodenal flexure (Fig. 17-4). Such elongation has no clinical significance but it may be mistaken for a deformed bulb caused by an ulcer.

DUODENUM INVERSUM

As an anomaly of rotation, the duodenum may loop to the right rather than to the left so that the descending and ascending portions tend to overlie one another; or, the ascending portion may actually lie to the right of the descending crossing to the left, at or above the level of the pylorus to its point of junction with the jejunum (Fig. 17-4).

The jejunum is in normal position and the rest of the small bowel is usually in normal situs.

RIGHT-SIDED DUODENUM

As part of a more extensive rotation anomaly, the duodenum together with the jejunum and the ileum may lie largely to the right of the midline with the colon on the left side of the abdomen (nonrotation of the bowel: see Chapter 18).

DUPLICATIONS

Congenital duplication of the duodenum is a rare anomaly but corresponds essentially to the same type of lesion that may be found in any other part of the gastrointestinal tract. It consists of a closed cystic mass of variable size that develops in the wall of the duodenum. The coats of the cyst reproduce the coats of the duodenum or some other part of the intestinal tract. Thus the lining of the cyst may be gastric or colonic mucosa instead of duodenal. The cystic mass may be submucosal intramural, or subserosal. When large it is impossible to determine the exact nature of such a mass from its roentgen features and it generally shows only the characteristics of an intramural tumor, with a smooth-surfaced mass bulging into the duodenal lumen but with mucosa intact over the surface. The lesion, if of any appreciable size, may cause obstruction. The small duplications are usually asymptomatic. Roentgen diagnosis, if at all possible, is usually limited to that of an intramural mass and an etiologic diag-

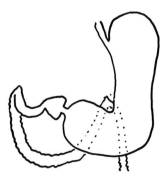 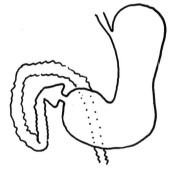

Fig. 17-4. Diagram illustrates two common anomalies involving the duodenum. *Left,* Redundancy of the superior portion of the duodenum. *Right,* Duodenum inversum.

nosis is hardly possible. Duplications are apt to give rise to symptoms rather early in life because of the increasing size of the mass as fluid accumulates within it. This is also true of those involving other parts of the gastrointestinal tract.

DISEASES OF THE DUODENUM

DUODENAL ULCER

Duodenal ulcer is the most frequent organic lesion encountered in the upper gastrointestinal tract. The ratio of duodenal to gastric ulcers is on the order of 4 or 5 to 1. Most duodenal ulcers develop in the first portion of the duodenum, the duodenal bulb. A less common site is at the junction of the first and second portions or in the immediate proximal part of the descending portion; these are called postbulbar ulcers. Below this level ulcers in the duodenum are extremely rare. Ulcers in the duodenal bulb may form on any wall or surface, although they are somewhat more frequent on the posterior wall and along the lesser curvature than elsewhere.

Roentgen Observations

THE ULCER CRATER. The demonstration of the ulcer crater is as important in the diagnosis of a duodenal ulcer as it is in the recognition of a gastric ulcer and represents the one positive roentgen sign of the lesion. When visualized on edge the ulcer crater projects as a niche, similar to the niche of a gastric ulcer except for its smaller size (Fig. 17-5). Frequently the crater is not seen directly on edge but rather is visualized *en face,* and is brought out to best advantage by applying compression over the bulb. As the barium content is expressed out of the more pliable portion of the bulb, the crater remains filled because of its rigid walls and appears as a dense round spot (Fig. 17-6). If a proper amount of compression is used so that a thin coating of barium remains on the mucosa, the folds can be seen to radiate outward from the crater as they do with gastric ulcers. The crater usually is small and less than 1 cm in diameter. Infrequently a very large crater, several centimeters in diameter, may be present (giant crater) (Figs. 17-7 and 17-12). Such a

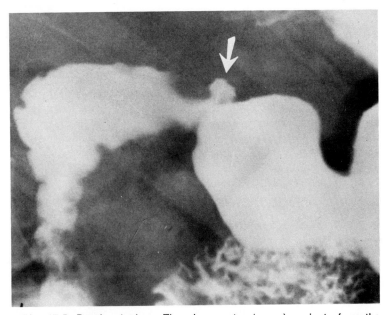

Fig. 17-5. Duodenal ulcer. The ulcer crater (**arrow**) projects from the superior surface near the base of the bulb.

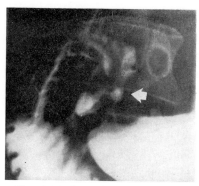 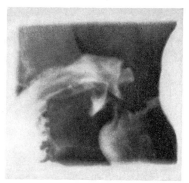

Fig. 17-6. Duodenal ulcer. Serial roentgenograms illustrates healing of an ulcer crater. *Left,* Spot roentgenogram of the pyloric end of the stomach and proximal duodenum made during fluoroscopy with compression applied over the duodenum. This brings out the crater of an ulcer (**arrow**) situated in the central part of the posterior wall of the duodenal bulb. Mucosal folds radiate outward from the base of the crater. *Right,* Progress examination after a period of medical treatment. Similar compression spot roentgenogram as shown on the *left.* The crater has disappeared but the distortion of mucosal folds remains.

crater may be so large as completely to replace the bulb and may actually be mistaken for a normal bulb. The constancy of its shape and persistent retention of barium with inability to express barium out of it on manual palpation are significant findings. The crater of a duodenal ulcer may be difficult to visualize when the general contour of the bulb is extremely irregular and deformed by scar tissue and it may be impossible to state at times whether an ulcer crater is present or whether the deformity is only the result of scar-tissue formation from a previous ulcer. With an acute duodenal ulcer the bulbar outline may be normal and only when compression is used will the lesion be identified. This is particularly true when the crater is directly on the anterior or the posterior wall, where it may be difficult to bring the lesion into relief so that the projecting niche becomes visible.

MARGINAL DEFORMITY. Regardless of the site of the ulcer crater, the margins of the duodenal bulb usually show some irregularity in contour as a result of one or more incisurae. These are similar to the incisurae that are prone to develop on the greater curvature opposite a gastric ulcer on the lesser curve, and in the early stages are spastic in nature; later on they become fixed as a result of scar tissue. In the presence of an acute ulcer, marginal deformity may be slight or entirely absent and what deformity is present is caused by spasm. This may be inconstant and vary during the examination. With more chronic ulcers deformity becomes fixed and as fibrosis and scarring develop the normal contours of the bulb become completely lost. Once this stage is reached, the deformity is permanent even though the ulcer heals (Fig. 17-8). One of the common deformities seen in chronic duodenal ulcer is that which resembles a collar button. The apex of the bulb is constricted, leaving rounded projections at the base adjacent to the pylorus. The appearance resembles that of a collar button very closely and this type of deformity is characteristic of a chronic ulcer involving the apex of the bulb (Fig. 17-9).

POSTBULBAR ULCER. Duodenal ulcers occurring distal to the bulb usually develop on the inner side at the junction of the bulb and the descending duodenum. The crater projects as a niche and an incisura forms on the opposite side, causing a rather classic deformity (Fig. 17-10). The incisura represents an indrawing

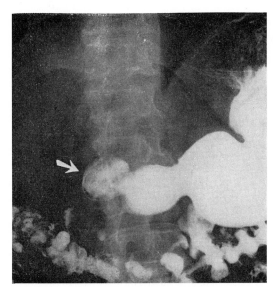

Fig. 17-7. Duodenal ulcer with giant crater. The **arrow** points to the crater of the duodenal ulcer, which has completely replaced the normal bulb and mimics the appearance of a normal bulb.

of the lateral wall of the duodenum that tends to become fixed and permanent as a result of scar tissue. Because of the location, an ulcer at this site is easily obscured by the overlapping shadows of the bulb and the descending duodenum. The right lateral position is best for demonstrating this lesion.

EXAMINATION FOR THE DETECTION OF AN ULCER IN THE PRESENCE OF RECENT BLEEDING. Bleeding is, ordinarily, not a contraindication to roentgen examination of the gastrointestinal tract provided that it is done with gentleness and that palpation of the abdomen is largely avoided. Posterior wall craters are a frequent source of bleeding and they often can be demonstrated by rotating the patient into a left posterior oblique position after the stomach has started to empty. Barium tends to remain in the crater in this position since it is dependent. Because the pyloric end of the stomach will be higher than the cardia the gastric air will pass through the pylorus into the duodenum. The air distention of the bulb plus the retained barium in the crater often produce a very good demonstration of the

lesion in "double contrast" without the need for compression (Hampton technique).[7] The use of arteriography for the demonstration of the site of bleeding from the gastrointestinal tract is discussed in the section on "Abdominal Arteriography in Gastrointestinal Bleeding," Chapter 16 (Fig. 17-11).

OBSTRUCTION. Duodenal ulcer is the most frequent cause of pyloric obstruction. When only a partial obstruction exists, the stomach may empty itself within a normal period of time or there may be a small amount of retention after overnight fasting. Fluoroscopically peristaltic waves are vigorous, they are increased in depth, and one wave follows another at relatively close intervals. In this stage the antrum often appears somewhat enlarged during the period of antral diastole but contracts promptly as a result of peristalsis. The periods of peristaltic activity may last for a minute or two and alternate with periods of quiescence. With increase in the degree of obstruction the stomach is unable to empty itself within the usual time and gastric retention is found at the time of roentgen examination. Hyperactive peristalsis may still occur, but the periods of activity are shortened and the stomach becomes more and more atonic. Eventually the obstruction may increase to the point where little emptying occurs through the pylorus and large amounts of fluid accumulate within the stomach. The stomach may become huge and in the upright position hang down into the lower abdomen or pelvis. At this stage the muscular activity has become greatly diminished and the stomach is, in fact, decompensated. Roentgenologic examination of such a stomach is hampered greatly by its size and by the retention of the fluid and food. Preliminary gastric aspiration and lavage may remove some of the material but seldom empties the stomach completely. Unless there is some passage of the barium mixture through the pylorus, it may not be possible to determine the cause of the obstruction. If the pylorus and duodenal bulb are visualized, the cause usually is apparent and it can be decided whether a duodenal ulcer is responsible or whether the lesion is on the gastric side of the pylorus (e.g.,

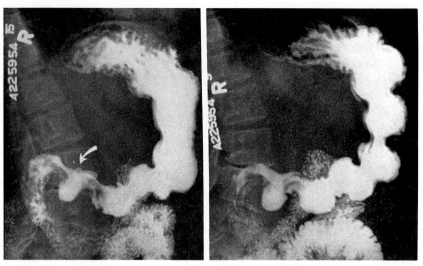

Fig. 17-8. Duodenal ulcer. *Left,* The duodenal bulb is deformed in outline and there is a small crater projecting as an ulcer niche on the lesser curvature side (**arrow**). *Right,* Same patient after therapy for ulcer. The crater has disappeared but the contour deformity of the duodenal bulb remains because of scar tissue formation.

a gastric ulcer or carcinoma). In difficult cases reexamination after a period of several days, during which time repeated aspirations or continuous gastric suction is carried out, may allow a more definitive examination to be done.

PERFORATION. Some of the roentgen findings in perforation of the gastrointestinal tract are described in Chapter 13, in the section entitled "Pneumoperitoneum" where the escape of gas and its detection in roentgenograms of the abdomen is discussed. The most frequent cause of so-called "spontaneous pneumoperitoneum" is rupture of an ulcer. A posterior-wall duodenal ulcer may perforate into the lesser omental sac and the gas and fluid may accumulate and be loculated in this area. Air from a perforated posterior-wall ulcer may dissect along the retroperitoneal fascial planes and be visualized as linear streaks or bubbles along the psoas sheaths or as a more localized accumulation of gas bubbles in the posterior abdominal wall.

In roentgenograms demonstrating a spontaneous pneumoperitoneum, Frimann-Dahl has called attention to the fact that at times gas within the duodenal bulb may clearly outline the deformity caused by an ulcer or even show the crater of the ulcer; in these instances the diagnosis of the cause of the perforation can be made without a barium-meal examination.

If the roentgen examination is not done for a period of 5 or 6 hours after the perforation has occurred, a certain amount of adynamic ileus is almost always present. Gas accumulates in loops of small intestine and in the colon although the distention is seldom very severe. Evidence of free fluid may be suggested by blurring of the inferior edge of the right lobe of the liver which, normally, can be seen. These latter signs, of course, are not specific for perforation.

A perforated ulcer may become walled-off and later, when the patient is examined by means of a barium meal, a sinus tract may be demonstrated as it fills with the barium. An example of this is shown in Figure 17-12.

HEALING OF DUODENAL ULCER. If an ulcer crater has been demonstrated at the initial examination, its progress can be followed by serial studies. Disappearance of the ulcer crater indicates healing of the ulcer. The general contour deformity of the bulb usually does not change since it is, in most instances, caused by scarring and fibrosis. The importance of crater demonstration therefore becomes obvious, because bulbar deformity alone may give no clue as to the presence of an active ulcer (see Figs. 17-6 and 17-8).

DIVERTICULA OF THE DUODENUM

Duodenal diverticula are found very frequently during roentgen examination of the upper gastrointestinal tract. They are acquired lesions that may form in any part of the duodenum but with the most common site being along the inner side of the descending duodenum close to the ampulla of Vater. Duodenal diverticula vary greatly in size from those that measure on the order of 1 cm in diameter to an occasional large one which measures from 8 to

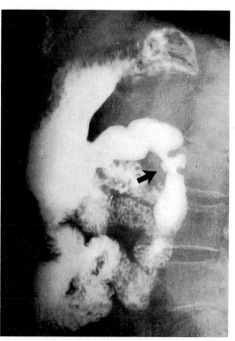

Fig. 17-10. Postbulbar duodenal ulcer. Lateral roentgenogram of the stomach and duodenum. The ulcer is situated along the inner anterior surface of the descending portion of the duodenum just distal to the bulb (**arrow**) with two incisurae on the opposite wall. The duodenal bulb is slightly dilated above the level of the lesion but it is not obstructive to any significant degree.

10 cm in size. Usually considered to be asymptomatic lesions of no clinical significance, an occasional, very large diverticulum, by retention of food, may cause symptoms of partial upper gastrointestinal obstruction. In rare instances ulceration within a diverticulum has been reported and the lesion has been a rare cause of upper gastrointestinal tract bleeding. A single diverticulum is the rule but occasionally two or more are found and in an infrequent patient multiple diverticula of the duodenum are present, associated with multiple diverticula of the jejunum.

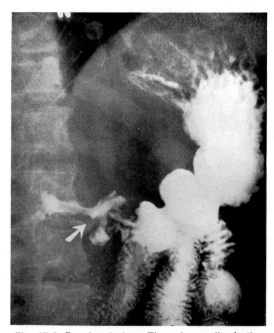

Fig. 17-9. Duodenal ulcer. There is a collar-button type of deformity of the duodenal bulb with a fairly concentric narrowing of the apical portion. **Arrow** points to the ulcer crater, which is visible as a small dense spot along the inferior surface near the constricted area.

Roentgen Observations

Diverticula of the duodenum resemble those occurring elsewhere in the gastrointestinal tract. The diverticulum consists of a projecting

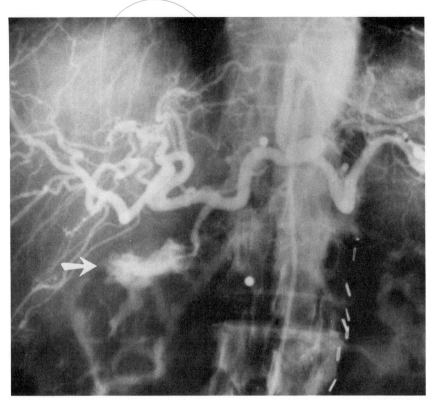

Fig. 17-11. Bleeding duodenal ulcer demonstrated by arteriography. The gastroduodenal artery, arising as a branch of the hepatic artery, leads to a dense accumulation of extravasated contrast material in the duodenal bulb (**arrow**).

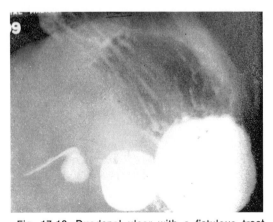

Fig. 17-12. Duodenal ulcer with a fistulous tract secondary to previous rupture. The rounded accumulation of barium represents a large ulcer crater that is almost as large as a normal bulb. The fistulous tract extends laterally beneath the undersurface of the liver for a distance of several centimeters.

sac and when filled with barium mixture it results in a pouchlike projection that is connected by a narrow neck to the duodenal lumen (Fig. 17-13). The diagnosis is made without difficulty. Diverticula in the distal part of the duodenum may be obscured by barium in the stomach; also, when the stomach is palpated or compressed over a diverticulum a false impression of an ulcer crater in the gastric wall may be obtained. A diverticulum can be distinguished from a duodenal ulcer by the smooth, rounded, pouchlike appearance, the absence of spasm, and the lack of distortion of mucosal folds about the orifice. At times an accumulation of gas or nonopaque food material may be found within the diverticulum, causing a filling defect. This is usually inconstant and may disappear or otherwise change in appearance during observation. At times it may be necessary to repeat the examination to be certain that one

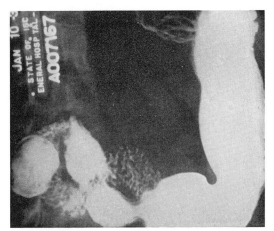

Fig. 17-13. Diverticulum of the second portion of the duodenum.

is not dealing with a neoplasm developing within the diverticulum. As a rare occurrence, a diverticulum of the duodenum may be entirely intraluminal. It is visualized as a pocket-like accumulation of barium projecting within the duodenal lumen. It occurs in the region of the ampulla of Vater and may be a cause of partial obstruction. It is, in a sense, a form of congenital duplication.[14]

TUMORS OF THE DUODENUM

Considered as a group, neoplasms of the duodenum are rare lesions. Primary tumors are less frequent than secondary invasion of the duodenum by carcinoma of the pancreas, the common bile duct, or other contiguous structures.

DUODENAL POLYPS

Benign polyps or adenomas originating in the duodenum are rare. The roentgen signs are similar to those of polyps elsewhere in the gastrointestinal tract. The polyp causes a sharply circumscribed, rounded filling defect in the barium shadow (Fig. 17-14). Air bubbles and food particles can be excluded by noting the constancy of the defect. Occasionally a repeat examination is needed to be certain that one is dealing with an organic lesion. The polyp often has a pedicle and it may

move over some distance under the effect of peristalsis. The pedicle may be visualized as a stalklike shadow and at its point of attachment an inward tenting of the wall may be caused as the stalk is put under tension by a peristaltic wave. Occasionally a pedunculated polyp of the gastric antrum will prolapse intermittently through the pylorus and the head of the polyp may be found in the duodenal bulb (see Fig. 16-22). Such a prolapsing polyp may lead to the signs and symptoms of intermittent pyloric obstruction.

INTRAMURAL TUMORS

A tumor that forms within the duodenal wall beneath the mucosa is called an intramural-extra-mucosal tumor. A variety of benign tumors occur in the duodenum but as a group they are uncommon. The most frequently encountered are leiomyomas, lipomas, adenomatous polyps, and Brunner's gland adenomas. Less common lesions include ectopic pancreas, neurofibromas, angiomas, hamartomas, and duplication cysts. Of these lesions, lipomas may change shape under the influence of peristalsis because of the usual softness of the tumor. This may be a helpful differential sign but a few cases of duplication cysts also have been reported showing a similar finding so that it probably is not completely specific for lipoma. The defect caused by an intramural lesion is characterized by the fact that mucosal

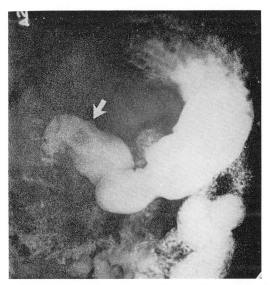

Fig. 17-14. Benign polyp of the duodenum (**arrow**).

folds are visualized over its surface. The defect forms a smooth, convex bulge into the lumen, and usually a fairly sharp angle is formed by the junction of the defect and the normal duodenal wall. Ulceration may develop on the surface of the tumor and the ulcer crater may fill and be visualized as a dense, round shadow representing the barium-filled pocket, the "target sign." Occasionally the tumor develops largely beneath the serosa and the major portion of it may project outside of the duodenal lumen, so that little narrowing of the lumen or evidence of obstruction is present. The roentgen diagnosis of aberrant pancreatic nodules has been considered in the section dealing with these lesions in Chapter 16. Only the larger nodules that measure at least a centimeter in diameter are likely to cause sufficient deformity of the duodenal lumen to be visualized roentgenologically and it usually is impossible to determine the histologic nature of such a lesion from roentgen examination alone. The usual diagnosis is that of an intramural lesion, type undetermined (Fig. 17-15). A sign that may be of value

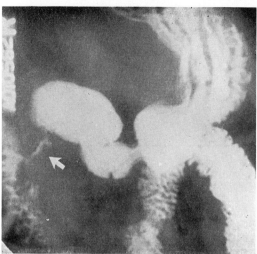

Fig. 17-16. Carcinoma of the second portion of the duodenum (**arrow**). The lesion is annular and encircles the lumen of the duodenum just below the bulb. It causes an irregular constriction similar to the type of defect produced by carcinoma elsewhere in the gastrointestinal tract. Note the dilatation of the duodenal bulb in spite of the fact that barium passes through the lesion into the distal duodenum and jejunum so that obstruction is minimal.

in differential diagnosis consists in the demonstration of a fine, hairline extension of barium from the duodenal lumen into the defect caused by the mass. This has been interpreted as evidence of a pancreatic duct opening from the nodule into the duodenal lumen. Closed duplications of the duodenum or so-called "enterogenous cysts" also may reveal roentgen signs indistinguishable from those of other intramural masses.

CARCINOMA OF THE DUODENUM

Primary carcinoma of the duodenum causes a filling defect that is usually annular and of relatively short length. The mucosal pattern is absent over the surface of the lesion and the defect is constant, fixed, and rigid, resembling essentially the same type of defect encountered in carcinoma elsewhere in the gastrointestinal tract (Fig. 17-16). Some degree of obstruction is the rule and the duodenum above the lesion will be dilated. Gastric retention and moderate gastric dilatation often are noted.

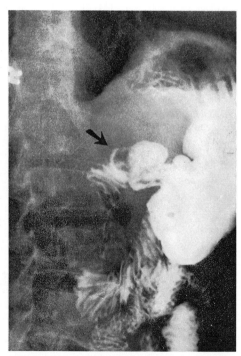

Fig. 17-15. Aberrant pancreatic nodule in the duodenum (**arrow**). There is a small dimple on the bulbar side of the defect probably representing the orifice of the duct.

annular pancreas — longer filling defect

PERIAMPULLARY CARCINOMA

The term "periampullary carcinoma" is used to include those lesions arising from the ampulla of Vater or the distal part of the common bile duct, those developing primarily in the duodenum near the region of the ampulla, and those that are primary in the head of the pancreas but invade the duodenum secondarily and obstruct the ampulla. The roentgen findings in periampullary carcinoma have been described and illustrated in Chapter 13 in the section entitled "Carcinoma of the Pancreas."

DUODENITIS

Duodenitis is a frequent accompaniment of duodenal ulcer. As a separate entity without associated ulceration it probably is infrequent and the diagnosis can hardly be made on roentgen examination. The clinical signs and symptoms are essentially those of ulcer.

The roentgen findings that have been described include (*1*) irritability of the duodenal bulb, (*2*) inconstant deformity of the bulbar outline, and (*3*) coarsening of the mucosal folds. However, these signs can occur in the normal and they cannot be depended upon as evidence of duodenitis.

REGIONAL DUODENITIS (CROHN'S DISEASE)

The duodenum is an infrequent site of regional enteritis. The findings are similar to those noted in the jejunum. There is loss of motility and alteration in the appearance of the mucosa. The folds become thickened and a cobblestone relief may develop. Later there is obliteration of the folds.

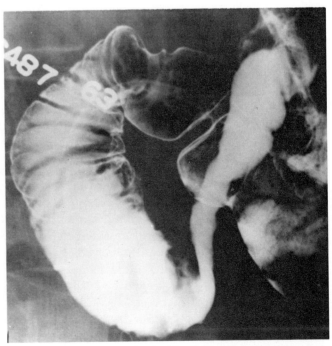

Fig. 17-17. Regional duodenitis demonstrated by hypotonic duodenography. The bulb and descending duodenum are dilated and atonic. There is a long, smooth, stricturelike narrowing of the ascending duodenum representing the stenotic phase of the lesion.

Narrowing of the involved segment develops as a result of fibrosis and the end result is a relatively long and smooth stenotic area with proximal dilatation (Fig. 17-17) and, often, some degree of gastric retention. The diagnosis is aided if there are similar areas of disease elsewhere in the small intestine, particularly in the terminal ileum. Involvement of the gastric antrum is present occasionally.

OTHER CONDITIONS

HYPERTROPHY OF BRUNNER'S GLANDS

Infrequently the duodenal glands of Brunner may become enlarged sufficiently so that they cause nodular defects in the bulbar outline. Hypertrophy of these glands usually follows and is associated with gastric hyperacidity; it is thought to be a protective response against hyperacidity. Roentgenologically the enlarged glands cause multiple nodular defects in the bulbar shadow, giving it a mottled or cobblestone appearance. The walls of the bulb remain pliable and its motility is undisturbed. The process may be mistaken for a polyposis of the duodenum. Occasionally, a single gland will undergo hypertrophy causing a small, solitary, intramural mass which cannot be distinguished from other intramural tumors.

PERIDUODENAL ADHESIONS

Inflammatory adhesions, particularly between the gallbladder and the duodenum, are frequent. These may cause a distortion in the outline of the bulb or a flattening of its superior surface. The duodenal bulb may form a sharp angle with the pyloric antrum or there may be an unusually sharp angulation between the bulb and the descending portion of the duodenum. At times the deformity caused by adhesions may resemble that of a duodenal ulcer rather closely and differentiation may be difficult. As noted in the section on "Duodenal Ulcer," the demonstration of the ulcer crater is a highly reliable sign and in its absence the diagnosis of duodenal ulcer often is presumptive.

PROLAPSE OF GASTRIC MUCOSA THROUGH THE PYLORUS

When the mucosa of the gastric antrum is redundant it may prolapse through the pylorus under the influence of active peristalsis. Slight degrees of mucosal prolapse are observed frequently during gastrointestinal examinations. There has been a difference of opinion concerning the significance of this finding. Some have believed it to be a frequent cause of symptoms related to the upper gastrointestinal tract and have considered it to be a cause for bleeding. Other observers have stated that in the majority of patients demonstrable prolapse of mucosa through the pylorus has little if any significance as far as symptoms are concerned. While the lesion may be a cause for gastrointestinal bleeding, this is probably an unusual complication. Evidence has been presented to show that the same type of defect can be

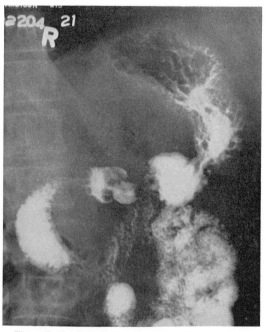

Fig. 17-18. Prolapse of gastric mucosa through the pylorus. There is a peristaltic wave in the gastric antrum that has almost reached the pylorus. Redundant and prominent folds of mucosa bulge through the pylorus into the base of the duodenal bulb.

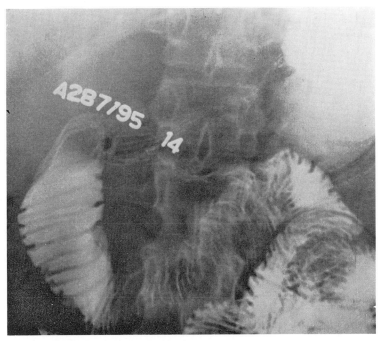

Fig. 17-19. Intramural hematoma of the duodenum occurring in a patient with hemophilia. The lesion is in the transverse and ascending portions of the duodenum. Note the "picket fence" arrangement of the folds and the lack of sharp definition of the margins of the defect.

demonstrated in individuals who are having no gastrointestinal symptoms and one should be cautious about attributing too much significance to its presence.

Roentgen Observations

Typically, prolapse of the gastric mucosa results in a lobulated filling defect in the base of the duodenal bulb leading to an irregular concavity of the base of the bulb (Fig. 17-18). Mucosal folds in the prepyloric area of the stomach usually can be traced through the pylorus and can be seen to be continuous with the small nodular defects in the base of the bulb. The resulting defect has been likened to that of an open umbrella. When the prolapse is extensive, the folds may fill the major portion of the bulb as a gastric peristaltic wave passes through the antrum. As the wave relaxes the folds tend to return into the antrum and the defect in the base of the bulb will diminish or completely disappear. The defect caused by mucosal prolapse resembles in some ways that resulting from hypertrophy of the pylorus. It is distinguished from the latter by the inconstancy of the defect and its intensification by peristalsis in the antrum, by the nodular type of filling defect, and by a lack of narrowing or elongation of the pyloric canal on the gastric side. Prolapsed mucosa can be differentiated from the defect caused by a prolapsing gastric polyp by the continuity of folds in the antrum with those in the bulb and by the multiplicity of nodulations in the defect (umbrella sign) rather than a single mass.

INTRAMURAL HEMATOMA OF THE DUODENUM

Hematoma of the duodenum usually follows abdominal trauma, or else it occurs in patients subject to bleeding tendencies such as in hemophiliacs or in those receiving anticoagulants.

Roentgen examination reveals evidence of an intramural mass without sharply demarcated margins. The valvulae conniventes appear stretched, producing a "coiled-spring" appearance (Fig. 17-19). Also, the pointed projections of the valvulae have been likened to a picket fence. In other patients the hematoma forms a more circumscribed intramural mass with well-defined margins. Obstruction of some degree is usually present and may be complete. The hematoma regresses spontaneously and re-examination in a few days to a week will show the improvement. Because of the hazards associated with surgery in hemophilia and other causes for spontaneous bleeding, accurate diagnosis is very important. In traumatic cases there is a predilection for hematomas to occur in the retroperitoneal or fixed portion of the duodenum. In hemophiliacs and others with bleeding tendencies the hematoma may occur elsewhere in the gastrointestinal tract.

REFERENCES AND SELECTED READINGS

1. BROWN, C. H., and STRITTMATTER, W. C.: Obstructive lesions of the duodenum distal to the bulb. *Radiology 70:* 720, 1958.

2. DODD, G. D., FISHLER, J. S., and PARK, O. K.: Hyperplasia of Brunner's glands. Report of two cases with review of the literature. *Radiology 60:* 814, 1953.

3. DODD, G. B., and NAFIS, W. A.: Annular pancreas in the adult. *Am. J. Roentgenol. Radium Ther. Nucl. Med. 75:* 333, 1956.

4. EATON, S. B., BENEDICT, K. T., JR., FERRUCCI, J. T., and FLEISCHLI, D. J.: Hypotonic duodenography. *Radiol. Clin. North Am. 8:* 125, 1970.

5. FELDMAN, M., and WEINBERG, T.: Aberrant pancreas: A cause of duodenal syndrome. *JAMA 148:* 893, 1952.

6. FREE, E. A., and GERALD, B.: Duodenal obstruction in the newborn due to annular pancreas. *Am. J. Roentgenol. Radium Ther. Nucl. Med. 103:* 321, 1968.

7. HAMPTON, A. O.: A safe method for the roentgen demonstration of bleeding duodenal ulcers. *Am. J. Roentgenol. Radium Ther. Nucl. Med. 38:* 565, 1937.

8. HYATT, H. W.: Neonatal duodenal obstruction caused by annular pancreas in two mongoloid children. *JAMA 180:* 1128, 1962.

9. JONES, C. W., JR.: Regional enteritis with involvement of the duodenum. *Gastroenterology 51:* 1018, 1966.

10. MARTEL, W.: Hypotonic duodenography without intubation. *Radiology 91:* 387, 1968.

11. ROBERTS, S. W., and HAMILTON, W. W.: Regional enteritis of the duodenum. *Radiology 86:* 881, 1966.

12. SENTURIA, H. R., SUSMAN, N., and SHYKEN, H.: The roentgen appearance of spontaneous intramural hemorrhage of the small intestine associated with anticoagulant therapy. *Am. J. Roentgenol. Radium Ther. Nucl. Med. 86:* 62, 1961.

13. SERRANO, J. F., and McPEAK, C. J.: Primary neoplasms of the duodenum. *Surgery 59:* 199, 1966.

14. WIOT, J. F., and SPIRO, E.: Intraluminal diverticulum. A form of duplication. *Radiology 80:* 46, 1963.

18

THE MESENTERIC SMALL INTESTINE

ANATOMY AND PHYSIOLOGY

The mesenteric small intestine begins at the duodenojejunal junction and ends at the ileocecal valve. When coated with a thin layer of barium the jejunum shows a prominent mucosal pattern. The folds stand out clearly as a network of crisscrossing lines and with finely serrated edges. This pattern is produced by the folds of Kerkring or valvulae conniventes and resembles that seen in the duodenum distal to the bulb. The mucosal surface of the ileum is much smoother and even mild distention tends to obliterate what folds are present. In the jejunum, on the other hand, the folds of Kerkring are not obliterated even when there is severe distention of the bowel.

The junction between the jejunum and ileum is not distinct, the folds gradually becoming fewer. The jejunum usually occupies the upper central, left side, and lower central portions of the abdomen; the ileum is found in the right lateral abdomen and within the pelvis. There is much variation, however, in the location of the different parts of the small intestine and there often seems to be a change in the same individual at different times. Because of its mesentery the loops of small intestine move freely and often change considerably in position in serial films (Fig. 18-1).

The junction of ileum and colon forms an anatomic landmark that can be recognized without difficulty by the roentgenologist. The lips of the ileocecal valve project into the lumen of the cecum for a short distance and the superior lip is more prominent than the inferior (see Fig. 19-3). Occasionally the valve stands out more clearly than usual and causes a circular filling defect along the cecal margin. At times the ileocecal valve is situated on the posterior wall of the cecum and if the valve is a prominent structure, pressure over it causes it to appear as a round filling defect in the barium-filled cecum that may be mistaken for a polypoid tumor. Usually there will be a small amount of barium caught in the opening of the valve and this results in a dense shadow in the center of the translucent area. This is usually elliptical in shape and crevices between folds may radiate outward from the center in a spokelike manner. This configuration is typical of a thickened ileocecal valve when it is visualized *en face*.

Peristalsis in the jejunum is active and rapid. Propulsive movements begin in the duodenum and may progress into the jejunum for a considerable distance within a matter of seconds before they gradually cease. Such peristaltic rushes may transport a bolus of barium for a considerable distance along the small intestine and it is common to find barium in most of the jejunum in a matter of several minutes after the meal has begun to leave the stomach. In addition to peristaltic rushes, areas of segmental contraction occur that do not serve to propel the intestinal contents but rather seem to be a

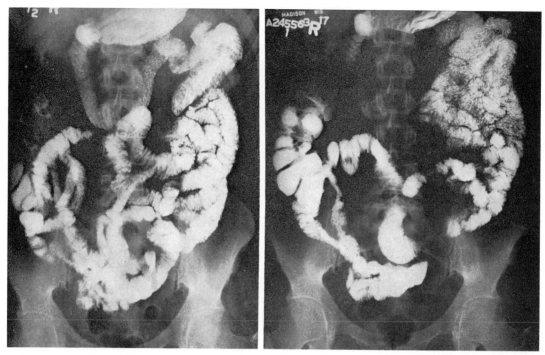

Fig. 18-1. Normal small intestine. *Left,* Half-hour and *Right,* 1-hour roentgenograms after barium meal. Note the change in distribution of the coils of small intestine and the change in the mucosal pattern from jejunum to ileum. At the end of 1 hour the head of the meal has reached the upper ascending colon.

mechanism for mixing and bringing the fluid into intimate contact with the absorbing surfaces of the bowel.

Peristalsis in the ileum is much slower, the gradient of course being a gradual one. Propulsive waves are relatively infrequent, at least as compared to the jejunum, and they move at a slower rate. Thus the progress of a meal, after an initial rapid propulsion through the upper and midportions of the jejunum, decreases considerably in the lower small intestine and it often requires from 1 to 1½ hours or even longer for a barium-water meal to reach the cecum. So much normal variation occurs, however, that it is difficult to set a limit for the transit time through the small intestine. To be noted also is the fact that the times given are for a barium-water mixture. Food leaves the stomach at a much slower rate and small-bowel progress also is much slower.

If food is given after the stomach is empty of the barium-water mixture, or nearly so, there usually is a prompt acceleration of small-bowel motility and a rapid propulsion of the mixture into the colon if it has not already reached the large bowel. The small-bowel transit time can be affected by many other factors. Drugs such as morphine may cause a pronounced delay in motility. Fear, excitement, nausea, etc. may affect motility adversely. Patients with severe or poorly controlled diabetes often show a considerable delay in gastric emptying and in small-bowel motility. One should use considerable caution before interpreting minor degrees of variation in the appearance of the small intestine as evidence of derangement of function or as a sign of organic disease.

METHODS OF EXAMINATION

SCOUT FILMS OF THE ABDOMEN

As discussed in Chapter 13, preliminary or scout films of the abdomen are the method of choice for the study of small-bowel obstructions of acute nature and this aspect of small-intestine roentgenology will not be discussed further in this section. In the presence of a partial chronic obstruction of the small intestine there may be little or no accumulation of gas above the site of obstruction and the diagnosis then will depend upon contrast visualization. The lesions of non-obstructive character will ordinarily not be recognized until contrast study of the tract is done.

CONTRAST VISUALIZATION

Contrast visualization of the small intestine is to a large extent only a continuation of the roentgen study of the upper gastrointestinal tract as detailed in previous sections. The same barium-water mixture is used. It is essential that a non-flocculating barium sulfate containing a suspending agent be used in order to bring out satisfactory mucosal detail. It usually is preferable to increase the amount of the mixture if small-intestine study is to be done and an additional 90 to 120 ml may be given after completion of the fluoroscopic study of the stomach and duodenum. Mixing of the barium sulfate with ice-cold normal saline solution instead of plain water has been recommended by some to hasten the transport of material through the small intestine and thus shorten the time needed for the examination.

Among the drugs that increase small-intestinal motility, *neostigmine* has been preferred by some. It is given intramuscularly in doses of from 0.5 to 0.75 mg for an average-sized adult after completion of fluoroscopy of the upper intestinal tract. Another drug, introduced more recently, which has been found useful in increasing gastric, duodenal, and jejunal peristalsis and relaxation of the pylorus is *metoclopramide*.[18] It is given intravenously in a dose of 20 mg. Within minutes, increase in gastric peristalsis is seen, the pylorus relaxes, and there is rapid filling of the small intestine. The mean small-intestinal transit time was found by Harper to be 55 minutes.[15] The drug is of low toxicity.

The addition of 10 ml of Gastrografin to the routine barium mixture also has been advocated as a means of acclerating the small-bowel transit time.

The routine small-intestine study consists of a series of roentgenograms of the abdomen made at certain intervals after the ingestion of the barium mixture (Fig. 18-1). While this will vary among patients, depending upon the particular clinical problem at hand, and to some extent on the initial fluoroscopic observations of gastric and duodenal motility, the roentgenograms usually are made at the end of 30 minutes, 1 hour, and 1½ hours. If the barium-water meal has made a normal progress and has reached the colon the examination is discontinued. If the head of the barium column remains in the small intestine, the patient is allowed to eat a small meal and another roentgenogram is made 2 hours later. Usually the stimulation of peristalsis following eating will have caused a general advance of the barium mixture into the colon at this examination.

When time and facilities warrant it, fluoroscopy can be substituted for film examination or it can be done in conjunction with film study. We have found that, as a rule, the more simplified study as outlined above can be used as a survey examination and will exclude disease with considerable accuracy or demonstrate a lesion if one exists. If more information is needed or if the routine roentgen study does not demonstrate a lesion when the clinical evidence suggests that one may be present, examination can be repeated with fluoroscopic observation carried out at frequent intervals. Palpation then can be used to separate overlying loops and occasionally a small lesion will be visualized that cannot be seen in the routine roentgenograms. There is no doubt that the accuracy of the method is increased by the use of fluoroscopy but routine roentgen study will serve a useful purpose if its limitations are kept in mind and there is recourse to reexamination when necessary. In general, the accuracy of detection of disease in the mesenteric small intestine by roentgen methods is less than that in other parts of the gastrointestinal tract. This is caused by the multiplicity of loops of bowel, the difficulty in separating them and visualizing individual segments clearly, and by the fact that in many individuals, particularly those of an asthenic habitus, much of the small intestine lies deep in the pelvis and cannot be palpated nor can the loops be otherwise separated from one another. In spite of these drawbacks, roentgen examination of the small intestine is an extremely useful procedure and a great deal of information can be obtained from it.

WATER-SOLUBLE CONTRAST AGENTS

The use of water-soluble iodinated compounds has been recommended for the study of the small intestine when obstruction is present or suspected.

However, investigative and clinical experience has shown that barium does not become inspissated above a small-bowel obstructive lesion and does not change a partial obstruction into a complete one. The water-soluble compounds are hypertonic and become considerably diluted in the lower small bowel. The mucosal pattern is difficult to identify. A barium sulfate mixture, therefore, can be employed safely and allows better visualization even when obstruction is present.

INTUBATION METHODS

A double-lumen tube of the Miller-Abbott or Harris type can be passed into the small intestine and the opaque mixture injected directly into the bowel. At times this is done when the tube has been used to decompress the bowel above an obstruction. When the tip of the tube has progressed as far as it will go, the barium is injected under fluoroscopic control. In this way the exact site and the nature of the obstructing lesion sometimes can be identified.

Schatzki recommended the use of a small-intestinal enema for examining this part of the intestinal tract. The method consists in the passing of a single lumen tube into the upper jejunum and then allowing a barium-water mixture to flow slowly but steadily into the bowel. As a result the entire length of the small intestine can be filled at one time. The method may be of some value in difficult diagnostic cases but is not very satisfactory for routine use because of the necessity for passage of a tube.

REFLUX METHOD

It is possible in some patients and with suitable technique to fill most or all of the small intestine by reflux of a barium enema through the ileocecal valve.[24] The filling is done under fluoroscopic control. We have had no personal experience with this method which has been used primarily for the detection of organic filling defects.

ARTERIOGRAPHY

In some patients selective superior mesenteric or celiac axis arteriography may give useful information if routine barium studies have been negative. The method is particularly valuable if there has been acute or chronic bleeding from the gastro-intestinal tract and a source of blood loss cannot be found. In some cases of acute hemorrhage the bleeding point may be localized because of leakage of contrast material into the lumen (see Fig. 17-11). In other patients the lesion responsible may be identified, such as an hemangioma or arteriovenous malformation. Other tumors, particularly if they show abnormal tumor vessels or a tumor stain or blush, can be visualized. Some investigators have recommended that, in cases of acute hemorrhage, gastrointestinal arteriography be done as the initial procedure to be followed by barium studies if necessary. In most patients, however, it is preferable to do the barium studies first as they may obviate the need for vascular opacification. Selective injection of vasopressor substances has been used to control bleeding, at least on a temporary basis, after the bleeding point has been localized.

ANOMALIES OF THE SMALL INTESTINE

DUPLICATIONS

In the chapters dealing with other parts of the gastrointestinal tract mention has been made of congenital duplications. This malformation is also found in the small intestine, somewhat more frequently in the ileum than elsewhere. The duplication may or may not communicate with the intestinal lumen. If it does it usually is of tubular shape, paralleling the normal gut and lying between the layers of the mesentery. A closed duplication is in the nature of a cyst. If small the cyst may lie within the wall of the gut; a larger lesion usually lies within the mesentery. The mucosal lining of the duplication may be that of any part of the gastrointestinal tract; gastric mucosa is present frequently. Associated anomalies such as spina bifida, hemivertebra, and meningocele are common.

If the duplication communicates with the intestinal lumen, a barium meal may cause opacification of it but its recognition probably would be very difficult because of surrounding barium-filled intestinal loops and the tendency for these loops to overlie one another. The closed cystic type gives roentgen signs of a circumscribed soft-tissue mass displacing segments of bowel and perhaps compressing them. Those duplications that lie within the wall resemble other intramural tumors and may cause the roentgen signs of partial or high-grade obstruction. It is hardly possible to state the nature of such a lesion from the roentgen findings.

Duplication may be associated with atresia. Sometimes, calcification occurs in the duplicated segment. The finding of a small area of calcification associated with the signs of jejunal or ileal atresia may suggest the diagnosis. Otherwise, it can be made only at the time of operation or at postmortem.

An unusual type of duplication of the small intestine, with a part of the duplicated segment lying within the thorax, has been reported infrequently. In the patient described by Snodgrass, the duplicated segment formed a mass along the right posterior mediastinum.[28] After a barium meal, the contrast material was found within the mass and it was demonstrated to communicate with the small intestine within the abdomen. This lesion is rare but must be considered in the differential diagnosis of lesions of cystic nature found within or along the mediastinum.

ERRORS OF ROTATION

Embryologists divide the gut into three parts, the foregut (mouth to duodenojejunal junction), the midgut (duodenojejunal junction to the midtransverse colon), and the hindgut (midtransverse colon to the anus). The important segment concerned in errors of rotation is the midgut. This part of the tube grows very rapidly during the first weeks of life and in order to have room, it herniates into the umbilical cord. Rotation of the midgut begins about the eighth week, during the period in which it lies outside the celomic cavity. The first stage is one of counterclockwise rotation with the superior mesenteric artery as the axis. The rotation is one of 180°, which brings the postarterial segment toward the front. The second stage of rotation is of short duration and consists in a return of the gut to the abdomen and a further counterclockwise rotation of 90°, making a total of 270°. This occurs about the tenth week of life. The jejunum is the first part to return to the abdomen, followed by the

ileum, cecum, ascending and transverse colon. The small intestine collects in the left side of the abdomen and the cecum and ascending colon, the last parts to enter the abdomen, come to lie in the right hypochondrium. The third or final stage is completed at about the time of birth or shortly thereafter with completion of descent of the cecum into the right lower quadrant. Fixation of the cecum, ascending colon, and the duodenum take place during the third stage. The anomalies of rotation that may occur depend upon the stage at which rotation was arrested.

FIRST-STAGE ARREST

This results in an omphalocele, a persisting herniation of the midgut into the umbilical cord. Occasionally other abdominal structures are present in the hernia such as the liver, spleen, or stomach. The diagnosis is a clinical one.

SECOND-STAGE ARREST

NONROTATION. The gut may return into the abdomen without rotating. The small intestine is found in the right side of the abdomen and the colon in the left. This is an infrequent malformation and often is asymptomatic. On roentgen examination the distribution of the bowel is characteristic (Fig. 18-2). The entire colon lies to the left of the midline. The cecum is often near the midline but the ileocecal valve opens on the right side. A barium-meal examination will show the stomach and the first and second portions of the duodenum to be in normal position but the duodenojejunal flexure is absent; instead the entire jejunum is found to the right of the midline.

REVERSAL OF ROTATION. This is a very rare anomaly in which rotation occurs in a clockwise manner. The duodenum comes to lie in front of the superior mesenteric artery and the transverse colon behind it. Obstruction from compression by peritoneal bands or from volvulus may occur.

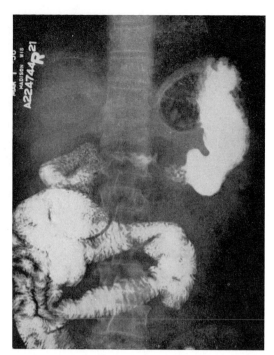

Fig. 18-2. Congenital nonrotation of the bowel. Roentgenogram after a barium meal demonstrates the stomach and first portion of the duodenum to be in normal position but the remainder of the duodenum and the jejunum lie almost entirely to the right of the midline. On barium enema the colon was found on the left side of the midline.

THIRD-STAGE ARREST

Anomalies of fixation occur as a part of third-stage arrest and these are much more frequent than complete failure of rotation (second-stage arrest). The attachment of the mesentery may be very short, while the length of the mesentery is abnormally long. This predisposes to volvulus of the entire midgut with or without compromise of its blood supply (see Fig. 17-3). There may be a failure of fixation of the cecum and the ascending colon; this predisposes to volvulus of the cecum (see Chapter 19). There also is a tendency to persistence of peritoneal bands or veils in these patients, with the possibility of compression or kinking of the bowel. Peritoneal bands may compromise the lumen of the duodenum and be a cause for high-intestinal obstruction in the newborn. One of the most frequent defects is a

failure of complete descent of the cecum, which remains along the inferior surface of the liver. The appendix often remains in a retrocecal position with its tip pointing upward behind the cecum.

MECKEL'S DIVERTICULUM

Meckel's diverticulum is reported to occur in from 1 to 2 per cent of the population and is three times as frequent in males as in females. The cause is a failure of obliteration of the vitelline duct. Usually asymptomatic, Meckel's diverticulum may be a cause of hemorrhage, obstruction, intussusception, acute inflammation, or perforation. Heterotopic islands of gastric mucosa may be present in the diverticulum; ulceration may result and be the source of the blood loss. Roentgen demonstration of a Meckel's diverticulum is difficult and often requires meticulous technique and careful observation. As a rule the diverticulum is located in the lower part of the ileum where overlapping of loops of small intestine make it difficult to visualize all segments clearly; those loops lying within the pelvis cannot be separated by palpation. Because of the usual shape of the diverticulum, elongated and tubular with a wide ostium, it does not retain the barium very well and even when completely filled can easily pass for a segment of bowel.

Occasionally a Meckel's diverticulum is demonstrated by retrograde filling of the ileum during a barium enema. More often the lesion is discovered during a small-bowel study (Fig. 18-3). Those that are visualized usually are saclike rather than elongated and tubular and have a narrow neck and ostium. The saclike character of the lesion causes it to retain barium after the rest of the meal has progressed into the colon. Upright roentgenograms may demonstrate a gas-fluid level within the sac. *Scan c̄ Sodium pertechnetate*

ATRESIA

Congenital atresia may involve the small intestine as well as other parts of the gastrointestinal tract. The signs of bowel obstruction develop in the immediate postnatal period and roentgen examination is useful in establishing the level of the lesion. The diagnostic findings have been

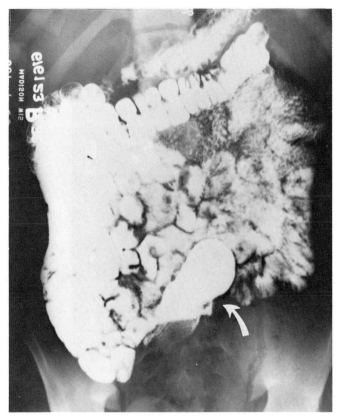

Fig. 18-3. Meckel's diverticulum demonstrated during a small-intestine study (**arrow**). Elevation of bowel out of the pelvis is caused by a distended urinary bladder. The presenting complaint was bleeding and an ulcer in heterotopic gastric mucosa was found at time of operation.

considered in Chapter 19 in conjunction with atresia of the colon. Figure 18-4 illustrates an example of small intestinal atresia. A few cases of small-bowel atresia have been reported in which the ileum distal to the atresia opened directly into the peritoneal cavity, indicating possible danger from barium-enema studies if the obstruction is in the distal ileum. Atresia may be a complication of meconium ileus.

DISEASES OF THE SMALL INTESTINE

NEOPLASMS

A variety of neoplasms may develop in the small intestine, including carcinomas, carcinoids, leiomyomas, leiomyosarcomas, lymphosarcomas, etc. In the Mayo Clinic series[14] leiomyoma was the most frequent type. Other tumors included adenomas, lipomas, fibromas, myxomas, and their malignant counterparts. Many of these lesions present as localized, polypoid filling defects and resemble one another in their roentgen appearances and in their tendency to cause intussusception. Hemangioma also is found in the small intestine and is sometimes recognized because of the presence of calcified phleboliths—calcified thrombi in the dilated vascular spaces. As a group neoplasms of the small intestine are uncommon. The clinical manifestations usually result from the development of obstruction or are caused by bleeding or a combination of the two.

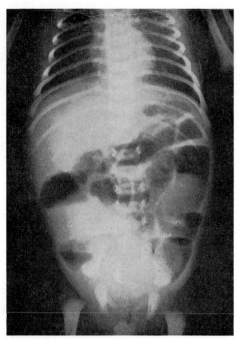

Fig. 18-4. Congenital atresia of the jejunum in a newborn infant. There is gas distention of bowel throughout the abdomen. It is difficult to determine if there is gas in the colon or not at this age period because the mucosal pattern of the small intestine, particularly in the lower jejunum and in the ileum, is very scanty and when the bowel becomes appreciably distended its margins become smooth and resemble colon. To locate the level of obstruction more accurately a barium enema often is necessary in a case of this type. This will exclude the colon as the site of obstruction.

ROENTGEN OBSERVATIONS

SIGNS OF OBSTRUCTION. Obstruction may result in the accumulation of abnormal amounts of gas and gas distention of loops of small bowel with gas-fluid levels present when roentgenograms are made with the patient upright or in a lateral decubitus position. These signs have been described in Chapter 13. As a rule the obstruction must be fairly severe in order to produce these changes. Because obstruction caused by small-bowel tumors often is intermittent in character with asymptomatic periods, roentgen examination done during the time when symptoms are present may give valuable information. The temporary nature of the obstructive signs is probably the result of episodes of intussusception. If roentgen examination is done during a period when there is complete absence of obstructive symptoms it may be difficult to detect the lesion. When a barium-water meal is given, obstruction is demonstrated by the obvious dilatation of the barium-filled loops of bowel above the level of the lesion. When obstruction is minimal or early this may be the first clue to the presence of the tumor (Fig. 18-5). The gastric emptying rate may be delayed and the progress of the meal through the small bowel slowed. The wide range of normal should be kept in mind and unless there is dilatation of the bowel as well as a delay in progress, the diagnosis of an obstructive lesion is hardly justified. If the examination is done during a period of intussusception, the diagnosis may be made during contrast filling. The intussusception causes a local dilatation of the bowel. The barium mixture caught in the crevices of the dilated intussusceptum produce a "coiled-spring" appearance. This is always highly suggestive of intussusception when it occurs in any part of the gastrointestinal tract. Frequently, there is complete obstruction associated with the intussusception and the nature of the lesion responsible may not be obvious.

FILLING DEFECT. If the lesion has caused a complete obstruction or a nearly complete one so that the barium mixture does not extend through the area of the lesion and outline its lumen, the roentgen diagnosis may be limited to that of an obstructing process. If obstruction is incomplete the filling defect of the tumor may be visualized (Fig. 18-6). In general such defects resemble those caused by similar tumors in the esophagus, stomach, and colon. Thus, carcinomas are likely to encircle the lumen, producing an annular constriction with irregular narrowing of a short segment and with the margins of the lesion sharply demarcated from the normal and with overhanging edges. An intramural mass, such as a *leiomyoma*, causes a smooth-surfaced filling defect with intact mucosa over the surface except where ulceration may possibly have developed

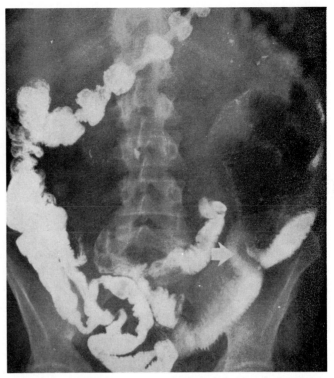

Fig. 18-5. Partial obstruction of the jejunum caused by a malignant polyp. The **arrow** points to the site of the lesion, which is only partially obstructive. The bowel proximal to it is dilated and contains gas. The barium mixture has passed through the area to fill the lower small intestine and proximal portion of the colon, and these segments are of normal caliber.

(Fig. 18-7). A leiomyoma may become very large and bulky and result in a sausage-shaped mass projecting into the intestinal lumen. Because the bowel wall is not completely fixed or infiltrated by the tumor, obstruction may be relatively moderate even when the tumor is large. Occasionally a leiomyoma or its malignant counterpart may grow almost completely extrinsic to the bowel lumen and thus cause little or no deformity in the barium outline. Such a tumor can hardly be identified as arising from the bowel wall unless it does develop to the point where it causes obstruction. Small tumors may not cause any signs of obstruction and the only clinical symptom may be that of bleeding. Very careful investigation with multiple roentgenograms, fluoroscopy, and spot films may be required to locate such a lesion. It is in some of these patients that selective superior mesenteric arteriography can often provide diagnostic information by demonstrating the bleeding site.

Lymphosarcoma involving the small intestine may appear in several forms. In one, the lesion presents as a discrete, polypoid, intramural mass. In another, the lesion is more infiltrating, causing a ragged, irregular defect. Ulceration and excavation may occur so that the lumen through the lesion is actually larger than the normal. Fistulous communication with adjacent loops of bowel is not uncommon. In still another type the disease occurs in the form of multiple, small, nodular defects, causing a coarse scalloping of the bowel wall. The disease is most frequent in the ileum where the greatest amount of lymphoid tissue is present.

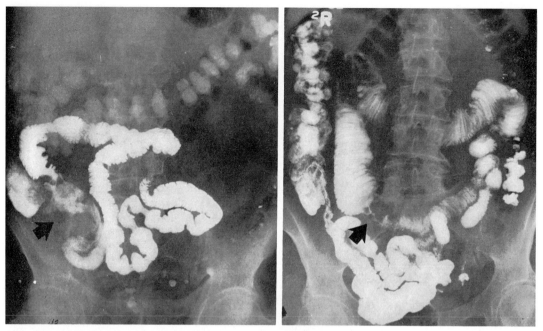

Fig. 18-6. Neoplasms of the small intestine. *Left,* Primary adenocarcinoma of the ileum (**arrow**). The lesion causes an irregular filling defect but is not obstructive. *Right,* Reticulum cell sarcoma of the jejunum (**arrow**). The lesion is annular and has caused a considerable irregular constriction of the jejunal lumen with a moderate dilatation above it. Note the stacked-coin appearance of the dilated barium-filled jejunum above the lesion.

Gastric and colonic lesions may accompany the small intestinal disease. In some patients lymphosarcoma presents as a malabsorption syndrome with diffuse infiltration of multiple segments of bowel and mesentery.[22] Segmentation and flocculation similar to that seen in sprue occur in some patients. The lesion may be very difficult to distinguish from some of the other causes of the malabsorption syndrome but there often are nodules projecting into the lumen suggesting the neoplastic nature of the process.

Carcinoid tumors are relatively uncommon affecting the small intestine but in some series they have been reported as being the most frequent tumor. If small the tumor may cause only a localized filling defect; larger lesions may cause intussusception or obstruction. The tendency for carcinoid to invade the contiguous mesentery and to cause fibrosis is to be noted. This may cause an angulation and kinking of the bowel, aggravating the obstruction. In contrast to carcinoids of the appendix, those in the small intestine are often malignant. In some cases there results a so-called *carcinoid syndrome* consisting of chronic diarrhea, flushing and cyanosis of the skin, respiratory distress, and right-sided cardiac disease. These clinical signs in association with roentgen evidence of a small-intestinal tumor are highly suggestive of the diagnosis.

Adenomas, lipomas, and *fibromas* resemble one another. The lesions may be single or multiple and cause a sharply outlined, polypoid-type filling defect of variable size. They often cause intussusception.

THE PEUTZ-JEGHERS SYNDROME. This entity consists of multiple, polypoid lesions in the gastrointestinal tract associated with a peculiar oral pigmentation. The pigment is melanin. The intestinal lesions are most commonly

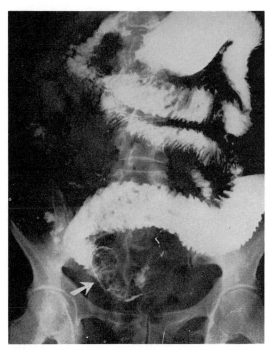

Fig. 18-7. Leiomyoma of the lower jejunum (**arrow**). The lesion forms a smooth oval-shaped filling defect that is partially obstructive and is causing dilatation of the bowel above it.

found in the small bowel but also occur in the colon and stomach. They represent hamartomas rather than true polyps. Often they are very small and difficult to identify in roentgenograms particularly in the jejunum where there is a rich fold pattern. They resemble other polypoid lesions and may be sessile or pedunculated. Their multiplicity and small size are suggestive signs and the diagnosis is confirmed by the presence of oral pigmentation.

Carcinoma, metastatic to the bowel, is usually multiple. A wide variety of roentgen appearances have been described depending on whether the lesion involves the wall of the intestine or the mesentery or both, the presence or absence of obstruction and of ulceration, and the size of the individual mass. *Metastatic malignant melanoma* is likely to cause multiple, nodular or polypoid filling defects. Central necrosis and ulceration may occur causing a "target deformity," a dense, barium-filled central crater surrounded by the sharply marginated nodular mass.[22] The tendency for this tumor to metastasize to the intestinal tract has been noted frequently.

Hodgkin's disease involving the small intestine resembles lymphosarcoma except that narrowing and stricture formation tend to be more severe owing to the fibrotic reaction associated with this disease.[10] Also extensive necrosis and excavation are less likely to occur. Multiple lesions are common and the stomach and colon may be involved.

REGIONAL ENTERITIS; CROHN'S DISEASE

Regional enteritis is an inflammatory disease of the small intestine, the cause of which is unknown. Because it develops most frequently in the terminal portion of the ileum, it is often referred to as "terminal ileitis." The same disease can involve the proximal part of the ileum, the jejunum, and even the duodenum and the stomach. The term "regional enteritis" is preferred since it recognizes the wide distribution of the disease throughout the small intestine. In the colon the disease has been called *granulomatous colitis* or *Crohn's disease* (see page 626). Cases also have been reported where the disease involved the duodenum and stomach[7] and, rarely, the esophagus. An acute form of ileitis is seen, particularly during childhood. The patients often are operated upon because of an erroneous diagnosis of acute appendicitis. Based on study of resected specimens, some authors believe that this is an acute exacerbation of chronic disease which may have been relatively asymptomatic previous to the acute episode. In many patients, however, there is spontaneous improvement with disappearance of symptoms, and the disease does not recur. The roentgen changes resemble the early findings in regional enteritis. It should be noted that in children, particularly during adolescence, there may normally be hyperplasia of lymphoid follicles in the distal ileum causing numerous tiny projections on the mucosal surface or a fine, cobblestone mucosal relief. This should not be misinterpreted as evidence of early regional enteritis.

Roentgen examination of a patient suspected of having regional enteritis should be initiated by means of a barium enema. If the lesion involves the terminal ileum, this segment may fill by reflux through the ileocecal valve and it can be studied to good advantage during fluoroscopy. If the terminal ileum does not fill an oral barium meal and a small-bowel study, as described previously, should be done. This procedure also is essential for the detection of lesions in the more proximal part of the small intestine and for determination of the presence or absence of obstruction. Because the terminal ileum is the most frequent site of the disease the following discussion refers mainly to regional ileitis.

Roentgen Observations

PRESTENOTIC PHASE. When filled by reflux during a barium enema the ileum is seen to be normal in caliber or irregular and slightly narrowed. The mucosal folds may be blunted or thickened. Later, ulceration develops, the normal fold pattern is lost, and the mucosal surface develops a rough cobblestone appearance. Linear ulcers, if present, are seen as longitudinal crevices filled with barium. Spastic contractions, an indication of irritability may be noted fluoroscopically. If filling occurs proximal to the area of involvement, the change from an abnormal to a normal ileal pattern is abrupt.

Following an oral barium meal, there often is an initial delay in progress through the lower ileum. The head of the barium column will not move into the colon until food is given; then it moves rapidly through the involved segment.

STENOTIC PHASE. As the disease becomes more chronic it is characterized by marked inflammatory induration of the wall of the bowel and of the mesentery (Fig. 18-8). The segment has a fixed, rigid appearance as shown in serial roentgenograms. The internal surface becomes smoother or finely irregular with complete absence of a mucosal fold pattern. The diam-

eter of the lumen is narrowed, sometimes uniformly, at other times in a more irregular manner. Apparently owing to irregular fibrosis and contraction, diverticulumlike outpouchings called pseudodiverticula may form. With increasing fibrosis the lumen may be narrowed to a diameter of only a few millimeters in size. When the segment is filled with barium the appearance resembles a string and is known as "the string sign" (Fig. 18-9). This now is the stenotic phase of the disease. The length of the involved segment is variable but may extend for a foot or more. Skip areas also are common, that is, two or more involved segments separated by normal bowel.

Fistula formation is common in regional enteritis. The fistulas may be between adjacent segments of small intestine or between small bowel and colon, vagina, urinary bladder, or skin surface. Perianal fistulas are frequent. The tracts often can be identified in roentgenograms. Abscess formation owing to extension of the disease beyond the confines of the bowel also occurs with some frequency. The thickened bowel wall and mesentery, enlargement of regional lymph nodes, and the formation of abscesses results in an inflammatory mass that displaces loops of bowel away from the area of disease (Fig. 18-10). A soft-tissue space, therefore, will surround the involved bowel where normally there would be other segments of small intestine. The medial wall of the cecum often shows a concave indentation caused by the inflammatory mass surrounding the terminal ileum. Because of its rigidity the terminal ileum often develops a goosenecked shape as it curves downward into the pelvis from the ileocecal valve. The lips of the valve become thickened and cause characteristic biconcave filling defects in the medial wall of the cecum.

Although the bowel may be markedly stenotic, obstructive signs may be minimal. When it does occur the bowel above the lesion becomes dilated with excess fluid and gas present.

JEJUNAL DISEASE. The same lesion may affect a segment of bowel above the terminal ileum

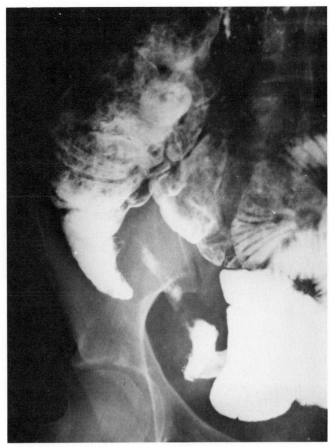

Fig. 18-8. Regional ileitis. The terminal ileum is narrowed with loss of normal mucosal pattern. The segment is surrounded by an inflammatory mass which displaces adjacent loops of bowel and causes a concave indentation on medial wall of cecum.

and the roentgen findings may be similar. Sometimes this occurs as a skip lesion above a diseased terminal ileum. At other times the jejunum is the primary site of disease. The early mucosal changes are similar to those noted in the ileum. During the stenotic phase there often are multiple constricted areas with dilated segments in between. Fistula formation is less frequent with jejunal disease. A long, stringlike area of narrowing is also less frequent; rather, areas of constriction alternate with area of dilatation. The strictures usually have a smooth lumen with tapering ends. Occasionally ulceration may cause irregularity to the margins. Duodenal involvement is un-common and is manifested by stricture formation with proximal dilatation.

After surgical resection and anastomosis there is a great tendency for the disease to recur in the bowel adjacent to the anastomosis.

NODULAR LYMPHOID HYPERPLASIA

Hyperplasia of the lymphoid follicles may affect the small intestine, the colon, or both. Mention is made on page 579 of hyperplastic follicles in the terminal ileum in older children as a normal finding. When it occurs in other

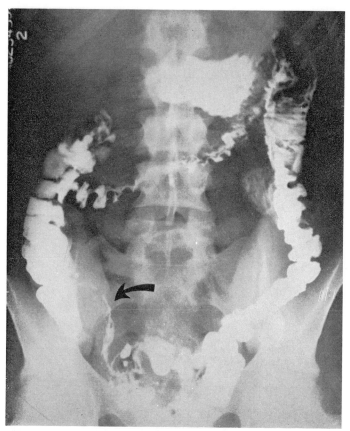

Fig. 18-9. Regional enteritis involving the terminal ileum. The lesion is advanced and has caused a typical "string sign" (**arrow**).

parts of the intestinal tract or during other age periods than adolescence it is called *nodular lymphoid hyperplasia*. It may be associated with dysgammaglobulinemia,[16] the patients are susceptible to infections and *giardiasis* involving the bowel is said to be common. Other authors report it as an essentially benign condition and consider that the lymphoid hyperplasia is the result of a variety of stimuli. The increased incidence during childhood and adolescence has been noted. The roentgen findings consist of numerous tiny nodular projections on the mucosal surface (Fig. 18-11). The individual lesions usually measure from 1 to 3 mm in diameter and are so small that they are difficult to identify in the jejunum where mucosal folds are most prominent. The lesions

may be widespread or limited to a shorter segment of bowel. A localized area of inflammatory disease resembling regional enteritis may be found in the duodenum or jejunum owing to giardiasis. In the small intestine, *systemic mastocytosis* may cause a fine nodulation in some cases closely resembling lymphoid hyperplasia. The clinical manifestations may allow differentiation. In the colon the nodules resemble the lesions of *familial polyposis* and biopsy is necessary to distinguish the two conditions. In the nodular form of lymphosarcoma the lesions usually are larger. The same is true of *metastatic melanosarcoma* and other metastatic tumors. Other diseases to be considered in differential diagnosis include the *Puetz-Jeghers syndrome* and *Gardner's syndrome*.

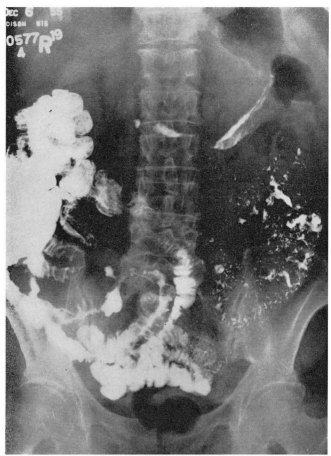

Fig. 18-10. Regional enteritis involving a long segment of the ileum. The lumen is narrowed irregularly and there are several small extensions of barium representing early fistula formation. The adjacent loops of small intestine are displaced away from the involved area because of the inflammatory mass associated with the disease. The lesion is not causing significant obstruction.

TUBERCULOSIS

The incidence of tuberculous ileocolitis has decreased considerably in recent years and it has become an uncommon disease in general hospital radiologic practice. Tuberculosis of the intestinal tract is usually localized to the distal part of the ileum, the cecum, and the proximal part of the ascending colon. While the lesions may be limited either to the ileum or to the colon, most often both are involved. Since intestinal tuberculosis may be secondary to pulmonary disease, evidence of lung involvement is important in establishing the diagnosis and in distinguishing tuberculosis from other diseases, particularly regional enteritis.

Roentgen Observations

After the oral administration of barium there may be an initial delay in progress through the lower part of the small intestine but, after several hours, occasionally only following the taking of food, there will be noted a

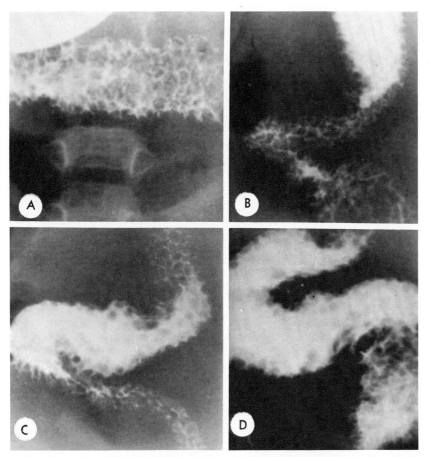

Fig. 18-11. Nodular lymphoid hyperplasia. *A,* Segment of transverse colon. *B–D,* Portion of sigmoid colon in varying degrees of filling and contraction. Note the multiple tiny, nodular projections on the mucosal surface. The colon contracts well. When the small intestine is involved, the changes are similar. (From Wolfson, J. J., Goldstein, G., Krivit, W., and Hong, R. *Am. J. Roentgenol. Radium Ther. Nucl. Med. 108:*610, 1970. *Reproduced with the permission of the authors, Editor, and Publisher.*)

rapid propulsion of the barium through the ileocecal area. Serial roentgenograms or fluoroscopy may demonstrate temporary filling but the tendency is for the inflamed segments to remain empty. One finds, as a result, barium filling of proximal ileal loops, filling of the colon distal to the ascending portion, but a very incomplete filling of the terminal ileum and cecum. If, normally, barium remains in the upper ileum and the head of the column is in the colon, filling is continuous or nearly so between the two areas. A similar phenomenon may be seen in regional ileitis, particuarly the

acute form of the disease, and it is not specific for tuberculosis (*Stierlin's sign*).

When examination is by means of a barium enema, the cecum and often the entire ascending colon are found to be very irritable. Only in very chronic disease is such irritability absent. The bowel fills momentarily, only to undergo a mass contraction with propulsion of the mixture from the ascending into the distal colon, and the patient may be unable to retain the enema. The terminal ileum is difficult to fill and once filled does not tolerate the barium very well.

In the later stages of the disease irritability is less pronounced. Deep and large ulcers may form. These, combined with scarring and fibrosis, cause the lumen to become very irregular (Fig. 18-12). If limited to a small area, the lesion may have a superficial resemblance to carcinoma. The margins of the defect, however, are not as sharply demarcated from the normal bowel; there are no overhanging edges or sharp angular junctions between the filling defect and the bowel wall. It is unusual to have cecal disease without involvement of the terminal ileum. More often the disease is so extensive and predominantly ulcerative that its resemblance to carcinoma is remote. There is a tendency for it to skip areas leaving normal bowel in between sites of disease. The smooth, uniform, stringlike constriction often seen in regional ileitis does not develop; instead irregularity in width of the ileal lumen is the rule. In difficult cases the presence or absence of pulmonary tuberculosis may be a very important factor in diagnosis.

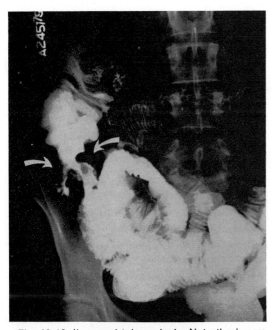

Fig. 18-12. Ileocecal tuberculosis. Note the irregular contraction of the cecum and irregularity of the margin of the ileum adjacent to the ileocecal valve (**arrows**).

MALABSORPTION AND RELATED SYNDROMES

Abnormal changes in the small intestine were first described in sprue by Snell and Camp but subsequently a number of other entities were found to cause similar alterations. These are now generally grouped under the designation of the *malabsorption syndrome*. The main fault in this syndrome is defective absorption of carbohydrate, protein, and fat from the small bowel. The result is steatorrhea with passage of bulky, foul-smelling, high-fat content stools. Various deficiency states may thus be induced, including osteomalacia and rickets, with loss of weight and anemia among the clinical signs. Marshak and Lindner[22] have listed over 20 diseases which may cause the malabsorption syndrome.

Harper[15] has listed the following causes:

1. Idiopathic steatorrhoea (sprue, nontropical sprue, celiac disease)

2. Pancreatic disease (pancreatitis, mucoviscidosis, tumors, pancreatectomy)

3. Obstructive jaundice, portal hypertension, and cardiac failure

4. Small-intestinal parasitic infestation

5. Pathologic conditions of the small intestine and mesentery (regional enteritis, tuberculosis, caseating mesenteric glands, diverticula, amyloidosis, systemic sclerosis, Whipple's disease, mesenteric vein thrombosis)

6. Toxic effects of drugs, nephrosis, hypoproteinemia and exudative enteropathy, diabetes, and hypogammaglobulinemia

7. Dermatitis herpetiformis

Some investigators[17] have not been able to find any specific signs which would allow differentiation between one of these entities and the others on roentgen study. Other writers, however, believe that differentiation can be made in many cases based upon the alterations in the small-bowel patterns.[22] The changes seen in sprue form a classic pattern for this syndrome (Fig. 18-13). In addition, a few of the more important diseases that enter into

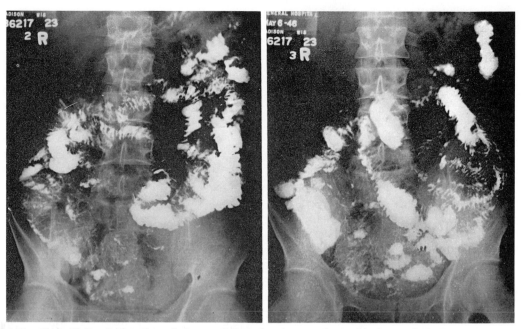

Fig. 8-13. Motor dysfunction of the small intestine in a patient with sprue. *Left,* Two-hour, and (*right*) 3-hour roentgenograms after barium meal, demonstrating extensive segmentation of the small intestine with a coarsening of the mucosal pattern in areas and unusual smoothness in others. There is moderate flocculation.

the differential diagnosis of sprue will be considered including Whipple's disease, amyloidosis, and scleroderma. Other diseases such as regional enteritis and lymphosarcoma will be discussed elsewhere in the sections entitled "Regional Enteritis: Crohn's Disease" and "Neoplasms."

SPRUE

Celiac disease in children and nontropical sprue in adults are generally considered to be the same disease. Tropical sprue may be a different entity but the roentgen findings in the gastrointestinal tract are similar to the other two diseases.[22] The changes described below are related to one another and are usually all present in any individual patient although varying in degree.

DILATATION. This is present in practically all patients and tends to be most severe in the lower half of the jejunum. However the extent and severity of dilatation varies among patients. The width of the lumen may be two or three times the normal width or even more. Narrowed segments also are seen. Serial roentgenograms show considerable variation in the width of the same segments and peristaltic waves or other motor activity may account for the narrowing.

SEGMENTATION. This is another important finding in sprue and refers to the accumulation of barium mixture in segments of variable length and separated by empty segments containing no barium mixture. Segmentation may involve much of the small intestine but tends to be more severe in the ileum in milder degrees of involvement. It is accompanied by an excessive amount of fluid.

CHANGES IN MUCOSAL FOLDS. The folds tend to be thinned and often are decreased in height. In some patients, however, the folds appear thickened and the valleys between the folds are widened. The fine, crinkled appearance of the normal valvulae conniventes is lost. Some segments of jejunum often show a complete absence of folds, the margins being quite smooth and tubular. This appearance has been termed the "moulage sign" and is one of the significant findings in sprue. It is associated with segmentation and dilatation. Simple distention will not completely obliterate the folds, even though it is severe.

HYPERSECRETION. Increased fluid content in the bowel lumen is shown by a tendency for the barium to be scattered in flecks and blotches (flocculation) and by the presence of air-fluid levels in upright roentgenograms.

ALTERATIONS IN MOTILITY. The transit time of barium mixture through the small intestine may be normal, decreased, or accelerated. Because of the wide range of transit times in the normal, this finding often is difficult to interpret unless the motility—increased or decreased—is clearly abnormal.

TRANSIENT INTUSSUSCEPTION. It is not uncommon in sprue to find the characteristic appearance of intussusception in one or several segments. It is nonobstructive and transient and the cause is not known. The diagnosis is based on the findings of a localized filling defect with stretched and thinned valvulae conniventes overlying it (i.e., the coiled-spring appearance).

DIFFERENTIAL DIAGNOSIS. In addition to other causes for the malabsorption syndrome, differential diagnosis includes mechanical small-intestinal obstruction. Irregular dilatation, segmentation, flocculation, and the moulage sign are characteristic of sprue. In obstruction, the bowel is dilated uniformly above the obstructing lesion and the barium column tends to be continuous. Also the loops of bowel appear to be under tension forming arched curves across the abdomen; in sprue the intestinal loops are flaccid and atonic. If the obstruction is partial the bowel distal to the block is normal in cali-

ber or collapsed and the transition from dilated to collapsed bowel is abrupt.

WHIPPLE'S DISEASE

Patients with Whipple's disease have steatorrhea, diarrhea, abdominal pain, weight loss, and arthralgia. Lymphadenopathy and polyserositis are present on physical examination. The basic and characteristic histologic lesion is the presence in the lamina propria and in lymph nodes of macrophages which are Sudan-negative and periodic acid-Schiff (PAS) positive. The wall of the intestine, along with the mesentery, is thickened and edematous. The roentgen findings in the gastrointestinal tract are similar to those of sprue and some authors have noted difficulty in differentiation. Marshak and Lindner,[22] stress the findings of thickened mucosal folds, more than in sprue, and a lesser degree of dilatation, segmentation and flocculation. The latter findings may be absent altogether. The thickened folds are more prominent in the jejunum. Also, the folds may be slightly nodular and have a "wild" and redundant appearance (Fig. 18-14). The lumen may be normal or slightly dilated. Similarity to intestinal lymphangiectasia and amyloidosis has also been noted. Correlation with clinical findings and biopsy is essential in most cases.

SCLERODERMA (PROGRESSIVE SYSTEMIC SCLEROSIS)

Involvement of the esophagus is common in scleroderma but other parts of the gastrointestinal tract also may be affected. The major histologic alteration is atrophy of the muscularis and replacement by fibrous tissue. In the small intestine the changes of a malabsorption syndrome may be seen. As in the esophagus, atony and hypomotility occur with varying degrees of dilatation (Fig. 18-15). The delayed transit time plus the dilatation may be severe enough to strongly suggest a small-bowel obstruction. Usually the mucous membrane folds are not greatly altered but in more advanced

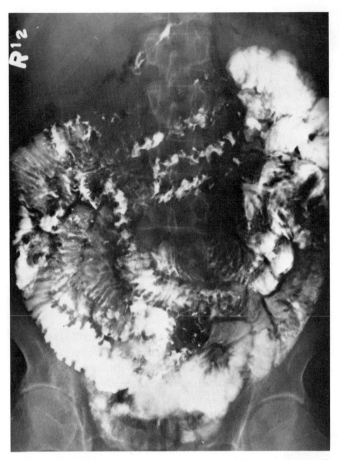

Fig. 18-14. Whipple's disease. The mucosal folds of the small intestine are thickened and irregular and some segments of the bowel are moderately dilated. The barium mixture is diluted in areas by increased fluid content and there is some segmentation.

disease the formation of saccules or pseudo-diverticula is characteristic. This also is seen in the colon. The other findings seen in sprue such as segmentation, flocculation and hypersecretion are uncommon. The occurrence of *pneumatosis intestinalis* (intramural gas) in scleroderma has been documented. Small-bowel changes in *dermatomyositis* are similar to those of scleroderma except that dilatation of the bowel often is more severe.

AMYLOIDOSIS

Amyloid infiltration of the gastrointestinal tract is frequent in amyloidosis. The most sig-

nificant roentgen finding in the small intestine is a thickening of the mucous membrane folds which may involve the entire small bowel. If there is an associated malabsorption syndrome there may be a mild degree of segmentation, flocculation, and dilatation but changes in the folds remain the most obvious abnormality. The differentiation from Whipple's disease is difficult and often impossible on roentgen study.

INTESTINAL LYMPHANGIECTASIA

This entity, first described about 10 years ago, is one of the diseases that causes loss of

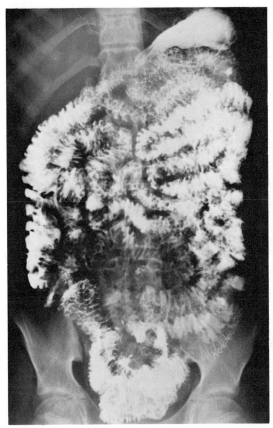

Fig. 18-15. Scleroderma of the small intestine. The mucosal folds are thickened particularly in segments in the lower abdomen.

protein from the gastrointestinal tract with resulting hypoproteinemia. Some patients develop malabsorption. Study of microscopic sections reveals edema and dilatation of lymphatics throughout the mucosa and submucosa. The disease may be present in infants and is thought to be congenital in such patients. When it develops later in life it apparently is acquired but the pathogenesis is uncertain. Chylous ascites if often present, particularly in infants. The most characteristic roentgen change is a diffuse, symmetric thickening of the mucosal folds owing to edema. Hypersecretion also is noted but the other changes seen in the "sprue pattern" such as segmentation and dilatation are usually minimal or absent. The differentiation from Whipple's disease and amyloidosis

may be difficult on roentgen study. The same is true of the other entities that may cause intestinal edema (see section entitled "Hypoproteinemia: Intestinal Edema.")

INTUSSUSCEPTION

In the presence of an uncomplicated intussusception occurring during infancy or childhood, scout roentgenograms of the abdomen may reveal either an essentially normal gas pattern or a moderate dilatation of gas-filled loops. Because of the rather wide variation in the amount of gas normally present in the small intestine of an infant or a young child, this finding may be difficult to evaluate. If the complications of gangrene and peritonitis develop, the roentgen signs of adynamic ileus and fluid become apparent.

The administration of a barium enema, not only for establishing or confirming the diagnosis of intussusception but also for treatment of it, is a valuable procedure. As the barium column reaches the site of obstruction, the end of the column assumes a concave or cup-shaped form as it surrounds the intussusceptum. Thin ringlike shadows of barium may mark the limit of the column, representing material caught in the haustral crevices as they surround the mass of intussuscepted bowel. As the hydrostatic pressure of the enema becomes effective it will be noticed that the barium column moves proximally, the concavity of its end being maintained (Fig. 18-16). If successful, the intussusception may be reduced completely, the entire colon filling and barium refluxing through the ileocecal valve into the ileum.

Although there has been objection to the use of this method for the nonoperative reduction of intussusception, the majority opinion seems to be in favor of it, at least as a preliminary measure of treatment. The objections raised have included the danger of rupture of the friable bowel by manipulation during the procedure, the possibility of incomplete reduction being overlooked (persisting ileoileal intussusception

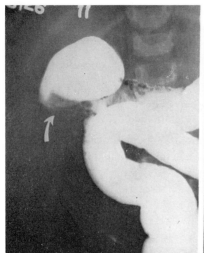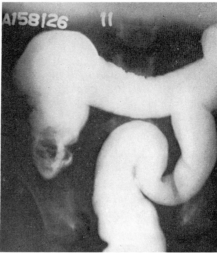

Fig. 18-16. Ileocolic intussusception in a young child. *Left,* Roentgenogram made during barium enema, showing the intussusception partially reduced. The obstruction was encountered in the distal transverse colon but gradually reduced to the point shown here. The concavity of the barium column (**arrow**) marks the intussusceptum. *Right,* Second roentgenogram made shortly after the one on the left shows further reduction of the intussusception but this still is not complete and the mass of intussuscepted ileum can be seen projecting into the cecum.

after the reduction of the ileocolic phase), and the possibility of missing a lesion that might have been a causative factor, such as a Meckel's diverticulum. These are not serious objections provided that certain precautions are observed. The enema container should not be elevated more than 3 feet above the level of the table and only hydrostatic pressure should be used; manual palpation in an attempt to facilitate the reduction should be avoided; free filling of the terminal ileum must be obatained. In addition there should be disappearance of any mass previously palpable and a prompt subsidence of the clinical signs of obstruction. In uncomplicated intussusception there usually is little evidence of obstruction in plain-film roentgenograms of the abdomen. If there is demonstrated dilated, gas-filled loops of bowel, thickening of the bowel wall, or other signs of significant obstruction or inflammation, hydrostatic reduction should not be attempted since these findings usually indicate that complications such as gangrene, obstruction, and peritonitis are present. If these precautions are observed there is little danger in the procedure as shown by published statistics of large series of cases.

In the adult, intussusception of the small intestine most often develops as a result of a polypoid tumor and this is true of intussusception of the colon as well. This may be a polypoid carcinoma or an intramural lesion, such as a lipoma or leiomyoma, which forms an intraluminal mass, sometimes with a pedicle. The roentgen findings are hardly different from those encountered during infancy. Occasionally the polypoid mass of the tumor may be recognized as the barium column surrounds the intussusception. The tumor mass usually is situated at the leading edge of the intussusceptum and thus will be surrounded by barium mixture. In many patients, however, the defect of the tumor cannot be identified clearly and only the mass of bowel projecting into the lumen is recognizable. Frequently, the mucosal folds stretched over the intussusceptum may be coated with barium, resulting in an appearance likened to a coiled spring. This is a highly significant finding in intussusception (see Fig. 19-11).

HYPOPROTEINEMIA; INTESTINAL EDEMA

There are a number of diseases that can cause excessive loss of protein from the gastrointestinal tract with resulting hypoproteinemia. These include such entities as Menetrier's disease (page 537), intestinal lymphangiectasia (page 588), regional enteritis (page 579), ulcerative colitis (page 622), lymphosarcoma (page 577) and Whipple's disease (page 587). These diseases have frequently been listed under the term *protein-losing enteropathies*. The hypoproteinemia causes noninflammatory intestinal edema. The roentgen findings in edema consist of generalized and uniform thickening of the mucosal folds (Fig. 18-17), interference with normal motor activity of the bowel, thickening of the wall of the intestine and, in some, ascites.[22] Some dilatation of the intestinal lumen often is seen but segmentation and flocculation are absent. Because the intestinal walls are thickened, some widening of the soft-tissue spaces between adjacent loops may be seen. The uniformly thickened folds with a continuous column of barium in the lumen has been likened to a stack of coins. The changes often are seen to best advantage in the jejunum.

Hypoproteinemia also occurs as a result of kidney or liver disease (cirrhosis) and the roentgen signs of edema of the bowel become apparent. It also has been found in a variety of other conditions such as congestive heart failure, burns, allergy, the Zollinger-Ellison syndrome, sprue, neoplasms, histoplasmosis of the small intestine with giant villi and secondary protein-losing enteropathy, the Cronkite-Canada syndrome and constrictive pericarditis, among others. A correlation with the clinical findings is helpful in evaluating the roentgen findings of intestinal edema. The symptoms are those of the primary disease and not of the intestinal edema. The primary disease (e.g., regional enteritis, Menetrier's disease, lymphosarcoma) often can be identified with considerable assurance from the roentgen appearances but, in other instances, the signs are only those of edema. Many of the diseases that cause intestinal edema also cause a malabsorption syndrome and it has been speculated that some of the changes seen in malabsorption are the result of edema.

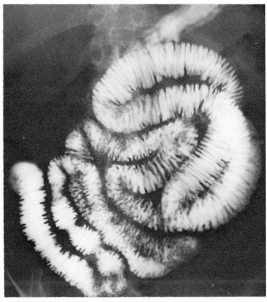

Fig. 18-17. Intestinal edema. The patient had a carcinoma of the pancreas with dissemination. The uniform thickening of mucosal folds is characteristic and was shown at autopsy to be caused by submucosal edema.

DIVERTICULOSIS

Diverticulosis of the jejunum is an uncommon but not rare entity characterized by a few or many diverticular outpouchings. The sacs vary in size from tiny ones up to some measuring 2 cm or more. Occasionally they are very numerous and often are associated with diverticula of the duodenum. They show the roentgen characteristics of diverticula elsewhere in the gastrointestinal tract and consist of a smooth-walled sac communicating with the lumen through a narrow neck. In some patients there is an associated *malabsorption syndrome*. Isolated diverticula also occur in the terminal ileum. Acute infection of the diverticulum may cause the symptoms and signs simulating acute appendicitis.

MESENTERIC VASCULAR OCCLUSION

ACUTE MESENTERIC OCCLUSION

The occurrence of acute obstruction of the superior or inferior mesenteric arteries or veins owing to embolus or thrombosis results in an acute, severe illness with infarction of the bowel, necrosis, peritonitis and, usually, death. Most patients are too ill for barium studies to be performed. The plain-film findings in acute mesenteric occlusion have been discussed in Chapter 13 under the heading "Acute Mesenteric Vascular Occlusion."

SEGMENTAL ISCHEMIA

If the vascular occlusion occurs gradually and there is an adequate collateral blood flow infarction may not develop and there are no positive roentgen changes. Also if the occlusion involves a small branch vessel and perforation does not occur, the patient may survive and later show roentgen findings that become fairly characteristic. This has been called segmental ischemia or, depending on the location, ischemic jejunitis, ileitis, or colitis.

Abdominal roentgenograms may reveal positive signs of the disease in some patients. One or several segments of small intestine will be outlined by gas in the lumen. Thickening of the bowel wall can be identified if two segments lie adjacent to one another. The luminal surface may become smooth with effacement of the normal fold pattern (or haustral sacculations in the colon). The segments appear rigid and the appearance does not change significantly in serial films taken over a period of several days. If necrosis of the intestinal wall develops, intramural gas sometimes is seen as thin, radiolucent, gas stripes paralleling the bowel lumen (i.e., *pneumatosis intestinalis*). Gas in the portal vein branches within the liver is found infrequently but carries a grave prognosis, most patients succumbing to the disease. The combination of intramural gas and portal vein gas form a significant roentgen diagnostic complex for intestinal necrosis. If a small-bowel barium study is done the involved segment shows thickening of mucosal folds and nodular indentations along the margins called "thumbprinting" or "scalloping" owing to submucosal hemorrhage or edema. As the edema increases the folds become greatly thickened. If diffuse ulceration develops the folds become effaced and the lumen becomes smooth. This is more obvious in the jejunum because of the greater number of folds present normally. With healing and fibrosis one wall may become flattened and shortened and multiple sacculations or pseudo-diverticula form on the opposite border. Further fibrosis leads to a rigid tubular appearance followed shortly by stricture formation and dilatation of the bowel above the stricture. The strictured area is usually several inches long and is characterized by smooth tapering ends and a concentric lumen. The entire gamut of these changes occurs rapidly, often only a matter of several weeks from onset to stricture formation. Similar changes occur in the colon when it is involved by segmental ischemia. In the earlier stages the appearance resembles intramural hemorrhage. When stricture formation develops, regional enteritis must be considered in differential diagnosis.

INTESTINAL PARASITES

The demonstration of roundworms in the intestinal tract is possible when a small-intestine study is carried out. The worm may be visualized as an elongated, tubular filling defect in the barium-filled loop of bowel (Fig. 18-18). Because the worm may ingest some of the barium, it is not uncommon to find a thin, dense, stringlike shadow centrally situated within the filling defect produced by the body of the worm. This stringlike shadow represents the barium-filled gastrointestinal tract of the worm. Follow-up roentgenograms after the bowel has emptied itself of the barium mixture (3 to 5 hours after ingestion) may then show the persisting string of barium, which may remain for some hours. The usual location for these defects is in the distal jejunum and proximal portion of the ileum. Only occasionally are worms recognized in the colon.

Tapeworms also can occasionally be demonstrated in the small intestine as long, linear

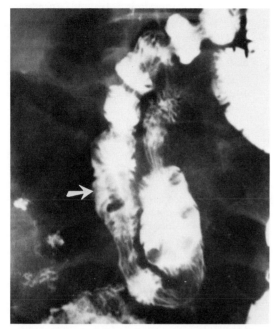

Fig. 18-18. Ascaris in the small intestine. A loop of bowel is shown. The worms are seen as elongated, linear defects (**arrow**) or as round translucencies when the worm is visualized on end.

translucencies. A tapeworm is differentiated from a roundworm because of its greater length and by the absence of the stringlike barium shadow outlining the intestinal tract of the worm as the tapeworm does not have an alimentary canal. Other parasitic infestations are rare in this country. They often produce changes in the duodenum and jejunum that can hardly be distinguished from regional enteritis. These include infestation with *Giardia lamblia* and *Strongyloides stercoralis*. Parasitic disease can be a cause of the malabsorption syndrome.

DISACCHARIDASE DEFICIENCY

Because they are necessary for the digestion of sugars, deficiency of lactase, sucrase, or fructase may give rise to symptoms of abdominal discomfort and distention, flatulence, and diarrhea. Lactase deficiency is said to be the most common abnormality of the small intestine. Normally, it is present in the epithelial cells of the small bowel. Suitable roentgen study may demonstrate signifi-

cant changes. The patient is given a nonflocculating barium mixture to which has been added 25 to 50 gm of lactose. Interval films of the small intestine will show a dilution of the barium in the small bowel, dilatation of loops, and an increased transit time so that the head of the barium column will be in the colon at the end of 1 hour or sooner. These signs are accompanied by abdominal cramps and diarrhea. It has been recommended that lactose be added to the barium mixture for all small-bowel examinations since it does not alter the quality of the study if there is no lactase deficiency.

INTRA-ABDOMINAL HERNIAS

Hernias affecting the intestinal tract may be either external or internal. The diagnosis of external hernia is essentially a clinical problem and roentgen examination is used chiefly to determine the contents of the hernial sac and to demonstrate how much, if any, obstruction is present. The roentgen aspects of external hernia are considered in Chapter 19 and will not be repeated here.

In internal hernias the intestinal protrusions are entirely within the peritoneal cavity. The abnormal sac or pouch may have been caused by trauma. More frequently the rent in the mesentery or peritoneum follows a surgical procedure. Also, some internal hernias develop on the basis of congenital defects with the formation of abnormal pouches or fossae. The incidence of intra-abdominal hernias in clinical practice is low. The congenital hernias, in particular, may exist without producing symptoms. When symptoms are caused by an internal hernia they are usually those of bowel obstruction.

Of the congenital types of internal hernia, those involving the paraduodenal fossae are generally considered to be the most important; left paraduodenal hernia is about four times as frequent as the right-sided type. When complete obstruction of the intestine is caused by an internal hernia, the roentgen findings are those of bowel obstruction (q.v.), and the nature of the causative lesion seldom can be stated. In those lesions causing only partial obstruction the diagnosis is possible in some cases. The same is true of the asymptomatic hernias. The roentgen findings depend upon the site of the hernia and the amount of bowel involved but, in general, consist in the visualization of an abnormal accumulation of the barium-filled loops of small intestine into a sac-like

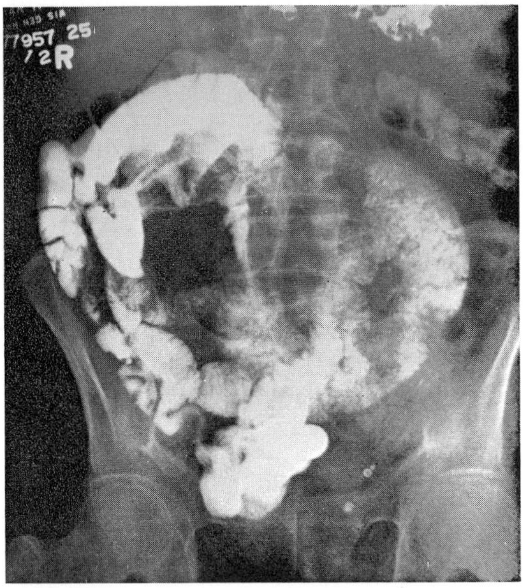

Fig. 18-19. Internal abdominal hernia into the left paraduodenal fossa. A large portion of the jejunum lies within the hernia sac. The margins of the sac are rather clearly identified.

configuration (Fig. 18-19). The afferent and efferent loops may be identified as they enter and leave the sac. There may be an abnormal retention of barium within the herniated loops and, if partial obstruction is present, the bowel above the level of the hernia will be dilated. The colon often is found in an abnormal position and the relationships of the colon and small intestine may be distinctly abnormal.

REFERENCES AND SELECTED READINGS

1. BAKER, H. L., and GOOD, C. A.: Smooth-muscle tumors of the alimentary tract: Their roentgen manifestations. *Am. J. Roentgenol. Radium Ther. Nucl. Med. 74:* 246, 1955.

2. BALIKIAN, J. P., NASSAR, N. T., SHAMMA'A, M. H., and SHADID, M. J.: Primary lymphomas of the small intestine including the duodenum. *Am. J. Roentgenol. Radium Ther. Nucl. Med. 107:* 131, 1969.

3. BISCHOFF, M. E., and STAMPFLI, W. P.: Meckel's diverticulum: With emphasis on the roentgen diagnosis. *Radiology 65:* 572, 1955.

4. BLUTH, I.: Gastrointestinal carcinoid tumors: Roentgen features. *Radiology 74:* 573, 1960.

5. CLEMETT, A. R., FISHBONE, G., LEVINE, R. J., JAMES, A. E., and JANOWER, M.: Gastrointestinal

lesions in mastocytosis. *Am. J. Roentgenol. Radium Ther. Nucl. Med. 103:* 405, 1968.

6. CLEMETT, A. R., and MARSHAK, R. H.: Whipple's disease. Roentgen features and differential diagnosis. *Radiol. Clin. North Am. 7:* 105, 1969.

7. COHEN, W. N.: Gastric involvement in Crohn's disease. *Am. J. Roentgenol. Radium Ther. Nucl. Med. 101:* 425, 1967.

8. COHEN, W. N.: Intestinal lymphangiectasis. *Radiology 89:* 1080, 1967.

9. CROHN, B. B., and JANOWITZ, H. D.: Reflections on regional ileitis, twenty years later. *JAMA 156:* 1221, 1954.

10. DEEB, P. H., and STILSON, W. L.: Roentgen manifestations of lymphosarcoma of the small bowel. *Radiology 63:* 235, 1954.

11. FERRUCCI, J. T., BENEDICT, K. T., PAGE, D. L., FLEISCHLI, D. J., and EATON, S. B.: Radiographic features of the normal hypotonic duodenogram. *Radiology 96:* 401, 1970.

12. GOLDEN, R.: Amyloidosis of the small intestine. *Am. J. Roentgenol. Radium Ther. Nucl. Med. 72:* 401, 1954.

13. GOLDSTEIN, H. M., POOLE, G. J., ROSENQUIST, C. J., FREIDLAND, G. N., and ZBORALSKI, F. F.: Comparison of methods for acceleration of small intestinal radiographic examination. *Radiology 98:* 519, 1971.

14. GOOD, C. A.: Tumors of the small intestine. Caldwell lecture, 1962. *Am. J. Roentgenol. Radium Ther. Nucl. Med. 89:* 685, 1963.

15. HARPER, R. A. K.: "New Advances in Radiology of the Gastrointestinal Tract," in *Modern Trends in Diagnostic Radiology-4,* ed. by J. W. McLaren. New York, Appleton-Century-Crofts, 1970.

16. HODGSON, J. R., HOFFMAN, H. N., II, and HUIZENGA, K. A.: Roentgenologic features of lymphoid hyperplasia of the small intestine associated with dysgammaglobulinemia. *Radiology 88:* 883, 1967.

17. ISBELL, R. G., CARLSON, H. C., and HOFFMAN, H. N., II: Roentgenologic-pathologic correlation in malabsorption syndromes. *Am. J. Roentgenol. Radium Ther. Nucl. Med. 107:* 158, 1969.

18. JAMES, W. B., and MELROSE, A. G.: Metoclopramide in gastrointestinal radiology. *Clin. Radiol. 20:* 57, 1969.

19. LAWS, J. W., SPENCER, J., and NEALE, G.: Radiology in the diagnosis of disaccharidase deficiency. *Br. J. Radiol. 40:* 594, 1967.

20. LING, J-T.: Intussusception in infants and children with emphasis on the recognition of cases with complications. *Radiology 62:* 505, 1954.

21. MARSHAK, R. H., KHILNANI, M., ELIASOPH, M.,

and WOLF, B. S.: Intestinal edema. *Am. J. Roentgenol. Radium Ther. Nucl. Med. 101:* 379, 1967.

22. MARSHAK, R. H., and LINDNER, A. E.: *Radiology of the Small Intestine.* Philadelphia, Saunders, 1970.

23. MIERCORT, R. D., and MERRIL, F. G.: Pneumatosis and pseudo-obstruction in scleroderma. *Radiology 92:* 359, 1969.

24. MILLER, R. E.: Reflux examination of the small bowel. *Radiol. Clin. North Am. 7:* 175, 1969.

25. PAUL, L. W., and WINSTON, M. C.: Focal constricting inflammatory lesions of the small intestine. *Am. J. Roentgenol. Radium Ther. Nucl. Med. 81:* 616, 1959.

26. POCK-STEEN, O. CH.: Roentgenologic changes in protein-losing enteropathies. *Acta Radiol. (Diag.) 4:* 681, 1966.

27. RAVITCH, M. M., and McCUNE, R. M.: Intussusception in infants and children: Analysis of 152 cases with discussion of reduction by barium enema. *J. Pediat. 37:* 153, 1950.

28. SNODGRASS, J. J.: Transdiaphragmatic duplication of the alimentary tract. *Am. J. Roentgenol. Radium Ther. Nucl. Med. 69:* 42, 1953.

29. TOD, P. A.: Radiological facets of malabsorption. *Australas. Radiol. 12:* 121, 1968.

30. WERBELOFF, L., BANK, S., and MARKS, I. N.: Radiological findings in protein-losing gastroenteropathy. *Br. J. Radiol. 42:* 605, 1969.

31. ZBORALSKI, F. F., and AMBERG, J. R.: Detection of the Zollinger-Ellison syndrome: The radiologist's responsibility. *Am. J. Roentgenol. Radium Ther. Nucl. Med. 104:* 529, 1968.

19

THE COLON

METHODS OF EXAMINATION

PRELIMINARY ROENTGENOGRAMS

It is good practice to obtain a scout roentgenogram of the abdomen prior to the introduction of contrast material into any part of the gastrointestinal tract. In the examination of the colon the conditions in which plain roentgenograms are of value include (*1*) obstructing lesions, (*2*) perforations, and (*3*) foreign bodies. These and other abnormalities have been discussed in Chapter 13 and the reader is referred to it for further details.

CONTRAST VISUALIZATION

THE ORAL MEAL

Barium given orally and followed through the gastrointestinal tract by means of serial roentgenograms is of limited value for the detection of organic lesions of the colon. This method may give some information in functional abnormalities of the bowel and it is useful in the investigation of errors of rotation. If obstruction of the colon is known to be present or is suspected, barium sulfate should not be given by mouth because of the likelihood of its becoming impacted above the obstruction. In general the roentgen study of the colon for the

detection of organic disease depends upon a barium-enema examination.

BARIUM-ENEMA EXAMINATION

PREPARATION OF THE COLON. For satisfactory examination it is necessary that the colon be cleansed thoroughly of fecal matter. This is most important if a search is being made for a source of bleeding. The accurate identification of small polyps is possible only when there are no confusing shadows caused by retained fecal lumps. The routine procedures used in the preparation of the adult colon are as follows:

1. Castor oil is given at bedtime the evening before the examination. The dose varies from 1 to 2 ounces, with the larger amount being preferred. Castor oil catharsis is contraindicated in the presence of acute intra-abdominal inflammatory disease, when bowel obstruction is believed to be present, and when there has been recent severe hemorrhage. Saline cathartics should not be used because they leave a residue of fluid in the colon. Some of the newer laxatives such as bisacodyl (Dulcolax) also give good results as a substitute for castor oil.

2. Food should not be taken on the morning of the examination. This is done to avoid stimulating small-bowel peristalsis and the movement of small-intestine contents into the colon.

3. A cleansing enema of warm tap water is

given from 1 to 2 hours before fluoroscopy. Soapsuds should not be used in the enema because of the tendency for it to cause a fluid residue in the colon.

4. Proctoscopic examination done immediately preceding the barium enema often leaves a large amount of air within the colon and this interferes with fluorscopic study. It is helpful in these cases to use a cleansing enema of tap water after completion of the proctoscopic examination and about an hour before fluoroscopy is to be done. This procedure aids in eliminating the gas and improves the preparation for barium-enema examination.

The preparation of the infant colon is generally similar to that for the adult patient, particularly if the examination is being done for the detection of polyps. Less drastic procedures are adequate for most other conditions, such as the identification of errors of rotation, partial or complete obstruction, and megacolon. *The introduction of a large quantity of water into the colon should be avoided in megacolon because of the danger of causing water intoxication.* In those cases in which castor oil is not used, one or two cleansing enemas of warm tap water will suffice.

When ulcerative colitis is known to be present or when diarrhea is a significant symptom, castor oil or other cathartics should be omitted. In these cases we have found it advantageous to use warm, normal saline solution for the cleansing enema. This should be given slowly to avoid overdistention of the colon and the quantity of the enema should be reduced. Frequently 200 to 300 cc of solution are sufficient to remove fecal residues and accumulations of mucus and allow good visualization of the mucosal surface.

BARIUM MIXTURES. The standard enema mixture used by us consists of 300 gm of barium sulfate powder added to each 1000 cc of tap water. It is better to weigh the barium sulfate rather than to measure it by volume since this assures a more accurate control of the density of the mixture and a uniform consistency from day to day.

In the past it was common practice to add "fluffy" tannic acid powder to the barium mixture to promote evacuation of the barium enema and give a better mucosal pattern in the post-evacuation study. However because of some evidence that tannic acid might be toxic particularly to the liver its use was banned a few years ago by the Federal Food and Drug Administration. Recently the use of a substance called Clysodrast has received approval. This contains a bisacodyl salt of tannic acid and can be added to the barium mixture in the amount of two packets per 2000 ml of mixture. It promotes colonic peristalsis and precipitates mucus that might otherwise cling to the mucosa. The result is an improved post-evacuation study. Present contraindications include: 1) patients under 10 years of age, 2) pregnancy, and 3) known or suspected ulcerative disease.

Gianturco has advocated the use of high kilovoltage technique in roentgenography of the filled colon in order to visualize small polyps more easily. Roentgenograms made with kilovoltages above 100 often allow one to "see through" the dense barium shadow and small filling defects are not likely to be obscured by the layer of barium overlying them. Potter[36] and others have recommended the use of a thin barium-water mixture to accomplish the same purpose. Unfortunately, with a thin mixture fluoroscopic visualization is very unsatisfactory. Because we consider it to be a very important part of the examination our own preference is for a thicker suspension.

TECHNIQUE OF EXAMINATION. The barium mixture is introduced into the colon by gravity, using a disposable barium enema unit. The container is placed from 2 to 3 feet above the top of the fluoroscopic table. The mixture is allowed to flow into the colon slowly in order to avoid overdistention of the rectum which may precipitate defecation. If difficulty is encountered or expected a small Foley type of balloon catheter can be used in place of the hard rectal tip, the balloon being inflated with no more than 30 cc of air. This is useful also in examining the colon after colostomy. If ulcerative colitis is present or if there is a rectal stricture a balloon should not be used because of the danger of rupture of the rectum.

The flow of mixture is observed by fluoroscopy from the moment it enters the rectum until satisfactory filling of the colon has been obtained or the examination is discontinued for other reasons. The patient is rotated into various positions to bring the flexures and the loops of sigmoid into profile. Manual palpation with the lead-glove-protected hand or a palpating spoon is used to separate overlying loops, to determine the pliability of the walls, and to bring out small intraluminal defects. When the barium column reaches the cecum the flow is discontinued. Ordinarily there will be reflux into the terminal ileum either when the cecum fills or later during evacuation of the enema. When the ileum fills, this segment of the small intestine can be examined; also it locates the ileocecal valve and this is an anatomic landmark that assures that the entire colon has been filled. At times ileal filling is a disadvantage because the barium-filled loops may obscure some part of the colon that is under suspicion or in which a lesion has been found. The sigmoid often is hidden in this way. Filling of the ileum should be avoided if a double-contrast examination is to be done, as described in a later paragraph. Sometimes ileal filling can be prevented by stopping the flow of mixture when the head of the column has reached the hepatic flexure. The pressure that has been built up in the distal colon, combined with manual palpation, may cause the ascending colon and cecum to fill. A slow administration of the enema and avoidance of too much distention of any part of the colon also may prevent reflux, at least until after the patient has been allowed to evacuate the enema.

During filling, spot roentgenograms are made of suspicious areas or of any region that is difficult to visualize in standard roentgenograms, such as the flexures and the sigmoid loops. We have no fixed pattern for spot filming but vary our procedure from patient to patient, depending upon the nature of the problem.

After completion of fluoroscopy a roentgenogram of the abdomen is exposed with the patient in a prone position; evacuation of the mixture then is allowed and a postevacuation roentgenogram obtained. Variations from this more or less routine procedure are available. Lateral roentgenograms are helpful at times and fluoroscopy after the patient has evacuated the mixture may be useful.

In searching for small polyps a double-contrast examination can be done (Fig. 19-1). In this procedure barium and air are combined as contrast media. While a number of different techniques for this procedure have been described, including methods that combine a regular barium enema

with the double-contrast examination, we prefer to do it as a separate procedure and only when the regular examination has not given all the information desired. The double-contrast examination is time-consuming and expensive. A complete fluoroscopic study of the entire colon and the terminal ileum cannot be done very well if a double-contrast procedure is to follow because filling of the right side must be avoided during fluoroscopy. Thorough preparation of the colon is very necessary because fecal lumps and small accumulations of mucus may simulate polyps very closely and unless the colon is free of such material the examination usually is unsatisfactory no matter what method is used. Castor oil catharsis and preparatory cleansing enemas are given as described previously. For filling of the colon we use the same mixture as for the regular barium enema. The use of one of the fine, micropulverized barium sulfate powders is recommended for double-contrast examination of the colon. A better adherence of the mixture to the mucosa results and there is less tendency for the barium to clump, leaving large areas of the surface of the mucosa without a barium coating. Filling should be discontinued when the barium column reaches the midpart of the transverse colon. The patient is asked to evacuate the mixture. As soon as this has been accomplished, fluoroscopy of the abdomen again is performed. Usually a small amount of the barium will be found distributed throughout the colon, the ideal being a thin uniform coating of the mucosa. If too much barium remains, the patient is requested to attempt further evacuation. When it appears that a satisfactory distribution of the residual barium has been obtained, air is injected under fluoroscopic control until the entire colon has been moderately distended. This part of the examination should be done without too much delay for otherwise the barium tends to separate from the mucosa and a satisfactory double contrast is not obtained. For the air injection a rubber rectal tube and a hand-operated bulb are used. After completion of the air injection a series of roentgenograms is made (Fig. 19-1). Usually these are made with the patient prone and supine and turned into right and left oblique positions. In some cases stereoscopic roentgenograms are made; these are useful when redundant loops overlie one another. Right and left lateral decubitus views may be obtained in place of the oblique projections.

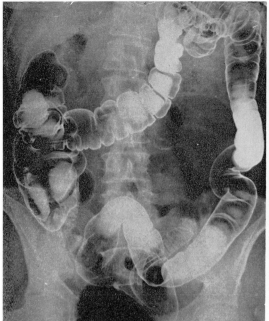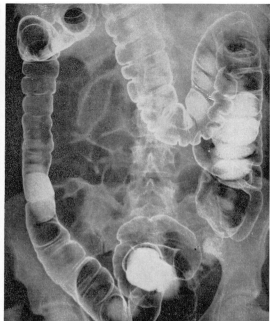

Fig. 19-1. Double contrast examination of the colon. Two roentgenograms of a series. *Left,* Roentgenogram made with the patient prone. *Right,* Patient in a supine position. Oblique and lateral decubitus projections are also valuable; multiple positions cause shifting of residual barium and a different distribution of gas in various segments to allow better visualization. (*Courtesy Dr. Ames W. Naslund, Minneapolis, Minn.*)

OTHER METHODS

A number of special methods have been introduced which can be used in particular circumstances.[29]

AEROSOL-FOAM ENEMA. This is similar to the double-contrast examination but with the introduction of aerosol shaving cream after barium has been administered by rectum.

WATER ENEMA. This is used to show the increased radiolucency of a lipoma, once the lesion has been identified as a mass on regular barium-enema study.

ARTERIOGRAPHY. Arteriography of the mesenteric arteries, preferably by selective catheterization of the vessels has been used to locate bleeding sites in the colon that cannot be detected by more conventional means. Some tumors can be identified particularly if they are highly vascular. However, many tumors are not and routine barium enema study may be more reliable in these patients.

THE NORMAL COLON

ANATOMY AND PHYSIOLOGY

The discussion to follow deals mainly with the appearance of the colon, (*1*) when fully distended by means of a barium enema, and (*2*) when contracted after the barium enema has been expelled. These are the conditions under which most roentgenograms of the colon are obtained (Fig. 19-2). Only those aspects of anatomy and physiology of particular interest from a roentgen point of view will be included and the reader is referred to standard texts dealing with these subjects for more basic information.

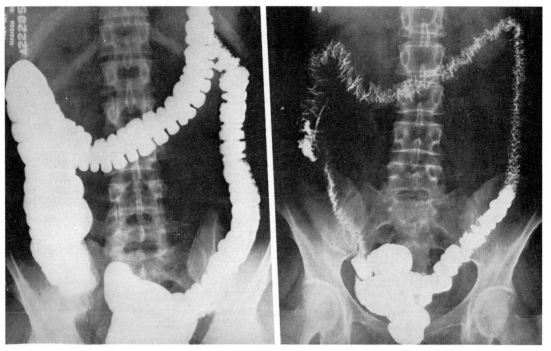

Fig. 19-2. Normal colon. *Left,* Roentgenogram of the barium-filled colon with patient in a prone position. *Right,* Roentgenogram made after evacuation of the barium mixture, showing the colon contracted and the mucosa thrown into fine crinkled folds. In this postevacuation roentgenogram there has been reflux of the barium into the terminal ileum. Note the retrocecal position of the appendix.

THE DIVISIONS OF THE COLON

The usual anatomic divisions of the colon can be recognized in most patients and ordinary anatomic usage is followed in the description of roentgenograms.

ILEOCECAL VALVE, CECUM, AND APPENDIX. The junction of the ileum and cecum is a most important roentgen landmark. While considerable variation exists in the structure of the normal valve, the studies of Fleischner and Bernstein and of Lasser and Rigler indicate the following roentgen features to be of significance.

Of the two lips forming the valve the superior is the longer. As they project into the filled cecum from the medial side and are viewed in profile, these lips cause filling defects, one above the other and separated by a small extension of barium that may, if ileal reflux has occurred, be continuous with the barium-filled lumen of the ileum. The lips seen in this manner measure from 2 to 5 mm in width (Fig. 19-3).

If the ileocecal valve is on the posterior surface

and compression is applied over the cecum the valve appears as a transverse, spindle-shaped filling defect with a small pocket of barium in the center representing the opening of the valve (see Fig. 19-3, *right*).

Thickening of the valve lips is not infrequent. In some patients this is caused by an accumulation of fatty tissue; in others hypertrophy of the muscle coats is responsible; in still other patients it is caused by a protrusion of ileal mucosa beyond the valve lips. This latter condition resembles closely the protrusion of gastric mucosa through the pylorus, which has been discussed in Chapter 17 under the heading "Prolapse of Gastric Mucosa through the Pylorus." The significance of these conditions is doubtful but the defect in barium filling caused by a prominent valve may resemble a polypoid or an intramural tumor. The correct interpretation depends upon establishing its relationship to the filled ileum, the smoothly rounded contour of the mass with a small accumulation of barium in the center indicating the valve opening, the occasional stellate radiation of mucosal folds from the center of the defect,

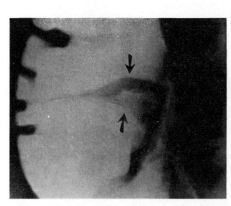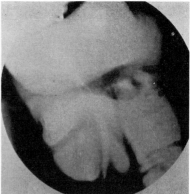

Fig. 19-3. The ileocecal valve. *Left,* Compression roentgenogram of the ileocecal area made during fluoroscopy, showing the terminal ileum projecting downward from the medial side of the cecum and the lips of the valve forming a spindle-shaped translucency in the medial aspects of the cecum (**arrows**). *Right,* Spot roentgenogram of the filled cecum and ileum of another patient in whom the ileocecal valve is situated on the posterior wall of the cecum and is seen *en face.* Note also the filling of the appendix, demonstrating it to be in a retrocecal position.

and by changes in shape of the defect during examination when it is caused by mucosal prolapse.

The appendix arises from the base of the cecum on the side of the ileocecal valve. When the valve is on the posterior surface of the cecum the appendix almost always is in a retrocecal position. The ileocecal valve therefore serves as a fairly good indicator of appendiceal location. Following appendectomy and inversion of the appendiceal stump, a small polypoid defect in the base of the cecum may be visualized. This is caused by the invaginated stump and may resemble the defect of a true polyp. A history of previous appendectomy and the location of the defect aid in identifying it correctly (see Fig. 19-4).

The cecum is surrounded completely by peritoneum and thus has a fair degree of mobility. A portion of the ascending colon also may be surrounded by peritoneum and, in some individuals, there may be a distinct mesentery. In these the cecum and ascending colon are unusually mobile and the position of the cecum may vary widely from time to time. It is in these patients that volvulus of the cecum can develop.

THE ASCENDING COLON. Except for that portion immediately adjacent to the cecum, the ascending colon ordinarily is retroperitoneal in location and is covered by peritoneum only on the anterior surface. At the hepatic flexure the colon turns toward the midline and forward to form the beginning of the transverse portion, and it acquires a mesentery. The length of the ascending colon is variable. In some persons it is very long and the cecum is situated within the pelvis.

THE TRANSVERSE COLON. This part of the colon has a mesentery and is freely movable. It is displaced easily by manual palpation and by masses within the abdomen. It varies in length from one individual to another. In persons of asthenic habitus it may extend into the pelvis and overlie the sigmoid. The flexures also may be unusually low in such individuals. The position of the colon has little to do with its function in most cases and the diagnosis of visceroptosis should carry no implication that functional derangement must be associated. The transverse colon and the hepatic flexure occasionally are found interposed between the liver and the diaphragm. As a rule this displacement is a transient one and usually has no clinical significance.

THE DESCENDING COLON. The splenic flexure is one of the most fixed parts of the gastrointestinal tract, being held to the diaphragm by the phrenicocolic ligament. The flexure and the entire descending colon are retroperitoneal in position and there usually is no mesentery. Infrequently this is not true and a mesentery is present allowing a certain amount of medial and lateral movement.

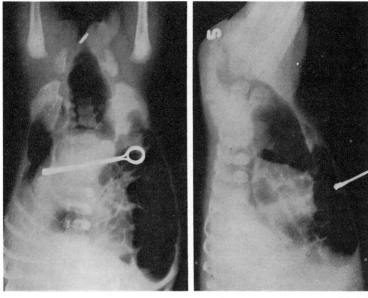

Fig. 19-4. Imperforate anus. Anteroposterior (*left*) and lateral (*right*) roentgenograms with the patient inverted at the time the exposures were made and with a lead marker placed over the anal dimple. Gas, ascended into the rectum, demonstrates that the atretic segment is short, no more than a centimeter.

The junction of the descending colon and the sigmoid is indicated anatomically by the emergence of the colon from the retroperitoneal space and the development of a mesentery for the sigmoid portion. This occurs just below the iliac crest within the left fossa. This junction is usually not very distinct in roentgenograms and can be located only approximately.

THE SIGMOID COLON. Having a long mesentery, the sigmoid colon is freely movable. The length is variable but usually the sigmoid executes one or two loops within the pelvis. It may be very long and extend upward on the left side as high as the splenic flexure. In other patients it curves to the right side as far as the cecum before turning back toward the midline and then to the left to its junction with the descending portion. Extreme elongation and mobility of the sigmoid predispose to volvulus.

THE RECTUM. The junction of the rectum and the sigmoid is not an abrupt one in roentgenograms, although anatomically it represents a change from the colon with a mesentery to the rectum, which has none and lies in the retroperitoneal space. Proctoscopy is the method of choice for examination of the rectum and routine roentgen methods used in examining the colon should not be relied upon for diagnosis. Many rectal lesions, such as fungating carcinomas and ulcerative colitis, can be demonstrated clearly by roentgen examination but at other times significant lesions are not identified. This is caused chiefly by the great distensibility of the rectum. During the administration of the enema it is filled with a large amount of barium and small lesions may be covered completely. The rectum being situated within the pelvis cannot be palpated during fluoroscopy and this aid to roentgen diagnosis is not available.

THE COLON AS A WHOLE

The colon is characterized by the presence of haustral sacculations and by the taeniae coli; these give it an appearance distinct from the remainder of the gastrointestinal tract. The taeniae are three longitudinal muscle bands that extend from the tip of the cecum to the lower part of the sigmoid and constitute the majority of the longitudinal musculature of this portion of the tract. The haustra are saclike pouches separated by crescentic folds made up of all the layers of bowel wall.

The sacculations vary from 1 to 5 cm in length and are most constant in the right half of the colon. Haustra are variably present in the lower part of the descending colon and sigmoid, although usually demonstrable in these areas. The haustra are not completely fixed and serial roentgen studies carried out over a period of minutes show a constant change in the depth of the crescentic folds and in the width of the sacculations. This leads to a certain amount of forward and backward movement, known as haustral churning. The diameter of the colon decreases from the cecum to the rectosigmoid junction.

The length of the colon varies greatly in the newborn and during infancy. Elongation of the sigmoid is the rule but the rest of the colon may be unusually redundant. The elongation tends to diminish as the child grows older but even in the adult one must allow a wide range of variation for the normal before considering that abnormal elongation is present.

After evacuation of the barium mixture, a thin coating usually remains on the mucosal surface. When contracted the mucous membrane is thrown into a network of folds, giving it a fine, crinkled relief (see Fig. 19-2). Occasionally in the lower part of the descending and sigmoid areas the folds are more or less parallel and run in the direction of the long axis of the bowel. Otherwise parallel folds of this type usually are seen only momentarily and in short lengths of the bowel; they are caused by the presence of a mass peristaltic contraction.

During the process of evacuation the colon contracts in length as well as in breadth; if redundant loops are present in the filled colon, they often are reduced in length or disappear completely in the contracted state.

MOVEMENTS OF THE COLON

The forward movement of contents in the cecum and ascending colon often seems to be the result only of the constant addition of material from the small intestine. Serial studies often show only a gradual forward movement of the head of the barium column, which may continue until it is well along in the transverse colon. The chief means of movement of fecal material into the distal part of the colon is by mass peristaltic contractions. In the normal these probably occur only a few times a day. During a barium enema examination when the colon has been made irritable by catharsis and by the distention from the enema, mass contractions are seen occasionally. Usually in these cases the contraction wave begins in the ascending colon, moving with moderate speed and pushing the colonic content before it. Within a few seconds the wave will have reached the descending colon or occasionally the sigmoid. In some it may stop before reaching the splenic flexure. Once forward progress of the contraction has been halted the colon relaxes and usually refills. In some patients, while the contraction is in progress the desire to defecate is strong and the enema may be expelled.

Reference has been made to haustral churning movements in a previous paragraph. These are very slow movements and can be visualized only by exposing serial roentgenograms at intervals of from 15 to 30 seconds over a period of several minutes. They are studied to best advantage when the colon has been filled by means of a barium meal. The haustral movements are not believed to play any part in the forward propulsion of colonic content; rather the type of motion suggests that they are a means of constantly changing the material that is in contact with the colonic mucosa.

CONGENITAL MALFORMATIONS

ERRORS OF ROTATION

During its development the intestinal tract is described as consisting of the foregut, the midgut, and the hindgut. During early fetal life the midgut grows so rapidly that it cannot be contained within the abdominal cavity and it herniates into the umbilical cord. In time it returns into the abdominal cavity. During this process of herniation and return the gut undergoes a rotation of 270° counterclockwise on the axis of the mesenteric artery. The process of rotation may be arrested at any stage. Faulty rotation of the gut during its development involves not only the colon but the small intestine as well. This condition is also discussed in Chapter 18.

REVERSAL OF ROTATION

Rotation in a clockwise direction is extremely rare and results because the postarterial rather than the prearterial segment enters the abdominal cavity first, passing behind the superior mesenteric artery from left to right. The transverse colon then comes to lie behind the duodenum.

COMPLETE FAILURE OF ROTATION

This is relatively infrequent. When this happens the jejunum and ileum are found in the right side of the abdomen and the colon in the left. The cecum may overlie the sacrum or even be to the left of the midline; the ileocecal valve is situated on the right side of the cecum. The diagnosis is made without difficulty on barium-enema examination if the colon is filled completely and the ileocecal valve identified. Serial roentgenograms after a barium meal will show the absence of a normal duodenal loop, the third portion of the duodenum turning downward and the jejunum being entirely on the right side of the abdomen. The condition usually is not a cause of symptoms.

INCOMPLETE ROTATION (MALROTATION)

This condition is common and is always associated with a defect in peritoneal attachment that is of greater clinical significance than the faulty rotation. The cecum is unusually mobile; the ascending colon is surrounded by peritoneum and may have a mesentery. The attachment of the mesentery can be unusually short. These conditions predispose to volvulus. On barium-enema examination the cecum is found in an abnormal position or, if normally situated, it is found to be abnormally mobile. If volvulus develops, the diagnosis often can be made by plain roentgenograms of the abdomen without the use of contrast material. Roentgen findings in volvulus are described in Chapter 13.

DUPLICATION OF THE COLON

Duplication of the colon is a rare anomaly. The duplicated segment may form a cystic mass without communication with the normal colonic lumen. The nature of the lesion can hardly be recognized on roentgen examination. Rarely there is an open duplication that communicates with the colonic lumen. A case of this type in which the colon was found to have double lumen has been reported by Weber and Dixon.[42]

IMPERFORATE ANUS

Imperforate anus is responsible for about 5 per cent of cases of intestinal obstruction in the neonatal period. Roentgen examination is useful in determining if the lesion is "high" or "low" and the presence and nature of the frequently associated anomalies.

For many years the *inverted view* has been used to determine the length of the atretic segment (Fig. 19-4). This consisted of anteroposterior and lateral views of the inverted infant with a radiopaque marker placed on the perineum. The distance from the end of the rectal gas column to the marker was supposed to indicate the length of the atresia. There are, however, several possible sources of error: (*1*) it requires from 6 to 8 hours for swallowed air to reach the rectum. If the examination is done too soon after birth an erroneous result may be obtained; (*2*) an accumulation of meconium in the rectum may prevent gas from entering it; and (*3*) another area of atresia higher up in the gastrointestinal tract may make the examination of no value as far as the rectum is concerned. For these and other reasons the inverted view is no longer recommended as a means for determining the length of the atresia.[2] It can be used, however, to show (*1*) air in the bladder in male patients with rectourethral and rectovesical fistulas; (*2*) the mass of a dilated vagina (filled with fluid, air, or both) in the rare female cloacal anomaly; and (*3*) lumbosacral spinal anomalies that correlate well with urologic malformations that are found in two-thirds of male and female "high" lesions and one-third of male "low" atresias.

Berdon and associates[2] divide imperforate anus into four major groups, according to sex and whether there is a "high" or a "low" lesion. If there is a detectable perineal fistula, the atresia is classified as "low." If there is no detectable perineal fistula, it is considered a "high" lesion. More than 50 per cent of males with a high atresia will show air in the bladder from a fistula to the urethra or bladder. If air cannot be demonstrated, voiding cystourethrography can be done to outline the fistula.

The spinal anomalies are mostly errors of segmentation. Kurlander[27] found that more than 70 per cent of imperforate anus patients with anomalies of the sacrum had urologic anomalies. Because many of these anomalies are of a serious nature diagnosis should be made as soon as possible, i.e., within the first week of life. The urologic anomalies in addition to those mentioned, include crossed ectopy, crossed fused ectopy, renal agenesis or nonfunction, hydronephrosis, and vesicoureteral reflux.

ATRESIA AND STENOSIS OF THE COLON

Atresia of the colon above the level of the rectum is infrequent. The atresia may be a complete discontinuity or, more rarely, an internal veil or diaphragm that occludes the lumen completely. In the first type the segments may be connected by a fibrous band or have no connection. There may be multiple areas of atresia with isolated blind segments joined by fibrous strands. The passage of meconium does not exclude atresia but when cornified epithelial cells are absent in the meconium it is fairly good evidence that atresia exists.

Roentgen Findings

Plain-film roentgenograms of the abdomen may reveal the site of obstruction because of gas distention above it. It requires 6 to 8 hours after birth for swallowed air to reach the lower part of the colon. When atresia exists, the bowel gradually becomes distended with gas and fluid. It often is difficult to distinguish gas-distended loops of colon from small intestine in the infant because both become smooth-walled and tubular when distended. The persistence of haustra in the colon and of the valvulae conniventes in the jejunum, which are distinguishing features in the adult, even when the

bowel becomes greatly distended, is not true during infancy. The position of the segments becomes important, the colon situated along the circumference of the abdomen and the small intestine within the central part. If there is doubt about the location of the obstruction a barium enema can be given. The colon below the atresia invariably has a small lumen. This has been referred to as "microcolon." If the atresia is in the small intestine and located in the duodenum or proximal jejunum the caliber of the colon may be normal. In distal jejunal or ileal obstructions the entire colon has a very small caliber. Microcolon occurs only when the colon has not been used—i.e., when no meconium has passed through it. This should not be construed as the cause of the patient's difficulty; it is merely the normal appearance of bowel below the level of a congenital obstruction.

According to Berdon et al.[3] atresia of the small intestine can occur if there has been volvulus of a segment of small bowel in utero. The volvulated segment undergoes infarction and necrosis and may eventually be absorbed leading to atresia at the site of the obstruction. Meconium ileus is a frequent cause of the volvulus.

Incomplete obstruction or stenosis of the colon also is a rare condition. Symptoms depend upon the severity of the stenosis and are related to the degree of obstruction. Cornified epithelial cells usually can be found in the meconium, since swallowed amniotic fluid can pass through the gastrointestinal tract. Plain-film roentgenograms will show gas distention above the level of stenosis if it is at all severe. If these are not diagnostic, a barium enema can be given to outline the site and degree of stenosis.

MEGACOLON

Megacolon usually is considered as being of three types, organic, functional, and congenital. Because congenital megacolon is the most important the condition will be considered in this section.

ORGANIC MEGACOLON

Any lesion that causes a chronic partial obstruction of the colon may lead to a gradual enlargement of the bowel above the level of obstruction to a size where it may properly be called megacolon. Because it requires a period of time for development, the lesions that cause it usually are benign. They include adhesive bands, chronic volvulus, congenital and acquired strictures, etc. In our experience adhesions and chronic or recurrent volvulus have been the most frequent causes. The diagnosis of organic megacolon and its differentiation from the congenital type depend upon the history and the demonstration of the causative lesion. In congenital megacolon the onset of symptoms usually dates from birth; in organic megacolon the onset is later in life. The characteristic findings in congenital megacolon will be described subsequently and the diagnosis can be made without difficulty when they are present. The dilatation of the colon usually is less in organic megacolon and the site of obstruction may be higher than the rectosigmoid. Megacolon caused by volvulus usually is recognized because of the demonstration of the volvulus or by the unusually redundant and mobile sigmoid if examined during a nonobstructive period.

FUNCTIONAL MEGACOLON

Functional megacolon results from faulty bowel habits in children and not infrequently in psychotic adult patients. The onset of symptoms may be early in life but usually they do not date from birth. On digital examination the rectum is found filled with feces, in contrast to congenital megacolon in which the rectum usually is empty. Barium enema demonstrates dilatation of the entire colon, including the rectum. Enlargement of the rectum may be especially great and when distended with the barium enema it may fill the entire pelvis. The dilatation of the rest of the colon usually is not as pronounced as it is in congenital megacolon, the amount of impacted feces is less, and relief often is obtained at least temporarily by repeated enemas.

CONGENITAL MEGACOLON (HIRSCHSPRUNG'S DISEASE)

Congenital megacolon is defined as a pronounced dilatation of the colon or a portion of it with hypertrophy of the walls of the dilated portion and with a normal-sized or narrowed segment in the rectum or the rectosigmoid region. Within the narrowed portion there is a marked diminution or a complete absence of the ganglion cells in the myenteric plexuses. The dilated colon is filled with a large amount of feces at all times.

According to current concepts the difficulty arises from a failure of development of the ganglion cells in the myenteric plexuses in the rectum and sigmoid. In turn this causes an interruption of peristalsis. There is an absence of the defecation reflex and a retention of feces above the aganglionic segment results. The proximal colon undergoes a gradual enlargement. The aganglionic segment usually is in the lower sigmoid and rectum but a long segment of bowel may be involved, even the entire colon. Rarely there is more than one aganglionic segment. Hypotonia of the urinary bladder frequently is present, indicating abnormality of parasympathetic innervation to the bladder as well as to the distal colon.

Congenital megacolon is much more common in males than females, approximately 80 per cent of patients being males. The symptoms begin at birth or shortly thereafter with constipation, abdominal distention, and vomiting. At first the distention may be relieved by enemas but eventually these become ineffective. The distention may vary from time to time. In some patients the development of symptoms is insidious but eventually the more or less typical pattern characteristic of the condition develops. In the older child it is usual to find the colon filled with masses of feces that can be palpated through the thin abdominal wall. Peristaltic waves may be observed. The patients often are malnourished and anemic.

Roentgen Observations

PLAIN-FILM ROENTGENOGRAMS. The diagnosis of megacolon often can be made from a simple roentgenogram of the abdomen. The widely dilated colon filled with fecal matter and gas results in a mottled shadow that is diagnostic of fecal impaction. The abdomen is distended and the diaphragm is elevated. In order to outline the aganglionic segment a barium enema is necessary.

BARIUM-ENEMA EXAMINATION. A number of cases of sudden death following tap-water enemas have been reported in patients with Hirschsprung's disease. The cause of death is uncertain although some believe it is the result of water intoxication. Megacolon has a much larger absorptive surface than the normal and the superficial ulcerations frequently present contribute to rapid absorption of hypotonic solutions. The high pressure sometimes used to fill a dilated colon also may contribute to rapid absorption of water. Because there is a known hazard, certain precautions should be observed[39]: (1) Normal saline solution should be used for the barium enema and for preparatory enemas. (2) As much of the fluid should be recovered as possible by siphoning or suction; (3) Avoid using high pressure, an elevation of the enema container 2 to 3 feet above the table top being sufficient; and (4) as soon as the aganglionic segment has been out-lined, the procedure should be stopped and there should be no attempt to fill the dilated segment.

As the barium is introduced the rectum is found to be of essentially normal caliber. At some place in the upper part of the rectum or the distal sigmoid the lumen may decrease slightly in caliber for a short distance or it may remain fairly normal. The transition from the normal or narrowed area to grossly dilated bowel is abrupt and the barium column passes through it without difficulty. If examination is continued the barium is seen to enter the dilated bowel, passing around fecal masses or intermingling with the fecal material (Fig. 19-5). In patients with a long aganglionic segment, difficulty in diagnosis may be experienced because of some variation in caliber of this segment. In some patients it may be larger than normal but comparison with the greatly dilated proximal colon will indicate that, although the aganglionic segment is long and dilated, the dilatation above it is greater and the transition between the two is abrupt. The

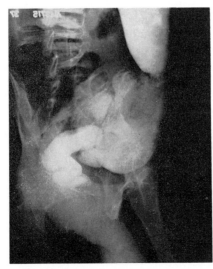
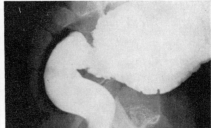

Fig. 19-5. Congenital megacolon. Two patients illustrate the characteristic change from a normal or narrowed rectal segment to the dilated lower sigmoid. *Left,* Oblique roentgenogram after filling of the distal colon with barium demonstrates a normal-sized rectum and an abrupt transition into a greatly dilated sigmoid, which contains fecal residue. *Right,* Spot roentgenogram made during fluoroscopy with the patient in a lateral position, shows the transitional segment between the normal rectum and dilated sigmoid.

difference in caliber and the sudden change are the important criteria in these cases. In some patients only the upper sigmoid colon is dilated and elongated with the rest of the bowel relatively normal in caliber. In others the entire colon above the aganglionic area is greatly dilated. It can be seen, therefore, that appearances will vary somewhat among patients.

It is essential that the barium filling of the colon be done under fluoroscopic guidance. The transition between normal or narrowed bowel to dilated colon is seen to best advantage with the patient rotated to the left into a left posterior oblique position. Otherwise the dilated colon often overlies the rectum and in routine roentgenograms may completely hide the significant lesion. Spot roentgenograms are useful to record the condition on film and they can be made with the patient in whatever position is found best to delineate the area.

In the newborn and the very young infant the classic signs of the disease may not be evident on roentgen examination, the aganglionic segment distending during the barium enema. Evans and Willis have called attention to the importance of stasis of barium in these cases. Twenty-four- to 72-hour roentgenograms after barium enema will show residual barium in the colon above the rectal level, the rectum being empty. This finding is less significant in the older infant or the child because simple constipation may also cause colonic stasis. However, in constipation the barium tends to collect in multiple masses or boli rather than being more uniformly distributed as seen in Hirschsprung's disease. Also, the rectum may be empty in the latter condition and is usually full of barium in constipation.

Hope et al.[21] have described the occurrence of irregular, disorganized, spastic contractions in the aganglionic area which they consider to be significant in diagnosis in the neonatal period. However, the most important sign at this age period, if a transition zone cannot be demonstrated, is colonic stasis. Twenty-four- and 48-hour roentgenograms should be obtained if Hirschsprung's disease is a consideration and they may simplify an otherwise difficult diagnostic problem.

DISEASES OF THE COLON

CARCINOMA

Published statistics indicate that the majority of carcinomas of the large intestine can be visualized during proctosigmoidoscopic examination. Approximately 60 per cent are found in the rectum and in the rectosigmoid region, another 10 per cent in the remainder of the sigmoid, and the final 30 per cent in the rest of the colon. The diagnosis of lesions in the rectum and distal part of the sigmoid should be made by proctosigmoidoscopy rather than by roentgen examination and a negative barium enema is not considered adequate to exclude a lesion in this area unless special procedures are used. Above the level of proctoscopic vision roentgen examination is the method of choice.

From the roentgen point of view carcinoma of the colon occurs in three major types: (1) polypoid or fungating, (2) infiltrative or annular, and (3) completely obstructive. In general, carcinoma of the colon has roentgen features similar to those of cancer elsewhere in the gastrointestinal tract that have been discussed in appropriate sections. Carcinoma stiffens the bowel wall and causes a fixed defect, it destroys the mucosal pattern or alters it markedly, and it is prone to narrow the lumen and cause obstruction.

POLYPOID OR FUNGATING CARCINOMA

When the colon has been filled with barium mixture a polypoid carcinoma is seen as an intraluminal mass or filling defect of variable size attached to the colonic wall by a broad base (see Figs. 19-6 and 19-7). Characteristically the surface of the defect is somewhat irregular or lobulated; the edges of the lesion form an acute angle with the normal colonic wall; the mucosal pattern is lost completely over the surface of the defect. The larger bulky lesions often are described as fungating, a term that indicates a more advanced stage of growth. Areas of necrosis develop frequently in

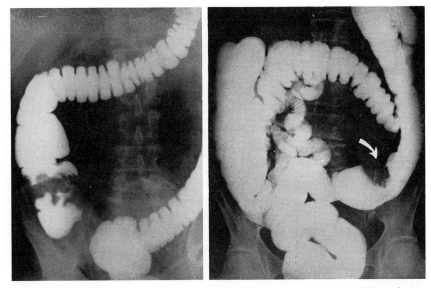

Fig. 19-6. Polypoid or fungating carcinoma of the colon. *Left,* Polypoid carcinoma of the cecum. Although large, the lesion has not prevented filling of the cecal tip. It shows the overhanging edges characteristic of carcinoma. *Right,* Small lesion attached to the wall of the sigmoid, projecting into the lumen and causing a typical polypoid defect (**arrow**).

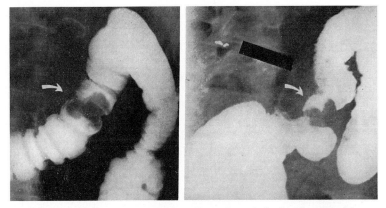

Fig. 19-7. Polypoid carcinoma of the colon. *Left,* Small polypoid carcinoma in the distal part of the transverse colon causing a lobulated filling defect (**arrow**). *Right,* Polypoid carcinoma that has become annular, surrounding the lumen but showing the essential features of a polypoid lesion (**arrow**).

these large tumors and result in pocketlike accumulations of barium within the necrotic cavities. Small polypoid carcinomas resemble sessile benign polyps and often it is impossible to state from roentgen evidence whether such a lesion is benign or malignant. Polypoid carcinomas occur in all parts of the large intestine but it is the predominant type in the cecum and ascending colon. In this location the tumor often reaches a large size before it causes enough symptoms to lead to the diagnosis; not infrequently the patient is examined only because of a refractory anemia or an unexplained fever or loss of weight. Polypoid carcinomas are not as likely to cause obstruction as the annular type but bleeding is a common and often an early symptom.

INFILTRATING OR ANNULAR CARCINOMA

This type of carcinoma is characterized by infiltration of the wall rather than by a bulky intraluminal mass. It narrows the bowel lumen and when it has reached the stage of an annular growth, constriction is invariably present. The length of colon involved by an annular carcinoma seldom exceeds 4 to 6 cm. The edges of the lesion tend to overhang and form acute angles with the bowel wall. This is one of the features of carcinoma in all parts of the gastrointestinal tract. The constriction caused by the tumor usually is concentric and in some cases only a few centimeters long, which gives an appearance that has led to the designation of "napkin-ring carcinoma" (Figs. 19-8 through 19-10). The folds of mucosa are completely absent within the area of the lesion. The defect

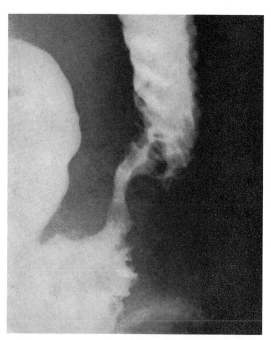

Fig. 19-9. Annular carcinoma of the lower part of the descending colon. Spot roentgenogram made during fluoroscopy centered over the lower descending colon, show the characteristic defect of an annular carcinoma.

is constant and rigid and a mass often is palpable.

OBSTRUCTIVE CARCINOMA

Either of the above types may cause complete obstruction although the annular is more prone to do so. When obstruction to the retrograde flow of barium is complete, the information obtained by outlining the channel through the tumor is no longer available. Often the abrupt termination of the barium column and the evidence of overhanging edges at the distal border of the lesion can be identified. In other cases a partial outlining of the channel is obtained. In many, however, the appearance of the end of the barium column is not distinctive and the roentgen diagnosis must be limited to that of an obstructive lesion.

It is rather common to find complete or nearly complete obstruction to the retrograde flow of enema mixture and yet to have few of

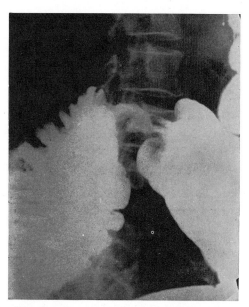

Fig. 19-8. Annular carcinoma of the hepatic flexure of the colon. The lesion completely surrounds the lumen, giving a napkin-ring type of defect.

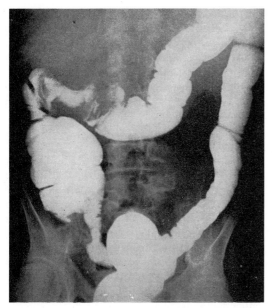

Fig. 19-10. Carcinoma of the hepatic flexure of the colon. The lesion is extensive and shows both polypoid and annular or infiltrating characteristics. While somewhat extensive and with narrowed lumen through the lesion, it has not prevented filling of the proximal colon and terminal ileum.

the clinical signs and symptoms of bowel obstruction. In these patients peristalsis apparently is able to keep semisolid material passing through the narrowed area but when an enema is given the retrograde flow and the hydrostatic pressure used closes the narrow orifice. Even though these patients may be unobstructed clinically it is very unwise to give barium by mouth because the chance for causing impaction is considerable. As the water is absorbed by the colon there is left the insoluble barium sulfate to form a hard, rocklike mass. An acute obstruction may be precipitated in such a case; at the least the impacted barium may be impossible to remove and adds to the surgical difficulties when resection is attempted or it may complicate the postoperative period.

FURTHER OBSERVATIONS

Sinus Tracts and Fistulas. Sinus tracts extending into contiguous tissues or fistulous communications with other abdominal viscera

are rather frequent complications of advanced carcinoma of the colon. During filling of the colon with barium mixture there may be noted extension of contrast material into a loop of small intestine through a direct fistulous communication. Similar fistulas may form between the colon and the urinary bladder, the gallbladder, or the stomach. It may be impossible in some of these cases to determine from which structure the tumor arose.

Other Inflammatory Changes. The development of inflammatory changes other than sinus tracts or fistulas is relatively common and at times the inflammatory aspect may overshadow the neoplastic. Inflammatory thickening or abscess formation adds to the mass characteristics of the cancer but also changes the roentgen features. The defect is increased in length and one or both ends of it may taper gradually rather than have an abrupt demarcation from the normal bowel. Thus, one of the characteristic signs of gastrointestinal carcinoma is lost. Fortunately, this usually affects only one end of the lesion and at the other the typical overhanging edges of a carcinoma defect remain. When an annular defect of more than 6 cm in length is found it is probable that there is an intramural or pericolic inflammatory mass associated with the carcinoma.

Intussusception. Intussusception in the adult usually is caused by a tumor of sessile or pedunculated nature. Some are the result of lipomas or leiomyomas. Intussusception as a complication of colonic carcinoma occurs chiefly with the polypoid type involving the right side of the colon. The signs of intussusception predominate in the roentgen picture. As the barium column reaches the obstruction it widens out and the end of the column develops a concave or cup-shaped appearance as it surrounds the intussusceptum. The tumor responsible for the obstruction ordinarily forms the leading edge of the intussusceptum. In many cases, however, it cannot be clearly identified. Characteristically, ringlike shadows of barium mark the termination of the column representing barium caught in the haustra of the intussuscipiens (Fig. 19-11). As the hydrostatic pressure of the enema becomes effective, the head of the barium column will move proximally for some distance but the concavity of its end is maintained. The intussusception may be reduced completely by this method and the defect of the tumor then becomes clearly apparent. At other times reduction is incomplete and filling of the colon proximal to the obstruction is not obtained.

DIFFERENTIAL DIAGNOSIS

INFLAMMATORY MASSES. The most important lesion from the standpoint of differential diagnosis is a localized inflammatory mass and this usually is the result of diverticulitis with or without a frank abscess in the colonic wall or pericolic tissues. The inflammatory changes cause a narrowing of the lumen and this may be severe enough to result in complete obstruction. As the lesion

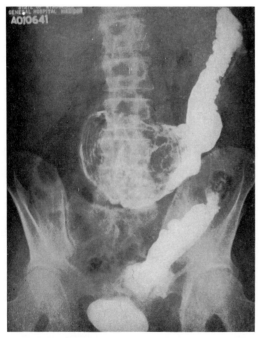

Fig. 19-11. Intussusception of the transverse colon caused by a polypoid carcinoma of the cecum. Note the ringlike appearance of the mucosal folds as they are stretched over the intussusceptum, which forms a large filling defect projecting into the end of the barium-filled colon.

encroaches upon the lumen a filling defect is produced when the colon is filled with barium. The differential signs are discussed on page 620.

Other inflammatory lesions that may be confused with carcinoma are infrequent. Hyperplastic tuberculosis in the cecum and ascending colon has been reported as causing a defect somewhat similar to carcinoma but this lesion is rare in general radiologic practice. An area of granulomatous colitis may resemble to some degree the defect of an annular carcinoma. However, this lesion usually involves a longer segment of bowel, the lumen may not be narrowed too greatly, the mucosal surface has a granular appearance, and the ends of the defect taper gradually, a characteristic of all inflammatory lesions. Infrequently, a nonspecific inflammatory granuloma is found in the colon and it may cause roentgenologic findings very similar to those of carcinoma. Because they are rare these lesions seldom enter into the differential diagnostic picture.

Amebic disease of the colon may present as a localized mass known as *ameboma*. In areas where this disease is endemic it has been suggested that most patients with a localized filling defect in the colon have a course of emetine therapy prior to any surgical procedure. This is because the lesion may mimic carcinoma very closely. If due to amebiasis, the lesion will improve promptly under adequate therapy.

BENIGN POLYPS. With larger polyps it may be difficult to determine if the lesion is benign or not from its roentgen features. Small polyps, those less than 1 cm in diameter, usually can be kept under observation with reexamination at intervals of 3 to 6 months unless the lesion is a source of bleeding. The same is true of a polyp with a pedicle. The presence of a pedicle indicates that the lesion is not invading the bowel wall. The demonstration of a pedicle, therefore, is of considerable importance from the standpoint of treatment as well as diagnosis.

EXTRINSIC MASSES. A variety of masses within the abdomen may cause pressure defects on the colon. As a rule the defect is a smooth one and often changes during the examination or can be made to disappear by altering the position of the patient or by the effect of manual palpation. The mucosa is intact, an important point in differential diagnosis because mucosal folds are not seen over the surface of a carcinoma defect. A malignant tumor from a neighboring structure may invade the colon and often it is difficult if not impossible to determine whether such a lesion is primary in the colon or not. If only the external wall is involved and the mucosa is intact, the demonstration of mucosal folds through the area of defect is significant.

INTRAMURAL TUMORS. Tumors arising from elements of the bowel wall other than the mucosa are relatively infrequent. They include such lesions as lipomas, leiomyomas, and leiomyosarcomas. The roentgen features of a small, extramucosal, intramural tumor resemble those of a sessile polyp. The larger tumors of this nature often suggest polypoid carcinoma. The visualization of mucosal folds over the surface of the mass is of importance in establishing the intramural nature of the mass, but it may be difficult to be certain about this finding. Lipomas of the cecum are said to be a common cause of intussusception in the adult and in some cases a lipoma may actually develop a pedicle because of peristaltic pressure. If large enough, a lipoma may appear unusually translucent because of its fat content. In our experience, polyps and polypoid carcinomas have been more frequent causes of intussusception in the adult.

POLYPS

The term "polyp" often is used to include inflammatory as well as neoplastic lesions. Roentgenologists frequently use the term "polypoid lesion" because of inability to determine the histologic nature of many of the small masses that have similar gross features. Polyps of the colon are slightly more common in males than in females; multiple tumors are frequent. Their distribution in the various parts of the colon and the age incidence are similar to carcinoma. From 60 to 75 per cent occur in the rectum or lower part of the sigmoid and are accessible to proctoscopic examination. The incidence of colonic polyps in routine autopsy series has been given as 7 per cent by Swinton[40] and 9.5 per cent by Helwig. An even higher incidence has been reported by others, and apparently the care with which a search is made results in some variation in the reported incidence of these tumors. Swinton reports finding polyps of the rectum and sigmoid in 5 per cent of all patients over 35 years of age undergoing proctoscopic examination. The incidence of polyps of the colon above the rectosigmoid level and detected by roentgen examination also has varied in published reports. In asymptomatic individuals Stevenson found polyps in only 0.4 per cent of patients having a barium enema examination. However, this figure rose to 5 per cent when limited to patients with bleeding from the colon, polyps found at proctoscopy, or those with a history of previous polyp removal.

The majority of colonic polyps are adenomas. The lesion may be sessile and attached to the colonic wall by a broad base but the larger ones often have a pedicle caused by peristaltic pressure. The pedicle may be as much as 4 or 5 cm in length. Polyps vary greatly in size from tiny wartlike excrescences on the mucosal surface to lesions that measure several centimeters in diameter. The relation of polyps to carcinoma is an interesting one and opinions have been expressed repeatedly in the literature that a high percentage of carcinomas of the colon and rectum originate in preexisting polyps. Others, however, have disputed this and evidence has been presented to indicate that most polyps of the colon do not become malignant. As noted before, the demonstration of a stalk, roentgenologically, is an important finding, since it indicates a lack of invasiveness on the part of the lesion.

Roentgen Observations

If the head of the advancing barium column is watched closely during fluoroscopy the defect of a polyp often is seen momentarily as the barium flows around it. If the polyp is small it soon becomes obscured as the segment fills more completely. Palpation with the lead-glove-protected hand helps to bring out the defect more clearly; or compression cones and similar devices found on most modern fluoroscopes can be used to approximate the colonic walls. Sufficient pressure is used to squeeze most of the barium from the area, leaving a thin layer within which the small defect of the polyp will be visible.

A polyp causes a rounded, negative (translucent) filling defect in the barium shadow (Fig. 19-12). The edges are smooth and the margins sharply defined. If sessile, the defect does not move at any time during the examination. If it has a pedicle, the head of the polyp may move during filling and evacuation of the enema or be displaced by palpation. Occasionally a pedicle of considerable length is present and the polyp can move a distance twice the length of the pedicle. The pedicle may be visualized as a stalklike defect and its point of attachment is indicated by a slight indrawing of the colonic wall (Fig. 19-13).

The postevacuation roentgenogram is an important part of the roentgen examination for the detection of polyps. In the contracted state a thin layer of barium usually coats the mucosal surface, which then is seen as a network of fine folds. The polyp also is coated with barium and appears as a rounded mass displacing or replacing the normal mucosal relief (Fig. 19-14). The minimum size of a polyp that can be detected regularly on roentgen examination is variable, but is usually considered to be on the order of 0.7 to 1 cm. Practically all polyps of this size should be demonstrated, provided that proper cleansing of the colon has been obtained. Polyps smaller than this are often visualized if preparation has been good and if other factors, including location in an area accessible to visualization, are favorable. The identification of tiny polyps is accomplished most often when multiple lesions are present.

Double-contrast studies (see page 598) are of value and this method of examination finds its greatest usefulness in the detection of polyps. When surrounded by air a polyp forms a positive shadow as it projects into the colonic lumen because it is of greater radiographic density than air. The surface usually is coated with a thin layer of barium, which is continuous with that coating the contiguous intestinal wall.

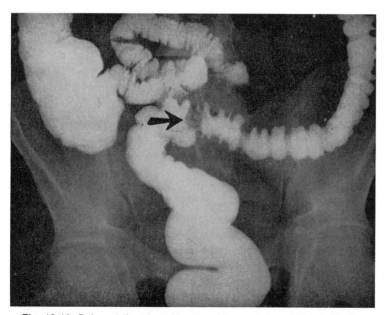

Fig. 19-12. Polyp of the sigmoid colon. The lesion is seen as a smooth, round filling defect in the lumen of the barium-filled sigmoid (**arrow**).

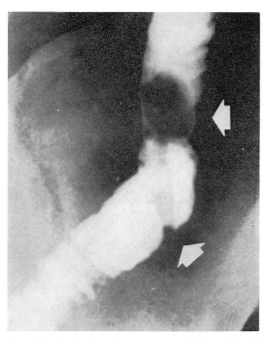

Fig. 19-13. Pedunculated polyp of the sigmoid colon. Spot roentgenogram made during fluoroscopy, shows a segment of the upper sigmoid colon filled with barium and clearly outlines the head and stalk of a pedunculated polyp. **Upper arrow** points to the head of the polyp and the **lower arrow** to its point of attachment on the outer wall of the colon.

DIFFERENTIAL DIAGNOSIS

FECAL LUMPS. Small lumps of nonopaque fecal matter offer the greatest difficulty in differential diagnosis. A lump of feces may move extensively as the mixture flows through the colon; it may disappear completely in postevacuation roentgenograms; or it may disintegrate while being palpated. The constancy of a polyp defect is one of its characteristic features. When there is doubt, re-examination is required and this should be done without hesitation whenever any question exists. Visualization of a pedicle, when one is present, is an extremely important finding and allows a diagnosis of polyp to be made with assurance (see Fig. 19-13).

DIVERTICULA. A diverticulum may resemble a polyp to some extent in double-contrast roentgenograms if seen *en face* rather than in profile. If the diverticulum contains a nonopaque fecalith or air and has only a coating of barium on its sur-face, it will appear as a ringlike shadow. Also a diverticulum when seen *en face* may appear as a double ring, the inner one formed by the barium coating of the neck and the outer ring by the sac of the diverticulum. The air-filled sac of the diverticulum stands out with a greater translucence than the adjacent bowel, while a polyp causes a shadow denser than the surrounding air (Fig. 19-15).

INTRAMURAL TUMORS. A sessile polyp may resemble an extramucosal intramural tumor very closely and the differentiation often is impossible on roentgen examination, particularly when the lesions are small. Actually, some intramural tumors become to all intents and purposes polyps in their gross features and may develop a pedicle.

PSEUDOPOLYPS. In some cases of chronic ulcerative colitis, the coalescence of small ulcers into larger and deeper ulcerations with undermined edges may leave islands or tags of inflamed but otherwise intact mucosa. These tags cause small, round translucent defects in the barium shadow that resemble true polyps very closely. In most cases it is impossible to distinguish a pseudopolyp from a true one and both may be present in the same patient (see Fig. 19-29).

FAMILIAL POLYPOSIS OF THE COLON

Familial polyposis or adenomatosis of the colon is a rare disease of hereditary or familial nature. In most patients the onset is during the second decade of life, but cases have been reported in which the disease has been found during early childhood. The familial aspects of the disease have been thoroughly studied by Dukes and by others. Apparently it represents a gene mutation which, if carried as a Mendelian dominant, appears in succeeding generations; if as a recessive, it may skip a generation unless both parents carry the gene. The only possibility of cure lies in a total colectomy; otherwise the usual course is the development of carcinoma of the colon unless death from other causes supervenes. During barium-enema examination routine fluoroscopy may fail to reveal evidence of the disease because the polyps often are very small. Even in roentgenograms of the filled and contracted colon it may be difficult to visualize the lesions. The margins of the filled colon usually show a fine

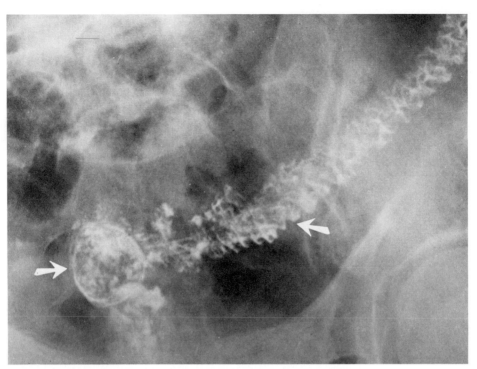

Fig. 19-14. Pedunculated polyp of the sigmoid colon. Postevacuation roentgenogram. **Left arrow** points to head of polyp coated with barium. **Right arrow** indicates point of attachment of stalk to wall.

roughening, representing the defects of small polyps seen in profile (Fig. 19-16). Postevacuation roentgenograms may show the larger polyps but the small ones may be lost in the crinkling of mucosal folds when the bowel contracts. The ideal method for roentgen demonstration is by means of double-contrast studies. Properly done, double-contrast roentgenograms reveal the innumerable tiny polyps as small nodules along the mucosal surface of the colon (Fig. 19-17). Some of the tumors may be larger than others and easily seen by routine methods. Carcinomatous degeneration is often present in some of these even at the time the patient is first examined. The differentiation of familial polyposis of the colon from pseudo-polyposis or polyposis developing during ulcerative colitis is not difficult since in the former the bowel is otherwise normal while in the latter condition the extensive changes of ulcerative disease are apparent. When ulcerative colitis has "healed," leaving only pseudopolyps, the differentiation may be more difficult. In the diffuse form of lympho-sarcoma involving the colon, the thickened folds may suggest multiple polyps.

PUETZ-JEGHERS SYNDROME. This entity consists of multiple polyposis of the colon, the small intestine, or both, associated with a peculiar oral pigmentation. The pigment is melanin. The lesions usually are very small and best identified in double-contrast study. They represent hamartomas rather than true polyps. The diagnostic clue is the oral pigmentation. Otherwise the appearances simulate familial polyposis (also see Chapter 18 under the section entitled "Puetz-Jeghers Syndrome").

GARDNER'S SYNDROME. This syndrome consists of colonic polyposis associated with osteomas of the skeletal system and various soft-tissue tumors.[23] The osteomas may occur in any bone but are most frequent in the calvarium, mandible, and other facial bones. They vary considerably in size from small areas of cortical thickening to larger, distinct masses having the density of cortical bone.

NODULAR LYMPHOID HYPERPLASIA. The condition known as *benign* or *nodular lymphoid hyperplasia* of the colon may present findings very similar to those of familial multiple polyposis in air-contrast

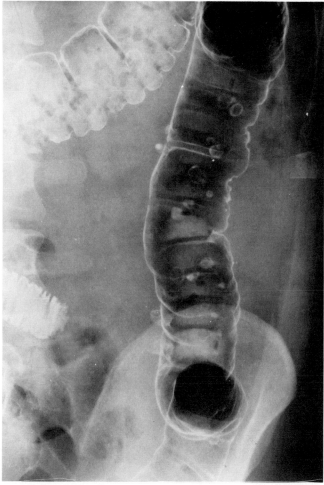

Fig. 19-15. Diverticula of descending colon in double-contrast enema. When seen *en face* some of the diverticula appear as dense spots, others as rings owing to coating of the wall only.

studies of the colon. The roentgen observations and clinical findings are similar to those seen when the process involves the small intestine as discussed on page 581. In some cases small, central dimples on the surface of the nodules (umbilication) have been noted, a finding that has proved helpful in their differentiation from familial polyposis and other polypoid lesions of the colon. The umbilication is seen as a tiny fleck of barium in the center of the round, translucent defect of the nodule.

CRONKHITE-CANADA SYNDROME. This rare syndrome consists of non-familial diffuse gastrointestinal polyposis (stomach, small intestine and colon) with ectodermal changes and pigmentation. Usually there is severe protein loss and it is generally considered to be one of the protein-losing enteropathies (see under "Hypoproteinemia," Chapter 18).

JUVENILE POLYPS

Polyps of the colon occurring in children have a different histologic appearance than the usual adenomatous polyp found in adults. They are benign lesions with no reported instance of malignant degeneration. The presenting complaint usually is that of bleeding from the rectum or an anemia from chronic blood loss. Occasionally the

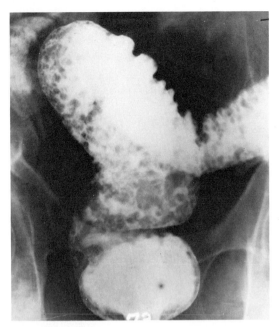

Fig. 19-16. Multiple familial polyposis of the colon. The rectum and lower part of the sigmoid are shown. The polyps appear as numerous round translucent defects.

radiolucent than the water and soft tissues around it. Larger lipomas can be identified at times by this procedure. Theoretically the demonstration of an intact mucosa over the surface of a mass should be good evidence of its nonmucosal origin. Actually, this is a difficult decision to make in tumors of the colon for the mucosa over an intramural mass may be stretched and flattened so that folds cannot be identified. Roentgen findings usually limit the diagnosis to that of a polypoid mass or lesion. Some intramural tumors even develop a pedicle because of the effects of peristalsis.

Lymphosarcoma of the colon may occur as a discrete tumor simulating carcinoma, or as a diffuse involvement of considerable lengths of

lesion may cause obstruction because of intussusception. The roentgen findings are similar to those of polyps of the colon in adults but their occurrence in children and the fact that they apparently do not become malignant are significant factors. Excisional biopsy is reported to be curative provided that the clinical findings are sufficiently severe to warrant a surgical procedure.

OTHER TUMEFACTIVE LESIONS

As is true in other parts of the gastrointestinal tract, a variety of tumors of extramucosal, intramural nature is found in the colon but as a group these tumors are not common lesions. They include lipomas, leiomyomas, and leiomyosarcomas. Lipomas are found most frequently in the right side of the colon (Fig. 19-18). With the larger lipomas the tumor may appear unusually translucent. If a mass has been found on routine barium-enema examination the use of a water enema has been recommended. If the mass is a lipoma it will be more

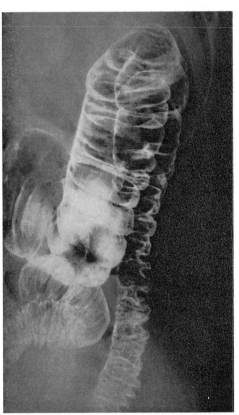

Fig. 19-17. Familial polyposis of colon. Roentgenogram of the splenic flexure and descending colon of a patient with numerous tiny polyps throughout the large intestine. The double-contrast examination demonstrates the polyps as tiny translucent defects in the barium coating the mucosal surface.

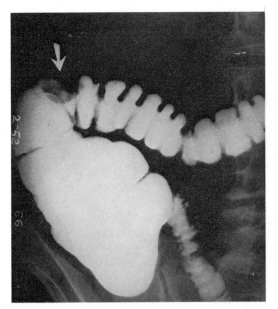

Fig. 19-18. Intramural tumor (lipoma) at the hepatic flexure of the colon. The **arrow** points to the defect caused by the tumor.

colon, or with multiple nodules. The diffuse form is characterized by extensive submucosal infiltration, leading to thickening of the mucosal folds somewhat similar to that seen when this disease involves the stomach. The thickened tortuous folds give the appearance of multiple polypoid protrusions. The terminal ileum is often involved in association with the colonic disease and gastric lesions also are common.

ENDOMETRIOSIS

The occurrence of implants on the peritoneal surface consisting of islands of tissue having the characteristics of normal endometrium is termed *endometriosis*. This condition is relatively common in women during active menstrual life. Endometrial implants in the wall of the rectum or sigmoid may lead to an inflammatory reaction since each implant functions as a miniature uterus during menstrual periods. This causes a fibrotic reaction and leads to the development of a constricting process that may cause the symptoms and signs of bowel obstruction. As pointed out by Jenkinson and Brown,[22] the important clinical features of endometriosis include: (*1*) age range

usually between 25 and 45 years; (*2*) high incidence of menstrual irregularities; (*3*) absolute or relative sterility; (*4*) long history of symptoms suggesting bowel obstruction with frequent exacerbations at the time of menstruation; (*5*) absence of cachexia of weight loss; (*6*) infrequent evidence of bleeding from the bowel; (*7*) high incidence of benign uterine tumors. The roentgen findings in their cases included; (*1*) a filling defect approximately 4 to 7 inches in length; (*2*) a sharp demarcation from normal to narrowed bowel similar to carcinoma; (*3*) an essentially intact mucous membrane; and (*4*) fixation and tenderness to palpation during fluoroscopy (Fig. 19-19). While these features are characteristic, we have seen small defects that were difficult if not impossible to distinguish from carcinoma. Correlation of roentgen and clinical observations is extremely important in these cases.

VILLOUS ADENOMA

This unusual tumor is found chiefly in the rectum and rectosigmoid in patients of middle age or older. It is characterized pathologically by a soft, velvety mass made up of a large number of villi or frondlike projections from the base of the tumor. It is usually benign, but some observers believe that malignant degeneration occurs rather frequently. Clinically, there is an excess of mucus leading to frequent watery or mucuslike stools.

On barium-enema examination the lesion may be of variable size from a few centimeters to those that are large and bulky, encircling the lumen and causing an extensive filling defect. The appearance of the tumor may vary considerably in the filled and evacuated state of the colon as seen in barium enema. Characteristically, the margin is rough and serrated. There may be many streaks of barium where it has extended between the numerous villi (Fig. 19-20). In other cases the surface has a cobblestone appearance. These findings, taken in association with the clinical signs and symptoms, may allow a preoperative diagnosis.

DIVERTICULA

Diverticula are very common lesions in the adult colon and the incidence increases above the age of 40; most elderly persons have at

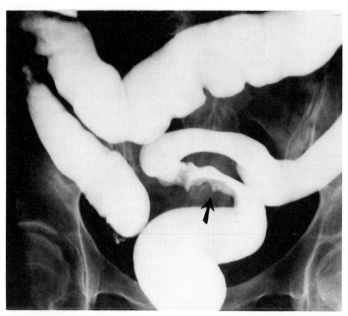

Fig. 19-19. Endometriosis. **Arrow** points to a mass from an endometrial implant.

least a few. Diverticula of the colon are acquired and form at points of anatomic weakness, usually at the sites where blood vessels perforate the muscular coat. The sigmoid colon is most frequently involved but in some patients diverticula are found throughout the length of the large intestine. Isolated diverticula have been described as occurring in the cecum and elsewhere. As a rule, however, multiple diverticula are present and very large numbers are often seen. Diverticula vary in size from tiny ones no more than 1 or 2 mm in diameter to some that measure several centimeters; the majority of them do not measure more than a centimeter.

Roentgen Observations

The presence of diverticula without the signs of inflammation is designated as *diverticulosis;* when inflammation is present the condition is termed *diverticulitis.* Diverticula may be filled with fecal matter and not be visualized at all during a barium-enema examination. In others the sac may contain a fecalith but enough

barium will enter to coat the wall; the diverticulum then appears as a ring shadow (see Fig. 19-15). When the entire diverticulum fills with barium and is seen along the margin of the colon it forms a budlike shadow projecting beyond the confines of the barium-filled colonic lumen. If seen *en face* it appears as a dense round spot. Diverticula once filled with barium often retain the contrast material for days. Such retention does not appear to be harmful. Many times they become visible only after the barium has been given orally and the barium meal often demonstrates the extent of a diverticulosis of the colon more clearly than the barium enema.

DIVERTICULITIS

Inflammatory reaction in a diverticulum may be limited to the sac and the pericolic tissues, and the wall of the colon not be affected to any appreciable degree. The roentgen signs of inflammation often are meager in these cases. According to some investigators,[12] localized inflammation results from rupture of

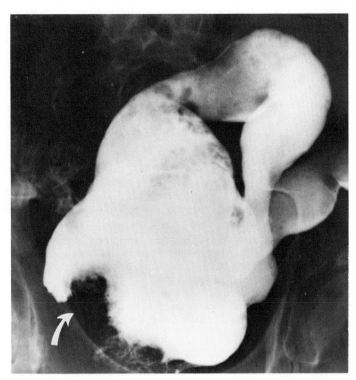

Fig. 19-20. Villous adenoma of the rectum. The lesion presents as a filling defect (**arrow**) with a ragged surface and with thin, linear extensions into the tumor mass near the anal canal.

a diverticulum. This may be a microperforation and the associated inflammation correspondingly mild. Even larger perforations may be sealed over rapidly leading to a localized abscess in the pericolic tissues of variable size. Multiple perforations may occur and the accompanying abscesses may communicate with each other. A fistulous tract usually can be seen extending into the abscess and the abscess cavity may partially fill with barium (Fig. 19-21).

On barium-enema study a small perforation may be visualized as a small, cloudy area of barium density around the site of the diverticulum. Local swelling from inflammation of the pericolic tissues as well as the wall of the colon leads to formation of a mass. This causes a localized filling defect in the barium column. Larger abscesses cause correspondingly larger defects and the inflammatory reaction may be sufficient to cause partial or complete ob-

struction to retrograde filling. The inflammatory mass may surround the lumen causing narrowing of a short segment (Fig. 19-22) or appear as a unilateral filling defect encroaching upon the bowel lumen. Particularly in the early stages, spasm is usually present and the area is irritable as seen under the fluoroscope. An acute diverticulitis is tender to palpation. However this also may be found in carcinoma, particularly if there is much of an inflammatory element associated.

If there is complete perforation which does not become sealed off, pneumoperitoneum often can be demonstrated and, later, the signs of local or general peritonitis including adynamic ileus and exudate separating loops of bowel. Diverticular perforation also may cause fistulous communications between the colon and urinary bladder or colon and vagina in females.

The differentiation from carcinoma may be

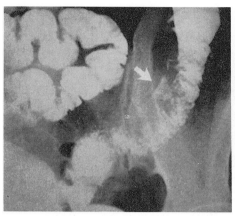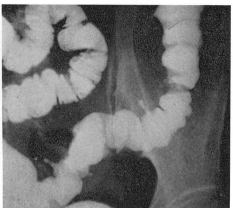

Fig. 19-21. Diverticulitis of the sigmoid with perforation and fistula formation. *Left,* Appearance of the lower descending and upper part of the sigmoid colon at the initial examination. There is an irregular defect on the medial wall of the colon but mucosal folds can be seen throughout the area. There is an extension of contrast material beyond the lumen, caused by a fistula that has perforated into the wall and extracolonic tissues (**arrow**). Note the few filled diverticula above the area of the lesion. *Right,* Same patient several months later. The inflammatory reaction has subsided and the caliber of the bowel is fairly normal. Numerous diverticula are visible. There is only a tiny spikelike projection of barium at the site of the previous fistula.

difficult. The presence of overhanging edges at the margins of the filling defect, and the irregular eccentric stricture seen in carcinoma are significant. (Fig. 19-23). The signs of walled-off perforation including the defect due to inflammatory mass, the demonstration of one or more fistulous tracts, the presence of diverticula in or adjacent to the filling defect, and spasm and irritability of the involved area are findings pointing to inflammatory disease. In many patients the diagnosis can be confirmed by progress examinations done over a period of a few weeks which will show a gradual subsidence and eventual disappearance of the signs of inflammation. If barium has extravasated into the abscess, a small amount may be trapped and continue to be visible for some time as a small fleck or patch of barium.

CHRONIC IDIOPATHIC ULCERATIVE COLITIS

In the majority of cases, chronic idiopathic ulcerative colitis begins in the rectum or lower part of the sigmoid and the diagnosis can be made by proctoscopy. In these cases roentgen examination is useful to determine the extent and the severity of the disease above the level of proctoscopic vision. Less often the disease begins in the left side of the colon above the rectosigmoid and infrequently it has its origin in the right side of the colon. Ulcerative colitis sparing the rectum is infrequent.

Most cases of chronic ulcerative colitis have a subacute onset, subsiding gradually into a chronic course, but occasionally the onset is abrupt and the course is that of an acute, severe, fulminating infection. In still other cases the onset is so insidious that the nature of the disease is not recognized for some time. Pathologically it begins as a mucosal inflammation that in time spreads to involve all coats of the bowel wall. However, the inflammation remains most intense in the mucosa and submucosa. Small and superficial ulcers are a feature of this stage. In chronic disease the entire or the major part of the mucous coat may be denuded or there may be left islands of inflamed and hypertrophied mucosa. The wall becomes stiffened by fibrosis.

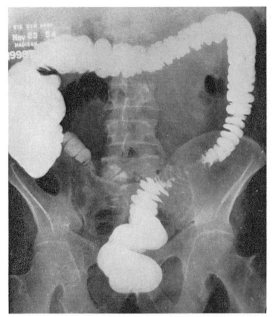

Fig. 19-22. Diverticulitis of the sigmoid colon. There is considerable narrowing of the lumen of the sigmoid through the area of involvement but the defect shows tapering edges both above and below and small diverticula are visible in the distal part of the area. There was tenderness to palpation over the region during fluoroscopy.

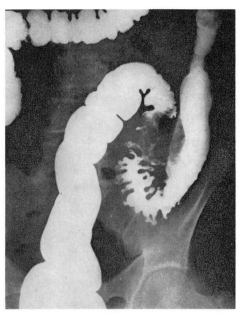

Fig. 19-23. Carcinoma and diverticulosis of the sigmoid colon. There are numerous diverticula in the sigmoid colon but there also is a localized filling defect and evidence of a mass associated with it that causes pressure deformity on the contiguous segment of descending colon. This defect shows the features of polypoid carcinoma.

Roentgen Observations

EARLY CHANGES. During the early stages of the disease roentgen findings may be meager and the diagnosis can be established more readily by proctoscopy, unless the disease has begun above the rectosigmoid level. Usually the involved segment of colon is more irritable than normal as observed under the fluoroscopic screen. It may be difficult to keep it filled with barium and the patient suffers more distress from the enema than is usual. Otherwise fluoroscopy may show little in the way of abnormality. Roentgenograms of the filled colon demonstrate a persistence of haustral sacculations but the haustra are irregular in width and the septa separating them are thickened. The postevacuation roentgenogram often gives important information. Instead of the mucosa forming a crisscrossing network of fine folds, the folds are thickened and tend to course in a longitudinal direction (Fig. 19-24).

The thin coating of barium on the surface appears finely stippled because of the innumerable tiny ulcers. When seen along the edges, the ulcers cause numerous, tiny, spikelike projections. Rather similar tiny projections are seen occasionally in the normal colon and are thought to result from barium filling of the colonic glands. The other signs of inflammatory disease, of course, are absent. If only part of the colon is involved, the demarcation between the diseased and normal bowel is not distinct. In the lower descending portion longitudinal folds are sometimes seen in the normal individual during the postevacuation phase. However, the folds are finer than those seen in cases of ulcerative colitis and there is no stippling of the barium coating caused by the tiny ulcers. Normally, when distended, there are few if any haustra in the lower descending colon and this should be taken into account when early ulcerative colitis is a possibility. The appearance of the mucosa is the significant

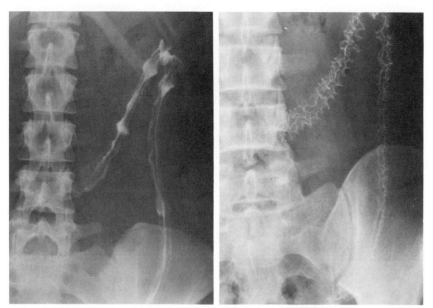

Fig. 19-24. Chronic ulcerative colitis. *Left,* Postevacuation roentgenogram of a patient with chronic ulcerative colitis to show the appearance of the contracted colon. The roentgenogram includes only the splenic flexure area, distal transverse, and upper part of the descending colon. The mucosal folds are coarsened and thrown into longitudinal folds. Contrast with *right,* appearance of a normal colon in a contracted state after barium enema. The folds of mucosa are finely crinkled and form no specific pattern.

feature in differentiation along with the presence or absence of the other signs of inflammation.

In the acute fulminating cases, roentgen findings during the early stages are even more difficult to evaluate. Some patients are critically ill and yet show a minimal amount of ulceration and inflammation on direct inspection; the severity of clinical signs and symptoms, therefore, does not always bear a direct relationship to the severity of pathologic changes. As a rule it is unwise to do a barium enema on a patient with acute fulminating disease because of the danger of perforation and the toxicity and prostration caused by the disease. If it is done, usually within a short time after onset, the margins of the barium-filled colon begin to appear rough and shaggy because of the presence of deep ulcers. Excess secretions are present. Haustra may persist but the septa are thickened and vary in depth. In other cases an

acute fulminating disease develops during the course of chronic ulcerative colitis. The disease is often accompanied by a *toxic dilatation of the colon.* A striking feature in abdominal roentgenograms in these patients is the marked colonic dilatation. The most severe involvement tends to be localized to the transverse colon (Fig. 19-25) Even when the entire colon is involved, the maximum dilatation is likely to be in the transverse segment. The diagnosis often can be made from plain roentgenograms. The mucosal surface, as outlined by the gas, is roughened with a cobblestone appearance. Haustral markings are either absent or irregular in width and depth and the wall of the colon is thickened. Polyps or pseudopolyps cause rounded projections on the luminal surface of the affected bowel (Fig. 19-26), adding to the generally roughened appearance of the mucosal surface. Perforation of the colon is one of the major complications and may be recognized roentgenographically by the demonstration of free gas within the abdominal cavity (see Chapter 13 under "Pneumoperitoneum").

LATER CHANGES. As the disease becomes more advanced and more chronic the roentgen pattern becomes characteristic. Haustra diminish in depth and eventually disappear. The lumen of the colon becomes uniformly narrowed and the bowel is shortened (Fig. 19-27). When the disease is of segmental distribution, as in right-sided colitis, the ends of the area of involvement taper gradually and the transition to normal bowel is not abrupt. The margins of the barium-filled lumen are finely roughened as a result of the miliary ulcerations. In the post-evacuation roentgenogram, when the colon is contracted, mucosal folds are absent; instead the surface coated with barium residue has a granular appearance.

In still later stages the colon develops the characteristic "lead-pipe" appearance (Fig. 19-28). It fills very rapidly with only a few ounces of the mixture. The lumen is diffusely narrowed and the colon is greatly shortened. Occasionally one or more areas of smooth stricture formation are present.

Occasionally ulcerative colitis begins in the right side of the colon. When it does the appearance is hardly different from that seen in cases that originate in the distal part of the colon.

When the cecum is involved by chronic ulcerative colitis, the ileocecal valve usually is widely patent and rapid filling of the terminal ileum results. The ileum may be dilated but otherwise normal. Involvement of the terminal ileum, the so-called "backwash ileitis," occurs in about 10 per cent of cases of generalized ulcerative colitis. The appearance resembles regional enteritis except that the changes are less severe. Thickening of mucosal folds owing to edema, and spasm and irritability of the segment are the main findings. Narrowing usually is not pronounced and a string sign is not seen. If changes in the terminal ileum are the same as is seen in regional enteritis, the colonic disease is most likely granulomatous colitis rather than ulcerative disease.

PSEUDOPOLYPOSIS. During the later, occasionally earlier, stages of chronic ulcerative colitis polypoid or pseudopolypoid changes become frequent. The coalescence of small ulcers into larger and deeper ones with undermined edges may denude large areas of mucosa but leave islands or tags of inflamed or hypertrophied mucosa. These cause small, rounded translucent defects in the barium shadow that resemble those caused by true adenomatous polyps (Fig. 19-29). In fact, during procto-scopic examination such tags may be misinterpreted as true polyps.

Pseudopolyposis secondary to ulcerative colitis presents a typical roentgen appearance. In addition to the usual changes of narrowing, shortening, and loss of haustrations characteristic of ulcerative disease, numerous translucent defects will be seen. Those situated along the margin of the colon cause it to appear roughened (see Fig. 19-29).

CARCINOMA. Carcinoma of the colon is one of the complications of chronic ulcerative colitis. The roentgen appearance in most cases is hardly different from when the carcinoma develops without preexisting ulcerative disease.

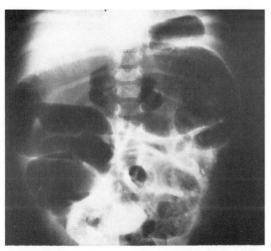

Fig. 19-25. Toxic megacolon in ulcerative colitis. The ascending and transverse portions of the colon are greatly distended with gas.

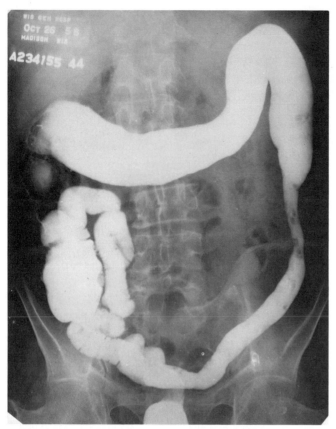

Fig. 19-26. Chronic ulcerative colitis. The entire colon is involved including the rectum with loss of haustra. A portion of the descending colon is greatly narrowed and a few pseudopolyps are seen in this area.

An occasional exception is seen where the lesion develops as a smooth, concentric narrowing with tapering ends that resembles the appearance of an inflammatory stricture very closely. Any stricture of the colon encountered under these circumstances should be viewed with suspicion and it warrants the consideration of surgical exploration.

GRANULOMATOUS COLITIS

This form of colitis is also known as Crohn's disease of the colon because it now is recognized as being the same disease as regional enteritis involving the small intestine. In contrast to ulcerative colitis, granulomatous disease tends to be right-sided and segmental and usually spares the rectum. Associated involvement of the terminal ileum is frequent and skip lesions are common. Fistula formation and sinus tracts occur as in regional enteritis. Carcinoma as a complication has not been reported and free perforation into the peritoneal cavity is rare.

Roentgen Observations

The roentgen changes in the colon are similar to those seen in regional enteritis. In the early stages the involved segment is stiffened and rigid. Mucosal folds are thickened. The small ulcers may be difficult to visualize but when seen appear as tiny spikes or projections from the lumen. Later, the wall

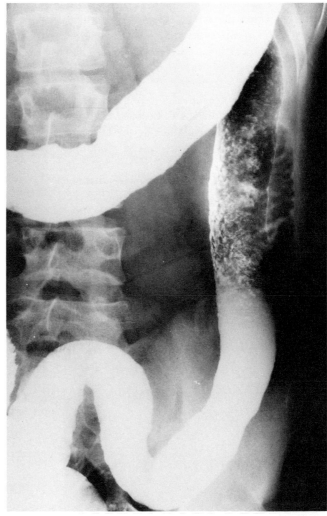

Fig. 19-27. Chronic ulcerative colitis. The left side of the colon is shown. There is complete absence of haustra and of a normal mucosal pattern. The combination of air and barium in the upper descending colon shows the mucosa to be denuded and with a coarse, granular appearance.

becomes greatly thickened and the lumen becomes narrowed. Deep ulcers develop giving the luminal margin a shaggy appearance (Figs. 19-30 and 19-31). Longitudinal ulcers also develop and are a characteristic of the disease. Transverse fissures also occur and the surface develops a cobblestone appearance. Pseudo-diverticula may develop on one wall because of eccentric involvement, the opposite wall having undergone fibrosis and contraction (Fig.

19-32). Finally the narrowing progresses to stricture formation (Fig. 19-33). The mucosa may be entirely denuded owing to the extensive ulceration. Fistulous communication to other segments of intestine may be demonstrated. Extracolonic abscesses may cause pressure defects on the bowel.

If the terminal ileum is involved, the changes are those characteristic of regional enteritis. The diagnosis at this stage then is dependent on the demonstration of single or multiple strictures, often the latter, because of the tendency to skip involvement, the presence of fistulas or sinus tracts, the smooth or cobblestone mucosal relief, the right-sided distribution, and the typical changes of regional enteritis in the ileum. The differentiation from ulcerative colitis is made on the basis of these factors and is usually possible. If the stricture is short, carcinoma may be a consideration. The sharply marginated and overhanging edges, the eccentric and irregular channel through the lesion and the complete loss of mucosal pattern favor carcinoma. Other diseases that may enter the differential diagnosis include diverticulitis and segmental infarction.

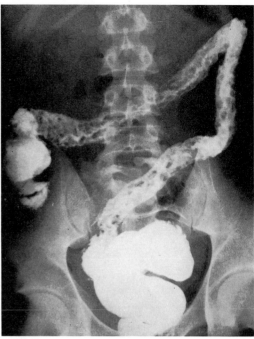

Fig. 19-29. Chronic ulcerative colitis with pseudo-polyposis. In addition to the characteristic changes of advanced chronic ulcerative colitis, there is an extensive nodular type of defect in the barium coating of the colon, indicating the presence of pseudopolyps.

OTHER INFLAMMATORY DISEASES

TUBERCULOSIS

Tuberculosis of the colon usually is associated with disease of the terminal ileum and it has been discussed in Chapter 18 under the section on "Tuberculosis."

AMEBIASIS

The diagnosis of acute intestinal amebiasis depends almost entirely upon the demonstration of *Entamoeba histolytica* in the stool. In chronic, localized disease (ameboma) those lesions in the rectosigmoid area can be biopsied. Serologic tests for amebiasis also have been found helpful by some investigators. Roentgen examination may reveal changes in the colon but in the majority of patients with

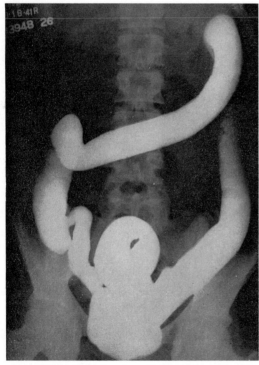

Fig. 19-28. Chronic ulcerative colitis. The disease is of considerable duration and advanced. It involves the entire colon with complete loss of normal haustral sacculations. The colon has a tubular appearance and not only is narrowed in caliber but somewhat foreshortened in length. There is a fine roughening of the mucosal surface where it is visualized in profile.

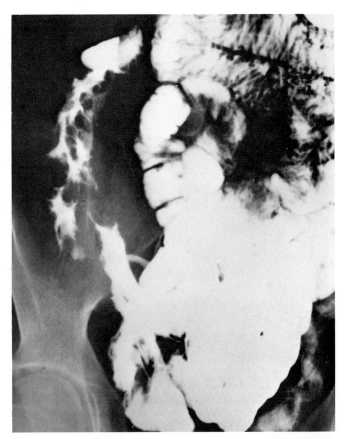

Fig. 19-30. Granulomatous ileocolitis (Crohn's disease) with involvement of terminal ileum and right side of colon as seen on a small-bowel study. The ascending colon is contracted with loss of haustra and normal mucosal pattern. There are large, irregular, and longitudinal ulcerations. The terminal ileum shows the changes of regional enteritis. There is moderate dilatation of the small intestine proximal to the terminal ileum.

amebiasis the findings are essentially normal. Pathologically the cecum, appendix, and ascending colon are involved initially in most patients. The next most frequent site is the rectosigmoid region. It is unusual to have the colon in between these areas affected unless there is an overwhelming infection. According to Faust and Jung[10] the most striking feature of amebic disease is the lack of inflammatory reaction in the mucosa unless there is secondary infection or a pronounced dysentery. Characteristically the ulcers are pinhead in size and separated from one another by normal

mucosa. As the disease progresses the ulcers become deeper, larger, and confluent with undermining of their edges.

In some patients with amebiasis, barium-enema examination will demonstrate a deformity of the cecum. It has been reported that cecal deformity occurs in approximately one-third of patients whose stools are positive for *E. histolytica* and it is much more frequent when the disease is symptomatic; thus carriers who are asymptomatic are not very likely to show changes on roentgen examination. The cecal deformity is one of concentric narrowing

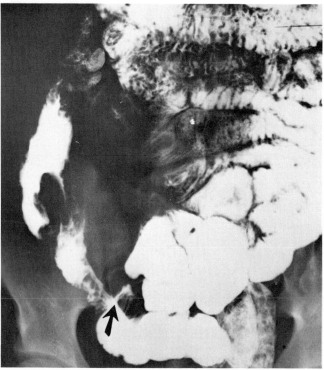

Fig. 19-31. Granulomatous ileocolitis (Crohn's disease). The ileum shows areas of constriction and dilatation. **Arrow** points to small fistulous tract arising from ileum. The ascending colon is contracted with loss of haustra. Note marked narrowing of ileum adjacent to ileocecal valve and indentation on the medial wall of the cecum owing to an inflammatory mass.

and shortening with loss of haustral indentations (Fig. 19-34). The cecum often assumes a cone-shaped appearance. The cecum usually is tender to palpation. The deformity of the cecum is believed to be caused by fibrosis from secondary infection and long-continued spasm.

Lesions in the rectosigmoid portion of the colon are even more difficult of evaluation, unless they occur in association with the rather typical cecal deformity. Stenotic narrowing is the rule but there is little to distinguish it from other lesions, particularly carcinoma. A localized, granulomatous, inflammatory mass, called an ameboma, is an occasional manifestation of the disease. According to Faust and Jung,[10] it may develop in either the cecum or the rectosigmoid area and closely resemble

carcinoma in its gross features. The roentgen differentiation may be difficult if not impossible. They recommend that preoperative stool examinations be done on all patients with a colonic mass; if amebae are found, that emetine therapy be carried out. An ameboma will decrease in size, as a rule, within 5 days under this treatment.

Tuberculosis can be distinguished from amebiasis without difficulty in most patients by the almost universal involvement of the terminal ileum as well as the cecum. The cecal deformity of amebiasis bears little resemblance to right-sided idiopathic ulcerative colitis that usually affects a much longer segment of the bowel.

A short segment of granulomatous colitis

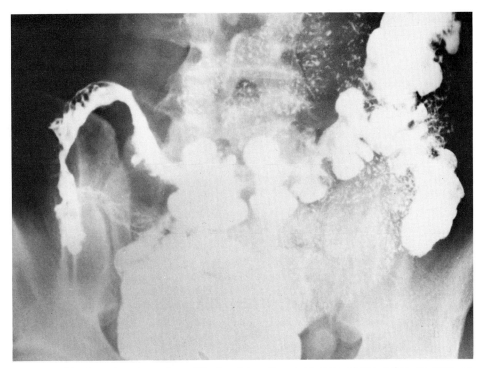

Fig. 19-32. Granulomatous ileocolitis involving the right side of the colon as seen on small-intestinal study. The terminal ileum also is involved.

may offer some difficulty in diagnosis but usually the changes of granulomatous disease are sufficiently characteristic to allow differentiation.

POSTRADIATION FIBROSIS

Following heavy doses of radiation to the pelvis, usually given for the treatment of cervical carcinoma, an intense inflammatory reaction may develop in the rectum and sigmoid. The acute reaction is followed by fibrosis and scarring and occasionally this becomes of sufficient severity to cause a stenosis of the bowel. The lesion is seen as a relatively long and smooth stricture affecting the upper rectum or sigmoid. The bowel may appear stiffened and fixed. The defect differs from that caused by an annular carcinoma by being of greater length and by the gradual tapering of its edges. The history of previous radiation to the pelvis of sufficient degree to cause damage to the bowel is important in diagnosis.

NECROTIZING ENTEROCOLITIS

This serious, usually fatal disease generally occurs in premature infants or in those with intestinal obstruction and in Hirschsprung's disease. The mucosal surface becomes denuded from extensive ulceration. On barium enema the appearance closely resembles severe ulcerative colitis. There is a complete absence of normal mucosal folds which are replaced by the extensive ulcerations. Intramural gas often is present, seen as gas bubbles within the wall of the bowel or as linear lucent streaks paralleling the lumen (Fig. 19-35). Gas in the portal venous system within the liver occasionally is noted, a finding which indicates a grave prognosis, although there have been reports of occasional survival.

SEGMENTAL ISCHEMIA; INTRAMURAL HEMORRHAGE

Segmental ischemia may involve the colon as it does the small intestine. The clinical and roentgen

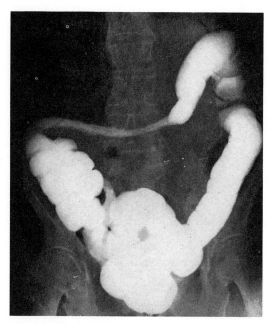

Fig. 19-33. Segmental or granulomatous colitis involving the proximal part of the transverse colon. The lesion has progressed to stricture formation. The normal mucosal pattern through the area is completely lost. The rectum and lower descending colon are uninvolved.

progress of the lesion is similar and if perforation of the colon does not occur, the end result usually is stricture formation.

Intramural hemorrhage also may occur in the colon following trauma to the abdomen, in patients taking anticoagulants, or in those suffering from a hematologic disorder such as hemophilia.

The early roentgen changes may be similar in these conditions owing to intramural bleeding in both. Characteristically on barium filling there are multiple, concave indentations or filling defects along one or both walls of the involved area, called "thumb printing" or "scalloping." It may be impossible at this stage to determine which of these lesions is present based solely on roentgen findings except that thumb printing tends to be more severe in intramural hemorrhage. However, progressive examinations usually show a prompt regression of these findings in uncomplicated hemorrhage and an eventual return to normal in contrast to the usual progressive changes in ischemia (also see page 592).

LYMPHOGRANULOMA VENEREUM

Lymphogranuloma venereum is a venereal disease spread sexually and is found most frequently in Negro women. Involvement of the rectum leads to an inflammatory fibrous stricture. According to Wright, Freeman, and Bolden[47] the length and location of the stricture are variable but the lesion usually is cylindric. The mucosal surface may be ulcerated and rectal fissures, perianal fistulas, and condylomata are often present. The Frei test usually is positive and offers a means for identification of the lesion in most cases.

INFLAMMATION OF APPENDICES EPIPLOICAE

The appendices epiploicae are small, pedunculated, fat pads along the surface of the colon, covered by the visceral peritoneum of the colon. Cases of inflammation of one or more appendices have been reported. There may be torsion with gangrene, acute inflammation with suppuration, chronic inflammation, or (rarely) intussusception. In cases reported by Kirsh and Drosd[26] the inflammatory process resembled a carcinoma in one patient; in another the appearance suggested an extrinsic mass; in a third patient there was spasm and edema of folds in the involved areas; and in a fourth patient there was only evidence of a reflex ileus. Calcification in the appendices has also been reported; it is a rare cause of intra-abdominal calcification.

HERNIAS INVOLVING THE COLON

Herniation of a loop of colon into an inguinal or femoral hernial sac is very frequent. In left-sided lesions the sigmoid colon is the portion usually involved. The hernia can be demonstrated by barium enema and its reducibility determined during fluoroscopic examination. Occasionally a large scrotal hernia will contain a long segment of the bowel. On the right side hernial sacs usually contain small intestine; infrequently the cecum will be present in the hernia. It is often impossible to distinguish an inguinal from a femoral hernia by roentgen examination; inguinal hernias are apt to be larger than femoral hernias. A volvulated loop of colon incarcerated within

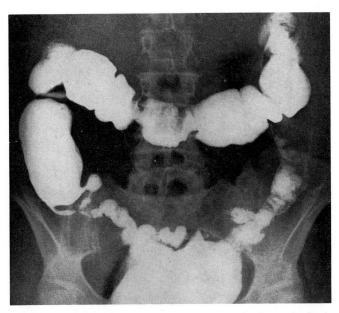

Fig. 19-34. Amebiasis of the cecum. The cecum is much short-ened but the ileum has filled readily and there also has been fill-ing of the appendix. This deformity is believed to be the result of fibrosis.

a hernia may be visualized at times because of the gas accumulation within the segment. In other patients it will contain only fluid and the roentgen signs will be those of bowel obstruction.

Herniation of colon into an anterior abdominal wall sac is another common condition. The diagnosis of abdominal hernia is essentially a clinical one and roentgen examination only serves to determine the nature of the hernial contents and to demonstrate the signs of obstruction if such exist. Lateral roentgenograms of the abdomen are useful to show the presence of gas-filled loops of bowel within the hernia when incarceration of bowel is suspected.

Lumbar hernia is an infrequent lesion that usually follows trauma but occasionally occurs spontaneously. The hernia projects posterolaterally and the diagnosis is readily made on barium enema. Plain roentgenograms of the abdomen may show a gas-filled loop of colon within the hernia. Oblique projections to bring the area into profile show the lesion to best advantage.

The colon is affected indirectly in many internal hernias but the major alteration most frequently is in the small intestine and these lesions are discussed in Chapter 18.

FUNCTIONAL DISTURBANCES

Examination of the colon by means of a barium enema is of little value in the study of most functional disturbances. The use of castor oil catharsis and cleansing enemas for preparation often make the bowel very irritable and spasm may be fairly intense. This method of examination has for its prime purpose the detection of organic disease rather than functional disturbances. An oral barium meal followed through the intestinal tract by means of serial roentgenograms may give some information concerning colonic stasis but the findings must be interpreted with considerable caution. Barium sulfate is not a food, it is insoluble in the gastrointestinal tract, and because of absorption of water from the colon the barium tends to become hardened. Because of this a colon that may function normally under ordinary circumstances may show evidence of barium stasis after an oral meal. As a general rule, therefore, the appearance of the colon after a barium meal cannot be relied upon for

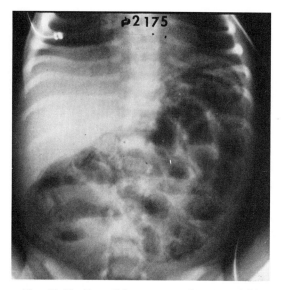

Fig. 19-35. Necrotizing enterocolitis. In addition to gas distention there are fine streaks of intramural gas in many of the segments. The presence of gas in the portal veins was suggested in the original roentgenogram.

the diagnosis of disturbed colonic function. Clinically, the terms "irritable colon," "mucous colitis," "spastic constipation" and similar designations are employed rather frequently. These clinical states do not have associated gross pathologic findings and roentgen examination does not lend itself to the clarification of these problems.

THE COLON AFTER PROLONGED CATHARTIC INGESTION

Roentgen examination occasionally demonstrates rather pronounced changes in the appearance of the colon and terminal ileum in patients who have been habitual users of irritant cathartics. In the milder cases there is shortening of the cecum, which develops a conical shape resembling somewhat the deformity seen in some cases of amebiasis. The ileocecal valve lips are shortened and the valve is gaping. In the more severe cases the colon distal to the cecum shows diminution in haustral sacculations and becomes quite smooth; the lumen may be narrowed or enlarged, and, in the con-

tracted state the mucosal folds assume a linear arrangement rather than a crisscross pattern. On the whole the appearance resembles in many ways idiopathic ulcerative colitis. The bowel, however, is not as stiffened, as it is in long-standing chronic ulcerative colitis, there is no history of diarrhea or bloody stools; instead there is a history of ingestion of irritant cathartics over a period of many years (Fig. 19-36).

In other patients who have developed the enema habit, using a daily or almost daily enema of soapsuds in order to obtain a bowel movement, a rather similar alteration in the appearance of the bowel has been observed by us. It is well to keep in mind these conditions when changes of this nature are found during barium-enema examination because they may be misinterpreted as evidence of chronic ulcerative colitis. As noted in the preceding paragraphs, correlation with the clinical history and findings is important.

THE POSTOPERATIVE COLON

Preparation of the postoperative colon for barium-enema examination depends to a large extent upon the nature of the operative procedure. If this has consisted of local excision of a polyp or resection with end-to-end anastomosis, the same preparation is used as for the standard examination, including castor oil catharsis and cleansing tap-water enemas. When a colostomy is present it usually is sufficient to irrigate the bowel through the colostomy opening, using a balloon catheter. If the rectum has not been removed as part of the operative procedure, the distal part of the colon is cleansed by means of tap-water enemas given in the usual manner.

For the barium enema, if a colostomy is present, the balloon catheter is inserted into the colostomy opening with the balloon inflated with no more than 20 to 30 cc of air. This forms an efficient plug so that filling of the proximal colon occurs without difficulty in most cases and the balloon prevents escape of material through the colostomy. The balloon is left in place and inflated until fluoroscopy is completed and roentgenograms of the filled colon have been made. If the rectum has not been removed, the lower part

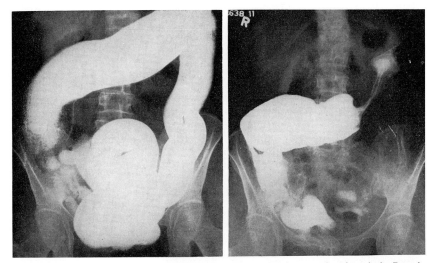

Fig. 19-36. The colon after prolonged ingestion of irritant cathartics. *Left,* Roentgenogram of the barium-filled colon and *right,* same patient after evacuation of the mixture. The appearance of the filled colon resembles that of chronic ulcerative colitis except that the caliber is not narrowed but rather dilated. In the postevacuation roentgenogram, emptying is very incomplete with only the left side contracted. The mucosal folds appear grossly abnormal and again suggest ulcerative colitis. Correlation of the roentgen findings with the clinical history is important in these patients.

of the bowel can be examined by barium enema given rectally, and if obstruction is not present the entire segment from the anus to the colostomy is examined in this manner. If the bowel above and below the colostomy is to be examined at one sitting it is preferable to fill the proximal part first by means of the balloon catheter; with this still in place an ordinary rectal tube can be inserted and the bowel distal to the colostomy filled. In this manner the entire colon can be examined, if obstruction is not present, without undue spilling of contents onto the skin surface.

END-TO-END ANASTOMOSIS

For lesions in the lower part of the descending colon and in the sigmoid area, local resection with end-to-end anastomosis often is performed. The roentgen appearance of such an anastomosis varies somewhat with the time interval after surgery. Usually after a period of several months there will have been subsidence of the postoperative edema and after this period the appearance of the anastomosis does not change significantly. In many cases the site of the anastomosis is difficult to detect. When the segment is completely distended, a thin ringlike constriction may be visualized, but in some cases there is no change in the width of the lumen. Frequently a distinct and abrupt change in the mucosal pattern and the haustral indentations will indicate the site of the resection. Occasionally the postevacuation roentgenogram demonstrates these changes to better advantage than when the colon is completely distended. Because the normal findings may vary somewhat, Fleishner and Berenberg[13] have recommended that a postoperative barium enema be done on every patient who has had resection and end-to-end anastomosis for carcinoma within several months after the operation. This preliminary examination will serve as a reference for later studies and will be of aid in detecting early recurrences. They point out that any irregularity or nodular defect along the suture line, no matter how small, should be viewed with suspicion unless a similar irregularity was seen in the immediate postoperative period. Only by careful observation

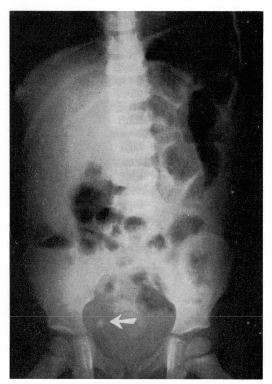

Fig. 19-37. Acute appendicitis with perforation. Upright roentgenogram of the abdomen of a child showing the presence of gas in the intestinal tract having the pattern of an adynamic ileus. The **arrow** points to a calcified appendiceal fecalith. Note fluid level in cecum.

and serial examinations is it possible to detect recurrent carcinoma at the site of resection when it still is in an early stage. After the lesion becomes more advanced the roentgen findings are no different from those seen in primary carcinoma of the colon. It is also important to remember that multiple tumors of the colon are not infrequent and that follow-up examinations are very useful in detecting early polyp formation and carcinomatous degeneration in polyps in other parts of the colon.

RESECTION OF THE COLON

Resection of the proximal colon and ileo-transverse colostomy is another common operative procedure performed for disease involv-ing the right side of the colon. The roentgenologist should be informed of the presence of an anastomosis between the ileum and colon before the barium-enema examination is begun. Otherwise there may be rapid extension of the barium mixture through the anastomosis with rapid flooding of loops of small bowel so that the site becomes obscured. This may happen while the examiner's attention is centered elsewhere and by the time he becomes aware of the presence of an anastomosis the field may be hidden completely and the examination will be unsatisfactory. Recurrence of carcinoma in the stump of the resected colon is relatively uncommon. In these patients recurrences are more likely to develop in the tissues at the site of the original lesion, in the draining lymph nodes, or as a metastatic spread to the liver. Barium-enema examination of the postoperative colon in these patients, therefore, is of value chiefly in demonstrating the patency of the ileotransverse colostomy and in the detection of possible new tumors in the colon that remains. These patients should have thorough preparation so that fecal matter is eliminated from the colon insofar as possible.

THE APPENDIX

Filling of the appendix occurs frequently during barium-enema examinations of the colon and it also can be demonstrated when delayed roentgenograms (i.e., at 6, 24, and 48 hours) are obtained after the oral administration of barium. Failure of visualization of the appendix by either method is no indication that it is diseased. If the appendix does fill, some idea of its size, position, and mobility can be obtained. It is not uncommon to find the appendix remaining visible because of barium filling for days after the examination and it is doubtful if the demonstration of such stasis has any clinical significance. The diagnosis of chronic appendicitis cannot be made from roentgen findings. The retrocecal position of the appendix often can be established if the structure fills with barium; even if it does not the posterior position of the ileocecal valve usually indicates a posterior location of the appendix as well.

ACUTE APPENDICITIS

Roentgen examination in acute appendicitis is usually limited to scout roentgenograms of the abdomen. Barium-enema examination should be avoided when possible in the presence of an acute inflammatory process within the abdomen and there seldom is any reason for doing a barium meal study of the upper gastrointestinal tract and small intestine in these patients. Within a few hours after the onset of acute appendicitis, scout roentgenograms often will show the presence of one or several short loops of gas-filled ileum in the right lower quadrant. As a rule the distention is slight and fluid levels, in upright roentgenograms, are either absent or short and inconspicuous. A fluid level may be demonstrated in the cecum in upright or left lateral decubitus views (Fig. 19-37). This is an important sign when taken in conjunction with other findings, provided an enema has not been given prior to the examination and there is no obstruction in the distal colon. In the presence of the latter, the entire colon will be distended rather than distention being limited to the cecum and ascending colon. In the presence of a spreading inflammation the signs of a more generalized ileus may develop. In later stages the soft-tissue spaces between the loops may be thickened as a result of spread of the inflammation and the presence of exudate on the serosal surfaces of the bowel. In some cases blurring of the properitoneal fat line (see page 412) along the right lower abdominal wall is observed. This finding is difficult to interpret because visibility of the line varies considerably in normal individuals and as an isolated observation its value in the diagnosis of acute appendicitis is limited. Indistinctness in the outline of the lower part of the psoas shadow and a scoliosis, concavity to the right, may be

seen in some patients, but these signs alone are also difficult to evaluate.

Whenever the diagnosis of acute appendicitis is being considered, careful observation of the right lower quadrant of the abdomen for evidence of a calcified fecalith in the appendix should be done. The fecalith is seen as a round or ovoid shadow of calcium density and may be laminated (Fig. 19-37). The size varies but usually is on the order of 0.5 to 1 cm. The fecalith frequently overlies the ilium and may be difficult to visualize because of the density of the bone. In some cases the fecalith is extruded from the appendix as a result of rupture and comes to lie within an abscess cavity. The fecalith may be visualized low in the right side of the pelvis when the ascending colon is long and the cecum abnormally low in position. It may resemble an ordinary phlebolith in the pelvic veins. Appendiceal fecaliths (coproliths) will be found in approximately one-fourth of cases of acute appendicitis in children and in about one-half of the patients plain films of the abdomen will suggest an inflammatory process in the abdomen.

If the appendix ruptures and a more extensive peritonitis develops, the roentgen signs become those of an adynamic ileus with evidence of peritoneal exudate separating the gas-filled loops of bowel. Rupture of the appendix rarely leads to pneumoperitoneum (Frimann-Dahl) and the demonstration of free gas in the peritoneal cavity in upright or lateral decubitus roentgenograms is not to be expected.

APPENDICEAL ABSCESS

During the acute stage of an appendiceal abscess roentgen findings are usually limited to those of (1) adynamic ileus (see Fig. 13-33), (2) evidence of an ill-defined mass of soft-tissue density in the lower right quadrant with an absence of gas shadows in the area, (3) occasional identification of a calcified concretion or fecalith in the area, and (4) in some cases gas may form within the abscess visualized as small flocculent translucencies within the mass of the abscess (see page 439 and Fig. 13-34). After subsidence of the acute phase, some patients are examined by means of a barium-enema because the clinical signs have been atypical and the diagnosis remains in doubt. In these cases a barium-enema examination often will show evidence of a mass adjacent to the tip of the cecum deforming it and causing a filling defect in the cecum (Figs. 19-38 and 19-39). There is local tenderness, the cecum is fixed in position, and careful study of roentgenograms will show mucosal folds and deformed but intact haustra. If the ileum fills by reflux through the ileocecal valve it will be displaced by the mass; its lumen may be narrowed irregularly and its mucosal folds thickened. In some of these patients the demonstration of a calcified fecalith within the mass is the most convincing diagnostic sign. The history of a recent episode of acute nature, the tender mass, and the location immediately

adjacent to and fixed to the cecum are helpful corroborative signs.

TUMORS OF THE APPENDIX

MUCOCELE

Mucocele of the appendix is an uncommon lesion, its frequency in routine autopsies being reported as from 0.2 to 0.5 per cent. It is generally considered to arise as a result of a gradual occlusion of the appendiceal lumen with the development of a cystlike mass filled with a pseudomucinous material. In addition to this benign type of lesion, there is a malignant form that is in fact a mucoid papillary adenocarcinoma of a low degree of malignancy. This tumor resembles a benign mucocele in its gross features but differs in behavior. Should rupture of a malignant mucocele occur, there may be implantation of epithelial cells on the surface of the peritoneum. These cells continue to produce mucus and give rise to the condition known as pseudomyxoma

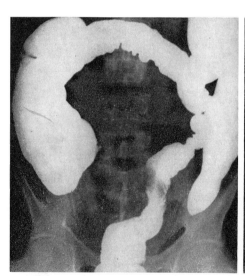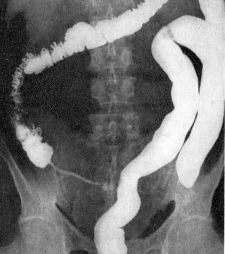

Fig. 19-38. Appendiceal abscess. *Left,* Roentgenogram of barium enema at the time of admission about a week after the onset of clinical symptoms. There is a mass below and medial to the cecum that is deforming the contiguous portion of the sigmoid and rectum. A small ring-contoured calcification could be seen over the midportion of the sacrum in the original roentgenogram. *Right,* Same patient several months later. Postevacuation barium-enema roentgenogram now shows the appendix, having filled with barium, extending to overlie the sacrum. The barium has surrounded the fecalith, which now can be seen to lie in the tip of the appendix. The mass of the abscess has decreased considerably. Patient was operated upon and the diagnosis confirmed.

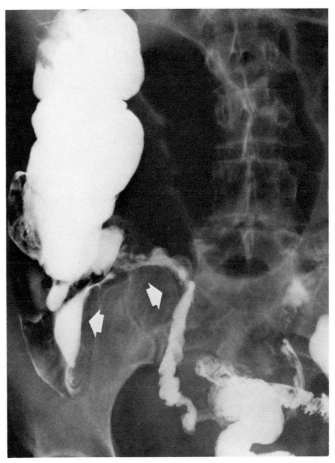

Fig. 19-39. Appendiceal abscess. Residual barium in the colon after barium enema demonstrates a mass pressing on the cecum and terminal ileum (**arrows**).

peritonaei, which is described in Chapter 13 under the heading "Pseudomyxoma Peritonaei."

The roentgen diagnostic features of appendiceal mucocele were outlined by Åkerlund[1] in 1936 and reemphasized by Euphrat[8]:

1. A sharply outlined round or ovoid soft-tissue mass in the right lower quadrant, usually having a fair degree of mobility. On barium-enema examination the mass is found to be attached to the cecum and to move with it (Fig. 19-40).

2. The cecum is displaced to some extent by the mass. It may be displaced laterally or medially, depending upon the position of the appendix.

3. Calcium deposits are common in the wall of the mucocele.

4. The appendix does not fill.

5. The mass may cause no cecal deformity if small; if larger, a smooth, pressure type of defect is seen with intact but distorted mucosal folds.

Intussusception of a mucocele into the cecum is a rare complication. When this happens the defect resembles that of a polypoid cecal tumor and the diagnosis of a mucocele cannot be made unless there is calcification in its wall.

ADENOCARCINOMA

Mention has been made in a previous paragraph of the mucoid papillary type of adenocarcinoma or malignant mucocele. There also is a solid so-called

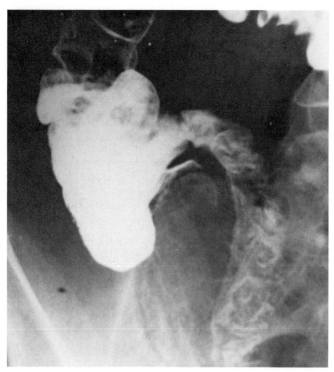

Fig. 19-40. Mucocele of the appendix. There is a thin shell of calcification partially outlining the mass which displaces the ileum medially and causes pressure indentation on the cecum.

"colonic" type of adenocarcinoma arising in the appendix but it is a very rare lesion. This tumor soon invades the cecum and then it comes to resemble a primary carcinoma of the cecum in its clinical and roentgen features.

CARCINOID TUMORS

Carcinoid tumors are not limited to the appendix although they occur most frequently in this location. It is known that this tumor may develop in any part of the gastrointestinal tract. It is generally accepted that carcinoids arise from the silver-staining cells known as Kultschitzky's cells that are found in the crypts of Lieberkühn. Because of silver-staining properties the tumor also is known as an *argentaffin tumor* or *argentaffinoma*. Current opinion also stresses the fact that carcinoids, particularly those arising elsewhere than in the appendix, in addition to being locally invasive, may metastasize and their malignant characteristics seem to be definitely established. Carcinoids of the appendix are more likely to be single lesions and they show less tendency to metastasize than do carcinoids arising elsewhere in the gastrointestinal tract. In the small intestine, invasion of the wall and infiltration of the tumor into the mesentery leads to fibrosis, angulation of the loop, and an adherence of peritoneal surfaces. Miller and Hermann found the combination of sharp angulation and a filling defect to be an important roentgen sign of carcinoid of the small intestine. In the appendix, the roentgen diagnosis is hardly possible. The tumors often are small and situated in the tip of the appendix. Only in the event that the lesion invades contiguous structures, particularly the mesentery and ileum or cecal tip, is it likely to produce any roentgen signs. (Also see Chapter 18).

APPENDICEAL STUMP DEFECT

After appendectomy, invagination of the appendiceal stump may produce a polyplike filling defect in the tip of the cecum, and which may resemble a polyp very closely (Fig. 19-41). The

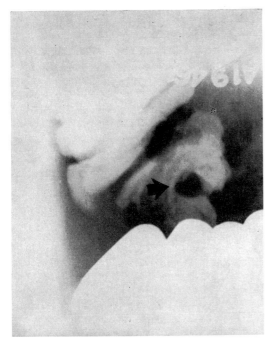

Fig. 19-41. Appendiceal stump defect. Spot roentgenogram of the cecum made during fluoroscopic examination and with compression applied over the abdominal wall. This brings out the defect of an inverted appendiceal stump as it projects into the base of the cecum (**arrow**).

history of previous appendectomy and the location of the defect are important aids in establishing its nature.

REFERENCES AND SELECTED READINGS

1. ÅKERLUND, A.: Mukozele in der appendix roentgenologisch diagnostizierbar. *Acta Radiol. 17:* 594, 1936.

2. BERDON, W. E., BAKER, D. H., SANTULLI, T. V., and AMOURY, R. A.: The radiologic evaluation of imperforate anus. *Radiology 90:* 466, 1968.

3. BERDON, W. E., BAKER, D. H., SANTULLI, T. V., AMOURY, R. A., and BLANC, W. A.: Microcolon in newborn infants with intestinal obstruction. *Radiology 90:* 878, 1968.

4. BRAHME, F.: Granulomatous colitis. Roentgenologic appearance and course of the lesions. *Am. J. Roentgenol. Radium Ther. Nucl. Med. 99:* 35, 1967.

5. CAPITANIO, M. A., and KIRKPATRICK, J. A.: Lymphoid hyperplasia of the colon in children: Roentgen observations. *Radiology 94:* 323, 1970.

6. CASTLEMAN, B., and KRICHSTEIN, H. I.: Do adenomatous polyps of colon become malignant? *N. Engl. J. Med. 267:* 469, 1962.

7. DUNBAR, J. D., and NELSON, S. W.: Nonangiographic manifestations of intestinal vascular disease. *Am. J. Roentgenol. Radium Ther. Nucl. Med. 99:* 127, 1967.

8. EUPHRAT, E. J.: Roentgen features of mucocele of the appendix. *Radiology 48:* 113, 1947.

9. FARMAN, J.: Vascular lesions of the colon. *Br. J. Radiol. 39:* 575, 1966.

10. FAUST, E. C., and JUNG, R. C.: Protozoan and metazoan parasitoses of the intestinal tract. *Ped. Clin. North Am.,* Feb. 1956, pp. 169–190. Philadelphia, Saunders.

11. FIGIEL, L. S., FIGIEL, S. J., and WIETERSEN, F. K.: Is surgical removal of every colonic polyp necessary? *Am. J. Roentgenol. Radium Ther. Nucl. Med. 88:* 721, 1962.

12. FLEISCHNER, F. G.: "Diverticular Disease and the Irritable Colon Syndrome," in *Alimentary Tract Roentgenology,* ed. by A. R. Margulis and H. R. Burhenne. St. Louis, Mo., Mosby, 1967, p. 784.

13. FLEISCHNER, F. G., and BERENBERG, A. L.: Recurrent carcinoma of the colon at the site of the anastomosis. Roentgen observations. *Radiology 66:* 540, 1956.

14. FLEISCHNER, F. G., and BERNSTEIN, C.: Roentgenanatomical studies of the normal ileoceal valve. *Radiology 54:* 43, 1950.

15. FRANKEN, E. A., JR.: Lymphoid hyperplasia of the colon. *Radiology 94:* 329, 1970.

16. FRYE, T. A.: Villous adenomas of the sigmoid colon. *Radiology 73:* 71, 1959.

17. GIRDANY, B. R., BASS, L. R., and SIEBER, W. K.: Roentgenologic aspects of hydrostatic reduction of ileocolic intussusception. *Am. J. Roentgenol. Radium Ther. Nucl. Med. 82:* 455, 1959.

18. HEILBRUN, N., and BERNSTEIN, C.: Roentgen abnormalities of the large and small intestine associated with prolonged cathartic ingestion. *Radiology 65:* 549, 1955.

19. HILL, M. C., and GOLDBERG, H. I.: Roentgen diagnosis of intestinal amebiasis. *Am. J. Roentgenol. Radium Ther. Nucl. Med. 99:* 77, 1967.

20. HODGSON, J. R., and SAUER, W. G.: The roentgenologic features of carcinoma in chronic ulcerative colitis. *Am. J. Roentgenol. Radium Ther. Nucl. Med. 86:* 91, 1961.

21. HOPE, J. W., BORNS, P. F., and BERG, P. K.: Roentgenologic manifestations of Hirschsprung's disease in infancy. *Am. J. Roentgenol. Radium Ther. Nucl. Med. 95:* 217, 1965.

22. JENKINSON, E. L., and BROWN, W. H.: Endometriosis. *JAMA 122:* 349, 1943.

23. JONES, E. L., and CORNELL, W. P.: Gardner's syndrome. Review of the literature and report on a family. *Arch. Surg. 92:* 287, 1966.

24. KAYE, J. J., and BRAGG, D. E.: Unusual roentgenologic and clinicopathologic features of villous adenomas of the colon. *Radiology 91:* 799, 1968.

25. KERRY, R. L., and RANSOM, H. K.: Volvulus of the colon. Etiology, diagnosis and treatment. *Arch. Surg. 99:* 215, 1969.

26. KIRSH, D., and DROSD, R. E.: Roentgen changes in diseases of the appendices epiploicae. *Am. J. Roentgenol. Radium Ther. Nucl. Med. 81:* 640, 1959.

27. KURLANDER, G. J.: Roentgenology of imperforate anus. *Am. J. Roentgenol. Radium Ther. Nucl. Med. 100:* 190, 1967.

28. LILJA, B., and PROBST, F.: Intestinal endometriosis. *Acta Radiol. (Diag.) 4:* 545, 1966.

29. MARGULIS, A. R.: "Examination of the Colon," in *Alimentary Tract Roentgenology,* ed. by A. R. Margulis and H. J. Burhenne. St. Louis, Mo., Mosby, 1967.

30. MARSHAK, R. H., and LINDNER, A. E.: "Ulcerative and Granulomatous Colitis," in *Alimentary Tract Roentgenology,* ed. by A. R. Margulis and H. J. Burhenne. St. Louis, Mo., Mosby, 1967, p. 742.

31. MARSHAK, R. H., MOSELEY, J. E., and WOLF, B. S.: The roentgen findings in familial polyposis with special emphasis on differential diagnosis. *Radiology 80:* 374, 1963.

32. MIKITY, V. G., HODGMAN, J. E., and PACINILLI, J.: Meconium blockage syndrome. *Radiology 88:* 740, 1967.

33. MOERTEL, C. G., DOCKERTY, M. B., and JUDD, E. S.: Carcinoid tumors of the vermiform appendix. *Cancer 21:* 270, 1968.

34. PARKS, T. G., CONNELL, A. M., GOUGH, A. D., and COLE, J. O. Y.: Limitations of radiology in the differentiation of diverticulitis and diverticulosis. *Br. Med. J. 2:* 136, 1970.

35. POCHACZEVSKY, R., and SHERMAN, R. S.: Diffuse lymphomatous disease of the colon: Its roentgen appearance. *Am. J. Roentgenol. Radium Ther. Nucl. Med. 87:* 670, 1962.

36. POTTER, R. M.: Dilute contrast media in diagnosis of lesions of the colon. *Radiology 60:* 500, 1953.

37. REEVES, B. F., CARLSON, H. C., and DOCKERTY, M. B.: Segmental ulcerative colitis versus segmental Crohn's disease. *Am. J. Roentgenol. Radium Ther. Nucl. Med. 99:* 24, 1967.

38. SAMUEL, E.: Gastrointestinal manifestations of vascular disease. *Proc. R. Soc. Med. 60:* 839, 1967.

39. STEINBACH, H. L., ROSENBERG, R. H., GROSSMAN, M., and NELSON, T. L.: The potential hazard of enemas in patients with Hirschsprung's disease. *Radiology 64:* 45, 1955.

40. SWINTON, N. W.: Polyps of rectum and colon. *JAMA 154:* 658, 1954.

41. SWISCHUK, L. E.: Meconium plug syndrome: A cause of neonatal obstruction. *Am. J. Roentgenol. Radium Ther. Nucl. Med. 103:* 339, 1968.

42. WEBER, H., and DIXON, C. F.: Duplication of the entire large intestine (colon duplex). *Am. J. Roentgenol. Radium Ther. Nucl. Med. 55:* 319, 1946.

43. WICHULIS, A. R., BEAHRS, O. H., and WOOLNER, L. B.: Malignant lymphoma of the colon. A study of 69 cases. *Arch. Surg. 93:* 215, 1966.

44. WOLF, B. S., and MARSHAK, R. H.: "Toxic" segmental dilatation of the colon during the course of fulminating ulcerative colitis: Roentgen findings. *Am. J. Roentgenol. Radium Ther. Nucl. Med. 82:* 985, 1959.

45. WOLFSON, J. J., GOLDSTEIN, G., KRIVIT, W., and HONG, R.: Lymphoid hyperplasia of the large intestine associated with dysgammaglobulinemia. *Am. J. Roentgenol. Radium Ther. Nucl. Med. 108:* 610, 1970.

46. WOOLNER, L. B.: Carcinoma of the appendix. Comments on pathology. *Proc. Staff Meet. Mayo Clin. 28:* 17, 1953.

47. WRIGHT, L. T., FREEMAN, W. A., and BOLDEN, J. V.: Lymphogranulomatous strictures of the rectum: A résumé of four hundred and seventy-six cases. *Arch. Surg. 53:* 499, 1946.

48. YOUNG, B. R., and SCANLAN, R. L.: Roentgen demonstration and significance of the pedicle in polypoid tumors of the alimentary tract. *Am. J. Roentgenol. Radium Ther. Nucl. Med. 68:* 894, 1952.

Section IV

THE URINARY AND
FEMALE GENITAL TRACTS

20

THE URINARY TRACT

METHODS OF EXAMINATION

THE PLAIN-FILM ROENTGENOGRAM

Roentgen examination of the urinary tract should begin with a plain film of the abdomen taken with the patient in a supine position. This roentgenogram includes the kidneys, ureteral and bladder areas, and is commonly termed a KUB or scout film. If the patient is tall, an extra roentgenogram of the bladder is necessary. In this plain-film examination the renal shadows can be seen and their size, shape, and position noted. The presence of calcium in cysts, tumors, or stones can be detected along with vascular or lymph-node calcification in the area. Psoas muscle shadows are usually well outlined and asymmetry or other abnormalities can be noted. The ureters cannot be defined but radiopaque calculi may be detected along the course of the ureter. The shadow cast by the urinary bladder can often be identified. Vesical calculi can be outlined. Vascular calcifications, including phleboliths and arterial plaques, are frequently seen in the pelvis and must be differentiated from urinary calculi. This often requires special examinations. These conditions are discussed more fully in Chapter 13.

EXCRETORY UROGRAPHY

PREPARATION OF THE PATIENT

Excretory or intravenous urography is a relatively simple method of outlining the excretory system and is used widely for detection of disease involving it. Preparation for the examination consists of castor oil catharsis the evening before the study to remove gas and fecal matter from the colon, since this tends to obscure the renal areas. Mild dehydration is obtained by omitting fluids from 10 P.M. the evening before the examination. Breakfast also is omitted. Many variations of the above method are in use and satisfactory urography often can be obtained with no preparation, particularly in ambulatory out-patients.

In infants and small children a carbonated beverage can be given to distend the stomach with gas. This displaces the bowel enough to allow visualization of the renal shadows through the gas-filled stomach.

CONTRAST MEDIA

The contrast media are organic iodides which depend on their iodine content for radiopacity. Those generally used in intravenous urography include the following:

1. Conray (meglumine iothalamate) in 60% concentration provides 28.2% iodine. Angio-conray is an 80% concentration of the same drug, used chiefly for angiocardiography and aortography.

2. Hypaque Sodium (sodium diatrizoate) in 50% solution contains approximately 30% iodine. Hypaque is also available in 75 and 90% concentrations for angiography.

3. Renografin-60 (meglumine diatrizoate) in 60% solution contains approximately 29% iodine. Renografin-76, a 76% solution, is also available for urography and angiography. Renografin-DIP (14% iodine) is used for infusion studies.

4. Renovist (sodium and meglumine diatrizoates) provides 35% sodium diatrizoate and 34.3% meglumine diatrizoate. It can be used for angiography as well as for excretory urography.

Because new contrast media are introduced at frequent intervals, the above list very likely will be altered within the next few years. At the present time we are using 50 ml of Renovist and find it a very satisfactory medium. This dose is somewhat larger than has been used in the past, but we find that the urograms are better with no more reactions.

Drip-infusion urography is used in patients with renal insufficiency when the BUN is over 40 mgm %. We have been able to get reasonably good studies when the BUN is between 40 and 80 mgm %. When the BUN is in the range of 80 to 120 mgm %, gross anatomic features of the renal collecting system can usually be defined in cases where such information is vital to the care of the patient. We use Renografin-DIP (42.3 gm of iodine per 300 cc) for this examination. It may be necessary to take a series of delayed films—often for several hours after the infusion.

Contraindications to intravenous urography are: (1) hypersensitivity to iodine or to the salts of diatrizoic acid, (2) the presence of combined renal and hepatic disease, (3) oliguria, (4) a BUN level over 100 to 120 mgm %, and (5) multiple myeloma (unless the patient can be kept well hydrated during and after the study). All of these contraindications are relative and the value of potential information to be obtained must be weighed against the risk in each patient.

In children high-dose urography is also used commonly to avoid the necessity of doing retrograde studies. Using either meglumine (Renografin-60) or sodium (Hypaque 50) diatrizoate, a dosage of 3 cc per kilogram of body weight at birth, 2 cc per kilogram of body weight in older infants and 1 to 2 cc per kilogram of body weight in children to 10 years is satisfactory. The following guidelines may also be used: below 2500 gm weight—use 5 to 8 cc; for full-term newborn use 10 cc; for those 1 to 6 months in age, use 12 to 15 cc; for those 6 to 12 months, use 15 to 18 cc; for ages 1 to 2 years, use 18 to 25 cc; for ages 2 to 5 years, use 25 to 30 cc, and for those 5 to 10 years of age, use 30 to 45 cc.

The contrast media usually are injected intravenously but intramuscular injection can be used in infants and children. The media are all organic iodides, which are filtered rapidly by the kidney. They may all produce reactions of varying severity so that certain precautions should be taken before their use. Sensitivity tests are not reliable and are not in general use except as a medicolegal precautionary measure. Intravenous, subcutaneous, and conjunctival tests can be used and directions for these tests are printed by the manufacturer and enclosed with the ampules of the contrast material. Even though a sensitivity test has been done it is advisable to inject a very small amount of the contrast substance intravenously and wait for 1 or 2 minutes before injecting the remainder. If there is a reaction to the test dose, the procedure should be discontinued. The most common symptoms are flushing, arm pain, nausea, vomiting, urticaria, asthma, allergic rhinitis, and other allergic manifestations. Severe reactions with vasomotor collapse and convulsions occur occasionally and deaths have been reported.

Treatment of reactions is usually symptomatic. Anoxia is almost always present and can be treated by the administration of 100% oxygen using a mask and bag. If necessary an intratracheal airway may be used. Oxygen and the necessary equipment for its administration should be available in departments where intravenous injections of these substances are performed.

Hypotension can be treated by injection of Neo-synephrine Hydrochloride intravenously in doses of 0.2 to 0.5 mg. Epinephrine may produce ventricular fibrillation in the presence of anoxia owing to reaction of some of the media and should not be used. If hypotension persists for more than a few minutes, a continuous infusion of Levophed Bitartrate should be started (4 cc of 0.2% solution in 500 cc of 5% dextrose).

Convulsions should be treated by administration of a short-acting barbiturate intravenously. Allergic phenomena are treated by intravenous Benadryl (1 to 5 cc) or by any of the other antihistaminic agents. The prophylactic use of antihistamines has been advocated by some, and we use them occasionally.

TECHNIQUE OF EXAMINATION

Following injection of the contrast substance it is desirable to use some method to hold the material in the kidneys in order to outline the pelvis and calyces. We use a compression band under which a blood pressure cuff has been placed; when a pressure of 90 to 100 mmHg is used the ureters are obstructed sufficiently to produce satisfactory filling. The band is placed just above the symphysis pubis so that the ureters are partially compressed as they pass over the pelvic brim. This method is simple and effective but there are other methods of compression that may be used and a variety of special divided compression devices are available. The Trendelenburg position is of some use when the patient cannot tolerate a compression device. Compression is not necessary in patients with obstruction and may be inadvisable when the examination is being done for a suspected ureteral calculus. When the examination is done as a functional study it is also inadvisable to use compression. In patients with hypertension of suspected renal origin the early films are taken without compression. Then compression may be applied after the 5-minute film to produce complete filling for anatomic study. In patients with suspected aortic aneurysms or similar masses the use of compression is unwise.

The first roentgenogram is taken approximately 5 minutes after injection and a second is obtained at 15 minutes. The compression band then is released and a third roentgenogram is made. Additional exposures of the bladder area may be necessary in some instances. Oblique films are of value in patients with suspected ureteral calculi and in those in whom questionable calyceal abnormalities are observed on the anteroposterior films. When it is important to visualize the ureters, a film in the prone position is useful, since the ureters fill better in the prone than in the supine position. In some institutions one roentgenogram in the prone position is taken routinely; others take an upright film routinely. It is important to inspect each film to determine what additional films are needed. Fluoroscopy is sometimes useful to determine renal motion and study ureteral function. If excretion of contrast material is delayed it may be necessary to obtain roentgenograms for periods up to several hours after injection. In patients with acute ureteral obstruction, such as is frequently present when a ureteral calculus is being passed, there is often a delay in excretion on the involved side. Delayed roentgenograms may show opacification of the renal pelvis and ureter down to the level of obstruction when the immediate roentgenograms will reveal only increased density of the renal parenchyma. Delayed roentgenograms are of value whenever there is delay in excretion. Special methods are used in patients with hypertension of possible renovascular origin. These are described on page 690.

RETROGRADE UROGRAPHY

Retrograde urography is another method used in the examination of the upper urinary tract. It is generally used to confirm findings suspected on intravenous urography and can also be used when the excretory urogram has been unsatisfactory or inconclusive. Cystoscopy and catheterization of the ureters is necessary for this examination. Roentgenograms are taken following direct instillation of contrast material into the pelves via the catheters. Media available are Pyelokon-R (20% solution of sodium acetrizoate), Retropaque (20% solution of methiodol sodium with 4.2% neomycin sulfate), and Retrografin (30% solution of sodium and methylglucamine diatrizoate with 2.5% neomycin). Occasionally air is used as a contrast substance, particularly when a radiolucent calculus is suspected and is not visible on excretory urography or on retrograde study using an opaque. Ten to 15 cc are slowly injected via ureteral catheter into the renal pelvis and roentgenograms are taken. The catheters are withdrawn and another roentgenogram is exposed. Oblique views and delayed frontal views may also be necessary in some patients. The chief advantage of retrograde pyelography is that a dense contrast substance can be injected directly under controlled pressure so that visualization is good. The extent of impairment of renal function that may be present does not influence the degree of visualization. Excretory urography is a simpler and easier procedure because cystoscopy is not necessary. This is particularly important in children and it also has advantages in patients with renal injury and with anomalies such as duplication of the ureters. The excretory method also serves as a test of renal function, particularly of comparative function of the two kidneys. Its chief disadvantage is incomplete visualization owing to failure of filling of portions of the excretory system. With the newer contrast media, excretory films of a quality comparable to retrograde studies can be obtained in many patients, eliminating the need for ureteral catheterization.

RENAL ANGIOGRAPHY

There are several methods for the radiographic study of the renal arteries. Translumbar aortography is one. The use of a catheter, introduced percutaneously into the femoral artery by the Seldinger technique or by direct arterial cut-down of the femoral or ulnar artery, permits more variability in techniques than the translumbar method. A midstream aortic injection is made first using 30 to 40 cc of Renovist or Renografin 76. This survey examination indicates location and number of renal arteries and may define abnormal lumbar vessels in patients with metastatic tumor (Fig. 20-1A). Then selective renal arteriograms are done by manipulation of the catheter tip under fluoroscopic control into the desired renal artery followed by injection of small amounts (6 to 10 cc of Renografin 60 or similar opaque material) into the artery. This has the advantage of dense opacification of the renal artery and its branches that is needed in a detailed study of the vessels. The main disadvantages are that a small accessory

vessel may be missed and multiple injections are required when multiple vessels are present. Simultaneous study of both renal arteries can be done by placing the catheter equipped with multiple side holes at the proper level in the aorta. Injection of 30 to 40 cc of 90% Hypaque or a similar medium usually results in satisfactory filling of both renal arteries. This method has the advantage of filling accessory arteries that may be present, as well as affording simultaneous visualization allowing comparison of the renal vessels on the normal and abnormal sides.

TRANSLUMBAR AORTOGRAPHY

This examination has been largely supplanted by the Seldinger technique of percutaneous transfemoral catheterization which permits aortography and selective renal arteriography at the same time. The translumbar approach is used only in patients with advanced arteriosclerotic disease when catheterization is hazardous or impossible. A long needle is inserted directly into the abdominal aorta from a point just below the twelfth rib on the left. After making certain that the needle is in the aorta, the contrast medium is injected and roentgenograms are made using automatic changers (Fig. 20-1B).

NEPHROTOMOGRAPHY

The term "nephrotomography" was introduced in 1954 by John A. Evans and his colleagues[29] to define a method of radiographic examination that has since been used extensively in the study of the kidneys. The basic technique consists of intravenous injection of a large amount (50 ml of one of the organic iodides (we use a rapid drip infusion of 300 ml of Renografin-DIP). Roentgenograms are then taken at suitable intervals to secure visualization of the arterial supply of the kidneys (arterial phase). This is followed by a nephrogram phase during which tomograms are obtained at predetermined levels. The nephrogram phase is relatively easy to obtain; timing is more critical for the arterial phase. We no longer study the arterial phase in nephrotomography, preferring to use selective renal arteriography for this purpose. Excretory tomograms can then be made in projections and sections needed to solve the problem at hand. Nephrotomography is used ex-

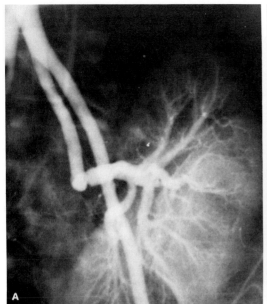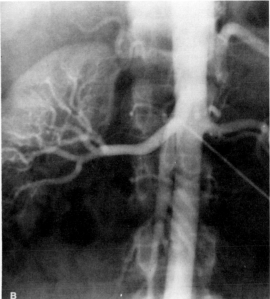

Fig. 20-1. *A*, Aortogram. This demonstrates the use of the percutaneous catheter technique in a patient with a renal transplant. The renal artery has been anastomosed to the internal iliac artery. *B*, Normal translumbar aortogram. The needle tip is near the orifice of the right renal artery which is well filled. There is some filling of the left renal, the splenic, hepatic, and the superior mesenteric arteries as well as the aorta.

tensively as an adjunct to intravenous urography whenever a questionable defect or shadow is observed. Examples of the use of this technique will be indicated in the sections entitled "Simple Cysts, and Tumors of the Kidney."

VOIDING CYSTOGRAPHY OR CYSTOURETHROGRAPHY

The examination is used largely in the study of patients suspected of having lower urinary tract obstruction, vesicoureteral reflux, and in children with persistent or recurrent urinary tract infection in whom vesicoureteral reflux is a possibility. In essence, the examination consists of filling the bladder with radiopaque material (sodium or meglumine diatrizoate), usually to the point of producing discomfort.

The patient is examined before, during, and after urination. The examination should be done on unanesthetized patients who have not had recent instrumentation. Bladder filling is checked during this part of the procedure. Fluoroscopy using image intensification is necessary to obtain an adequate examination. In addition, multiple spot films (70- or 90-mm or conventional spot films) are used to record the findings. The fluoroscopy can also be recorded on video tape if desired, since no additional radiation is used. Cinefluorography is not needed and its use entails unnecessarily high radiation exposures. The bladder, ureters, and sometimes renal pelves and calyces (when reflux is present), and urethra are examined during micturition.

CYSTOGRAPHY

Retrograde cystography is another method of studying the bladder. Following voiding, a catheter is inserted and the bladder is filled with opaque material, usually an organic iodide. Among the indications for this technique are the study of patients with bladder tumors, diverticula, and calculi. Air is sometimes used in amounts of 100 to 200 cc to study the bladder wall. Double contrast may also be used for the study of the bladder mucosa. One such method is the instillation of a 15% suspension of sterile barium sulfate (100 to 150 cc) into the bladder; the patient is allowed to void, then air, carbon dioxide, or nitrous oxide is instilled as a double-contrast agent. If barium refluxes into the kidney it is a potential cause of damage, so it is probably safer to use an organic iodide. Aqueous Dionosil has been used in amounts of 7 to 10 cc followed by one of the gases, but we prefer to use one of the diatrizoates or iothalamate. Films are taken in prone, supine, oblique, and decubitus positions. Filling can be monitored by fluoroscopy using image intensification; additional films may be obtained, depending upon the situation.

EXTRAPERITONEAL PNEUMOGRAPHY

Extraperitoneal (retroperitoneal) pneumography can be employed to outline any retroperitoneal tumor or organ, but is used most frequently in the examination of the kidneys and adrenal glands. The presacral area is preferred as the injection site since single puncture can be used for examination of both sides and the risk of embolism is much less than when the lumbar injection site is used. The method was first described by Ruiz Rivas in 1950 and it has largely replaced the earlier method of bilateral lumbar retroperitoneal insufflation.

TECHNIQUE

The patient lies on his right side with knees drawn up. The skin surrounding the tip of the coccyx is prepared and a local anesthetic agent is injected into the skin at a point 1 to 2 cm below the coccyx. Then a spinal needle is inserted and, with the aid of a finger in the rectum, is directed upward along the anterior sacral wall for 3 or 4 cm. A vinyl catheter then may be inserted through the needle and anchored in place. This will allow additional gas to be injected as indicated during the procedure. Oxygen or carbon dioxide may be used as the contrast substance. Carbon dioxide is preferred because of its solubility which avoids the possibility of gas embolism. After checking to see that the needle is not in a vein, 2 or 3 cc of the gas is injected. It should flow easily. If not, the needle should be moved slightly. If perineal emphysema appears, the needle should be inserted at least 2 cm farther. Then a total of 500 to 800 cc of oxygen or 750 to 1500 cc of carbon dioxide can be injected at a pressure of 15 to 20 cm H_2O. The side to be examined should be elevated

and if both sides are to be examined half of the gas is injected in each lateral decubitus position. Roentgenograms are taken on completion of injection. Then additional films can be made as indicated. Two hours is the optimum time for visualization of the retroperitoneal abdominal viscera when oxygen is used, but carbon dioxide is absorbed rapidly, so filming must be done quickly after injection (Fig. 20-2). The examination is relatively simple and safe since there are no large vessels in the retrorectal space. It is not an easy examination, however, and should be undertaken only when other methods have failed to determine the cause for the patient's symptoms or signs. This method may be combined with intravenous urography or aortography if necessary.

ROENTGEN ANATOMY

THE KIDNEY

The normal kidney is a bean-shaped structure that lies on either side of the lower thoracic and upper lumbar spine, usually between the upper border of the eleventh thoracic and the lower border of the third lumbar vertebrae. In the upright position, the kidney descends 2 or 3 cm. The right kidney lies approximately 2 cm lower than the left and both move slightly with respiration and with change in position. The long axis is directed downward and outward, parallel to the lateral border of the psoas muscle on either side. In the lateral view the axis is directed downward and anteriorly, so that the lower pole is 2 to 3 cm anterior to the upper pole. Renal size varies; the average length of the right kidney is from 12 to 12.7 cm while the left is 3 to 5 mm longer with an upper limit of a 1.5 cm variation in length. There is a relation between body height and renal length; as a general rule the kidney length in adults is 3.7 ± 0.37 times the height of the second lumbar vertebra measured on the same film using the posterior margins of the vertebral body. In children between 1½ and 14 years the renal length is equal to the length of the first 4 lumbar bodies including the three intervening discs ±1 cm. In infants renal size is relatively greater. In children the normal differ-

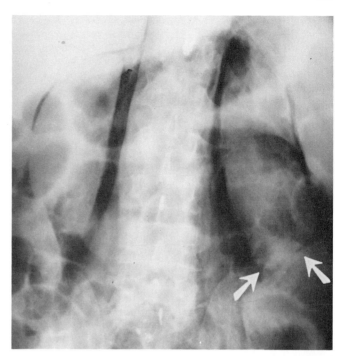

Fig. 20-2. Retroperitoneal pneumogram. Note the normal outline of the right kidney and the irregular enlargement of the lower pole of the left kidney (**arrows**). On the intravenous urogram, the outline of the lower pole of the left kidney was indistinct. The air clearly outlines the lower pole mass, which is a renal carcinoma.

ence in renal length on the two sides may be up to 1 cm.

There is some variation in renal shape, particularly on the left side. Fetal lobulations may persist on one or both sides, producing rather clearly defined indentations or notches along the lateral aspect of the kidney. The left kidney may be generally triangular in shape with a local bulge or convexity along the left midborder sometimes termed a "dromedary hump." This may be related to the position of the spleen or may be a form of fetal lobulation or both (Fig. 20-3). The kidney is visualized in roentgenograms mainly because of the presence of perirenal fat (Fig. 20-3). The increased radiotransparency of fat gives soft-tissue contrast so that the outline of the kidney stands out from the surrounding soft tissues. The renal outline is better visualized in obese individuals than in thin persons and if there has

been much wasting caused by chronic illness or malnutrition, the renal outlines may be very indistinct or completely invisible in roentgenograms of the abdomen.

THE URETERS

The ureters normally course straight downward from the most dependent portion of the pelves to the midsacral region, then turn posterolaterally and course in an arc downward and then inward and anteriorly to enter the trigone of the bladder on either side of the midline. A slight amount of redundancy is common and alteration in size is frequently noted. Therefore, it is necessary to exercise care in making the diagnosis of ureteral stricture, displacement, or dilatation. There are three areas where normal narrowing of the ureter can be

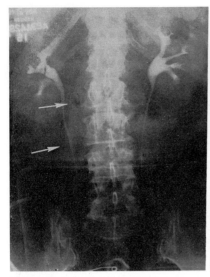 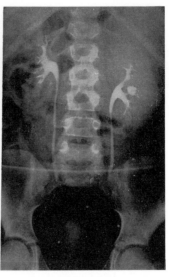

Fig. 20-3. Normal intravenous urogram. *Left,* In adult. *Right,* In child. Note the bean-shaped kidneys, which are better outlined in some areas than in others, depending upon the adjacent structures. The slight lobulation of the left kidney noted on both patients is not abnormal. The right psoas shadow is clearly defined (**arrows**) in the adult.

observed when it is filled with radiopaque material: the ureteropelvic junction, the uretero-vesical junction, and at the bifurcation of the iliac vessels.

THE BLADDER

The normal urinary bladder is an oval or round sphere, the inferior aspect of which normally projects 5 to 10 mm above the symphysis pubis. Its floor parallels the superior aspect of the pubic rami, while its dome is rounded in the male and flat or slightly concave in the female owing to the presence of the uterus above it. The size and shape of the normal bladder vary considerably. The wall of the bladder is smooth as outlined by opaque material used in urography or cystography. The bladder is in a higher position in children than in adults and is slightly higher in males than in females. The bladder is relatively larger in children than in adults. It should not be considered pathologically significant in children when the enlargement is symmetrical and the

longitudinal diameter is greater than the transverse.

THE NORMAL UROGRAM

The renal pelvis varies considerably in size and shape but is usually roughly triangular with the base parallel to the long axis of the kidney. It may be conical with the apex contiguous to the upper ureter. The range of normal is wide; some pelves are long narrow tubes while others are large and globular. There is also a considerable variation in position of the pelvis in relation to the kidney. It may be almost completely within the renal outline (intrarenal) or almost completely extrarenal. The former is usually small while the latter is large. The average normal pelvis is partially intra and partially extrarenal. Bifurcation or duplication of the pelvis is very common and is considered an anatomic variant rather than a congenital anomaly.

The calyceal system consists of major calyces that begin at the pelvis and extend into the kidney to the junction with the minor calyces. Each major calyx may be divided into a base adjacent to the pelvis, and an infundibulum that is more or less tubular and extends from the base to the apex, or distal portion, from which one or more minor calyces project. The minor calyx consists of a body or a calyx proper beginning at the junction with the major calyx, and the fornix that surrounds the conical renal papilla and into which the latter appears to project. The anatomic shape of the minor calyx is fairly constant, but since this structure is projected in various planes in the urogram there is considerable apparent variation. When viewed *en face,* it resembles a circular life preserver with a dense periphery and a relatively radiolucent center. In profile the appearance is somewhat triangular with the apex of the triangle pointing toward the major calyx, the base points away from it and is sharply concave or cupped. In contrast there is marked variation in the shape of the major calyces, which can be long and narrow or short and broad (Figs. 20-4 and 20-5). There are usually two major calyces and six to 14 minor calyces, but the number can vary widely. The calyceal system is not always bilaterally symmetric, which makes interpretation difficult in some instances. In the lateral projection the calyces are viewed obliquely and in the normal do not project anterior to the anterior aspect of the lumbar vertebral bodies.

There is a coordinated peristalsis that begins in the calyceal system of the kidney. These alternately fill and contract and it is this activity that accounts for the variable appearance of the collecting system during intravenous urography. When compression of the lower ureters is used, as described in the section entitled "Technique of Examination," peristaltic contractions are not frequently observed. The discharge of urine from the pelvis into the ureter is accompanied by ureteral peristalsis. These occur as broad waves at variable intervals (from four to 12 per minute). Ureteral peristalsis causes the ureter to have a variable caliber in different portions at the same time and a variation in contour in serial roentgenograms. The waves are visible as smooth areas of constriction or complete absence of filling that may separate one or more areas of slight dilatation. The effects of calyceal and ureteral peristalsis must be taken into account in the interpretation of intravenous urograms. Serial roentgenograms and fluoroscopy are of value in showing the rather wide variation in appearances of these structures from moment to moment.

RENAL BACKFLOW

The term "backflow" was initially applied to the escape of contrast material from the renal pelvis and calyces during retrograde pyelography as a result of an increase in intrapelvic

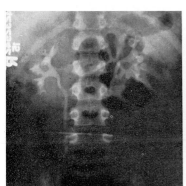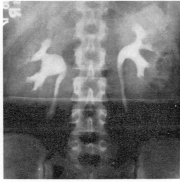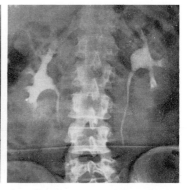

Fig. 20-4. Examples of normal intravenous urograms. The compression band causes slight calyceal dilatation. Note the variation in pelves and major calyces.

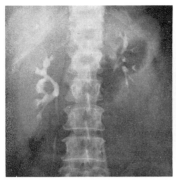
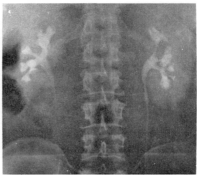
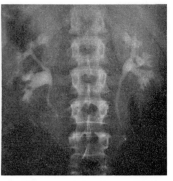

Fig. 20-5. Normal intravenous urograms. Note lack of bilateral symmetry here and in Figure 20-4.

pressure. The pressure is increased in intravenous urography by the use of compression devices. Acute ureteral obstruction also results in an increase of intrapelvic pressure. Since similar phenomena occur in these instances the term "backflow" has been carried over to describe changes observed in excretory urography. Backflow occurs in the normal kidney and its recognition and differentiation from diseases of the kidney are therefore important.

There are two major types, pyelotubular and pyelosinus or pyelointerstitial. Pyelolymphatic and pyelovenous backflow are merely stages of the pyelointerstitial form. Pyelotubular backflow is the most frequent type; when it occurs in intravenous urography it probably represents stasis in the tubules in the papilla rather than actual backflow. Roentgen findings consist of a brushlike tuft of opacity radiating into the papilla from the minor calyx (Fig. 20-6). Pyelointerstitial (pyelosinus) backflow begins with minute rupture (painless) of the fornix of a calyx permitting the escape of contrast material or urine into the renal sinus, which is the loose adipose and connective tissue surrounding the pelvis and calyces that support a venous plexus. When the amount of extravasation increases it extends medially into the peripelvic area, into the perirenal fat within Gerota's fascia, and downward along the ureter. The extravasated material may enter the lymphatics to produce pyelolymphatic backflow. A much less common occurrence is pyelovenous backflow in which, presumably, the material enters the arcuate and other veins. There is some con-

troversy as to whether or not this is ever demonstrated. Some investigators claim that the arcuate shadows observed in this condition are produced by perivascular extension of pyelosinus extravasation. All of the forms of backflow may be observed at one time (Fig. 20-6).

The roentgen findings in the early extravasation of the pyelointerstitial backflow consist of a hornlike projection of opaque medium extending from the fornix away from the papilla into the renal substance. As more material is extravasated it extends medially to the hilum and along the upper ureter, producing poorly defined densities in these areas. Pyelolymphatic backflow is manifested by opacification of lymphatic channels that extend from the hilum of the kidney medially toward the periaortic nodes. These channels tend to be redundant, somewhat tortuous, and branched (Fig. 20-7).

Extravasation of medium into the renal parenchyma also results when the catheter penetrates a calyx in retrograde pyelography. The roentgen appearance is variable, depending upon the amount and distribution of the extravasated material.

ARTERIAL AND VENOUS IMPRESSIONS

Arterial impressions or indentations on the renal pelvis and infundibula were found in 18 per cent of 150 patients studied by Nebesar, Pollard, and Fraley.[66] They occur three times more often on the right than on the left. The most common site is the superior infundibulum on the right. They consist of smooth transverse or oblique impressions on the infundibulum or pelvis. A slight delay in emptying of the upper pole calyces may be manifested by an apparent early opacification on the excretory urogram. Most of the involved vessels are ventral to the collecting system. They usually cause no symptoms and are significant only in that they must be differentiated from pathologic processes (Figs. 20-8 and 20-9). Occasionally, some infundibular obstruction is produced, leading to dilatation of calyces, pain, and occasionally to infection. Oblique as well as frontal projections are needed to make the diagnosis. Confirmation by angiography may be necessary when other causes are suspected.

Venous impressions on the superior infundibulum are not as common as those produced by arteries. Urographic findings are quite characteristic[61] and include a wide, smooth filling defect of the proximal part of the superior

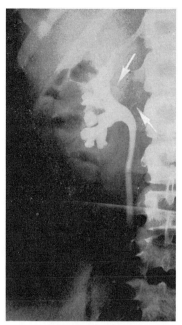

Fig. 20-7. Pyelolymphatic backflow (**arrows**). Intravenous urogram with compression band in place.

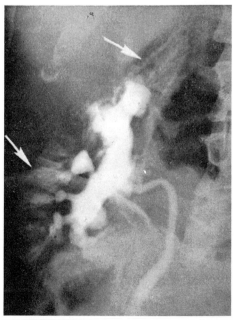

Fig. 20-6. Backflow. This retrograde pyelogram shows a marked amount of pyelolymphatic backflow (**upper arrow**). There is a considerable amount of pyelotubular backflow (**lower arrow**). Interstitial backflow occurs above and below ureteropelvic junction.

infundibulum that is usually horizontal or nearly so, and usually best shown on the prone film. Venography can be used to confirm the diagnosis.

THE NORMAL CYSTOGRAM

The normal cystogram outlines the smooth-walled, rounded or oval bladder. The urinary bladder is usually filled to some extent during excretory urography and this examination is often sufficient to outline gross lesions. When additional study of the bladder is indicated by roentgen means, cystography is used (Fig. 20-10). Films are taken in frontal, lateral, and oblique projections and, if necessary, upright and postvoiding roentgenograms may be taken as indicated earlier.

ANOMALIES

Anomalies of the kidney and ureter result from errors in development. The kidneys arise

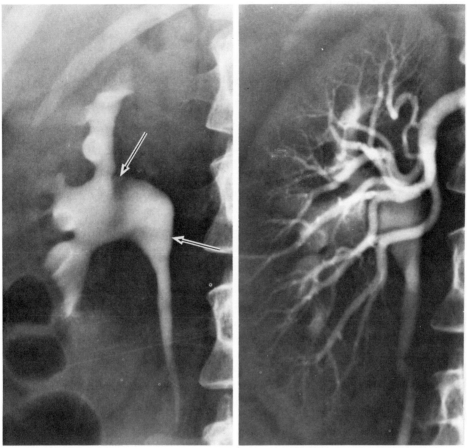

Fig. 20-8. *Left,* Urogram shows arterial indentations producing a vertical lucency on the lateral aspect of the pelvis (**upper arrow**) and horizontal pelvis indentations superiorly and inferiorly (**lower arrow**). *Right,* Selective renal arteriogram and urogram show relationship of the arterial branches to the collecting system.

from a mass of renal mesenchyme at the upper end of the ureteral buds, which in turn arise from the lower end of the mesonephric (wolffian) ducts. The mesonephron is the excretory organ lower in the phylogenetic scale and, in the human, it functions for a short time in early embryologic development before becoming a part of the male genital system. The ureteral buds grow dorsally, lying close together as the renal mesenchyme differentiates. Each bud bifurcates into an upper and lower sprout to form the major calyces. The ureter is anterior to the kidney as the latter ascends from the upper sacral area to its posi-

tion in the lower thoracic–upper lumbar region. As it ascends the kidney rotates to bring it lateral to the ureter in the midlumbar region. The renal blood supply is attained after the kidney reaches its normal adult position. The lower end of the ureter loses its relation to the wolffian duct and opens into the bladder in a higher and more lateral position. The wolffian duct migrates distally and its orifices eventually are situated in the distal portion of the floor of the prostatic urethra to become the ejaculatory ducts in the male. They become vestigial structures in the female.

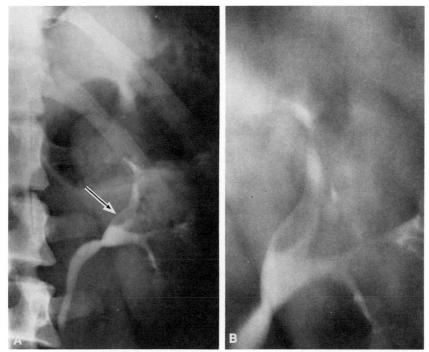

Fig. 20-9. *A,* Unusual vascular indentation causing a persistent elongated defect in the upper pole infundibulum on the left (**arrow**). *B,* Close-up of the defect which was persistent. Subsequent selective arteriogram showed a renal arterial branch causing the defect.

ANOMALIES IN NUMBER

SINGLE KIDNEY

The occurrence of a single kidney is a rare anomaly and great care must be taken when making a radiographic diagnosis of unilateral renal agenesis since a nonfunctioning kidney may not be readily visible. The single kidney tends to be larger in patients with agenesis of one kidney than in patients with secondary compensatory renal hyperplasia. Radiographic signs are an absence of a renal shadow on one side with an unusually large kidney on the other. The trigone is usually deformed with the ureteral orifice missing on the involved side, so that cystoscopy will confirm the diagnosis. Angiography confirms absence of renal artery. Surgical exploration is necessary at times to make certain of this anomaly.

SUPERNUMERARY KIDNEY

Supernumerary kidney is also a rare anomaly. The usual finding is that the third kidney is small and rudimentary, and the other kidney on the same side is often smaller than the normal kidney on the opposite side. The presence of a separate pelvis, ureter, and blood supply is necessary to make this diagnosis. Intravenous urography can be used to outline the excretory system of the supernumerary kidney if it is functioning and an abdominal aortogram will show the blood supply if that is necessary to confirm the diagnosis.

ANOMALIES IN SIZE AND FORM

HYPOPLASIA

Anomalies of renal size and form are much more common than anomalies in number. Hypoplasia on one side is usually associated with hyperplasia on the other. The hypoplastic or infantile kidney functions normally so that it can be seen on excretory urograms. It must be differentiated from the acquired atrophic kid-

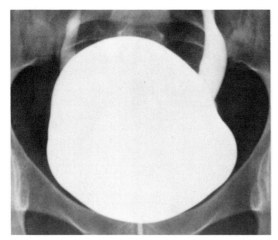

Fig. 20-10. Cystogram showing bilateral vesico-ureteral reflux. The bladder is normal.

ney which is small and contracted secondary to vascular or inflammatory disease that has resulted in a decrease of renal parenchyma. In congenital hypoplasia the calyceal system and pelvis are small, and there is a normal relationship between the amount of parenchyma and the size of the collecting system (Fig. 20-11). In the secondarily contracted kidney, the pelvis and calyces tend to be normal in size so that the decrease in renal size is due to a parenchymal deficit. Furthermore, the function of the latter tends to be impaired. Despite these differences, it is often very difficult to distinguish between these two conditions without the use of renal arteriography.

HYPERPLASIA

The other anomaly in size, hyperplasia, is associated with agenesis or hypoplasia on the opposite side. Enlargement of the kidney is usually caused by conditions other than agenesis or hypoplasia, however. Obstructive hydronephrosis, polycystic disease, other cystic or dysplastic disorders, neoplasm, renal vein thrombosis, acute infection, glomerulonephritis, uric acid nephritis, Kimmelstiel-Wilson disease, sickle cell disease, glycogen storage disease (von Gierke's), hereditary tyrosinemia, total lipodystrophy, and amyloidosis may cause enlargement. Usually it is bilateral however, and there are clinical and laboratory findings and urographic findings which help to make the dif-

ferentiation. Renal biopsy may be necessary in some instances.

FUSION ANOMALIES

Fusion anomalies represent an alteration in form of the kidneys and can often be recognized or at least suspected on plain roentgenograms of the abdomen (KUB films).

HORSESHOE KIDNEY. The horseshoe kidney is the most common type of fusion anomaly. In this condition the lower poles of the kidney are joined by a band of soft tissues, the isthmus, which varies from a thick parenchymatous mass as wide as the kidneys themselves to a thin stringlike band of fibrous tissue. Rarely the upper poles of the kidneys are united in this manner. In the usual situation when lower poles are involved, the long axis of the kidney is reversed in this anomaly so that the lower pole is nearer the midline than the upper. There is also an associated rotation anomaly on one or both sides that varies in degree. The calyces are directed backward or posteromedially rather than laterally. As a result they are seen on end or obliquely, which alters their appearance considerably (Fig. 20-12). The ureters tend to be somewhat stretched over the isthmus and partial obstruction on one or both sides is common. This leads to dilatation of the pelvis (pyelectasis) and calyces (caliectasis) and may also lead to chronic inflammatory disease and the formation of calculi.

CROSSED ECTOPY. Crossed ectopy with fusion, the unilateral fused kidney, is an anomaly of form that is much less common than the horseshoe kidney. It consists of fusion of the kidneys on the same side; the lower one is ectopic and its ureter crosses the midline to enter the bladder normally on the opposite side. Both kidneys are often lower in position than normal and various rotation anomalies as well as a wide variation in shape and type of fusion are noted. This anomaly is also frequently associated with partial obstruction, which results in inflammation and often in calculus formation.

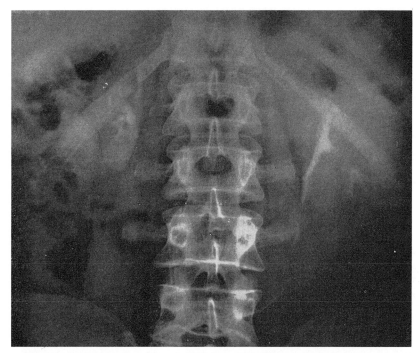

Fig. 20-11. Hypoplasia of the right kidney. Note the marked difference in size of the kidneys on the two sides. Function on the right is present despite its small size.

The "caked" kidney is a variation in which there is fusion of both upper and lower poles; with failure of rotation the calyces are directed posteriorly. The renal mass lies in or near the midline and is low in position, often overlying the sacrum. The ureters enter the bladder normally. A number of descriptive terms have been applied to other rare forms of fusion; all of them tend to result in obstruction, which in turn causes hydronephrosis, infection, and calculus formation.

ANOMALIES IN POSITION

Anomalies of renal position are common. Malrotation has been described above as being almost constantly present in fusion anomalies, but it also occurs as a single anomaly (Fig. 20-13). It results from incomplete or excessive rotation and urographic study will indicate the degree of anomaly. Rotation anomalies are usually of little clinical significance unless associated with obstruction but it is important to recognize them as anatomic variations that do not produce symptoms and are innocuous lesions. Retroperitoneal tumor masses may displace the kidneys and produce an alteration in rotation that must be differentiated from congenital rotation anomalies. Crossed ectopy may occur without fusion and the findings are similar to those described in the preceding section except for the lack of fusion. The ectopic kidney is lower than the normal one in position and is usually described as a sacral or pelvic kidney, depending upon its position. Failure to visualize the kidney in its normal position should lead one to suspect ectopy and to look for it, since agenesis of a kidney is very rare. In many instances the kidney can be visualized only when contrast material outlines it, so that intravenous urography or retrograde pyelography may be necessary to indicate its position. Characteristically the ureter of an ectopic kidney is only long enough to reach from the renal pelvis to the bladder and this aids in

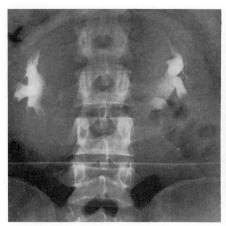 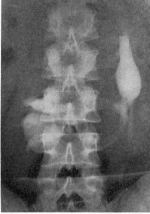

Fig. 20-12. Horseshoe kidney. *Left,* Note the reversal of the long axis of the kidneys with very little rotation anomaly. *Right,* Marked rotation anomaly, fusion inferiorly. Note considerable abnormality in position of the right kidney.

distinguishing displacement of a normal kidney downward from one that developed in an abnormally low position. Superior ectopia of the kidney or thoracic kidney is probably more common than reports in the literature would indicate. The possibility of intrathoracic kidney should be considered in the differential diagnosis of masses of appropriate size projecting into the posterior thorax from below. This anomaly may be associated with herniation through the foramen of Bochdalek or a congenital eventration of the diaphragm posteriorly. Intravenous urography will readily identify the position of the kidney in these cases.

"Nephroptosis" is the term applied to abnormal downward displacement of the kidney. Roentgenograms taken in the upright position normally show downward displacement of the kidney equal to the width of a lumbar vertebra. When it is displaced more than this, ptosis is said to be present. The condition is more common on the right side than on the left; it is frequent in females but rare in males. It is of doubtful clinical significance since obstruction ordinarily is not produced and surgical intervention is rarely, if ever, indicated. Roentgen demonstration of this condition can be accomplished by taking an additional exposure during urography with the patient in an upright position. In the low position the kidney often rotates on its horizontal axis; the

lower pole then lies more anterior than normal. Oblique views are necessary to measure true renal length when this occurs.

OTHER ANOMALIES

DUPLICATION OF THE PELVIS AND URETER

Incomplete double ureter is formed when the renal bud divides too early or the division extends into the ureter. The division varies from an exaggeration of the length of major upper and lower pole calyces to duplication of the ureter for most of its length. Complete duplication of the ureter may also occur. Each ureter has its own vesical orifice and the upper ureter usually drains the upper third of the kidney, while the ureter that drains the lower pelvis drains the lower two-thirds of the kidney (Fig. 20-14). The ureter that drains the upper pole is ventral to the lower one but crosses over and empties into the bladder in a lower and more medial position, and when one of the ureters empties in an extravesical location it is the one that drains the upper pelvis. Urographic recognition of duplication is simple when both pelves and ureters are opacified and should be suspected if only one of them fills since there

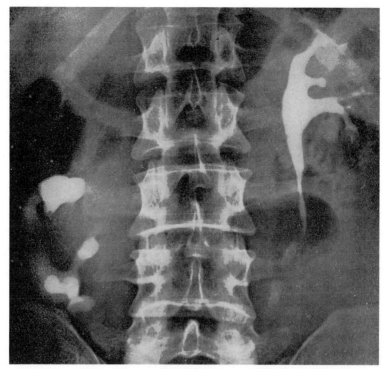

Fig. 20-13. Ectopic and malrotated right kidney. Note dilatation of calyces as compared to the normal kidney on the *left*.

will then be a segment of kidney without drainage. These anomalies of the pelvis and ureter may be unilateral or bilateral, with a tendency to be asymmetric. Occasionally multiple budding will result in multiple short upper pelves and ureters that are extrarenal in type. In this anomaly each of several major calyces will have its own pelvis and upper ureter, which usually joins with the others to form a common lower ureter. It is not infrequent for one-half of a double ureter to be obstructed. Triple ureter has also been reported.

ANOMALIES IN POSITION OF URETERAL ORIFICE

There are several possible anomalies in position of the ureteral orifice and this variation is usually better studied by cystoscopy than by radiographic means. In the male, the ureter may open into the seminal vesicles, the vas deferens, the ejaculatory duct, or the posterior urethra. In the female, the abnormal ureter may open into the urethra, beneath the urethral orifice near the hymen, or into the lateral vulvar wall, the uterus, or the vagina.

URETERAL JET PHENOMENON. The ureteral jet phenomenon is caused by a jet of opaque medium propelled by ureteral peristalsis, which may occasionally extend across the base of the bladder to the opposite side. The jet maintains the caliber of the ureter and simulates an anomalous ureter that opens on the opposite side of the trigone (Fig. 20-15). When there is any question as to the cause of the apparent anomaly, another film will reveal a normal lower ureter in these patients.

RETROCAVAL URETER

Postcaval or retrocaval ureter is limited to the right side. It is caused by failure of the right posterior cardinal vein to atrophy; it persists as the adult vena cava. Normally, the right subcardinal vein persists as the vena cava. The abnormal relationship may cause partial obstruction, leading to hydronephrosis, infection and calculus

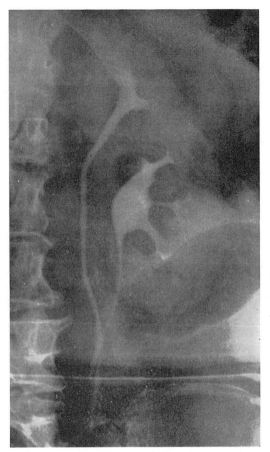

Fig. 20-14. Duplication of the pelvis and ureter. The upper pelvis drains the upper pole while the lower pelvis drains the remainder of the kidney.

formation. The ureter passes to the left behind the inferior vena cava, then turns toward the right and courses downward in its normal position. In some cases there is redundancy of the ureter proximally, so that an S type, or fishhook or inverted J type of deformity is produced. The site of narrowing or obstruction, if present, is proximal to the vena cava and is probably at the lateral edge of the psoas, and caused by the pressure of the retroperitoneal fascia over the muscle. In others, with no redundancy, obstruction is less common and when present coincides with the lateral margin of the inferior vena cava.

The diagnosis can usually be made on urography. In addition to the abnormal course of the right ureter in the frontal projection, its posterior position in the lateral view can be ob-

served. The diagnosis can be confirmed by inferior vena cavography with an opaque catheter in the ureter. Retroperitoneal masses with ureteral displacement must be differentiated.

URETEROCELE

There are two types of ureterocele, simple and ectopic. The simple ureterocele consists of an intravesical dilatation of the ureter immediately proximal to its orifice in the bladder. It usually results from a combination of ureteral orifice stenosis and a deficiency in the connective tissue attachment of the ureter to the bladder. It varies in size from a scarcely perceptible dilatation to one that is moderately large and resembles a cobra head in shape. There may be partial obstruction resulting in hydroureter. In general this type is smaller than the ectopic ureterocele. It occurs with equal frequency in males and females and is usually discovered in adults. The ectopic type is four or five times more frequent, is usually discovered in childhood, and is much more common in females than in males. It is more likely to be associated with severe hydronephrosis, hydroureter, and infection than the simple type. Both types tend to occur in the presence of duplication of the ureter; the ectopic type is almost always associated with this anomaly. It consists of the submucosal passage of the distal portion of the involved ureter within the vesical wall to terminate in the urethra rather than in the bladder as in the simple type. The submucosal portion of the ureter dilates and bulges anteriorly into the bladder to form the ureterocele. It may prolapse through the urethra to form a vulval cyst and usually extends posterior to the vesical neck and proximal urethra. It invariably involves the ureter from the upper pole of the kidney.

The roentgen appearance depends on whether the opaque medium fills the ureterocele. If it is filled the lesion is outlined by a radiolucent wall that stands out in contrast to the filled bladder as well as to the filled, dilated, distal ureter. When it is not filled with opaque material it presents as a radiolucent mass within the opacified bladder in the region of the ureteral orifice. The shape is typically somewhat fusiform with a narrow lower end resembling a cobra head. The larger ones tend to be more rounded in shape. When a calculus is present in the ureterocele, it is noted to lie on one

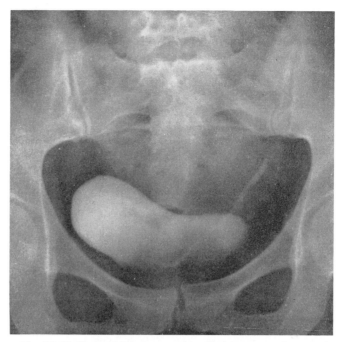

Fig. 20-15. Ureteral jet phenomenon. Ureter apparently extends across the midline. Cystoscopy revealed normal position of the ureteral orifice on the left.

side of the midline and remains there despite changes in position of the patient (Fig. 20-16).

Ectopic ureteroceles are larger than the simple ones and often extend to the anterior bladder wall when viewed in the lateral projection. The contact with the floor of the bladder is broad and extends to the internal urethral orifice. Obstruction of the other ureter is frequent and the extravesical portion ' may distort the bladder. Intravenous urography is the roentgen method of choice in diagnosis of this condition.

PATENT URACHUS AND URACHAL CYST

The urachus probably represents the intra-abdominal remnant of the allantois or caudal extension of it, which is continuous with the vesical portion of the urogenital sinus in embryologic development. Normally it constitutes the middle umbilical ligament. The allantois extends from the primitive urinary bladder through the umbilicus to the placenta. There are four types of anomalies possible: (1) Complete patency; (2) patency at umbilical end or blind external type; (3) patency at vesical end or blind internal type; and (4) patency between bladder and umbilicus, which gives rise to urachal cyst. The blind external type and complete patency are usually recognized on inspection when the umbilical cord sloughs off but may be suspected earlier. Roentgen visualization can be obtained by using any of the organic iodides mentioned earlier as contrast materials that can be injected into the umbilical end of the urachus. Cystography is needed to demonstrate the internal type. The findings are those of a smooth-walled tubal structure lying in the anterior midline which extends into the plane of a line between umbilicus and the bladder. The bladder may be distorted and elevated. The cyst may extend from the bladder to the umbilicus or end blindly when it begins at either end. When a cyst of the urachus is present without internal or external communication the roentgen findings depend upon its size. If large, it may be noted as a midline, soft-tissue mass lying between the bladder and the umbilicus in the anterior abdominal wall. Gas-filled small intestine may be displaced

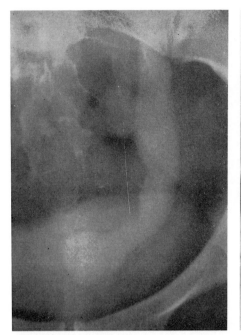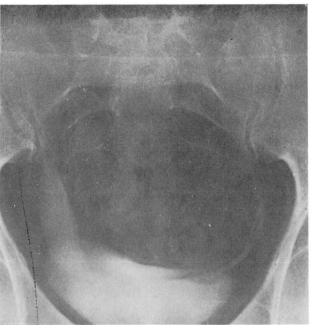

Fig. 20-16. Ureteroceles. *Left,* Note bulbous ureteral dilatation overlying the bladder representing a simple ureterocele. *Right,* Bilateral small simple ureteroceles; the one on the left is more easily visualized because of radiolucency produced by displacement of the opaque medium in the bladder.

and study of the small bowel by means of barium meal will show comparable displacement. Rarely calculi may form in a patent urachus or urachal cyst.

HYDRONEPHROSIS

Regardless of its cause, chronic obstruction of the urinary tract leads to hydronephrosis, which indicates dilatation of the pelvis and calyces with progressive destruction of renal parenchyma. The terms "pyelectasis," "caliectasis," "ureterectasis," or "hydroureter" are more accurate in localizing the dilatation. The obstruction that produces hydronephrosis may be unilateral or bilateral, depending on the site of the lesion producing it. Unilateral obstruction is caused by a lesion at or above the ureterovesical junction, while bilateral obstruction may be caused by a lesion distal to that point. Bilateral obstruction above the ureterovesical junction is not uncommon, however, particularly in congenital anomalies, and in such patients the hydronephrosis is usually asymmetric.

NONOBSTRUCTIVE HYDRONEPHROSIS

There are several nonobstructive conditions which may cause dilatation of the renal pelvis and calyces and also the ureters. Diabetes insipidus may be associated with relatively moderate hydronephrosis. Nephrogenic diabetes insipidus tends to cause a more severe degree of dilatation, often with tortuosity of the ureters in addition to the dilatation. In this condition there is a tubular abnormality with insufficient absorption of water, leading to a large volume of hypotonic urine.[64] Urinary tract infection tends to cause segmental or generalized dilatation (ileus) of the ureter with poor or reversed peristalsis leading to hydronephrosis. This may be augmented by vesicoureteral reflux which is commonly found in urinary infections. The changes may decrease or disappear when the infection is successfully treated. Hydronephrosis in the absence of urinary tract abnormality may also be caused by chronic constipation of the functional variety. Fecal masses in the rectum may displace and compress the base plate of the bladder resulting in anterior displacement of the urethra. This may cause hydronephrosis and vesicoureteral reflux.[87]

CONGENITAL HYDRONEPHROSIS

Congenital hydronephrosis is caused by a variety of lesions. In anomalies of position it is usually caused by the abnormal relationship of the upper ureter to the kidney. Congenital strictures, bands, aberrant vessels, and valves may also produce hydronephrosis. In addition, there are instances of congenital hydronephrosis in which the cause is obscure; many of these are "neurogenic" in that they are associated with lesions of the spinal cord and with congenital megacolon. The dilatation is usually bilaterally symmetrical in the latter patients.

ACQUIRED HYDRONEPHROSIS

Acquired hydronephrosis is caused by a variety of lesions also; among them are tumors, calculi, strictures, operative procedures, and prostatic enlargement. Ureteropelvic junction obstruction is the most common type of bilateral obstruction above the bladder. It may be asymmetric, however. Congenital valves appear to be the most common cause of the obstruction, but an aberrant artery may contribute to obstruction or may cause it in some instances. Pregnancy is often associated with hydronephrosis which tends to be more severe on the right than on the left. Ureters are dilated to the pelvic brim. This is probably caused by mechanical pressure. Hydrocolpos and hydrometrocolpos tend to cause ureteral obstruction. Abdominal aortic aneurysm may compress the ureter or retroperitoneal bleeding, associated with aneurysm, may cause fibrosis leading to ureteral stricture and hydronephrosis. Granulomatous disease of the small intestine and colon (Crohn's disease) or both

occasionally cause ureteral obstruction. There are all degrees of dilatation and progression of the changes can be noted on serial examinations if the obstruction is not relieved.

UROGRAPHIC FINDINGS

The earliest urographic change in hydronephrosis is a flattening of the normal concavity of the calyx and blunting of the sharp peripheral angle produced by the papilla as it juts into the calyx. This change is reversible and is readily produced by a small increase in pressure. It is noted in normal patients when a compression band is in place during urography. The pelvis enlarges gradually with increasing or prolonged obstruction but pelvic and calyceal dilatation are not necessarily parallel. The next calyceal change is that of "clubbing," in which the concavity produced by the papilla is reversed (Figs. 20-17 through 20-19). Calyces then gradually enlarge with progressive destruction of parenchyma and enlargement of the collecting system of the kidney until it becomes a nonfunctioning hydronephrotic sac in which the normal anatomy is obliterated (Fig. 20-20). Renal function may be greatly diminished in severe hydronephrosis and there is accumulation of opaque material in the parenchyma adjacent to the grossly dilated calyces. This forms crescentic areas of faint opacification termed the "crescent" sign of hydronephrosis (Fig. 20-21). Later there may be faint opacification of the calyces themselves. Infec-

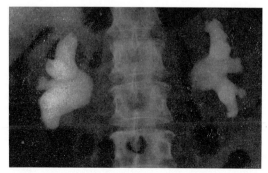

Fig. 20-17. Minimal bilateral hydronephrosis. The pelves are not greatly enlarged but there is definite blunting of the calyces.

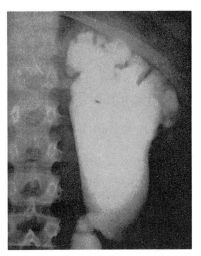

Fig. 20-18. Hydronephrosis and hydroureter as seen on a retrograde pyelogram. Chronic infection is present with resultant loss of parenchyma. A thin rim of renal parenchyma can be visualized superiorly.

tion may be a complicating factor, tending to accelerate parenchymal destruction. When present, it produces more irregularity in the dilated calyces than is seen in uncomplicated hydronephrosis.

RENAL AND URETERAL CALCULI

Urinary tract calculi are formed in the pelvis, often in the region of the papillae, and calyces. The calculus may remain within the pelvis and gradually increase in size to form a cast of the pelvis and calyces. This represents what is known as the staghorn calculus (Fig. 20-22). In other patients multiple calculi may form within the calyceal system and they may be similar in size or may vary considerably in size. Calculi tend to be asymptomatic until they cause obstruction. Then the typical renal or ureteral colic is produced. Most renal calculi contain enough calcium to be visualized on roentgenograms. Calcium phosphate, calcium oxalate, and magnesium ammonium phosphate stones are the most common and they are usually mixed since pure stones are relatively rare. Cystine, urate and xanthine stones are rare. Urinary stasis is the most important single causative factor in the formation of calculi. In-

fection is usually associated with stasis and becomes an additional factor. Hyperparathyroidism and other conditions with hypercalcemia, including some which cause dissolution of bone, may also be associated with calculi. They include osteolytic metastases, leukemia, multiple myeloma, and sarcoidosis. There is some evidence to indicate that calculi may also result from renal artery stenosis; the vascular insufficiency may cause parenchymal injury leading to calculus formation.

ROENTGEN FINDINGS

The roentgen findings are those of an opacity of varying size and shape overlying the urinary tract. Often the plain-film diagnosis is rather simple, particularly when the calculus forms a cast of the pelvis or calyces or both. Intravenous urography is usually indicated to make certain of the localization and to determine the condition of the calyceal system. Oblique and lateral views may be necessary in addition to frontal projections in order definitely to localize a calculus. Urography is also necessary to find radiolucent calculi. They appear as negative shadows displacing the opaque medium. In patients with renal or ureteral colic there is usually delayed excretion by the involved kidney. The diatrizoates and other triiodinated media in the large doses used in urography are excreted almost entirely by glomerular filtration. With the acute obstruction produced by the passage of a ureteral stone, the intrapelvic pressure increases to the point where there is little or no glomerular filtration. Despite this, increasing density of the kidney (demonstrated by nephrogram) indicates accumulation of iodide, probably a result of tubular excretion, and eventually there is usually some opacification of the calyces, pelvis, and ureter. It is therefore important to take films until opacification is adequate to make the diagnosis. If the routine films show a nephrogram on the involved side, it is likely that films taken at 30-minute intervals will show enough opacification to localize the site of the obstructing ureteral calculus and confirm its

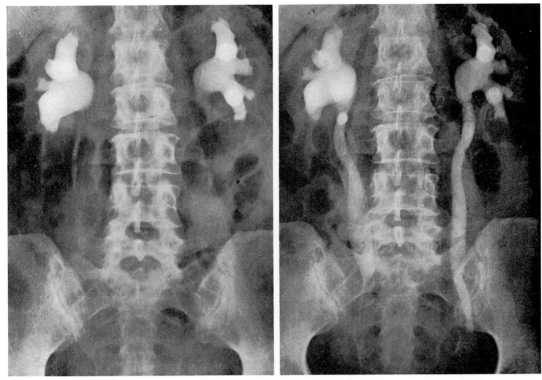

Fig. 20-19. Bilateral hydronephrosis. This examination shows the value of delayed films. The roentgenogram on the right is a delayed film taken 90 minutes after injection of the contrast material. It indicates that the obstruction is in the lower ureters and not at the ureteropelvic junction as would be expected on the roentgenogram on the left.

presence within the ureter (Fig. 20-23). If this method fails, an opaque catheter can be passed and the calculus localized in relation to it by means of frontal, oblique, and lateral roentgenograms. The most common site for ureteral calculi to lodge is at or above the ureterovesical junction in the pelvic portion of the ureter. Occasionally a calculus will have passed before the examination is completed and no obstruction is then visible. When the calculus has lodged at the ureterovesical junction for any length of time, it is not uncommon to note a localized radiolucent indentation on the bladder owing to edema above the ureteral orifice, even though the calculus may have been passed. Ureteral calculi are small in size (1 to 3 mm in diameter). In general these small stones pass quickly down the ureter to lodge at or near the ureterovesical junction. They tend to be parallel to the course of the ureter

when they are oval or elongated. Most of them lie above a line drawn through the ischial spines. However, it should be recognized that angulation of the roentgen-ray tube or alteration of position of the pelvis may project these calculi lower in position. Larger calculi are not so likely to leave the renal pelvis and to become lodged in the ureter. Ureteral calculi tend to be round or oval in shape. If the calculus remains within the ureter for any length of time it may become elongated and increased in size; large stones found within the ureter usually indicate that they have been present for a considerable period of time (Fig. 20-24).

It is not uncommon to observe a single loop of gas-filled small bowel usually in the left upper quadrant in patients with acute renal colic. The site of the loop is not necessarily related to the position of the stone. Occasionally, extensive adynamic ileus may occur.

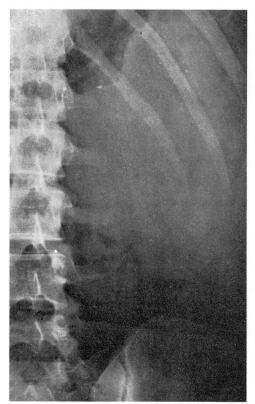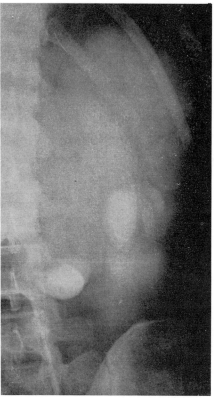

Fig. 20-20. Severe hydronephrosis. *Left,* Plain film showing a mass in the left renal area. *Right,* Urogram shows faint outlines of grossly dilated pelvis and calyces.

DIFFERENTIAL DIAGNOSIS

Suspected renal or ureteral calculus must be differentiated from all other calcifications that may occur in the renal areas and along the course of the ureters. Gallstones are usually multiple, tend to be faceted, and often exhibit typical concentric rings of calcium. Oblique roentgenograms will show their anterior position. Common duct and cystic duct stones may be opaque but they also lie anterior to the kidney and ureter. Calcification of costal cartilages is common and usually readily identified. Oblique projections will show the relationship of such shadows to the anterior lower thoracic wall if there is any doubt about the nature of the densities. Calcified mesenteric nodes and calcifications in the appendices epiploica usually move enough from one time to another to be differentiated from urinary calculi. The same is true of opaque material in the gastrointestinal tract, but it is frequently necessary to take more than one roentgenogram to make

the differentiation. Pancreatic calculi usually conform to the shape of the portion of pancreas and can be identified readily, but occasionally it is necessary to examine the stomach and duodenum by means of a barium meal to make certain of the position of the calculi. Calcification in cysts and tumors of the kidney and elsewhere in the abdomen must also be differentiated. The contour of the cyst wall can usually be identified and when calcified tumor is present, it is usually large enough to be visualized as a soft-tissue mass. Occasionally the lateral tip of a transverse process of one of the lumbar vertebrae may be easily visible in comparison to the remainder of the process and resemble a ureteral calculus; close inspection will suffice to make the differentiation. Vascular calcification, either in pelvic arteries or in veins (phleboliths) are generally the most difficult problems. Arterial calcification is usually along the course of a large artery and tends to be elongated as well as to outline both walls of the artery. Phleboliths often have a fairly typical ap-

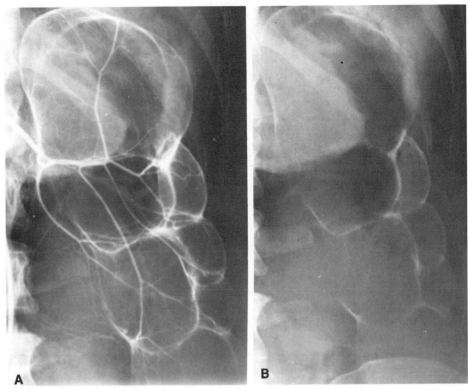

Fig. 20-21. Hydronephrosis, the crescent sign. *A,* Selective left renal arteriogram shows grossly stretched, narrow vessels with very few branches. Note the vessels stretched over the large renal pelvis medially. *B,* Later film shows the crescent sign caused by opacification in the thin rim of remaining renal tissue. Surgical removal confirmed the diagnosis of severe hydronephrosis. (Courtesy *Dr. Thomas L. Carter and Dr. Richard Logan).*

pearance with a radiolucent central area and tend to be more rounded in contour than calculi. Phleboliths may have a central calcific nidus surrounded by a zone of lesser density, which in turn is surrounded by a more dense periphery. Roentgenograms taken in anteroposterior and oblique projections are often sufficient to exclude urinary calculus as the cause for the density or densities present. If not, excretory urography with oblique and special views as needed, including delayed roentgenograms, usually is diagnostic. If there still is doubt concerning the diagnosis, cystoscopy with introduction of a radiopaque catheter into the ureter usually solves the problem. The ureteral stone stays in relation to the contrast in all projections. In any patient having symptoms suggestive of ureteral colic, importance should be attached to any calculus density, no matter how small, occurring along the course of the ureter, particularly if it is found in the region

of the distal part of the ureter. Conversely, in a patient with no symptoms at all suggestive of ureteral colic, small rounded calcifications in the lateral aspect of the pelvis can usually be disregarded as representing only phleboliths. Occasionally a ureteral calculus may cause no pain, so that catheter studies may be indicated if the density closely resembles a ureteral stone in a patient without pain.

NEPHROCALCINOSIS

"Nephrocalcinosis" is the term used to describe calcium deposits within the renal parenchyma. Calcium is usually concentrated in the medullary pyramids but may be scattered rather diffusely throughout the entire renal parenchyma and the amount of calcification may vary considerably. This lesion is found in several diseases charac-

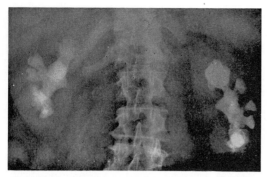

Fig. 20-22. Staghorn calculus. Note the calcification forming a cast of the pelvis and calyces. No contrast material has been administered.

terized by abnormally high concentrations of calcium or phosphorus resulting in precipitation of calcium phosphate in healthy renal tissue. Primary hyperparathyroidism is the best example of this group and nephrocalcinosis occurs in approximately 25 per cent of patients with the disease but renal lithiasis is more common than calcinosis. When the latter occurs, tiny calcifications confined to the medulla are usually present, with occasional larger calcifications occurring in the renal pyramids. Hypercalciuria of undetermined etiology, hyperchloremic acidosis, hypervitaminosis D, milk-alkali syndrome, sarcoidosis and idiopathic hypercalcemia are other conditions producing nephrocalcinosis. Another group comprises patients with renal disease in which calcium is precipitated in damaged tissue. Normal blood calcium levels are usually present in the latter group, which includes such renal diseases as chronic pyelonephritis, chronic glomerulonephritis, lower nephron nephrosis, and injury of distal convoluted tubules owing to various causes. In chronic pyelonephritis unequal distribution of relatively large deposits occurs. Calcinosis is rare in chronic glomerulonephritis; when present the findings of tiny granular calcifications scattered throughout the cortices of small kidneys are very suggestive of the diagnosis. Medullary deposits are found in "sponge kidney."

Roentgen findings depend on the extent of calcification. This varies from faintly visible, milky, granular densities to stippled calcification in the renal papilla and cortex (Fig. 20-25). The finding is relatively rare and it has been shown that there are many instances of histopathologically proved renal calcification in which the calcium cannot be visualized radiographically in the living subject.

INFECTIONS AND RELATED CONDITIONS

ACUTE PYELONEPHRITIS

There are no specific roentgenologic findings in the presence of acute pyelonephritis. Intravenous urography is often contraindicated during the acute phase, but a plain film may reveal some enlargement of the kidneys, particularly in severe acute infection.

Emphysematous pyelonephritis is a special form of acute pyelonephritis affecting diabetics or patients with urinary tract obstruction. The finding of gas in and around the kidney in an acutely ill patient suggests the diagnosis. The affected kidney usually does not function. Gas-forming organisms recovered include *Escherichia coli* and *proteus vulgaris*. Emphysematous pyelonephritis should be regarded as a complication of a severe necrotising infection, usually indicating extensive destruction of renal parenchyma, and having a poor prognosis.

RENAL ABSCESS

Acute suppurative infection of the renal parenchyma is usually hematogenous in origin and begins in the cortex. The most frequent causative organism is the staphylococcus. When one or more small cortical abscesses develop in the parenchyma, no roentgen findings are present. If these small abscesses coalesce to form a large abscess, a plain-film roentgenogram often shows local enlargement of the kidney. The term "carbuncle of the kidney" is also used for coalescent cortical abscesses which result in local or generalized renal enlargement. The perirenal fat is blurred in the area of involvement so that the renal outline tends to be indistinct. The involved kidney is fixed during inspiration and expiration. The psoas muscle is often indistinct. There may be scoliosis with the concavity

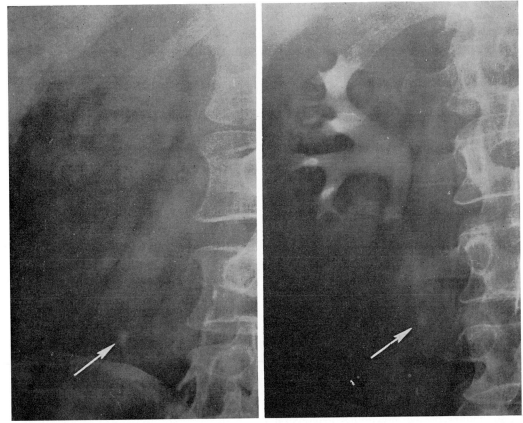

Fig. 20-23. Right ureteral calculus. *Left,* Note density (**arrow**) just above the right iliac crest. *Right,* Urogram shows slight dilation of the ureter, extending down to the site of the calculus. This also shows the value of delayed film in patients with acute ureteral obstruction. The early films did not show any excretion. This roentgenogram taken at 90 minutes shows excretion and outlines the ureter to localize the calculus within it.

toward the involved side; this suggests the complication of perirenal abscess. Excretory urography is of value if there is enough function to outline the calyceal system. The findings are those of compression and displacement or obliteration of the calyces owing to the tumor-like mass produced by the abscess.

Clinical signs of infection may not be present in some patients, particularly when the course is prolonged and the infection is chronic. Therefore, the differentiation from tumor may be difficult and renal angiography is useful. Angiographic findings include late increased vascularity at the margin of the lesion, local stretching of the vessels over the mass, enlarged stretched capsular vessels if perirenal

extension is present, absence of tumor vessels (no arteriovenous shunting), lucent defect at site of lesion noted in the nephrogram, and a blush in the late capillary-early venous phase. The findings may simulate those of a necrotic, renal-cell carcinoma, however, so clinical findings are of great importance in the differential diagnosis.

PERIRENAL ABSCESS

Hematogenous infection may also result in perirenal inflammatory disease and abscess formation. The infection may actually arise in the perirenal area in addition to extending there as a complication of cortical abscess. Plain-film

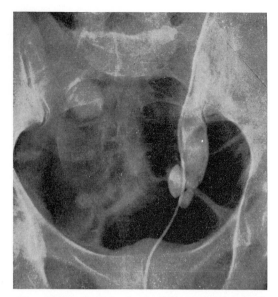

Fig. 20-24. Multiple large left ureteral calculi. Opaque catheter indicates the position of these calculi in relation to the ureter. The bladder is outlined by air.

roentgenograms of perirenal abscess will show an absence of the perirenal fat shadow causing an indistinctness of the renal margin. Fixation of the kidney by the infection is demonstrated on upright roentgenograms that show a failure of the normal descent in this position. The psoas muscle shadow is enlarged and its margin blurred adjacent to the area of infection. Lumbar scoliosis with convexity away from the side of the lesion results from muscle splinting and is usually present. The diaphragm is often slightly elevated with areas of linear atelectasis in the basal lung manifested by small horizontal densities in the basal lung parenchyma.

Psoas abscess may displace the kidney and ureter, but does not ordinarily spread to involve the kidney (Fig. 20-26).

CHRONIC PYELONEPHRITIS (ATROPHIC PYELONEPHRITIS)

Chronic bacterial infection of the kidneys usually starts as a focal process in the medulla, causing a localized area of fibrosis or scarring. As it progresses, the infection causes further scarring, resulting in loss of renal parenchyma, irregularity of the renal surface, and distortion of the calyx in the involved area. The calyces involved become clubbed. Renal tissue between involved areas is normal or hypertrophied. Parenchymal loss may progress to the point where there are only a few millimeters of scar tissue between the capsule and the calyx. Unless there is obstruction or significant reflux the distribution of the lesions is uneven (Fig. 20-27).

According to Hodson[43] the disease usually begins in childhood, but it may not be recognized until early adult life. The earliest roentgen sign is a decrease in the amount of renal parenchyma, often in one pole of the kidney. Later the adjacent calyx or calyces exhibit clubbing. As the disease progresses, the findings become more generalized and are often bilateral but usually not symmetric.

Hydronephrotic atrophy or obstructive atrophy of the kidney also causes progressive blunting of the calyces and narrowing of the renal parenchyma. However, this tends to be very symmetric in contrast to the irregular distribution of the scars of pyelonephritis. A similar appearance may be observed in patients with vesicoureteral reflux. Infection may be present in both of these conditions and it also can cause the focal parenchymal scarring which is found in pyelonephritis. When the disease begins in adult life, there is less scarring of the parenchyma, but the calyceal blunting is similar.

Renal angiography is frequently employed to assess the blood supply and is helpful in differential diagnosis. In pyelonephritis there is bilateral asymmetry of blood supply with decrease in caliber corresponding to the extent of the renal disease. The nephrogram phase outlines the irregularity of the cortical margin of the kidney. The intrarenal arteries are obliterated at the sites of severe disease and tend to be tortuous in areas of lesser involvement (Fig. 20-28).

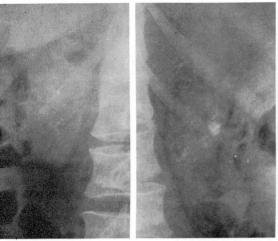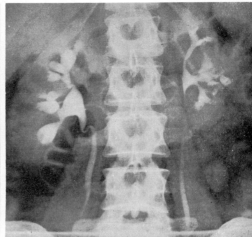

Fig. 20-25. Nephrocalcinosis. Note stippled calcific densities overlying both renal areas in the preliminary roentgenograms. On the urogram film, the calcifications on the right are not clearly defined but those on the left are visible. Some of them are definitely within the renal parenchyma.

XANTHOGRANULOMATOUS PYELONEPHRITIS

This is a form of severe chronic inflammation of the kidney found predominantly in adult females. The clinical findings consist of a history of easy fatiguability and low-grade fever that may antedate urinary symptoms of dysuria, frequency, and a dull, aching flank pain sometimes associated with palpable flank mass. Recurrent attacks may occur. Calculi are common, but there is no parenchymal calcification. The disease is usually unilateral, but the opposite kidney is often involved by pyelonephritis. The pathologic process consists of granulomatous involvement of the fatty tissue in Gerota's fascia leading to production of a fixed renal mass. Similar granulomas arise in the renal parenchyma, associated with foam cells, cholesterol slits, extensive fibrotic changes, and atrophic glomeruli. The process may be localized or involve the entire kidney; at times it may extend to produce a periureteric mass in the upper ureteral region. Ureteropelvic junction obstruction may be a significant etiologic factor with secondary infection. *B. proteus* is commonly found in the urine but may not be the etiologic agent. Urographic findings consist of calyceal dilatation and blunting with irregularity of papillae, decreased cortical thickness, ureteral deformity and stricture which may resemble extensive tuberculosis. In others, no function may be present. The kidney and psoas outlines may be indistinct. When obstructed, retrograde studies reveal dilatation and gross distortion of pelves and calyces. Angiography reveals displacement and stretching of intrarenal arteries with absence of small peripheral branches. Capsular and ureteric branches may be prominent. The nephrogram phase resembles that of hydronephrosis.

PYELITIS OF PREGNANCY

This term is applied to renal infection which sometimes accompanies pregnancy. Most pregnancies are associated with some degree of hydronephrosis, usually more marked on the right than on the left. This is believed to be from mechanical obstruction caused by increased uterine size; it usually clears promptly following delivery. When infection occurs, however, urinary symptoms result from the combination of obstruction and infection.

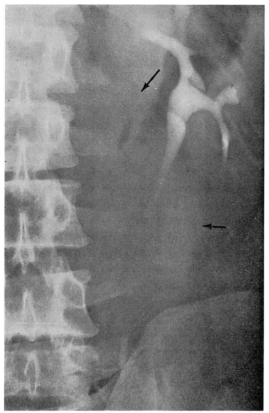

Fig. 20-26. Psoas abscess. Note the large psoas mass (**arrows**) which displaces the left kidney and upper ureter and also compresses the ureter. This is a chronic abscess which is well localized, so that the psoas shadow is clearly defined.

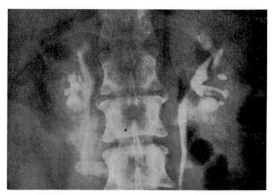

Fig. 20-27. Bilateral pyelonephritis. Most of the calyces are blunted but the involvement is not uniform. Some of the infundibula are slightly narrowed. The right kidney is small, secondary to chronic inflammatory disease. The lower pole of the left kidney is small, indicating loss of parenchyma there.

Urograms will outline the dilated calyces and there usually is associated dilatation of the ureter down to the brim of the pelvis (Fig. 20-29). Infection, when present, is usually of recent origin, so that there are no anatomic changes directly related to it unless the patient has had repeated infections in the past or has a chronic pyelonephritis.

RENAL PAPILLARY NECROSIS

Renal papillary necrosis, or necrotizing renal papillitis, is characterized by infarction of renal papillae, resulting in necrosis with demarcation and sloughing of the involved tissue. The necrotic material may be passed in fragments or as a single mass or it may remain in the calyx. When it remains it may calcify peripherally to form a rather typical concretion. The cause of the necrosis is not clear. It is usually bilateral and may involve few or many papillae. It is more frequent in females than in males.

Formerly it was thought to be an acute fulminating disease occurring mainly in patients with diabetes mellitus or with obstructive hydroenphrosis. It is now known to occur much more frequently as a chronic condition in which renal infection is present. Pyuria is nearly always present in the chronic forms. Excessive use of phenacetin over prolonged periods (i.e., 8 to 12 months) is also associated with the disease and probably causes it. It may also occur in renal vein thrombosis. Sickle-cell disease is another cause of renal papillary necrosis. In these patients, hematuria is a common symptom. Intravascular stasis leading to thrombosis is thought to lead to necrosis. Infection is not a prominent feature in necrosis associated with sickle-cell disease or with phenacetin abuse. In the acute fulminating form the diminished renal function may make excretory urography useless, but in most instances the diagnosis can be made with this examination. Therefore, retrograde pyelography is seldom necessary to make the diagnosis.

Roentgen findings are quite characteristic. Cavity formation is the major finding, but it is preceded by local impairment of function and

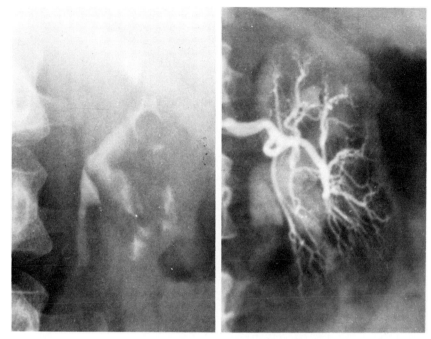

Fig. 20-28. Chronic pyelonephritis. *Left,* Urogram shows poor filling and some distortion of calyces and pelvis. *Right,* Selective arteriogram shows tortuosity of arteries which appear pruned because the small branches are obliterated.

irregularity and blurring of papillary contour. The cavities are formed as a result of the sloughing of necrotic tissue. Two types are found. In the medullary type, the necrosis starts centrally and the cavity forms within the papilla; it communicates with the calyx via the tip of the papilla. A thin layer of parenchyma separates the cavity from the fornix of the calyx. In the second type, the papillary form, the entire papilla sloughs off, leaving a cavity which may extend rather deeply into the adjacent pyramid. No remaining fornix is observed and the cavity is a direct extension of the calyx. A triangular radiolucent shadow ringed with the dense opaque, the "ring shadow," may be observed when the necrotic papilla remains in the calyx. Eventually, a typical concretion may develop; it consists of a dense, calcified shell surrounding a radiolucent center. Late in the disease, scarring may result in some distortion. Ureteral involvement varying from slight irregularity to stricture formation is found occasionally. The diagnosis can be histopathologically confirmed if some of the sloughed material is passed and recovered from the urine. The increased incidence

of the disease in recent years is attributed to its recognition as a chronic condition and possibly to increasing abuse of phenacetin.

BILATERAL RENAL CORTICAL NECROSIS

This disease is characterized by bilateral, symmetric, ischemic necrosis of the renal cortex, with sparing of the medullary portion of the kidney and a thin rim of subcapsular cortex. It is a cause of acute renal failure which has terminated fatally in most instances. It may be associated with a number of antecedent conditions such as severe burns, multiple fractures, internal hemorrhage, severe infections, transfusions of incompatible blood, peritonitis, and others. It occurs frequently in pregnancy, often associated with abruptio placentae. With the advent of modern treatment, including hemodialysis, a number of patients have recovered partially from the disease and certain roentgen findings have been observed which suggest the diagnosis.

Initially the kidneys are usually enlarged. This

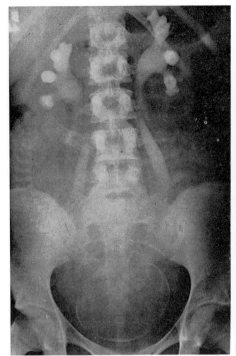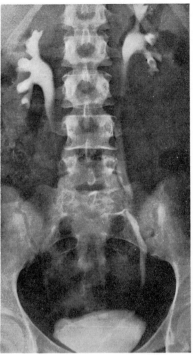

Fig. 20-29. Hydronephrosis in pregnancy. The patient had upper urinary tract infection; this combination is sometimes termed "pyelitis of pregnancy." *Right,* Taken 2 months after delivery shows almost complete return to normal.

is followed by a decrease in size of varying degrees. Faint cortical calcification in the form of a thin shell-like rim around the periphery of the kidney appears in 50 to 60 days following the onset. This is so faint that tomograms may be necessary for adequate visualization in patients suspected of having the disease. Tram-line or double-line calcification has also been reported. The calcification may extend into the interlobular septa. The renal contour may be irregular and the calcification interrupted, depending upon the distribution of the disease. The renal pelvis and calyceal system appear normal but function is usually decreased following recovery from the acute phase of the disease.

PYELOURETERITIS CYSTICA, PYELITIS CYSTICA, AND URETERITIS CYSTICA

Pyeloureteritis cystica and ureteritis cystica are special manifestations of chronic inflammatory disease in which small cysts arise from the ure-

teral wall and sometimes from the wall of the renal pelvis and bladder. These cysts appear as small radiolucent defects along the course of the ureter when it has been opacified by contrast substance. The appearance of multiple, small, mucosal filling defects is pathognomonic. The defects are usually more numerous in the upper ureter than elsewhere. They may become large enough to produce partial ureteral obstruction. Signs of pyelonephritis are often present in these patients. The condition is commonly noted in the bladder at cystoscopy, but is relatively rare in the ureters and renal pelvis.

TUBERCULOSIS

PATHOLOGY

The kidney is involved by tuberculosis in a manner comparable to involvement of other organs. The infection is hematogenous. One or several organisms are filtered out by the glomeruli and migrate from the cortex to the region of the renal papilla where tubercles are formed, leading to destruction of medullary tissue and ulceration. These early lesions are often multiple, but do not involve all the papillae. As the disease progresses, involvement of adjacent infundibula often leads to obstruction. Similar stricture formation leading to obstruction is found when there is ureteral involvement. The disease does not heal spontaneously and the destruction continues, producing irregular cavities adjacent to the calyces. Eventually this leads to virtual destruction of the entire kidney. If ureteral obstruction is not a factor the kidney may gradually decrease in size or remain normal in size and gradually fill with caseous material along with some calcium to form the so-called "putty kidney." If ureteral obstruction occurs before the kidney is destroyed and functionless, a large hydronephrotic kidney results, in which there are irregular cavities adjacent to the calyces. These anatomic changes are visible on urography and form the basis for the roentgen diagnosis of renal tuberculosis. This should always be confirmed, as in pulmonary tuberculosis, by demonstration of the organisms in the urine from the involved kidney.

ROENTGEN FINDINGS

The roentgen findings on plain-film examination are those of alteration in size of the kidney and calcification within it. These are nonspecific findings but may be suggestive, particularly if cloudy flocculent calcification outlines most of the renal shadow, indicative of extensive destruction of parenchyma. The calcification may be dense and irregular and lie within the renal outline, often in the cortical area. In the early stages of cortical involvement, no urographic findings are present and it is possible to have considerable parenchymal involvement without urographic change. The earliest finding is a slight irregularity of the involved calyx caused by ulcerative papillary lesions (Fig. 20-30). Further destruction is manifested by loss of the normal papilla and

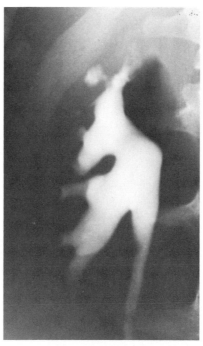

Fig. 20-30. Renal tuberculosis. The upper pole calyces are involved and are irregular as a result of adjacent parenchymal destruction.

irregular ragged cavity formation (Fig. 20-31). Often this is associated with a narrowing of the infundibulum to the affected calyx. The infundibulum may later become completely obstructed, so that the diseased area is not visible on retrograde pyelography. In this event there may or may not be enough function to visualize the cavity on intravenous urography. Therefore, a careful evaluation of calyceal distribution in relation to the renal outline is necessary in all patients with suspected renal tuberculosis. When the renal pelvis is involved, the mucosa is irregular owing to ulceration. Local constriction caused by fibrosis is also common and dilatation results when there is obstruction at or below the ureteropelvic junction. Ureteral involvement may result in stricture formation, which is often multiple; and mucosal infection can also produce small local nodules that appear as filling defects along the ureteral wall. In advanced involvement of the ureter it is common to find the ureter unusually straight, ex-

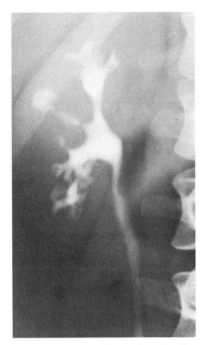

Fig. 20-31. Renal tuberculosis. There is extensive involvement with cavity formation noted superiorly and centrally. There is also infundibular narrowing of one of the central calyces.

tending in a direct line downward from the renal pelvis to the pelvic brim without the usual slight curves seen in the normal ureter. The bladder, seminal vesicles, and vas deferens may also be involved in patients with renal tuberculosis. Irregular mottled calcification in these structures is a roentgen finding which suggests the diagnosis.

Urography is used in renal tuberculosis as a method of making an anatomic diagnosis, to be confirmed by bacteriologic study. It is also of value in following the renal lesion during treatment and in outlining the opposite kidney.

DIFFERENTIAL DIAGNOSIS

Differential diagnosis of calcium deposits must include renal calculi and nephrocalcinosis as well as cyst and tumor calcification. Calculi are usually more discrete and rounded than the calcification seen in tuberculosis. Tumor calcification often extends beyond the border of the kidney and tends to be less hazy and flocculent in appearance

than in tuberculosis. Calcification in cysts occurs in the wall and tends to outline it in an arcuate form of varying size. This calcification also tends to extend beyond the shadow of the normal kidney. Urographic changes in chronic pyelonephritis consist of calyceal abnormality that may resemble early tuberculous involvement, but the change is usually more general than in tuberculosis. The same is true in renal papillary necrosis, which is usually bilateral and tends to be more extensive than renal tuberculosis.

TRAUMA

The kidney lies in a well-protected area and is not frequently injured. In patients with chronic renal disease, however, relatively minor trauma may cause considerable damage. Direct force over the renal area is the usual cause of injury. Trauma to the kidney is manifested by hematuria, which may be gross or microscopic. When found after injury, blood in the urine indicates some type of renal damage or injury to the lower urinary tract. There is a difference of opinion as to how patients with kidney injury should be handled. The trend is toward examination by means of intravenous urography, which is done as soon as possible after injury. This is a safe procedure and may lead to a definitive diagnosis of the extent of renal injury relatively soon after the trauma. The intravenous urogram is the most commonly used study in patients with renal trauma. The excretory nephrogram (1- to 2-minute film) is a good indicator of renal function. It is possible to check the presence and condition of the contralateral kidney if surgical removal of the injured kidney is contemplated. However, there are instances where extravasation is not shown on the intravenous study. Retrograde pyelography is indicated when excretion is poor or absent. The use of renal angiography in the posttraumatic period is indicated if there is diminution of renal function, since renal artery involvement with resultant thrombosis is not uncommon following renal trauma. It is the only method that will yield accurate information regarding damage to the blood supply. Renal arteriography is indicated whenever significant renal damage is present or suspected. Immediate surgical correction of the vascular lesion may prevent permanent renal damage in some instances. The anatomic and physiologic alterations produced by trauma may be caused by occlusive renal arterial change much more often than is now realized.

The severity of parenchymal injury may vary from rupture of a calyx with extravasation into the parenchyma to more extensive fracture of parenchyma with subcapsular and parenchymal extravasation. When the injury is more severe the capsule may rupture with perirenal extravasation of urine as well as perirenal hemorrhage. Immediate surgical extirpation of the kidney may be needed in some instances when there is extensive fracture with retroperitoneal and intraperitoneal hemorrhage. The opposite kidney should always be studied by means of excretory urography before nephrectomy.

Roentgen findings depend upon the extent of injury. If perirenal hemorrhage is present the renal shadow and sometimes the psoas shadow is obliterated or enlarged. At times the hemorrhage remains localized in the perirenal area and produces a localized or generalized enlargement of the kidney that may simulate tumor. Rarely, calcification of a hematoma in or around the kidney may be seen as a late finding in renal trauma. Hemorrhage within the renal capsule may also produce a local or generalized enlargement of the kidney. Accessory signs on plain-film roentgenograms are scoliosis, convexity to the opposite side indicating muscle spasm, gas in the small bowel in the vicinity of the injury caused by localized adynamic ileus, and fracture of an adjacent rib, vertebral body, or vertebral process. Urography demonstrates the amount of extravasation and may show calyceal compression and distortion caused by parenchymal and subcapsular accumulations of blood, urine, or both (Fig. 20-32). The amount of extravasation is not necessarily proportional to the parenchymal or vascular damage, however. Because posttraumatic distortion and stricture are important, urographic studies should also be

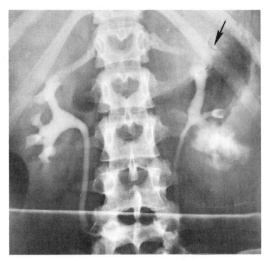

Fig. 20-32. Interstitial extravasation of opaque medium in the lower pole of the left kidney, caused by trauma. Note fracture of the left eleventh rib (**arrow**).

carried out during or following convalescence to outline any residual deformity.

RENAL CYSTIC DISEASES

The classification of renal cystic diseases is difficult and there is much confusion in the literature because of many disagreements among pathologists. For our purposes the classification of Bernstein and Meyer[9] as modified by Elkin and Bernstein[24] is most useful.

RENAL DYSPLASIA

MULTICYSTIC KIDNEY

Congenital multicystic disease of the kidney is an uncommon disorder usually considered to be a severe form of renal dysplasia. The bilateral form results in renal nonfunction, while the unilateral form which is more common, carries a good prognosis if uncomplicated by other anomalies. There is absence of normal renal parenchyma, the pelvis is small or absent, and the ureter is hypoplastic, stenotic, or

TABLE 20-1. Classfication of Renal Cysts

I. Renal Dysplasia
   A. Multicystic kidney
   B. Focal and segmental cystic dysplasia
   C. Multiple cysts associated with lower urinary tract obstruction
II. Polycystic Disease
   A. Infantile polycystic disease
      1. Polycystic disease of the newborn
      2. Polycystic disease of childhood
         a. Congenital hepatic fibrosis
         b. Medullary tubular ectasia
   B. Adult polycystic disease
III. Cortical Cysts
   A. Trisomy syndromes
   B. Tuberous sclerosis complex
   C. Simple cysts
      1. Solitary
      2. Multiple
   D. Multilocular cysts
IV. Medullary Cysts
   A. Medullary sponge kidney
   B. Medullary cystic disease
   C. Medullary necrosis
   D. Pyelogenic cyst
V. Miscellaneous Intrarenal Cyst
   A. Inflammatory
      1. Tuberculosis
      2. Calculous disease
      3. Echinococcus disease
   B. Neoplastic-cystic degeneration of carcinoma
   C. Traumatic intrarenal hematoma
VI. Extraparenchymal Renal Cysts
   A. Parapelvic cyst
   B. Perinephric cyst

Based on classification of Bernstein, J., and Meyer, R.[9] and Elkin, M., and Bernstein, J.[24]

atretic. The nephrons which are present are hypoplastic with arrested development. The blood supply is variable. The kidney consists of a mass of cysts of varying size and is usually very large. At times the involved kidney is small and is distinguishable from aplastic kidney only by the presence of cysts. The disease usually presents as a unilateral flank mass in a healthy appearing infant. The mass may be visible on the plain film. Excretory urography shows no function of the affected kidney and a normal appearance of the contralateral kidney. When the affected kidney is small it may be undetected until adult life.

MULTIPLE CYSTS ASSOCIATED WITH LOWER URINARY TRACT OBSTRUCTION

A number of conditions causing urinary obstruction in fetal life may lead to renal dysplasia. The most common occurrence is in infant males with posterior urethral valves. On excretory urography the dilated bladder, hydroureter, and hydronephrosis are observed if renal function is satisfactory. The cysts are not demonstrated, but their presence may distort the calyces and pelvis.

POLYCYSTIC DISEASE

INFANTILE POLYCYSTIC KIDNEY

Infantile sponge kidney (polycystic disease of the newborn) is a rare condition, is genetically autosomal recessive, and involves both kidneys and usually the liver. Most patients die in infancy with only an occasional one living into childhood, usually afflicted with hypertension and increasing renal insufficiency. The cortex and medulla are filled with radially oriented cysts.

There is bilateral renal enlargement which is easily detected on palpation of the abdomen in the newborn infant. Roentgen findings include massive renal enlargement which can be seen on the plain film. The nephrographic phase of the urogram is usually delayed and when it appears, tends to present a peculiar fuzzy, streaky, or striated appearance. Concentration is usually poor, so that the collecting system is faintly visualized at best. The kidneys retain the contrast medium for some time. Renal outlines are smooth and there is very little calyceal distortion.

ADULT POLYCYSTIC DISEASE

The pathogenesis of renal polycystic disease is not completely understood, but it is transmitted as an autosomal dominant trait and is associated with cystic disease of the liver and occasionally of the pancreas and with berry aneurysms of the cerebral vessels. It is most likely a congenital anomaly of structure resulting from failure of union between collecting tubules and the metanephrogenic anlage, which results in cyst formation when excretion begins. The cysts are numerous and often vary in size up to several centimeters. This sometimes results in marked renal enlargement and a lobulation or irregularity of renal outline is often present. Involvement is bilateral in 90 per cent of patients, but is not necessarily symmetric, so that renal enlargement is often unequal. The disease tends to be progressive, often leading to renal failure and death. When the diagnosis is made in infancy, it usually means that the condition is severe and the prognosis is poor. In adults the prognosis is generally fair unless there is marked renal failure. Urographic findings are usually characteristic enough to be diagnostic (Fig. 20-33). In addition to the general renal enlargement there is extensive elongation of infundibula and calyces and irregular enlargement of calyces, but no calyceal clubbing is present. The infundibula often appear partially to surround the

cysts of varying size and the calyces also are noted to stretch around the smaller cysts. This results in multiple, crescentic contours of the filled calyces and their infundibula and in elongation and thinning of infundibula. The minor calyces are often separated, but no irregularities are noted such as are found in infiltrating tumors. On plain-film roentgenograms the renal outlines are often indistinct despite the enlargement, owing to a decrease in perirenal fat. The bilaterality of the findings is of considerable aid in differential diagnosis. Angiographic findings consist of stretching of vessels around the cysts and a decrease in density of the areas of involvement during the nephrographic phase of the examination. The latter finding is quite characteristic and can also be seen on nephrotomography.

CORTICAL CYSTS

TUBEROUS SCLEROSIS

Renal cysts are usually small and of tubular origin. Rarely, cortical cysts large enough to

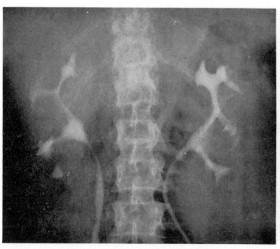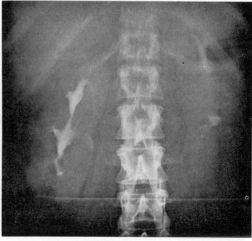

Fig. 20-33. Polycystic kidneys. *Left,* Note the poor definition of renal outlines in addition to the enlargement, which is more marked on the left than on the right. Calyces and infundibula are typically stretched, particularly on the left side. *Right,* The changes are less marked and the left kidney is noted to be more severely involved than the right, where the major changes are noted to be in the lower pole. The changes are therefore bilateral but not symmetric.

produce distortion have been reported. Angiomyolipoma of the kidney is found frequently in tuberous sclerosis. This tumor or hamartoma is described in the section on "Benign Tumors."

SIMPLE CYSTS

The simple renal cyst is often a silent lesion of little or no clinical importance. Cysts sometimes bleed and may become large enough to be noted as masses that can be palpated through the abdominal wall. In the latter instance they may cause renal damage by reason of their size, particularly if situated in a region where obstruction of the excretory system can occur. These lesions are usually unilateral and they may be solitary but often there are two or more. The roentgen findings depend on the location. The chief importance of the simple cyst is that it may simulate a tumor in its appearance. Plain-film roentgenograms outline a smooth, local enlargement of the kidney. Occasionally there is a thin shell of calcium

outlining the cyst wall or a portion of it (Fig. 20-34). It is much more common to see curvilinear calcifications in tumors of the kidney than in cysts. The cysts may reach massive size and actually dwarf the kidney (Fig. 20-35). Urographic findings consist of crescentic defects and stretching of the infundibula and calyces when the lesion arises close to the calyces. When the cyst arises further away, there is less calyceal change and when the cyst is in a subcapsular position there is little or no pressure deformity on the pelvis or calyces. The changes caused by a cyst are usually less marked than those produced by a tumor of similar size and location. There is often less distortion of calyces with cysts than with tumor.

The "claw" sign is thought by many to be very valuable in the identification of renal cysts. It consists of a triangular claw-like projection of renal parenchyma observed on the nephrographic phase of the renal angiogram or on nephrotomography (Fig. 20-36). Angio-

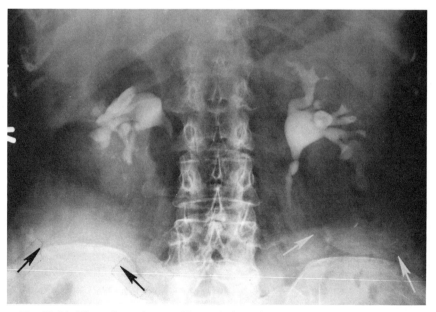

Fig. 20-34. Bilateral renal cysts. Note relatively large size of cysts with calcification in their walls, which produce very little deformity of the calyces. **Arrows** indicate the outline of the cysts and the calcification.

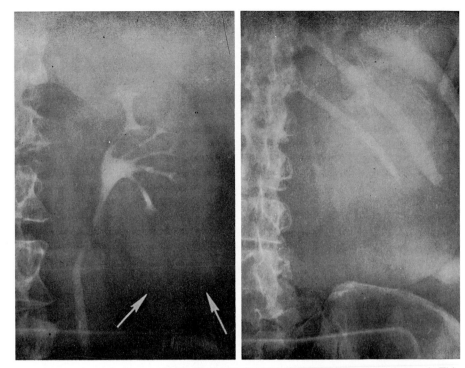

Fig. 20-35. *Left,* Moderate-sized cyst in the lower pole of the left kidney (**arrows**). This cyst produces no significant alteration in the lower pole calyces. *Right,* Large cyst, which is two or three times the size of the left kidney. Excretory urogram shows poor filling and indicates considerable compression of the pelvis and calyces by the cyst.

graphic findings include displacement of vessels around a clearly defined, smoothly rounded, thin-walled mass, nonopacification of the mass during the nephrogram phase, and absence of abnormal ("tumor") vessels. For further discussion on the differentiation of cysts and tumors see page 695.

MULTILOCULAR CYSTS

This condition is very rare. It consists of unilateral solitary cysts which contain several loculi which do not intercommunicate or connect with the renal pelvis. This abnormality is usually found in childhood. Abdominal mass is the major presenting complaint. Roentgen findings resemble those of simple cyst and include visible mass on the plain film. Distortion of the pelvis and calyces depending on the size and location of the cystic mass is noted on the

urogram. Arteriography shows the mass to be avascular and vessels around it may be stretched.

MEDULLARY CYSTS

MEDULLARY SPONGE KIDNEY

This condition is a form of cystic disease involving the medulla of the kidney. It has also been called precalyceal canalicular ectasia, renal tubular ectasia, cystic disease of the renal pyramids, cystic dilatation of the collecting tubules, and multiple cysts of the renal medulla. The changes are confined to the renal medulla and consist of dilatation and cyst formation involving the collecting tubules in the renal pyramids. Calculi are frequently found in the cysts. It may be limited to a single pyramid,

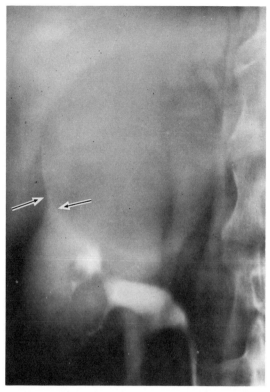

Fig. 20-36. Claw sign of renal cyst (**arrows**). Nephrotomogram clearly outlines smooth wall of the radiolucent cyst adjacent to the density of the opacified parenchyma.

but is usually more extensive. Renal enlargement may be present when the lesions are general. The disease is thought by some to be a congenital disturbance of fusion of nephrogenic tissue and the wolffian ducts. Others believe that it is an unusual form of polycystic disease or related to it. Some think a heterogeneous group of conditions including renal tubular acidosis may be included. Function is usually preserved and the disease does not appear to progress. However, there may be morbidity caused by infection and colic or both when calculi are passed. In the advanced disease, the extensive cyst formation in the medulla resembles a sponge. Microscopically the rounded, elongated, or irregular cysts present a varied appearance. The epithelium varies from transi-

tional to squamous or columnar, normal tubules are reduced or absent and some degree of inflammatory change is usually present. The cysts may contain calculi or masses of calcified debris.

The disease is usually discovered in middle age, but has been found in children. Clinical symptoms may be absent, but recurrent infection results in pyuria and fever. Hematuria is common and renal colic may be the presenting symptom.

The roentgen findings are quite characteristic, even though the extent of the disease varies considerably. The plain film demonstrates the calculi when present. Their position and appearance is often diagnostic. The calculi are usually multiple, small, smoothly rounded or oval and occur in clusters or in a fanlike arrangement in the renal pyramids (Fig. 20-37). Intravenous urography is a better method of examination than retrograde pyelography, since the dilated tubules may not fill in a retrograde manner. In the urogram the dilated tubules are opacified unless infection has impaired renal function. Minimal dilatation produces a fine striated appearance; with increasing dilatation the appearance becomes more cystlike, with rounded or elongated cavities enlarging and often distorting the papilla and minor calyx (Figs. 20-37 and 20-38). Adjacent calyces may show a considerable difference in the degree of involvement. There is usually no difficulty in the roentgen diagnosis of typical sponge kidney, but in some instances pyelotubular backflow, renal tuberculosis, renal papillary necrosis, and nephrocalcinosis must be considered in the differential diagnosis.

MEDULLARY CYSTIC DISEASE (NEPHRONOPHTHISIS)

Nephronophthisis (familial juvenile nephronophthisis, medullary cystic disease of the kidney) is a rare disorder of unknown etiology usually found in children and young adults. Anemia, polydipsia, polyuria, salt-wasting, and progressive uremia develop insidiously. Growth

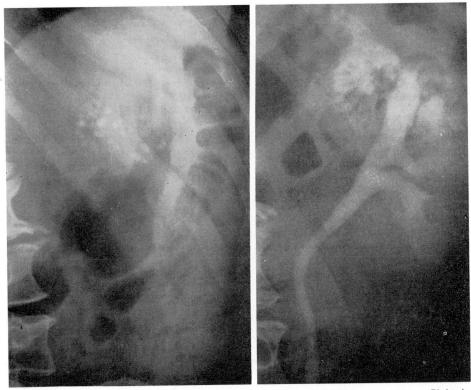

Fig. 20-37. Sponge kidney. *Left,* Note calculi in the upper pole of the left kidney. *Right,* In the urogram, the contrast medium now outlines dilated tubules and obscures the calculi within them. The calyces are considerably distorted.

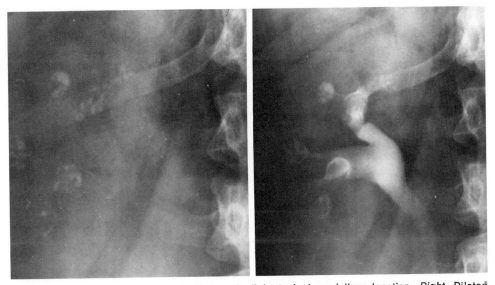

Fig. 20-38. Sponge kidney. *Left,* Note calculi in typical medullary location. *Right,* Dilated tubules in renal papillae are present in addition to the calculi there.

retardation, bone deformities, and hypocalcemic tetany occur in young patients. Urine has a low, fixed specific gravity with absence of protein or formed elements. Histopathologic findings consist of alternating areas of cystic dilatation and atrophy in the proximal and distal tubules with marked thickening of the basement membrane. Interstitial fibrosis with round-cell infiltration is prominent. Glomeruli show minor focal thickening early, progressing to sclerosis and periglomerular fibrosis.

Urographic study has been of limited value because of poor function but with high-dose urography, minor calyceal blunting and uniform contraction of the kidneys are visible. If these changes are correlated with the clinical and laboratory findings, the diagnosis should be suggested.

RENAL MEDULLARY (PAPILLARY) NECROSIS

See section on Infections and Related Conditions.

PYELOGENIC OR CALYCINE CYSTS

The term "pyelogenic" or "calycine" cyst (calyceal diverticulum) refers to the small cystlike spaces that often communicate with a calyx, but that occasionally are observed to opacify on urography despite no apparent connection with the adjacent calyx. This lesion is a true congenital cyst, but cystlike structures of similar appearance may result from inflammatory destruction of parenchyma adjacent to a calyx or from inflammatory obstruction of a calyx. The diagnosis is made on intravenous urography when a small, rounded space fills with opaque material (Fig. 20-39). The cysts are filled by their own tubules and so are visible despite lack of apparent communication with the calyceal system. In contrast to the cysts in the renal pyramids as found in sponge kidney, the calycine cysts apparently arise from the fornix of the calyx and occur laterally rather than centrally in relation to the papilla. Calculi are frequently formed in the cysts and are visible on plain roentgenograms. Rarely

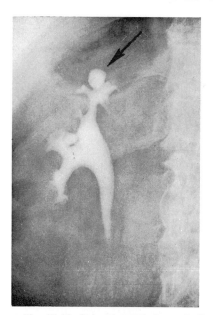

Fig. 20-39. Calycine cyst. **Arrow** indicates calycine cyst in the upper pole of the right kidney. This cyst communicates with one of the upper pole calyces.

milk of calcium is observed, with a fluid level present on an upright film (Fig. 20-40).

EXTRAPARENCHYMAL RENAL CYSTS

PARAPELVIC CYSTS

Parapelvic cysts are relatively rare and unlike the simple renal cysts, they do not lie within the renal parenchyma. They are located and probably originate in the hilus of the kidney in close proximity to the pelvis and major calyces. Their origin is obscure. Some authors believe them to be of lymphatic origin; others believe that they are congenital cysts which arise from embryonic rests or from remnants of the wolffian body or from mesonephric remnants.

Roentgen findings are those of a mass in the renal hilus which causes compression and displacement of the pelvis and distortion and displacement of the major calyces and infundibula. Mild local caliectasis may result from partial obstruction resulting from compression. They do not contain calcium. The renal vascu-

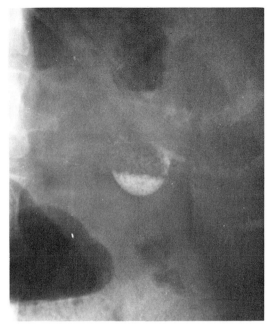

Fig. 20-40. Milk of calcium in a renal cyst. This upright film shows calcium to be largely dependent.

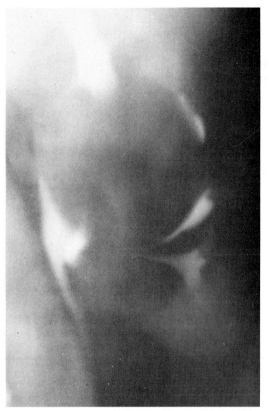

Fig. 20-41. Halo sign of parapelvic cyst. Nephrotomogram shows ill-defined radiolucency caused by compressed renal sinus fat surrounding the smoothly rounded cyst in the renal hilus.

lar pedicle may be displaced and distorted by the mass. They resemble lipoma of the renal hilus or lipomatosis when the latter results in a hilus mass.

Since there is no renal parenchymal interface with this type of cyst, the nephrographic phase of arteriography or nephrotomography is somewhat different than that seen in the simple cyst. The parapelvic cyst appears as a spherical mass of lesser density than the opacified renal parenchyma adjacent to it surrounded by a halo of fat which is more radiolucent than the cyst. When this halo of fat can be clearly seen to outline a smooth, round mass, the diagnosis can be made with a high degree of certainty (Fig. 20-41).

PERINEPHRIC CYST (PARARENAL PSEUDOCYST; URINOMA)

Pararenal pseudocyst is a term used to describe a complication of renal or ureteral injury. Pararenal pseudohydronephrosis, hydrocele renalis, hygroma perirenalis, perirenal cyst, and perinephric cyst are synonyms. Persistent extravasation of urine or blood or both following accidental trauma or surgery may produce a vicious cycle of extravasation, compression of the pelvis or upper ureter and resultant hydronephrosis which may lead to eventual loss of renal function. Roentgen findings consist of a mass adjacent to the kidney, usually below it. The mass often displaces the kidney upward and rotates it. Usually a definite line of separation between the mass and the kidney is observed. Intravenous urography may opacify the mass (if contrast extravasates into it) and will reveal the displacement of the ureter and kidney or both. Retrograde study may be necessary to confirm the diagnosis. This complication is rare, but is one reason why it is necessary to do follow-up urography in patients with renal trauma.

MISCELLANEOUS INTRARENAL CYSTS

ECHINOCOCCAL (HYDATID) CYSTS

The kidney may be involved in patients with echinococcal infestation with formation of cysts similar to those noted in the liver and other parenchymatous organs. The cysts may have a calcified wall visible on plain-film study. Calcification occurs in 50 to 80 per cent of patients. The calcification may be similar to that found in tumors or cysts or may resemble renal calculi. Cysts are pear-shaped or round and may be closed, although most of them eventually open into a calyx and can be outlined by opaque medium upon urography and pyelography. Often the large cyst contains daughter cysts that are smaller and resemble a grapelike cluster of masses extending into the larger cyst. The cysts deform the renal outline and calyceal system in a manner similar to the deformity produced by simple cyst. They do tend to obliterate the minor calyces and deform the major calyces to a somewhat greater extent, however. They may reach very large proportions, and result in considerable compression of renal parenchyma and distortion of calyces. The discharge of daughter cells into the renal pelvis can produce colic. This discharge can be retroperitoneal and intraperitoneal also. The findings are those of renal mass and are not pathognomonic.

The cystlike lesions found in tuberculosis, neoplasms, etc., are described in the appropriate sections.

RENAL VASCULAR ABNORMALITIES

RENAL ARTERY ANEURYSM

Aneurysms of the renal artery are not common, but are well known to radiologists because they have been observed to contain calcium in a high percentage of reported cases. In recent series where angiography has been used to study the renal artery, the figure has changed. It is likely that no more than 25 to 30 per cent of these aneurysms contain enough calcium to be roentgenographically visible. The diagnosis can usually be made on plain-film studies in the calcified group. The rounded, ring-contoured, calcified aneurysm maintains a constant relationship to the renal pelvis in various projections. About two-thirds are located at the bifurcation of the renal artery and one-third in the segmental branches. Systemic hypertension is present in about 15 per cent of patients with aneurysm of the renal artery. Angiography can be used for confirmation and is the only means of diagnosis when the aneurysm is not calcified. Bilateral renal aneurysms are relatively common, so arteriography is indicated on the opposite side when an aneurysm, either calcified or noncalcified, is found on one side. In general the calcified aneurysms do not tend to rupture, but the incidence of rupture of uncalcified aneurysms is in the range of 25 per cent. Because of the threat of rupture, renovascular hypertension, arterial thrombosis, or renal infarction, patients with noncalcified renal artery aneurysms should be considered for surgical repair.

POLYARTERITIS NODOSA

Multiple, small, intraparenchymal renal aneurysms are observed in polyarteritis nodosa. Renal involvement occurs in 80 to 100 per cent of patients. Similar microaneurysms are present in other viscera involved by this disease. In the kidney the multiple, small aneurysms involving the interlobar and arcuate arteries are associated with scarring which results from thromboses and infarctions. The aneurysms may rupture to produce perirenal hemorrhage. The infarcts produce pain and hematuria. Renal angiography outlines the aneurysms and its use is essential to make the diagnosis.

RENAL ARTERY OCCLUSION

Renal arterial occlusion is most commonly caused by embolism in patients with cardiac disease. Thrombosis also occurs, most often secondary to atherosclerosis, but sometimes caused by trauma. Regardless of cause, when a renal artery is occluded function is lost. Partial function may occasionally return in a year or more. The roentgen findings in acute renal arterial occlusion consist of urographic evidence of a nonfunctioning kidney of normal size in which retrograde pyelography is normal. Acute segmental infarction may cause either complete nonvisualization on intravenous urography or a local failure of calyceal filling. Following total renal infarction without infection the kidney decreases in size and usually remains nonfunctioning. Retrograde study reveals decrease in size of the calyceal system consistent with renal size. The late findings in segmental infarction are those of local decrease in size which may distort the kidney locally and cause an irregular contour. Renal arteriography is used to confirm the diagnosis in all types of arterial occlusion.

RENAL VEIN THROMBOSIS

Thrombosis of the renal vein occurs more frequently in children than in adults. In adults, direct invasion or extrinsic pressure by tumor, and thrombosis of the inferior vena cava are among the more frequent causes. Ileocolitis is considered the chief cause in children. The diagnosis is difficult from a clinical standpoint so radiographic methods are of prime importance. The roentgen findings depend on the rapidity of the occlusion and its relation to the development of venous collaterals. In the acute, complete thrombosis with infarction and perirenal hemorrhage, the kidney is enlarged and intravenous urography shows no function. The renal arteriogram shows delayed flow through narrow, stretched, interlobar arteries. Opacification of the parenchyma is poor and the nephrogram phase is prolonged. Venous drainage cannot be identified. When the acute occlusion is partial, the kidney also becomes enlarged. Function as demonstrated by excretory urography is gradually regained in about 2 weeks as venous collaterals develop. In gradual occlusion, collateral circulation has time to develop and the roentgen picture may be entirely normal. When renal arteriography is done, the venous phase may show extensive venous collaterals.

When renal vein thrombosis is suspected, excretory urography should be done. If the diagnosis is supported by absence or decrease of function and increase in renal size, renal arteriography should be the next step in the radiographic study of the patient. Evaluation of the renal arterial supply, intrarenal pathology, venous collaterals, or absence of renal vein filling and possibly demonstration of the actual obstructive site can all be accomplished with proper timing of the examination (Fig. 20-42).

RENOVASCULAR HYPERTENSION

Renal arterial disease resulting in decreased arterial blood supply to the kidney long has been recognized as a cause of hypertension. Advances in vascular surgery have focused attention on this cause of hypertension, since surgical correction may relieve or diminish the severity of the disease. It is estimated that there are correctable renal lesions in 3 to 5 per cent of hypertensive patients.

Certain clinical features have been used to indicate that renal artery stenosis is the cause of hypertension. They include (1) unexplained hypertension in a child or young adult or in a patient over age 50, especially if there is no family history; (2) sudden onset of malignant hypertension in a patient known to have been mildly hypertensive in the past; (3) hypertension in a patient with known atheromatous disease; (4) the presence of an upper abdominal bruit; and (5) history of unexplained flank pain or renal trauma which suggests the possibility of renal vascular accident. However, the only finding which appears consistently in patients with renovascular hypertension is an upper abdominal bruit. Roentgen methods are essential in the study of patients with suspected renovascular hypertension. The excretory urogram and the isotope renogram are used as screening tests. There is some difference of opinion as to their relative value but most investigators use the urogram and find the renogram of little value. However, the radioiso-

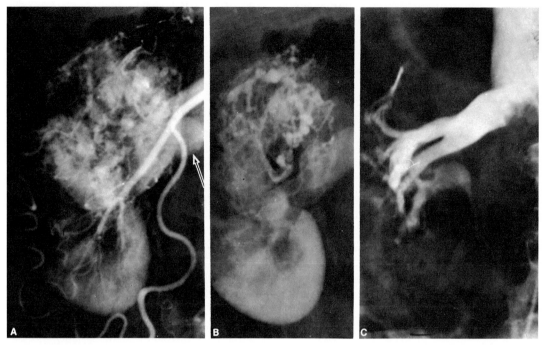

Fig. 20-42. Renal vein thrombosis. *A*, Renal arteriogram (at 2 seconds) shows large vascular mass in the upper pole of the right kidney. Note renal vein below the artery (**arrow**). *B*, Five-second film shows continued opacification of the tumor and clear definition of the renal vein with faint opacification of the vena cava. *C*, Renal venogram. The tumor thrombus is clearly defined and the vena cava is now outlined. The renal vein is partially obstructed and no collaterals are visible.

topic renogram may be used to detect decreased or delayed renal vascular flow and decreased functioning renal mass. (The reader is referred to references 3 and 99 for information relating to this method.) If the excretory urogram is positive, renal arteriography is indicated.

The intravenous urogram is modified in order to make it a more useful test in unilateral renal artery stenosis. The most common modification is the rapid-sequence method, with films every minute for 5 minutes after injection; the 1-minute film can be omitted without suffering a loss of diagnostic potential, which is 85 to 90 per cent accurate. The injection of the contrast substance should be rapid and no compression device is used. After the 5-minute film a compression band may be used for a 10- and 15-minute study, then removed if later films are indicated. Another modification

is the urea washout study in which a rapid saline infusion with a diuretic (urea) is used to "wash out" the medium in the normal kidney and accentuate the persistent concentration on the abnormal side. Although a number of reports indicate the value of this method, we have found it to add no significant information to that obtained by the rapid intravenous urogram.

The following urographic findings are significant in the diagnosis of renovascular hypertension and the presence of any one or a combination of them constitutes a positive study: (*1*) a difference in renal size of 1.5 cm if the right is larger than the left or of 2 cm if the left is larger than the right kidney; (*2*) appearance time: delay in appearance or a distinct decrease in volume of medium excreted; (*3*) the presence of vascular indentations on the upper ureter or pelvis or both which indicates development of collateral circulation; (4) hyperconcentration observed on the later films; and (5) local atrophy (caused by segmental infarct), often best visualized on tomography as areas of decreased concentration in the parenchyma. Even in patients with bilateral renal artery disease the above findings are pertinent, since the stenosis is usually more severe on one side than on the other.

When any of the screening tests are positive or suggestive, anatomic localization of the renal artery lesion by means of arteriography is indicated. This permits the study of the arteries on the "normal" side as well. Actually, the obstructed kidney is protected by the low pressure resulting from the stenotic lesion and is often more normal than the contralateral one.

Arteries may be studied by:

1. Translumbar aortography—direct aortic puncture. This method is rarely used in our department.

2. Catheter techniques in which the percutaneous transfemoral method of Seldinger or direct arterial cut-down may be used. The opaque medium is injected into the aorta near the renal artery orifices. This is the best method for detecting multiple renal arteries. This is followed by selective renal arteriography in which the renal artery is catheterized and a small amount of medium is injected directly into it.

Arteriosclerotic disease is the most common cause of renal artery obstruction. Atheromatous plaques in the aorta may encroach on the orifice of the renal artery. When the renal artery is involved single or multiple defects may be visible. Usually the lesion occurs in the proximal portion of the renal artery, very near its origin. It may cause a concentric or eccentric constriction of the artery. Poststenotic dilatation is common and aneurysm may be present. Diffuse involvement results in multiple irregularities in the lumen. The lesions are more common in males (60 per cent) than in females (Fig. 20-43). The left renal artery is more often involved in a ratio of 3 to 2 when

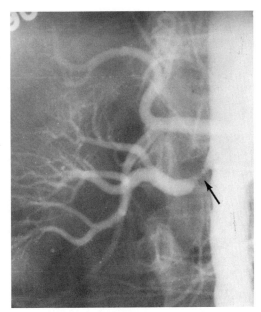

Fig. 20-43. Translumbar aortogram and renal arteriogram showing an arteriosclerotic stenotic lesion (**arrow**) in the right renal artery in a 63-year-old male with hypertension. Note the poststenotic dilatation of the renal artery.

unilateral. Approximately one-third of patients have bilateral artery disease.

The other major cause of stenosis leading to renovascular hypertension is fibromuscular dysplasia (hyperplasia). This disease may be seen at any age, but is most common in young adult females (55 per cent of the focal form and 85 per cent of the multifocal disease is found in females). The lesions are bilateral in nearly 50 per cent of patients. When unilateral, the right renal artery is involved in approximately 75 per cent of patients. The process tends to involve the main renal artery and extend into its branches. The characteristic sites are in the middle and distal portions of the renal artery in contrast to the atherosclerotic involvement which is at or very near the origin of the artery (Fig. 20-44). Fibrous stenosis involves either intima or perivascular tissues while fibromuscular stenosis involves the media.

Kincaid et al.[48] classify fibromuscular dys-

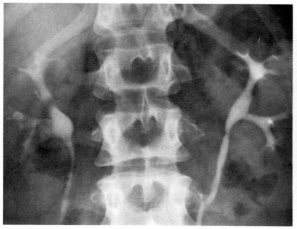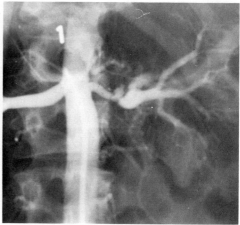

Fig. 20-44. Fibromuscular dysplasia in an 18-year-old female with hypertension. *Left,* Urogram shows slight hyperconcentration on the left. There are a few minor indentations on the upper ureter suggesting the possibility of collateral vascular indents. *Right,* Renal arteriogram shows normal right renal artery. On the left multiple constrictions with poststenotic dilatation and aneurysm formation are present (multifocal type). Perfusion of the left kidney is delayed. Note collateral arteries in and below the renal hilus.

plasia into the following gross morphologic forms:

1. Multifocal (62.4 per cent of 125 patients); "string of beads" appearance caused by alternate areas of narrowing and mural aneurysms

2. Focal (7 per cent); solitary stenosis less than 1 cm in length

3. Tubular (13.6 per cent); elongated, smooth concentric stenosis

4. Mixed (16.8 per cent; two or more of the above forms

All multifocal and most tubular lesions in their study were of the medial type. A few of the tubular and focal lesions were intimal and two of the tubular were periarterial. In the multifocal form, there were rings of extreme hyperplasia of the fibrous components and rarely of the muscular elements of the media. They alternated with zones of extensive medial degeneration resulting in mural aneurysms. In the tubular form, mural aneurysms were not observed. The mural aneurysms may become very thin-walled, and enlarge beyond the perimuscular wall to become true aneurysms. Renal artery dissection may occur; there is a tendency to extend into primary or secondary branches of the renal artery and produce focal infarction. Occasionally renal artery aneurysm may cause partial obstruction leading to renovascular hypertension.

The presence of a renal vascular lesion does not mean that it is the cause of hypertension, since there are a number of factors involved in the production of this disease. Furthermore, there are many normotensive patients with severe renal artery disease. One likely hypothesis is that normotension is present when there is a balance between the available blood supply and the amount of functioning renal parenchyma. If the blood supply is reduced more than the functioning parenchyma, the resultant ischemia may cause hypertension. When major renal arterial disease is present, there may be associated arteriolosclerosis of smaller renal vessels and other factors decreasing the amount of functioning renal parenchyma; this also reduces demand for blood, so that no ischemia is present and hypertension is not produced. It is therefore very difficult to assess hemodynamically significant stenosis. It is generally agreed that the presence of collateral vessels indicate significant stenosis. The principal value of pressure measurements across a stenotic area lies in exclusion of a gradient; this saves the patient from unnecessary exploratory surgery. Demonstration of a gradient indicates a significant stenosis, but it does not follow that the hypertension is curable by removal of the lesion causing the gradient. As a general rule a stenosis of 70 per cent with a lumen of 2 mm or below indicates a significant vascular lesion. Renal vein renin determinations and split-function studies are used in conjunction with renal arteriography in the assessment of patients with possible renovascular hypertension as candidates for surgery.

TUMORS OF THE KIDNEY

BENIGN TUMORS

Benign renal tumors are rare and usually asymptomatic. Histologic types include adenoma, fibroma, lipoma, leiomyoma, hemangioma, and hamartoma. When they are small, no roentgen signs are produced. If they attain sufficient size a plain-film roentgenogram will reveal enlargement of the renal shadow at the site of the tumor. Urography may then show distortion of the calyceal system enough to make the diagnosis of renal tumor. It is also possible for one of these benign lesions to project into the pelvis locally enough to be recognized as a space-occupying mass. The chief importance of these benign renal tumors lies in differentiation between them and malignancies of the kidney. This usually cannot be made with certainty on excretory urography. Rarely, a leiomyoma arising in the renal capsule will contain calcium resembling that observed in leiomyoma elsewhere. With the exception of hemangioma, the benign renal tumors are noted to be avascular on angiography.

RENAL ANGIOMYOLIPOMA

Renal angiomyolipoma (hamartoma) often can be differentiated from other benign tumors and from malignant renal tumors. It usually

occurs in patients with tuberous sclerosis. It is a mixed mesodermal tumor composed of adipose, smooth muscle, and blood vessels in varying proportions. The tumors may be single or multiple, unilateral or bilateral. They occur without other lesions of tuberous sclerosis, but then may be a "forme fruste" of the condition. Clinical manifestations include signs of infection, pain, hematuria, or an asymptomatic abdominal mass. Urographic findings are those of a mass which enlarges the kidney, and distorts and displaces the pelvis and calyces. If there is much fat present, the radiolucent areas within the mass suggest the diagnosis. If multiple and bilateral, they may simulate polycystic disease. Renal angiography is the method used to differentiate this tumor from polycystic disease and from renal carcinoma. The most striking finding is the presence of many, peculiar, small, regular outpouchings of the interlobar and interlobular arteries resembling berry aneurysms. In some patients the interlobular arteries terminate in the "aneurysms" resembling a cluster of grapes, in contrast to the irregular size and contour of the tumor vessels of hypernephroma. This appearance is present in the arterial phase and is obscured by the nephrographic phase. Later there is irregular puddling indistinguishable from malignant tumor. The venous phase is normal, not early as in hypernephroma. Differentiation from renal cell carcinoma may be very difficult, however. Polycystic disease is readily differentiated by means of angiography.

LIPOMATOSIS OF THE RENAL SINUS

This condition is also called fibrolipomatosis, fatty replacement, fatty transformation, lipomatous paranephritis, and lipoma diffusum renis. It consists of an excessive amount of fat in the renal sinus which distorts the renal pelvis, infundibula, and calyces to varying degrees. It is usually found as a replacement process in renal atrophy whatever the cause, but may occur in simple obesity. It is found in older age groups, usually in those over 50. The roentgen appearance may simulate renal tumor, peripelvic cyst, or polycystic disease. It is therefore important that differentiation be made since lipomatosis is not a surgical problem.

Roentgen Observations

The condition can usually be suspected on intravenous urography but nephrotomography is the examination which best outlines the changes and permits a positive diagnosis. The pelvis is flattened or irregularly indented on its lateral aspect, the infundibula are elongated, narrow, and often appear stretched. The calyces may be relatively normal but may be blunted and dilated in patients with pyelonephritis. At times the deposition of fat is localized so that tumor or cyst may be simulated, while the more diffuse type may resemble polycystic disease. The process may be unilateral or

bilateral. When bilateral it is not necessarily symmetric. The infusion method of urography in conjunction with nephrotomography is usually diagnostic when this condition is suspected. This method of examination combines a good nephrographic phase with filling of calyces to bring out in sharp relief the relationship of the radiolucent fat to the opacified pelvis, calyces, and renal parenchyma (Fig. 20-45).

RENAL PSEUDOTUMOR

The kidney is capable of hypertrophy and hyperplasia. When local, a mass (pseudotumor) may result which is difficult to differentiate from tumor. There may be compression of the pelvis and calyces, splaying of the calyces, and local enlargement with protrusion from renal surface. The calyces do not regenerate, so

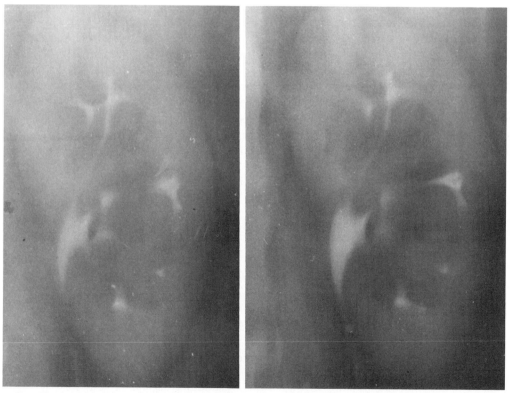

Fig. 20-45. Lipomatosis of the renal sinus.Nephrotomograms show the radiolucent fat in the renal sinus. Infundibula are narrow and elongated. Thickness of the fat varies inversely with parenchymal thickness.

the masses do not contain these structures. In addition to the demonstration of a mass, excretory urography may reveal the signs of the renal disease which results in the regeneration of renal parenchyma including nonobstructive caliectasis and irregular thinning of cortex. On nephrotomography, parallel linear streaks of density similar to normal medullary pattern aids in the diagnosis. Angiography reveals spreading of the arteries, but no tumor vessels or arteriovenous shunts are present, so there is no early venous filling. The capillary blush equals or exceeds that of the remaining renal parenchyma and there is no evidence of a wall or capsule.

MALIGNANT TUMORS

Malignant tumors of the kidney are of five general types: (1) adenocarcinoma (hypernephroma); (2) embryoma (embyronal adenosarcoma, Wilms' tumor); (3) carcinoma of the renal pelvis; (4) sarcoma; and (5) malignant lymphoma, including leukemia. The adenocarcinoma or hypernephroma is the most common renal malignant neoplasm. This tumor usually arises in the upper or lower pole of the kidney and may attain great size before causing symptoms.

ADENOCARCINOMA (HYPERNEPHROMA)

Plain-film roentgen findings consist of local or general enlargement of the kidney which varies with the size of the tumor. The renal outline tends to be preserved even though it may be lobulated, distorted, and irregular. This is because the lesions are limited by the renal capsule until far advanced. It is not unusual to note calcification within the tumor. The calcification may be irregularly scattered or curvilinear within the tumor. It may also be curvilinear or rimlike, outlining the periphery of the tumor. Displacement of neighboring organs occurs when the tumor attains sufficient size. This may be apparent on a plain-film roentgenogram but it is often necessary to outline the

colon and small intestine by means of a barium enema and small bowel study to determine the amount and direction of displacement.

Urographic changes are due to the distortion produced by the tumor mass. Calyces are elongated, distorted, narrowed, or obliterated. The renal pelvis may be altered in a similar manner. As a rule, hypernephroma produces more disruption of the normal pattern than a cyst of similar size. Distortion of the calyces is particularly significant because cysts can elongate and compress them and cause a stretching of the infundibula. Filling defects in the pelvis can simulate epithelial tumors arising there, but the latter do not usually produce calyceal deformity. Large tumors may cause considerable displacement of the upper part of the ureter and may also partially obstruct the pelvis or upper ureter (Fig. 20-46). There is usually enough function to visualize the pelvis and calyces on excretory urography, in contrast to the loss of function often noted in hydronephrosis, which may also produce renal enlargement. Occasionally infiltrating hypernephroma can cause renal enlargement without much distortion of the calyces, and subcapsular tumors can also reach considerable size without much distortion.

The malignant renal tumor must be differentiated from renal cyst. This differentiation may be impossible on excretory urography because tumor may simulate cyst. Excretory urographic findings[80] show the following characteristics:

Renal Cyst

1. Kidney is normal in size.

2. Mass is attached to periphery of the kidney in many cases; sharp outlines, permitting measurement of diameter of mass; may be less dense than kidney tissue and produce a "double shadow."

3. Calcification may be curvilinear, but very rare.

4. Renal pelvis may be displaced or compressed.

5. Calyceal elongation is sometimes found

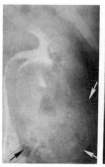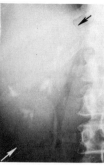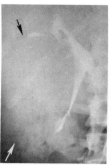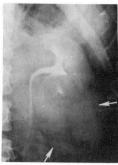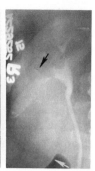

Fig. 20-46. These excretory urograms indicate the various findings produced by renal carcinoma. Note the considerable distortion of the calyces associated with soft-tissue mass. The **arrows** indicate the tumor in each case.

usually in combination with calyceal displacement or compression.

6. Calyceal displacement often takes the form of "crowding" together of calyces.

7. Calyceal compression is common, particularly with centrally located cysts.

8. Calyceal amputation is rare.

9. Simple types of calyceal deformity are noted.

10. No calyceal deformity may be seen, particularly if cyst is subcapsular.

11. "Claw-sign" is present in nephrographic phase.

Renal Tumor

1. Kidney is enlarged.

2. Mass is contiguous with body of kidney; indistinct outlines; mass often is denser than kidney and may obliterate psoas shadow.

3. Calcification is central, eccentric, or peripheral in location—curvilinear or amorphous.

4. Renal pelvis may be displaced, compressed, or invaded.

5. Calyceal elongation is sometimes found, often in combination with calyceal amputation.

6. Calyceal displacement often takes the form of separation of calyces.

7. Calyceal compression is common, particularly with centrally located tumors.

8. Calyceal amputation is very common.

9. Complex or bizarre types of calyceal deformity are seen.

10. No calyceal deformity may be seen if tumor is peripheral in location.

It is generally agreed that renal angiography is an essential part of the roentgen study of patients with renal masses. Nephrotomography in conjunction with infusion urography is useful, but does not replace angiography (Figs. 20-47 and 20-48). In addition to its value in differentiating cysts and benign neoplasms from malignancy, angiography yields valuable information regarding the extent of the tumor, its blood supply, and the venous drainage in many instances. Some investigators advise cavography and direct catheterization of renal veins to get precise evidence of major renal vein invasion. Others advise selective catheterization of the small retroperitoneal arteries (e.g., inferior phrenic, middle adrenal, lumbar, and gonadal) to aid in the demonstration of extracapsular extension. Epinephrine injected into the renal artery a few seconds preceding the injection of contrast is a valuable adjunct, especially in small tumors. The normal arteries contract and the tumor vessels which do not respond are more clearly outlined. This differential constriction may sometimes be observed in renal abscess or carbuncle, which makes the

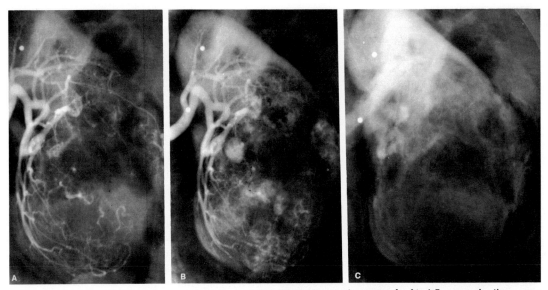

Fig. 20-47. Hypernephroma as seen on a selective renal arteriogram. *A,* At 1.5 seconds there are abnormal "tumor" vessels within the lower pole mass while arteries surrounding it are stretched. *B,* At 3 seconds, more puddling and arteriovenous shunting is visible. *C,* At 16 seconds, the renal vein is opacified. Note also abnormal veins lateral to the mass, outside of the kidney.

differential diagnosis difficult in these cases. Also, there may not be a differential effect in metastases to the kidney.

Another examination which is in wide use in the differentiation of renal masses is percutaneous cyst puncture. When there is a reasonable certainty on arteriography that a mass is cystic, it can be punctured directly under fluoroscopic control. Fluid is aspirated and checked for cells. Then an opaque material is injected and the cyst walls outlined. In the benign cyst, the aspirate is clear, the wall is smooth, and the Papanicolaou smear is negative. The wall is outlined by placing a contrast medium (Pantopaque, Hypaque, etc.) or air or both within the cyst. Methylene blue can be used to outline the needle tract if a tumor is suspected and surgery contemplated. Pantopaque seems to aid in regression or disappearance of the cyst.

The evaluation of renal masses should include the following roentgen procedures in the order given:

1. Scout film
2. Intravenous urogram

3. Nephrotomogram may be done in conjunction with the urogram or if deemed useful, with the angiogram

4. Angiography with selective renal arteriogram

5. Aspiration of suspected cyst

We rarely do a nephrotomogram as a separate procedure in these cases. In some institutions, renal scans are used. Angiography with cyst puncture in questionable cases approaches 100 per cent in accuracy.

The radiographic findings in cyst consist of a thin wall, sharp margination, avascularity, stretched and displaced vessels, no abnormal vascularity, pooling or abnormality of venous filling. In renal cell carcinoma there may be (1) relative avascularity of the entire tumor or a portion of it, (2) increased vascularity with irregular pooling, arteriovenous communications with early venous fill, (3) abnormal circulation via capsular or extrarenal vessels, (4) lack of constrictor response to epinephrine in tumor vessels, and (5) venous collaterals and abnormal peripheral venous channels around the mass.

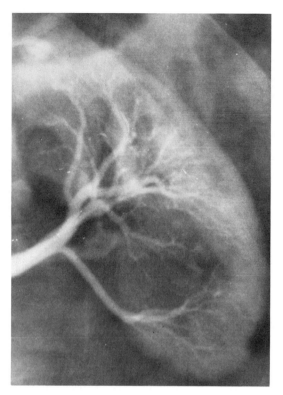

Fig. 20-48. Renal cyst. Selective renal arteriogram shows normal vessels stretched around the radiolucent intrarenal mass.

WILMS' TUMOR

The malignant embryoma or Wilms' tumor is the most common abdominal neoplasm of infancy and childhood. The majority arise in the first 5 years of life, but this tumor is rarely present at birth in contrast to fibromyomatous hamartoma of the kidney or to neuroblastoma. Wilms' tumor arises from embryonic renal tissue and tends to become very large. Visible enlargement of the abdomen is often the presenting complaint. Scout roentgenograms show the outline of the mass with displacement of neighboring structures and elevation of the diaphragm on the side of the lesion. These tumors rarely contain calcium, in contrast to neuroblastoma, which also causes a large tumor mass in infants and children. Urographic findings are those of a large tumor that distorts the pelvis and calyces and often displaces and partially obstructs the ureter. The distortion of the

calyces tends to be less than with hypernephroma of similar size but is greater than in neuroblastoma, which often arises adjacent to the kidney and produces pressure upon it. Renal function may be impaired but there is usually enough to outline some of the calyces on urography and to differentiate this tumor from hydronephrosis causing massive renal enlargement (Fig. 20-49). Wilms' tumor tends to metastasize to the lungs and periaortic nodes and may also extend locally by direct invasion. Angiography has been done in a few reported cases. Tumor stain is not common and no arteriovenous shunts are present to produce pooling or puddling. The tumor vessels are long and tortuous, resembling a creeping vine; they tend to be discrete, of large caliber, and an irregular diameter.

TUMORS OF THE RENAL PELVIS

Tumors of the renal pelvis are of epithelial origin and present a different roentgen picture from adenocarcinoma of the renal parenchyma. There are two major types of malignancy, the transitional cell and the squamous cell epithelioma. Transitional cell tumors comprise nearly 90 per cent of malignant tumors of the renal pelvis. They tend to be somewhat less invasive than the squamous cell type. The latter is very commonly associated with chronic infection, leukoplakia, or calculi. On the plain film, there may be no sign of tumor. Because hematuria is an early sign, the patients are usually examined when the lesion is small and therefore difficult to detect. The tumor causes a filling defect in the pelvis or calyx that may be smooth or irregular and may be large or small. These defects are outlined on urograms as radiolucent areas projecting into the opacified pelvis or calyx (Fig. 20-50). Malignant tumors are generally more irregular than benign papillomas of the pelvis, but roentgen differentiation of the various cell types of renal pelvis tumors is not possible. The roentgen evidence of an infiltrating type of tumor may be minimal, but it may become very large and produce major alterations in the renal pelvis (Fig. 20-51). Blood clots and radiolucent

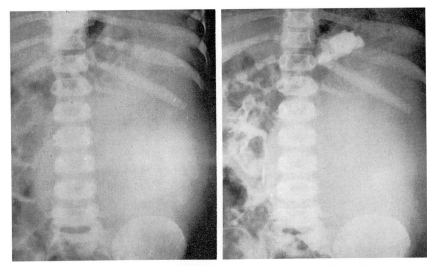

Fig. 20-49. Wilms's tumor. A huge mass is noted in the left side of the abdomen. The excretory urogram shows some function on the left side with several dilated calyces above the major mass. The right kidney is normal but the right ureter is displaced slightly by the tumor, which extends across the mid-line. *Left,* Preliminary film. *Right,* Excretory urogram.

calculi can produce similar defects. For this reason, it is common practice to follow intravenous urography by retrograde pyelography when a filling defect is noted. If a blood clot or calculus has caused the defect, the second examination will show disappearance or alteration in size or position of it. Calcification may occur within this type of tumor but is uncommon. Ureteral and bladder implants occur frequently and they produce small defects similar to those caused by primary tumor in the kidney. Occasionally a tumor may invade and infiltrate the adjacent parenchyma to simulate renal cell carcinoma. There are angiographic differences which may be helpful. The tumor is relatively hypovascular, there is no pooling or arteriovenous shunting or neovascularity. The residual parenchymal vessels are occluded or encased by tumor and narrowed. These angiographic findings may also be present in metastatic tumors of the kidney.

SQUAMOUS METAPLASIA OF THE RENAL PELVIS

Leukoplakia or squamous metaplasia of the renal pelvis is probably caused by infection or chronic irritation of other source. It is included here because it may resemble carcinoma of the pelvis. Infection is found in 80 per cent of patients and 40 per cent have had renal calculi. The patient may describe passing tissue or gritty material and the diagnosis is established by finding keratinized squamous epithelium in the urine. The condition is usually unilateral.

Radiographic findings are varied. Irregular areas in the renal pelvis partially surrounded by contrast material, large laminated masses presenting an onion-skin appearance, irregular plaques or bands producing linear striations, and roughening or wrinkling of the renal pelvis may be found. Any of the above findings should suggest the diagnosis, but lucent calculi, hematoma, and particularly carcinoma of the renal pelvis must be differentiated.

SARCOMA

Sarcoma arising from the connective tissue elements of the kidney is rare. Often retroperitoneal sarcoma arising in or near the kidney becomes so extensive that it is not possible to determine the site of origin even at autopsy. Roentgen findings are those of a mass in the renal area that is

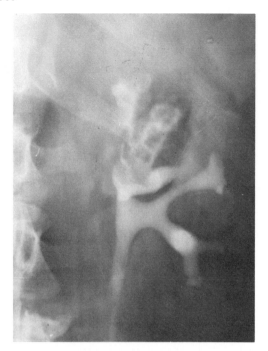

Fig. 20-50. Carcinoma of the renal pelvis. Note the irregular filling defects of the upper pole calyces and infundibula. The lesion was a transitional cell carcinoma.

often difficult to outline clearly and may obliterate the psoas shadow in its superior aspect. Urograms tend to show somewhat less distortion of the pelvis and calyces than is noted in a hypernephroma of similar size (Fig. 20-52).

MALIGNANT LYMPHOMA AND LEUKEMIA

Involvement of the kidneys in patients with chronic leukemia may occur late in the disease. In children with acute leukemia, renal involvement is more common than in the chronic form. The leukemic infiltrate tends to be largely cortical in location. The plain-film finding is that of renal enlargement, usually bilateral. Urographic signs in addition to bilateral enlargement consist of enlargement of the renal pelvis without dilatation or evidence of obstruction, calyceal and infundibular elongation, and irregularity of renal outline. The findings may be caused either by leukemic in-

filtration or by edema and hemorrhage secondary to the disease.

The distribution of disease is somewhat more varied in the malignant lymphomas. Diffuse infiltration causing renal enlargement, with distortion, elongation, and compression of the calyces, is the most common form of involvement. The disease may also be manifested by single or multiple tumor nodules or by perirenal masses resulting in displacement or distortion of the kidney. The solitary tumor nodules resemble masses produced by primary renal tumors and cannot be differentiated on the basis of roentgen findings alone. Multiplicity of tumor nodules should suggest the possibility of malignant lymphoma, however. The kidney is involved by lymphosarcoma and reticulum cell sarcoma somewhat more fre-

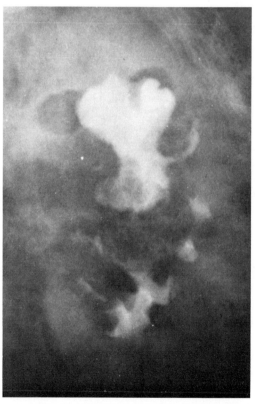

Fig. 20-51. Infiltrating carcinoma (transitional cell) of the renal pelvis. Note gross distortion of infundibula and calyces; the pelvis was filled with tumor and does not opacify.

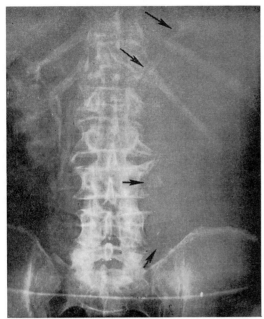

Fig. 20-52. Fibrosarcoma arising in or adjacent to the left kidney. A huge mass in the left abdomen is noted to elevate the few calyces that can be visualized and displace the left upper ureter to the right. **Arrows** indicate approximate size of the mass and site of the renal pelvis and upper ureter.

quently than by Hodgkin's disease. There are a few reports of angiography in these conditions. Some resemble renal cell carcinoma; others contain tumor vessels with a straight palisade-like appearance.

TUMORS OF THE URETER

Tumors of the ureter are rare, but benign papilloma, hemangioma, and epithelial carcinoma may arise there. Most tumors occur in the lower one-third of the ureter. Epithelial carcinoma arising in the renal pelvis may implant in the ureter. The roentgen findings do not differentiate the various types. Ureteral obstruction is common, leading to hydronephrosis, and an intraluminal tumor mass may be visible in addition to the signs of ureteral obstruction. Occasionally an infiltrating carcinoma may result in local narrowing of the lumen simulating benign ureteral stricture

(Fig. 20-53). In some cases there is no dilatation above the neoplasm, even though it is relatively large. The ureter apparently dilates locally as the tumor grows, so that obstruction does not develop. In these instances it is important to visualize the entire ureter in order to make the diagnosis, since the only roentgen sign is the intraluminal mass, which must be outlined by the contrast material to be seen. A localized dilatation of the ureter immediately below the tumor has been described. When retrograde pyelography is attempted, the catheter tip may coil in this area of dilatation; its upward progress is impeded by the intraluminal mass, which is outlined when contrast material is injected. This coiling of the catheter is then a sign of ureteral tumor, since the local dilatation does not occur below ureteral calculi (Fig. 20-54). Metastatic tumor may also in-

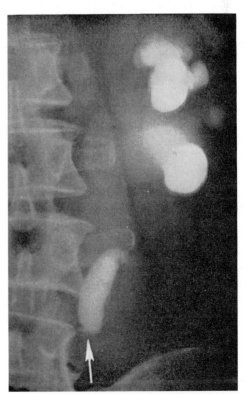

Fig. 20-53. Carcinoma of the left ureter indicated by the **arrow** has produced partial obstruction of the left ureter with hydronephrosis and hydroureter above it.

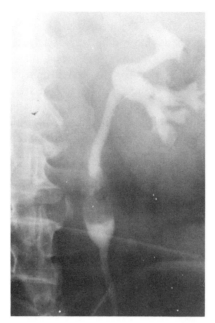

Fig. 20-54. Ureteral carcinoma produces a filling defect in the left ureter and demonstrates dilatation below the tumor.

volve the ureter. It may produce local involvement without extrinsic mass; or the ureter may be caught in a large retroperitoneal mass, displaced, and narrowed. Selective arteriography is sometimes useful in identifying ureteral tumor and differentiating it from stricture.

RETROPERITONEAL FIBROSIS

This condition was originally called periureteral fibrosis. The term "retroperitoneal fibrosis" is better because the disease may involve vascular and lymphatic structures in addition to the ureters. The disease is characterized by a fibrosing inflammatory process of unknown etiology in the retroperitoneal space, which may extend from the kidneys down to the pelvic brim and spread laterally to involve the ureters. In addition to the idiopathic cases, a number have been reported in patients with migraine who have been on long-term methysergide (Sansert) therapy. In many of them, discontinuance of the drug causes regression of the process. Fibrosis of the orbit, duodenum, rectosigmoid, common bile duct, and pancreatic duct system has been reported in asso-

ciation with retroperitoneal fibrosis involving the ureters. Involvement of the splenic vein, vena cava, celiac axis, superior mesenteric artery or iliac artery may also be associated with this condition. It is much more frequent in males than in females and is usually bilateral. The most common symptom is dull, indefinite backache. The radiographic findings may suggest the diagnosis. The normal fat lines may disappear, so that the outlines of the psoas muscle are not visible on the plain film. Intravenous urography may show delayed excretion with varying degrees of hydronephrosis or absence of excretion caused by obstruction. If the ureters opacify a local narrowing of the ureters is demonstrated in which there is a gradual tapering to the area of maximum stenosis. The involved segment is often 4 to 5 cm in length and usually deviates sharply toward the midline. The common site of involvement is opposite the fourth and fifth lumbar vertebrae. Some slight redundancy may be observed in the ureter above the stenotic segment. Despite a rather severe degree of obstruction there is often noted a paradoxical ease of retrograde passage of ureteral catheters. Lymphangiography may be helpful in diagnosis, since lymphatic obstruction is common. Inferior vena cavography may reveal narrowing and medial displacement of the vena cava at the site of involvement. Early recognition and surgical ureterolysis is important to preserve renal function in idiopathic disease.

THE URINARY BLADDER

CONGENITAL ANOMALIES

Exstrophy of the bladder is of radiologic interest only because of the wide separation of the pubic bones anteriorly at the symphysis that accompanies this defect. The symphysis is separated approximately the width of the sacrum and this leads to a rather square appearance of the pelvis (Fig. 20-55). Exstrophy consists of an absence of the anterior wall of the bladder and of the lower anterior abdominal wall. The diagnosis is made on observation, so that roentgen study is not necessary but is useful to study the kidneys and ureters, since ureteral obstruction is often associated. Wide separation of the pubic bones is also noted in some patients with epispadias.

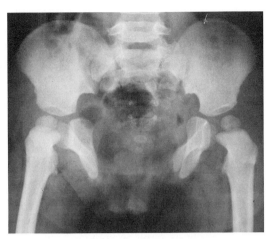

Fig. 20-55. The pelvis in exstrophy of the bladder. Note the wide separation of the symphysis pubis.

Duplication of the urinary bladder is extremely rare and is usually associated with urethral duplication (Fig. 20-56). Incomplete duplication may also occur, in which a septum partially divides the bladder and a multilocular bladder has been described. Occasionally there may be a partial horizontal septum, sometimes resulting in an hourglass appearance. The ureters empty into the lower compartment.

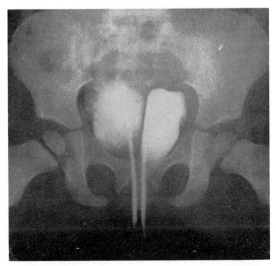

Fig. 20-56. Duplication of the urinary bladder. Cystogram outlines the duplication with each bladder drained by its own urethra.

Cystography is necessary to outline the anomaly.

Congenital enlargement of the bladder with hydronephrosis and hydroureter is found in association with congenital absence or hypoplasia of the abdominal muscles. This is a rare condition which occurs almost exclusively in males. No obstruction can be demonstrated to account for the dilatation. Associated abnormalities include nondescent of the testes, malrotation of the intestine, and, more rarely, persistent urachus, dislocated hips, clubfoot, harelip, spina bifida, hydrocephalus, and cardiac malformations. The abdomen is distended and the skin wrinkled; so the name "prune belly" has been applied to this condition.

"Bladder ears," lateral protrusions of the bladder caused by extraperitoneal herniations through the internal inguinal ring into the inguinal canal, have been observed. They are usually observed in infants and are associated with a high incidence of clinical inguinal hernia. This is not a true bladder anomaly, but is rather a bladder deformity secondary to a large internal inguinal ring. The term "bladder ears" has been used in preference to hernia because the deformity does not usually persist beyond infancy. Roentgen findings at cystography or urography consist of anterolateral protrusion of the bladder into the inguinal canal which is usually bilateral. The protrusion is most often observed in the partially filled bladder and tends to disappear when the bladder is filled. Oblique or lateral views bring out the anterior extent of the protrusion.

VESICAL CALCULI

Obstruction and infection are the chief causes of vesical calculi. Many of them are radiopaque and can be easily seen on plain-film roentgenograms (Fig. 20-57). Others contain small amounts of calcium and are poorly visualized on the plain film.

Cystography with air or with an opaque medium can be used to outline radiolucent stones. Calculi may be single or multiple and

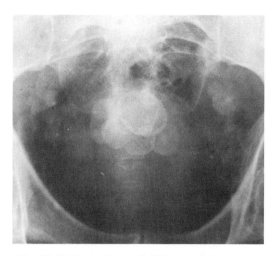

Fig. 20-57. Vesical calculi. This roentgenogram of the pelvis taken without the use of contrast material outlines five partially calcified bladder stones. Note their midline position.

tend to lie in the midline except when contained in a bladder diverticulum, in which case the position of the calculus depends on the site of the diverticulum. Bladder calculi must be differentiated from calcification in lymph nodes, fecaliths, calcification in uterine fibroids, and from prostatic and seminal vesicle calculi. Radiopaque bladder calculi are often laminated and very dense; when multiple, they may be faceted. Lymph-node calcification usually is higher in position and the nodes are mottled and not as uniformly dense as calculi. Uterine leiomyomas that contain calcium are often higher in position than bladder calculi and have a rather characteristic mottled appearance. Fecaliths of the sigmoid are rare but may simulate bladder calculi closely in texture and position. Oblique views and barium enema will permit differentiation. Prostatic calculi are usually multiple and produce a mottled density in contrast to the uniform or laminated appearance of vesical calculi; they are also lower in position. The same is true of calculi in the seminal vesicles. The position of bladder calculi in the midline is an important differential point.

Cystography and cystoscopy may be necessary to differentiate bladder calculi from other

causes of calcification. A foreign body within the bladder may act as a nidus for deposition of calcium and other salts to form a calculus. Foreign bodies may be introduced by the physician via the urethra during treatment or by the patient. They also may be introduced via penetrating wounds or left in or near the bladder during surgery. The shape of the calculus then is dependent upon the foreign body, which can often be visualized on scout roentgenograms.

Calculi in the prostate usually occur in the form of small granular deposits and these are visualized overlying or directly above the level of the symphysis pubis in standard anteroposterior roentgenograms of the lower abdomen. They offer little difficulty in differential diagnosis as a rule because of the position, characteristic small size, and multiplicity of the calculi (Fig. 20-58).

INFECTIONS OF THE BLADDER

Acute inflammation of the urinary bladder does not produce changes that can be recognized and diagnosed on cystography. Chronic cystitis results in a decrease in bladder size. The wall may be smooth but sometimes is serrated and when this serration is present along with the major contrac-

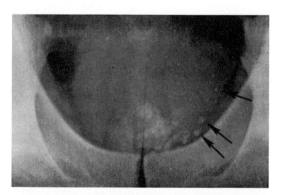

Fig. 20-58. Prostatic calculi. The mottled densities above the symphysis pubis are characteristic of prostatic calculi. Their distribution indicates probable prostatic enlargement. The calcifications to the left and above the prostatic area (**arrows**) are phleboliths.

tion at the dome, the so-called "Christmas tree bladder" of chronic cystitis is formed. Cystoscopy is a more useful method of examination in bladder infections, however, then cystography. Various types of bladder inflammation are defined according to the gross anatomic changes found at cystoscopy and need not be discussed here.

Of interest roentgenologically is the condition known as *cystitis emphysematosa* (emphysematous cystitis). This is an inflammatory disease of the bladder in which there is gas in the vesical wall. It is caused by gas-forming bacteria and in nearly 50 per cent of the reported cases it has occurred in patients with diabetes mellitus. The gas may be present for only a short time, which probably accounts for its low reported incidence. Roentgen findings are characteristic. A ring of radiolucency outlines the bladder wall or a part of it. There is often gas within the bladder as well. The zone of gas expands and contracts with the bladder and is a transient finding unless the infection fails to respond to therapy.

SCHISTOSOMIASIS

Schistosomiasis (bilharziasis) is caused by a group of blood flukes, *Schistosoma mansoni, Schistosoma japonicum* and *Schistosoma haematobium*. The lower urinary tract is involved mainly by *S. haematobium*. Large numbers of ova are deposited in the submucosa of the blad-

der wall. The wall becomes thickened, ulcerated and papillomas may be formed. In chronic disease, the distal ureters may be involved, leading to stricture, hydronephrosis, and renal damage. Calcification in the bladder wall, which occurs in chronic cases, has a characteristic appearance. When the bladder is empty, thin parallel lines of density are observed. The appearance is similar to that of the postvoiding bladder on excretory urography, in which a thin coating of opaque medium outlines the bladder wall. When the bladder is full of opaque medium, a very thin radiolucent line representing the thickened mucosa separates the opacified bladder lumen and the thin rim of submucosal calcification (Fig. 20-59). Bladder capacity eventually is reduced. The distal ureters may be calcified in a manner similar to that noted in the bladder. Calculi in the bladder, ureters, and kidneys are common.

OBSTRUCTION OF THE BLADDER

Bladder obstruction may be caused by congenital or acquired lesions. Benign prostatic hyperplasia is the most common cause. Prostatic enlargement is difficult to assess radiographically. However when elevation of the

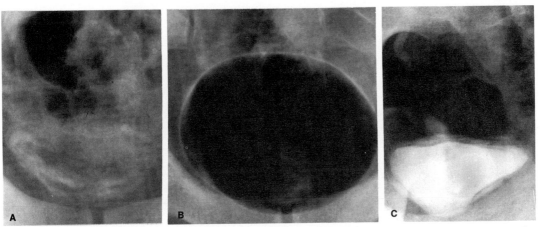

Fig. 20-59. Schistosomiasis (bilharziasis) of the bladder. *A,* Plain film showing parallel lines of calcific density in the wall of the empty bladder. (No opaque had been used.) *B,* Air cystogram showing thin rim of calcium in the bladder wall. *C,* Renografin cystogram showing thin rim of calcium separated from lumen by a lucent line representing thickened mucosa.

bladder floor is accompanied by "J-shaped" or hockey-stick appearance of the distal ureters, prostatic enlargement is indicated. Prostatic carcinoma, acquired urethral stenosis, urethral valves, and neurogenic dysfunction (cord bladder) are other causes. The first change in the bladder wall resulting from obstruction is hypertrophy of the muscles. This can often be observed as a soft-tissue shadow of several millimeters thickness paralleling the opaque shadow of the inner bladder wall in excretory urography or cystography. The normal bladder wall does not ordinarily produce a visible soft-tissue shadow. As the muscle bundles enlarge they cause irregular interlacing bands known as trabeculae. The intervening depressions are called cellules (Fig. 20-60). Trabeculation becomes more prominent as obstruction continues and the cellules may enlarge until diverticula are formed. There also may be reflux of medium into one or both ureters with development of hydronephrosis (see section on hydronephrosis). It is more likely that these findings are caused by infection, however.

As obstruction develops the bladder may become decompensated, increasing in size and containing increasing amounts of residual urine, until it presents as a large lower abdomi-nal mass on physical examination and on roentgen study. The scout roentgenogram will demonstrate a large soft-tissue mass extending out of the pelvis, often displacing the bowel upward and posteriorly. Cystography will outline the large bladder with trabeculations standing out in a somewhat reticular manner, with more or less cellule or small diverticulum formation.

Cystourethrography is used to examine patients with suspected bladder or urethral obstruction as well as in patients (usually children) with chronic or recurrent urinary infection. There is a great deal of controversy regarding the incidence, cause, and roentgen findings in bladder neck obstruction. Shopfner[88] believes that a roentgen diagnosis of bladder neck obstruction is no longer tenable, since there are changes in diameter during various stages of voiding. He also thinks that similar variation occurs in the diameter of the meatus and distal urethral segment during voiding, and has not encountered pathologic urethral narrowing. The most common abnormalities he encountered on cystourethrography were trabeculation and cellules of the bladder which he attributes to infection. Vesicoureteral reflux, also caused by infection, was the second most

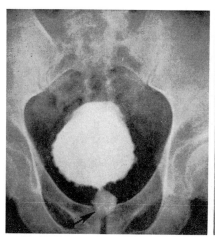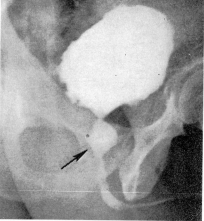

Fig. 20-60. Trabeculation of the bladder. Note the irregularity of the inferior and lateral bladder walls in the cystogram. In this patient the obstruction was caused by prostatic enlargement. Transurethral prostatectomy has been done. The opaque material outlines the enlarged prostatic urethra secondary to the resection (**arrows**).

common lesion. Other abnormalities include urethritis, urethral valves, bladder, and urethral diverticula.

DIVERTICULUM OF THE BLADDER

A diverticulum of the bladder is a localized herniation of mucosa, usually having a narrow neck. These defects may be single or multiple and vary in size from a small cellule to a large sac having a capacity greater than the bladder itself. Chronic obstruction is a frequent cause, but some diverticula are of congenital origin. Infection is also a factor in many cases. If they are small and empty completely they are usually of no clinical significance. Large diverticula that do not empty completely, however, are often the site of infection that is fostered by stagnation. Calculus formation is also common in this type of large diverticulum and when a density resembling vesical calculus is visualized outside the usual position of the bladder, this condition should be suspected and may be confirmed by means of cystography. Roentgen findings are confined to those noted at cystography or excretory urography unless the diverticulum is large enough to produce an actual

mass shadow on a plain-film roentgenogram, and then the nature of the mass must be determined by means of cystography or cystoscopy. When the bladder is examined by means of cystography the diverticulum is outlined by the opaque substance and its size, shape, and position, as well as the width of its neck, can be determined (Fig. 20-61). It is often of importance to assess the presence of and the amount of urinary retention in a large diverticulum and a roentgenogram taken following voiding is usually sufficient for this purpose. If the bladder still contains enough opaque material partially to obscure the diverticulum, a second roentgenogram may be taken following catheterization of the bladder. Occasionally a tumor may occur in a diverticulum; this lesion is often difficult to visualize, but presents as a filling defect on the otherwise smooth wall of the diverticulum. Double-contrast cystography is very useful when such a lesion is suspected.

NEUROGENIC BLADDER

Disease or injury involving the spinal cord or peripheral nerves supplying the bladder results in changes in bladder function that may produce

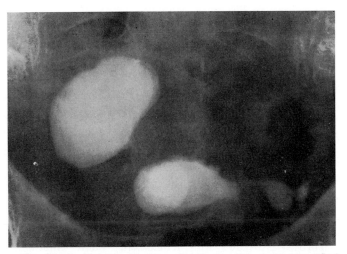

Fig. 20-61. Multiple bladder diverticula. The large opacified diverticulum on the right has a smooth wall in contrast to the trabeculation in the bladder. Note the small diverticulum on the left.

either incontinence or retention of urine. The type of neurogenic bladder is dependent upon the site of the lesion producing it. The autonomous bladder is caused by involvement of the second, third, and fourth sacral segments which form the spinal center for micturition. The bladder functions autonomously; it is hypertonic, contracted, and trabeculated with a hypertrophied wall. The automatic (reflex) bladder is caused by cord lesions above the sacral segments. The bladder is distended and does not empty completely. It is large, trabeculated, and has a thick wall. The atonic bladder is associated with lesions of the posterior roots; no sensory stimuli from the bladder reach the cord. The bladder is large, overdistended, thin and smooth-walled. The causative lesion, such as anomalies of the spine, pelvis, or sacrum, injury of the spine, and disease of the spine, may be visible on the urogram. The diagnosis of exact abnormality is difficult and is based on extensive study, including neurologic examination, cystoscopy, cystometric studies (measurement of intravesical pressures), and cystography. The cystographic study will determine vesical size, presence or absence of trabeculation, reflux into the ureters, retention or lack of it, vesical neck dilatation, and the presence of any other associated gross anatomic changes.

VESICOURETERAL REFLUX

Infection is the most common cause of vesicoureteral reflux. It is also found in patients with obstruction in the lower urinary tract. The causative lesions include posterior urethral valves, urethral stricture, and median bar enlargement. Neurogenic disorders which result in neurogenic bladder may also cause reflux. Congenital anomalies such as ectopic ureter and other anomalies of the distal ureter and trigone may also produce reflux.

The roentgen study used for the detection is the voiding cystourethrogram. If reflux is present it is manifested by retrograde filling of one or both ureters. The ureters may dilate considerably and there may be marked hydronephrosis associated with reflux. Any child with unexplained recurrent urinary tract infection should have a complete urologic study including cystourethrography. The evidence of reflux is sometimes fleeting so fluoroscopic examination is important.

THE MEGACYSTIS SYNDROME

The term "megacystis" refers to a large, smooth, thin-walled bladder accompanied by vesicoureteral reflux and dilated ureters and recurrent or persistent urinary tract infection. It is usually discovered in childhood and is much more frequent in females than in males. The trigone is usually much larger than normal and the intramural portion of the ureters is shortened and widened. The nature of the underlying disorder leading to the megacystis syndrome is not clear, but it is believed to be a congenital disproportionate increase in size of the vesical base leading to reflux and infection. Cystography demonstrates the large bladder and the large trigone with vesicoureteral reflux on one or both sides. Lalli and Lapides[52] described 21 patients who voided infrequently (*the infrequent voider*). Roentgen signs are bladder enlargement, increased bladder capacity, no evidence of obstruction, and ability to empty the bladder normally. They believe that this is the same condition as the megacystis syndrome.

VESICAL TUMORS

Most tumors of the bladder arise in the region of the trigone and tend to obstruct the ureteral or urethral orifices. The benign papilloma is the most common tumor and is often multiple, but so small as to be difficult if not impossible to visualize on cystography. Radiographic detection of this tumor depends upon its size. The diagnosis is best made by cystoscopy.

Carcinoma of the bladder is usually of the transitional cell type. Cystographic finding is that of an irregular filling defect, usually at the base, often resulting in ureteral obstruction. The size and shape of the tumors vary widely

(Fig. 20-62). Double-contrast cystography is useful for the study of the bladder mucosa in patients with intravesical tumors. Angiography using bilateral femoral artery catheterization is useful for staging bladder tumors. Cystoscopic confirmation is necessary since tumor type cannot be determined without biopsy. Occasionally the bladder may be involved by direct extension of prostatic carcinoma, rectal carcinoma, or by extension of uterine neoplasms in the female. Pelvic tumors, retroperitoneal sarcoma, and malignant lymphoma may also involve the bladder and deform it. Rhabdomyosarcoma occasionally arises in the bladder. This tumor usually presents in the first 3 or 4 years of life. It may originate in the submucosal or superficial layers, usually at the base. The tumor tends to become large enough to displace the ureters laterally and to bulge upward into the bladder to form a lobulated filling defect in it. The tumor nodules may also force their way downward into the urethra, forming a cone of dilatation in the posterior urethra. Urinary retention is the most common symptom. Intravenous urography often shows ureteral displacement as well as deformity and displacement of the bladder. There is nothing distinctive which will help in differentiating the tumor type in these patients.

TRAUMA OF THE BLADDER

Rupture of the bladder may result from a direct blow to the distended bladder as a single injury or may be associated with more extensive injury such as pelvic fracture, penetrating war wounds, or gunshot wounds. Instrumentation may also cause rupture of the bladder or urethra. The rupture may be intra- or extraperitoneal. There is now a trend toward early cystographic examination to establish the diagnosis. Intraperitoneal rupture results in extravasation of urine into the peritoneal cavity and the opaque medium also enters the peritoneal cavity to outline the smooth outer wall of the pelvic and lower abdominal viscera as well as the smooth serosal surface of the pelvic walls. The actual site of rupture may not be visible on the roentgenogram because of overlapping shadows. Extraperitoneal rupture of the bladder produces a more varied pattern, depending upon the site of rupture. The medium is extravasated, outlines the tissue planes of the pelvic floor, and extends varying distances into the perivesical soft tissues in an irregular, streaky manner. Pelvic and lower abdominal trauma may also result in perivesical hematoma without rupture. Cystography will then show displacement of the bladder, which varies with the size and location of the hematoma.

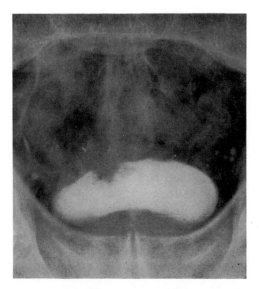

Fig. 20-62. Carcinoma of the bladder. Note the irregular filling defect in the dome of the bladder just to the right of the midline.

FOREIGN BODIES

Foreign bodies in the bladder are usually identified on plain-film roentgenograms when they are radiopaque. Oblique and lateral views may be necessary, however, to verify the position of the foreign body in relation to the bladder. Cystography will outline radiolucent foreign bodies and demonstrate associated changes in the bladder wall. Various oblique and lateral projections are usually necessary to make certain of the location. Cystoscopy is used for both diagnosis and treatment. Foreign body in the bladder is usually introduced by the patient and is therefore found in children and in adults who are perverted or psychotic. Occasionally foreign bodies are introduced at the time of surgery or instrumentation and they may also result from penetrating wounds. A foreign body may serve as a nidus for the deposition of calcium salts and the formation of a bladder calculus.

URETHROGRAPHY AND SEMINAL VESICULOGRAPHY

The urethrogram is the radiographic method for examination of the urethra. It consists of injection of a relatively viscous radiopaque oil or jelly into the urethra, following which films are made in various projections as the occasion demands. It is used in the female to demonstrate diverticula that may be missed at cystoscopy. In the male, diverticula, strictures, abscess cavities, fistulas, and abnormalities caused by prostatic enlargement may be outlined. Further descriptions of the method can be found in urology texts listed in the bibliography at the end of this chapter. Seminal vesiculography is a specialized urologic-radiologic method of examining the seminal vesicles by means of radiopaque material injected into the ejaculatory ducts and is beyond the scope of this book.

POSTERIOR URETHRAL VALVES

Posterior urethral valves produce varying degrees of obstruction leading to infection, vesicoureteral reflux, and hydronephrosis, with more or less destruction of the kidneys unless corrected They are found almost exclusively in males Eneuresis is a common symptom. The "valve' is located on the ventral aspect of the urethra lumen in the vicinity of the verumontanum. Voiding cystourethrography is the roentgen method used to demonstrate this lesion.

Roentgen fiindings consist of a thin membrane arising anteriorly which partially obstructs the urethra. The posterior urethra must be filled in order to distend the valve; otherwise it may not be visible. A true lateral projection is also necessary in order to identify the anterior position of the valve. The valve stretches in sail-like fashion to obstruct the urethra. A complete description can be found in the book by Kjellberg, Ericcson, and Ruhde.[50]

VAS DEFERENS CALCIFICATION

Calcification of the vas deferens is occasionally present in diabetic males, rarely it occurs in nondiabetics. It probably represents a degenerative phenomenon in these patients. Roentgen findings are the presence of densely calcified bilaterally symmetrical tubular shadows about 3 mm in diameter in the low midpelvis (Fig. 20-63).

THE ADRENAL GLANDS

The adrenal glands lie upon the upper pole of the kidneys within the perirenal fascia of Gerota. The right adrenal is a long thin triangle or wedge while the left is wider, shorter, and is somewhat crescentic in shape. They are small, the combined average weight being 11 to 12 gm.

Calcification in the adrenal glands is usually an incidental finding and is of no clinical sig-

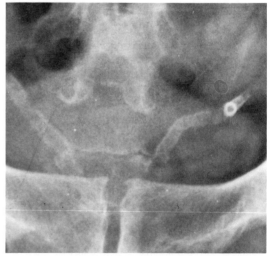

Fig. 20-63. Calcification in the vas deferens of a 45-year-old male with diabetes for over 20 years.

nificance. The most frequent cause is believed to be hemorrhage, often associated with birth trauma. There is a high incidence of abnormal obstetric history, including prematurity and forceps and breech deliveries in children with adrenal calcification. Occasionally, in adults stippled areas of calcification are found in one or both adrenals without any signs or symptoms of adrenal insufficiency. The cause in these cases remains obscure. Oblique roentgenograms may be needed to prove the constant relationship of the calcium to the upper pole of the kidney upon which the adrenal rests. Tuberculosis of the adrenal glands (Addison's disease) results in calcification within the gland in about one-third of the patients with this disease. The calcification may outline the entire gland or appear as amorphous granular density within it.

Cysts of the adrenal glands may also contain calcium. These lesions are rare. The incidence is 50 per cent higher in females than in males. They occur in equal numbers on right and left sides. Approximately 20 per cent of them contain roentgenologically visible calcification which characteristically is located peripherally, forming a thin rim of density outlining the cyst wall. When present in a suprarenal mass, the calcification is strongly suggestive of cyst. Cysts that do not contain calcium simulate tumor and are not visible on plain film unless they become large (Fig. 20-64). Calcification in tumors is discussed below.

ADRENAL CORTICAL TUMORS

Tumors of the adrenal gland are divided according to their origin into cortical and medullary types. The cortical lesions are glandular in type and are mesodermal in origin. Benign adenoma and carcinoma are the two types found. Both of these tumors as well as hyperplasia of the adrenal cortex may result in a disturbance of function of both cortex and medulla. The symptoms are varied and may be caused by an excess of androgens, excess of estrogens, or excess of other hormones. Sex changes and Cushing's syndrome may be

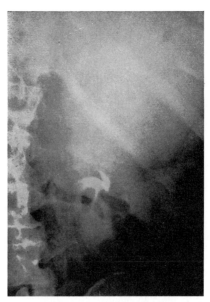

Fig. 20-64. Cyst of the left adrenal gland. Note the large mass above and partially overlying the upper pole of the left kidney. The kidney is depressed but not deformed.

present. In some patients no hormonal disturbance is noted. Occasionally the tumor is large enough to be visualized as a mass above the kidney. The hyperplastic gland is enlarged and retains its normal shape, whereas tumors tend to be round or oval and produce an alteration in the contour of the adrenal. The diagnosis of adrenal hyperplasia must be made with caution, because the fat surrounding the gland cannot be differentiated from the glandular tissue. Arteriography is being used extensively in the study of patients with suspected adrenal tumor or hyperplasia. In some instances aortography will clearly outline the adrenal and demonstrate a tumor involving it. If not, selective arteriography is necessary; some believe that a selective study should be done in nearly all patients. Others use adrenal venography extensively. Retroperitoneal pneumography can then be reserved for the patient with suspected tumor in which angiography fails to demonstrate the adrenal. The angiographic signs are similar to those of tumor elsewhere and consist of dilated and displaced vessels,

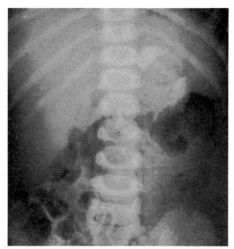

Fig. 20-65. Neuroblastoma arising in the left adrenal gland. Note the calcification in the left upper abdomen, which is somewhat granular and mottled, and is typical of the calcification often present in neuroblastoma.

tortuous vascular patterns, and arteriovenous shunts.

ADRENAL MEDULLARY TUMORS

Medullary tumors are ectodermal in origin. The benign pheochromocytoma often results in paroxysmal hypertension, while the ganglioneuroma that is also benign usually causes no symptoms. If large, these tumors may be visible on scout roentgenograms. If not angiography, venography, and retroperitoneal pneumography can be used as indicated in the preceding paragraph.

NEUROBLASTOMA

The malignant tumor of adrenal medullary origin is the neuroblastoma, which is usually found in childhood. It may arise in cells of the sympathetic nervous system as well as the adrenal medulla, so that this type of tumor may be found below as well as above the kidney. The tumor is highly malignant and may attain great size before discovery. The presence of calcification in the mass is common (Fig. 20-65), while in Wilms' tumor, from which it

must be differentiated, there is rarely any calcium. The kidney may be displaced and the tumor may fill most of the abdomen. Metastases to the liver, lungs and bone are common.

REFERENCES AND SELECTED READINGS

1. ABRAMS, H. L.: The response of neoplastic renal vessels to epinephrine in man. *Radiology 82:* 217, 1964.

2. ALLEN, R. P., and CONDON, V. R.: Transitory extraperitoneal hernia of the bladder in infants (bladder ears). *Radiology 77:* 979, 1961.

3. AMPLATZ, K.: Assessment of curable renovascular hypertension by radiographic technics. *Radiology 83:* 816, 1964.

4. AREY, L. B.: *Developmental Anatomy.* Philadelphia, Saunders, 1936.

5. BAILEY, H.: Cystitis emphysematosa. *Am. J. Roentgenol. Radium Ther. Nucl. Med. 86:* 850, 1961.

6. BATESON, E. M., and ATKINSON, D.: Circumcaval ureter; a new classification. *Clin. Radiol. 20:* 173, 1969.

7. BECKER, J. A.: Xanthogranulomatous pyelonephritis. A case with angiographic findings. *Acta Radiol. 4:* 139, 1966.

8. BERGMAN, H., FRIEDENBERG, R. M., and SAYEGH, V.: New roentgenologic signs of carcinoma of the ureter. *Am. J. Roentgenol. Radium Ther. Nucl. Med. 86:* 707, 1961.

9. BERNSTEIN, J., and MEYER, R.: "Parenchymal Maldevelopment of the Kidney," in *Brennemann-Kelley Practice of Pediatrics.* Hagerstown, Md., Harper & Row, 1969, vol. 3, pp. 1–28.

10. BOIJSEN, E., WILLIAMS, C. M., and JUDKINS, M. P.: Angiography of pheochromocytoma. *Am. J. Roentgenol. Radium Ther. Nucl. Med. 98:* 225, 1966.

11. BOOKSTEIN, J. J.: Appraisal of arteriography in estimating the hemodynamic significance of renal artery stenosis. *Invest. Radiol. 1:* 281, 1966.

12. BRODEUR, A. E., GOYER, R. A., and MELICK, W.: A potential hazard of barium cystography. *Radiology 85:* 1080, 1965.

13. CAFFEY, J.: *Pediatric X-ray Diagnosis,* 5th ed. Chicago, Year Book Publishers, 1967.

14. CAMIEL, M. R.: Calcification of vas deferens associated with diabetes. *J. Urol. 86:* 634, 1961.

15. CAPLAN, L. H., SIEGELMAN, S. S., and BOSNIAK, M. A.: Angiography in inflammatory space-occupying lesions of the kidney. *Radiology 88:* 14, 1967.

16. COOPERMAN, L. R., and LOWMAN, R. M.: Fetal

lobulation of the kidneys. *Am. J. Roentgenol. Radium Ther. Nucl. Med. 92:* 273, 1964.

17. Correa, R. J., Jr., Stewart, B. H., and Boblitt, D. E.: Intravenous pyelography as a screening test in renal hypertension. *Am. J. Roentgenol. Radium Ther. Nucl. Med. 88:* 1135, 1962.

18. Crummy, A. B., Jr., Barquin, O. P., and Wear, J. B., Jr.: Renal sinus lipomatosis. *J. Urol. 96:* 127, 1966.

19. Crummy, A. B., Jr., and Madsen, P. O.: Parapelvic renal cyst: The peripheral fat sign. *J. Urol. 96:* 436, 1966.

20. Currarino, G.: Roentgenographic estimation of kidney size in normal individuals with emphasis on children. *Am. J. Roentgenol. Radium Ther. Nucl. Med. 93:* 464, 1965.

21. Deliveliotis, A., Kehayas, P., and Varkarakis, M.: The diagnostic problems of the hydatid disease of the kidney. *J. Urol. 99:* 139, 1968.

22. Dorst, J. P., Cussen, G. H., and Silverman, F. N.: Ureteroceles in children, with emphasis on the frequency of ectopic ureteroceles. *Radiology 74:* 88–91, 1960.

23. Dubilier, W., Jr., and Evans, J. A.: Peripelvic cysts of the kidney. *Radiology 71:* 404, 1958.

24. Elkin, M., and Bernstein, J.: Cystic diseases of the kidney—radiological and pathological considerations. *Clin. Radiol. 20:* 65, 1969.

25. Elkin, M., Meng, C. H., and de Paredes, R. G.: Roentgenologic evaluation of renal trauma with emphasis on renal angiography. *Am. J. Roentgenol. Radium Ther. Nucl. Med. 98:* 1, 1966.

26. Elliott, C. B., Johnson, H. W., and Balfour, J. A.: Xanthogranulomatous pyelonephritis and perirenal xanthogranuloma. *Br. J. Urol. 40:* 548, 1968.

27. Emmett, J. L., and Witten, D. M.: *Clinical Urology,* 3rd ed. Philadelphia, Saunders, 1971.

28. Ericsson, N. O.: Ectopic ureterocele in infants and children. *Acta Chir. Scand. Suppl. 197,* 1954.

29. Evans, J. A., Dubilier, W., Jr., and Monteith, J. C.: Nephrotomography. *Am. J. Roentgenol. Radium Ther. Nucl. Med. 71:* 213, 1954.

30. Faegenburg, D., Bosniak, M., and Evans, J. A.: Renal sinus lipomatosis. *Radiology 83:* 987, 1964.

31. Faingold, J. E., Hansen, C. O., and Rigler, L. G.: Cystitis emphysematosa. *Radiology 61:* 346, 1953.

32. Felson, B., and Moskowitz, M.: Renal pseudotumors: The regenerated nodule and other lumps, bumps, and dromedary humps. *Am. J. Roentgenol. Radium Ther. Nucl. Med. 107:* 720, 1969.

33. Friedenberg, M. J., Eisen, S., and Kissane, J.: Renal angiography in pyelonephritis, glomerulonephritis and arteriolar nephrosclerosis. *Am. J.*

Roentgenol. Radium Ther. Nucl. Med. 95: 349, 1965.

34. Friedenberg, R. M., and Ney, C.: The radiographic findings in neurogenic bladder. *Radiology 76:* 798, 1961.

35. Gelford, G. J., Wilets, A. J., Nelson, D., and Kroll, L. L.: Retroperitoneal fibrosis and methysergide. *Radiology 88:* 976, 1967.

36. Gowdey, J. F., and Neuhauser, E. B. D.: The roentgen diagnosis of diffuse leukemic infiltration of the kidneys in children. *Am. J. Roentgenol. Radium Ther. Nucl. Med. 60:* 13, 1948.

37. Grossman, H., Winchester, P. H., and Colston, W. C.: Neurogenic bladder in childhood. *Radiol. Clin. North Am. 6:* 155, 1968.

38. Gwinn, J. L., and Landing, B. H.: Cystic diseases of the kidneys in infants and children. *Radiol. Clin. North Am. 6:* 191, 1968.

39. Handel, J., and Schwartz, S.: Value of the prone position for filling the obstructed ureter in the presence of hydronephrosis. *Radiology 71:* 102, 1958.

40. Hemley, S. D., and Finby, N.: Renal trauma. *Radiology 79:* 816, 1962.

41. Herschman, A., Blum, R., and Lee, Y. C.: Angiographic findings in polyarteritis nodosa. *Radiology 94:* 147, 1970.

42. Hinman, F., Jr.: Peripelvic extravasation during intravenous urography, evidence for an additional route for backflow after ureteral obstruction. *J. Urol. 85:* 385, 1961.

43. Hodson, C. J.: The radiological contribution toward the diagnosis of chronic pyelonephritis. *Radiology 88:* 857, 1967.

44. Inman, G. K. E., and Mitchell, J. P.: The radiological appearances of bilateral ureterocele. *Br. J. Radiol. 27:* 350, 1954.

45. Kahn, P. C.: Selective venography in renal parenchymal disease. *Radiology 92:* 345, 1969.

46. Kahn, P. C., and Wise, H. M., Jr.: The use of epinephrine in selective angiography of renal masses. *J. Urol. 99:* 133, 1968.

47. Kikkawa, K., and Lasser, E. C.: "Ring-like" or "rim-like" calcification in renal cell carcinoma. *Am. J. Roentgenol. Radium Ther. Nucl. Med. 107:* 737, 1969.

48. Kincaid, O. W., Davis, G. D., Hallermann, F. J., and Hunt, J. C.: Fibromuscular dysplasia of the renal arteries. Arteriographic features, classification and observations on natural history of the disease. *Am. J. Roentgenol. Radium Ther. Nucl. Med. 104:* 271, 1968.

49. King, R. L., Tucker, A. S., and Persky, L.: Congenital hypoplasia of the abdominal muscles. *Radiology 77:* 228, 1961.

50. KJELLBERG, S. R., ERICCSON, N. O., and RUHDE, U.: *The Lower Urinary Tract in Childhood.* Chicago, Year Book, 1957.

51. LAGERGREN, C., and LINDVALL, N.: Medullary sponge kidney and polycystic diseases of the kidney: Distinct entities. *Am. J. Roentgenol. Radium Ther. Nucl. Med. 88:* 153, 1962.

52. LALLI, A. F., and LAPIDES, J.: The infrequent voider. *Radiology 92:* 1177, 1969.

53. LANDES, R. R., and RANSOM, C. L.: Presacral retroperitoneal pneumography utilizing carbon dioxide. *J. Urol. 82:* 670, 1959.

54. LICH, R., JR.: The obstructed ureteropelvic junction. *Radiology 68:* 337, 1957.

55. LINDBLOM, K.: Percutaneous puncture of renal cysts and tumors. *Acta Radiol. 27:* 66, 1946.

56. LINDVALL, N.: Roentgenologic diagnosis of medullary sponge kidney. *Acta Radiol. 51:* 193, 1959.

57. LINDVALL, N.: Renal papillary necrosis. *Acta Radiol. Suppl. 192,* 1960.

58. LLOYD-THOMAS, H. G., BALME, R. H., and KEY, J. J.: Tram-line calcification in renal cortical necrosis. *Br. Med. J. 1:* 909, 1962.

59. LOITMAN, B. S., and CHIAT, H.: Ureteritis cystica and pyelitis cystica. *Radiology 68:* 354, 1957.

60. LUSTED, L. B., BESSE, B. E., JR., and FRITZ, R.: Intravenous urogram in acute leukemia. *Am. J. Roentgenol. Radium Ther. Nucl. Med. 80:* 608, 1958.

61. MCALISTER, W. H., and NEDELMAN, S. H.: The roentgen manifestations of bilateral renal cortical necrosis. *Am. J. Roentgenol. Radium Ther. Nucl. Med. 86:* 129, 1961.

62. MENG, C. H., and ELKIN, M.: Angiographic manifestations of Wilms' tumor. *Am. J. Roentgenol. Radium Ther. Nucl. Med. 105:* 95, 1969.

63. MENG, C. H., and ELKIN, M.: Venous impression on the calyceal system. *Radiology 87:* 878, 1966.

64. MILLER, S. M., and WINSTON, M. C.: Nephrogenic diabetes insipidus. *Radiology 87:* 893, 1966.

65. MOELL, H.: Kidney size and its deviation from normal in acute renal failure. A roentgendiagnostic study. *Acta Radiol. Suppl. 206,* 1961.

66. NEBESAR, R. A., POLLARD, J. J., and FRALEY, E. E.: Renal vascular impressions. *Am. J. Roentgenol. Radium Ther. Nucl. Med. 101:* 719, 1967.

67. NICHOLS, R. W., and LOWMAN, R. M.: Patent urachus. *Am. J. Roentgenol. Radium Ther. Nucl. Med. 52:* 615, 1944.

68. NOYES, W. E., and PALUBINSKAS, A. J.: Squamous metaplasia of the renal pelvis. *Radiology 89:* 292, 1967.

69. OLSSON, O.: Studies on backflow in excretion urography. *Acta Radiol. Suppl. 70,* 1948.

70. OLSSON, O., and WEILAND, P. O.: Renal fibrolipomatosis. *Acta Radiol. 1:* 1061, 1963.

71. ORMAND, J. K.: Bilateral ureteral obstruction due to envelopment and compression by inflammatory retroperitoneal process. *J. Urol. 67:* 476, 1952.

72. OTTOMAN, R. E., WOODRUFF, J. H., JR., WILK, S., and ISAAC, F.: The roentgen aspects of necrotizing renal papillitis. *Radiology 67:* 157, 1956.

73. PALUBINSKAS, A. J.: Medullary sponge kidney. *Radiology 76:* 911, 1961.

74. PALUBINSKAS, A. J., CHRISTENSEN, W. R., HARRISON, J. H., and SOSMAN, M. C.: Calcified adrenal cysts. *Am. J. Roentgenol. Radium Ther. Nucl. Med. 82:* 853, 1959.

75. PALUBINSKAS, A. J., and WYLIE, E. J.: Roentgen diagnosis of fibromuscular hyperplasia of the renal arteries. *Radiology 76:* 634, 1961.

76. PAQUIN, A. J., JR., MARSHALL, V. F., and MCGOVERN, J. H.: The megacystis syndrome. *J. Urol. 83:* 634, 1960.

77. PETEREIT, M. F.: Chronic renal brucellosis: A simulator of tuberculosis. *Radiology 96:* 85, 1970.

78. PITT, D. C.: Retrocaval ureter. *Radiology 84:* 699, 1965.

79. REUTER, S. R., BLAIR, A. J., SCHTEINGART, D. E., and BOOKSTEIN, J. J.: Adrenal venography. *Radiology 89:* 805, 1967.

80. REYNOLDS, L., FULTON, H., and SNIDER, J. J.: Roentgen analysis of renal mass lesions. *Am. J. Roentgenol. Radium Ther. Nucl. Med. 82:* 840, 1959.

81. RIESZ, P. B., and WAGNER, C. W., JR.: Unusual renal calcification following acute bilateral renal cortical necrosis. *Am. J. Roentgenol. Radium Ther. Nucl. Med. 101:* 705, 1967.

82 ROONEY, D. R.: Vesicoureteral reflux in children. *Am. J. Roentgenol. Radium Ther. Nucl. Med. 86:* 545, 1961.

83. SAULS, C. L., and NESBIT, R. M.: Pararenal pseudocysts. Report of four cases. *J. Urol. 87:* 288, 1962.

84. SENGPIEL, G. W.: Renal backflow in excretory urography. *Am. J. Roentgenol. Radium Ther. Nucl. Med. 78:* 289, 1957.

85. SHAPIRO, J. H., RAMSAY, C. G., JACOBSON, H. G., BOTSTEIN, C. C., and ALLEN, L. B.: Renal involvement in lymphomas and leukemias in adults. *Am. J. Roentgenol. Radium Ther. Nucl. Med. 88:* 928, 1962.

86. SHOPFNER, C. E.: Nonobstructive hydronephrosis and hydroureter. *Am. J. Roentgenol. Radium Ther. Nucl. Med. 98:* 172, 1966.

87. SHOPFNER, C. E.: Urinary tract pathology associated with constipation. *Radiology 90:* 865, 1968.

88. SHOPFNER, C. E.: Cystourethrography: Methodology, normal anatomy and pathology. *J. Urol.* *103:* 92, 1970.

89. SIAO, N. T., SWINGLE, J. D., and GOSSET, F.: Nephronophthisis. *Radiology 95:* 649, 1970.

90. SIMON, A. L.: Normal renal size: An absolute criterion. *Am. J. Roentgenol. Radium Ther. Nucl. Med. 92:* 270, 1964.

91. SUTTON, D., BRUNTON, F. J., and STARER, F.: Renal artery stenosis. *Clin. Radiol. 12:* 80, 1961.

92. TARABULCY, E. Z.: The radiographic aspect of urogenital schistosomiasis (bilharziasis). *J. Urol. 90:* 470, 1963.

93. VAUGHAN, J. H., SOSMAN, M. C., and KINNEY, T. D.: Nephrocalcinosis. *Am. J. Roentgenol. Radium Ther. Nucl. Med. 58:* 33, 1947.

94. VESTBY, G. W.: Percutaneous needle puncture of renal cysts. New method in therapeutic management. *Invest. Radiol. 2:* 449, 1967.

95. VIAMONTE, M., JR., RAVEL, R., POLITANO, V., and BRIDGES, B.: Angiographic findings in a patient with tuberous sclerosis. *Am. J. Roentgenol. Radium Ther. Nucl. Med. 98:* 723, 1966.

96. WEGNER, G. P., CRUMMY, A. B., FLAHERTY, T. T., and HIPONA, F. A.: Renal vein thrombosis. *JAMA 209:* 1661, 1969.

97. WEIGEN, J. F., and THOMAS, S. F.: Reactions to intravenous organic iodine compounds and their immediate treatment. *Radiology 71:* 21, 1958.

98. WEINTRAUB, H. D., RALL, K. L., THOMPSON, I. M., and ROSS, G., JR.: Pararenal pseudocysts. *Am. J. Roentgenol. Radium Ther. Nucl. Med. 92:* 286, 1964.

99. WHITLEY, J., WITCOFSKI, R. L., QUINN, J. L., III, and MESCHAN, I.: The radiologic diagnosis of renovascular hypertension. *Radiology 78:* 414, 1962.

100. ZANCA, P., BARKER, K. G., PYE, T. H., FU, W-R., and HAGG, E. L.: Ureteral jet stream phenomenon in adults. *Am. J. Roentgenol. Radium Ther. Nucl. Med. 92:* 341, 1964.

21

OBSTETRIC AND GYNECOLOGIC ROENTGENOLOGY

ROENTGEN DIAGNOSIS IN OBSTETRICS

There are a number of conditions arising during pregnancy in which roentgen examination of the abdomen and pelvis may be indicated and useful. This method of examination is used in: (*1*) the examination of the maternal pelvis, including pelvimetry and cephalometry (measurement of the pelvis and fetal head), (*2*) estimation of the duration of pregnancy and the stage of maturity of the fetus, (*3*) determination of fetal death, (*4*) determination of fetal malformations and malpositions, (*5*) determination of presentation, position, and multiple pregnancy, (*6*) localization of the placenta and (*7*) to aid in localization of the fetal abdomen for intrauterine transfusions.

In view of the possible genetic effects of irradiation on the fetus as well as the mother, the roentgen examination of the pregnant woman is not to be undertaken without a firm indication for its use. The use of roentgen pelvimetry as a routine in all primiparous women cannot now be justified. The method should not be discarded, however, because it still has a place in the examination of patients in whom there is equivocal clinical evidence of cephalopelvic disproportion. In other types of roentgen

examination, the dosages to the gonads are not as high as in pelvimetry; the possible harmful genetic effects to the mother and fetus must be weighed against the danger to them should the examination be omitted, and against the usefulness of the information to be obtained.

THE FEMALE PELVIS

CLASSIFICATION OF PELVIC TYPES

The female pelvis has been classified by Caldwell and his associates into four major types, determined chiefly by the shape of the pelvic inlet. The characteristics of more than one of the basic types are often present in a group of intermediate types. The classification is as follows: (*1*) gynecoid (round), (*2*) anthropoid (long oval), (*3*) android (wedge-shaped), and (*4*) platypelloid (flat).

GYNECOID

This is the average female pelvis that is found in approximately 42 per cent of human females. The inlet is round, the sacrum is usually curved posteriorly so that its anterior border presents a rounded concave contour.

The sacrosciatic notch is average to wide in size; the ischial spines are small and the pelvic side walls are relatively straight. The average ratio of the anteroposterior diameter of the pelvic inlet (true conjugate) to the transverse diameter is 11 to 13. Even though this type of pelvis may be somewhat small, there is usually very little difficulty in labor caused by cephalopelvic disproportion.

ANTHROPOID

This type of pelvis occurs in approximately 23 per cent of white and 40 per cent of Negro females. It is characterized by a long narrow inlet; the transverse diameters of the pelvis are decreased, while the anteroposterior diameters are increased in comparison to the gynecoid type. The sacrum tends to be more flat than in the gynecoid type and the sacrosciatic notch is usually wide and shallow. The inlet is often steeply inclined as the result of lordosis.

ANDROID

This type of pelvis occurs in approximately 32 per cent of white and 16 per cent of Negro females. It is a female pelvis in which masculine characteristics predominate. The inlet is triangular or wedge-shaped with a narrow anterior portion. The widest transverse diameter is near the sacral promontory and lies farther posteriorly than in the gynecoid and anthropoid types. The pelvic side walls tend to converge and the sacrum is flat. The sacrosciatic notch is small and the ischial spines are often large. These characteristics have led to the use of the descriptive term "funnel" pelvis. The android pelvis is a poor obstetric pelvis, and midpelvic or outlet dystocia may be anticipated frequently.

PLATYPELLOID

The flat pelvis is characterized by short anteroposterior and wide transverse diameters. The sacrosciatic notch is wide and tends to be deeper than in the gynecoid type.

ANOMALOUS PELVIC TYPES

GENERALLY CONTRACTED PELVIS

The shape of the pelvis including the sacral curve, inlet, and sacrosciatic notches may be normal but the measurements are all decreased.

RACHITIC FLAT PELVIS

The rachitic type of pelvis is rare in this country and consists of loss of the normal concave curve of the anterior aspect of the sacrum. When the change is severe, the anterior sacrum may be convex.

OBLIQUELY CONTRACTED PELVIS (NAEGELE)

This is caused by underdevelopment of the wing of the sacrum on either side. It results in considerable pelvic deformity, which is usually incompatable with normal delivery.

TRANSVERSELY CONTRACTED PELVIS

In this anomaly, both sacral wings are small or absent. This causes a marked decrease in the transverse diameter.

OTHER DEFORMITIES

The pelvis may be deformed as the result of injury. Generalized osseous dysplasias may also be accompanied by a considerable amount of pelvic deformity. In many of these deformities and anomalies, the birth canal is so distorted that normal delivery is out of the question, and pelvic measurements by roentgen methods are unncessary.

ROENTGEN PELVIC MEASUREMENT

The amount of enlargement of an object measured on a roentgenogram depends upon its distance from the film in relation to its distance from the target of the roentgen-ray tube. This enlargement is termed "divergent distortion." All the methods of roentgen pelvimetry are directed toward correcting for this distortion or eliminating it by increasing the target-film distance. There is often no actual necessity for elaborate methods of pelvic mensuration. During the last month of gestation, a single lateral roentgenogram taken with the patient upright may be sufficient to indicate the absence of disproportion. The head frequently engages in this position even though it may be floating in the supine position. When the head is engaged in the upright view and an additional anteroposterior film reveals that the pelvis is gynecoid in shape, there is no disproportion. If it is desirable to measure the anteroposterior diameters in the upright lateral view, a strip of lead notched at 1-cm intervals attached to or parallel with the intergluteal fold is used. The centimeter scale is distorted to the same degree as the anteroposterior pelvic diameters because it is the same distance from the film.

ROENTGEN PELVIMETRY

INDICATIONS, LIMITATIONS, AND VALUE OF PELVIMETRY

Adequate clinical examination and measurements permits the obstetrician to classify his patients into three general groups; (1) pelvis adequate for normal delivery, (2) pelvis obviously distorted or contracted to such an extent that normal delivery is impossible, and (3) intermediate group in whom some disproportion may exist. Roentgen pelvimetry is not indicated in groups 1 and 2 but may be indicated in the intermediate group 3 in which disproportion is suspected. The major indications are history of protracted labor in a previous pregnancy in which cephalopelvic disproportion was the likely cause; and arrest of the head despite strong uterine contractions. Less strong indications are malpresentation, the elderly primigravida, failure of the fetal

head to engage in primigravida, particularly if the external measurements are borderline.

The value of pelvimetry is limited by inability to forecast the uterine forces or the effect of the soft tissues upon the fetus. The size of the fetus must also be taken into account. The radiologist should realize that although roentgen pelvimetry yields accurate information regarding the measurements and contours of the bony pelvis and may yield information relating to bony cephalopelvic disproportion, it does not give information regarding all of the remaining factors in labor. Therefore, in reporting the results it is important to include only the conclusions that can be based on the presence or absence of bony disproportion.

There is information to be gained in addition to the measurements of the pelvis and fetal head. This includes the shape of the pelvis, the relation of the presenting part to the pelvic inlet, the position of the placenta (in many cases), and the presence of gross fetal anomalies.

The roentgen measurement of the pelvis should be done in labor for maximum information regarding the relative size of the fetal head and maternal pelvis. Both mother and fetus are exposed to irradiation in antepartum pelvimetry. Unless care is used in shielding and coning, fetal as well as maternal gonads may be included in the direct beam. Shielding can be used in the anteroposterior projection to protect the fetus, including most, if not all of the fetal head; thus the only fetal exposure is to scattered irradiation. The only maternal gonadal irradiation is also by scatter in the body if this method of shielding is used. Shielding can be nearly as effective in the lateral projection.[20] Actual radiation dosages differ considerably, but maternal gonadal doses of 0.090 to 0.600 R and fetal gonadal doses in the range of 0.150 R or less can be obtained if coning and shielding is effectively used.

High voltages used to reduce skin dose to the mother do not have any significant advantage so far as gonadal dose is concerned, particularly if filtration is used. The range of 60 to 70 kVp using added filtration of 2 mm of aluminum produces the best detail and is recommended for the anteroposterior projection. Higher voltages in the range of 100 to 120 kVp are needed for the lateral view.

FETAL SKULL MEASUREMENTS (CEPHALOMETRY)

Cephalic measurements can be made on the same roentgenograms, but the measurements are not as accurate as those for the maternal pelvis. Rotation of the head and inability to determine the exact distance of the head from the film contribute to the difficulty in making accurate measurements. The method of Ball[2] is the most widely used in cephalometry. Borell and Fernstrom[6] measure the biparietal diameter of the head and consider 9.0 cm to be small, 9.5 cm medium, and 10.0 cm a large head.

GENERAL CONSIDERATIONS

Most of the numerous methods described for measurement of the pelvis are reasonably accurate. The anteroposterior diameters are readily measured because they all lie in the same plane. This plane can be determined by direct measurement on the patient because it lies in the midline. The transverse pelvic diameters are at varying distances from the film and cannot be measured directly on the patient; most of the methods have been devised to measure these diameters. The various methods of pelvimetry are described in the books and articles listed in the bibliography.

MEASUREMENT OF SAGITTAL DIAMETERS

Since these diameters are in the midline, measurements can be made directly using a centimeter scale. The sagittal diameters are measured on a lateral film taken in the upright position if possible, since sagittal diameters in this position are similar to those during delivery in the supine position with the thighs and knees in flexion. A centimeter scale placed in the midline between the thighs can be used in the direct measurement of these diameters. The patient is held firmly against the table top or cassette and the centimeter scale is held parallel to the cassette and at a right angle to the central ray. Voltages ranging from 100 to 120 kVp are used.

It is also simple and accurate to use a mathematical correction factor for the divergent distortion in measuring sagittal diameters. This is based on the geometric rule that the bases of similar triangles are proportional to their altitudes. If the distance of an object (e.g., one of the sagittal pelvic diameters) from the film and the distance of the target of the tube from the film are known, it is possible to calculate the actual size of the object after measuring its image directly on the roentgenogram. Since the sagittal diameters are in the midline, the distance from the symphysis to the film is measured. This can be checked by comparing it to one-half of the transverse diameter of the patient measured at the trochanters. This method of measurement is illustrated in the accompanying diagram shown in Figure 21-1.

In pelvimetry, to simplify calculation a target-film distance of 100 cm can be used. The pelvic diameter to be measured is *CD* in the diagram; its image on the film is *AB*.

The distance of the object from the film for the anteroposterior diameters is measured on the patient at the time the lateral roentgenogram of the pelvis is made. Subtracting this distance from 100 gives the tube-object distance.

MEASUREMENT OF TRANSVERSE DIAMETERS

The orthometric[32] or orthodiagraphic[7] method is described here because it is simple and accurate. The anteroposterior view is taken in the supine position with the knees flexed and the thighs abducted about 90° to prevent medial soft tissues from obscuring the ischial spines. The object-film distance is shortened by placing a cassette directly under the patient's buttocks. The light-beam diaphragm is adjusted to an area 20 x 10 cm[32] or 13 × 6 cm[7] projected on the film. The tube may be angled 20° cephalad, but some prefer a

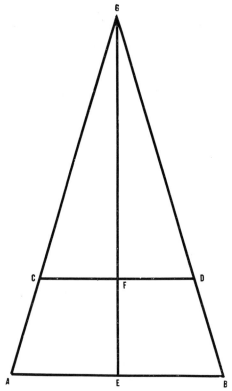

Fig. 21-1. Diagram used to indicate calculation and measurement in pelvimetry. In this diagram *GE,* target-film distance (known); *GF,* target-object distance (measured); *FE,* object-film distance (measured; and *CD,* object size (to be calculated).

$$CD \times GE = AB \times GF$$
$$CD = \frac{AB \times GF}{GE}$$

sured. This results in a slight decrease in measured diameters as compared to actual diameters below 10 cm and a slight increase in measured diameters as compared to actual diameters above 10 cm. The 10-cm tube shift is used because it represents the average interspinous diameter, which is the most important transverse measurement made in this examination. The errors are very small; if the beam is inaccurately centered by 1 to 2 cm, the interspinous diameter is only 1 to 2 mm in error as measured on the film. When the diameters are smaller than 8 cm, disproportion is obvious, so accurate measurement is not essential. When the diameters are over 12 cm, no bony disproportion is present, so accurate measurement of the larger diameters is not essential.

PELVIC LANDMARKS IN MAKING THE MEASUREMENTS

The discussion of landmarks below refers to the diameters marked on Figures 21-2, 21-3, and 21-4.

On the lateral roentgenogram, the following measurements (Figs. 21-2 and 21-3) are made:

1. The sagittal (anteroposterior) diameter of the inlet—a line from the upper inner margin of the symphysis pubis to the point on the

vertical tube angle with the patient's back arched by a pillow. The beam is centered at the upper border of the symphysis. Two exposures are made without moving the patient or film; the tube is 5 cm to the left of the midline on one and 5 cm to the right of the midline on the other. To obtain the best detail, voltages in the range of 55 to 60 kVp are used with high-speed screens and rapid film. The dose to the maternal and fetal gonads is only 0.2 mR if presentation is cephalic. The only factor producing distortion when this method is used is the difference between the tube shift (10 cm) and the length of the dimension to be mea-

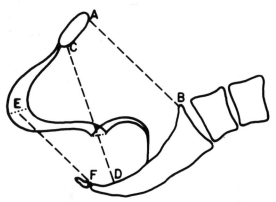

Fig. 21-2. Diagram of the pelvis indicates diameters measured on the lateral roentgenogram. **AB,** Anteroposterior diameter of the inlet; **CD,** anteroposterior diameter of the midpelvis; **EF,** posterior sagittal diameter.

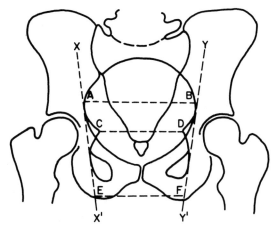

Fig. 21-3. Diagram of pelvis shows measurements made on the anteroposterior roentgenogram. **AB,** transverse diameter of the inlet; **CD,** transverse diameter of the midpelvis (interspinous); **EF,** transverse diameter of the outlet (bituberous); x–x' and y–y' mark lateral pelvic walls.

sacrum where the two iliopectineal lines intersect (*CE*).

2. The sagittal (anteroposterior) diameter of the midplane of the pelvis—a line from the lower inner margin of the symphysis through the midpoint between the tips of the ischial spines to the sacrum. If this line falls below the last fixed sacral segment, then the latter point is used as the sacral termination of the diameter (*FH*).

3. The posterior sagittal diameter (anteroposterior diameter of the outlet)—a line from the midpoint between the ischial tuberosities to the top of the last fixed sacral segment (*IJ*).

The following measurements are made on the anteroposterior roentgenogram (see Fig. 21-3):

1. The transverse diameter of the inlet—a line connecting the points of widest separation of the right and left iliopectineal lines (*AB*).

2. The interspinous diameter (transverse midpelvic diameter)—measured from the tip of one ischial spine to the other (*CD*).

3. The bituberous diameter (transverse diameter of the outlet)—measured from one ischial tuberosity to the other (*EF*). Lines are

drawn downward outlining the inner aspect of the pelvic side wall on either side; the transverse distance between them is measured at the level of the ischial tuberosities. There is some disagreement in the literature regarding the range of normal pelvic measurements. Those given by Snow[34] are listed in Table 21-1.

TABLE 21-1. Average Pelvic Measurements in Centimeters

	Small	Medium	Large
Inlet			
Anteroposterior	Below 10.5	10.5–11.5	Above 11.5
Transverse	Below 11.5	11.5–12.5	Above 12.5
Total	Below 22.0	22.0–24.0	Above 24.0
Midpelvis			
Anteroposterior	Below 11.0	11.0–12.0	Above 12.0
Interspinous	Below 10.0	10.0–11.0	Above 11.0
Total	Below 21.0	21.0–23.0	Above 23.0
Outlet			
Posterior sagittal	Below 6.5	6.5–8.0	Above 8.0
Bituberous	Below 9.5	9.5–10.5	Above 10.5
Total	Below 16.0	16.0–18.5	Above 18.5

Based on Snow, W.[34]

THE FETUS

FETAL AGE AND DURATION OF PREGNANCY

Reasonably accurate estimation of fetal age is useful in a number of situations. Determination of the earliest safe date for the termination of pregnancy may be necessary in diabetics, preeclamptic states, maternal hypertension, in patients with Rh problems, in cephalopelvic disproportion, and in patients who have had previous cesarian sections. Fetal age may also be important in patients who are presumably overdue and in cases where there is discrepancy between size of the fetus and uterus or both and the given dates.

In the early weeks of pregnancy the fetal skeleton is not visible, so that roentgen examination is of no value in determining fetal age. The skeleton is usually visible at 12 weeks. The

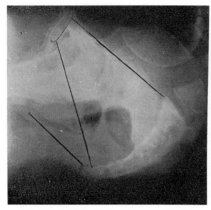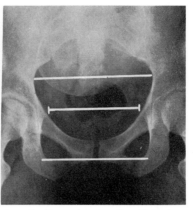

Fig. 21-4. Pelvimetry. Frontal and lateral projections showing the diameters indicated in Figures 21-2 and 21-3.

ossification centers for the vertebral bodies are usually the first visible skeletal parts; ribs are also ossified at 12 weeks. The date and appearance of different skeletal parts can be used to estimate maturation within 1 or 2 months. Films of good quality are necessary and the various ossification centers may then be identified. For example, the semicircular canals are well outlined at the 20th week but are partially obscured by ossification around them by the 24th week and are almost completely obscured by the 40th week. The parietal bones ossify frequently by the 20th week and invariably by the 24th week. The calcaneus appears between the 24th and 26th week and the talus between the 26th and 28th week. The distal femoral epiphysis is present by the 36th to 37th week in females and in some males. The center for the upper end of the tibia appears at 38 weeks. There is individual variation, so the appearance of the various ossification centers gives only a rough approximation of fetal age.

Hodges[18] has compiled a series of graphs for computation of fetal age in weeks using various measurements of the fetus. They include the occipitofrontal diameter of the skull, the biparietal diameter of the skull, the average corrected circumference of the skull, the length of the calcified portion of the shaft of the femur and the net vertebral length. It is usually possible to obtain one or more of these diameters, or lengths, so that findings for these

measurements can be correlated on the various graphs. They were based on the original measurements and equations of Scammon and Calkins[31]. Stockland and Marks[36] use combined measurements of fetal skull, body length, and uterine diameters to determine body weight. A graph with body weight plotted against gestation period is then used to determine approximate fetal age. They believe that averaging the multiple measurements introduces an "equalizing factor" which increases accuracy. Their error was less than 15 per cent in 91 per cent of patients.

The crown to breech measurement is also a reliable index of fetal age. In utero, the crown to breech measurement can be made from the crown to the proximal end of the femur since the coccyx is not ossified. When the patient is placed in the prone position, the fetus is near the film and the fetal spine is nearly parallel to the table top. The distortion using a focal-film distance of 40 inches can be corrected by using a factor of 0.9. Occipitofrontal diameter can also be measured. Maturity is then obtained by reference to the table reported by Zuppinger as found in Bishop's book.[3] A number of determinants have been described, but it is often difficult to get satisfactory films to show fetal extremities. If several measurements and observations as seen on single anteroposterior and lateral films can be correlated, the estimation is reasonably reliable, particularly if the

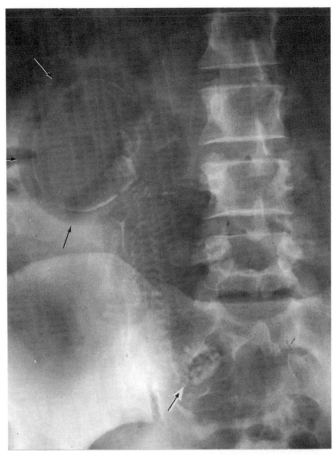

Fig. 21-8. Erythroblastosis fetalis. Fetal hydrops demonstrated by amniography. The thick, edematous scalp is easily defined (**arrows**). Opaque medium in the intestine (**lower arrow**) indicates that the fetus is alive. Note the large fetal abdomen.

made. The halo sign, previously reported in this disease, is not observed and is of no value.

PRESENTATION, POSITION AND MULTIPLE PREGNANCY

Fetal presentation and position are easily demonstrated by means of roentgenograms of the abdomen in frontal and lateral projections. The diagnosis of multiple pregnancy is also easily made and the position and presentation of each fetus can usually be determined without difficulty.

THE PLACENTA

PLACENTA PRAEVIA

Roentgen examination is used in the study of patients with painless uterine bleeding in the third trimester of pregnancy. The roentgen diagnosis of placenta praevia and the localization of the placenta are fairly accurate. Various methods are available for this examination and can be used if the occasion demands. The placenta measures approximately 20 cm in diameter and 4 to 6 cm in thickness. The inner surface is not visible because the radiographic density of the placenta is the same as that of the amniotic fluid. Its location can be surmised by the width of the soft-tissue shadow between the nearest part of the fetus and the outer uterine wall. The external surface of the uterus usually is clearly defined because of gas in the intestinal tract of the mother and the intra-abdominal fat that outline the relatively dense uterus. When the fetal parts are within a few centimeters of the external surface of the uterus, the presence of placenta in that particular area can be excluded. If there is an increase in the amount of amniotic fluid (hydramnios) the location of the placenta is difficult to determine. The placenta can be demonstrated on the lateral roentgenogram of the uterus in over 90 per cent of pregnancies, so this projection should be obtained first. Rossi et al.[27] use a cassette loaded with three films for this lateral view. The middle film is protected from the intensifying screens and is used for anterior uterine wall-soft tissue detail. One of the outer films is used for good visualization posteriorly where tissues are more dense. The other outer film can be kept in the cassette and reused, since it acts only as a filter to absorb a part of the fluorescence of the intensifying screen. This eliminates the need for wedge filters or multiple films. When the placenta can be identified in this projection, no further study is necessary unless it is demonstrated to lie below the equator of the uterus. If it is not clearly outlined or is found to lie in a low position, further examination is necessary. The fetus is heavier than amniotic fluid and will sink to the lowest part of the uterus in the upright. This is sometimes called the gravitational method. The bladder should be catheterized before taking the films; voiding is not adequate. A small amount (30 to 40 cc) of diatrizoate or other organic iodide may be injected into the bladder if desired. The normal space between the fetal head and the opaque is 1 cm or less. Roentgenograms are then obtained in frontal and lateral projections in the upright position. These films will show the relative position of the presenting part of the fetus to the sym-

physis, the bladder, and the sacral promontory. In the normal patient, the fetal head should lie equidistant from the pelvic side walls and nearly equidistant from the anterior and posterior walls of the pelvic inlet, particularly if the head is engaged. The findings are not as precise in breech presentations, but breech presentation with complete placenta praevia is rare. If the head is more than 3 cm from the pubis or more than 1.5 cm, from the sacral promontory when the head is engaged, some degree of placenta praevia is likely (Fig. 21-9). If the head is unduly small in relation to the maternal pelvis, the range of the normal measurements is increased.

There is approximately 1 cm of soft tissue between the bones of the fetal cranium and the bladder lumen in the normal. Any soft-tissue separation greater than this is suggestive of placenta praevia. When the bladder is partially distended with contrast material the fetal head

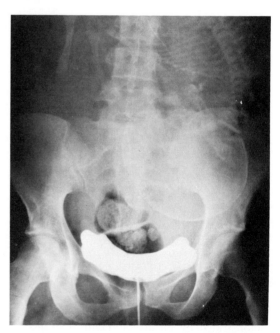

Fig. 21-9. Placenta praevia. Cystogram with the patient in the upright position. Placenta previa is indicated by the eccentricity of the fetal head in relation to the pelvis and the distance of the head from the dome of the bladder caused by the presence of soft-tissue between the fetal cranial vault and the bladder.

indents the dome of the bladder so that its margin forms a smooth, concave curve paralleling the curve of the skull adjacent to it.

In marginal placenta praevia the mass of the placenta causes an asymmetric thickening of the space between the bladder and the fetal skull. The fetal head usually extends into the pelvic inlet when the patient is standing, but will lie in asymmetric relationship to the symphysis pubis and sacral promontory or to the pelvic side walls, or both, depending upon the location of the placenta. The major part of the placenta may be visible above the level of the pelvic inlet in these patients.

In complete (or nearly complete) placenta praevia the head often may not enter the pelvis and the thick soft-tissue mass between the skull and the bladder is apparent.

In summary, the roentgen signs of placenta praevia are as follows:

1. Nonvisualization of the placenta in the fundus.

2. Placenta is visible but the greater part of its mass noted to be below the equator of the uterus.

3. Displacement of the fetal head from the midplane of the pelvis in either frontal or lateral projection with abnormal amount of soft tissue between it and the bony structures making up the pelvic inlet when the patient is examined standing.

4. Abnormally high position of the head.

5. Abnormal amount of soft tissue between the head and the bladder when the latter is outlined by contrast material.

SPECIAL METHODS OF PLACENTAL LOCALIZATION

AMNIOGRAPHY. This examination may be used for placental localization. After removal of 30 to 40 cc of amniotic fluid, a similar amount of contrast (one of the organic iodides) is injected into the uterine cavity. The placenta appears as a negative shadow in the opacified amniotic fluid. Soft tissue abnormalities of the fetus may also be recognized along with uterine deformities and tumors. Indications for the use of this procedure are limited.

ARTERIOGRAPHIC PLACENTOGRAPHY. Percutaneous femoral artery puncture is done using the Seldinger technique with insertion of a catheter into the lower abdominal aorta. Both uterine arteries can be filled by a single injection of 20 to 50 cc of renografin or another opaque agent. Only three or four exposures are necessary. The placenta is readily localized. The uterine arteries are large, placental branches are large and tortuous; the opaque medium quickly collects in the placental sinusoids and remains there for several seconds, so that timing of films is not critical. Placental filling can be augmented by applying pressure to the femoral arteries during the injection. The placental arteriographic pattern appears as early as the beginning of the third month of gestation and is the only reliable method of localizing the placenta at this early stage. The simpler roentgen methods outlined above are accurate after the 32nd week of gestation, but when placenta praevia is suspected earlier the other methods are not accurate and angiography may be used. The examination carries a slight amount of risk and should be used only when definitely indicated.

RADIOACTIVE ISOTOPE LOCALIZATION. Radioactive iodinated human serum albumin (RISA = ^{131}I), ^{51}CR = labeled erythrocytes or human serum albumin, and technicium (^{99m}) = labeled human serum albumen are used for placental localization. When the placenta is anterior, lateral, or fundal in position, localization is satisfactory. When posterior, the placenta is located by exclusion. However, when the placenta is low, interpretation of results is difficult. Therefore, at present, the method is one of exclusion of placenta praevia when the placenta can be located at some distance from the internal cervical os. Using ^{131}I a dose of 3 μCi is satisfactory. This gives a total radiation dose of 10 millirads to the mother and less than 4 millirads to the fetus.

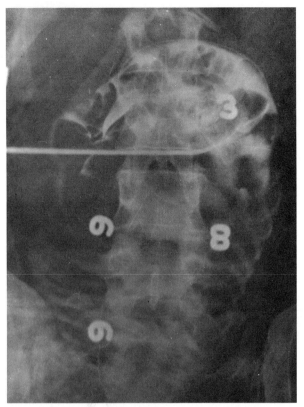

Fig. 21-10. Intrauterine transfusion. The opaque medium outlines the loops of bowel in the fetal peritoneal cavity. The needle and catheter remain in place. Lead numbers are used for localization.

PREMATURE SEPARATION OF THE PLACENTA

When the placenta is visible in the uterine fundus in patients with bleeding in the last trimester of pregnancy, placenta praevia is excluded. Then the question of premature separation of the placenta arises. Occasionally there is a localized bulge of the uterus, owing to accumulation of blood when it is confined between the placenta and the uterine wall and forms a hematoma there. This does not occur frequently and is not a reliable sign because a uterine fibroid or uterine asymmetry may cause similar change. Blood is not often trapped between the uterine wall and the placenta in an amount sufficient to cause local distortion. The diagnosis of this condition therefore is rarely possible by roentgen methods. However, when the placenta appears considerably enlarged and erythroblastosis can be excluded, premature separation of the placenta can usually be inferred. The diagnosis of placental hematoma may be made by means of pelvic arteriography. The opaque medium remains in the hematoma much longer than in the normal placenta and is more homogenous than the placental sinusoids and arteries.

INTRAUTERINE FETAL TRANSFUSION

This procedure is reserved for erythroblastotic babies who would probably die in utero before attaining sufficient maturity to have a reasonable chance of survival. This type of transfusion may result in salvage of a number of such infants who can be carried until they are mature enough to be delivered. The radiologist aids the obstetrician in localization of the position of the needle which is inserted into the fetal abdominal cavity through the maternal abdominal wall and uterus. A small amount (2 to 3 cc) of Hypaque or Renografin is injected. The pattern of the fetal abdominal cavity is characteristic (Fig. 21-10). Fluoroscopy using image intensification, or filming can be used. Markers on the abdominal wall aid in localization.

ULTRASOUND IN OBSTETRICS

There are no known adverse effects following the use of ultrasound to study the fetus or other intra-abdominal masses. Therefore this method of examination is of great interest to obstetricians and radiologists. An ultrasonic wave can be produced by substances (e.g., quartz, barium titanate, lead zirconate) which have the capability of changing mechanical energy into an electric signal and vice versa (piezo-electric effect). A wafer crystal of one of these substances energized electrically is used to send an ultrasound pulse. The return "echo" is received by the transducer and converted into electrical energy which is then recorded on an oscillograph.

An A-scan is a unidirectional technique used in measuring a diameter such as in detection of the position of midline structures in the brain. This is not generally applicable to the more complex problems of abdominal scanning. Therefore a multidimensional technique must be applied. This is termed the B-scan, which permits mapping of structures within the abdomen. Ultrasonic energy is almost totally reflected by tissue-gas interfaces so the transducer used must be closely applied to the body being studied. As a result, a number of inconveniences and technical difficulties must be overcome to make this method easily applicable to the examination of abdominal structures. Ultrasonic methods are now being used

for the study of the gravid uterus and the fetus, but the techniques and equipment need improvement. Instrumentation is being developed however and it is very likely that ultrasound techniques will be in general clinical use in obstetrics and many other areas in a few years. Further discussion is beyond the scope of this book.

ROENTGEN DIAGNOSIS IN GYNECOLOGY

PELVIC CALCIFICATIONS

Urinary tract calculi and appendiceal calcifications have been described in Chapter 20. Occasionally, calculi occur in a Meckel's diverticulum located in the pelvis. Phleboliths are very common. Rarely, calculi are formed in the fallopian tube; they usually result from infection and may be single or multiple. When multiple they resemble a string of beads; this appearance should suggest tubal calculi. Calcification in uterine fibroids is typical in distribution (p. 732). Calcification in ovarian dermoid cysts and psammoma bodies are discussed on pages 733 and 734). Calcification of an entire ovary and ovarian "stones" have also been reported. Ovarian fibromas may contain calcium and old areas of endometriosis may calcify. The diagnosis of the presumptive site of these calcifications is made by exclusion in most instances.

PELVIC CYSTS AND TUMORS

The roentgen examination consisting of films in the frontal and oblique positions may reveal abnormal pelvic masses, but with a few exceptions, the nature of the mass cannot be established by this method. Opacification of the colon and of the urinary bladder may aid in localization of masses.

Pelvic arteriography, with visualization of the uterine arteries, is of definite value in some cases. Those interested in this special examination are referred to the comprehensive monograph by Fernstrom.[10]

Gynecography (pelvic pneumography) is another special examination which can be used in the examination of pelvic organs. It consists of intraperitoneal injection of 1000 to 1,500 ml of nitrous oxide or carbon dioxide, followed by roentgenograms of the pelvis taken with the patient prone and tilted about 45° with the head down. The gas surrounds the pelvic organs, permitting ready visualization of abnormalities or masses involving them (Fig. 21-11).

UTERINE TUMORS

LEIOMYOMA

A large uterine leiomyoma produces sufficient opacity to be visible on the roentgeno-gram of the abdomen and pelvis and is outlined as a clearly defined, soft-tissue mass that may be smoothly rounded or lobulated. It may extend up out of the pelvis to lie in the lower abdomen (Fig. 21-12). These tumors may contain calcium which assumes a characteristic mottled appearance (Fig. 21-13). The calcium may outline all or part of one or more uterine fibroids.

OTHER UTERINE TUMORS

Occasionally a hydatid mole may result in gross enlargement of the uterus that is readily detected on a roentgenogram of the abdomen. Chorioepithelioma can cause enlargement also. Occasionally leiomyosarcoma or adenocarcinoma of the endometrium may result in sufficient enlargement so that the uterus is visible as a soft tissue mass in the pelvis. There is no way to differentiate these masses roentgenographically.

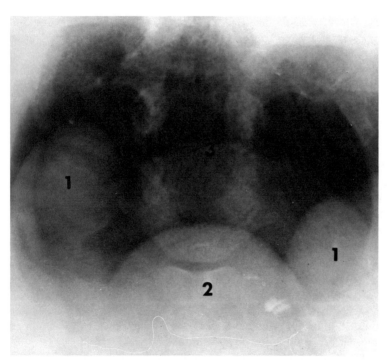

Fig. 21-11. Pelvic pneumogram. Gas within the pelvic peritoneum outlines the viscera. Numerals indicate the following: **1,** the ovaries; **2,** the urinary bladder; **3,** the uterus. These structures are normal.

OVARIAN CYSTS AND TUMORS

DERMOID OR TERATOMA

Approximately one-third of the dermoid cysts of the ovary contain some calcium, usually in a tooth or toothlike structure attached to one wall of a rounded pelvic mass. Rarely there is enough calcium in the wall of the cyst to visualize it. These dermoids vary in size and are often eccentric in position. There is usually enough lipid material within the mass to make it relatively radiolucent and when the combination of toothlike structure within a radiolucent pelvic mass is present, the diagnosis is almost certain. In the larger percentage of ovarian dermoids where no calcification is present, the radiolucency of the mass is a valuable diagnostic sign. The radiolucency is enclosed in a thin cyst wall more dense than the lipid material within it. When the typical radiolucent mass is found in the pelvis or lower abdomen surrounded by the smooth and clearly defined soft-tissue wall, which is of greater density, a

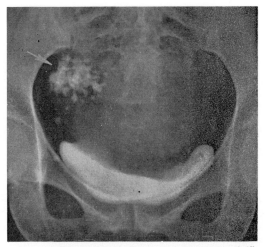

Fig. 21-13. Uterine leiomyoma. Mottled calcification characteristic of leiomyoma of the uterus indicated by **arrow**. Soft-tissue mass above bladder is the enlarged uterus. (Bladder opacified during excretory urography.)

diagnosis of ovarian dermoid cyst can be made with reasonable certainty (Fig. 21-14).

PSAMMOMA CALCIFICATION IN OVARIAN TUMORS

Psammoma bodies are frequently found on pathologic examination of papillary cystadenoma and papillary cystadenocarcinoma of the ovary. When there is enough calcification in the tumor it can be recognized roentgenographically. The psammoma bodies are small calcifications which are distributed widely in the tumor, resulting in a more uniform type of calcification than is noted in uterine fibroids. These tumors metastasize widely and calcification may be found in the metastases, which may be scattered throughout the abdomen and chest. The calcification has been noted in metastases to peripheral nodes. The findings are typical enough to make the diagnosis or strongly suggest it in most instances (Fig. 21-15).

OTHER OVARIAN CYSTS AND TUMORS

Ovarian cysts and tumors often attain great size before they are recognized by the patient

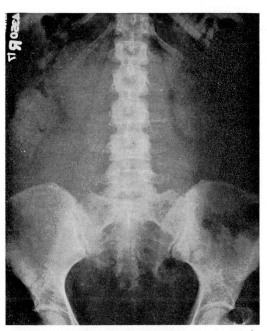

Fig. 21-12. Uterine leiomyoma. Note the large abdominal mass slightly to the right of the midline that extends to the level of the superior aspect of the first lumbar vertebral body.

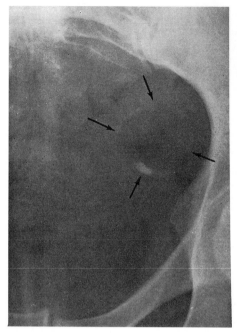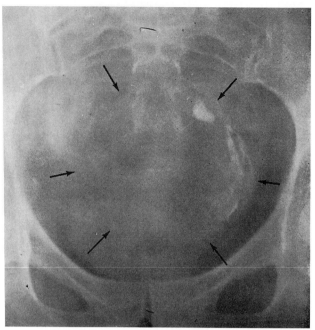

Fig. 21-14. Ovarian dermoid (teratoid) cysts. *Left,* Small cyst (**arrows**) containing a tooth and a small amount of calcification in its wall. *Right,* Large cyst (**arrows**) containing amorphous calcific material.

or her physician. When large, they are readily outlined radiographically and appear as oval or rounded masses in the pelvis. They are often large enough to extend out of the pelvis into the abdomen and are often noted to move with change of position of the patient. They may lie directly in the midline or slightly to one side and can therefore resemble large uterine tumors. The latter do not tend to be as freely movable with change in position, however. When malignant, the ovarian tumors are often associated with ascites, which causes general increase in abdominal density; this obscures the margins of the mass and makes it difficult or impossible to identify in the roentgenogram.

MEIGS' SYNDROME

This syndrome as originally described by Meigs[23] consisted of benign ovarian fibroma associated with ascites and pleural effusion. The fluid cleared on removal of the ovarian tumor. The term is now used by some to indicate the association of ascites and hydrothorax

with any benign ovarian tumor or with low-grade malignant ovarian tumor when the fluid clears soon after removal of the tumor. Roentgen findings are those of ascites and pleural effusion, which may be unilateral or bilateral. The ovarian tumor is small and is usually hidden by the fluid in the abdominal cavity. Exact diagnosis of Meigs' syndrome is not possible by roentgen methods.

HYSTEROSALPINGOGRAPHY

This examination consists of opacification of the uterus and fallopian tubes by means of opaque contrast material injected into the uterus. Enough pressure is applied to fill the uterus and the fallopian tubes with escape of medium into the abdominal cavity. There is considerable difference of opinion as to which of the media available is the best. Most investigators feel that water-soluble media are to be preferred to iodized oil. We use Sinografin which combines diatrizoate methylglucamine

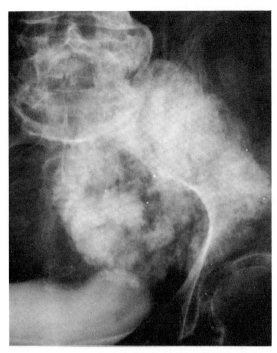

Fig. 21-15. Recurrent serous cystadenocarcinoma of the ovary. This film, taken during an excretory urogram, shows a large irregular, densely calcified tumor in the left pelvis. This represents psammomatous calcification of marked density.

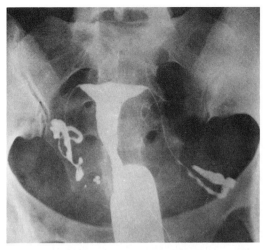

Fig. 21-16. Normal hysterosalpingogram. Uterus and tubes are well outlined and there is some opaque material in the peritoneal cavity on the right, indicating patency of the fallopian tube on that side. Some of the material on the left also appears to be free in the peritoneal cavity.

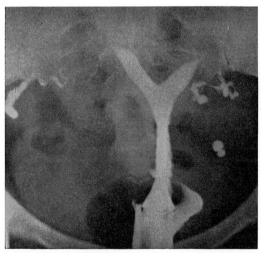

Fig. 21-17. Hysterosalpingogram showing bicornuate uterus. There is some free contrast material in the pelvis on the left, indicating that the left fallopian tube is patent.

(40%) and iodipamide methylglucamine (20%). This medium is water soluble and contains approximately 38% firmly bound iodine. It is absorbed within 1 hour, unless there is obstruction and dilatation of the fallopian tubes, when complete absorption may require up to 24 hours. Salpix is another satisfactory water-soluble medium now in use; it contains sodium acetrizoate and polyvinylpyrrolidone.

INDICATIONS

This examination has been used widely for a number of years in the study of the problem of sterility in females. The opaque material outlines the uterus and tubes and indicates the presence or absence of tubal patency. The indications in addition to infertility studies are not as widely accepted but in some areas it is being used to ascertain causes of abnormal uterine bleeding, to outline anomalies, and as an aid in identification of pelvic masses and intrauterine tumors. It is also used as an aid to the diagnosis of extrauterine pregnancy when the fetus is dead.

CONTRAINDICATIONS

Active infection of the genital tract, recent or active uterine bleeding, suspected pregnancy, genital tuberculosis, and severe systemic disease involving the cardiorespiratory system all contraindicate this procedure. Risks are minimal when water-soluble media are used.

TECHNIQUE

The examination is usually performed jointly by the gynecologist and the radiologist. A special type of cannula that occludes the external os of the cervix and prevents escape of material into the vagina is used. Several types of these instruments are available. The cannula is inserted and held firmly in place. Then 6 to 12 cc of the contrast material are injected, under fluoroscopic control using image intensification. The uterus and tubes can be visualized during the injection. Roentgenograms are taken as indicated during and after injection. If there is any doubt as to whether or not there is "spill" of the material into the abdominal cavity through one or both of the fallopian tubes, delayed films may be obtained.

ROENTGEN FINDINGS

When the tubes are patent there is opaque material in the pelvic portion of the peritoneal cavity. The size and shape of the uterine cavity are readily outlined and the anomalies present are also easily visualized (Fig. 21-16). When the fallopian tubes are occluded, they may be partially visualized. There may or may not be dilatation, indicating hydrosalpinx. When one or both tubes are patent, the material in the pelvic peritoneal cavity is readily recognized by the fact that it outlines the pelvic peritoneum and often loops of bowel within the pelvis (Fig. 21-17).

THE VAGINA

FOREIGN BODIES

The presence of an opaque foreign body within the vagina is readily detected roentgenologically. Localization is relatively simple, using a frontal and a lateral projection. These

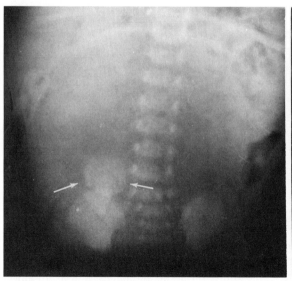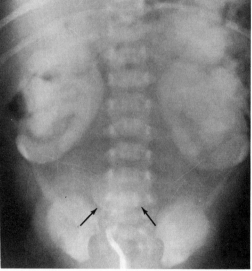

Fig. 21-18. Hydrometrocolpos. *Left,* Excretory urogram. Large central lower abdominal and pelvic mass displaces the bladder (**arrows**) upward and to the right and the gas-containing intestine upward and laterally. Excretion is too poor to clearly outline the renal pelves and calyces. *Right,* Retrograde pyelogram shows displacement of the bladder (**arrows**) and ureters and also reveals a considerable hydronephrosis.

foreign bodies are found most commonly in children.

HYDROCOLPOS AND HYDRO-METROCOLPOS

Imperforate hymen or atresia of the vagina may lead to distention of the vagina (hydrocolpos) or both vagina and uterus (hydrometrocolpos). This may also lead to obstruction of the urinary tract. The most consistent finding is a lower abdominal mass associated with a mass protruding from the vaginal introitus. The condition may be apparent in infancy or may not appear until puberty and the onset of menstruation. In the latter instance, hematocolpos or hematometrocolpos develops.

Roentgen findings on the plain film of the abdomen are those of a lower abdominal mass. Urograms may reveal hydronephrosis and hydroureter with distortion of the bladder and unusual separation of the lower ureters. If opaque material is injected into the vagina through the protruding vaginal membrane, the large distended vaginal and uterine cavities can be visualized. The diagnosis can be suggested when the abdominal mass is outlined and the urographic evidence of obstruction and distortion is present (Fig. 21-18).

VAGINOGRAPHY AND GENITOGRAPHY

Vaginography is occasionally used to confirm the diagnosis when hydrocolpos or hydrometrocolpos is suspected. Genitography is a term used to describe a more extensive study of all genital cavities in children with genital tract obstruction, imperforate anus, and an intersex problem. These conditions and their diagnosis are beyond the scope of this volume. The reader is referred to the monograph by Shopfner.[33]

REFERENCES AND SELECTED READINGS

1. Avnet, N. L., and Elkin, M.: Hysterosalpingography. *Radiol. Clin. North Am. V:* 105, 1967.

2. Ball, R. P., and Golden, R.: Roentgenographic obstetrical pelvicephalometry in the erect posture. *Am. J. Roentgenol. Radium Ther. Nucl. Med. 49:* 731, 1943.

3. Bishop, P. A.: *Radiologic Studies of the Gravid Uterus.* New York, Harper & Row, 1965.

4. Bishop, P. A.: The roentgenologic diagnosis of fetal hydrops. *Am. J. Roentgenol. Radium Ther. Nucl. Med. 86:* 415, 1961.

5. Borell, U., and Fernstrom, I.: The value of the "halo sign" in the diagnosis of intrauterine foetal death. *Acta Radiol. 48:* 401, 1957.

6. Borell, U., and Fernstrom, I.: Radiologic pelvimetry. *Acta Radiol. Suppl. 191,* 1960.

7. Borell, U., and Radberg, C.: Orthodiagraphic pelvimetry with special reference to capacity of distal part of pelvis and pelvic outlet. *Acta Radiol. 2:* 273, 1964.

8. Dedick, A. P., and Whelan, V. M.: Psammoma bodies in cystadenocarcinoma of the ovaries. *Radiology 64:* 353, 1955.

9. Diehl, J., and Fernstrom, I.: Radiologic pelvimetry with special reference to widest transverse diameter of pelvic inlet. *Acta Radiol. 4:* 557, 1966.

10. Fernstrom, I.: Arteriography of uterine artery. Its value in diagnosis of uterine fibromyomata, tubal pregnancy, adnexal tumor and placental site localization. *Acta Radiol. Suppl. 122,* 1955.

11. Germann, D. R.: Teleroentgenographic pelvimetry. *Radiology 58:* 548, 1952.

12. Graber, E. A., Barber, H. R. K., and O'Rourke, J. J.: X-ray pelvimetry. *Am. J. Obstet. Gynecol. 77:* 28, 1959.

13. Gruber, F. H.: Gas in the umbilical vessels as a sign of fetal death. *Radiology 89:* 881, 1967.

14. Hartley, J. B.: Radiological estimation of foetal maturity. *Br. J. Radiol. 30:* 561, 1957.

15. Heagy, F. C., and Swartz, D. P.: Localizing the placenta with radioactive iodinated human serum albumin. *Radiology 76:* 936, 1961.

16. Hill, A. H.: Fetal age assessment by centers of ossification. *Am. J. Phys. Anthropol. 24:* 251, 1939.

17. Hodges, P. C.: The role of x-ray pelvimetry in obstetrics. *Minn. Med. 32:* 33, 1949.

18. Hodges, P. C., and Dippel, A. L.: The use of x-rays in obstetrical diagnosis with particular reference to pelvimetry and fetometry. *Int. Abst. Surg. 70:* 421, 1949.

19. Isaacs, I.: Roentgen pelvimetry by differential divergent distortion. *Am. J. Roentgenol. Radium Ther. Nucl. Med. 63:* 669, 1950.

20. Kendig, T. A.: Reduction of fetal irradiation in pelvimetry. *Radiology 75:* 608, 1960.

21. LINSMAN, J. F., and CHALEK, J. I.: Placental calcification in the roentgen pregnancy study. *Am. J. Roentgenol. Radium Ther. Nucl. Med. 67:* 267, 1952.

22. MCDONALD, E. J.: Evaluation of placentography in late bleeding of pregnancy. *Radiology 64:* 826, 1955.

23. MEIGS, J. V., and CASS, J. W.: Hydrothorax and ascites in association with fibroma of the ovary. *Am. J. Obstet. Gynecol. 53:* 249, 1937.

24. MOLOY, H. C., and SWENSON, P. C.: "The Use of the Roentgen Ray in Obstetrics," in *Diagnostic Roentgenology,* ed. by R. Golden. Baltimore, Williams & Wilkins, 1956.

25. PARKINSON, C. E.: Traumatic rupture of the gravid uterus. *Am. J. Roentgenol. Radium Ther. Nucl. Med. 80:* 684, 1958.

26. ROBINS, S. A., and WHITE, G.: Roentgen diagnosis of dermoid cysts of the ovary in the absence of calcification. *Am. J. Roentgenol. Radium Ther. Nucl. Med. 43:* 30, 1940.

27. ROSSI, P., RIZZI, J., and DE SANTIS, V.: Simultaneous lateral placentography. *Radiology 74:* 298, 1960.

28. SAMUEL, E., and COHEN, J.: Prenatal radiological diagnosis of hydrops fetalis. *Br. J. Radiol. 23:* 225, 1950.

29. SAVIGNAC, E. M.: Roentgen amniography: A valuable and safe aid to obstetrical diagnosis. *Radiology 60:* 545, 1953.

30. SAVIGNAC, E. M.: The prenatal roentgen diagnosis of fetal hydrops. *Am. J. Roentgenol. Radium Ther. Nucl. Med. 80:* 673, 1958.

31. SCAMMON, R. E., and CALKINS, L. A.: *The Development and Growth of the External Dimensions of the Human Body in the Fetal Period.* Minneapolis, University of Minnesota Press, 1929.

32. SCHWARZ, G. S.: An orthometric radiograph for obstetrical roentgenometry. *Radiology 66:* 753, 1956.

33. SHOPFNER, C. E.: Radiology in pediatric gynecology. *Radiol. Clin. North Am. V:* 151, 1967.

34. SNOW, W.: *Roentgenology in Obstetrics and Gynecology.* Springfield, Ill., Thomas, 1952.

35. STEVENS, G. M.: Pelvic pneumonography. *Semin. Roentgenol. IV:* 252, 1969.

36. STOCKLAND, L., and MARKS, S. A.: A new method of fetal weight determination. *Am. J. Roentgenol. Radium Ther. Nucl. Med. 86:* 425, 1961.

37. TAGER, S. N.: A new roentgen sign of fetal death. *Am. J. Roentgenol. Radium Ther. Nucl. Med. 67:* 106, 1952.

38. TODES, J. V.: Advanced abdominal pregnancy. Its radiological diagnosis. *Br. J. Radiol. 31:* 28, 1958.

39. WHITEHOUSE, W. M., SIMONS, C. S., and EVANS, T. N.: Radiation hazards in obstetric roentgenography. *Am. J. Roentgenol. Radium Ther. Nucl. Med. 80:* 690, 1958.

40. WOLFE, J. N., and EVANS, W. A.: Gas in the portal veins of the liver in infants. *Am. J. Roentgenol. Radium Ther. Nucl. Med. 74:* 486, 1955.

Section V

THE CHEST

22

METHODS OF EXAMINATION, ANATOMY, AND CONGENITAL MALFORMATIONS

METHODS OF EXAMINATION

It is generally agreed that the radiographic examination of the chest is extremely important in the diagnosis of pulmonary disease and its value is equally great in the diagnosis of diseases of the mediastinum and bony thorax. The chest roentgenogram also serves as a record of the presence or absence of disease on the date it was taken, and follow-up examinations can serve to determine progress or development of disease. On the other hand, the chest roentgenogram should not supplant routine physical examination and clinical history even though it is well established that this method will demonstrate lesions that cannot be found in any other manner. It is possible to make positive diagnoses of a number of conditions on chest roentgenograms alone, while in other instances a lesion is disclosed, the nature of which must be ultimately determined by bacteriologic or cytologic studies. Cardiovascular disease can also be studied by radiographic and other roentgen methods and will be discussed in Chapter 32.

ROENTGENOGRAPHY

Routine roentgen examination of the chest varies in different institutions but should con-sist of at least posteroanterior and lateral projections. These are taken at a tube-film distance of 6 feet to minimize distortion and magnification as much as possible, and are made in moderately deep inspiraton. There is some difference of opinion regarding the proper density of chest roentgenograms. We prefer a moderately high-voltage technique (98 to 124 kV) that tends to reduce contrast so that the sharp black and white differentiation is reduced to varying shades of gray. This permits better penetration and visualization of retrocardiac and mediastinal structures than lower voltages. We also use a stationary grid and ionization chamber timing. It is desirable to visualize the upper thoracic vertebral interspaces and to define vascular markings behind the heart (Fig. 22-1).

A number of other views are used in special circumstances to outline local lesions or to visualize areas that are not well seen on the routine roentgenograms. Oblique projections are taken at approximately 45° angles and are named according to the side of the chest nearest the film and away from the roentgen-ray tube. For example, the designation "right anterior oblique" indicates that the patient is standing with the right anterior chest wall in contact with the cassette holder at an angle of 45° so that the left posterior chest wall is nearest the tube; the rays then traverse the

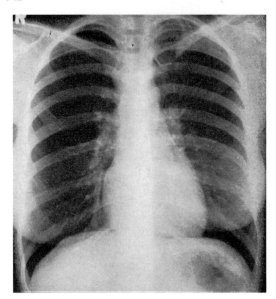

Fig. 22-1. Normal chest. This frontal roentgenogram is taken with a high-voltage technique. Note that the vascular markings at the left base are visible through the cardiac shadow. The upper thoracic intervertebral spaces are also visible.

thorax from posterior to anterior in an oblique direction. Greater or lesser degrees of obliquity may be used as desired. When small nodules below the level of the dome of the diaphragm are poorly visualized by routine methods, the tube may be angled upward or downward as necessary. Special views may also be taken tangential to lesions of the thoracic wall to define them. The apical lordotic view is used to visualize disease in the pulmonary apices, that is often obscured by the clavicle and first rib. This roentgenogram is taken in an anteroposterior direction with the patient leaning backward on the cassette holder. An anteroposterior upright projection with the tube angled cephalad 15° may also be used. It results in clear visualization of the lung apices because the clavicle and first rib are projected above the pulmonary apex (Fig. 22-2). Lateral recumbent views are sometimes indicated to outline fluid levels in cavities or in the pleural space and to determine the presence of pleural effusions in some instances. The films are taken with the roentgen-ray beam directed in a hori-

zontal plane with the patient lying on either the right or left side. When there is any question of obstructive emphysema involving a lung, lobe, or segment, a film in complete expiration is indicated, along with a film in inspiration. This combination can also be used to record diaphragmatic motion in conditions affecting the diaphragm on one or both sides.

Stereoscopic roentgenograms are preferred by many radiologists as a routine procedure and are particularly helpful in localizing small solitary nodular lesions and in the study of pulmonary tuberculosis where pulmonary infiltrates and cavities at varying depths can more readily be identified and visualized. Since there are two films, this method of examination also tends to eliminate the danger of misinterpreting an artefact. An automatic film changer is used and two films are taken in quick succession. The patient remains stationary and the tube is shifted approximately one-tenth of the distance between the anode of the roentgen ray-tube and the film.

The air-gap technique described by Jackson[21] uses a 10-foot distance from the focal spot of the tube to the film. The patient is separated from the film cassette a distance of 15 cm by a suitable frame. Moderately high voltages are used (average of 120 kV for adults). There is no need for a grid. Jackson prefers to use the anteroposterior position. The outstanding advantage is the clarity of vascular shadows in the lung. We have had no experience with this technique.

Direct magnification techniques are also being used by some. This is particularly valuable in the examination of the newborn chest.

FLUOROSCOPY

There are many indications for fluoroscopy of the chest; they are discussed under the various conditions for which fluoroscopy is used. The dynamics of the cardiovascular system and respiration can be studied to good advantage by this method and it is also particularly useful in obstructive emphysema. Conditions affecting diaphragmatic motion are also indications for fluor-

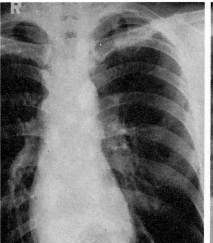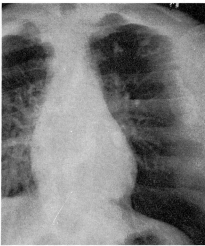

Fig. 22-2. The value of the lordotic view is demonstrated. *Left,* In the routine frontal projection the disease at the left apex is partially hidden by the clavicle and first rib. The lordotic view (*right*) shows the disease clearly outlined in the upper lung field and not obscured by the bony structures.

oscopy of the thorax; localized effusions can be studied to advantage.

Since there are radiation hazards to both patient and physician in the use of fluoroscopy, it is important to reduce radiation to a practical minimum. Image intensification is used to improve visualization and to decrease radiation. It is important to have chest roentgenograms available for study and to know as much as possible about the patient's problem before beginning fluoroscopy. This avoids unnecessary search for a lesion which is much better examined via radiographic methods. It is necessary to use the smallest possible aperture and to limit the total fluoroscopic time in order to reduce radiation exposure. A built-in timer that indicates the duration of radiation exposure is the best method to time fluoroscopy. We attempt to keep the total fluoroscopic time below 5 minutes.

The actual procedure used in fluoroscopy varies with the indication for it and with the examiner, but the examination should be systematic. For example, diaphragmatic motion is observed during normal and deep inspiration in the oblique as well as in the anteroposterior positions; slight weaknesses can often be detected by having the patient sniff. It is sometimes helpful to observe diaphragmatic motion in both lateral decubitus positions to detect small variations in motion on the two sides. The Valsalva maneuver (forced expiration with the glottis closed) can be used to increase the intrathoracic pressure to empty or decrease the size of veins, cardiac atria, and arteriovenous malformations. The Müller experiment (forced inspiration with the glottis closed) can be used to decrease intrathoracic pressure and thereby increase the size of these thin-walled vascular structures. At times it is necessary to examine the patient in the supine or recumbent position, particularly when pleural effusion tends to obscure the diaphragm on one or both sides.

BRONCHOGRAPHY

Bronchography is the study of the bronchial tree by means of the introduction of opaque material into the desired bronchus or bronchi, usually under fluoroscopic control. In general, this examination is done for three main reasons: (*1*) to map the entire bronchial tree of one or both lungs to outline the extent of known disease, such as bronchiectasis; (*2*) to determine the presence of disease that may have been suspected and to localize it; and (*3*) to aid in the diagnosis of abnormal shadows, the nature of which is uncertain. In this instance the examination may be localized to a single lobe or segment; in the first, complete mapping of one or both lungs is necessary.

INDICATIONS

BRONCHIECTASIS. To establish the presence of the disease and its extent. It is imperative to outline all the segments in both lungs before surgical removal of bronchiectatic lobes or segments is undertaken since unsuspected disease may be demonstrated by this method.

HEMOPTYSIS WITHOUT OBVIOUS CAUSE. It is not uncommon to observe patients in whom roentgen examination of the chest is negative despite the history of one or more episodes of hemoptysis. In some instances the diagnosis can be made by means of this examination when other methods have failed.

SUSPECTED BRONCHOGENIC TUMOR. When clinical findings and bronchoscopy are insufficient to make the diagnosis, bronchography may demonstrate sufficiently typical signs to establish the diagnosis.

PULMONARY TUBERCULOSIS. Bronchography is often indicated to outline involved bronchi and accurately localize the site of disease, particularly when there is considerable distortion secondary to fibrosis, and to determine the presence of bronchiectasis, which is a common finding in pulmonary tuberculosis.

ANOMALIES. Bronchography is the only method short of surgical exploration to determine the presence of various anomalies of bronchopulmonary segments as well as to confirm the presence of pulmonary hypogenesis and agenesis.

MISCELLANEOUS. Bronchography is sometimes useful in the examination of patients with postoperative complications following pulmonary resection. It is also useful in patients with cystic disease and is sometimes used as an additional diagnostic method in patients with pulmonary parenchymal shadows of uncertain nature, many of which turn out to be tumor while others represent inflammatory lesions of various types.

CONTRAINDICATIONS

RESPIRATORY INSUFFICIENCY. Is a contraindication to a degree related to its severity; e.g., severe forms completely rule out the possibility of doing bronchography.

ALLERGY. Patients with bronchial asthma often tolerate bronchography poorly and highly allergic individuals without asthmatic manifestations are also poor risks. The examination should not be done on these patients unless it is essential. Known iodine sensitivity and sensitivity to local anesthetic agents are also contraindications.

RECENT HEMOPTYSIS. Hemoptysis of 2 ounces or more contraindicates bronchography for a time but after the bleeding has stopped for 7 to 14 days it is usually possible to examine the patient. Minimal hemoptysis, even though repeated, is probably not a contraindication.

PULMONARY TUBERCULOSIS. The examination is contraindicated in active early exudative disease and is not ordinarily done until the tuberculosis has stabilized to the extent that surgery is contemplated; then bronchography may be done with little risk.

ACUTE INFECTIONS. Acute pulmonary parenchymal infections, including acute lung abscess, contraindicate bronchography and the examination should not be done in the presence of acute upper respiratory infections.

TECHNIQUE

Numerous methods of doing this procedure have been described and most of them are satisfactory in the hands of those who use them long enough to gain proficiency. The method described here is used in our department.

CONTRAST MATERIAL. Dionosil (3,5-diiodo-4-pyridone-N-acetic acid) is the contrast medium used extensively in this country. It contains 34% iodine and is available both as an aqueous and an oily suspension. Aqueous Dionosil is more irritating than Dionosil oily and both appear to be slightly more irritating than Iodochlorol. Dionosil is rapidly absorbed and does not remain to obscure disease in the lobe or lung in which bronchography is done. This material does not break down to form free iodine and is probably the best agent now available for bronchography.

Barium sulfate suspended in carboxymethylcellulose has been advocated as a safe contrast agent for bronchography. Our experience has been limited to its use in a few patients with iodine sensitivity. It evidently causes less pulmonary reaction than any of the other agents now in use.

PREPARATION OF THE PATIENT. The meal prior to the examination is withheld and the patient is not allowed to eat or drink for a period of 4 hours following bronchography. Premedication consisting of 100 mg of Seconal or Nembutal and 60 mg of codeine is administered an hour before the examinaton. If there is much bronchial secretion, 0.4 mg of atropine sulfate may be given an hour before the examination. In patients who have large amounts of sputum it is wise to employ postural drainage to decrease the amount of secretions because material in the bronchi interferes with the induction of anesthesia and with contrast filling of the bronchi.

ANESTHESIA. Proper anesthesia is essential for successful bronchography and the examination is almost invariably doomed to failure unless good anesthesia is attained. In infants and small children general anesthesia is used. This is administered by the anesthesiologist who inserts an endotracheal catheter. Under fluoroscopic control, the contrast material is then introduced into the desired lobe or segment via the catheter. In older children and adults, local anesthesia is used. Lidocaine hydrochloride (4% xylocaine hydrochloride) is the local anesthetic agent we use. The anesthetic agent is sprayed over the pharynx, hypopharynx, and tonsil areas and after a short wait, the pharynx, pyriform sinuses, and epiglottis are swabbed with the anesthetic solution, using a long forceps and gauze sponges or cotton pledgets. As a final measure, approximately 1 cc of the anesthetic solution is dropped into the glottis by means of a curved cannula; this usually initiates severe coughing that spreads the material over the glottis and upper trachea. There is considerable individual variation in patients; some are very easily anesthetized while others are extremely refractory. An intermittent positive pressure apparatus especially adapted for administration of local anesthetics in bronchography has now been developed.[28] It has many advantages over topical application and spraying and will probably be used extensively in the future.

TECHNIQUE OF OIL INJECTION. When satisfactory anesthesia has been achieved, a tracheobronchial catheter is inserted into the trachea or a desired bronchus and the opaque medium can be injected directly into the bronchus. When it is necessary to examine both lungs or portions of both lungs by this method, we prefer to do one side at a time and to allow an interval of several days between the two sittings. The direct method of injection by means of a needle puncture through the cricothyroid membrane is also used in our department. A total of approximately 15 to 20 cc of contrast material is usually required to map the bronchi of one lung. The procedure is usually started with the patient in the upright or semi-upright position on the table, which is then moved into the horizontal or Trendelenberg position. The patient is rotated until fluoroscopic observation indicates that the desired filling is obtained. When local obstruction or local disease is observed during fluoroscopy, spot films are exposed. It is important that the patient breathe deeply once the contrast has been introduced into the desired bronchi. He should also be encouraged to cough a few times to aid in complete distribution of the opaque into the smaller bronchi. A lateral roentgenogram is taken first with the examined side down, using a Bucky technique. Then an anteroposterior roentgenogram is obtained with the patient lying on the table in the supine position. The patient is turned into an oblique position and a third film is exposed using Bucky technique. For this projection the examined side is down with the opposite side elevated at a 45° angle. Then, with the patient in an upright position stereoscopic posteroanterior and lateral roentgenograms are exposed (Fig. 22-3). An appropriate oblique projection may also be taken if deemed necessary. Following the procedure, the patient is encouraged to cough and expectorate the contrast material, using postural drainage as an aid.

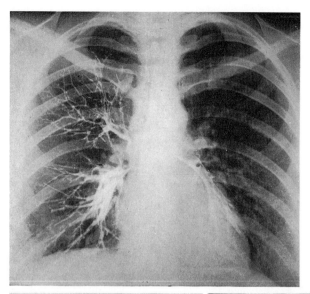

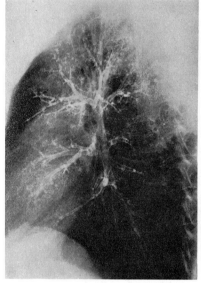
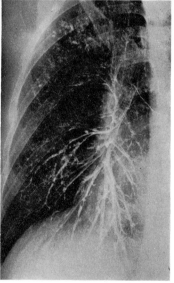

Fig. 22-3. Normal bronchogram. Note the iodized oil outlining the bronchi, which decrease in diameter toward the periphery and branch in a treelike manner.

HAZARDS

ANESTHETIC REACTIONS. The danger of anesthetic reactions can be reduced to a minimum by proper premedication and by keeping the total amount of Xylocaine used to less than 200 mg. This examination should be avoided in patients who have had previous local anesthetic reactions. Common symptoms are dizziness, restlessness, apprehension, confusion, and convulsive twitchings progressing to convulsive seizures. Cyanosis, dyspnea, respiratory arrest and cardiac failure may also occur. Treatment consists of administration of oxygen as soon as possible, making certain that the airway is maintained. Small doses of a short-acting barbiturate such as Pentothal sodium (Thiopental in a dose of 30 to 50 mg per minute) should be administered intravenously if convulsions occur. Artificial respiration may be necessary in the presence of respiratory failure, and thoracotomy with cardiac massage may be needed if cardiac arrest occurs.

IODIZED OIL REACTIONS. These reactions are infrequent and are usually allergic in type and relatively mild. Manifestations consist of bronchial asthma and urticaria; when these reactions are immediate they can be treated by the use of antihistaminic drugs. Late reactions owing to aggravations of existing inflammatory disease can be managed by administration of appropriate antibiotics. Local obstruction produced by the viscous contrast material is treated by encouraging postural drainage and cough. Oil granulomas have been reported as late complications when alveolar oil is retained but this complication is extremely rare.

OTHER COMPLICATIONS. Spread of tuberculous disease has been mentioned in the past but this is not an important factor at present with the use of antituberculous drugs and judicious timing of the procedure in relation to the activity of the tuberculous disease. Hemorrhage has also been reported but in our experience this is a rare complication and the amount of hemorrhage has never been of sufficient quantity to be a real hazard.

LARYNGOGRAPHY

Laryngography includes the study of the hypopharynx, the larynx, and the subglottic portion of the trachea. The technique consists of coating the structures to be examined with oily Dionosil. Premedication with large doses of atropine sulfate to decrease secretions is very important. We use 1 mg of atropine if the patient will tolerate it. We also use codeine to suppress the cough reflex. The pharynx and larynx are anesthetized using Xylocaine hydrochloride or Cetacaine spray or both. Then the oily Dionosil is administered by cannula over the back of the tongue. Using fluoroscopy to see that the hypopharynx and larynx are coated, spot films are taken in lateral and frontal projections during (1) quiet respiration, (2) pho-

nating "E," (3) Valsalva maneuver, and (4) modified Valsalva, with the mouth closed and the glottis open. Voltages in the range of 65 to 70 kV are optimal. This examination is very useful in the study of tumors of the supraglottic region, the larynx particularly in the evaluation of possible subglottic extension, and in determination of pyriform sinus involvement. We often use a combination of laryngography and tomography of the larynx in the study of disease in this region (Figs. 22-4 and 22-5).

TOMOGRAPHY

TECHNIQUE

Tomography is also known as body section radiography, planigraphy, laminagraphy, and stratigraphy. These terms refer to a method of radiographic examination by which it is possible to examine a single layer of tissue and to blur the tissues above and below the level by motion. This is accomplished by simultaneous motion of the roentgen-ray tube and the film cassette during the exposure by means of a connecting rod or bar. The tube and film move in opposite directions and the fulcrum of the bar or rod connecting the tube and film carrier is placed at the level to be examined (Fig. 22-6). The amount of blurring depends upon the distance of the object or tissue from the level of the fulcrum. The thickness of the plane of tissue examined is determined within certain limits by the distance traveled by the tube and film during the radiographic exposure. Zonography is a variation in which the thickness of the plane of tissue examined is increased by shortening the excursion of the tube. By raising or lowering the fulcrum one can then examine planes of tissue within the chest at various levels as desired. Most of the manufacturers of radiographic equipment also make or distribute attachments for body section radiography. A number of special deveices are now available which permit tomography in a number of planes.

Circular, elliptical, and hypocycloidal tomography is possible in addition to rectilinear. Transverse tomographic units are also available. As a general rule, rectilinear tomography is sufficient for most studies of the lungs and thorax. If needed, one of the other motions can be used.

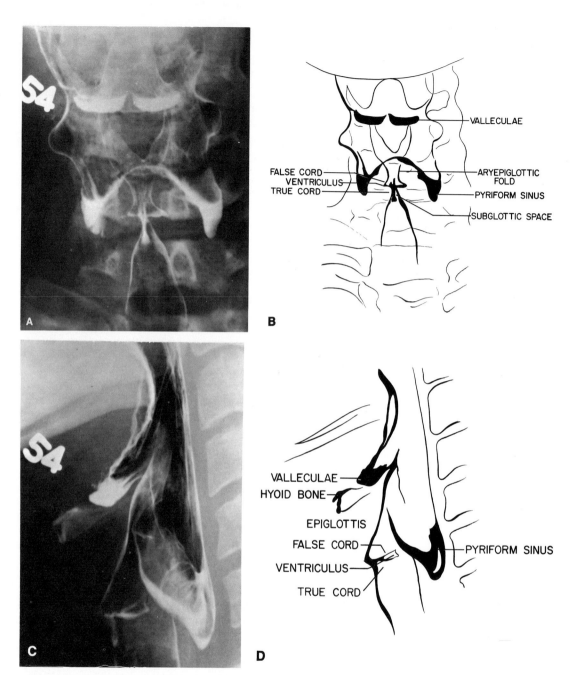

Fig. 22-4. Laryngogram. *A,* This anteroposterior film was taken with patient phonating "E." *B,* Diagram of *A* with anatomy labeled. *C,* Lateral film. *D,* Diagram of *C* with anatomy labeled.

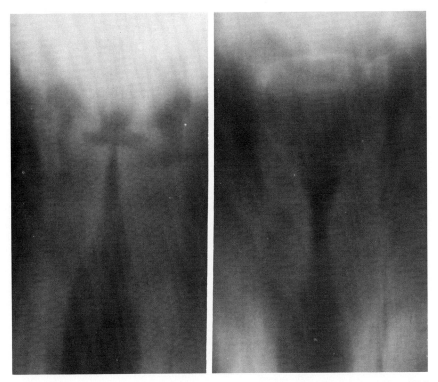

Fig. 22-5. Tomogram larynx. *Left,* Film was taken with patient phonating "E." Note the clear definition of the ventriculus and cords. There is subglottic stenosis of the trachea. *Right,* Film was taken in modified Valsalva maneuver (mouth closed, glottis open). The tracheal stenosis persists.

There is also available a multiple cassette holder that permits the simultaneous exposure of seven films so that multiple planes of thoracic tissue at 1-cm intervals can be examined on a single exposure. This reduces total radiation exposure and also decreases the time consumed in the examination, but it has not been very satisfactory in our hands.

INDICATIONS

There are many indications for tomography of the chest. It is used to outline detailed anatomy of the lung, mediastinum, or other thoracic structures in which an abnormality is observed on the chest film. It is also used to outline the vascular pattern and pulmonary pattern in diffuse processes such as emphysema, pulmonary hypertension, and pulmonary vascular anomalies. It is particularly useful in the study of patients with pulmonary tuberculosis. Cavities can be outlined that are not visible on routine roentgenograms and nodular infiltration can be more clearly defined than with any other type of examination. These studies are usually done in an anteroposterior position but lateral tomograms can be taken when necessary to show lesions not well seen in frontal projection. Bronchiectasis associated with tuberculosis can often be identified by means of tomography and the method is particularly useful in examining the compressed lung beneath a thoracoplasty. In patients with bronchogenic carcinoma, the mass of the tumor can be outlined and it is often possible to visualize the site of bronchial occlusion when this complication is present. Tomography also is useful in detecting calcium in small parenchymal nodules (Fig. 22-7) and in the study of lung abscess.

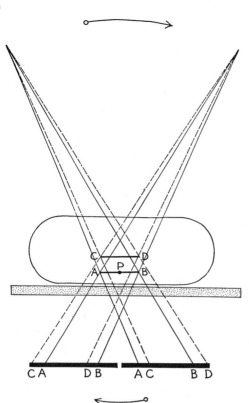

Fig. 22-6. Diagram illustrates the principles of tomography. The **upper arrow** indicates the direction of the tube shift. The fulcrum is at the level **P** on line **AB.** Note that the relationship of the projected image of **AB** remains the same on the initial and final position of the cassette, while the image of the line **CD** at some distance from the fulcrum has moved from right to left. Therefore, the tissues at the level of the fulcrum are clearly defined while those above and below it are blurred by motion.

PULMONARY ANGIOGRAPHY

TECHNIQUE

The purpose of this examination is to outline the pulmonary arterial system. This can be accomplished in several ways. The simplest is the injection of a large bolus of contrast medium (one of the organic iodides) intravenously using a needle. Timed films then show filling of the right heart and the pulmonary arteries. Properly timed filming will also show opacification of the pulmonary veins and left heart. Major disadvantages are less than optimal filling of the desired vascular structures. Catheter methods include injection into

the vena cava, right atrium, distal right ventricle, pulmonary artery or selectively into either right or left pulmonary artery or one of their branches (Fig. 22-8). The nature of the process for which the procedure is performed tends to determine the method used. The catheter methods result in better opacification and therefore better visualization of the vessels studied. For a complete discussion of angiocardiography see Chapter 32.

INDICATIONS

We use this method in conjunction with azygography in evaluating operability of lung carcinoma. The superior vena cava is included by placing the catheter in the proximal subclavian vein via the basilic. It is also used in the study of patients with suspected pulmonary arterial or venous anomalies or diseases, and most importantly, in the study of thromboembolic disease of the lungs.

BRONCHIAL ARTERIOGRAPHY

This examination requires selective catheterization of bronchial arteries which is very difficult. Its use in clinical medicine is very limited.

AZYGOGRAPHY

Azygos venography is a procedure used to outline the azygos system using the major tributaries, the intercostal veins. We use the intraosseous method, but direct catheterization via the femoral vein, right atrium, and superior vena cava can be done.

TECHNIQUE (INTRAOSSEOUS METHOD)

A No. 16 bone-marrow needle is used to hand inject 25 ml of methylglucamine diatrizoate (Renografin 60) into the marrow cavity of the eighth, ninth, or tenth rib laterally. Xylocaine is used to anesthetize the marrow space. Serial films are taken at one per second for 6 seconds after the end of the injection. The azygos system is filled via the right side and the hemiazygos via the left side; then the azygos fills via communications extending across the vertebral column (Fig. 22-9).

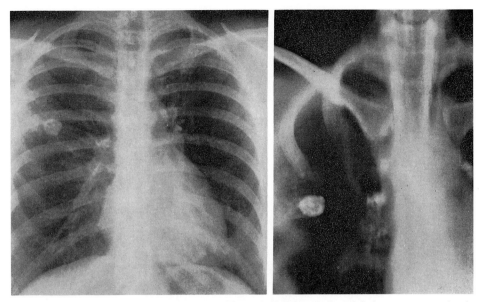

Fig. 22-7. Example of use of tomogram. The calcification and nodulation are more clearly defined on the tomogram (*right*) than on the routine roentgenogram on the *left*.

INDICATIONS

We use this method in evaluating operability of lung cancer and also of esophageal cancer. It is also used in the investigation of the cause of azygos vein enlargement.

ROENTGENKYMOGRAPHY

Roentgenkymography is a special method of examination of the chest in which motion of the intrathoracic structures can be recorded on film. The apparatus used for this examination consists of a lead grid in which parallel slits are cut at intervals of 12 mm. These slits are 0.4 mm in width. This grid is placed between the patient and the film. Since lateral motion is to be recorded in most instances, the slits in the grid are transverse. Motion parallel to the slits is recorded during roentgen exposure in which the film moves at uniform speed in a vertical direction at right angles to the slits for a distance equal to the width of the lead spacers. Motion parallel to the slits is then recorded on the film in the form of a wave as irregular lines or borders. The depth of the wave will indicate the amplitude of motion. Structures that are not moving will be indicated by a straight vertical line or border on the film (Fig. 22-10). This method of examination does not have wide use in examination of the chest but can be used to record motion of the heart, mediastinum, diaphragm, and expansile pulsation in vascular anomalies.

DIAGNOSTIC PNEUMOTHORAX

Diagnostic pneumothorax is occasionally used in examination of diseases of the chest. A measured amount of air or oxygen (100 to 300 cc) is introduced into the affected side and roentgenograms of the chest are taken in desired projections. Fluoroscopy of the chest can also be done following injection of the gas. This method of examination is useful in differentiating the soft-tissue masses or densities in the mediastinum, chest wall, or diaphragm from intrapulmonary lesions. It can also be used in differentiating pleural disease from disease of the diaphragm. Occasionally it is neces-

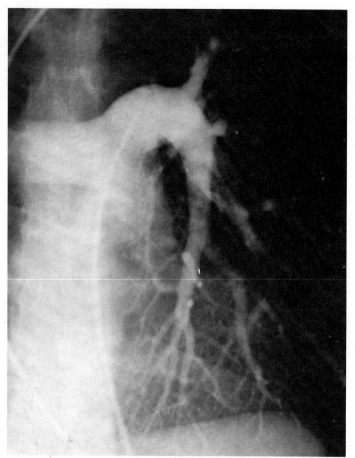

Fig. 22-8. Normal pulmonary arteriogram. This is an example of selective pulmonary arteriography. The catheter is in the left pulmonary artery.

sary to use diagnostic pneumoperitoneum in conjunction with pneumothorax to differentiate lesions producing soft-tissue densities in the diaphragm or those projecting upward from the abdomen.

DIAGNOSTIC PNEUMOMEDIASTINOGRAPHY

The introduction of a gas into the mediastinum for diagnostic purposes has been used for some time, chiefly in Europe. Recently this procedure has been advocated in this country by Berne et al.,[4] who use it in conjunction with scalene node biopsy. Three to 8 liters of carbon dioxide are introduced into the mediastinum via a catheter which is inserted at surgery. Films are then taken in desired projections. Usually there is good visualization of mediastinal structures and of any mass which may be present. Tomography may also be used in conjunction with this procedure. We have had no experience with this method.

BRONCHIAL BRUSH BIOPSY

Bronchial biopsy and aspiration of bronchial secretions for microscopic study have been used in conjunction with bronchography for a number of years. Recently, Fennessy[17] has developed the method of transcatheter brush biopsy. The opaque, Odman type of catheter is shaped in a manner which facilitates entry into the desired bronchus. The catheter with guide wire is inserted through the pharynx, larynx, and trachea using fluor-

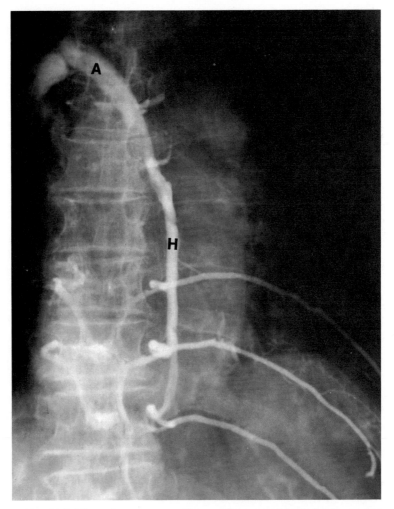

Fig. 22-9. Normal azygogram. The medium was injected into marrow cavity of the left ninth rib. There is good opacification of three intercostal veins, the hemiazygos vein **(H)**, and the azygos vein **(A)**. A small amount of medium is noted in the superior vena cava.

oscopy. Small brushes are passed through the catheter into the lesion. Microscopic slides are then prepared immediately from the brushes. We have had very little experience with this method which is used to examine peripheral lung lesions.

NEEDLE ASPIRATION BIOPSY

This method of examination used largely for local lesions in the periphery of the lung has become popular in the last 5 years. Percutaneous aspiration biopsy uses fluoroscopic localization. Thin-walled, No. 18 needles can be used. The major complication is pneumothorax, which is usually easily managed. We use this method in preference to bronchial brush biopsy because of its relative simplicity.

THE NORMAL CHEST

GENERAL CONSIDERATIONS IN CHEST INTERPRETATION

Interpretation of chest roentgenograms requires that the viewer first find the abnormal-

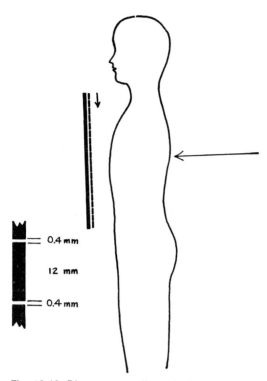

0.4 mm

12 mm

0.4 mm

Fig. 22-10. Diagram to outline principles of roentgen kymography. The **horizontal arrow** on the right indicates direction of the roentgen rays. The **vertical arrow** anterior to the patient indicates the direction in which the film moves. The film is indicated by the **solid black vertical line,** the grid by the **broken vertical line.** The *inset* on the left shows the relative size of the strips of lead and slits in the grid.

ity. It is useful to develop a method of studying the film to make certain that all areas are searched. The mediastinum including the heart, the lung fields, diaphragm, bony thorax, soft tissues of the thorax, and the subdiaphragmatic upper abdominal structure should be inspected. It is helpful for the student or trainee to compare the two lung fields interspace by interspace until he learns the normal thoroughly and can recognize variations and abnormalities. Once an abnormality is observed, interpretation of the changes follows. We find it valuable to make the initial examination of the film without knowledge of the clinical findings. Before reaching a decision, however, roentgen observations must be correlated with all of the available clinical information. Specific questions may arise, the answers to which may not be available on the chart. Additional information must then be sought from the referring physician or patient.

In the chapters to follow on chest roentgenology, the presentation is disease oriented. Patterns of pulmonary density of various types are observed. The terms interstitial and alveolar are used to describe the predominant pattern of pulmonary involvement. *Alveolar* or airspace disease is characterized by homogeneous density which may vary from a small area, just large enough to be recognizable to consolidation of an entire lobe or more. The alveoli are filled with exudate, transudate, blood or tissue which replaces the air. Classic pneumococcal pneumonia is a good example of alveolar disease. Bronchi may become visible when such consolidation occurs; the *air-bronchogram* is then observed, which indicates adjacent alveolar disease.

Interstitial disease is characterized by an increase in density of the perivascular, interlobular, and parenchymal interstitial spaces. Alveolar aeration is maintained and the interstitial tissues increase in volume. The process may be localized, as in viral pneumonia, or general as in extensive interstitial edema. The pattern may range from reticular or latticelike, to granular, to nodular, or to various combinations of these findings.

Combinations of interstitial and alveolar density may also occur. A common example of this is the patient with combined interstitial and alveolar pulmonary edema. Mycoplasmal and viral pneumonia are also frequently observed to have a combined pattern.

The localization and sometimes the recognition of pulmonary disease is dependent in many instances upon the *silhouette sign.* The term was coined by Felson, who credited Dr. H. Kennon Dunham with making the initial observations. Felson[15] defines this sign as follows: "An intrathoracic lesion touching a border of the heart, aorta or diaphragm will obliterate that border on the roentgenogram. An intrathoracic lesion not anatomically contiguous with a border of one of these structures will not obliterate that border." The principle defined above is very useful in a variety of chest conditions.

THE ADULT CHEST

The roentgenogram of the adult chest outlines the heart, lungs, bony thorax including the ribs and thoracic vertebrae, the diaphragm, all or part of the clavicles, and all or part of the scapulas. The soft tissues making up the chest wall also are included. The thorax is divided by the mediastinum into right and left compartments, each containing an air-filled lung that is recognized by its relative radiolucency as compared to the mediastinum, chest wall, and the upper abdominal viscera. The greater part of the trachea is also shown so that most of the lower respiratory tract is visible.

THE BONY THORAX

Roentgenography of the chest is done primarily for visualization of intrathoracic structures but the shoulder girdles, ribs, cervical and thoracic vertebral bodies and sternum are often well enough outlined so that disease or anatomic variation can be readily recognized. Therefore these structures should be examined on all chest roentgenograms. The shape of the thorax varies with age and with body habitus so that the range of normal is wide. The angulation of the ribs varies considerably with body type; downward angulation is minimal in short hypersthenic individuals and maximal in asthenic patients. The intercostal spaces are numbered according to the rib above them. In describing disease in relation to intercostal spaces, the interspace must be designated as either anterior or posterior because there is considerable difference in position of these interspaces in relation to the horizontal plane of the lung. The costal cartilages are not visible unless there is calcification within them; when calcification is present it assumes a rather characteristic mottled appearance (Fig. 22-11). The diaphragm in a normal adult is very slightly higher on the right than on the left and is at approximately the level of the posterior arc of the tenth rib or the fifth anterior rib or interspace in deep inspiration. The ribs below the level of the diaphragm are usually not as well visualized as those above it because of the greater density of the contents

of the abdomen. The rhomboid fossa is an irregularly rounded indentation on the inferior surface of the clavicle near its sternal end. It marks the attachment of the costoclavicular ligament and varies from slight roughening that may not be visible to a deep indentation. It should be recognized on the chest roentgenogram as an anatomic variant of no clincal significance (Fig. 22-12).

THE SOFT TISSUES

The soft-tissue structures covering the bony thorax also produce density on the chest roentgenogram and they can project over the lung and pleura in a manner that simulates disease. Skin folds in patients who have lost weight can produce linear shadows running in any direction. Breast shadows are usually not difficult to identify but do result in increase in density over the lower thorax, bilaterally. Nipple shadows may appear as rounded densities in the fourth anterior interspace or lower. They are usually bilaterally symmetric, but stereoscopic films or fluoroscopy may occasionally be necessary to differentiate

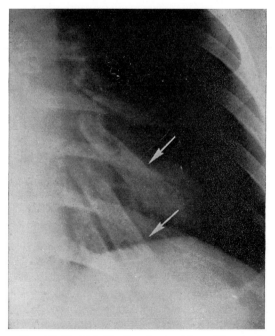

Fig. 22-11. Calcification in costal cartilages. An unusually large amount of calcification is noted in several of the costal cartilages, two of which are indicated by the **arrows**. The mottled appearance of the calcium is characteristic.

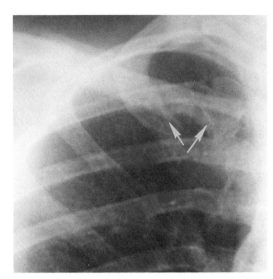

Fig. 22-12. Rhomboid fossa. **Arrows** indicate the irregular round indentation on the inferior aspect of the clavicle.

them from intrapulmonary lesions (Fig. 22-13). The skin and subcutaneous tissues over the clavicles produce a faint, soft-tissue shadow paralleling the clavicles. This measures from 2 or 3 mm up to 1 cm in thickness, but projects beyond the lung field so that it can be identified. Soft-tissue masses or nodules projected over the lung fields can simulate pulmonary nodules; lateral, oblique, or stereoscopic films must be employed in some instances to accurately localize such densities.

THE MEDIASTINUM

ANATOMIC DIVISION AND CONTENTS. The mediastinum is the space lying between the right and left pleurae in and near the median sagittal plane of the chest. It extends from the posterior aspect of the sternum to the anterior surface of the thoracic vertebrae and contains all the thoracic viscera except the lungs. It is divided into four parts, the superior, anterior, middle, and posterior mediastinum (see Fig. 22-19). The superior mediastinum lies between the manubrium sterni and the upper four thoracic vertebrae. It contains the aortic arch and its branches as well as the innominate veins, the upper half of the superior vena cava, the trachea, esophagus, thoracic duct, thymus,

lymph nodes, and various nerves. The anterior mediastinum is bounded above by the superior mediastinum, laterally by the pleura, anteriorly by the sternum, and posteriorly by the pericardium. It contains loose areolar tissue, a few lymph nodes, and some lymphatic vessels that ascend from the convex surface of the liver. The middle mediastinum contains the heart and the pericardium, the ascending aorta, the lower half of the superior vena cava and the azygos vein that empties into it, the bifurcation of the trachea, the main bronchi, the pulmonary artery and its two branches, and the bronchial lymph nodes. It is bounded in front by the anterior mediastinum and posteriorly by the posterior mediastinum. The posterior mediastinum lies behind the heart and pericardium, and extends from the level of the fourth to the twelfth dorsal vertebra. It contains the thoracic portion of the descending aorta, the esophagus, thoracic duct, the azygos and hemiazygos veins, lymph nodes, and several nerves.

THE LYMPH NODES. The mediastinal nodes are divided into three major groups. The anterior mediastinal nodes lie in the anterior portion of the superior mediastinum in relation to the innominate vein and the large arteries that arise from the aortic arch. The posterior mediastinal nodes lie behind the pericardium in the region of the descending aorta and esophagus. The tracheobronchial nodes consist of a chain of paratracheal nodes lying on either side of the trachea, the bronchial or bifurcation nodes lying between the lower trachea and bronchi, the bronchopulmonary or hilum nodes situated in the hilum of each lung, and the pulmonary nodes found in the lung substance adjacent to the larger bronchial branches (Fig. 22-14). Anatomists have recognized a greater number of lymph nodes associated with the right lung and a greater number of nodes associated with the right upper lobe bronchus than with the bronchi to the middle and lower lobes. The node adjacent to the azygos vein is termed the azygos node. Because of its location it may become visible even when only slightly enlarged.

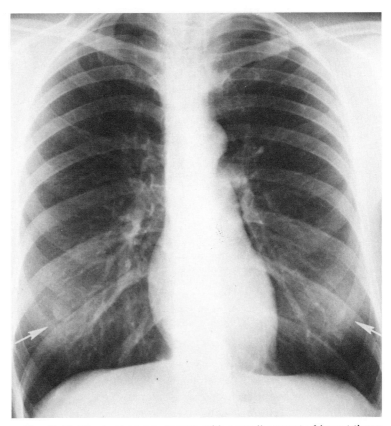

Fig. 22-13. Nipple shadows. Female with a small amount of breast tissue in whom nipple shadows appear as small rounded densities (**arrows**) in the sixth anterior interspace.

ROENTGEN FEATURES OF THE MEDIASTINUM. The trachea and main bronchi are usually visible in a chest roentgenogram of good quality. These structures lie within the mediastinum and the trachea is situated in the midline except for very slight deviation to the right at the level of the aortic arch. In older persons it may curve slightly to the left above the arch and then to the right as it passes the arch. It extends from the level of the sixth cervical vertebra downward to the level of the fifth thoracic vertebra or slightly lower, where it divides into the right and left main bronchial branches. It is identified on the roentgenogram as a band of radiolucency in the midline that extends from the lower cervical region downward to the point of bifurcation. The main bronchi are somewhat smaller in diameter (Fig. 22-15).

The right main bronchus continues downward more vertically than the left and divides into two main branches. The first branch is the upper lobe bronchus, which curves sharply upward above the right pulmonary artery and is termed the eparterial bronchus. The continuation downward is termed the hyparterial or common bronchus, which continues as the right lower lobe bronchus. The middle lobe bronchus arises from the hyparterial bronchus, extending downward and laterally from its point of origin. On the left side the main bronchus is somewhat longer than on the right and forms a greater angle with the trachea. In addition to a lateral angulation it curves outward in its distal porton and divides into a lower lobe bronchus and a left upper lobe bronchus that courses horizontally for a short

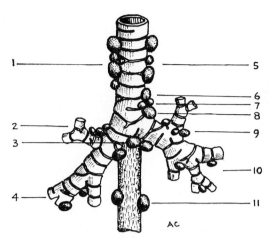

Fig. 22-14. The tracheobronchial lymph nodes. **(1)** Right paratracheal; **(2)** superior tracheobronchial (*right*); **(3)** inferior tracheobronchial (bifurcation); **(4)** right bronchopulmonary; **(5)** left paratracheal; **(6)** preaortic; **(7)** nodes of ligamentum arteriosum; **(8)** superior tracheobronchial (*left*); **(9)** superior bronchopulmonary (*left*); **(10)** bronchopulmonary; **(11)** paraesophageal.

distance before dividing. A continuation of the left main bronchus downward and laterally forms the lower lobe bronchus. It is usually possible to outline the main bronchi and portions of the upper and lower lobe bronchi in the normal patient. These structures have an appearance similar to that of the trachea, namely, a band of radiolucency but smaller in diameter.

In the frontal projection of the chest the mediastinum along with the sternum and thoracic spine form the dense central shadow as observed on the normal roentgenogram. On the right side the superior margin is formed by the innominate artery or vein, below which lies the superior vena cava. The ascending aortic arch is usually not border-forming but in cardiac diseases or aortic diseases that produce aortic dilatation it may be visualized. Immediately below the ascending aortic arch is the lung hilum. The smooth convex border of the right atrium forms the lower right mediastinal border. On the left side the left subclavian artery forms the superior aspect of the mediastinum. Below this the rounded convexity of the aortic arch is outlined. The pulmonary artery

and the hilum of the left lung lie immediately below the aortic arch and the left ventricle forms most of the left lower mediastinal border although a short segment of the pulmonary outflow tract may be visible below the hilum. In infancy the thymus is often a large structure that lies in the anterior portion of the superior mediastinum and extends down into the anterior mediastinum. When visible it produces widening of the mediastinum superiorly and this widening is often asymmetric; the thymus then forms the lateral border of the superior mediastinum on both sides. Classically, the inferior aspect of the enlarged thymus forms an acute angle on one or both sides, a configuration that has been likened to a ship's sail (Fig. 22-16). It is not unusual to note some lobulation of the thymus. When such superior mediastinal widening is present it is usually necessary to obtain a lateral projection in order definitely to ascertain that the shadow is in the anterior mediastinum and thus represents the thymus. Moderate widening of the superior mediastinal shadow is not considered abnormal in infancy; this portion of the mediastinum usually assumes its normal width during the first year of life.

The lungs approach the midline anteriorly in

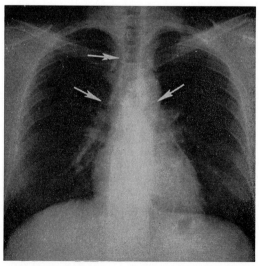

Fig. 22-15. Normal chest. **Arrows** indicate trachea and main bronchi.

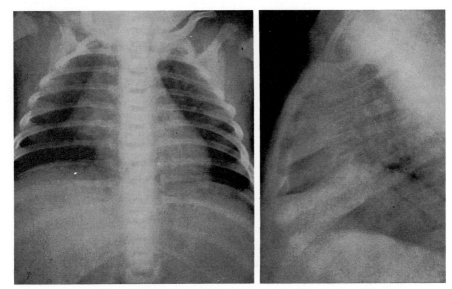

Fig. 22-16. Enlargement of the right lobe of the thymus. Note the angulation on the right, which represents the sail sign. *Right,* In the lateral view, anterior superior mediastinal density is produced by the thymus.

the anterior mediastinum. As a result the air in the lung on either side defines a vertical linear density sometimes called the anterior mediastinal line. It extends from a point near the level of the sternal angle superiorly to a point 3 or 4 inches below it. The "line" is visible on most roentgenograms of good quality. When one lung herniates across the midline, the line is displaced accordingly. The "line" thickens or diverges on either end.

The lungs also outline a "pleural" line in the paraspinal area on both sides. This is usually 2- to 5-mm thick, when measured from the lung to the lateral vertebral margin and is often most clearly defined on overexposed high-voltage films. A pleural line is also observed on the right in the lower thorax outlining the lateral esophageal wall; this is medial to the paraspinal pleural line in the normal.

The hilum of the lung contains the pulmonary artery, the pulmonary veins, the bronchus, the bronchial arteries and veins, as well as lymph nodes. In the normal chest the pulmonary arteries and veins produce most of the density outlined on the roentgenogram (Fig. 22-17). The left hilum is higher in position than the right because the left pulmonary ar-

tery extends above the left main bronchus while the right pulmonary artery crosses below the right upper lobe bronchus (Fig. 22-18). In the normal, the lymph nodes in the region of the hilum do not contribute enough to the hilar density to be identified but when enlarged or when these nodes contain calcium they can be recognized. The size of the hilum varies in the normal so that it is difficult to set a standard beyond which hilar size is abnormal. Since the size of the pulmonary vessels is related to pulmonary bloodflow, those vessels which make up the hila are increased when the bloodflow is increased and decreased in size in diseases that produce a diminution in pulmonary bloodflow. In addition to the variation in hilar size produced by the variability of caliber of the blood vessels, enlargement of hilar nodes may cause hilar enlargement; thus it is often difficult if not impossible to distinguish the cause for slight hilar enlargement. Fluoroscopy may be of some help in differentiating vascular from lymph node enlargement. When slight node enlargement does produce alteration in the hila it is often necessary to examine progress films to determine the presence or absence of actual enlargement.

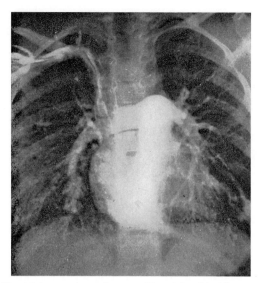

Fig. 22-17. Angiocardiogram. The right-sided heart chambers and the pulmonary arteries are opacified. The radiographic hilum on the left is somewhat higher and more prominent than on the right. There are some basal arteriovenous malformations bilaterally.

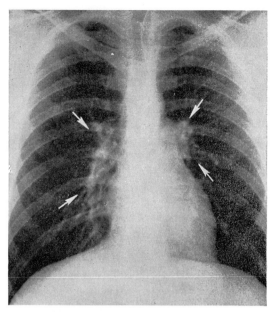

Fig. 22-18. Normal chest. Hila are well outlined and indicated by **arrows**. The difference in height is noted. Continuations of the hilar densities can be followed into the lung fields and are noted to branch in a treelike fashion. They represent pulmonary arteries.

In the lateral view of the chest the four anatomic divisions of the mediastinum are well demonstrated (Fig. 22-19). The anterior mediastinum is seen as an area of relative radiolucency between the sternum and the heart. It is roughly triangular in shape, with the apex pointing downward. The internal thoracic muscle may be seen as a flat, wedgelike, soft-tissue shadow immediately posterior to the lower sternum in the anterior mediastinum. This is more commonly observed in muscular males than in any other group. The superior mediastinum lies above it and the anterior aspect of the superior mediastinum is also radiolucent in the normal while the posterior portion is often somewhat opaque, owing to inability to elevate the soft parts of the shoulders and shoulder girdle enough to outline clearly this portion of the mediastinum. It is in the anterior mediastinum and anterior portion of the superior mediastinum that the enlarged thymus is noted as an area of density in infants. The middle mediastinum is clearly defined in a lateral roentgenogram, since it contains the heart and aorta. The posterior mediastinum is the area lying between the heart and the spine. It is visualized as a radiolucency of approximately the same density as that noted in the anterior mediastinum. The trachea is also visible in the lateral roentgenogram of the chest as a radiolucent structure that angles slightly posteriorly as it extends into the chest. The bifurcation is usually visible along with short segments of one or both bronchi. In this region an irregular, somewhat stellate density is noted that represents the vascular structures which produce the hila, the two being superimposed. In the examination of the mediastinum it is often of considerable value to opacify the esophagus by means of ingestion of thick barium paste. Then the relationship of the esophagus to the structures in the mediastinum can be determined and abnormalities can be clearly defined that would otherwise be very difficult to outline. The relationship of the esophagus to the trachea and its relation to the midline as well as to the heart can also be determined.

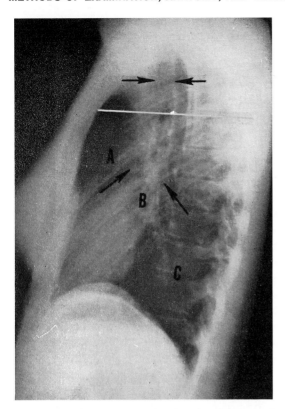

Fig. 22-19. Lateral chest showing the divisions of the mediastinum. The superior mediastinum lies above the line extending from the sternal angle to the fourth dorsal vertebra. **A**, the anterior mediastinum; **B**, the middle mediastinum; **C**, the posterior mediastinum. **Arrows** indicate the trachea in the superior mediastinum and the hila below it in the middle mediastinum.

THE LUNGS

LOBAR AND SEGMENTAL ANATOMY. The right lung is divided into three lobes, the upper, middle, and lower by two fissures. The major or primary interlobar fissure separates the lower lobe from the upper and middle, while the secondary (minor) fissure separates the middle from the upper lobe. On the left side there are two lobes separated by the major interlobar fissure. The major fissures are sometimes visible in the lateral roentgenogram in the normal and are readily visualized in this projection when there is a small amount of thickening of the interlobar pleura or small amount of fluid in the interlobar fissure. These fissures are visible in the frontal projection only when there is pleural disease or pleural thicken-

ing. The secondary interlobar fissure on the right is sometimes visible in the frontal projection in the normal (Fig. 22-20) and when pleural thickening is present can be easily identified in this projection as well as in the lateral view. It is horizontal and lies at the level of the anterior arc of the fourth rib or interspace. The major fissure on the right extends from the level of the fifth posterior rib downward and forward to the level of the sixth rib anteriorly while the left major fissure is slightly more vertical and extends from the level of the third to fifth posterior ribs down to the level of the seventh rib anteriorly. The levels are somewhat variable in the normal and in disease there may be marked variation in position. Occasionally, the major fissure on the right is directed slightly anteriorly into the sagittal plane in its lateral portion. It may then be visible as a "vertical" fissure line roughly paralleling the curve of the lower lateral chest wall. This is observed frequently in adults with small amounts of pleural fluid and has also been described in infants, particularly in those with cardiac enlargement.

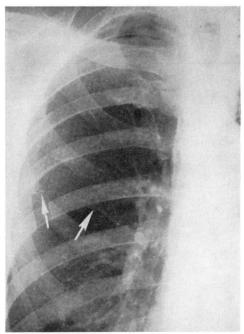

Fig. 22-20. Normal chest. **Arrows** indicate the secondary interlobar fissure on the right. It is slightly less horizontal in this patient than in the average and its lateral aspect is slightly higher in position. Note also small density in the fifth anterior interspace, representing nipple shadow.

The importance of bronchopulmonary segmental anatomy has increased now that advances in thoracic surgery have made segmental and subsegmental pulmonary resection a common procedure. These segments have been classified by a number of investigators, but the classification by Jackson and Huber[20] is now in general use and will be used here. The segments and subsegments are not strictly morphological units, since arteries may cross from one segment to another and the segments contain veins that drain adjacent segments. The bronchi to these lobes and segments are not outlined on the chest roentgenogram unless they are diseased. Therefore it is necessary to use bronchography if accurate localization of a small lesion to a segment is required. By means of lateral and oblique roentgenograms along with frontal film, it is often possible to be moderately accurate in localization of pulmonary parenchymal disease without bronchography. In chronic inflammations, however, it is common to have sufficient fibrosis and contraction to distort the involved segment as well as the adjacent segments to the point that localization is not accurate without bronchography. The positions and names of the bronchopulmonary segments are given in the accompanying roentgenograms and drawings (Figs. 22-21A through F).

ROENTGEN FEATURES. The normal lungs contain a considerable amount of air and since chest roentgenograms are taken in inspiration they appear much more radiolucent than other structures making up the thorax and its contents. There is a distinct radiographic pattern that is produced largely by the blood vessels as they extend from the hilum into the lungs. The large bronchi can often be visualized as radiolucent tubes in the hilum, adjacent to which are dense smooth-walled tubes that represent the pulmonary arterial branches. These vessels branch in a treelike manner and decrease in caliber rapidly as they extend into pulmonary parenchyma. This pattern is readily visible on the roentgenogram. The pulmonary arteries lie in close relationship to the bronchi and branch and subdivide the same as the bronchi. The pulmonary veins, on the other hand, have an anatomic distribution entirely separate from the bronchi.

The lung fields are often divided arbitrarily into zones, depending upon the size of the vessels. The inner zone or inner one third adjacent to the hilum contains the large main trunks. The middle zone contains intermediate-sized vessels and the peripheral one third of the lung or peripheral zone usually contains vessels that are less than 1 mm in diameter. The pulmonary veins cannot be differentiated from the arteries in the peripheral or middle zones but in the central zone the veins do not course near the arteries. They lie below the comparable arteries and empty into the left atrium at the lower margin of the hila. They rarely fuse into a single common trunk, so that there are usually two or more veins entering the atrium on either side. It is often difficult to outline them distinctly and differentiate them from arteries, but on tomograms they are visualized as smooth elongated densities extending into the region of the left atrium in the lower hilum on either side (Figs. 22-22 and 22-23). Occasionally they are clearly defined on a routine frontal chest roentgenogram. This is particularly true in patients with congenital cardiac defects resulting in high-volume, left-to-right shunts. In patients with venous congestion the upper lobe veins can often be visualized as hornlike structures extending into the lower hila from the medial aspects of the upper lobes.

The pulmonary vessels at the bases are generally larger than the vessels elsewhere and, since the right medial base is better visualized than the left, the trunks stand out more clearly in this region than elsewhere in the lung fields. The anteroposterior diameter of the chest is greater inferiorly than it is superiorly and this means that more vessels are superimposed at the bases than elsewhere. This factor also adds to the apparent difference in size and number of vessels between the upper and lower lung fields. The branched vascular markings tend to increase slightly in prominence with an increase in age of a given individual but there is marked variation in their size in the normal. Care is needed to avoid reading pulmonary disease into the chest roentgenogram of a patient in whom these vessels are slightly more prominent than usual. They can be identified by their smooth margins and decreasing caliber

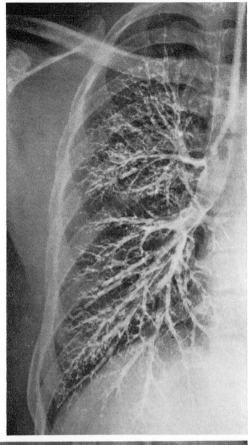

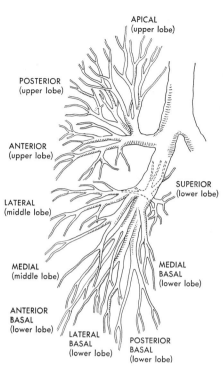

APICAL
(upper lobe)

POSTERIOR
(upper lobe)

ANTERIOR
(upper lobe)

SUPERIOR
(lower lobe)

LATERAL
(middle lobe)

MEDIAL
(middle lobe)

MEDIAL
BASAL
(lower lobe)

ANTERIOR
BASAL
(lower lobe)

LATERAL
BASAL
(lower lobe)

POSTERIOR
BASAL
(lower lobe)

Fig. 22-21**A**. Right lung. Bronchogram with diagram of the normal bronchopulmonary segments in the frontal projection. (*Courtesy Dr. J. Stauffer Lehman and Dr. Antrim Crellin, and Eastman Kodak Company.*)

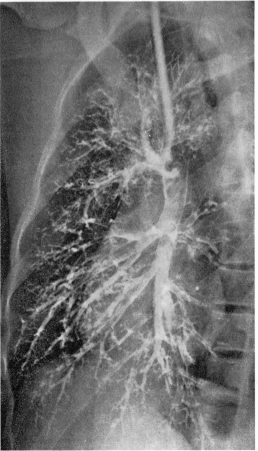

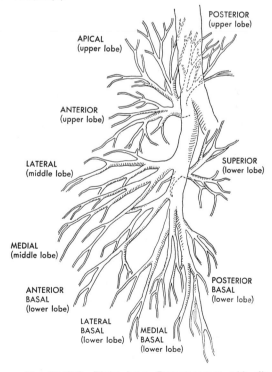

POSTERIOR
(upper lobe)

APICAL
(upper lobe)

ANTERIOR
(upper lobe)

LATERAL
(middle lobe)

SUPERIOR
(lower lobe)

MEDIAL
(middle lobe)

ANTERIOR
BASAL
(lower lobe)

POSTERIOR
BASAL
(lower lobe)

LATERAL
BASAL
(lower lobe)

MEDIAL
BASAL
(lower lobe)

Fig. 22-21**B**. Right lung. Bronchogram with diagram of the normal bronchopulmonary segments in the left anterior oblique projection. (*Courtesy Dr. J. Stauffer Lehman and Dr. Antrim Crellin, and Eastman Kodak Company.*)

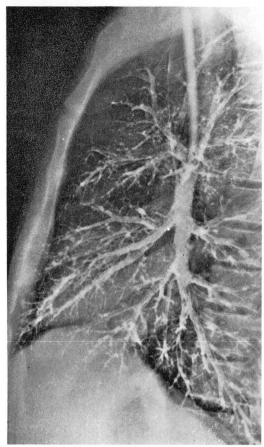

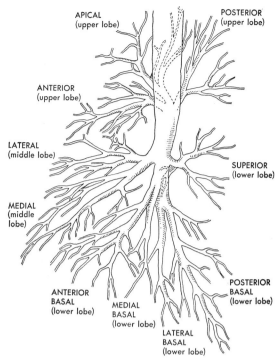

APICAL
(upper lobe)

POSTERIOR
(upper lobe)

ANTERIOR
(upper lobe)

LATERAL
(middle lobe)

SUPERIOR
(lower lobe)

MEDIAL
(middle
lobe)

ANTERIOR
BASAL
(lower lobe)

MEDIAL
BASAL
(lower lobe)

LATERAL
BASAL
(lower lobe)

POSTERIOR
BASAL
(lower lobe)

Fig. 22-21**C**. Right lung. Bronchogram with diagram of the normal bronchopulmonary segments in the lateral projection. (*Courtesy Dr. J. Stauffer Lehman and Dr. Antrim Crellin, and Eastman Kodak Company.*)

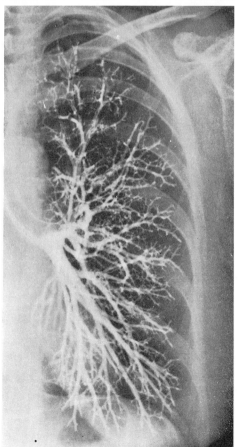

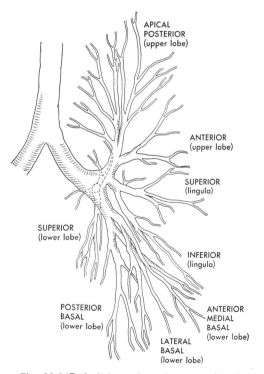

APICAL
POSTERIOR
(upper lobe)

ANTERIOR
(upper lobe)

SUPERIOR
(lingula)

SUPERIOR
(lower lobe)

INFERIOR
(lingula)

POSTERIOR
BASAL
(lower lobe)

ANTERIOR
MEDIAL
BASAL
(lower lobe)

LATERAL
BASAL
(lower lobe)

Fig. 22-21**D**. Left lung. Bronchogram with diagram of the normal bronchopulmonary segments in the frontal projection. (*Courtesy Dr. J. Stauffer Lehman and Dr. Antrim Crellin, and Eastman Kodak Company.*)

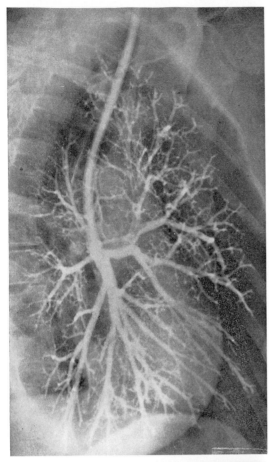

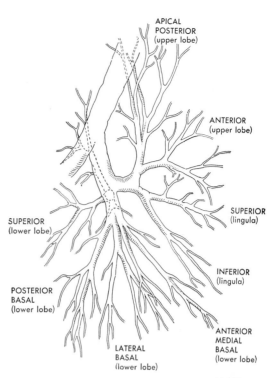

APICAL
POSTERIOR
(upper lobe)

ANTERIOR
(upper lobe)

SUPERIOR
(lingula)

INFERIOR
(lingula)

SUPERIOR
(lower lobe)

POSTERIOR
BASAL
(lower lobe)

LATERAL
BASAL
(lower lobe)

ANTERIOR
MEDIAL
BASAL
(lower lobe)

Fig. 22-21**E**. Left lung. Bronchogram with diagram of the normal bronchopulmonary segments in the right anterior oblique projection. (*Courtesy Dr. J. Stauffer Lehman and Dr. Antrim Crellin, and Eastman Kodak Company.*)

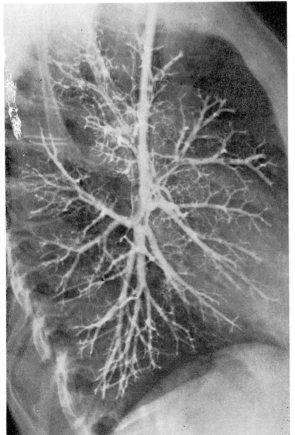

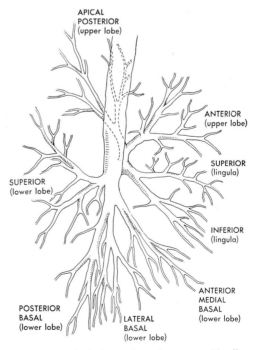

APICAL
POSTERIOR
(upper lobe)

ANTERIOR
(upper lobe)

SUPERIOR
(lingula)

INFERIOR
(lingula)

SUPERIOR
(lower lobe)

POSTERIOR
BASAL
(lower lobe)

LATERAL
BASAL
(lower lobe)

ANTERIOR
MEDIAL
BASAL
(lower lobe)

Fig. 22-21**F**. Left lung. Bronchogram with diagram of the normal bronchopulmonary segments in the lateral projection. (*Courtesy Dr. J. Stauffer Lehman and Dr. Antrim Crellin, and Eastman Kodak Company*).

as they leave the hilum along with the typical branching pattern.

In addition to the vascular markings in the lung fields, there are interstitial markings that are much less prominent. They produce a fine lacy or reticular pattern that is uniform throughout the lung fields and has a tendency to become more prominent with advancing age. These interstitial markings also stand out clearly in patients with emphysema and may be greatly increased in diseases that produce diffuse interstitial fibrosis in the lungs.

THE PULMONARY APEX. The lung apices occupy the portion of the thoracic cavity above the level of the clavicles as seen on the posteroanterior roentgenogram. Since pulmonary tuberculosis frequently begins in this area it is important to be able to differentiate pulmonary parenchymal disease from the various shadows representing normal soft-tissue structures that overlie the pulmonary apex. This portion of the lung is in the peripheral zone so that the markings due to vessels are very small and are often difficult to outline.

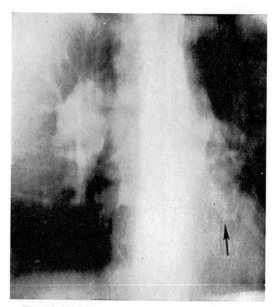

Fig. 22-23. Tomogram taken to outline mass involving the right hilum shows the pulmonary veins on the right; the pulmonary veins on the left are also moderately well shown (**arrow**). This also shows the value of tomography in outlining structures at a given level.

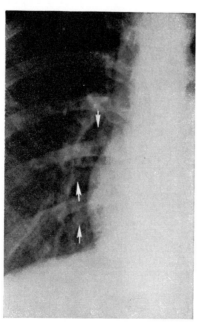

Fig. 22-22. Normal chest, with good visualization of the right pulmonary veins, which are indicated by **arrows**.

Several soft-tissue structures can be demonstrated on most chest roentgenograms in normal patients. The supraclavicular border or companion shadow is a linear band of soft-tissue density that parallels the clavicle and extends for 2 or 3 mm to 1 cm above it, depending upon the amount of subcutaneous tissue in the individual. It represents the skin and subcutaneous tissue visualized tangentially as they cover the superior clavicular margin. This shadow can be followed lateral to the pulmonary apex and can therefore be readily identified as being outside the lung. It often fades off medially with only a small lateral portion visualized or it may be apparent as far as the clavicular attachment of the sternocleidomastoid muscle. This muscle produces another soft-tissue density, which is a vertical shadow clearly defined laterally. It can be traced upward into the neck above the pulmonary apex and can thus be identified (Fig. 22-24). The muscle is not visible in all patients but is particularly well outlined in those who are old or emaciated. The medial

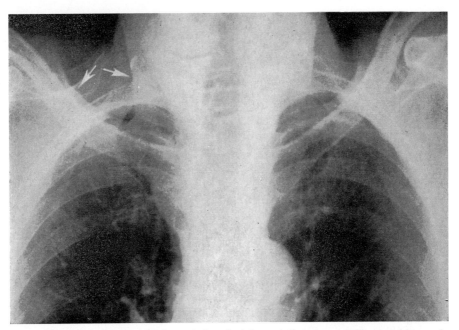

Fig. 22-24. Companion shadow of the clavicle and the sternocleidomastoid muscle are indicated by **arrows**.

borders of the pulmonary apices are formed by the superior mediastinum. The soft-tissue margin of the left mediastinal border is smooth and slightly concave owing to the curve of the left subclavian artery that forms it. On the right side the medial soft-tissue mediastinal demarcation is produced by the innominate artery or superior vena cava and is often slightly less distinct than on the left side, particularly in younger individuals. When the innominate artery becomes tortuous and dilated in patients with arteriosclerotic disease this margin may become more distinct and actually convex.

The posterior portions of the upper three and sometimes the fourth rib lie above the clavicle and the bony structures are readily identified. Companion or border shadows are sometimes visible along the inferior aspects of the upper two ribs and are identified as smooth linear bands from 1 to 3 mm in thickness. The densities are parallel to the inferior rib margins (Fig. 22-25). Occasionally a very thin border shadow will be noted in the same relationship to the posterior arc of the third rib. These findings are produced by the soft tissues beneath these ribs, which are at a tangent to the roentgen-ray beam. There is enough soft-tissue density made up of pleura, subpleural connective tissue, and intercostal arteries and veins to produce them.

The pleura at the extreme lung apex is often thickened and is recognized on the roentgenogram as a soft-tissue density. These shadows are commonly termed apical pleural scars or caps and represent thickened pleura, usually the result of inflammatory disease. It has been generally recognized that although a number of the lesions are definitely tuberculous in origin, many of them represent nonspecific pleural disease. It is possible that there are a number of these lesions that actually represent residues of tuberculosis in which the typical granulation tissue cannot be found, nor can the organisms be identified or cultured. It is likely that the scars are of more significance in relation to tuberculosis when present in young individuals than in patients of advanced age. Although this shadow of apical pleural thickening often presents as a soft-tissue density below the inferior aspect of the second rib, there are certain

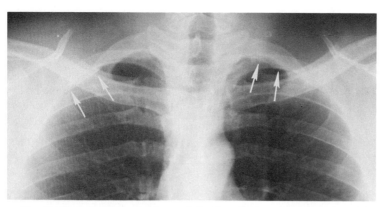

Fig. 22-25. Companion shadows of the first (*left*) and second ribs (*right*) are indicated by **arrows.**

characteristics that differentiate it from the companion shadow of this rib. In pleural scarring, the density is likely to vary somewhat and the thickness is often asymmetric on the two sides in contrast to the symmetry and homogeneous density of the companion shadows. Furthermore, the inferior surface of the pleural scar is likely to be somewhat irregular while that of the companion shadow is perfectly smooth in outline (Fig. 22-26).

THE DIAPHRAGM

The diaphragm is a muscular structure that separates the thorax from the abdomen. Its superior surface is covered by parietal pleura. There is a central membranous portion, called central tendon, in which there is no muscle. The diaphragm arches upward toward the central tendon to form a smooth, dome-shaped appearance on both sides. It is attached to the xiphoid process and lower costal cartilages anteriorly, the ribs laterally and the ribs and upper lumbar vetebrae posteriorly. In the roentgenogram, the upper surface of the diaphragm is clearly defined as a smooth, dome-shaped density that stands out in sharp contrast to the aerated lung above it. In the frontal projection the most inferior visible portion of the diaphragm meets the lateral chest wall at an acute angle. This is called the costophrenic angle or sulcus. It is sharply and clearly defined

in the normal but may be obliterated in diseases that produce pleural effusion, thickening, or adhesions. The position of the diaphragm varies considerably with the body habitus of the individual, with respiration, and with the position of the patient at the time the roentgenogram is taken. These factors should be known to interpret correctly alterations in height of the diaphragm. It is apparent, therefore, that there can be no accurate standard for position of the diaphragm but in the average adult during moderately deep inspiration the right dome of the diaphragm lies in the region of the fifth anterior interspace or at the level of the rib above or below it, while that on the left is slightly lower in position. The position of the

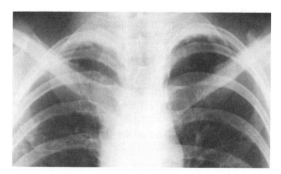

Fig. 22-26. Apical pleural thickening in a patient with minimal right upper lobe tuberculosis. Note the irregularity of the soft-tissue density at both apices. Note also the irregular nodular disease in the right second anterior interspace.

diaphragm in children and young adults is somewhat higher, while in the aged the diaphragm is usually lower in position. In the supine and recumbent positions the diaphragm is higher than in the upright.

In the lateral roentgenogram the right and left diaphragmatic domes are outlined as separate structures since they are usually not at the same level. The dome of the diaphragm is slightly anterior to the midpoint between the anterior and posterior chest walls. On the average the anterior aspect of the diaphragm is at the level of the anterior arc of the sixth rib or interspace while the posterior sulcus is at or slightly below the level of the twelfth rib. It is usually possible to identify the diaphragm on either side in the lateral roentgenogram even though it may be at or very near the same level, because the anterior aspect of the left dome is obscured by the heart above it while the anterior portion of the right side stands out clearly. In addition, there is often gas in the stomach or colon immediately beneath the left hemidiaphragm, which aids in its identification in this projection. There are several normal openings in the diaphragm as well as several weak areas that are indicated in Figure 31-20. Diaphragmatic hernia may present through these openings; these abnormalities are described in Chapter 31.

THE PLEURA

The pleura is a thin, serous membrane that is visible roentgenographically only when it is seen in contrast to adjacent structures that are more or less dense. Thus the visceral pleura is not often definitely visualized in the normal. When pneumothorax is present, it is outlined as the thin outer wall of the lung. It is also occasionally visible when a sufficient part of it is parallel to the roentgen-ray beam; e.g., the secondary interlobar fissure on the right, made up of the visceral pleura covering the inferior aspect of the upper lobe and the superior aspect of the middle lobe, is visible in approximately 20 per cent of patients as a thin, straight, horizontal line. The major fissures are occasionally visible on a lateral roentgenogram in the absence of disease. The parietal pleura covers the diaphragm and lines the thorax but it blends with the other structures of the chest wall and is not separately identified on roentgenograms. The relationships of visceral pleura to the bony thorax are shown in Figure 22-27.

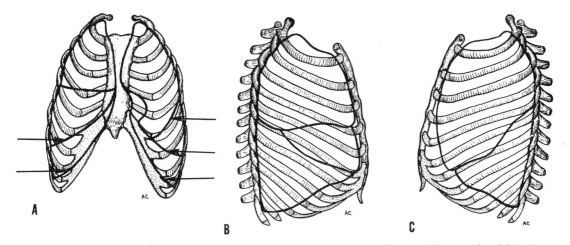

Fig. 22-27. *A,* Relation of the visceral pleura to the bony thorax in the frontal plane: on the right, **upper arrow** indicates the anterior inferior border, **lower arrow** the posterior inferior border. On the *left,* anterior (**upper and middle arrows**); posterior (**lower arrow**). *B,* Visceral pleura on the right as visualized in the left lateral projection. Note primary and secondary interlobar fissures separating the three lobes. *C,* Pleural outlines on the left as visualized in the right lateral position.

THE CHEST IN INFANCY AND CHILDHOOD

In the newborn infant the thorax is deep in its anteroposterior diameter as compared to the lateral diameter. The diaphragm is higher and this makes the vertical diameter of the thoracic cavity less than in the adult. With growth the chest becomes narrower in its anteroposterior diameter but the vertical and lateral diameters gradually increase. The ribs are nearly horizontal in position and they gradually angulate downward as the child grows. The sternum is incompletely ossified at birth and this structure ossifies in a segmental manner. There are two ossification centers lying side by side in each segment. The centers for the manubrium are united at birth but the remainder may not fuse for several years. The centers are of radiographic importance because they appear as small rounded densities that may overlie the lung fields in oblique or semi-oblique projections; they should be recognized as ossification centers and not be mistaken for lesions within the pulmonary parenchyma.

The thymus gland is often large enough in the newborn period or early infancy to produce widening of the superior mediastinum. The roentgen appearance has been described in the section on "Roentgen Features of the Mediastinum" (see Fig. 22-19). The appearance of the heart in the infant and child differs considerably from that in the adult. The heart in the newborn is globular in shape and relatively larger in comparison to the diameter of the chest than in adults. The left ventricle becomes more prominent with increase in age, resulting in downward displacement of the apex, and the relative heart size gradually decreases. These changes are discussed more fully in the chapter on cardiovascular disease.

The lung fields in the infant and child tend to be slightly more radiolucent than in the adult, since the interstitial markings are less prominent, but the relative size of the visible vascular trunks is comparable. The root of the lung making up the hilar shadow is relatively high and is usually situated at the level of the third dorsal vertebra. The tracheal bifurcation gradually descends and reaches the adult level (fifth dorsal vertebra) at about 10 years of age.

The diaphragm tends to be higher in infancy and childhood than in adult life and in the newborn it is not unusual to note a reversal of the adult situation with regard to relative height. The left hemidiaphragm is slightly higher than the right, probably because the stomach is frequently distended with air. There is considerable variation in position of the diaphragm in infancy and childhood and the same factors of position of the patient as well as habitus are involved as have been previously noted in the discussion of the adult diaphragm (Fig. 22-28).

THE CHEST IN ADVANCING AGE

There is gradual alteration in the shape of the bony thorax with advancing age. The amount of alteration varies widely and there is also a great individual variation in the age at which these changes appear and become marked. The tendency is for a gradual increase in the dorsal kyphotic curve, resulting in an increased anteroposterior diameter of the chest; it may approach or even exceed the transverse diameter in some instances. Varying amounts of decalcification may be noted in the bones visualized in the chest roentgenogram, because of senile osteoporosis. Rib irregularities from ancient healed fractures are commonly noted and more or less calcification may be seen in costal cartilages. This calcification varies greatly in amount and tends to appear earlier in females than males. Its roentgen appearance is that of calcific density outlining the cartilage and extending from the anterior rib edge toward the sternum.

The changes in the mediastinum with advancing age are largely caused by alteration in the aorta and its branches, which tend to become elongated and tortuous. As a result the right superior mediastinal border may become more prominent and clearly defined, because of increasing visibility of the innominate artery.

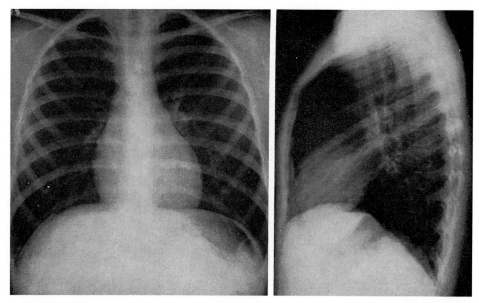

Fig. 22-28. The normal chest in a 10-year-old child. Note that the heart is somewhat globular and the anteroposterior diameter of the chest is relatively large in comparison to the transverse diameter.

The ascending arch of the aorta projects farther to the right and causes a definite convex shadow of soft-tissue density, the lower half of which overlies the right hilum. Similar prominence of the left upper mediastinum may be apparent with sclerotic changes in the left subclavian artery and the aortic knob tends to become increasingly prominent (Fig. 22-29). The presence of calcification in the aortic arch is common and calcification in the innominate and subclavian arteries is not rare. Pulmonary vessels making up the roentgenographic hilar shadows may become larger, particularly when emphysema or other pulmonary abnormality results in increased pressure within the lesser circulation.

Alteration in appearance of the lung fields varies widely with advancing age but there is a general tendency for the vessels in the mid and peripheral zones to be separated by hyperdistention of alveoli representing emphysema, and this is often associated with increase in size of the vessels in the midzones and hila. In addition, it is not uncommon to see linear shadows produced by residues of previous inflammatory disease in one or both bases and there is a tendency for the reticular interstitial pattern to become more pronounced. Small pulmonary parenchymal calcific foci are common along with calcification in hilar nodes. Apical pleural scarring producing irregular soft-tissue densities at the extreme apices is also found commonly in the aged and it is not uncommon to find one or both costophrenic sulci at least partially obliterated by previous basal pleural disease. The diaphragm tends to become lower and flatter with the alteration in the shape of the bony thorax and the appearance of senile emphysema. Irregularities of the diaphragm resulting from pleural inflammatory residuals is not uncommon. As the diaphragm becomes lower the dome becomes more horizontal and the costophrenic angles less acute.

CONGENITAL MALFORMATIONS

THE BONY THORAX

Minor developmental abnormalities are common in the ribs and are usually of no clinical significance, but should be noted and

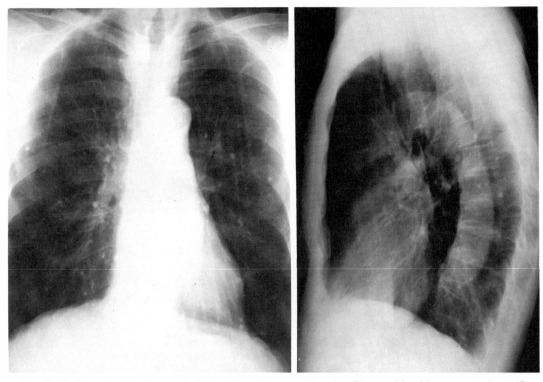

Fig. 22-29. The chest in the aged. Patient is a 71-year-old male with considerable amount of calcification in the aortic wall, aortic dilatation, and elongation. The lungs are slightly hyperlucent, the thoracic curve is increased, with resultant increase in anteroposterior chest diameter. Scattered parenchymal calcifications represent residues of previous histoplasmosis.

recognized as such on the roentgenogram. Cervical ribs are not uncommon and may be very small and difficult to outline or long and easily recognized as they project downward to overlie the pulmonary apex. Occasionally the transverse processes of the seventh cervical vertebra are unusually long and simulate short cervical ribs. One or both first ribs are often rudimentary in type. The most common anomaly of the remaining ribs is an anterior bifurcation, usually resulting in a broad, thin rib anteriorly that bifurcates in its anterior few centimeters. Complete fusion along the arcs of the ribs and pseudarthrosis between the ribs are other common anomalies. Intrathoracic rib is extremely rare. The anomalous rib usually arises from the posterior inferior margin of an otherwise normal rib or from a vertebral body, most often on the right side. The rib is sometimes

attached to the diaphragm by a fibrous band. It projects into the pleural space and may be surrounded by lung. Diagnosis is suspected on chest roentgenogram and confirmed by tomography or fluoroscopy.

Anterior protrusion deformities of the sternum resulting in the so-called "pigeon breast" are usually so mild that no significant abnormality is noted on the frontal projection and only on the lateral view can the diagnosis be made. In these patients the sternum protrudes anteriorly to a greater or lesser degree. The amount of protrusion is readily apparent on the lateral roentgenogram of the chest.

Funnel chest deformity or pectus excavatum produces changes that can usually be recognized on a posteroanterior roentgenogram. These alterations are described on page 1030. In the lateral projection the posterior displacement of the sternum is readily discerned. Congenital midline defect in the sternum is a rare anomaly. The sternum is divided into equal halves by the fissure, which is easily recognized on the roentgenograms. Rarely, small accessory ossicles are noted immediately above the manubrium in the region of the suprasternal notch. They are termed episternal or suprasternal bones; they may be single or paired and range from a few millimeters to more than a centimeter in diameter. They may be fused to the manubrium or articulate with it; or there may be no contact with the sternun.

Scoliosis is a frequent abnormality in the thoracic spine and may be congenital. Hemivertebrae and other vertebral anomalies occur in conjunction with scoliosis and often produce it. In many instances, however, no definite anomaly is noted involving the vertebral bodies. The deformity of the thorax is proportional to the severity of the scoliosis and when marked, the anatomic alteration produced in the heart and lungs may result in alteration in cardiac and pulmonary function. Kyphosis often accompanies scoliosis and adds to the thoracic deformity. Kyphosis of the thoracic spine may also occur as an isolated deformity. It results in an increase in the anteroposterior diameter and a decrease in the vertical diameter of the thorax.

PULMONARY AGENESIS AND HYPOGENESIS (HYPOPLASIA)

Aplasia of the lung is a rare anomaly, based on failure of one of the lung buds to appear in early embryonic development. It may be anatomically complete or there may be a small bronchus with or without a small amount of pulmonary tissue. The left lung is involved somewhat more frequently than the right; in the few reported cases the anomaly has been found in males more than females in a ratio of three to two. Roentgen findings on routine examination include a marked shift of the heart and other mediastinal structures to the involved side with decrease in size of that hemithorax; herniation of the normal lung across the midline; and evidence of increase

in volume of the normal lung, which is very likely due to a combination of hyperplasia and compensatory emphysema. Bronchography is necessary to visualize the bronchial tree and, on this examination, either a small bronchial stump or no bronchus at all is visualized. No lung is noted on the involved side except that which has herniated across the midline from the normal side. Angiocardiography can be used to outline the vascular system and will demonstrate the single pulmonary artery to the normal lung and thus confirm the diagnosis.

Pulmonary hypogenesis indicates incomplete development of the lung or a part of it and is also uncommon. All gradations from minor to severe degrees of hypoplasia may occur. Unless the anomaly is severe, there is usually very little alteration in the size of the affected hemithorax because some normal lung tissue remains; mediastinal shift along with elevation of the diaphragm on the involved side and compensatory emphysema on the opposite side all help to fill the hemithorax. One lobe may be completely missing or hypoplastic so that bronchography may be necessary for diagnosis. This condition must be differentiated from the results of previous inflammatory disease producing fibrosis and contraction of a lobe or portion of a lobe. The evidence of previous disease may be apparent, but if not, bronchography can be used to show the bronchial distribution.

ACCESSORY LOBES AND FISSURES

AZYGOS LOBE

The azygos lobe is formed when the arch of the azygos vein fails to migrate medially to lie in its normal position just above the right main bronchus. This vein remains lateral to its normal position and the small portion of the apex of the lung that lies medial to it early in development is deeply invaginated. The vessel carries two layers of visceral pleura and two layers of parietal pleura with it since it lies peripheral to the parietal pleura. As a result, the pleural fissure is visible as a thin curvilinear line extending upward toward the apex to end at the parietal pleura of the apex. This line is

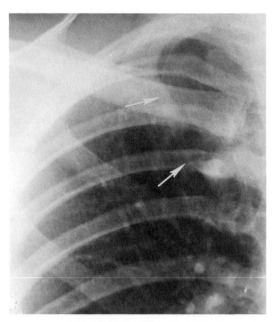

Fig. 22-30. Azygos lobe. Note the vein below the sternal end of the clavicle and the fissure (**arrows**) extending in an arc up to the central apex.

usually bowed outward and its base, formed by the vein itself, is comma-shaped with the tail of the comma pointing upward toward the fissure (Fig. 22-30). The size of the azygos lobe varies but it is seldom very large. It is a common anomaly said to occur in 0.5 per cent of the population and is usually of no significance.

THE INFERIOR ACCESSORY LOBE

The inferior accessory or cardiac lobe is the most common accessory lobe. The fissure may be complete or incomplete and is visualized on the posteroanterior roentgenogram as a faint line at the right medial base beginning at the diaphragm and extending upward toward the hilum. It arches somewhat with lateral convexity and there is often a very small upward projection at the diaphragmatic end of the fissure. This accessory lobe is usually supplied by a bronchus branching off the posterior basal segment of the lower lobe. The anomaly is less common on the left than on the right and is more difficult to see because it is often hidden by the cardiac shadow. It is of no particular

significance but occasionally becomes involved by disease and is then more readily identified (Fig. 22-31).

OTHER ACCESSORY LOBES

The left upper lobe may be divided in a manner similar to the division on the right producing an accessory middle lobe. In these instances the interlobar fissure that divides the upper and accessory lobes is in approximately the same position as the secondary fissure on the right. This is a rare anomaly and of no clinical significance.

The posterior lobe is produced when the superior segment of the lower lobe is separated from the basal segments of the lower lobe by a horizontal fissure. This accessory lobe is rarely identified radiographically unless it is involved by disease sufficient to outline the smooth fissure separating it from the base of the lower lobe. It is somewhat more common anatomically, however, than radiographic examination would indicate.

Supernumerary bronchi are also commonly found and can be recognized roentgenographically only on bronchography, since they result in supernumerary segments rather than lobes. The most common site is the right upper lobe where the anomalous bronchus arises from the lateral aspect of the right main bronchus above the upper lobe bronchus. Occasionally it arises from

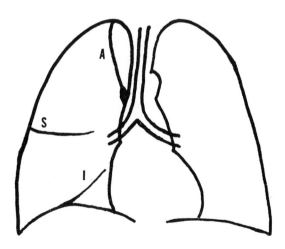

Fig. 22-31. Sketch shows position of the two most common accessory fissures: **A,** azygos; **I,** inferior accessory lobe fissure. The secondary interlobar fissure is also indicated as **S.**

the lower right trachea. Minor variation in origin of segmental bronchi is not uncommon and displacement of a bronchus is often difficult or impossible to differentiate from a supernumerary bronchus. Numerous minor variations of bronchial segmentation have been found in all lobes and are not uncommonly visualized on bronchographic examination. An entire lobe may be affected or there may be one or more segments involved (Fig. 22-32).

ABSENCE OF FISSURES

Variations of interlobar fissures are relatively common but since they occur without alteration in bronchopulmonary segmentation they produce no roentgenographic findings. In a study of 1200 lungs in cases of sudden death, Medlar[25] found the interlobar fissure on the left complete in 82 per cent while the major fissure on the right was complete in 69 per cent and the secondary fissure complete in only 37.7 per cent. In the remainder the fissures were absent or incomplete.

BRONCHOPULMONARY SEQUESTRATION

Intralobar sequestration of the lung or bronchopulmonary sequestration refers to a congenital anomaly in which a systemic artery arising from the lower thoracic or upper abdominal aorta extends into the lung on either side, where it supplies a portion of pulmonary tissue that is not connected with the normal bronchial tree and is therefore termed "sequestered." It is drained by the pulmonary venous system. This sequestered lung forms the site of a congenital cyst that may be uni- or multilocular. If it is uninfected, the lesion produces no symptoms. If it becomes infected and communicates with the bronchial tree, signs and

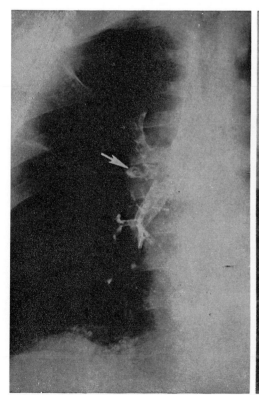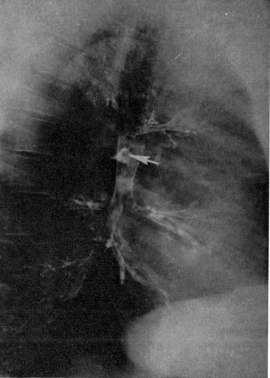

Fig. 22-32. Accessory lobe arising below the right upper lobe bronchus. This accessory bronchus is outlined on the bronchogram but its branches are not filled because of the presence of a small intraluminal lipoma (**arrows**) partially obstructing it.

symptoms are produced. It is almost entirely a lower lobe lesion and usually involves the posterior basal segment of the lower lobe; the number reported in each lower lobe is approximately equal. The lesions have been found somewhat more frequently in males than in females; the ratio is approximately two to one.

Roentgen findings depend upon the presence or absence of infection. In the patients in whom there is no infection, the condition is usually an incidental finding and presents as a round or oval mass in the posterior lung base on either side that may range up to 10 cm or more in diameter. It is usually found in the medial aspect of the lung base and occasionally a poorly defined, fingerlike projection extends toward the mediastinum from the medial aspect of the mass representing the artery supplying the tissue. When infection is present there is enough bronchial communication so that fluid levels and air are usually visible in a single cyst or in several adjacent cysts the walls of which are usually thin, if they are not obscured by infection in the adjacent lung. Even though there is evidence of bronchial commu-

nication manifested by the presence of air within the cysts, bronchography does not ordinarily demonstrate the communication and no oil enters the cysts. The lesion must be differentiated from lung abscess, acquired infected cysts, and chronic pulmonary inflammatory disease with cavitation. The asymptomatic type with no apparent connection with the bronchi must be differentiated from tumors and cysts of other origin. The location of these lesions is rather characteristic however and when a soft-tissue mass or an infected cyst is noted in the area, intralobar sequestration should be considered (Fig. 22-33). If this lesion is suspected, the diagnosis can be confirmed by aortography, sometimes with selective opacification of the anomalous artery.

Extralobar sequestration results when the sequestered tissue is contained in its own pleural covering between the lower lobe and the diaphragm, or even beneath the diaphragm. This form of sequestration is drained by the vena cava or azygos venous system. It is on the left side in 90 per cent. It is asymptomatic and is therefore an incidental roentgen finding. Associated congenital anomalies are common;

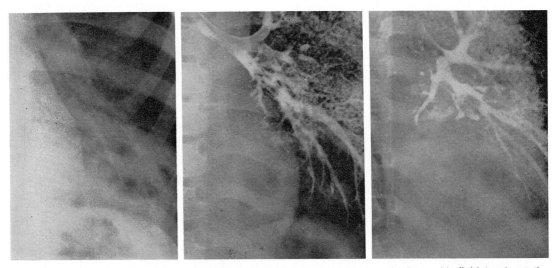

Fig. 22-33. Bronchopulmonary sequestration. *Left,* There are several cavitations with fluid levels at the left lung base in addition to density caused by inflammatory disease. The posteroanterior (*center*), and right anterior oblique (*right*) bronchograms show displacement of bronchi by the infected sequestration. (*Courtesy of Dr. Charles Benkendorf, Green Bay, Wisconsin.*)

eventration of the diaphragm being a frequent associated finding. In addition to an abnormal diaphragm, a mass representing the sequestered lung may be visible. Aortography can be used for confirmation when sequestration is suspected. The venous drainage differentiates it from the intralobar form.

BRONCHIAL (BRONCHOPULMONARY) CYSTS

Most cystic lesions of the lung are now believed to be acquired, but it is likely that the cysts occurring within the lung, lined by bronchial epithelium and resembling the bronchogenic cysts found in the mediastinum, represent congenital rather than acquired lesions. They are usually solitary and may occur anywhere within the lung. They present as rounded, clearly defined, intrapulmonary, soft-tissue masses. This lesion produces no symptoms and may be found on routine chest roentgenograms. If the cyst becomes infected and communicates with the bronchus, the roentgen findings are those of a thin-walled cavity containing gas and fluid that may be considerably obscured by inflammatory disease in the adjacent lung. The subject of cysts is discussed more fully in Chapter 24.

CONGENITAL CYSTIC ADENOMATOID MALFORMATION OF THE LUNG

This is a rare form of congenital cystic disease of the lung in which neonatal respiratory distress is often present. It usually involves a single lobe which is greatly enlarged and consists of a mass of disorganized tissue. The lobe is firm and rubbery and consists of multiple cysts of varying size, with no normal bronchial or lobular pulmonary pattern. Radiological findings are those of a pulmonary mass which displaces the mediastinum and heart and often herniates into the opposite hemithorax. The multiple cysts result in a coarse, honeycombed appearance. Irregular areas of density

often outline some of the cysts and form part of the enlarged lobe. Surgical removal is necessary to allow the remaining normal lung to expand.

CONGENITAL PULMONARY LYMPHANGIECTASIS

This is a rare congenital disease which causes neonatal respiratory distress. The lungs are large and lobulated with prominent subpleural lymphatics which are cystic. Lobular septae are enlarged by the cystic lymphatics. Roentgen findings are those of bilateral increase in density with some granularity which simulates the findings in hyaline membrane disease. Most affected infants survive for only a short time.

MISCELLANEOUS MALFORMATIONS

Congenital tracheoesophageal fistula is present in approximately 70 per cent of infants with esophageal atresia. This subject is discussed in Chapter 15, in the section on "Atresia of the esophagus." Tracheal atresia is a rare condition that is incompatible with life and need not be discussed here. Congenital stenosis of the trachea is also a rare anomaly that may involve a short portion or a relatively long segment of the trachea. It is usually associated with an anomaly of the tracheal cartilages ranging from absence of cartilages to complete cartilaginous rings. Congenital stenosis must be differentiated from tracheal narrowing caused by extrinsic pressure from thymic enlargement or other upper mediastinal or low cervical masses. In the latter, the causative mass is usually visible on the roentgenogram or can be noted fluoroscopically. It is important to realize that the trachea in the infant is relatively pliable even in the normal so that it may appear unusually narrow in a single roentgenogram in patients without stenosis. It is, therefore, important to fluoroscope these infants and determine tracheal size during the phases of respiration. Congenital vascular lesions such as hemangioma may also involve the trachea and produce enough obstruction to cause stridor. Radiographic findings are not specific but may show local narrowing at the site of the vascular lesion. These patients often have hemangiomata elsewhere, which aids in the diagnosis. Malformations of the pulmonary vascular system are discussed in Chapter 32.

REFERENCES AND SELECTED READINGS

1. ABLOW, R. C., GREENSPAN, R. H., and GLUCK, L.: The advantages of direct magnification technic in the newborn chest. *Radiology 92:* 745, 1969.

2. BENFIELD, J. R., BONNEY, H., CRUMMY, A. B., and CLEVELAND, R. J.: Azygograms and pulmonary arteriograms in bronchogenic carcinoma. *Arch. Surg. 99:* 406, 1969.

3. BERMAN, E. J.: Extralobar (diaphragmatic) sequestration of the lung. *Arch. Surg. 76:* 724, 1958.

4. BERNE, A. S., IKINS, P. M., STRAEHLEY, C. J., JR., and BUGDEN, W. F.: Diagnostic carbon dioxide pneumomediastinography. *N. Engl. J. Med. 267:* 225, 1962.

5. BOYDEN, E. A.: A synthesis of the prevailing pattern of the bronchopulmonary segments in the light of their variations. *Dis. Chest 15:* 657, 1949.

6. BOYDEN, E. A.: The distribution of bronchi in gross anomalies of the right upper lobe, particularly lobes subdivided by the azygos vein and those containing pre-eparterial bronchi. *Radiology 58:* 797, 1952.

7. BROCK, R. C.: *The Anatomy of the Bronchial Tree with Special Reference to the Surgery of Lung Abscess.* London, Oxford University Press, 1946.

8. BROWN, W. H.: Episternal bones. *Radiology 75:* 116, 1960.

9. CAFFEY, J.: *Pediatric X-ray Diagnosis,* 5th ed. Chicago, Year Book, 1967.

10. CARTER, R. W., and VAUGHN, H. M.: Congenital pulmonary lymphangiectasis. *Am. J. Roentgenol. Radium Ther. Nucl. Med. 86:* 576, 1961.

11. CIMMINO, C. V.: The anterior mediastinal line on chest roentgenograms. *Radiology 82:* 459, 1964.

12. CRAIG, J. M., KIRKPATRICK, J., and NEUHAUSER, E. B. D.: Congenital cystic adenomatoid malformation of the lung in infants. *Am. J. Roentgenol. Radium Ther. Nucl. Med. 76:* 516, 1956.

13. CRUMMY, A. B., WEGNER, G. P., FLAHERTY, T. T., BENFIELD, J. R., BRUNETTE, K. W., and FRANCYK, W. P.: Azygos venography, an aid in the evaluation of esophageal carcinoma. *Ann. Thorac. Surg. 6:* 522, 1968.

14. DAVIS, L. A.: The vertical fissure line. *Am. J. Roentgenol. Radium Ther. Nucl. Med. 84:* 451, 1960.

15. FELSON, B.: *Fundamentals of Chest Roentgenology.* Philadelphia, Saunders, 1960.

16. FELSON, B., and FELSON, H.: Localization of intrathoracic lesions by means of the posteroanterior roentgenogram. *Radiology 55:* 363, 1950.

17. FENNESSY, J. J.: Bronchial brushing in the diagnosis of peripheral lung lesions. *Am. J. Roentgenol. Radium Ther. Nucl. Med. 98:* 474, 1966.

18. FERGUSON, C. F., and NEUHAUSER, E. B. D.: Congenital absence of the lung and other anomalies of the tracheobronchial tree. *Am. J. Roentgenol. Radium Ther. Nucl. Med. 52:* 459, 1944.

19. FRASER, R. G., and PARÉ, J. A. P.: *Diagnosis of the Diseases of the Chest.* Philadelphia, Saunders, 1970, vols. 1 and 2.*

20. JACKSON, C. L., and HUBER, J. F.: Correlated applied anatomy of the bronchial tree and lungs with a system of nomenclature. *Dis. Chest 9:* 319, 1943.

21. JACKSON, F. I.: The air-gap technique, and an improvement by anteroposterior positioning for chest roentgenography. *Am. J. Roentgenol. Radium Ther. Nucl. Med. 92:* 688, 1964.

22. KRAUSE, G. R., and LUBERT, M.: Anatomy of the bronchopulmonary segments: Clinical applications. *Radiology 56:* 333, 1951.

23. LACHMAN, E.: The dynamic concept of thoracic topography. *Am. J. Roentgenol. Radium Ther. Nucl. Med. 56:* 419, 1946.

24. LARSEN, L. L., and IBACH, H. F.: Complete congenital fissure of the sternum. *Am. J. Roentgenol. Radium Ther. Nucl. Med. 87:* 1062, 1962.

25. MEDLAR, E. M.: Variations in interlobar fissures. *Am. J. Roentgenol. Radium Ther. Nucl. Med. 57:* 723, 1947.

26. MESCHAN, I.: *An Atlas of Normal Radiographic Anatomy.* Philadelphia, Saunders, 1951.

27. MICHELSON, E., and SALIK, J. O.: The vascular pattern of the lung as seen on routine and tomographic studies. *Radiology 73:* 511, 1959.

28. MOLNAR, W., and PRIOR, J. A.: Anesthesia for bronchography utilizing intermittent positive pressure breathing apparatus. *Am. J. Roentgenol. Radium Ther. Nucl. Med. 87:* 836, 1962.

29. MOUNTS, R. J., and MOLNAR, W.: The clinical evaluation of a new bronchographic contrast medium. *Radiology 78:* 231, 1962.

30. NELSON, W. W., CHRISTOFORIDIS, A., and PRATT, P. C.: Barium sulfate and bismuth subcarbonate

* This two volume work is extensively annotated, has a large bibliography, and is recommended as a complete reference on roentgen findings in chest disease. It is useful in further study of all chest diseases reported in this section.

suspensions as bronchographic contrast media. *Radiology 72:* 829, 1959.

31. PARKER, G. W., STURTEVANT, H. N., REED, J. E., and FLAHERTY, R. A.: Segmental localization of pulmonary disease. *Am. J. Roentgenol. Radium Ther. Nucl. Med. 83:* 217, 1960.

32. PENDERGRASS, E. P., and HODES, P. J.: The rhomboid fossa of the clavicle. *Am. J. Roentgenol. Radium Ther. Nucl. Med. 38:* 152, 1937.

33. SCHEFF, S., and LAFORET, E. G.: The internal thoracic muscle and the lateral chest roentgenogram. *Radiology 86:* 27, 1966.

34. SCOTT, W. G.: The development of angiocardiography and aortography. *Radiology 56:* 485, 1951.

35. STAUFFER, H. M., LA BREE, J., and ADAMS, F. H.: The normally situated arch of the azygos vein. *Am. J. Roentgenol. Radium Ther. Nucl. Med. 66:* 353, 1951.

36. STEINER, H. A.: Roentgenologic manifestations and clinical symptoms of rib abnormalities. *Radiology 40:* 178, 1943.

37. STEVENS, G. M., WEIGEN, J. F., and LILLINGTON, G. A.: Needle aspiration biopsy of localized pulmonary lesions with amplified fluoroscopic guidance. *Am. J. Roentgenol. Radium Ther. Nucl. Med. 103:* 561, 1968.

38. WEINSTEIN, A. S., and MUELLER, C. F.: Intrathoracic rib. *Am. J. Roentgenol. Radium Ther. Nucl. Med. 94:* 587, 1965.

39. WYMAN, S. M., and EYLER, W. R.: Anomalous pulmonary artery from the aorta associated with intrapulmonary cysts (intralobar sequestration of lung). *Radiology 59:* 658, 1952.

23

ACUTE PULMONARY INFECTIONS

Acute pulmonary infection may be caused by a variety of organisms. In some instances they produce a reasonably characteristic, gross pathological pattern and, therefore, a recognizable roentgen pattern. The findings can be classified as follows:

1. Alveolar (lobar) pneumonia: This is exemplified by pneumococcal pneumonia. There is alveolar exudation which produces peripheral homogenous consolidation. It spreads toward the hilum and tends to cross segmental lines.

2. Bronchopneumonia: This is often observed in staphylococcal infection of the lung. The disease originates in the airways and spreads to peribronchial alveoli. A variety of roentgen patterns may result, including a confluent consolidation resembling alveolar (lobar) pneumonia.

3. Interstitial pneumonia: This is observed in viral and mycoplasmal infections. Often the interstitial involvement is masked by alveolar exudate. A variety of roentgen patterns are observed.

4. Mixed: A combination of the above.

In the subsequent discussions we will try to point out the most common gross anatomic findings in the pneumonias of various etiologies as reflected in chest roentgenograms. However, in each instance it should be remembered that roentgen findings must be correlated with clinical and laboratory data to ascertain the correct etiological diagnosis upon which treatment is based.

THE BACTERIAL PNEUMONIAS

PNEUMOCOCCAL PNEUMONIA

The acute pulmonary infection caused by *Diplococcus pneumoniae* is commonly termed "lobar pneumonia." However it does not usually involve an entire lobe and is better termed "alveolar pneumonia." There are about 75 types of *D. pneumoniae,* but most of the pneumonias are caused by Types 1, 2, 3, 5, 7, and 8. Type 14 causes pneumonia in children, but rarely in adults. The organisms are aspirated in droplets of saliva or mucus, so the lower lobe and right middle lobe are most commonly involved. It occurs in individuals who are otherwise healthy and is frequently seen in children and adult males. The onset is sudden and the gross pathologic changes appear early in the disease, so that roentgen findings can be observed within 6 to 12 hours of the onset. Involvement begins peripherally and spreads centripetally with homogenous involvement which may cross segmental boundaries. The consolidation produced by the disease is manifested on the roentgenogram by homogeneous density. An entire lobe may be affected or there may be one or more segments involved. A peripheral, nonsegmental, sublobar consolidation is seen when peripheral spread across segmental boundaries occurs. This tends to separate the acute pneumococcal pneumonia from the pneumonias of segmental distribution, such as those caused by bronchial obstruction by tumor. The latter disease does not ordinarily cross the barrier formed by interlobar fissures and is, therefore, clearly defined by the fissure on either the frontal or lateral projection, depending upon the lobe or segment infected (Fig. 23-1). In pneumococcal pneumonia all of the elements in the diseased lobe except the larger bronchi are affected, resulting in complete airlessness. The larger bronchi can often be visualized as air-containing, radiolucent tubes within the otherwise homogeneous density. There is often enough pleural infection to result in elevation of the diaphragm on the affected side because of splinting, and a small amount of pleural fluid sufficient to obscure the depth of the costophrenic sulcus is not uncommon. The volume of the lobe or segment is not decreased significantly, so that the density caused by this disease can be differentiated from that produced by atelectasis, which causes considerable decrease in volume, manifested by shift of mediastinal structures to the involved side and elevation of the hemidiaphragm (Fig. 23-2). Resolution is usually fairly rapid if there are no complications and tends to start at the hilum and progress toward the periphery of the lobe or segment. The density becomes more irregular and patchy during resolution, in contrast to its homogeneous character earlier in the disease. Focal atelectasis often develops.

Complications are few since the disease responds well to antibiotics which are given at the first sign of respiratory infection in many instances. Complications include delayed resolution or nonresolution, empyema, and lung abscess. The roentgen findings in delayed resolution are those of persistence of density in the area, which becomes rather irregular and patchy but eventually clears. Very rarely the process clears incompletely, leaving some irregular fibrosis manifested by irregular strands

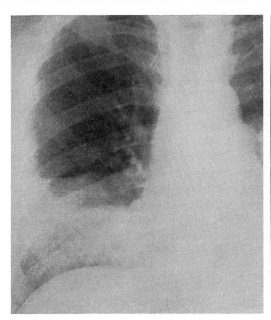 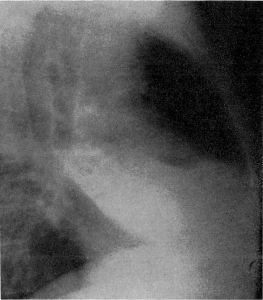

Fig. 23-1. Lobar pneumonia of the right middle lobe. Note the homogeneous density clearly defined by the secondary fissure in the frontal projection (*left*) and by the major fissure as well as the secondary fissure in the lateral view (*right*).

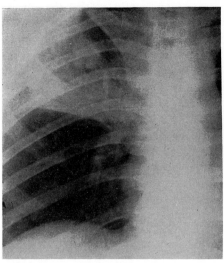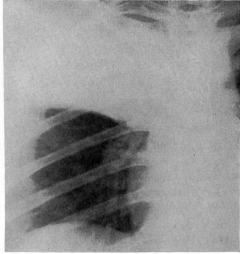

Fig. 23-2. Right upper lobe pneumococcus pneumonia. *Left,* Roentgenogram taken the day after onset of symptoms shows the disease clearly defined by the secondary interlobar fissure. Consolidation is not complete. *Right,* Three days later: complete consolidation of the right upper lobe. Note that the volume has not been significantly reduced.

of density in the segment or lobe with decrease in volume of the affected lung. The findings in empyema and lung abscess are discussed in other sections.

BRONCHOPNEUMONIA

Bronchopneumonia is an acute pulmonary infection, bacterial in origin, that usually occurs as a complication of various debilitating diseases, often at the extremes of life. Therefore, it is most commonly found in the very young or very old who are afflicted with another disease. The infection is often mixed so that several pathogenic bacteria can be isolated from the sputum. The disease originates in numerous adjacent areas, resulting in scattered foci of inflammation that vary in size and shape but produce enough density to be visible on the film. The roentgen findings in bronchopneumonia are varied, since this disease may be quite localized to a single lobe or segment or may be widespread and involve all lobes. The pneumonic consolidation causes densities of varying sizes that are usually rather small, poorly defined, and are best described as "mottled." The disease may progress so that these

small areas may coalesce to form large irregular patches of density. The location is usually basal but the disease may occur anywhere in the lung fields (Fig. 23-3). It often occurs as a complication of other pulmonary disease, which may obscure the pneumonia or vice versa. It is particularly difficult to define and diagnose when it occurs as a complication in cardiac failure with pulmonary congestion and edema, which also result in basal density. Occasionally the process may be extremely widespread and simulate miliary pulmonary disease, with small, poorly defined nodules scattered uniformly throughout both lung fields. Since bronchopneumonia causes a variety of roentgen patterns and is caused by a number of organisms, it is now used as a descriptive term rather than a definitive one as far as etiology is concerned. In contrast to lobar pneumonia it originates in bronchial airways and involves the surrounding parenchyma. As indicated, it may become confluent and then resemble alveolar pneumonia. It should be remembered that neoplasms can be masked by patchy focal pneumonia and if clinical symptoms persist unduly, progress roentgenograms as well as cytological studies should be carried out.

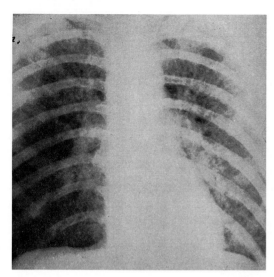

Fig. 23-3. Bronchopneumonia. Note widespread mottled density, which is most marked at the left base, but the disease can also be seen in the right upper lung field and at the right medial base.

ASPIRATION PNEUMONIA

Aspiration pneumonia is usually a mixed bacterial infection caused by aspiration of foreign material into the bronchial tree. The causes are numerous and range from aspiration of vomitus in a postsurgical or semicomatose patient to aspiration as the result of paresis or paralysis of the pharyngeal muscles. Tracheoesophageal fistula and various other esophageal lesions may also cause aspiration pneumonitis.

The radiographic findings vary with the extent of the disease and with its location. The right lower and middle lobes are the most frequently affected but left lower lobe involvement is not unusual. Irregular, poorly defined areas of increased density are visualized and may be extensive (Fig. 23-4). Early in the disease these infiltrates are focal but later they may become conglomerate. In some instances the disease is acute and clears rapidly as the patient recovers from the condition that produced the aspiration. In other instances the pneumonia results from a chronic disease and repeated aspiration leads to chronic basal pneumonitis, which causes patchy or linear basal density (Fig. 23-5). The roentgen find-ings are, therefore, varied and it may not be possible to differentiate this basal inflammatory disease from other nonspecific basal pneumonia and from the chronic pneumonitis associated with bronchiectasis. However, correlation of the history with clinical and roentgen findings usually leads to the proper diagnosis.

FRIEDLÄNDER'S (KLEBSIELLA) PNEUMONIA

Friedländer's pneumonia is a confluent alveolar type of pneumonia caused by *Klebsiella pneumoniae*. The disease occurs most frequently in elderly and debilitated patients. The onset is usually sudden and the illness is often fatal within a few days. It may begin as bronchopneumonia manifested by patchy areas of increased density, usually in one or both upper lobes, but spreads rapidly to become confluent. It may involve an entire lobe. The lung tends to increase in volume, resulting in convexity of the adjacent interlobar fissure. Extensive destruction of tissues leads to abscess formation in most of these patients and the abscess cavities are typically thin-walled, if a wall can be demonstrated (Fig. 23-6). Often the confluent pneumonia surrounding the cavity obscures its actual wall. At times the necrosis is very extensive and extremely large cavitation results when the necrotic material sloughs out. Pleural effusion is common. In the more chronic form, the disease tends to be more patchy, the cavitation is smaller, and the lesions may closely simulate tuberculosis.

The diagnosis should be suspected when a rapidly progressing confluent pneumonia is observed in one or both upper lobes in which cavitation forms quickly. When it progresses more slowly, the disease is often less confluent and its distribution in one or both upper lobes plus the presence of cavities often leads to a mistaken diagnosis of tuberculosis. Bacteriologic studies are then needed for differentiation. In patients who survive, a considerable amount of fibrosis may result, leading to contraction of the lobe with secondary changes in the thorax resulting from the loss of lung volume.

STAPHYLOCOCCAL PNEUMONIA

Staphylococcal pneumonia may be primary in the lungs or secondary in the lungs with a

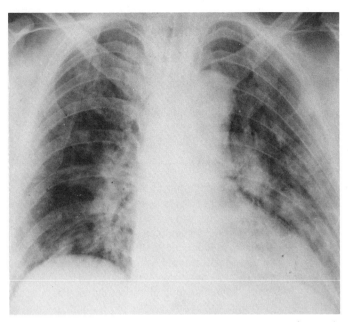

Fig. 23-4. Postoperative aspiration pneumonia. Note the scattered patchy density in the lower half of the left lung field with similar but less extensive change at the right base, along with a few areas of density in the upper lung field. This disease was acute but cleared quickly on treatment.

primary staphylococcal infection elsewhere in the body. In the latter instance there is hematogenous spread of the organism while in the primary type the pulmonary spread is usually bronchogenic. The disease usually occurs in debilitated adults and infants during the first year of life. The onset of the illness is usually abrupt, with severe prostration. Death may occur within 24 to 48 hours. Because some of the many areas of involvement occur adjacent to the pleura, it is not uncomon to have pleural infection with empyema and bronchopleural fistula.

In children the roentgen findings are rather characteristic and consist of dense areas of pulmonary involvement which may be segmental and local or diffuse. Consolidation rapidly spreads to involve a whole lobe; bronchi are usually obscured by exudate so air bronchogram is not ordinarily seen in this disease. Pleural effusion, empyema, and pneumothorax are common, and pneumatoceles are often noted. Abscess formation may also occur;

coalescence of small abscesses is frequent. The pneumatocele is distinguished from the abscess by its thin wall and rapid change in size. It is caused by a check-valve obstruction of a small bronchus. Multiple pneumatoceles may develop, usually in the first week of the disease. They may become very large. Accumulation of fluid with air-fluid levels is common during the active phase of the pneumonia. It may persist for months, but usually disappears completely (Fig. 23-7). In adults the findings are not as characteristic. Pneumothorax and pneumatocele are rare; pleural effusion and empyema are not as common as in children. Abscesses are slightly more frequent than in children and tend to coalesce (Fig. 23-8). The disease is usually bilateral and may be diffuse and somewhat nodular, but is seldom lobar in distribution. Rapid change and lack of correlation between severity of clinical symptoms and roentgen findings is often observed. Resolution is usually slow in both children and adults.

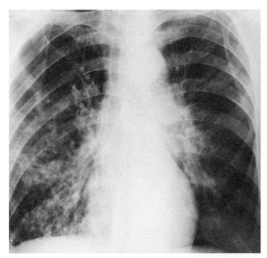

Fig. 23-5. Chronic aspiration pneumonia. Pneumonia in the right parahilar area and base is somewhat more stringy and clearly defined than in acute disease. This was secondary to partial esophageal obstruction.

STREPTOCOCCAL PNEUMONIA

Streptococcal pneumonia usually occurs following such acute infectious diseases as measles and influenza. This disease is now rare and is roentgenographically similar to staphylococcal pneumonia in the frequency of pleural involvement. The actual pulmonary involvement has a tendency to be more diffuse and interstitial in type, with fine densities radiating outward to the periphery from the hila. The combination of rapidly developing, hazy, nodular infiltration in an acutely ill patient and subsequent cavitation in many of the areas is highly characteristic of either staphylococcal or streptococcal pneumonia, with the former more likely.

TULAREMIC PNEUMONIA

Tularemia is an infectious disease caused by *Pasteurella tularensis*. It is a disease of small animals and may be spread to man directly from the animals. The most common mode of infection of this type is through the skin of hunters who dress small game animals. It may also be transmitted by means of tick bites and the bites of horse and deer flies. Pulmonary involvement in the form of pneumonia resulting from this organism is present in approximately 50 per cent of humans affected. The roentgen findings are not characteristic. The disease may produce unilateral or bilateral pulmonary inflammatory disease, which is usually poorly circumscribed. Occasionally the distribution is lobar, resulting in consolidation of an entire lobe. The infection is commonly a basal one and there is usually more disease on one side than the other so that it is asymmetric when bilateral. A small amount of pleural effusion is not uncommon and hilar lymph-node enlargement is also present in many instances. The time required for resolution varies widely. In some instances complete clearing may occur within a week or 10 days while in other patients the infiltrate may persist for 6 weeks. Since the roentgen picture is not characteristic, the diagnosis must be confirmed by laboratory methods. Organisms are difficult to isolate from the sputum but if the disease is suspected it can be proved by means of agglutination tests.

PULMONARY BRUCELLOSIS

Pulmonary involvement is uncommon in brucellosis and symptoms are usually mild. The roentgen findings are varied. This disease may produce strands of density radiating outward from the hila often associated with hilar adenopathy. The parenchymal infiltrates and the adenopathy may be bilateral. Pleural involvement with effusion is occasionally encountered. In other instances, widespread miliary disease is found that resembles miliary bronchopneumonia. Solitary, circumscribed, pulmonary nodules have also been described. The pulmonary roentgen changes appear quickly but tend to persist for long periods of time with very slow resolution. The diagnosis cannot be made on roentgen examination, but must depend on the results of bacteriologic studies, agglutination, and skin tests.

PERTUSSIS PNEUMONIA

Recently Barnhard and Kniker[1] have described central densities radiating into the pulmonary parenchyma from the hilar and low central pulmonary areas, resulting in blurring of the cardiac margins and producing an irregular appearance termed the "shaggy heart" pattern. This begins in the paroxysmal stage of the disease and extends into the resolution phase. They found the sign in 13 of a group of 32 patients who were either

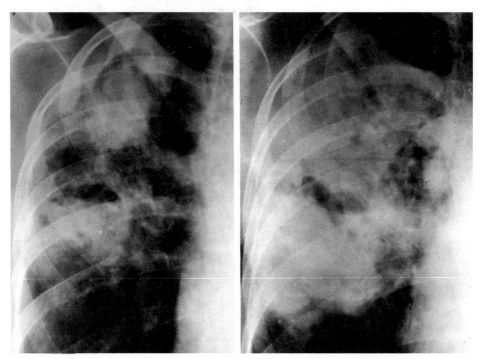

Fig. 23-6. *Klebsiella* pneumonia. *Left,* The disease is extensive, with evidence of cavitation containing masses of dense necrotic material. *Right,* Ten days later, the film shows rapid advance of the disease.

under 1 year of age or had serious respiratory difficulty or encephalopathy. The cause is uncertain; it may indicate a complicating bronchopneumonia. Atelectasis has also been described in older children, presumably caused by thick mucous plugs.

PSEUDOMONAS AERUGINOSA PNEUMONIA

There is an increasing incidence of pneumonia caused by *Pseudomonas aeruginosa* related to increasing use of immunosuppressive drugs, antibiotics, steroids, and cytotoxic drugs. Hospitalized patients are usually involved, and there is evidence that the widespread use of positive pressure breathing apparatus is a major factor. This organism is extremely difficult to eradicate, once pulmonary disease is established.

Several roentgen patterns of pulmonary involvement have been described by Joffe:[10] (*1*) bilateral pneumonic consolidation; patchy scattered disease progressing and coalescing to involvement of the major portions of both lobes; (*2*) extensive bilateral pneumonic consolidation with abscess formation; abscesses may be multiple and small or few and large; (*3*) diffuse nodular densities with or without abscess formation; and (*4*) unilateral pneumonia—similar to the coalescent bilateral pneumonia. Pleural effusion may occur, but is not a prominent feature of the disease.

RARE BACTERIAL PNEUMONIAS

Pneumonic involvement is found in typhoid fever and other *Salmonella* infections as well as in bubonic plague and anthrax. Pfeiffer's bacillus (*Hemophilus influenzae*) is also a rare cause of pneumonia. The roentgen findings are not characteristic in any of these diseases.

THE VIRAL, MYCOPLASMAL, AND RICKETTSIAL PNEUMONIAS

PRIMARY ATYPICAL PNEUMONIA

The primary atypical pneumonias are caused by various strains of virus including type IV

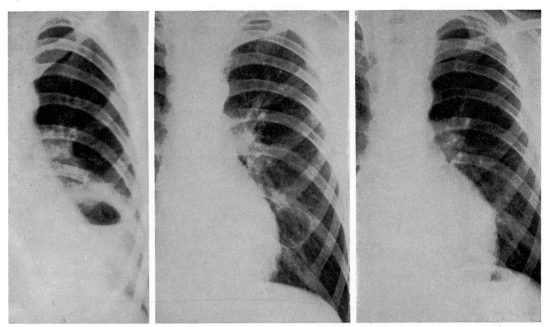

Fig. 23-7. Staphylococcal pneumonia in the left lower lobe, resulting in formation of a pneumatocele. *Left,* Note homogeneous density at the left base with a fluid level in the pneumatocele. A considerable amount of infection obscures the lung around the cavity so that its wall thickness cannot be ascertained. *Center,* Note that the inflammatory disease has cleared almost completely, leaving the thin-walled, cyst-like pneumatocele. This roentgenogram was taken 1 month after the initial one on the *left. Right,* The pneumatocele is no longer visible and there is only slight accentuation of markings in the area of earlier involvement. This roentgenogram was taken 3 months after the initial examination on the *left.*

adenovirus, influenza virus, parainfluenza, and respiratory syncytial viruses. *Mycoplasma pneumoniae* (the Eaton agent) is also responsible for a significant percentage of cases. The atypical pneumonias tend to occur in epidemics, as well as sporadically, so it is difficult to get meaningful figures as to relative frequency of the various etiologic agents. *M. pneumoniae* and type IV adenovirus are probably the most common, however. The disease usually occurs in young adults who are in good health. It is mild and self-limited in most instances, but may be severe with widespread pulmonary lesions. Occasional fatalities have been reported. The inflammatory exudate is more interstitial than in bacterial pneumonias but alveolar exudate may be present, which contains less cells and more fluid than in the bacterial type. The onset of symptoms is gradual and there is often a delay in appearance of visible pulmonary density on roentgen examination for 2 or 3 days.

Roentgen findings reflect the anatomic changes and are varied. Recognizable anatomic forms can be divided into several types:

1. Peribronchial type. The findings in the peribronchial type consist of streaky densities extending outward from the hilum following the pattern of the vascular markings limited to a single segment or affecting one or several lobes. Alveolar exudate may produce scattered patchy density as well as the linear shadows. This is the interstitial viral pneumonia[2] which may also produce a widespread reticular pattern (Fig. 23-9).

2. Bronchopneumonic type. The roentgen findings are similar to those described under bronchopneumonia and may be just as widespread. Densities that are usually poorly de-

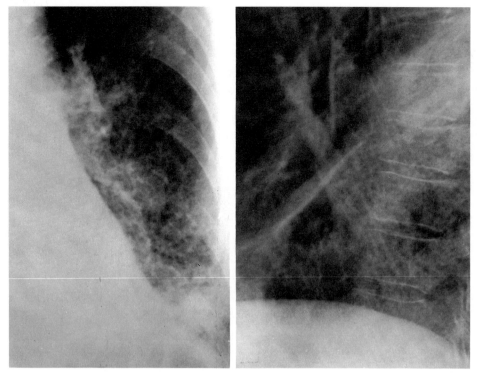

Fig. 23-8. Staphylococcal pneumonia. *Left,* Figure shows extensive left lower lobe disease. There is homogeneous alveolar density at the base and, in the area above it where the disease is less dense, there are numerous small round abscess cavities or pneumatoceles. *Right,* Lateral view shows mottled appearance produced by the small cavities or pneumatoceles.

fined and scattered may be noted in any lobe or segment and may be bilateral.

3. Segmental and lobar types. The findings are those of homogeneous density representing consolidation in a segment, several segments, or a lobe. The appearance of the consolidation is similar to that found in pneumococcal lobar pneumonia. This probably represents the pathologic process of localized hemorrhagic pulmonary edema, which may involve a segment or lobe (Fig. 23-10).

4. Extensive, severe viral pneumonia may occur in a perihilar distribution, resembling pulmonary edema. It is often associated with pleural effusion and often bilateral.

5. Miliary type. Widespread, small, poorly defined nodules are scattered throughout both lung fields. These patients are acutely ill and occasionally succumb to the disease. Conglom-

eration of the miliary infiltrates may occur to form larger densities.

6. Pleural exudation may be the predominant feature of the disease. There may also be pericardial involvement with effusion.

One or more of these gross anatomic types of the disease may be present in a patient. There is a tendency for the disease to clear in one area and spread in another, often in the opposite lung. Atelectasis is often produced by bronchial obstruction and is often lobular and focal in type. Occasionally a pneumatocele may result from check-valve obstruction and must be differentiated from lung abscess (see Fig. 23-7). Resolution is usually slow and it is common to see persistent roentgen lesions for a week or more after the clinical findings have disappeared. Occasionally the delay is considerably greater. Scattered atelectasis that is a

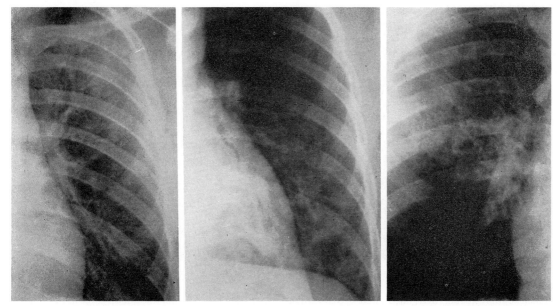

Fig. 23-9. Viral pneumonia. These three films illustrate diffuse involvement in the upper lung field (*left*), the lower lung field (*center*), and the central lung field (*right*).

result of obstruction by the interstitial infiltrate is a factor in the persistence of roentgen findings. Mycoplasmal pneumonia cannot be differentiated from the viral type (Fig. 23-11).

DIFFERENTIAL DIAGNOSIS. There are findings that help to differentiate this disease from bacterial pneumonia. They consist of the lack of pleural involvement manifested by absence of elevation of the diaphragm and absence of pleural fluid in most cases. The delay in appearance after clinical onset is also helpful. The tendency to clear in one area and spread in another is more common in this disease than in bacterial pneumonia. Bilateral involvement is more common than in bacterial pneumonias, with disease often in one lower lobe and the opposite upper or middle lobe. However, because the roentgen pattern may vary widely, the diagnosis must be substantiated by clinical and laboratory findings (Fig. 23-12).

PSITTACOSIS (ORNITHOSIS)

Psittacosis, or ornithosis, is primarily a disease of birds and is transmitted to man by members of the parrot family. It is also found in other domesticated and wild birds and may be transmitted to man by them. The roentgen findings are similar to those in primary atypical pneumonia. The disease tends to be multifocal and is often bilateral with a tendency to change rather rapidly in appearance and distribution. A transparent reticular pattern has also been reported. Enlargement of hilar nodes may also be present. Pleural involvement is uncommon. The roentgen changes tend to persist for a long time (6 to 9 weeks) after the initial symptoms. The diagnosis is confirmed by serologic and bacteriologic studies but can be suspected when this type of infiltrate is seen in a patient who has had contact with birds.

OTHER VIRAL PNEUMONIAS

Epidemic influenza, which is a virus disease, may be associated with virus infection of the pulmonary parenchyma in addition to involvement of the tracheobronchial tree. Roentgen signs are variable, with findings often bilateral and extensive. Especially in severe epidemics of the past, the pneumonia was often of the interstitial type with hazy, strandlike densities radiating outward from the hila. This results in a coarse appearance of the bronchovascular pattern and irregular hilar thickening. The diagnosis is often made from clinical findings during an epidemic. The roentgen changes are then largely confirma-

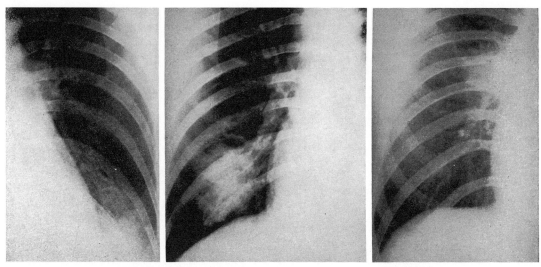

Fig. 23-10. Viral pneumonia. These three patients show a variety of radiographic manifestations. *Left,* Homogeneous basal consolidation not unlike that often noted in early lobar type of pneumococcal pneumonia. *Center,* Local and fairly well circumscribed consolidation resembling tumor. *Right,* Parahilar consolidation.

tory but roentgen examination is useful to observe the course of the pulmonary parenchymal disease. A complicating staphylococcal pneumonia may also occur, particularly in epidemics when influenza may be severe. Most of the fatalties are caused by this complication.

Pneumonia associated with chickenpox is believed by some to be viral in origin and has been reported occasionally. It usually occurs in adults. Roentgen findings consist of widespread nodular densities associated with increase in parahilar markings and occasional enlargement of the hilar nodes. Densities are most marked in the parahilar areas and at the bases. There is often considerable change in the roentgen findings from day to day, since the infiltrates are transitory. Clearing is generally slow, however. It is entirely possible for bacterial pneumonia to appear in patients with these various virus diseases and there is no way to differentiate etiology on roentgen study.

Measles is occasionally associated with pneumonia caused by the virus. Pneumonia caused by other organisms sometimes complicates measles however, so roentgen differentiation may not be possible. The measles virus causes reticuloendothelial involvement resulting in hilar and mediastinal adenopathy. The virus may also involve the lung to produce an interstitial process which is manifested as a widespread reticular type of reaction, with predilection for the bases. Consolidation of

lung with varying degrees of atelectasis is probably a complicating bacterial pneumonia in many instances.

Pneumonic involvement may occur with a number of other viral diseases including smallpox, lymphocytic choriomeningitis, and cytoplasmic inclusion disease in infants and children. There is nothing characteristic about the roentgen appearance of the pneumonia associated with these diseases.

RICKETTSIAL PNEUMONIAS

Q FEVER. This disease is caused by a rickettsia that is an intracellular parasite considered to be intermediate between the bacteria and virus. The causative organism is *Coxiella burnetii.* The roentgen findings resemble those in pneumococcal pneumonia with a tendency to dense, homogeneous, segmental, or lobar consolidation producing a uniform roentgen density in the area of involvement. Hilar involvement and small focal lesions are uncommon. Some pleural involvement occurs in approximately one-third of these cases. This is manifested by a small amount of pleural fluid. The roentgen findings appear within 48 hours of the onset of the disease in the usual instance and resolve rather slowly so that the pulmonary consolidation persists longer than in pneumococcal pneumonia. This disease does not exhibit the mi-

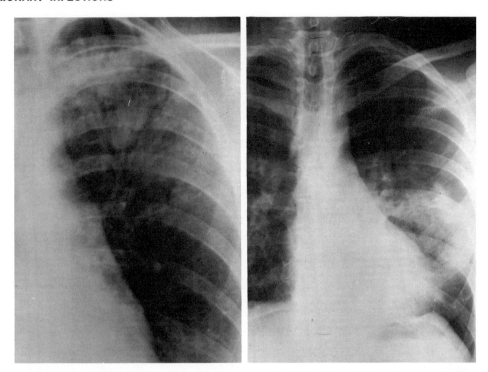

Fig. 23-11. Examples of mycoplasmal pneumonia. *Left,* The air bronchogram denotes alveolar disease, but there also appears to be some interstitial change in the upper central lung. *Right,* Alveolar pneumonia is seen in the left lower lobe.

gratory type of change often found in virus pneumonia. As in other pneumonias, the diagnosis depends on correlation of clinical, roentgen, and serologic findings.

OTHER RICKETTSIAL PNEUMONIAS. Pulmonary involvement has been reported occasionally in other rickettsial diseases such as Rocky Mountain spotted fever and severe cases of typhus. The roentgen findings are not characteristic in these diseases but the infiltrates are usually scattered and produce disseminated densities on the chest roentgenogram.

OTHER INFECTIONS

LUNG ABSCESS

When an acute suppurative pulmonary infectious process breaks down to form a cavity of greater or less size, it is termed "lung abscess." The majority of lung abscesses are bronchogenic in origin and result from aspiration of foreign material following dental operations, surgery of the respiratory tract and elsewhere, and various conditions that produce unconsciousness. This type of abscess may also result from stasis of secretions owing to various causes and from bronchogenic carcinoma or other endobronchial tumor resulting in incomplete drainage of the bronchial tree. Hematogenous lung abscess, which is usually produced by staphylococcus and occasionally by streptococcus, has been discussed in a previous section. The abscess formation in pneumonia produced by the Friedländer bacillus has also been discussed earlier. Cavitation occurs in approximately 5 per cent of patients with pulmonary infarction and when infected, an abscess is formed.

Because lung abscess is the result of aspiration of foreign material in many instances, it is usually found in areas in the lung that are dependent at the time of aspiration. Therefore the posterior segment of the upper lobe is the most

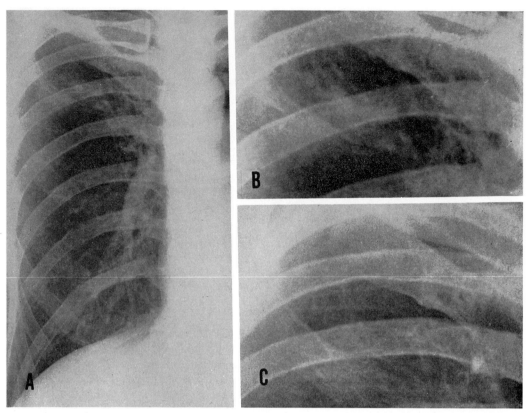

Fig. 23-12. Viral pneumonia simulating minimal tuberculosis. *A*, Chest roentgenogram showing an infiltrate in the right subclavicular area. *B*, Enlargement of the disease-bearing area. The infiltrate appears somewhat nodular in character. *C*, Enlargement of the same area 2 weeks later, which shows complete clearing of the disease.

common site, with the right side affected more than the left. The next most common sites are the superior segments of the lower lobes because these segments are dependent when the patient is in the supine position. The basal segments in the lower lobes are also commonly involved and abscess can occur in any segment of any lobe. The lesion is always peripheral in relation to the bronchopulmonary segment involved but on the frontal roentgenogram it may project in a central position. The pleura is inflamed adjacent to the abscess and there may be pleural effusion.

The early roentgen finding is that of consolidation producing density confined usually to one pulmonary segment. Characteristically, the lesion has a dense center with a hazy and poorly defined periphery and is often roughly circular in shape. When bronchial communication is established, the fluid contents of the cavity are replaced, at least in part, by air and the radiolucent abscess cavity will appear within the area of disease. It is usually incompletely drained so that an air-fluid level can be outlined within it. In these cases, the fluid produces homogeneous density inferiorly, which blends with the wall of the cavity. The drainage of the abscess may vary so that at times it may contain more or less air. When the necrotic lung tissue has not sloughed completely, it is not uncommon to observe a crescent-shaped radiolucency owing to air in the superior aspect of the partially filled cavity. In some patients several small cavities may appear within the area and may remain as separate lesions or may coalesce to form one or more larger cavities. These may be well outlined on the routine frontal and lateral roentgenograms but small cavities can be hidden by the surrounding pneumonic consolidation; when cavitation is suspected, tomography is indicated. It is not uncommon to see cavities on a tomogram that cannot be visualized in any other way. This examination also aids in localizing and in defining the inner and outer walls of the abscess cavity (Fig. 23-13). Tomography is also of value in differentiating lung abscess from bronchogenic carcinoma in which the central portion of the carcinoma has become necrotic and has sloughed out, leaving a central cavity. The wall of the lung abscess is usually relatively smooth on its inner aspect, whereas a carcinoma is usually irregular. In acute lung abscess the outer wall is poorly defined. As the abscess becomes more chronic the wall is thicker and its external surface more sharply marginated (Fig. 23-14). Complications are much less common now than before the use of antibacterial drugs, but empyema and spread of the infection locally or by aspiration of pus from the abscess into a more dependent portion of the lung may occur.

Differential diagnosis depends upon the stage of disease when the roentgenogram is obtained. In the early stage before excavation and communication with a bronchus has occurred, the process

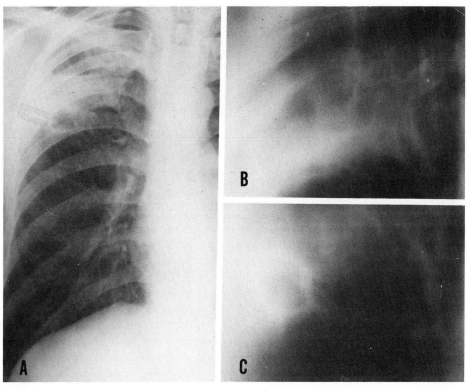

Fig. 23-13. Acute lung abscesses. *A*, Note the irregular radiolucency in the right subclavicular area in which a fluid level is present. Below it is a smaller cavity in the plane of the third anterior rib (**arrow**). *B*, Tomogram (enlarged) of the upper cavity, which lies posteriorly. The wall is very difficult to define and there is a considerable amount of inflammatory disease adjacent to the cavity. *C*, The smaller cavity is faintly defined on this enlarged tomogram. Its medial wall is visualized while inflammatory disease laterally produces homogeneous density and makes the wall more indistinct.

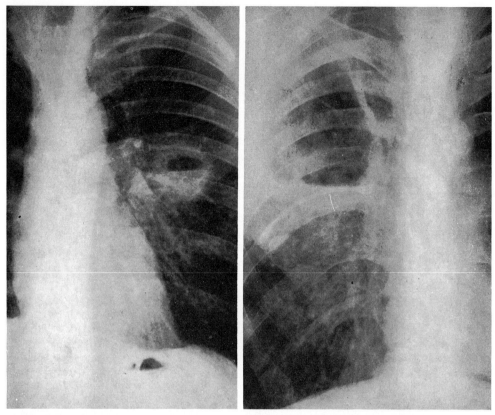

Fig. 23-14. Lung abscesses. *Left,* Chronic lung abscess with a thick wall and very little inflammatory disease surrounding the cavity. The fluid level is readily recognized. *Right,* Large chronic lung abscess in the right upper lung field. A fluid level is noted lateral to the right hilum and there is a considerable amount of scattered inflammatory disease throughout the lung.

cannot be differentiated from a segmental pneumonia. However, excavation usually occurs early and the abscess cavity can then be visualized on the roentgenogram if the examination is made with the patient upright. The clinical findings of profuse, foul-smelling sputum shortly after the onset of the acute process strongly suggest lung abscess and if the cavity is not visible on a plain film, tomography is indicated. Chronic lung abscess must be differentiated from cavitary tuberculosis, the fungal infections that produce cavitation, infected lung cyst, and bronchogenic carcinoma in which the central portion of the lesion has sloughed. This differentiation may be very difficult roentgenographically and examination of the sputum for bacteria and fungi along with appropriate cultures are used to confirm the diagnosis. Cytologic study of the sputum and bronchial aspirates is also indicated in these chronic abscesses, particularly in males over 40, because of the high incidence of bronchogenic carcinoma.

MIDDLE LOBE SYNDROME

The middle lobe syndrome is discussed here because the term appears frequently in the literature. It refers to recurrent pneumonitis in the right middle lobe caused by present or previous obstruction of the bronchus to this lobe. The middle lobe bronchus arises approximately 2 cm below the origin of the upper lobe bronchus and is relatively pliable; there are nodes adjacent to it that may produce compression of this bronchus when they become enlarged. When there is sufficient compression to cause partial obstruction, pneumonitis may result. The obstruction may persist or decrease

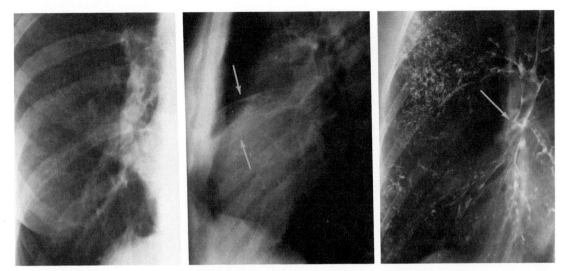

Fig. 23-15. Middle lobe syndrome; note the contracted middle lobe below the right hilum (*left*). The lateral view shows the contracted middle lobe indicated by arrows (*center*). The bronchogram (*right*) shows obstruction (**arrow**) of the middle lobe bronchus with filling of the upper and lower lobe bronchi.

leading to atelectasis, bronchiectasis, and chronic pneumonitis, or to temporary resolution of the process. Endobronchial disease at the site of the lymph node compression may result in gradually increasing stenosis of the middle lobe bronchus.

The initial obstruction may be caused by any inflammatory process that produces hilar node enlargement. This node enlargement may not be sufficient to be detected roentgenographically but when obstruction is produced, there are roentgen findings in the lung that are somewhat varied, depending upon the relative amount of pneumonitis and atelectasis. The lobe is usually decreased in size. This results in downward displacement of the secondary interlobar fissure and in increase in density below and lateral to the right hilum. This is sometimes difficult to visualize is the posteroanterior roentgenogram, although it will cause blurring of the right cardiac margin. It can usually be readily outlined on the lateral film. Then the middle lobe will be clearly defined as a wedge-shaped or triangular area of density sharply bounded above and below by normally aerated lung. The apex of the triangle is at the hilum and the base at the anterior inferior thoracic wall. When it is not clearly defined in

either projection, it can be well visualized in an anteroposterior lordotic view. When bronchiectasis is marked, the dilated bronchi may be visible in the lateral view as air-filled tubular structures within the consolidated lung. The hilar nodes producing the obstruction may contain calcium and can then be visualized. The relationship of these nodes to the middle lobe bronchus can be accurately determined by means of tomography, and bronchography is valuable in outlining the bronchi in these patients.

Bronchographic findings vary, depending upon the degree of bronchostenosis, the duration of the disease, and the presence or absence of bronchiectasis. There are three major bronchographic patterns that can be recognized:

1. The lobar bronchus is patent at the time of the examination and the iodized oil extends freely into the smaller bronchial branches. The bronchi are narrowed, closely approximated to one another, and surrounded by dense lung. There is no alveolar filling and no filling of the finer bronchioles. The bronchi have the appearance of the limbs of a tree completely devoid of leaves. The lobe is decreased in volume. When such a lobe is removed it will

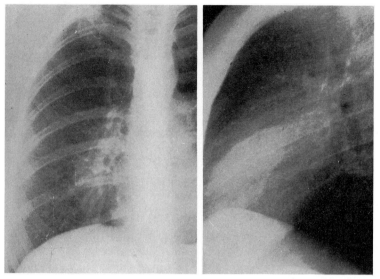

Fig. 23-16. Right middle lobe syndrome. *Left,* The density in the region of the middle lobe is readily noted at the right medial base. It is roughly triangular with its base toward the mediastinum and blurs the right lower cardiac margin. *Right,* Lateral view shows the density in the region of the middle lobe, which is reduced in volume.

reveal chronic pneumonia or, in long-standing cases, only fibrosis and atelectasis with the alveoli being completely obliterated.

2. The lobar bronchus is patent but may be concentrically narrowed at its point of origin by an inflammatory stricture. Filling of the segmental and subsegmental bronchi occurs and they are found to be dilated and involved by bronchiectasis, usually of the tubular type. Again, there is no alveolar filling and the lung surrounding the dilated bronchi is more or less solid because of atelectasis and chronic pneumonitis.

3. The lobar bronchus is more severely stenosed and little or none of the iodized oil will enter the lobe. The bronchus tapers gradually to a point. If any oil does extend beyond the lobar bronchus, bronchiectasis is usually apparent. Because bronchogenic carcinoma may cause somewhat similar findings, bronchoscopy, cytologic study of the sputum or the bronchial washings, or even surgical exploration may be required to settle the diagnosis in this type of disease (Figs. 23-15 and 23-16). Surgical removal is the usual treatment since

the bronchial changes are usually irreversible by the time the syndrome is recognized.

MUCOVISCIDOSIS (CYSTIC FIBROSIS OF THE PANCREAS) AND PULMONARY INFECTION

Mucoviscidosis is the term used to describe the generalized process of which fibrocystic disease of the pancreas is the most commonly recognized finding. It is a congenital and familial disease in which there is an abnormality involving the mucous glands. Obstruction by viscid mucus leads to atrophy and fibrosis of the gland or organ. It is probable that the condition involves all exocrine glands to some extent. The gastrointestinal changes have been described elsewhere. Pulmonary manifestations vary in degree but are almost invariably present if the child lives long enough to develop them.

The earliest roentgen change in fibrocystic disease of the pancreas is over-inflation (emphysema) which is diffuse and symmetrical. This is often difficult to recognize in children but films in inspiration and expiration, as well as chest fluoroscopy, will indicate the distended state of the lungs and the signs of poor respiratory exchange.

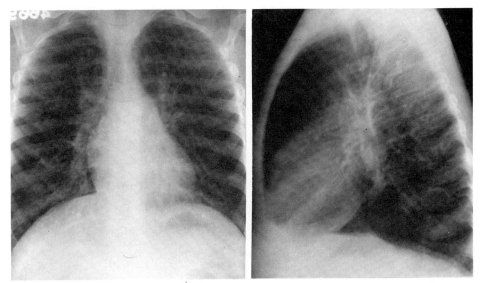

Fig. 23-17. Mucoviscidosis. Cystic fibrosis of the pancreas with chronic pulmonary inflammation causing scattered pulmonary densities. There is moderate overinflation of the lungs.

The degree of obstruction tends to increase to a different extent in various segments so that small areas of density resulting from focal atelectasis are visible as the disease progresses. These patients develop repeated pulmonary infection so that signs of pneumonia are superimposed. The infection is usually widespread and is peribronchial in distribution, which leads to a rather irregular stringy accentuation of markings extending outward from the hila on both sides. This is often associated with areas of poorly defined, hazy density caused by focal areas of pneumonitis in the parenchyma. Segmental or lobar collapse may also occur and the repeated infection leads to a considerable amount of fibrosis and often to bronchiectasis. The fibrosis and inflammatory disease produces irregular stringy and patchy density. The lung between the consolidated areas is emphysematous and hyperaerated, giving a characteristic roentgenographic picture in far advanced disease (Fig. 23-17). It is often possible to suspect the presence of mucoviscidosis early in the course of the disease when emphysema, which may often be associated with small areas of focal atelectasis and which is somewhat irregular in distribution, is noted in these infants. The diagnosis can then be confirmed by the sweat test —the finding of more than 50 mEq of chloride per liter of sweat and by demonstration of decreased amounts of pancreatic enzymes in duodenal contents.

CHRONIC GRANULOMATOUS DISEASE OF CHILDHOOD

Chronic granulomatous disease of childhood[26] (CGD) is another genetically determined disorder in which pulmonary infections begin early in life and persist or recur at intervals. Leukocytes phagocytize bacteria normally but do not destroy them properly.

REFERENCES AND SELECTED READINGS

1. BARNHARD, H. J., and KNIKER, W. J.: Roentgenologic findings in pertussis. Am. J. Roentgenol. Radium Ther. Nucl. Med. 84: 445, 1960.

2. CONTE, P., HEITZMAN, E. R., and MARKARIAN, B.: Viral pneumonia. Roentgen pathological correlations. Radiology 95: 267, 1970.

3. DENNIS, J. M., and BOUDREAU, R. P.: Pleuropulmonary tularemia. Radiology 68: 25, 1957.

4. EFFLER, D. B., and ERVIN, J. R.: The middle lobe syndrome. A review of the anatomic and clinical features. Am. Rev. Tuberc. 71: 775, 1955.

5. FRASER, R. G., and WORTZMAN, G.: Acute pneumococcal lobar pneumonia: The significance of non-segmental distribution. J. Can. Assoc. Radiol. 10: 37, 1959.

6. HARPER, C.: The middle lobe syndrome. *Arch. Surg. 61:* 696, 1950.

7. HARVEY, W. A.: Pulmonary brucellosis. *Ann. Intern. Med. 28:* 768, 1948.

8. HOLMES, R. B.: Friedländer's pneumonia. *Am. J. Roentgenol. Radium Ther. Nucl. Med. 75:* 728, 1956.

9. JACOBSON, G., DENLINGER, R. B., and CARTER, R. A.: Roentgen manifestations of Q fever. *Radiology 53:* 739, 1949.

10. JOFFE, N.: Roentgenologic aspects of primary *Pseudomonas Aeruginosa* pneumonia in mechanically ventilated patients. *Am. J. Roentgenol. Radium Ther. Nucl. Med. 107:* 305, 1969.

11. KEATS, T. E.: Generalized pulmonary emphysema as an isolated manifestation of early cystic fibrosis of the pancreas. *Radiology 65:* 223, 1955.

12. LEWIS, E. K., and LUSK, F. B.: Roentgen diagnosis of primary atypical pneumonia. *Radiology 42:* 425, 1944.

13. MEYERS, H. I., and JACOBSON, G.: Staphylococcal pneumonia in children and adults. *Radiology 72:* 665, 1959.

14. NEUHAUSER, E. B. D.: Roentgen changes associated with pancreatic insufficiency in early life. *Radiology 46:* 319, 1946.

15. PULLEN, R. L., and STUART, B. M.: Tularemia: Analysis of 225 cases. *JAMA 129:* 495, 1945.

16. QUINN, J. L., III: Measles pneumonia in an adult. *Am. J. Roentgenol. Radium Ther. Nucl. Med. 91:* 560, 1964.

17. REIMANN, H. A.: The viral pneumonias and pneumonias of probable viral origin. *Medicine 26:* 167, 1947.

18. DI SANT' AGNESE, P. A.: Pulmonary manifestations of fibrocystic disease of the pancreas. *Dis. Chest 27:* 654, 1955.

19. SCHULTZE, G.: Primary staphylococcal pneumonia in infants. *Am. J. Roentgenol. Radium Ther. Nucl. Med. 81:* 290, 1959.

20. SOUTHARD, M. E.: Roentgen findings in chickenpox pneumonia. *Am. J. Roentgenol. Radium Ther. Nucl. Med. 76:* 533, 1956.

21. STENSTROM, R., JANSSON, E., and WAGER, O.: Ornithosis pneumonia with special reference to roentgenological lung findings. *Acta Med. Scand. 171:* 349, 1962.

22. STUART, B. M., and PULLEN, R. L.: Tularemic pneumonia: Review of American literature and report of 15 cases. *Am. J. Med. Sci. 210:* 223, 1945.

23. TAN, D. Y. M., KAUFMAN, S. A., and LEVENE, G.: Primary chickenpox pneumonia. *Am. J. Roentgenol. Radium Ther. Nucl. Med. 76:* 527, 1956.

24. WEED, L. A., SLOSS, P. T., and CLAGETT, O. T. Chronic localized pulmonary brucellosis. *JAMA 161:* 1044, 1956.

25. WIITA, R. M., CARTWRIGHT, R. R., and DAVIS, J. G.: Staphylococcal pneumonia in adults. *Am. J. Roentgenol. Radium Ther. Nucl. Med. 86:* 1083, 1961.

26. WOLFSON, J. J., QUIE, P. G., LAXDAL, S. D. and GOOD, R. A.: Roentgenologic manifestations in children with a genetic defect of polymorphonuclear leukocyte function. *Radiology 91:* 37, 1968.

24

BRONCHIAL DISEASES

BRONCHITIS

ACUTE BRONCHITIS

This term usually refers to acute catarrhal bronchial inflammation associated with upper respiratory infection, which is not usually a severe illness when uncomplicated. There are no positive roentgen findings in this condition but roentgenograms are useful to indicate that there is no complicating pneumonitis in patients with acute respiratory infections in whom symptoms are unusually severe.

CHRONIC BRONCHITIS

Chronic bronchial inflammatory disease may occur in patients with chronic specific pulmonary inflammatory disease. This is not considered here. We include chronic nonspecific bronchial inflammation which results in chronic cough with sputum, often of several years duration. If etiologic factors persist, this disease progresses to pulmonary insufficiency, emphysema, and cor pulmonale. Several etiologic possibilities exist, with one or more or a combination of several of them operating in an individual patient. They include air pollution, smoking (particularly cigarettes), infection and hereditary weakness of bronchial walls in a few patients. It is not uncommon to see no

roentgen findings in patients with chronic bronchial disease. In these patients, the chest roentgenogram serves to exclude other diseases which could cause the same symptoms. When it results in thickening of bronchial walls and in peribronchial inflammation, these thick-walled structures may be visualized extending well into the parenchyma whereas the normal bronchi within the lungs are not outlined on the plain-film roentgenogram. The visualization of these bronchi, therefore, indicates thickening of bronchial walls and peribronchial disease, which is often associated with chronic bronchitis regardless of etiology. These findings are often best outlined on tomograms. Hyperinflation of the lung may also be manifested by increased lucency of the lungs and increased thoracic volume. Roentgen changes must be correlated with clinical findings. The presence of prominent basal markings does not necessarily indicate chronic bronchial disease since there is a wide variation in the normal. The roentgen diagnosis of chronic bronchitis is therefore made with great caution on plain-film study.

Although there are no reliable plain-film findings in chronic bronchitis, there are reasonably reliable bronchographic signs in this disease. Small diverticulum like projections are often observed along the inferior surfaces of the large bronchi. They represent dilated mucous gland ducts. Distal bronchial or bronchiolar occlusions are also found. Some of them are tapering occlusions, whereas in others there is a bulbous expansion distally (bronchiolectasia). Irregularity or "beading" of the bronchial lumen may also be present. Dilatation of

small bronchi on inspiration, with return to normal caliber on expiration, has been described in this disease, but we have not observed this alteration with respiration. In the absence of bronchiectasis, the presence of dilated bron-

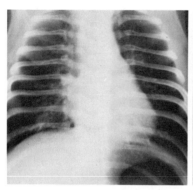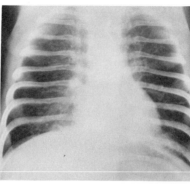

Fig. 24-1. Acute bronchiolitis. *Left,* Note relatively low diaphragm with hyperaerated lung and a small amount of density at the right medial base, representing early associated pneumonitis. *Right,* Emphysema slightly less marked but more pneumonitis, particularly on the right side. The patient was acutely ill, but recovered. The film on the *right* was taken 24 hours later than the one on the *left.*

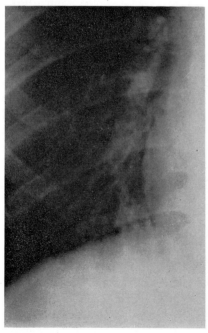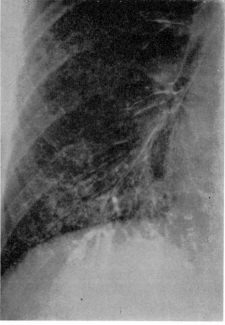

Fig. 24-2. Bronchiectasis of basal segments of the right lower lobe. Note the elongated densities in which radiolucencies representing dilated bronchi are present (*left*). Bronchogram outlines the dilated bronchi chiefly below the dome of the diaphragm (*right*).

chial glands, bronchiolectasia, and irregularity or beading of the bronchial lumen probably justifies the diagnosis of chronic bronchitis.

ACUTE BRONCHIOLITIS

Acute bronchiolitis refers to the acute purulent disease usually observed in small infants or in debilitated, elderly persons in which a widespread involvement of small bronchi and bronchioles is manifested by roentgen signs of emphysema with hyperaeration and low, flat diaphragm. The lungs appear clearer than in the normal and there is very little change on expiration. This is produced by a check-valve type of obstruction of the finer bronchioles by thick secretions. As the disease progresses, focal areas of alveolar involvement are manifested by scattered small densities, which may eventually resemble a very widespread, acute, miliary type of infiltrate (Fig. 24-1). The disease is less frequent than it was in the preantibiotic days. Then it was a serious disease, especially among infants, with a very high mortality rate.

BRONCHIECTASIS

Bronchiectasis refers to persistent dilatation of bronchi, which may vary widely in extent. It results from destruction of the elastic and muscle tissue of the bronchial walls. Descriptive adjectives such as cylindrical (tubular), varicose, saccular, and cystic are used to distinguish the various forms of dilatation. The cylindrical form of the disease is sometimes difficult to recognize, particularly when it is mini-

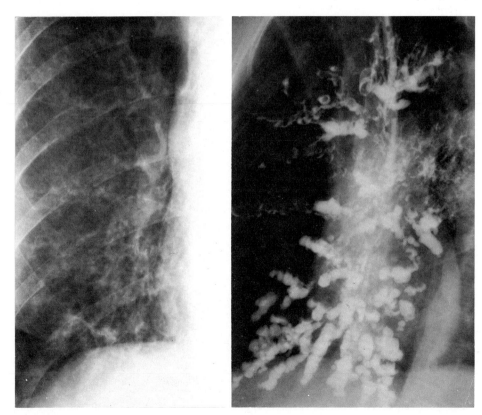

Fig. 24-3. Saccular bronchiectasis in right lung. *Left,* Extensive chronic interstitial disease in which some oval and elongated radiolucencies are present. *Right,* Bronchogram demonstrates extensive bronchiectasis.

mal. With progression, the bronchi tend to dilate further, making the diagnosis relatively easy on bronchography. The saccular and cystic forms are readily recognized. It may be local or general and is usually caused by obstruction and infection, but there is probably a congenital factor or a number of congenital factors in some instances; for example, the incidence of bronchiectasis associated with situs inversus is much greater than in the general population. The triad of situs inversus, paranasal sinus disease, and bronchiectasis is termed "Kartagener's triad" or syndrome. Bronchiectasis is also common in patients with mucoviscidosis. Immunologic defects such as agammaglobulinemia and dysgammaglobulinemia are also associated with bronchiectasis. The usual symptom of bronchiectasis is chronic productive cough, often associated with recurrent episodes of acute pneumonitis and hemoptysis.

It is often possible to make a presumptive diagnosis of bronchiectasis on plain-film study but it must be remembered that a negative roentgenogram of the chest does not exclude bronchiectasis. The findings that indicate this disease are accentuation of markings in the area of disease, often with associated patchy pneumonic densities in which linear or circular radiolucencies can be outlined (Fig. 24-2). It is sometimes possible to trace a thick-walled dilated bronchus well out into the periphery when there is enough peribronchial inflammatory disease so that the air-filled bronchus is visible. When severe saccular bronchiectasis is present, oval or circular radiolucencies may be outlined (Fig. 24-3) and it is not uncommon to see fluid levels in some of the larger cystlike dilatations. There is often decrease in volume of the lobe or segment associated with the chronic inflammation that produces fibrosis and atelectasis.

The fact that the presence of bronchiectasis can be determined on plain-film study in some cases and can be suspected in others does not mean that bronchography is unnecessary in

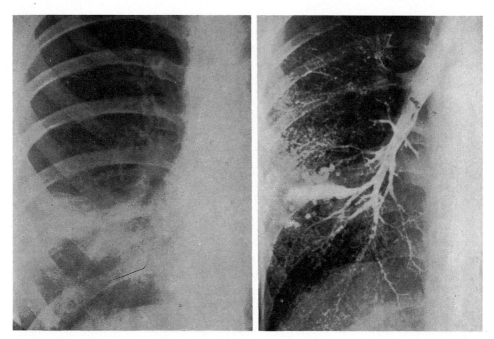

Fig. 24-4. Localized bronchiectasis. *Left,* Note inflammatory disease at the right base. *Right,* Note localized dilatation of a subsegment, which is cylindrical, along with several small saccular dilatations of other bronchi in the area.

these patients. Whenever surgical intervention is planned, complete bronchographic mapping of the bronchial tree is necessary in order that the surgery can be planned intelligently. In most instances the dilatation is either saccular or cylindrical or a combination of the two (Fig. 24-4). Saccular bronchiectasis is not difficult to define but unless there is good filling outlining the entire length of a bronchus, the presence of cylindrical bronchiectasis or the absence of it is sometimes difficult to ascertain and there is often some difference of opinion as to the presence or absence of dilatation. It is often possible to define small amounts of dilatation, however, by comparing the bronchus in question with an adjacent bronchus of a similar order.

Reversible bronchiectasis occurs in children and young adults, usually following acute pneumonia or atelectasis. In the postpneumonic group, the dilatation clears following complete resolution of the pulmonary disease. In the atelectatic group the bronchi decrease in caliber with reexpansion of the lung. Evidently the dilatation is reversible if the mucosa and musculoelastic elements of the bronchial wall are intact. The reversible disease is usually

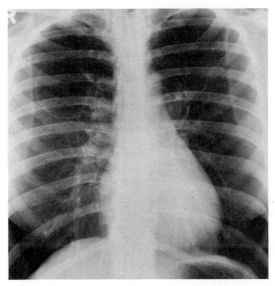

Fig. 24-5. Air-filled cyst, right upper lobe. Note thin wall with absence of infection in the area.

cylindrical or fusiform in type and there may be slight narrowing proximal to the dilatation caused by spasm secondary to inflammatory disease. The possibility of reversibility must be considered when surgical treatment is contemplated; a repeat bronchogram is the only accurate method of making a positive diagnosis of a return to normal.

The greatest dilatation of bronchi in nonspecific bronchiectasis is usually peripheral. In the bronchiectasis associated with pulmonary tuberculosis there is a somewhat different appearance since the peripheral portion of the involved bronchus is often obstructed and the dilatation is more central. This is not invariably true, however, and there are patients with pulmonary tuberculosis in whom upper lobe bronchiectasis extends far peripherally.

PULMONARY CYSTS AND CYSTIC DISEASE

There is considerable confusion in the literature as to the origin and classification of pulmonary cysts. It is now recognized that a number of lesions that were formerly thought to represent congenital cysts are actually acquired lesions, i.e., pneumatoceles resulting from inflammatory disease. This is usually caused by hyperinflation of a small pulmonary parenchymal segment secondary to one-way valve type of obstruction plus actual destruction of pulmonary parenchymal tissue in some instances. Such a lesion may persist for some time but will usually disappear eventually. The size may vary considerably and these acquired cysts may be single or multiple. Congenital pulmonary cysts may contain fluid or air and may or may not have an epithelial lining. A few cases of congenital cysts of lymphatic origin have also been reported.

CONGENITAL PULMONARY CYSTS

It is generally recognized that the differentiation between congenital and acquired pulmonary cysts is not possible in many instances even when histopathologic studies are available. The cysts may contain fluid or air and vary considerably in size. The roentgen findings depend on the presence or absence of fluid. The air-filled cyst is visualized as rounded radiolucency, which varies considerably in size (Fig. 24-5). Unless infected, its wall is rather thin. In some instances a small amount of fluid may be present and this produces an air-fluid level. The solitary cysts that contain only fluid are seen on roentgenograms as rounded masses that are usually very clearly circumscribed unless there is parenchymal infection in the area. When a cyst is acquired, there is often evidence of the inflammatory disease that initiated the lesion but it is also possible that inflammatory disease may appear surrounding a congenital cyst or the latter may become secondarily infected. The question as to whether the congenital cysts are all originally fluid-filled or air-filled has not been settled and it is possible that

there are both types (Fig. 24-6). Some of these cysts are definitely bronchogenic in origin and in others the lining is made up of mesothelium.

PNEUMATOCELE

A pneumatocele is produced when a one-way valve type of obstruction occurs in a small branch bronchus resulting in marked overinflation of the lung distal to the obstruction. The terms "regional obstructive emphysema" and "air cyst" have been applied to this lesion. It is usually the result of inflammatory disease and may be found in children and adults. It is not uncommon to see this type of lesion appear when a pneumonic process is resolving. The valve mechanism allows air to enter the segment on inspiration but does not allow the air to get out during expiration. The marked overexpansion produces disruption of alveolar

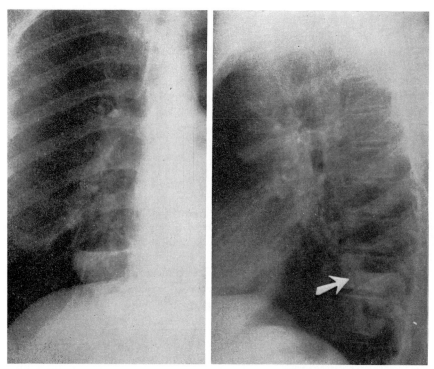

Fig. 24-6. Air and fluid in a cyst of the right lower lobe. *Left,* The fluid level is well outlined in the frontal projection. It is also visible (**arrow**) posteriorly in the lateral projection (*right*).

septa and the pneumatocele may become large enough to cause respiratory embarrassment because of its size. It is not unusual to see a small amount of fluid within the otherwise thin-walled, rounded, radiolucent defect and rapid change in size is common. These lesions usually clear if given enough time so that surgery is not often indicated. The term is usually applied to large, thin-walled cystic lesions but many of the smaller, acquired pulmonary cysts are also of similar origin and could, therefore, be termed pneumatoceles. This condition must be differentiated from lung abscess and from cavitation produced by suppurative or caseating types of pulmonary disease in which there is considerable destruction of pulmonary tissue. Serial roentgenograms along with bacteriologic studies and correlation with history and clinical findings are necessary (Fig. 24-7). The diagnosis is made on the roentgen findings of a thin-walled, air-filled cyst in the lung of a patient with a history of a recent acute pneumonic episode. Rapid change in the size is a characteristic finding.

CYSTIC DISEASE

A considerable difference of opinion is noted in the literature relating to cystic disease of the lung. Many authors believe that there is no such thing as congenital cystic disease while others disagree. Various terms are also used that apparently apply to the same condition; they include cystic disease, congenital cystic disease, cystic bronchiectasis, and polycystic lung. It is likely that this multicystic disease is not related to the solitary bronchopulmonary cyst. There are differences on bronchography in patients who have similar findings on routine roentgenograms. Multiple cysts are usually bilateral and cause numerous rounded radiolucencies with walls that are usually thin. Infection is common so that small fluid levels are often noted in some of these cysts and varying amounts of associated bronchial and parenchymal infection produce pneumonic changes in addition to the rounded air-filled spaces. There are no roentgen criteria to distinguish acquired from congenital types of cystic disease. Some

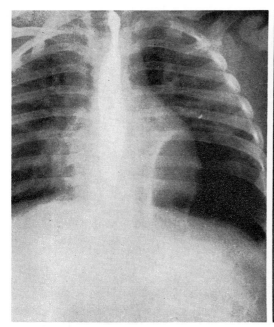
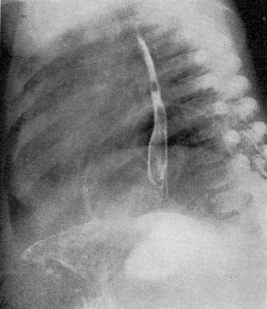

Fig. 24-7. Pneumatocele. Note large rounded radiolucent area at the left posterior base. This lesion resulted from an earlier pneumonia and cleared completely in 3 months.

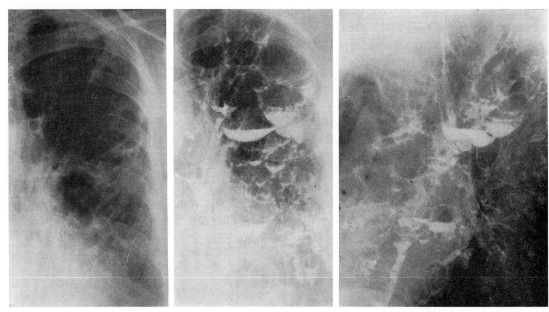

Fig. 24-8. Cystic disease or cystic bronchiectasis. Note large radiolucent "cysts," most of which fill with iodized oil on bronchography.

authors would distinguish between cystic bronchiectasis and cystic disease, or honeycomb lungs, by the bronchographic findings. In the latter disease there is very little filling of the cysts when iodized oil is introduced into the bronchial tree; in cystic bronchiectasis there is much more filling of the lesions, indicating more definite bronchial communication. Others point out that not all the cysts in cystic bronchiectasis fill with iodized oil and conversely some of those in cystic disease do fill. Furthermore Di Rienzo[2] describes a patient in whom the bronchographic findings were those of cystic bronchiectasis on one side and cystic disease or honeycomb lung on the other. The cysts appeared similar on the two sides on routine chest roentgenograms. It is therefore likely that the two conditions are the same or represent different aspects of the same disease. Certainly there is no positive differentiation on roentgen examination (Fig. 24-8).

Emphysematous bullae and blebs are also cystic spaces that are outlined as thin-walled areas of radiolucency on the roentgenogram.

They are described in Chapter 30 in the section on bullous emphysema.

REFERENCES AND SELECTED READINGS

1. Caffey, J.: On the natural regression of pulmonary cysts during early infancy. *Pediatrics 11:* 48, 1953.

2. Di Rienzo, S.: *The Radiologic Exploration of the Bronchus.* Springfield, Ill., Thomas, 1949.

3. Fleischner, F.: Reversible bronchiectasis. *Am. J. Roentgenol. Radium Ther. Nucl. Med. 46:* 166, 1941.

4. Gudbjerg, C. E.: Roentgenologic diagnosis of bronchiectasis. *Acta Radiol. 34:* 209, 1955.

5. Healy, R. J.: Bronchogenic cysts. *Radiology 57:* 200, 1951.

6. Koch, D. A.: Roentgenologic considerations of capillary bronchiolitis. *Am. J. Roentgenol. Radium Ther. Nucl. Med. 82:* 433, 1959.

7. Maier, H. C.: Pulmonary cysts. *Am. J. Surg. 54:* 68, 1941.

8. Miller, R. F., Grant, M., and Pashuck, E. T.: Bronchogenic cysts. *Am. J. Roentgenol. Radium Ther. Nucl. Med. 70:* 771, 1953.

9. Nelson, S. W., and Christoforidis, A.: Reversible bronchiectasis. *Radiology 71:* 375, 1958.

10. PAUL, L. W.: Roentgenologic diagnosis of acute bronchiolitis (capillary bronchitis) in infants. *Am. J. Roentgenol. Radium Ther. Nucl. Med. 45:* 41, 1941.

11. PIERCE, C. B., and DIRKSE, P. R.: Pulmonary pneumatocele. *Radiology 28:* 651, 1937.

12. SCHENCK, S. G.: Congenital cystic disease of the lungs. *Am. J. Roentgenol. Radium Ther. Nucl. Med. 35:* 604, 1936.

13. STUART-HARRIS, C. H., REID, L., and SIMON, G.: Chronic bronchitis and emphysema. A symposium. *Br. J. Radiol. 32:* 286, 1959.

14. STURTEVANT, H. N., and KNUDSON, H. W.: Bronchiolar ectasia. *Am. J. Roentgenol. Radium Ther. Nucl. Med. 83:* 279, 1960.

25

PULMONARY TUBERCULOSIS

GENERAL CONSIDERATIONS

In spite of the public health measures, photofluorographic chest surveys, and the use of specific antibacterial drugs that have reduced its death rate, pulmonary tuberculosis continues to be a common disease of great economic and social importance. The tubercle bacillus *mycobacterium tuberculosis* injures the tissues, resulting in an alveolar exudate termed "tuberculous pneumonia." The disease may advance rapidly and cause a poorly defined roentgen shadow of varying size and density. This is usually homogeneous when the lesion is small. If the process is halted by means of antibacterial drugs before caseation necrosis occurs, complete clearing of the process can occur. A chest roentgenogram does not permit a positive diagnosis of exudative tuberculosis but the findings are often typical enough that the diagnosis of an exudative type of lesion can be suggested. Subsequent complete clearing then tends to substantiate the impression. In other patients or in other areas the lesion may be productive in type with formation of tubercles consisting of epithelioid cells, lymphocytes, and Langhans' giant cells. These may coalesce to form large nodules that are visible as oval or rounded shadows on the roentgeno-

gram. They are usually more clearly defined than the exudative type of lesion. Caseation necrosis may occur in these areas or there may be gradual fibrous tissue replacement without necrosis. When liquefaction occurs in the necrotic area the material is extruded via a bronchus, leaving a tuberculous cavity; these may vary considerably in size.

Dissemination of the tubercle bacillus is of three types: bronchogenic, hematogenous, and lymphatic. Bronchogenic dissemination occurs when exudate from a cavity or small area of caseation drains into a bronchus and is aspirated into previously uninfected areas either on the same or on the opposite side. This type of spread occurs frequently after bleeding and when there is a cavity emptying into a bronchus. Hematogenous dissemination leads to miliary tuberculosis and to extrapulmonary lesions throughout the body. Acute massive hematogenous spread causes miliary tuberculosis, while chronic spread in smaller amounts usually results in the chronic extrapulmonary foci. Lymphogenous dissemination is common in primary infection. It is responsible for involvement with subsequent enlargement of hilar and mediastinal nodes that is often seen in children and in young adult Negroes

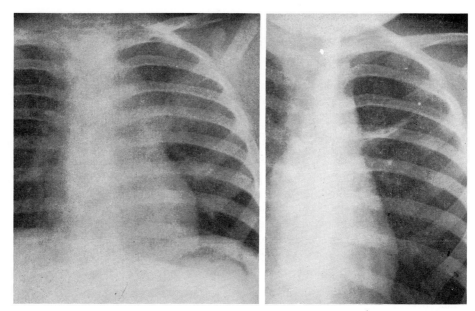

Fig. 25-1. Primary tuberculosis. *Left,* The primary infiltrate is noted in the left lung field lateral to the hilum. It consists of poorly defined density in the parenchyma associated with some enlarged hilar nodes. *Right,* Roentgenogram taken 12 months later. The primary parenchymal infiltrate remains as a clearly defined strand of density in the left second anterior interspace and the enlarged nodes have regressed.

CLASSIFICATION*

EXTENT OF DISEASE

The total extent and the location of pulmonary lesions are decided from examination of the chest roentgenograms. The posteroanterior single film may be sufficient but, in addition, stereoscopic, lateral, oblique, lordotic, overexposed, Bucky, or planigraphic films may be necessary to establish the extent, distribution, and character of the disease, and the presence or absence of cavity.

Minimal. Minimal lesions include those of slight to moderate density, but which do not contain demonstrable cavitation. They may involve a small part of one or both lungs, but the total extent, regardless of distribution, should not ex-

* The classification of pulmonary tuberculosis has been developed by the National Tuberculosis and Respiratory Disease Association and is published in *Diagnostic Standards and Classification of Tuberculosis* on pages 68–69. The last edition was published in 1969 and may be obtained by writing to the National Tuberculosis and Respiratory Disease Association at 1740 Broadway, New York City, New York 10019.

ceed the volume of lung on one side which is present above the second chondrosternal junction and the spine of the fourth or the body of the fifth thoracic vertebra. The term minimal is not to be interpreted as minimizing the activity or hazards of the disease in this stage. This classification also applies to lesions that cannot be seen on the roentgenogram but are associated with the confirmed finding by culture of tubercle bacilli from sputum or gastric aspirates.

Moderately advanced. Moderately advanced lesions may be present in one or both lungs, but the total extent should not exceed the following limits: disseminated lesions of slight to moderate density which may extend throughout the total volume of one lung, or the equivalent in both lungs; dense and confluent lesions that are limited in extent to one-third the volume of one lung; total diameter of cavitation, if present, must be less than 4 cm.

Far advanced. This term is used to describe lesions that are more extensive than moderately advanced.

The extent of pulmonary lesions following any method of therapy must be reestimated from time to time. The original extent of disease should always be noted; the change in extent should be noted; but the least extent that can be listed after chemotherapy, resection, or collapse procedures is minimal, even though a lesion can no longer be seen by roentgenography.

Examples of extent include "pulmonary tuberculosis, far advanced"; "pulmonary tuberculosis, minimal (after resection)."

It is recognized that the above criteria often make it impossible to determine activity on the basis of a single roentgen study but it is possible to suggest probable activity in some instances on the basis of poorly defined infiltrate, the edges of which are irregular and difficult to outline and that do not contain calcium. In patients with cavitation and with extensive disease it is not difficult to recognize that the disease is active. It is rarely possible to determine from a single roentgen study that the disease is inactive, despite the fact that the appearance may be that of clearly defined nodular disease, often with calcium noted in the nodules, because it is well known that these lesions may harbor tubercle bacilli for a long period and may become active at any time.

The roentgen findings in pulmonary tuberculosis are often typical enough to permit almost certain diagnosis, particularly when the disease is moderately advanced or far advanced. Despite typical roentgen findings, the diagnosis must be confirmed by bacteriologic study. Minimal tuberculosis, which often appears as a hazy or poorly defined shadow in the lung apex, must be differentiated from numerous other conditions causing shadows in these areas ranging from anatomic variation and artifacts to acute pneumonitis. The disease in all its forms must also be differentiated from other chronic pulmonary inflammatory diseases, many of which are caused by fungi. It is important to realize that bronchogenic carcinoma can simulate tuberculosis and that it is not rare in patients with tuberculosis. Bronchogenic carcinoma should be suspected in patients with pulmonary tuberculosis when unilateral hilar enlargement develops, when a density increases in size during antituberculous therapy, and when a homogeneous nodular lesion is observed in contrast to the more mottled appearance of nodular tuberculous dis-

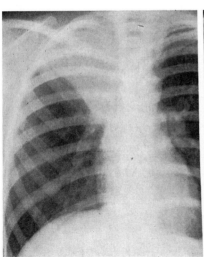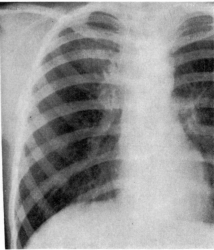

Fig. 25-2. Primary tuberculosis with atelectasis. *Left,* Note the homogeneous density in the right upper lobe with considerable elevation of the fissure, indicating atelectasis. There is a slight convexity of the lower border medially at the hilum, caused by hilar node enlargement. *Right,* Roentgenogram taken 5 weeks later shows that the upper lobe has reexpanded. The primary infiltrate is now visible in the subclavicular area and the enlarged hilar nodes are readily outlined on the right side.

ease. Numerous other diseases involving the lymphatic and vascular structures as well as the pulmonary parenchyma can also resemble pulmonary tuberculosis.

PRIMARY TUBERCULOSIS

Primary or first-infection tuberculosis occurs when the living tubercle bacilli produce a local inflammatory process in the lung in a patient who has not been previously infected. This disease is often overlooked since there are few clinical symptoms. If a roentgenogram is taken in the early phase, the infiltrate resembles that noted in any other segmental pneumonic process in that it is a poorly defined density, usually limited to a relatively small subsegment. The lymphatic spread of the disease to the hilar nodes results in enlargement of these nodes, which may be recognizable roentgenographically. The changes produced in the lymphatics may occasionally be sufficient to appear as streaks of increased density between the primary pneumonic infiltrate and the hilum. If serial films are obtained, slow resolution will be noted over a period of 6 months to a year. At times the original lesion disappears so completely that it cannot be recognized on later roentgenograms, but there is often a small nodule that later becomes calcified. The calcification within the hilar nodes along with the parenchymal calcification then remain as the only residues of primary tuberculosis. This combination of primary infiltrate plus regional node involvement is termed a primary complex and the parenchymal nodule is called a Ghon tubercle. The diagnosis cannot be made on roentgen study alone but in many patients the appearance is so typical that the diagnosis is relatively certain. Progress roentgenograms tend to substantiate the conclusion and the tuberculin skin test can be used to confirm it (Fig. 25-1).

The primary pulmonary parenchymal focus is usually solitary but may be multiple. There are a number of variations from the typical findings described. In some patients the primary parenchymal infiltrate is so small as to be invisible on a roentgenogram while node enlargement in the hilum in the same patient may be considerable. The reverse may be true in which no visible hilar node enlargement is demonstrated. Occasionally the first manifestation is pleural effusion and pleural disease, which may hide the parenchymal infiltrate.

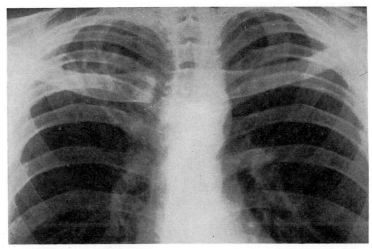

Fig. 25-3. Minimal tuberculosis, right upper lobe, which is considerably obscured by the clavicle and first rib. The disease is mottled and several nodules appear to be present.

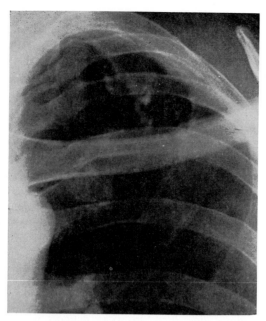

Fig. 25-4. Minimal tuberculosis of the left apex. This disease is clearly defined, and contains some calcium. Calcified nodes are also noted in the left upper hilum, which is included. There is no roentgen evidence of activity in this single film. There is a slight amount of pleural thickening at the lateral apex.

Pleural effusion is more common in adults than in children as a manifestation of the primary disease. Many patients who develop primary tuberculosis follow an uncomplicated course, which accounts for the relatively high incidence of tuberculin sensitivity in the general population, most of whom cannot recall any illness that could be interpreted as previous tuberculosis. When an active primary infiltrate along with lymphadenopathy is found, however, treatment with antibacterial drugs is indicated.

COMPLICATIONS OF PRIMARY TUBERCULOSIS

ATELECTASIS

A major cause of the density that is sometimes associated with primary tuberculosis is now known to be atelectasis, which usually results from com-

pression of a bronchus by the large hilar nodes. Complete occlusion may occur when there is an added factor of bronchial infection or edema, so that the atelectasis may appear and disappear from time to time, producing homogeneous density and decrease in volme of the involved lobe or segment. If the atelectasis persists despite treatment with antituberculous drugs it usually indicates bronchostenosis. It may then become necessary to resort to surgical removal of the involved lobe. The more usual course, however, is for the atelectasis to clear as the inflammatory process improves in the nodes and in the bronchial wall. Thus roentgen findings may vary from time to time in these patients. They consist of the hilar node enlargement plus varying amounts of density in the involved lobe depending on the amount of atelectasis present in addition to the actual infiltrate. The parenchymal infiltrate remains when the atelectasis clears (Fig. 25-2). Bronchiectasis may also result from this type of disease and can be outlined on bronchography.

HEMATOGENOUS DISSEMINATION

Widespread hematogenous dissemination of tuberculosis as the result of primary infection is uncommon but is a very serious complication as it may lead to metastatic involvement of many extrapulmonary structures including the meninges. This occurs in infants under 2 years and is much less common in older children. The pulmonary manifestations of this type of complication are discussed later under the heading "Hematogenous Tuberculosis."

REINFECTION TUBERCULOSIS

Reinfection or adult tuberculosis occurs when tubercle bacilli produce pulmonary inflammatory disease in an individual who has been previously sensitized to tuberculin. Unlike primary tuberculosis, this condition tends to be a progressive lesion leading to symptomatic pulmonary disease unless treated. Lymph node involvement is much less common than in primary disease and there is a considerable tendency for the secondary or reinfection form of the disease to localize in the upper lobes.

There is no certain way to distinguish between the two types on roentgen study, however.

THE EARLY TUBERCULOUS INFILTRATE

The upper lobes are the most common site and the parenchymal disease is most often found in the apical and posterior segments of the upper lobe. The right side is affected somewhat more frequently than the left. It is not uncommon to see the initial infiltrate in the superior segment of the lower lobe on either side but the basal segments of the lower lobe are not often the site of origin in reinfection pulmonary tuberculosis. The disease is asymptomatic in its early stages and a chest roentgenogram often indicates a lesion before the onset of subjective symptoms and before physical findings can be elicited on examination of the chest. For this reason, population surveys for the detection of pulmonary tuberculosis have been conducted, using chest roentgenograms or photofluorograms. As far as the roentgen findings are concerned, there is nothing characteristic about an early tuberculous infiltrate except its upper lobe location, which is usually fairly well peripheral in relation to

the hilum. Characteristically it appears as an area of mottled density that varies considerably in size; the limits of the lesion are usually poorly circumscribed. The hazy character and poor definition of the lesions causes them to be described as "soft," a term often used to denote a pneumonic or exudative process regardless of cause. It is not uncommon for this infiltrate to be obscured to a greater or lesser extent by the clavicle or by one of the upper ribs and thus escape attention unless the roentgenogram is examined carefully (Figs. 25-3, 25-4, and 25-5). In other patients the disease may be undetected until it is well advanced so that it is not unusual to find extensive disease with cavitation and bronchogenic spread to the opposite lung or to the lower lobe of the same lung. In others the initial chest roentgenogram will reveal a large area of segmental or lobar consolidation representing tuberculous pneumonia. Because there is a wide variation in the susceptibility of individuals, the virulence and number of organisms, and in the gross pathologic response to the disease it is not surprising that roentgen study of tuberculosis should outline a wide variation in the appearance of the disease. In a large number of patients the location and appearance of the initial tuber-

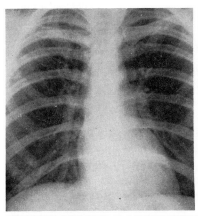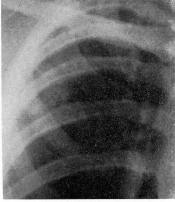

Fig. 25-5. Minimal tuberculosis. *Left,* There is hazy density in the right lateral subclavicular area, extending down as far as the anterior arc of the third rib. *Right,* Enlargement of the right upper lung field shows the hazy density to better advantage. It is in the typical peripheral location and its haziness and poor definition are compatible with active disease.

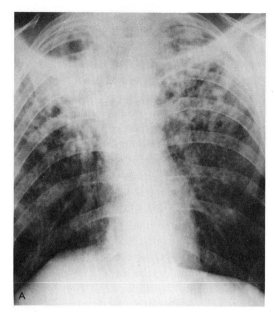

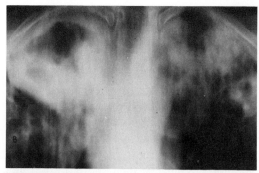

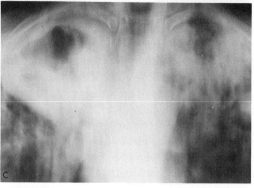

Fig. 25-6. *A*, Chest roentgenogram shows far-advanced bilateral pulmonary tuberculosis. The radiolucency above the right clavicle represents a large cavity and there are several suspected cavities on the left. Both hila are elevated and the trachea is shifted slightly to the right.

Fig. 25-6. *B* and *C*, Tomograms of the same patient show the apical cavity on the right to be readily identified along with the tracheal shift to the right. Note several smaller cavities on the left that were not clearly defined on the roentgenogram of the chest.

culous process are characteristic enough for the roentgenologist to make a presumptive diagnosis of pulmonary tuberculosis but this should always be confirmed by bacteriologic study of sputum or of gastric washings.

BRONCHOGENIC SPREAD

When there is enough necrosis produced by the action of the tubercle bacillus, a cavity is formed and when the necrotic material is extruded through a bronchus the cavity appears on the roentgenogram as a rounded or oval area of radiolucency, usually surrounded by a moderately thick wall and often by a considerable amount of disease in the same area. Exudate from this cavity can be coughed up and expectorated or in other cases it may be aspirated resulting in infection of other parts of the same lung or of the opposite lung. New foci of infection are then set up that in turn may undergo eventual cavitation. Small foci of tuberculous pneumonia are started by these

bronchogenic aspirates. All these lesions may heal, some may heal, others go on to caseation and cavitation, while still others become productive lesions resulting in the formation of a considerable amount of granulation tissue and eventual fibrosis.

CAVITATION

The presence of cavitation in a patient with pulmonary tuberculosis is common and is often readily detected roentgenographically since the cavity is large enough to produce a distinct rounded or oval radiolucency with a moderately thick wall surrounding it. From the standpoint of management of the patient, the presence of cavitation is of great importance and it is often necessary to use a number of methods of roentgen examination to ascertain the presence of cavity and to localize it. Stereoscopic views are often of considerable value and films in lateral and oblique projections will sometimes outline cavities not clearly defined in frontal projection. It is in the detection of such lesions that tomography has its greatest use in pulmonary tuberculosis. It is frequently possible to detect cavitation on tomograms that is not suspected on any other roentgenogram. Bronchography is of limited value in detection of cavitation since most cavities do not fill with iodized oil during this examination.

There is wide variation in appearance of tuberculous excavation just as there is considerable variation in the appearance of the disease from one patient to the next. They all appear as radiolucent areas that vary widely in size but are generally round or oval in shape. The walls are usually moderately thick except in tension cavities, which become fairly large and may exhibit thin walls. A tension cavity develops because of a check-valve type of obstruction of the bronchus leading to it, allowing air to enter the cavity more freely than it can escape. This type of cavity may disappear very quickly when treatment is instituted because the bronchial obstruction that contributed to its size may be relieved quickly to permit the cavity to collapse. Thick-walled cavities, on the other hand, often show little tendency to close, or may close or decrease in size very slowly when treatment is instituted. In general the walls of the cavities are noted to decrease in thickness and become less distinct as the disease regresses under treatment. Fibrosis, with contraction of the previously involved lung, and emphysema may result in production of irregular or oval radiolucencies that may simulate cavities very closely. In these instances it is often difficult and sometimes impossible to differentiate between a thin-walled cavity and an area of emphysema unless the disease has been well documented by repeated roentgenograms during its course. In these patients tomography is often of considerable value (Figs. 25-6*A, B,* and *C*).

BRONCHIECTASIS

Endobronchial involvement in pulmonary tuberculosis is very common and leads to bron-

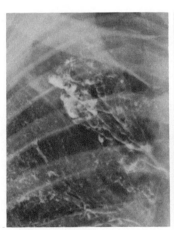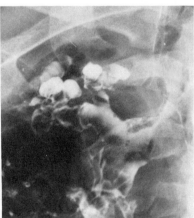

Fig. 25-7. Bronchiectasis in tuberculosis. *Left,* Note the dilatation of the upper lobe bronchi, which is partially saccular and partially cylindrical. The lobe is contracted. There is no alveolar filling and the distal bronchi are obstructed. The latter finding is typical of tuberculosis. *Right,* Far-advanced, long-standing tuberculosis of the right upper lobe. The bronchogram outlines saccular dilatation of the bronchi without any parenchymal filling. The bronchi are distorted and the trachea is deviated to the right.

chiectasis in a number of instances. The presence of bronchiectasis in patients with tuberculosis can often be diagnosed or at least suspected on routine roentgenograms because the thick-walled bronchi filled with air stand out in contrast to the diseased lung surrounding them. In other instances a diagnosis can be made with a fair degree of certainty on tomograms, particularly in patients with far-advanced disease. Bronchography, however, remains the best method for the detection or exclusion of bronchiectasis associated with tuberculosis, as it is in bronchiectasis of nonspecific origin. Bronchiectasis in patients with pulmonary tuberculosis may be saccular or cylindrical and is found in the lobe or segment involved by the disease. Occasionally it will be detected in an area where there is no obvious parenchymal involvement. Presumably the bronchiectasis was caused by tuberculous disease which has resolved to the point where no roentgen evidence remains. Therefore many investigators consider that bronchography is indicated before segmental surgery is undertaken in patients with pulmonary tuberculosis. There is some difference in the appearance of bronchiectasis in tuberculosis from that in the nonspecific type. In tuberculosis there is often peripheral obliteration and more fibrosis with greater distortion of bronchi (Fig. 25-7). We have found a very high incidence of bronchiectasis in lobes compressed beneath a thoracoplasty, which probably accounts for the persistence of tubercle bacilli in the pulmonary secretions of many of these patients. This can often be detected readily on tomography because the compressed lung serves as a contrast to the air-filled bronchi. However, in these patients, as well as others, accurate delineation and segmental distribution must be determined by bronchography.

TUBERCULOMA

This term refers to the round, focal, tuberculous lesion that may be solitary or multiple. There are many inflammatory nodules in which tubercle bacilli cannot be found. The histo-

pathologic findings are nonspecific. They are best termed chronic nonspecific granuloma, not tuberculoma. The tuberculous nodules vary in size from a few millimeters to 5 or 6 cm but usually range from 1 to 3 cm. They may or may not contain calcium and usually contain caseous debris. When present, calcium tends to form a more or less complete shell or ring in or near the outer wall of the nodule. It is not unusual to see several concentric rings of calcium and a central nidus of calcium is often present. The pathogenesis is varied and the nodule may represent either the primary or reinfection type of disease. Sometimes it results when a cavity is sealed by obstruction of its draining bronchus. All these lesions are potentially dangerous, since they may contain viable tubercle bacilli for long intervals and may break down at any time with resultant dissemination of the disease. They may remain constant in size or may grow very slowly over a period of years.

The roentgen finding is that of a round parenchymal nodule. If concentric rings of calcium are visible, the lesion is almost certainly a tuberculoma or other chronic inflammatory

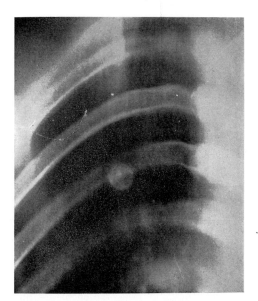

Fig. 25-8. Tuberculoma. Tomogram of the right upper lung field outlines the typical calcification with ring-contoured calcium deposition peripherally and a central nidus of calcium.

granuloma (Fig. 25-8). If no calcium is demonstrated on the routine roentgen study of the chest, tomography is indicated. Calcium can often be seen on the tomogram when its presence is not detected on the preliminary film. If no calcification is found, there is no way to differentiate the tuberculoma or other infectious granuloma from bronchogenic carcinoma, other lung tumors, or from solitary pulmonary metastasis. In the patient with a small, solitary nodule the lesion is usually benign, particularly in the female, but resection must be considered in all patients when no calcification is present unless previous films going back over a period of years indicate that the lesion has been present for a long time and is unchanged.

HEALING OF PULMONARY TUBERCULOSIS

In general, pulmonary tuberculosis heals slowly, so that it is possible by means of serial roentgenograms to follow the gross anatomic changes in the disease. Differences can be noted in the manner of healing, which very likely depend on the type of involvement and the susceptibility

of the tubercle bacilli to the antituberculous drugs as well as the response of the patient. Complete resolution often occurs in some areas and it is a common observation that this is likely to occur and be most striking in patients with relatively acute disease where the process is presumed to be largely exudative (Fig. 25-9). This accounts for the decrease in the thickness of the walls of cavities often noted in patients undergoing treatment. The exudative portion of the process making up the cavitary wall resolves, resulting in a decrease in thickness. In most patients the disease has progressed to the point of necrosis, and complete resolution is not possible. In these patients, fibrosis with contraction of the scars results in shrinkage in the volume of the involved lobe or segment and a decrease in the size of the hemithorax. The mediastinal structures are retracted to the side of involvement. The hilum is elevated in upper lobe disease and sometimes the diaphragm is raised. The tubercles that contain granulation tissue as well as caseation and are often noted as poorly defined nodules will show gradual reduction in size. The individual nodules tend to become more clearly defined on the roentgenogram, evidently also because of contraction and fibrosis. This type of lesion often is the site of calcium deposition and in some instances becomes densely calci-

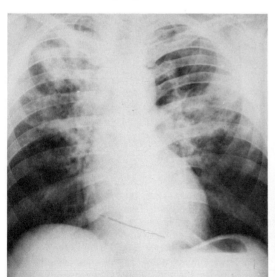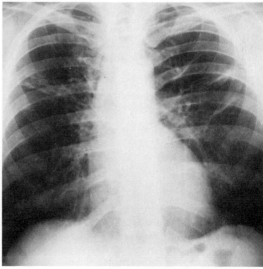

Fig. 25-9. Far-advanced, bilateral pulmonary tuberculosis. *Left,* The roentgenogram demonstrates a large amount of disease on both sides. *Right,* Roentgenogram of the same patient taken 9 months later shows marked regression of the disease as the result of treatment with antituberculous drugs. The remaining disease consists largely of fibrous strands with a few nodules noted in each lung. Much of the disease was exudative in type, which accounts for the marked clearing.

fied with the passage of time. Many of these lesions contain central areas of necrosis in which viable organisms can be found after long periods of apparent inactivity. In summary, as visualized roentgenographically, there is considerable difference in the healing process from one patient to another but it is rare to see the disease disappear entirely (Fig. 25-10). Tomograms are very helpful in demonstrating nodular residuals that cannot be clearly defined on routine chest roentgenograms. Examination of surgical specimens has demonstrated that it is very difficult to be certain on roentgen examination that no residual disease is present.

COMPLICATIONS OF REINFECTION TUBERCULOSIS

PLEURAL EFFUSION

Because pulmonary tuberculosis is a peripheral lesion, pleural involvement is not uncommon (Fig. 25-11); effusion may be found in patients without an obvious pulmonary lesion. In some instances the density produced by the fluid obscures the parenchymal disease. In others, pleural effusion may be the only roentgen manifestation and, even when the fluid has been removed or absorbed, no definite pulmonary parenchymal focus is roentgenographically visible. In some patients the fluid disappears spontaneously or can be successfully aspirated while in others tuberculous empyema may result. Occasionally the pleural space may be involved by secondary infection. The tuberculous empyema is similar to the empyema of nonspecific origin in its roentgen appearance. It is usually loculated and may become very large. If present and undrained for a long period of time, calcification may occur, producing marked radiographic density outlining the wall. Bronchopleural fistula may also occur with drainage of all or part of the contents of the empyema and entrance of air into it.

BRONCHOSTENOSIS

Narrowing of a bronchus may result from pressure of an enlarged lymph node that is involved by tuberculosis or it may be caused by

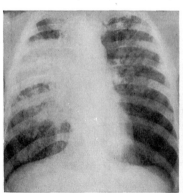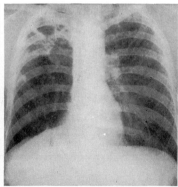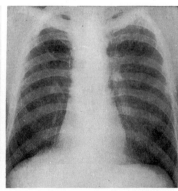

Fig. 25-10. Far-advanced pulmonary tuberculosis shows healing. *Left,* Far-advanced disease is noted on the right, with a large cavity at the apex. A marked amount of scattered disease is also noted on the left. *Center,* Roentgenogram of the same patient taken 9 months later, shows marked regression following treatment. Note that the upper lobe has contracted with a considerable amount of fibrosis but that cavitation persists. The exudative disease in the central and lower lung field has largely cleared. In the left lung there has been comparable clearing with only a few nodules noted in the subclavicular area. *Right,* Roentgenogram taken 16 months after the original film on the *left.* Bilateral resectional surgery was done in the interval. The right upper lobe and the superior segment of the right lower lobe were removed and the apical posterior segment of the left upper lobe was resected. A moderate amount of compensatory emphysema is noted on the right and there are a few strands of density in the second anterior interspace on that side and in the left subclavicular area that are probably secondary to the surgery.

endobronchial inflammation and granuloma formation or fibrosis. Roentgen findings are not evident until the obstruction is sufficient to cause either atelectasis or obstructive emphysema and the findings in either of these conditions are similar to those described in Chapter 30.

BRONCHOLITHIASIS

Occasionally a calcified node adjacent to a bronchus will erode into the bronchus and the material from the node will be extruded into the bronchus. This may produce very few symptoms or it may rarely result in bronchogenic spread of tuberculous disease or hemorrhage; or the calcification may cause bronchial obstruction with emphysema or atelectasis. This complication may also occur in patients with calcified nodes secondary to lesions other than pulmonary tuberculosis. Radiographic findings vary with the situation. The calcified nodes are often visible and their relation to the bronchus can be determined by tomography or bronchography.

TUBERCULOUS PNEUMOTHORAX

When pneumothorax complicates pulmonary tuberculosis it creates the hazard of widespread pleural involvement leading to tuberculous empyema and bronchopleural fistula, because the pneumothorax often results from rupture of a caseous subpleural focus into the pleural space in advanced disease. It is also possible for a small subpleural bleb to rupture leading to a simple pneumothorax that will resolve quickly without further complication. The roentgen appearance is similar to that noted in pneumothorax owing to other causes, but the tuberculous disease is visible and there may be a considerable amount of adhesive pleuritis resulting in irregular or loculated pneumothorax. This is an uncommon complication of tuberculosis.

DISSEMINATION TO OTHER ORGANS

Patients with pulmonary tuberculosis occasionally develop disease in other organs and systems such as the larynx, ileum and cecum, urogenital organs, and skeletal system. Gastrointestinal and laryngeal disease are frequently the result of contact with sputum and only rarely indicate a hema-

togenous spread. On the other hand, renal tuberculosis as well as skeletal involvement indicates hematogenous or lymphatic spread. These lesions are discussed under the organ or system involved.

HEMATOGENOUS TUBERCULOSIS

Hematogenous pulmonary tuberculosis includes several types of disease. When the organisms enter the bloodstream it is possible to get hematogenous involvement of numerous other organs and systems. The actual mode of dissemination is difficult to determine in any specific instance but may occur via the lymphatics and into the bloodstream through the thoracic duct, by direct rupture of a caseous focus into a vessel or by formation of a subintimal tubercle that serves as a source of organisms. The invasion of the bloodstream may occur in any stage of tuberculosis. When hematogenous dissemination develops, numerous factors have a bearing on the resultant disease. These aspects are beyond the scope of this discussion but include the following: The age of the patient, the number and virulence of the organisms entering the bloodstream, the individual and racial susceptibility and the general health of the patient, as well as the state of allergy and immunity at the time of the invasion. Prompt treatment with antibacterial drugs, of course, alters the disease considerably in a favorable manner.

MILIARY PULMONARY TUBERCULOSIS

Two clinical types of miliary tuberculosis are recognized, acute miliary tuberculosis and subacute or chronic miliary pulmonary dissemination. Acute miliary tuberculosis follows massive bloodstream invasion, producing a severe acute illness with frequently fatal termination before the use of antituberculous drugs. In infants and children it usually results from a spread from a primary complex and produces severe clinical manifestations. In adults, particularly in the older age group, the disease may be very insidious and extremely difficult to

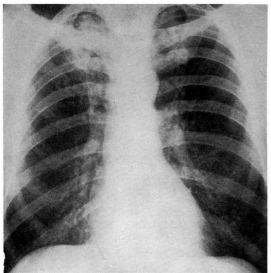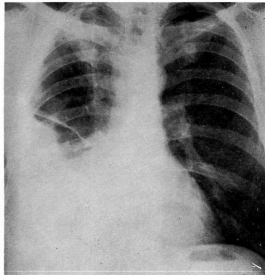

Fig. 25-11. *Left,* Bilateral upper lobe tuberculosis. No evidence of pleural fluid is noted on either side. *Right,* Roentgenogram taken 4 weeks later, showing a large pleural effusion on the right. The parenchymal disease has regressed on both sides.

recognize. Findings on chest roentgenograms depend on the size and number of miliary tubercles. The actual densities visualized on a roentgenogram are the result of superimposition of many small parenchymal lesions that create sufficient density to be recognized as a small nodule. In the typical patient the appearance is that of a fine granularity or tiny nodulation scattered uniformly throughout both lung fields. At times the lesions are rather clearly defined as innumerable fine nodules, each sharply delineated; in other patients they are less sharply outlined, with hazy margins (Fig. 25-12). In some patients with miliary pulmonary tuberculosis, no lesions can be seen on roentgen examination. Pleural involvement is common, resulting in unilateral or bilateral pleural effusion that varies considerably in amount. The individual lesions are largely exudative and when treatment with antibacterial drugs is effective, the widely scattered foci may disappear completely.

The differential diagnosis of miliary tuberculosis is often extremely difficult from a roentgen standpoint because numerous other diseases produce widespread scattered and miliary type of nodulation in both lung fields. Correlation of clinical and roentgen findings is necessary in all instances. There are several acute processes that cannot be differentiated from miliary tuberculosis on a single chest roentgenogram. Miliary bronchopneumonia, which may be of viral or bacterial etiology, and bronchiolitis in children, resulting in widespread miliary nodulation, may closely resemble miliary tuberculosis. In other diseases such as sarcoidosis, the pneumoconioses, and miliary pulmonary carcinomatosis, the history and clinical course usually permits differentiation. Felson[2] lists 40 conditions including miliary tuberculosis that are capable of producing acute, diffuse miliary lesions in the lung. They include, in addition to those mentioned, other bacterial infections such as staphyloccal and streptococcal pneumonia, viral and rickettsial infections such as chickenpox and Q fever, mycotic infections such as histoplasmosis and blastomycosis, and parasitic infestations such as schistosomiasis. He also includes the noninfectious diseases, acute berylliosis, fat embolism, miliary hemorrhages, and acute, diffuse, interstitial fibrosis as described by Hamman and Rich. It

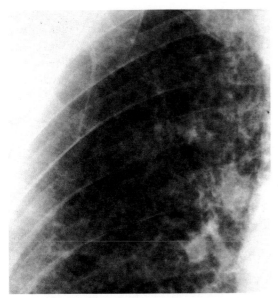

Fig. 25-12. Miliary tuberculosis. Close-up of right upper lung shows extensive small densities which were scattered throughout both lungs.

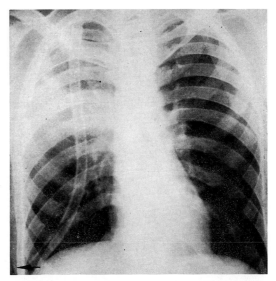

Fig. 25-13. Bedside film following segmental resection of the apical and posterior segments of the right upper lobe. A large drainage tube extends up to the apex. There is some hazy density representing a combination of fluid in the pleural space and exudative reaction at the surgical site. No definite pneumothorax is noted and there is very little subcutaneous emphysema (**arrow**).

is therefore evident that the roentgen findings must be correlated with the results of clinical and laboratory examinations and that in many instances serial roentgenograms, spaced over a period of days or even weeks, are necessary to establish the diagnosis.

SUBACUTE AND CHRONIC HEMATOGENOUS PULMONARY DISSEMINATION

Although this condition is produced by hematogenous dissemination of tubercle bacilli, it is a somewhat different clinical entity from miliary tuberculosis in that it is often asymptomatic. Repeated small episodes may occur so that lesions, although widespread and distributed rather uniformly throughout both lung fields, are likely to be somewhat more variable in size than in the acute miliary process. When this type of dissemination is widespread, the roentgen findings are similar to those in the acute type of miliary tuberculosis but there is considerable difference in the clinical course. In other instances the hematogenous pulmonary dissemination may be relatively localized,

producing small, poorly defined, rounded or oval areas of density in a segment or lobe. Some of these nodules may regress while others may coalesce to form larger nodules and they may heal in a manner similar to that described earlier in the discussion of reinfection type of tuberculosis. In patients with far-advanced pulmonary tuberculosis and a considerable amount of cavitation there is often hematogenous spread to the lower lobes or to the opposite lung, resulting in scattered lesions that cannot be differentiated from the secondary lesions produced by bronchogenic spread of the disease.

ATYPICAL MYCOBACTERIA

There is a group of mycobacteria that may cause pulmonary disease which is similar to tuberculosis caused by *Mycobacterium tuberculosis* from the standpoint of roentgen findings. They are termed atypical, anonymous,

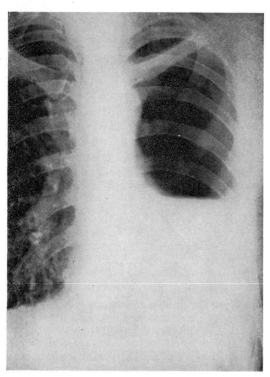

Fig. 25-14. Left pneumonectomy. There has been no rib resection. There is pneumothorax on the left, surmounting a fluid level. The fluid obscures the left lower border of the heart and the diaphragm.

chromogenic, or unclassified mycobacteria. The most important are *M. kansasii* which has caused a number of pulmonary infections in the Chicago area, Dallas, Houston, and New Orleans; and the Battey strain found chiefly in the Southeast. The roentgen findings are similar to those of *M. tuberculosis* infection except that there is a greater tendency to cavity formation and the cavity walls are thinner. Dissemination is rare. These organisms do not respond well to antituberculous therapy, so surgical removal is usually necessary if it is feasible.

SURGICAL MEASURES IN PULMONARY TUBERCULOSIS

Despite the undoubted value of the various antibacterial drugs now available for the treat-

ment of tuberculosis, a number of patients either fail to close cavities or continue to discharge tubercle bacilli in pulmonary secretions. Others continue to have considerable residual disease after long-term treatment. These patients then become possible candidates for surgery. The surgery is usually resectional with removal of the disease.

PULMONARY RESECTION

The roentgen appearance of the chest following pulmonary resection varies with the type of resection. There is also considerable variation, depending upon the ability of the remaining lung to expand and fill the hemithorax. Immediately following lobar or segmental resection, the roentgenogram often outlines pneumothorax that varies in amount and position, depending upon the volume of pulmonary tissue removed. The diaphragm on the operated side is usually elevated and there is often a mediastinal shift to that side. A drainage tube is left in place and this is visible along with some emphysema in the lateral chest wall that often extends up into the neck. Emphysema is manifested by streaks of radiolucency within the soft tissues (Fig. 25-13). There is often some fluid in the soft tissues along with air. This produces fluid levels that may overlie the lung parenchyma. These accumulations in the wound space can usually be differentiated from loculated pockets of air and fluid in the pleural space by their position in relation to the chest wall. A segment of rib is sometimes resected and surgical section or fracture of a rib above or below the missing rib is often observed. It is not unusual to note some diffuse density at the surgical site, even on roentgenograms taken very shortly following completion of the procedure. This is caused by a combination of edema and possibly hemorrhage at the surgical site, along with some fluid in the adjacent pleural space. It varies considerably with the type of resection, being most commonly observed when a segmental resection is carried out. Within 24 hours there usually is fluid in

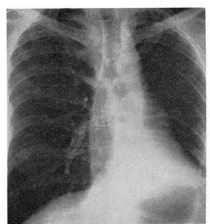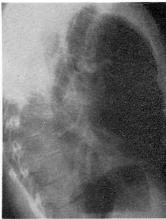

Fig. 25-15. Left pneumonectomy. These frontal (*left*) and lateral (*right*) roentgenograms show a remarkable shift of the right lung into the left hemithorax through the anterior mediastinum. The heart is noted to be displaced posteriorly in the lateral view and its anterior margin is clearly defined by the air in the herniated lung. The amount of diaphragmatic elevation and mediastinal shift is minor. The right lung is hyperaerated, indicating compensatory emphysema.

the pleural space at the base and surrounding the remaining lung. The amount of pneumothorax is often decreased in that period of time. It is not unusual to observe some atelectasis in the remaining lobe that often clears within 24 hours, with resultant increase in lung volume and decrease in the size of the pneumothorax. Subsequent roentgenograms show gradual decrease in the size of the residual pneumothorax and increase in expansion of the remaining lung. The subcutaneous emphysema usually disappears in a week or 10 days. Occasionally a severe subcutaneous emphysema is noted that extends into the neck on both sides and into the soft tissues of the opposite hemithorax as well as into the mediastinum. This requires a longer time to clear. Eventually the pneumothorax and fluid disappear, leaving a relatively small amount of residual pleural thickening or perhaps some irregular adhesive tenting of the diaphragm manifested by local elevation of it. When segmental resection is done and no rib is removed, it is often difficult, or impossible, to detect recognizable residues on the resected side after a period of 6 months. (See Fig. 25-10.)

Pneumonectomy is sometimes necessary in the treatment of tuberculosis and following this operation there usually is a large amount of pneumothorax noted in the immediate postoperative film along with subcutaneous emphysema as in the segmental and lobar resections. Rib removal and surgical section can also be recognized. As time goes on, fluid accumulates in the hemithorax and this gradually replaces the air (Fig. 25-14). Elevation of the diaphragm and shift of the mediastinal structures to the surgical side varies considerably but is almost always present, along with some herniation of the normal lung across the midline (Fig. 25-15).

Complications may occur and can be recognized on the roentgenograms. Bronchopleural fistula is manifested by continuing pneumothorax for an unusually long period of time or by sudden increase in the amount of pneumothorax along with decrease in fluid without aspiration. When lobar or segmental resections are done, the remaining segments or lobes may collapse. These atelectatic areas are recognized as areas of increased density because of the airlessness of the pulmonary parenchyma.

The roentgen findings following pulmonary

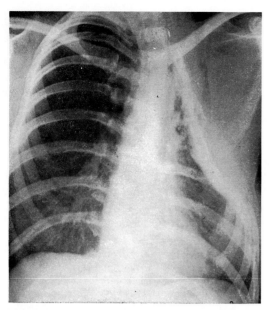

Fig. 25-16. Thoracoplasty. There has been a seven-rib thoracoplasty on the left. The lung is compressed and there is considerable regeneration of ribs, forming a solid bony plate along the left upper lateral chest wall. The scoliosis to the left commonly results from thoracoplasty.

resection for disease other than tuberculosis are similar to those described above.

OTHER SURGICAL PROCEDURES

THORACOPLASTY

Thoracoplasty is an operative procedure on the chest wall in which a number of ribs are resected for the purpose of decreasing the volume of the thorax. This operation has been superseded by resectional therapy to a large extent. It is also used following pneumonectomy to obliterate the pleural space and after lobectomy or segmental resection when the remaining lung fails to expand enough to fill the hemithorax. In time there is regeneration of bone along the sites of the resected ribs, which may form a rather heavy bony plate at the operative site (Fig. 25-16). When rib regeneration is not desired the periosteum is destroyed.

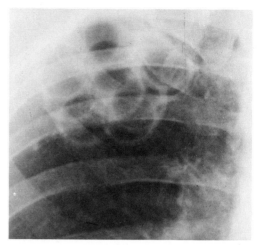

Fig. 25-17. Lucite-ball plombage. The round lucite balls used to compress the lung are clearly visible at the apex.

PLOMBAGE

This is another surgical procedure that has been used to decrease the size of the thorax. It consists of placing foreign material into a space of desired size either extrapleurally or extraperiosteally. Roentgenograms will show the site of plombage and the material used can often be visualized (Fig. 25-17). This procedure has been abandoned in recent years.

CAVERNOSTOMY OR CAVITY DRAINAGE

This is another surgical procedure used in tuberculosis, often as a last resort in a patient with a large cavity that cannot be resected and does not drain adequately. Roentgen findings are as expected and consist of visualization of the cavity with a drainage tube extending into it. A short overlying segment of rib is often resected and this will be visible.

REFERENCES AND SELECTED READINGS

1. BIRKELO, C. C.: Roentgen diagnosis of the primary tuberculous infection. *JAMA 118:* 350, 1942.
2. FELSON, B.: Acute miliary diseases of the lung. *Radiology 59:* 32, 1952.
3. FRIEDENBERG, R. M., ISAACS, N., and ELKIN, M.: The changing roentgenologic picture in pulmonary tuberculosis under modern chemotherapy.

Am. J. Roentgenol. Radium Ther. Nucl. Med. 81: 196, 1959.

4. GOOD, C. A., CARR, D. T., and WEED, L. A.: Positive roentgenograms plus positive sputum smears do not always equal pulmonary tuberculosis. *Am. J. Roentgenol. Radium Ther. Nucl. Med. 81:* 187, 1959.

5. JACOBSON, H. G., and SHAPIRO, J. H.: Pulmonary tuberculosis. *Radiol. Clin. North Am. 1:* 411, 1963.

6. KELLER, R. H., and RUNYAN, E. H.: Mycobacterial diseases. *Am. J. Roentgenol. Radium Ther. Nucl. Med. 92:* 528, 1964.

7. STEAD, W. W.: The iceberg of medicine: Tuberculosis. *Radiol. Clin. North Am. 3:* 299, 1965.

26

FUNGAL DISEASES AND OTHER
CHRONIC INFLAMMATIONS

The inflammatory diseases discussed in this chapter are caused by a variety of organisms, many of which are capable of producing acute, fulminating, generalized disease in which there is associated involvement of the lungs. These organisms may also cause disease, usually chronic, limited primarily to the lungs. The diseases must be differentiated from each other as well as from pulmonary tuberculosis and occasionally from lung tumor. The ultimate diagnosis depends upon demonstration of the causative agent in bronchial secretions or in sections of the lung. In many instances this is very difficult, so that other bacteriologic studies based on immunologic reactions are used. These consist of skin tests, agglutination, complement fixation, and precipitation reactions.

The gross anatomic changes in pulmonary disease produced by these varied organisms may be similar. On the basis of roentgen examination it is often possible to indicate only that the lesion is a chronic inflammatory disease of unknown etiology. At other times it is possible to make the diagnosis with a considerable degree of accuracy on the basis of clinical findings correlated with roentgen manifestations. In the paragraphs to follow these diseases are classified according to their etiology

and brief descriptions of the major roentgen changes are given.

FUNGAL DISEASES OF THE LUNGS

ACTINOMYCOSIS

This disease is caused by an anaerobic fungus called *Actinomyces bovis* in animals. In humans it is probably caused by *A. israeli*. The disease may affect any part of the body but is found most frequently in and about the jaw. Pulmonary infection occurs in approximately 15 per cent of patients with the disease. It is characterized by its tendency to produce suppurative sinus tracts and its ability to cross tissue planes that provide a barrier to the usual infections. The roentgen findings vary greatly. The disease may be unilateral or bilateral but tends to be unilateral unless widely disseminated throughout the body. It produces a dense, confluent opacity in the affected lung in which cavitation may be present (Fig. 26-1). Frequent pleural involvement results in varying amounts of pleural thickening and fluid. Infection of the chest wall causes soft-tissue swelling and destruction of ribs with sinus tract forma-

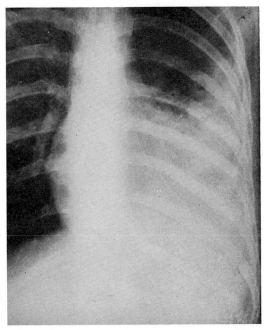

Fig. 26-1. Actinomycosis. The dense confluent consolidation in the left lower lung obscures the diaphragm and heart. Patient has a chest-wall mass with sinus tracts typical of this disease.

tion; this is characteristic of the disease. When these findings are noted on the chest roentgenogram, the disease may be strongly suspected. Another roentgen pattern is that of a fan-shaped consolidation near the hilum or radiating from it into the superior segment of the lower lobe. Actinomycosis must be differentiated from tuberculosis and from other chronic fungal infections by bacteriologic and histologic examinations.

NOCARDIOSIS

Nocardia asteroides is the most common of several species of *Nocardia* that may cause disease. Nocardia is an aerobic gram-positive, acid-fast fungus with finely branched hyphae. It is recognized increasingly as a secondary infection in patients with underlying chronic debilitating disease, particularly in those who have undergone therapy with immunosuppressive or cytotoxic agents or steroids. Pulmonary roentgen findings

consist of homogeneous segmental or lobar consolidation; cavitation is common. Pleural involvement with empyema is also frequent. Single nodular lesions may also occur and may progress to cavitation. The disease is frequently bilateral. This disease crosses fissures and anatomic barriers, but not as frequently as actinomycosis. The roentgen alterations in the lungs persist for long periods of time, frequently with little change. The organism is difficult to isolate in many instances so that the diagnosis is often obscure until material is obtained by lung biopsy for histologic study. It is not unusual for the disease to run a protracted course with very little variation in the appearance of the pulmonary lesions and very few symptoms. Pleural involvement with empyema, extension to involve ribs with production of chest-wall abscess is not as frequent as in actinomycosis. In addition to differentiating this disease from tuberculosis, the other mycotic lesions of the lungs must be included in the differential diagnosis. Identification of the causative agent is necessary to confirm the diagnosis (Fig. 26-2).

COCCIDIOIDOMYCOSIS

This is caused by the fungus *Coccidioides immitis*. It is an endemic pulmonary disease in the arid southwestern part of the United States and, particularly, in the San Joaquin Valley in California. The initial infection produces an acute pneumonia associated with symptoms of an acute pulmonary disease including fever, malaise, headache, and cough. Erythema nodosum is a frequent clinical manifestation during the acute febrile illness and, in the San Joaquin Valley, this clinical syndrome is known as Valley fever. The primary form is usually asymptomatic and may be discovered incidentally on the chest film. Roentgen findings are those of segmental pneumonitis resulting in homogeneous density that is poorly circumscribed. Hilar node enlargement is present very frequently. The roentgen findings in this type of involvement simulate those of other acute, atypical pneumonias. The pneumonia of coccidioidomycosis may be localized to one segment but wider dissemination has also been reported, with multiple areas of pneumonic

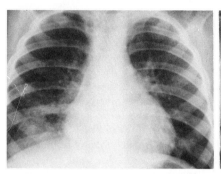 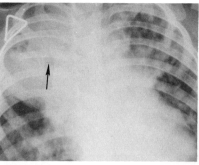 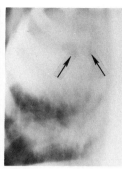

Fig. 26-2. Nocardiosis. *Left,* Small amount of poorly defined density is noted at the right base with a very minor amount on the left. Its appearance and distribution are not characteristic of any specific disease. *Center,* Roentgenogram taken 9 months later shows marked progression of the disease with scattered large nodules and patchy densities in both lung fields, along with the consolidation of the right upper lobe (**arrow**). There has been rib resection with open drainage of the pleural space at the right upper anterolateral chest wall. *Right,* Tomogram outlines the dense consolidation but also indicates the presence of several cavities within the disease (**arrows**).

consolidation. Occasionally the adenopathy in the hilar and mediastinal nodes is the predominant feature and in these patients there may or may not be evidence of pulmonary parenchymal involvement. Multiple nodular parenchymal lesions have also been reported but are not as common as the more localized pneumonitis. Cavitation within the area of disease is not uncommon. The cavities are usually small and may disappear quickly in the primary type of infection. Occasionally small pleural effusion is the only evidence of the disease noted on the chest roentgenogram; massive effusion is rare.

Dissemination occurs rarely when the initial infection fails to become localized. This is very uncommon in the white race but dark-skinned races are more susceptible. Clinically this is a continuation and progression of the primary infection and is often manifested by exacerbation of symptoms. Radiographic findings vary considerably from universal hematogenous spread of disease resembling miliary tuberculosis to local spread confined to the lungs. There is often bronchogenic dissemination to the opposite lung or other lobes resulting in scattered involvement of varying extent. Large cavities may appear, along with pleural involvement leading to empyema. Associated with the extensive pulmonary infiltrates in this form of the

disease there is often spread to abdominal viscera, skeletal system, lymph nodes, and sometimes to the brain and meninges. The disseminated type of involvement is extremely lethal.

Residual pulmonary coccidioidomycosis results when the acute primary disease subsides without widespread dissemination. The primary disease may clear completely but when there is disease remaining within the lung it usually assumes one of three general radiographic types. They are: (*1*) cavitation; (*2*) nodules which may be single or multiple; and (*3*) pulmonary infiltration, which may be relatively focal and occur in a single area or in several areas. The residual type of cavitation in coccidioidomycosis often is thin-walled and may remain unchanged in size and shape for years. There usually is some fibrotic disease in the area of cavitation but this is not always true. Studies of large numbers of patients have shown that the thin-walled cavity that was originally thought to be characteristic of the disease occurs in only 50 to 60 per cent of patients, while the remaining cavities have relatively thick walls. Cavitation in this disease must be differentiated from pulmonary tuberculosis and from other mycotic infections. This is usually not possible on roentgen examination alone but as a general rule the residual cavity in coccidioidomycosis has less pulmonary infiltrate around it than is seen in pulmonary tuberculosis, since bronchogenic spread is much less common in coccidioidomycosis than in tuberculosis. This finding is important in the differential diagnosis in untreated patients with chronic pulmonary disease in which there is persistent cavitation (Fig. 26-3).

The nodular residuals of coccidioidomycosis vary considerably in size and in number. They may, or may not, contain calcium. When single, they must be differentiated from other diseases that cause solitary pulmonary nodulation including primary bronchogenic tumor. When multiple, the lesions must be differentiated from other mycotic disease and pulmonary tuberculosis. These differentiations are not possible on roentgen examination and must be made on the basis of skin tests with coccidioidin and by means of serologic studies. The infiltrative fibrotic type of residual disease is similar to the fibrotic residues of numerous other inflammations, so that there is nothing in the roentgenogram to indicate the nature of the original disease. Pleural thickening and effusion are occasionally noted as the end results of this disease but there is nothing characterisic about these findings. Cavities are often peripheral and tend to rupture into the pleural space, resulting in empyema.

HISTOPLASMOSIS

Histoplasmosis is caused by the fungus known as *Histoplasma capsulatum*. It was originally thought to be a rare and fatal disease but it is now known that the disseminated form, which may be fatal, is only one of several types of the disease. The primary form is much more common. It is endemic in the Mississippi and Ohio valleys and along the Appalachian Mountains. In many areas histoplasmin-skin sensitiv-

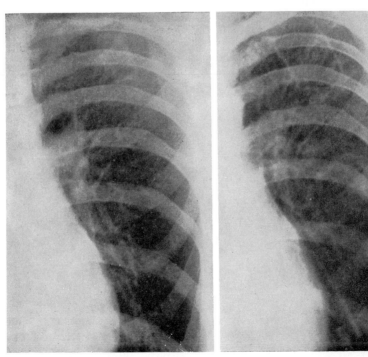

Fig. 26-3. Coccidioidomycosis. *Left,* Note the cavity in the left subclavicular area. The wall is moderately thick but there is very little disease other than a few strands of density in the area of cavitation. *Right,* One year later the cavity is larger and the wall is thinner. Again very little disease is noted in the parenchyma, considering the size of the cavity.

ity is almost universal in the young, adult lifetime residents, indicating previous infection. It is less common elsewhere in the United States but is found in nearly all states, as well as in Mexico and Panama.

The *primary form* of the disease is usually relatively benign and passes unnoticed in most instances (95 per cent). The roentgen changes found in the acute benign disease are varied with single or multiple areas of pneumonic consolidation. It cannot be distinguished from primary tuberculosis roentgenographically. It is often segmental in distribution and may be accompanied by hilar node enlargement. The hilar node involvement may be more prominent than the parenchymal disease in some cases (Fig. 26-4) particularly in children. In addition to the localized pneumonic consolidation, there is a more widespread form. Nodular lesions are scattered throughout both lung fields (Fig. 26-5). At first they are poorly defined. Later they become more clearly outlined, rounded nodules varying in size up to a centimeter. With healing, some of the nodules

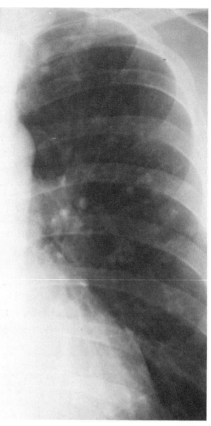

Fig. 26-5. Disseminated pulmonary histoplasmosis. Note the small nodules scattered throughout the lung.

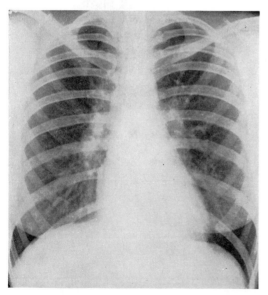

Fig. 26-4. Histoplasmosis. The parenchymal disease is minor and consists of a small amount of patchy density above the right hilum, but there is a considerable amount of hilar node enlargement, particularly on the right.

may disappear completely while others may gradually decrease in size and become calcified (Fig. 26-6). Calcification often occurs in the involved hilar nodes as well. Studies of large groups of people in endemic areas have shown that the amount of calcification in parenchymal nodules and in hilar nodes is greater in histoplasmosis than in tuberculosis as a general rule. The primary form of the disease may clear and leave no pulmonary residuals that can be recognized on roentgenograms. However, in others solitary calcified parenchymal nodules with or without calcified hilar nodes may be present (Fig. 26-7). Miliary parenchymal calcifications scattered throughout the lungs and large "mulberry" calcified hilar nodes are usually associated with histoplasmin

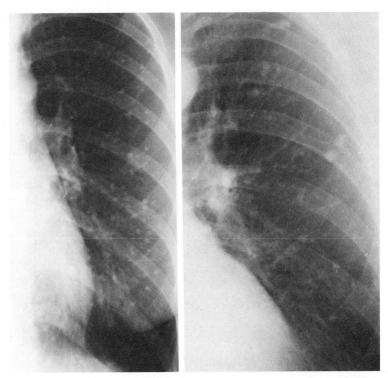

Fig. 26-6. Histoplasmosis. These are examples of calcified pulmonary parenchymal nodules resulting from this disease.

sensitivity rather than tuberculin sensitivity.

The *acute epidemic form* of histoplasmosis reported in a number of localities in the endemic regions probably represent a heavy exposure that results in more pulmonary parenchymal involvement than in the usual primary form of the disease. Often a miliary spread throughout both lungs is observed. The residuals are similar to those of the benign primary form, except that there may be more scattered, calcific, parenchymal foci in the severe acute epidemic form.

Fatal disseminated histoplasmosis is a progressive disease with dissemination not only to the lungs but also to other organs, including the bone marrow. The course may be extremely rapid and fulminating or slowly progressive, leading to cachexia and anemia. Marked variation has been found in the roentgen manifestations of disseminated pulmonary histoplasmosis, ranging from widespread granular nodula-

tions throughout both lung fields, which is the most common, to lobar type of pneumonic consolidation. Scattered involvement simulating other types of pneumonia is also noted and occasionally there is massive pleural effusion. In infants under 1 year the acute disseminated form is often fatal; hepatosplenomegaly is common in addition to extensive pulmonary involvement.

There is an *intermediate form* of histoplasmosis resulting in chronic active pulmonary disease and resembling reinfection tuberculosis clinically and radiographically. Cavitation along with local infiltration and nodulation similar to that noted in chronic pulmonary tuberculosis is often found. Pleural involvement, fibrosis, and contraction of the involved lobe or segment with alteration in the size of the thorax and mediastinal deviation may also be produced (Fig. 26-8). Histoplasmosis involving hilar nodes adjacent to bronchi may

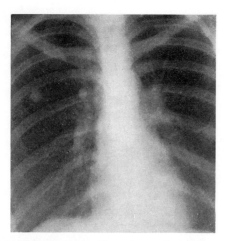

Fig. 26-7. Histoplasmosis. There is a solitary, partially calcified parenchymal nodule in the right upper lung field just below the anterior arc of the second rib. A number of partially calcified nodes are visible in the right hilum. Left hilar nodes are enlarged but no definite calcification is noted.

cause collapse of the middle lobe (middle lobe syndrome) or of other pulmonary segments. It may also be the cause of broncholithiasis.

Mediastinal involvement resulting in a chronic fibrosing process leading to superior vena caval obstruction has also been reported in this disease. The primary disease may have been quite asymptomatic, but the resultant fibrotic mediastinitis may produce pulmonary arterial and venous obstruction, and pericarditis and encroachment on the esophagus in addition to caval obstruction. Any or all of these findings may be present to greater or lesser degree.

The sole manifestation of the disease may be a solitary pulmonary nodule, the histoplasmoma. This lesion may be associated with calcified hilar nodes and there may be a few satellite nodules in the lung. Calcification may or may not be present in the lesion which may vary from 1 to 3 cm or more in diameter. The calcification may be laminated, or annular, solid or stippled, and may be central with a laminated or annular peripheral ring. Skin testing, complement-fixation studies, and mycologic studies are required to differentiate this

disease from pulmonary tuberculosis; occasionally both diseases may be present in the same patient.

CRYPTOCOCCOSIS (TORULOSIS)

This disease is caused by *Cryptococcus neoformans* (*Torula histolytica*). Pulmonary lesions are rare in cryptococcosis, which usually involves the central nervous system. As in other chronic pulmonary infections, several roentgen forms are found and the diagnosis cannot be made from roentgenograms alone (Fig. 26-9). Three general types of radiographic change have been described. The first is a fairly well circumscribed, rounded mass usually occurring in the lower half of either lung field, which must be differentiated from neoplasm as well as from other chronic pulmonary granulomas. The second is a pneumonic type of lesion consisting of a somewhat irregular density resembling the patchy infiltrate of tuberculosis but more likely to appear in the lower lobes than in the upper. This type of disease may extend across interlobar fissures. The density is often massive; cavitation and hilar node enlargement are rare. The third type is a widespread miliary type of nodulation often found in conjunction with severe central nervous system infection. This disease is frequently found associated with such chronic processes as Hodgkin's disease, leukemia, and lymphosarcoma, or is found to occur after steroid or antibiotic therapy. Although the diagnosis cannot be made on the basis of roentgenographic findings, the combination of signs of meningeal irritation and pulmonary lesions resembling those described is suggestive.

NORTH AMERICAN BLASTOMYCOSIS

This disease is confined to the continent of North America and is caused by the yeastlike fungus, *Blastomyces dermatitidis*. There are two general types of the disease, cutaneous and disseminated. In the disseminated form, the portal of entry is usually the respiratory tract and 95 per cent of patients have some form of pulmonary involvement. The roentgen findings in pulmonary disease produced by this organ-

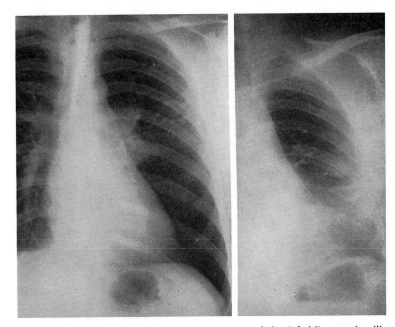

Fig. 26-8. Histoplasmosis. *Left,* Enlargement of the left hilum and a little associated parenchymal disease in the lung lateral to the hilum. The diaphragm is normal and the costophrenic angle is clear. *Right,* Five years later there is more conglomerate disease in the central and basal lung. This slow progression of disease is somewhat unusual.

ism are not characteristic. They vary from large, dense, pneumonic masses to widespread miliary nodules. Bilateral linear densities have also been reported in this disease. Most of the patients we have observed have had large, dense, pneumonic consolidations which are indolent and respond very slowly to treatment with amphotericin B. In these patients, bronchogenic spread to another lobe or to the opposite lung, may be present, resulting in scattered, poorly defined, patchy densities in the areas involved (Figs. 26-10 and 26-11). Pulmonary cavitation occasionally develops; the cavities tend to be small with poorly defined, irregular walls. Occasionally hilar and mediastinal node enlargement predominates to such an extent that the roentgen findings simulate those of malignant lymphoma involving these structures. Rounded, poorly defined, intrapulmonary masses have also been reported that may resemble pulmonary tumor (Fig. 26-12). The changes seen in this disease are similar to those noted in other mycotic infections as well as tuberculosis and neoplasm, so that the diagnosis must be based on mycologic studies.

SOUTH AMERICAN BLASTOMYCOSIS

This disease, caused by *Blastomyces brasiliensis,* is found most commonly in Brazil but has also been reported in the other South American countries. Pulmonary involvement is said to occur in 80 per cent of the patients with the visceral type of the disease. The portal of entry is apparently the intestinal tract in this disease so that the pulmonary lesions are secondary and are widespread and nodular in type.

ASPERGILLOSIS

Pulmonary aspergillosis is rare despite the fact that fungi of the genus *Aspergillus* are ubiquitous. It is often a secondary process in patients

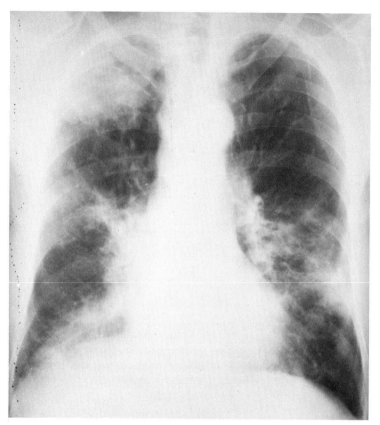

Fig. 26-9. Pulmonary cryptococcosis. There is rather extensive disease in the left lower lung which is poorly defined with some areas of strandlike density along with homogeneous consolidation. On the right there is similar but less extensive disease in the central and lower lung fields and a large homogeneous consolidation in the right apex. Findings are nonspecific.

who have been treated with antibiotics and in those with debilitating disease. It does occur as a primary disease, however. Three clinical and roentgen types of the primary disease have been described.

1. An acute bronchopneumonic form with scattered multiple areas of pneumonic consolidation, some of which break down to form cavities. This disease may progress with severe invasive destructive pulmonary disease eventually leading to death. This invasive form occurs in infants. There is often enough hilar node enlargement to be recognized as such on the roentgenograms.

2. A more chronic and milder form is one with irregular and rounded nodular infiltrates closely resembling those seen in pulmonary tuberculosis. The clinical course of this disease is less severe

than that of tuberculosis but the diagnosis must be made on the basis of identification of the organism in the sputum.

3. This type of aspergillosis has been described by Doub[9] in four patients in whom there were fairly widespread pulmonary nodules that at first were poorly circumscribed. They became more clearly defined and eventually calcified from 2 to 4 years following the onset, leaving multiple calcified parenchymal nodules along with some calcified hilar nodes as residuals. During the acute phase there were symptoms of a respiratory infection and all the patients had some hilar node involvement early in the course of the disease. It appears that aspergillosis may occasionally account for scattered calcified pulmonary parenchymal nodules.

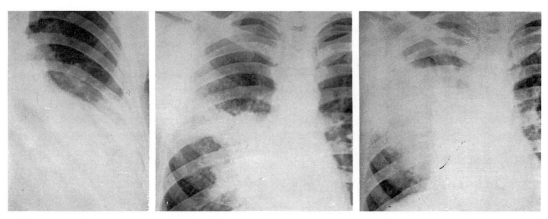

Fig. 26–10. North American blastomycosis. *Left,* Note dense pneumonic consolidation at the left lung base. *Center,* Dense consolidation above the minor fissure on the right and below the right hilum. Scattered patchy infiltration is noted adjacent to the more dense disease. *Right,* Massive consolidation occupying 50 per cent or more of the right lung. These three patients indicate the nonspecificity of roentgen findings.

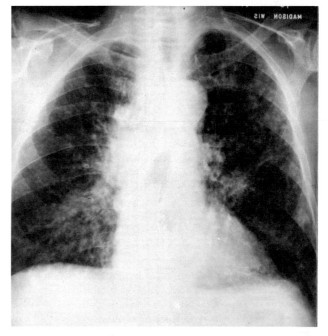

Fig. 26-11. North American blastomycosis. Numerous disseminated nodules are noted which are rather poorly defined and range up to a 1 cm or more in diameter. They are confluent in some areas. Adenopathy in the right hilum is possible. None is identified on the left.

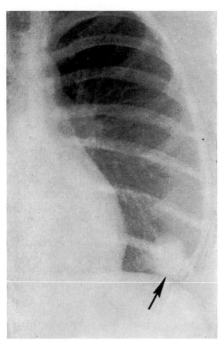

Fig. 26-12. North American blastomycosis. The large round mass at the left base that resembles tumor (**arrow**) was resected and proved to be blastomycosis.

Secondary aspergillosis is found in two forms, the aspergilloma (mycetoma) and a more diffuse form. The diffuse form is found in patients with severe debilitating disease and malignancies, and in those on cytotoxic drugs, steroids or immunosuppressive agents. Roentgen changes depend somewhat on the type of other pulmonary disease present. As a rule, there is diffuse consolidation with poorly defined margins in single or multiple areas. Cavitation may occur. In these patients, the immediate cause of death may be aspergillosis.

The aspergilloma (mycetoma) or fungus ball consists of a localized round or ovoid mass made up of aspergillus hyphae, blood, cellular debris, fibrin and mucous, which occupies a cavity slightly larger than the mass. It is usually found in the upper lobe, probably because the primary disease, commonly tuberculosis, occurs in the upper lobe. A thin, radiolucent rim is observed surrounding the mass. This is caused by air which is between the cavity wall and the mass and is virtually pathognomonic. The mass moves within the cavity. This can be demonstrated on tomography which is

often helpful in the diagnosis when mycetoma is suspected (Fig. 26-13). Calcification may occur within the mass and may be extensive. Hemorrhage is common and may be severe.

It is apparent that aspergillosis can produce a wide variety of pulmonary lesions simulating other chronic inflammatory lesions and the aspergilloma can simulate tumor so that the diagnosis cannot be made on roentgen evidence alone.

MONILIASIS (CANDIDIASIS)

Candida (Monilia) albicans is a yeastlike fungus frequently present in the normal mouth and that may be occasionally mildly pathogenic for man. Since the organism is often present in the normal, it is difficult to document this disease. The literature is very confusing and many of the reported cases are probably examples of other diseases. However, most investigators agree that *Monilia* can produce bronchopulmonary disease. Roentgen findings are a rather fine, mottled miliary type of nodulation associated with some prominence of pulmonary markings or less commonly, segmental homogeneous consolidation. Cavitation is rare, but is simulated when the disease involves an area of lung in which there are preexisting emphysematous bullae. There may be some hilar node enlargement. As in the other fungus diseases, the diagnosis must rest upon identification of the organism. The bronchial secretions rather than sputum should be examined since the organism is a normal inhabitant of the mouth.

GEOTRICHOSIS

Geotrichum is a fungus frequently found in the mouths of healthy subjects but that occasionally becomes pathogenic and causes pulmonary as well as skin and mucous membrane infection. Pulmonary manifestations are not characteristic. Irregular patchy densities are noted, often in both lung fields. Cavitation may develop, the cavities having rather thin walls. Hilar node enlargement is frequent. The disease may closely resemble pul-

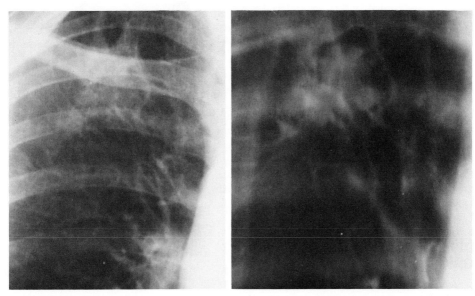

Fig. 26-13. Fungus ball. *Left,* There is an irregular mass somewhat obscured by the clavicle and first rib in the right apex. *Right,* Tomogram shows a somewhat irregular cavity filled with a mass separated from the wall by a radiolucent rim which is somewhat wider than is often observed in patients with aspergilloma.

monary tuberculosis (Fig. 26-14). The diagnosis is based on a positive skin test plus demonstration of the organism on repeated examination. Other fungal infections, as well as tuberculosis, must be excluded by appropriate studies since in this disease, as in moniliasis, the organism may be saprophytic rather than pathogenic.

OTHER MYCOSES

SPOROTRICHOSIS

This disease, produced by *Sporotrichum schenckii,* usually involves the skin, mucous membranes, and lymphatics. Occasionally it may cause pulmonary infection. There is nothing characteristic about the pneumonia it produces. Cavitation is often observed, however. It is sometimes found as a secondary invader in chronic pulmonary tuberculosis.

PENICILLIOSIS

Fungi of the genus *Penicillium* are capable of producing pulmonary infection. This disease is

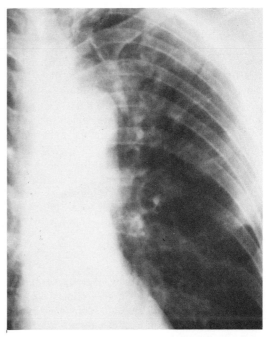

Fig. 26-14. Geotrichosis. Note the nodular disease in the left upper lung field, which resembles pulmonary tuberculosis. This disease was resected and proved to be geotrichosis.

very rare. This mold can cause lung abscess that cannot be distinguished from cavitation produced by other organisms, so that there are no roentgen signs that would lead to the specific diagnosis.

MUCORMYCOSIS (PHYCOMYCOSIS)

Mucor is a mold widely distributed in nature and is not usually pathogenic to man. Several cases of severe disseminated infection have been reported in diabetics, however. In some of these a widespread, rapidly fatal confluent pneumonia is present, which may cavitate, while in others meningitis has occurred.

DISEASES OF SPIROCHETAL ORIGIN

SYPHILIS

Involvement of the lungs in syphilis is very rare and the disease may simulate other chronic pulmonary disease symptomatically and radiographically. The diagnosis, therefore, depends upon exclusion of other diseases and upon laboratory studies as well as response to antiluetic therapy.

ROENTGENOGRAPHIC FINDINGS. Three radiographic types of pulmonary involvement have been described. (1) Interstitial fibrosis resulting in linear densities radiating into the lung fields from the hila; (2) a large solitary mass which may be clearly circumscribed and resemble pulmonary tumor or there may be some irregular inflammatory infiltrate surrounding it so that the lesion simulates other types of inflammatory disease; or (3) chronic lobar pneumonia with fibrosis and decrease in size of the diseased lobe. This type resembles chronic pulmonary tuberculosis.

LEPTOSPIROSIS

This disease is produced by a group of spirochetes called *Leptospira*. Several clinical forms have been described and pulmonary involvement is only a part of widespread disease in most instances. Occasionally hemorrhagic pneumonitis is an early or striking manifestation.

ROENTGENOGRAPHIC FINDINGS. The hemorrhagic pneumonitis usually results in widely disseminated small infiltrations. The individual lesions are poorly defined and hazy and resemble other acute, disseminated, pulmonary inflammations. The second type is a large confluent area of consolidation similar to lobar or segmental pneumonia. The third type consists of small patchy densities that resemble bronchopneumonia or a more linear infiltration such as is noted in virus pneumonitis. The diagnosis cannot be made on roentgen findings and depends upon bacteriologic studies.

PROTOZOAN DISEASES

AMEBIASIS

Amebic infection of the thorax is usually secondary to gastrointestinal involvement and often is associated with hepatic amebiasis. Rarely amebic lung abscess is found without other signs or symptoms of amebiasis.

The roentgen signs are somewhat different in the two types of disease. In the hematogenous pulmonary disease a lung abscess is formed that is similar to lung abscess produced by other organisms. When the abscess is evacuated into a bronchus, an air-fluid level can be demonstrated in upright views. The abscess cavity may become very large, and associated pleural effusion is not uncommon. These lesions do not respond to conventional therapy. When the pulmonary disease or pleural disease is secondary to hepatic involvement the appearance is somewhat more characteristic. The hepatic abscess causes elevation of the diaphragm. Fluid in the pleural space on the right is common. The lower and middle lobes adjacent to the diaphragm are involved by a confluent pneumonia in which cavitation may occur. In some instances the infection is confined to the pleural space in which case an amebic empyema is formed; this is often loculated at the base. In other instances there is a combination of pleural and pulmonary involvement with empyema and lung abscess. The diagnosis is confirmed by the presence of *Endamoeba histolytica* in the sputum.

TOXOPLASMOSIS

This disease is caused by the protozoan parasite *Toxoplasma*. The organism has an affinity for the central nervous system, the eyes, and the lungs. There is an infantile form in which it is not uncommon to find cerebral involvement, beginning in utero, resulting in scattered intracranial calcifications in the newborn. The disease behaves differently in the adult and involves the lungs primarily rather than the central nervous system. The roentgen findings in the lungs are similar to those noted in bronchopneumonia or viral pneumonia. Miliary dissemination produces miliary densities not unlike those noted in other acute miliary infections. If the disease becomes chronic, it may result in scattered areas of fibrosis and in scattered nodules, some or all of which may become calcified.

PNEUMOCYSTIS CARINII PNEUMONIA

This disease is caused by *pnuemocystis carinii,* a protozoan first observed in animals and thought to be a harmless saprophyte. However, epidemics and sporadic cases of the human disease have been reported in Europe since 1945. It has been apparently less frequent in the United States; the

first case was reported in 1955. Pneumocystis carinii pneumonia usually occurs in premature or debilitated infants, in infants or children with agammaglobulinemia or low gamma globulin levels, and in debilitated adults who have been on long-term steroid therapy, antibiotics, cytotoxic drug therapy, or immunosuppressive drugs. It is not infrequent in renal transplant patients.

The clinical onset may be either rapid or insidious, but there is usually a discrepancy between the physical findings in the chest, which are minimal, and the marked dyspnea and often extensive roentgen findings in the chest. Pathologic findings are those of interstitial pneumonia, with mononuclear cells infiltrating the interstitial tissues; very few polymorphonuclear cells are present. The alveoli and alveolar ducts tend to be compressed by the interstitial involvement; there is often enough obstruction to result in peripheral obstructive emphysema.

The roentgen findings are sometimes characteristic. The disease begins in the hilum and spreads peripherally; ultimately, it may involve the entire lung. There is an element of linear density spreading out from the hilum. The peripheral lungs are clear and may be "honeycombed" by local areas

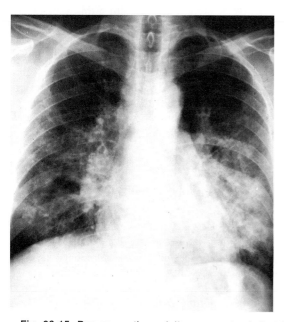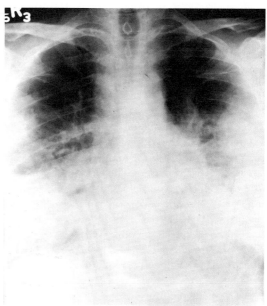

Fig. 26-15. Pneumocystis carinii pneumonia. *Left,* Bilateral parahilar inflammatory disease with considerable consolidation on the left and scattered disease in the right base. *Right,* One month later there has been extensive advance bilaterally. Again the disease is chiefly at the bases and in the central lung fields, sparing the upper lungs. The patient had lymphoma.

of emphysema and small areas of atelectasis. As the disease progresses, slight generalized involvement produces rather homogeneous density spreading outward from the hila. This may progress to the point of nearly total involvement, the lungs appearing virtually airless. No hilar adenopathy is observed. Pneumothorax and pneumomediastinum may occur. This progression is observed in children and sometimes in adults following renal transplantation. However, in many instances the pattern is not characteristic and the disease should always be considered when persistent and extensive pneumonic disease is found in adults with chronic disease (Fig. 26-15), posttransplant patients, and debilitated infants.

Needle biopsy is being used with increasing frequency in the patients suspected of having the disease, since the organism cannot be cultured.

PLATYHELMINTH (FLATWORM) INFESTATION

ECHINOCOCCOSIS (HYDATID DISEASE)

The small tapeworm, *Echinococcus granulosus,* is found in the intestinal tract of dogs. Its larval form is the cause of hydatid cysts. The ova are ingested by man and usually migrate to the liver, but may lodge in the lung where it produces a round or oval density that becomes massive in size. Since the cyst is readily molded as it grows, the shape may be varied, depending on its relation to the bony thorax. A wall is formed, composed of an external capsule caused by the host tissue. There is a double wall therefore, which may be separated by a thin lucent ring. The cyst may rupture into a bronchus and empty part of its contents, in which case an air-fluid level is noted. The cyst wall rarely calcifies in the lung in contrast to the hepatic lesions in which calcification is common. When the cyst ruptures there is a possibility of spread to other parts of the lung, giving rise to multiple, small daughter cysts. Occasionally many small cysts are scattered throughout the lungs. Rarely the cysts may form in the pleural space or may rupture into the pleural space, resulting in pleural effusion. When calcified hydatid cysts are present in the liver and the presence of a cyst in the lung is detected, the diagnosis can be made with a considerable degree of accuracy.

CYSTICERCOSIS

Occasionally humans can develop autoinfection when they have the pork tapeworm, *Taenia solium*. In these patients the cysticercus may be found scattered widely throughout the tissues, including the lungs, where they produce scattered soft-tissue nodular densities. When they die, calcification occurs and multiple oval or spindle-shaped calcifications measuring about 3 by 10 mm can then be noted, scattered in the lung fields and in other tissues as well. The disease is very rare in the United States.

PARAGONIMIASIS

The lung fluke, *Paragonimus westermani,* is distributed widely in the Far East, Africa, and in parts of South America, and has been further disseminated by the military. Hemoptysis is a frequent symptom, along with cough and chest pain. The organism causes an ill-defined consolidation in which eccentric cystic cavitation usually develops. The cyst is characteristic and is peculiar in that a corona effect is produced by a thick wall inferiorly or along one side with a thin wall superiorly. Tomography is useful in demonstrating this finding. Pleural thickening in the interlobar fissures is also observed and fleeting densities thought to represent Löffler's pneumonia often accompany the disease. Dense linear opacities are caused by burrows of the organism which can be demonstrated by bronchography to be independent of bronchi. They probably communicate with the cavities.

SCHISTOSOMIASIS

This disease is caused by three blood flukes, *Schistosoma mansoni, S. japonicum,* and *S. haematobium*. Several types of pulmonary reaction may occur. As the larval forms pass through the lungs, an apparent allergic response produces transient mottled densities. Ova reach the lungs from the veins of the bladder, intestine, and liver where they may implant in or around the arterioles producing necrotizing arteritis, and intra-arterial and peri-arterial granulomas, both of which obstruct the vessel. They rarely may cause multiple arteriovenous fistulas.

Roentgen findings in the chronic form consist of central enlargement of pulmonary arteries secondary to pulmonary hypertension, evidence of cor pulmonale, and a rather minimal amount of interstitial fibrosis causing accentuation of reticular lung markings. The multiple arteriovenous fistulas result in cyanosis with very little roentgen change; this is a rare phenomenon. Occasionally a circumscribed nodule or mass is produced by a granulomatous mass surrounding an adult worm. The wall (pericyst) gradually thickens as the cyst grows. The cyst is enveloped by a wall (endocyst). When air is introduced between the pericyst and the endocyst, a lucent air "halo" is visible, most clearly seen on tomography. When this appears, it often indicates impending rupture. This must be differentiated from mycetoma, but they are usually associated with other disease in the upper lobes, whereas hydatid cysts are usually found in the lower lobes as primary lesions.

NEMATHELMINTH (ROUNDWORM) INFESTATION

A number of roundworms cause pulmonary symptoms and transitory roentgen changes in the lungs as the larvae are carried to the lungs via the veins or lymphatics. As the larvae emerge from the alveolar capillaries into the bronchial tree they produce an allergic response, usually accompanied by eosinophilia. A combination of edema and hemorrhage causes radiographic findings of patchy areas of poorly defined density scattered throughout the lungs. They are transitory and their extent is related to the severity of the infestation. The following roundworms are among those which cause such a reaction: *Ascaris lumbricoides, Strongyloides stercoralis, Ancylostoma duodenale,* and *Necator americanus* (hookworm disease); *Filaria* or *Wuchereria bancrofti, malayi,* and *Loa loa* (filariasis); and *Trichinella spiralis* (trichinosis). In most of them the diagnosis is made by discovery of the larvae or mature worm in the stool specimen.

TROPICAL EOSINOPHILIA

Tropical eosinophilia or pulmonary eosinophilosis is manifested by mild symptoms of cough,

fever, lassitude, and sometimes dyspnea and weight loss associated with an elevation of the white blood count. There is a relative and absolute eosinophilia in the peripheral blood. Most of the reported cases originate in India and Ceylon but a few have been reported in the United States and elsewhere throughout the world. There have also been some cases reported in patients who have lived in India but who have been away more than a year before onset of symptoms. The disease is mild and self-limited but relapses may occur. Some of the cases are definitely caused by filarial infestation and the disease usually responds well to diethylcarbamazine, a drug effective in filariasis. In others, the cause cannot be established.

Roentgen findings are of several types. The most common appearance is that of increased pulmonary markings extending out from the hila, associated with mottled parenchymal disease which is rather general in distribution. The hilar nodes may be enlarged. Next in frequency is the addition of areas of patchy pneumonitis to the small mottled densities. Increased markings alone are nearly as frequent, and extensive scattered involvement by a pneumonialike process occurs occasionally.

SARCOIDOSIS

Sarcoidosis or Boeck's sarcoid is a granulomatous disease that may affect many organs and tissues in the body. The etiology is not clear. A number of theories have been advanced but none has been proved. It is known that most patients show no reaction or only slightly positive reaction to tuberculin and 10 to 20 per cent of patients with sarcoidosis develop frank tuberculosis. The lesion of sarcoidosis is a focal granuloma of epithelioid cells in which giant cells are usually present. Lymphocytes are generally noted around the periphery along with occasional eosinophils. The process resembles a tuberculous granuloma except that there is no central caseation necrosis. These lesions develop slowly and may resolve completely in some instances. They may also heal by a process of sclerosis leading to fibrosis and tissue distortion that may be extensive. Pulmonary involvement is frequent; the reported incidence ranges from 60 to 90 per cent. These figures include enlargement of hilar and paratracheal nodes as well as actual pulmonary parenchymal lesions.

ROENTGEN FINDINGS

Since this disease may be asymptomatic or nearly so for long periods of time, the roentgenographic changes produced by it are often noted for the first time in a survey film or on roentgenograms taken as a part of an examination prior to entrance into the armed services or industry. It is therefore somewhat difficult to be certain that the findings observed in these asymptomatic patients represent early disease.

Roentgen findings can be classified as follows:

1. Hilar and paratracheal adenopathy without parenchymal involvement (Fig. 26-16).

2. Adenopathy with parenchymal involvement. The parenchymal involvement includes a diffuse accentuation of interstitial markings resulting in a reticular pattern, a miliary nodular pattern, a reticular pattern plus miliary nodules (reticulonodular) or plus somewhat larger nodules (Fig. 26-17). The amount of general interstitial change may be varied when associated with nodularity.

3. The above parenchymal involvement without adenopathy.

4. Fibrotic change progressing to pulmonary insufficiency, with cor pulmonale. There may be extensive distortion with conglomerate areas of fibrosis and emphysema. This is the late irreversible form of the disease (Fig. 26-18). Large nodular densities which range up to 5 cm or more in size are occasionally found. They resemble hematogenous pulmonary metastases to some extent, but are not as clearly defined, since the periphery of the individual

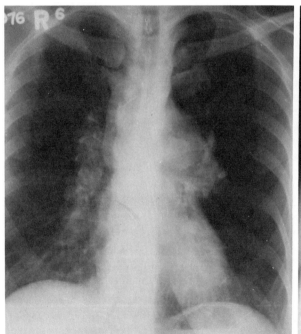
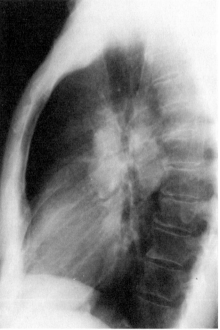

Fig. 26-16. Sarcoidosis. Hilar and right paratracheal adenopathy producing hilar enlargement and mediastinal widening; note the clearly defined enlarged nodes in the lateral view (*right*).

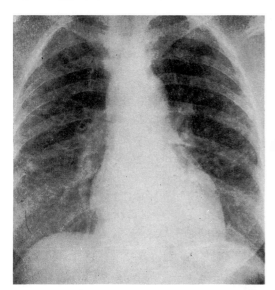

Fig. 26-17. Sarcoidosis. Diffuse pulmonary nodulation is noted, scattered in both lung fields. Hilar adenopathy is not marked.

nodules tends to be indistinct. They may become confluent. We have also observed a unilateral solitary nodular mass that resembled primary lung tumor in one instance. Late in the disease a somewhat cystic pattern may be observed, usually associated with extensive fibrosis which results in bullous emphysema. Pleural involvement is very rare.

All these manifestations can be seen at various times in a single patient and the mediastinal adenopathy has been observed to regress and reappear in patients with disseminated pulmonary lesions. The node enlargement is often massive but is usually symmetric in the hila and the descriptive term "potato" nodes has been applied to the large masses. The enlarged nodes form slightly lobulated masses extending throughout the lung hilum. Characteristically there is a relatively translucent space between the mass of nodes and the cardiovascular margin. This is more apparent on the right side, where the lung hilum normally is better seen than on the left (Fig. 26-19). In contrast, Hodgkin's disease, which is a frequent source of difficulty in differential diagnosis, is more likely to involve the more centrally situated nodes around the tracheal bifurcation in addition to those in the hila and the mass of nodes tends to merge with the cardiovascular silhouette.

The radiographic findings are of some prognostic significance since those patients in whom hilar and paratracheal adenopathy are observed without pulmonary parenchymal involvement often regress to complete disappearance of the large nodes over a period of months or years. Miliary nodular or reticulonodular disease with or without adenopathy also regresses completely in most patients. Steroids are used effectively in some patients, in others the process undergoes spontaneous regression.

The roentgen diagnosis of sarcoidosis can often be made with a considerable degree of certainty. The symmetry of the bilateral, hilar node enlargement along with the frequent associated enlargement of the right paratracheal nodes is characteristic. The pulmonary parenchymal involvement is often symmetric also and this is of diagnostic importance. The discrepancy between the extensive roentgen changes and the mild symptoms is the third finding of diagnostic significance. Finally, when progress roentgenograms are available, the long and slowly progressing or regressing nature of the process can be observed. The diagnosis must be confirmed by the presence of the typical granuloma in involved nodes; it is necessary to perform scalene node biopsy or a lung biopsy to secure positive proof of the disease. The fibrotic stage of the disease is probably irreversible to a certain extent but improvement has been obtained in some patients by the use of steroids.

DIFFERENTIAL DIAGNOSIS

Pulmonary lesions of sarcoidosis can simulate those of pulmonary tuberculosis to such a degree that bacteriologic and histopathologic studies are required to make differentiation. It is often possible, however, to be fairly certain of the diagnosis because of the relative lack of symptoms in the patient with sarcoidosis. The same is true in carcinomatosis, since the latter

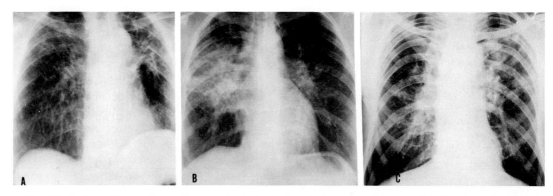

Fig. 26-18. Sarcoidosis. These three patients had chronic long-standing sarcoidosis. Note the fibrosis and contraction with elevation of the left hilum in *A*. The asymmetry of the disease in *B* is somewhat more marked than usual. In addition to the parenchymal fibrosis there appears to be some hilar adenopathy in *C*.

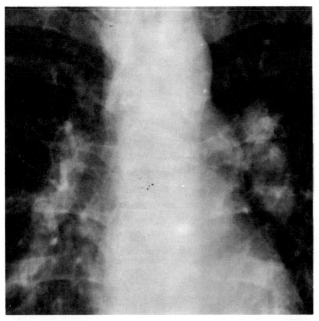

Fig. 26-19. Sarcoidosis. Bilateral hilar adenopathy. Nodes are clearly defined, somewhat lobulated, and there is a clear space between them and the cardiac shadow.

patients manifest the wasting and weakness usually noted in the disease and the presence of a known primary tumor along with clinical and roentgen findings makes the diagnosis of carcinomatosis almost certain. Hodgkin's disease and lymphosarcoma may result in mediastinal lymph node enlargement, which cannot be differentiated from that noted in sarcoidosis.

The malignant lymphomata usually produce more symptoms and the adenopathy is not as symmetric as in sarcoidosis. The more benign types of Hodgkin's disease, however, may be relatively asymptomatic and biopsy is then necessary to differentiate the two diseases. In general the nodes are larger in Hodgkin's disease than in sarcoidosis. Other chronic pulmonary lesions such as mycotic infections, the benign pneumoconioses, and a number of conditions producing interstitial pulmonary fibrosis may result in densities in the lungs similar to those noted in sarcoidosis. In these patients all clinical data must be evaluated along with the history in order to make the differentiation. Even then it is often necessary to obtain biopsy of available peripheral or scalene nodes, or of the lung. In some patients with the characteristic lesions and clinical symptoms of erythema nodosum, roentgen examination of the chest will reveal enlarged hilum nodes and, occasionally, linear and patchy infiltrations in the perihilar zones, resembling in all respects the changes of sarcoid disease. This does not necessarily indicate that the primary disease is sarcoidosis, but, in areas where coccidioidomycosis is not endemic, the combination of these findings is always very suggestive of this diagnosis.

REFERENCES AND SELECTED READINGS

1. BABBITT, D. P., and WAISBREN, B. A.: Epidemic pulmonary histoplasmosis. Roentgenographic findings. *Am. J. Roentgenol. Radium Ther. Nucl. Med. 83:* 236, 1960.

2. BIRK, M., and GERSTL, B.: Torulosis (cryptococcosis) producing solitary pulmonary lesion. *JAMA 149:* 1310, 1952.

3. BIRSNER, J. W.: The roentgen aspects of five hundred cases of pulmonary coccidioidomycosis. *Am. J. Roentgenol. Radium Ther. Nucl. Med. 72:* 556, 1954.

4. CHAIT, A.: *Schistosomiasis mansoni;* Roentgenologic observations in a nonendemic area. *Am. J. Roentgenol. Radium Ther. Nucl. Med. 90:* 688, 1963.

5. CHARTRES, J. C.: Radiological manifestations of parasitism by the tongue worms, flat worms and the round worms more commonly seen in the tropics. *Br. J. Radiol. 38:* 503, 1965.

6. CONANT, N. F., SMITH, D. T., BAKER, R. G., CALLAWAY, J. L., and MARTIN, D. S.: *Manual of Clinical Mycology.* Philadelphia, Saunders, 1954.

7. DICK, R.: The Cryptococcus reviewed. *Australas. Radiol. 9:* 212, 1965.

8. DONOHOO, C. M.: Bronchopulmonary aspergillosis. *Australas. Radiol. 10:* 225, 1966.

9. DOUB, H. P.: Miliary calcification of the lung: Etiologic aspects. *Radiology 51:* 480, 1948.

10. DRUCKMANN, A.: X-ray study of development of pulmonary echinococcus. *Radiol. Clin. 14:* 309, 1945.

11. ELLIS, K., and RENTHAL, G.: Pulmonary sarcoidosis. *Am. J. Roentgenol. Radium Ther. Nucl. Med. 88:* 1070, 1962.

12. FALKENBACH, K. H., BACHMANN, K. D., and O'LOUGHLIN, B. J.: *Pneumocystis carinii* pneumonia. *Am. J. Roentgenol. Radium Ther. Nucl. Med. 85:* 706, 1961.

13. FEINBERG, S. B., LESTER, R. G., and BURKE, B. A.: The roentgen findings in *Pneumocystis carinii* pneumonia. *Radiology 76:* 594, 1961.

14. FELD, D. D., and CADDEN, A. V.: Systemic blastomycosis. *Dis. Chest 16:* 473, 1945.

15. FELSON, B.: Less familiar patterns of pulmonary granulomas. *Am. J. Roentgenol. Radium Ther. Nucl. Med. 81:* 211, 1959.

16. FELSON, B.: Some less familiar roentgen manifestations of intrathoracic histoplasmosis. *Arch. Intern. Med. 103:* 54, 1959.

17. GREENING, R. R., and MENVILLE, L. J.: Roentgen findings in torulosis: Report of four cases. *Radiology 48:* 381, 1947.

18. GROSSMAN, C. B., BRAGG, D. G., and ARMSTRONG, D.: Roentgen manifestations of pulmonary nocardiosis. *Radiology 96:* 325, 1970.

19. GUNDERSON, G. A., and NICE, C. M., JR.: Nocardiosis: A case report and brief review of the literature. *Radiology 68:* 31, 1957.

20. HAWLEY, C., and FELSON, B.: Roentgen aspects of intrathoracic blastomycosis. *Am. J. Roentgenol. Radium Ther. Nucl. Med. 75:* 751, 1956.

21. HERLINGER, H.: Pulmonary changes in tropical eosinophilia. *Br. J. Radiol. 36:* 889, 1963.

22. HEUSLER, N. M., and CLEVE, E. A.: Chronic benign residuals of coccidioidomycosis. *Arch. Intern. Med. 98:* 61, 1956.

23. HOLLINGSWORTH, G.: Gumma of lung. *Br. J. Radiol. 24:* 467, 1951.

24. HOLT, J. F.: Roentgenologic pulmonary manifestations of fatal histoplasmosis. *Am. J. Roentgenol. Radium Ther. Nucl. Med. 58:* 717, 1947.

25. JACOBS, J. B., VOGEL, C., POWELL, R. D., and DEVITA, V. T.: Needle biopsy in *Pneumocystis carinii* pneumonia. *Radiology 93:* 525, 1969.

26. JACOBS, L. G.: Pulmonary torulosis. *Am. J. Roentgenol. Radium Ther. Nucl. Med. 71:* 398, 1958.

27. KUNSTADTER, R. H., MILZER, A., and WHITCOMB, F.: Bronchopulmonary geotrichosis in children. *Am. J. Dis. Child. 79:* 82, 1950.

28. LENCZNER, M., SPAULDING, W. B., and SANDERS, D. E.: Pulmonary manifestations of parasitic infestations. *Can. Med. Assoc. J. 91:* 421, 1964.

29. LEVIN, E. J.: Pulmonary intracavitary fungus ball. *Radiology 66:* 9, 1956.

30. LONGCOPE, W. T., and FREIMAN, D. G.: A study of sarcoidosis. *Medicine 31:* 1, 1952.

31. LULL, G. F., and WINN, D. F., JR.: Chronic fibrous mediastinitis due to *Histoplasma capsulatum. Radiology 73:* 367, 1959.

32. MARCHAND, E. J., MARCIAL-ROJAS, R. A., RODRIGUEZ, R., POLANCO, G., and DIAZ-RIVERA, R. S.: The pulmonary obstruction syndrome in *Schistosoma mansoni* pulmonary endarteritis. *Arch. Intern. Med. 100:* 965, 1957.

33. MAYER, J. H., and ACKERMAN, A. J.: Sarcoidosis. *Am. Rev. Tuberc. 61:* 299, 1950.

34. McGAVRAN, M. H., KOBAYASHI, G., NEWMARK, L., NEWBERRY, M., MILLER, C. A., and HARFORD, C. G.: Pulmonary sporotrichosis. *Dis. Chest 56:* 547, 1969.

35. NITTER, L.: Changes in the chest roentgenogram in Boeck's sarcoid of the lungs. *Acta Radiol. Suppl. 105, 1953.*

36. O'LEARY, O. J., and CURRY, F. J.: Coccidioidomycosis: A review and presentation of one hundred consecutively hospitalized patients. *Am. Rev. Tuberc. 73:* 501, 1956.

37. PALAYEW, M. J., FRANK, H., and SEDLEZKY, I.: Our experience with histoplasmosis: An analysis of seventy cases with follow-up study. *J. Can. Assoc. Radiol. 17:* 142, 1966.

38. PAUL, R.: Pulmonary "coin" lesion of unusual pathology. *Radiology 75:* 118, 1960.

39. REEDER, M. M.: RPC of the month from the AFIP (hydatid cyst). *Radiology 95:* 429, 1970.

40. REEVES, R. J.: Pulmonary histoplasmosis. *Am. J. Roentgenol. Radium Ther. Nucl. Med. 72:* 769, 1954.

41. RIGGS, W., JR., and NELSON, P.: The roentgenographic findings in infantile and childhood histoplasmosis. *Am. J. Roentgenol. Radium Ther. Nucl. Med. 97:* 181, 1966.

42. SCHWARZ, J., and BAUM, G. L.: Fungus diseases of the lungs. *Semin. Roentgenol. V:* 1, 1970.

43. SHAW, R. R.: Thoracic complications of amebiasis. *Surg. Gynecol. Obstet. 88:* 753, 1949.

44. SILVERSTEIN, C. M.: Pulmonary manifestations of leptospirosis. *Radiology 61:* 327, 1953.

45. SULLIVAN, B. H., JR., and BAILEY, F. N.: Amebic lung abscess. *Dis. Chest 20:* 84, 1951.

46. SUWANIK, R., and HARINSUTA, C.: Pulmonary paragonimiasis. *Am. J. Roentgenol. Radium Ther. Nucl. Med. 81:* 236, 1959.

47. TAYLOR, A. B., and BRINEY, A. K.: Observations on pulmonary cocciodioidomycosis. *Ann. Int. Med. 30:* 1224, 1949.

48. THOMAS, S. F., DUTZ, W., and KHODADAD, E. J.: *Pneumocystis carinii* pneumonia (plasma cell pneumonia). *Am. J. Roentgenol. Radium Ther. Nucl. Med. 98:* 318, 1966.

49. WARTHIN, T. A., and BUSHNEFF, B.: Pulmonary actinomycosis. *Arch. Intern. Med. 101:* 239, 1958.

50. WEBSTER, B. H.: Pleuropulmonary amebiasis. *Am. Rev. Resp. Dis. 81:* 683, 1960.

51. WEED, L. A., ANDERSEN, H. A., GOOD, C. A., and BAGGENSTOSS, A. H.: Nocardiosis: Clinical, bacteriologic and pathologic aspects. *N. Engl. J. Med. 253:* 1137, 1955.

27

DISEASES OF OCCUPATIONAL, CHEMICAL, AND PHYSICAL ORIGIN

THE "MALIGNANT" PNEUMOCONIOSES

The term "pneumoconiosis" refers to the group of conditions in which solid foreign substances are inhaled and stored in the lung. They form a group of occupational diseases of considerable economic importance. Many of these foreign materials are capable of producing fibrosis leading to decrease in pulmonary function. They are termed the malignant pneumoconioses, while those conditions produced by substances that do not cause significant fibrosis are termed benign. The malignant pneumoconioses include the following: (*1*) silicosis; (*2*) asbestosis; (*3*) talcosis; (*4*) bauxite fibrosis (shaver's disease); (*5*) coal worker's pneumoconiosis; (*6*) diatomite pneumoconiosis; and (*7*) berylliosis. (This condition is somewhat different from the others listed above and is more properly termed beryllium granulomatosis or beryllium poisoning. In addition, there is a large sensitivity factor. It is an occupational disease and is therefore related to the pneumoconioses and will be included in the present discussion.)

A number of substances may cause benign pneumoconiosis. They are: (*1*) coal dust (anthracosis); (*2*) iron oxide (siderosis); (*3*) barium sulfate (baritosis); and (*4*) tin (stannosis). Benign changes have also been reported with exposure to titanium oxide and tungsten carbide. Some of these dust diseases occur together and such terms as anthrasilicosis and siderosilicosis are then used.

SILICOSIS

This disease is caused by inhalation of particles of silicon dioxide that are less than 5 μ in diameter. The most active particles in producing the fibrotic reaction are those smaller than 3 μ. When these small particles are deposited in the alveoli, they are ingested by phagocytic cells that carry them into the perivascular lymphatics. Some investigators challenge this and indicate that the silica particles migrate and penetrate pulmonary interstitial structures without the aid of macrophages. Some of them remain in the peripheral lymphoid follicles while others reach the intrapulmonary, bronchial, hilar, and paratracheal nodes. The silica then produces a toxic reaction that is mechanical or chemical, or perhaps both. Chemical and physical theories have been supplanted by the immunologic theory. There is now some evidence to suggest that an adsorbed protein on the silica particle acts as an antigen which results eventually in an antibody reaction. This would explain the long latent period as well as progression of the disease long after the patient has been removed from exposure to silica. Whatever the cause, the formation of reticulum and collagen occurs, leading to fibrosis and formation of a silicotic nodule. Silicosis is found in a large number of industries including mining, foundries, and rock drilling, as well as grinding involving the production of silica dust. The development of fibrosis requires time. Even in the most dusty occupations the average time for development of disease in workers exposed to moderate concentrations of silica is 10 to 15 years. One or 2 years of exposure are required when the dust counts are unusually high.

Roentgen classification of silicosis and the pneumoconioses is difficult and a number of conferences and committees have presented new classifications from time to time. A classification has been published by a committee of experts under the auspices of the International Labour Office. The committee has made available a set of standardized films for comparison with roentgenograms of patients with pneumoconiosis. They have also introduced and defined standard descriptive terms. The one presented here (Tables 27-1 and 27-2) was published in 1970. The reader is referred to the original publication for additional information regarding it.[36] Of course these roentgen findings must be related to occupational history and to appropriate clinical and laboratory findings; this is true of all of the pneumoconioses.

Roentgen Observations

The earliest radiographic change produced by silicosis is slight exaggeration of the pulmonary interstitial markings. This is difficult to evaluate because many other conditions can cause the same change and the diagnosis of silicosis cannot be made on the basis of these early findings alone. Scattered pulmonary nodules are found somewhat later in the disease. At first the nodules are discrete and very small, on the order of 1 to 2 mm. At this stage,

an additive effect of multiplicity is necessary to make them visible. Superimposition is probably a factor also. They are usually distributed symmetrically and widely with some tendency to spare the apices and bases. Along with the presence of the scattered nodules, there is usually enough enlargement of hilar nodes to produce a radiographically recognizable increase in hilar size. As the pulmonary nodules increase in size, they tend to became conglomerate. The conglomeration and coalescence is usually accompanied by retraction toward the hilum, leaving the periphery of the lung relatively free of nodules and emphysematous. By the time this stage is reached there is often enough emphysema present to cause a downward displacement of the diaphragm and a decrease in diaphragmatic motion on respiration. There can be a considerable variation in the relative amounts of nodulation, hilar enlargement, and emphysema. The hilar nodes may undergo fibrosis and decrease in size by the time the nodular parenchymal lesions are large enough to be readily visualized. Occasionally there is actual calcification in the silicotic nodules. This is a manifestation of long-standing disease. In addition to the more extensive classifications given earlier which are used for industrial health purposes, the roentgen changes in simple silicosis have been classified into stages or degrees as follows:

Stage I (early nodular). Prominence or exaggeration of markings with faintly visible nodules (Fig. 27-1).

Stage II. Nodules 2 to 3 mm in size that tend to obscure linear markings (Fig. 27-2).

Stage III (Fig. 27-3). Nodules greater than 3 mm with coalescence.

The use of this classification does not indicate that the roentgen changes develop uniformly or that all patients eventually develop the lesions of third-stage silicosis. Therefore, descriptive terms such as early nodular, nodular, and conglomerate nodular are often used to describe the findings in simple silicosis. The hilar nodes are sometimes outlined because of the presence of a thin shell of calcium surrounding them. This has been termed "eggshell calcification" and when present is very suggestive of silicosis, but this type of calcification has also been described in patients with no exposure to silica or silicates (Fig. 27-4).

The diagnosis of silicosis can often be suspected on roentgen examination but the clinical history is of great importance, since the diagnosis cannot be accurately made unless there is a history of enough exposure to silica-containing dust to produce it. Because workers in dusty industries are often followed at intervals by means of chest roentgenograms, a review of these serial films will often lead to an accurate diagnosis. Extensive roentgen findings can be present without much alteration in pulmonary function; the reverse is also true in some instances, so there may be lack of correlation between roentgen appearance and pulmonary function.

SILICOTUBERCULOSIS

Silicosis appears to predispose to pulmonary tuberculosis. Massive areas of density representing conglomerate fibrosis are seen late in silicosis and some believe that infection is necessary to produce these large masses. The typical location for massive conglomerate fibrosis is above and lateral to the lung hilum in the infraclavicular part of the lung field. The masses are usually bilateral and relatively symmetric in size and location. Usually the mass does not reach to the periphery of the lung field; rather, a zone of emphysematous lung is to be seen lateral to the area of fibrosis, the emphysema developing as the involved lung shrinks because of the fibrosis. The typical configuration caused by these masses of fibrous tissue in relation to the central mediastinal shadow has been likened to the "wings of an angel." Atypical forms of conglomerate fibrosis are not uncommon. Thus a mass of fibrous tissue may be present in one lung and not in the other; the lesions may occur in areas other than the subclavicular zones; massive fibrosis may be present with little or none of the characteristic nodulation of silicosis in the rest of the lung fields. When massive fibrosis is observed in the presence of nodular silicosis, pulmonary tuberculosis should be suspected

(Fig. 27-5). Cavitation occurs in silicotuberculosis, but it is also observed in the absence of infection. Therefore, cavity per se is not diagnostic of silicotuberculosis. Bacteriologic confirmation is necessary. This is sometimes very difficult to obtain. In the absence of positive bacteriology, silicotuberculosis should be suspected when the roentgenograms reveal the large conglomerate masses in the upper lung fields, when cavitation is present, when the disease is asymmetric, and when there is a considerable amount of pleural disease. Such patients should be followed carefully by means of frequent chest roentgenograms and bacteriologic examination of sputum and gastric washings because of the high incidence of tuberculosis. Cavitation in conglomerate nodular silicosis is not always caused by tuberculosis, however, In one series of 182 patients with cavitation, 18 per cent were found to be nontuberculous. In these patients the cavity results from ischemic necrosis within the conglomerate mass.

ASBESTOSIS

Asbestos, a hydrated magnesium silicate, is a fibrous mineral used as an insulator against heat and cold and as a fireproofing material. The most important from the standpoint of pneumoconiosis is the serpentine mineral, chrysotile (white asbestos) which is magnesium silicate. This makes up 90 per cent of the total world production of asbestos. The other important forms are amosite (brown asbestos), an iron magnesium silicate; and crocidolite (blue), an iron sodium silicate which appears to have more carcinogenic properties than chrysotile, particularly in the causation of mesothelioma. Occupational exposure occurs in the manufacture and in the installation of insulating materials containing asbestos. The mechanical irritation of the long stiff fibers when they become lodged in the lungs is believed to account, at least in part, for the fibrosis that results. The autoimmune theory has been proposed as pathogenetic in this disease as in silicosis. However, there is some

TABLE 27-1. UICC/Cincinnati Classification of Radiographic Appearances of Pneumoconioses

		Codes	Definitions
Small opacities	Rounded profusion	0/- 0/0 0/1 1/0 1/1 1/2 2/1 2/2 2/3 3/2 3/3 3/4	The category of profusion is based on assessment of the concentration of opacities in the affected zones. The standard films define the midcategories. Category 0—small rounded opacities absent or less profuse than in category 1. Category 1—small rounded opacities definitely present but relative few in number. Category 2—small rounded opacities numerous. The normal lung markings are usually still visible. Category 3—small rounded opacities very numerous. The normal lung markings are partly or totally obscured.
	Type	p q r	The nodules are classified according to the approximate diameter of the predominant opacities. p—rounded opacities up to about 1.5 mm in diameter. q—rounded opacities exceeding about 1.5 mm and up to about 3 mm in diameter. r—rounded opacities exceeding about 3 mm and up to about 10 mm in diameter.
	Extent	Lung zones	The zones in which the opacities are seen are recorded. Each lung is divided into thirds—upper, middle, lower zones. Thus a maximum of six zones can be affected.
	Irregular profusion	0/- 0/0 0/1 1/0 1/1 1/2 2/1 2/2 2/3 3/2 3/3 3/4	The category of profusion is based on assessment of the concentration of opacities in the affected zones. The standard films define the midcategories. Category 0—small irregular opacities absent or less profuse than in category 1. Category 1—small irregular opacities definitely present but relatively few in number. The normal lung markings are usually visible. Category 2—small irregular opacities numerous. The normal lung markings are usually partly obscured. Category 3—small irregular opacities very numerous. The normal lung markings are usually totally obscured.
	Type	s t u	As the opacities are irregular, the dimensions used for rounded opacities cannot be used, but they can be roughly divided into three types. s—fine irregular or linear opacities t—medium irregular opacities u—coarse (blotchy) irregular opacities
	Extent	Lung zones	The zones in which the opacities are seen are recorded. Each lung is divided into thirds—upper, middle, lower zones—as for rounded opacities.
Large opacities	Size	A B C	Category A—an opacity with greatest diameter between 1 cm and 5 cm, or several such opacities the sum of whose greatest diameters does not exceed 5 cm. Category B—one or more opacities larger or more numerous than those in category A, whose combined area does not exceed one third of the area of the right lung. Category C—one or more large opacities whose combined area exceeds one third of the area of the right lung.
	Type	wd id	As well as the letter "A," "B" or "C," the abbreviation "wd" or "id" should be used to indicate whether the opacities are well defined or ill defined.

Other features		Right	Left			

Other features

Pleural thickening

costophrenic angle — Obliteration of the costophrenic angle is recorded separately from thickening over other sites. A lower-limit standard film is provided.

Other sites — (Right Left 1 2 3)
- Grade 0—not present or less than grade 1
- Grade 1—up to 5 mm thick and not exceeding one-half of the projection of one lateral chest wall. A lower-limit standard film is provided.
- Grade 2—more than 5 mm thick and up to one-half of the projection of one lateral chest wall *or* up to 5 mm thick and exceeding one-half of the projection of one lateral chest wall.
- Grade 3—more than 5 mm thick and extending more than one-half of the projection of one lateral chest wall.

Diaphragm

ill defined — (Right Left 1 2 3) The lower limit is one-third of the affected hemidiaphragm. A lower limit standard film is provided.

Cardiac outline

ill defined (shagginess) — (1 2 3)
- Grade 0—up to one-third of the length of the left cardiac border or equivalent.
- Grade 1—above one-third and up to two-thirds of the length of the left cardiac border or equivalent.
- Grade 2—above two-thirds and up to the whole length of the left cardiac border or equivalent.
- Grade 3—more than the whole length of the left cardiac border or equivalent.

Pleural calcification

diaphragm walls
other sites — (1 2 3)
- Grade 0—no pleural calcification seen
- Grade 1—one or more areas of pleural calcification, the sum of whose greatest diameters does not exceed 2 cm
- Grade 2—one or more areas of pleural calcification, the sum of whose greatest diameters exceeds 2 cm but does not exceed 10 cm
- Grade 3—one or more areas of pleural calcification, the sum of whose greatest diameters exceeds 10 cm

Other symbols

Obligatory

ca —suspect cancer of lung or pleura
co —a normality of cardiac size or shape
cp —suspect cor pulmonale
es —eggshell calcification of hilar or mediastinal lymph nodes
tba—opacities suggestive of active clinically significant tuberculosis
od —other significant disease. This includes disease not related to dust exposure, e.g., surgical or traumantic damage to chest walls, bronchiectasis, etc.

Optional

ax —coalescence of small rounded pneumoconiotic opacities
bu—bullae
cn —calcification in small parenchymal opacities
cv —cavity
di —marked distortion of the intrathoracic organs
em—marked emphysema
hi —marked enlargement of hilar shadows
ho —honeycomb lung
k —Kerley's (septal) lines
px —pneumothorax
rl —pneumoconiosis modified by rheumatoid process
tb —inactive tuberculosis.

From UICC/Cincinnati classification of the radiographic appearances of pneumoconiosis. *Chest 58:* 57, 1970.

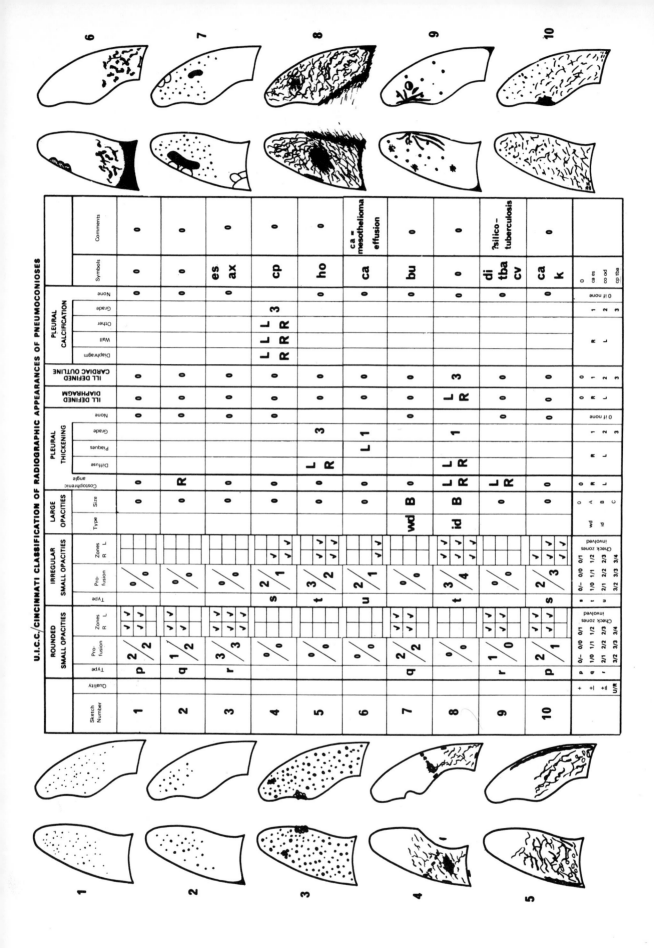

U.I.C.C./CINCINNATI CLASSIFICATION OF RADIOGRAPHIC APPEARANCES OF PNEUMOCONIOSES

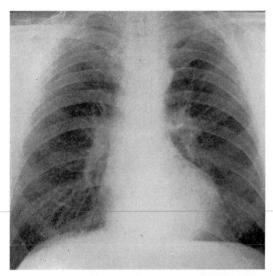

Fig. 27-1. Silicosis. There are scattered small nodules associated with a minimal prominence of interstitial markings. This represents an early nodular silicosis (category I, UICC).

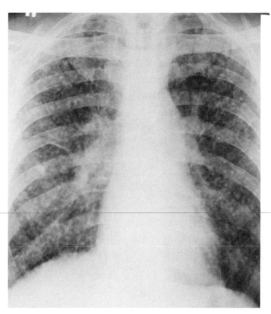

Fig. 27-2. Silicosis. Disease is more advanced here than in the patient shown in Figure 27-1. The nodules are larger and more profuse. There is some hilar node enlargement in addition to the scattered nodular change. This is similar to category III, or to the second stage in the old classification.

evidence to show that the pleural reaction is at least in part caused by mechanical irritation by the fibers which penetrate the visceral pleura. The disease does not develop unless there is a lengthy exposure, usually 10 years or more, to a fairly high concentration of dust. When the pulmonary lesion is established, it progresses even though exposure is not continued. The clinical findings are those of progressive dyspnea that is often out of proportion to the amount of roentgen change noted on the chest films. There is often cyanosis and cough with sputum in which asbestos bodies can be detected. However, many patients with asbestos fibers in the lungs are asymptomatic. The incidence of tuberculosis is not as high as in silicosis. There is an increased incidence of carcinoma of the lungs in patients with asbestosis and an increased incidence of pleural mesothelioma has also been established.

Roentgen Observations

The fibrosis produced by the foreign material results in nonspecific accentuation of pulmonary markings extending into the perihilar regions and bases in the earliest phase of the

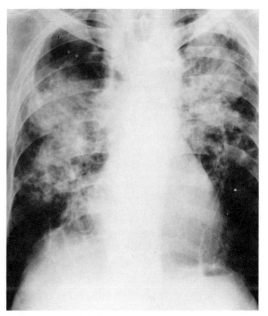

Fig. 27-3. Third-stage or conglomerate nodular silicosis. This is category C in the new classification. There is basal emphysema and hilar adenopathy was observed on the original film.

TABLE 27-2 (opposite)

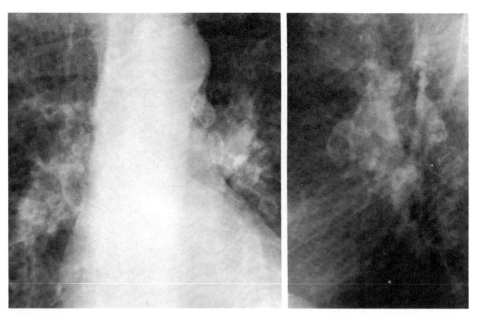

Fig. 27-4. Eggshell calcification in silicosis demonstrated on frontal (*left*) and lateral (*right*) projections.

disease. Later there is an increase in the basal fibrotic infiltrates, which usually appear stringy rather than nodular. The cardiac borders assume a shaggy appearance and the pleural surfaces may also appear shaggy. Pleural thickening, which may extend into the fissures, is common and may be the only roentgen finding. This often results in an irregular tenting of the diaphragm, giving it a shaggy appearance. Calcification also occurs in the areas of pleural involvement. Occasionally, areas of homogeneous density resembling pneumonic consolidation may appear. They may be unilateral or bilateral and are not necessarily symmetric. Pleural thickening is usually associated with this type of disease. When pleural thickening is the predominant feature, a homogeneous or ground-glass appearance may result. Pulmonary emphysema is usually present and may be severe. Pulmonary hypertension leads to hilar vascular prominence, but eggshell calcification of nodes is not a feature of this disease. As in silicosis, the diagnosis is based on correlation of the roentgen with the clinical findings plus an accurate occupational history of exposure to asbestos dust for long periods of time.

TALCOSIS

Talc is a hydrous magnesium silicate in which there is no free silica. It is reported to produce a malignant type of pneumoconiosis in workers exposed to it in mining and milling operations. The roentgen findings are similar to those in asbestosis. In severe cases plaques of calcium density are deposited in and adjacent to the pleura, usually at the bases and along the cardiac borders. This can occur in other pneumoconioses but is much more common in talcosis and when present suggests the etiology of the pneumoconiosis. Emphysema is also a prominent feature of this disease. The diagnosis, as in the other pneumoconioses, is based on correlation of historical, clinical, and radiographic findings.

BAUXITE FIBROSIS (SHAVER'S DISEASE)

This is a form of malignant pneumoconiosis that occurs in workers exposed to fumes containing fine particles of aluminum oxide and silica used in the manufacture of synthetic abrasives. The ore, known as bauxite, is fused in furnaces.

The radiographic findings consist of fibrosis with a slight increase in interstitial markings

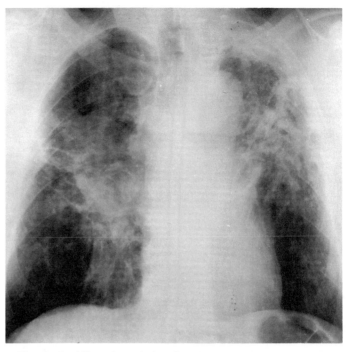

Fig. 27-5. Silicotuberculosis. Conglomerate disease is present bilaterally. Several cavities are noted in the left upper lobe. Tubercle bacilli were found in the sputum.

progressing to extensive fibrotic change. Emphysematous blebs are commonly observed and spontaneous pneumothorax is not infrequent. There is often a history of repeated spontaneous pneumothorax and in some patients there may be considerable pleural thickening. In severe disease the strands of fibrosis radiating from the hilum become coarse and produce mediastinal widening. In these late stages emphysema is usually marked. The diagnosis depends upon the history of exposure to the fumes of bauxite ore along with the clinical and roentgen findings. The disease is believed to be caused by the silica, but it is known that aluminum oxide can also induce pneumoconiosis under some conditions. There may be a sensitivity factor in the latter disease.

COAL WORKER'S PNEUMOCONIOSIS

This condition occurs in coal miners and also in those who work with coal elsewhere in extremely dusty conditions, such as in the hold of coal barges or ships. The condition is found chiefly in anthracite (hard coal) workers. The disabling or malignant pneumoconiosis is usually caused by silica and is, in reality, anthrasilicosis. Occasionally, a progressive form of the disease is found in bituminous (soft coal) workers; this is thought to be caused by exposure to extremely high concentrations of coal dust. This results in the accumulation of so much dust that the self-cleansing mechanism of the lung is overwhelmed and eventual damage leading to fibrosis and emphysema may take place. Roentgen findings are similar to those of silicosis. Progressive disease leading to massive fibrosis and conglomeration is probably caused by superimposed infection, often tuberculous in origin.

DIATOMACEOUS EARTH (DIATOMITE) PNEUMOCONIOSIS

Diatomaceous earth is used widely in filtration processes, as insulating material, as a catalyst carrier, and as an admixture for concrete. The crude diatomite contains amorphous silica. In certain types of processing, some of the amorphous silica is changed to crystalline silica in the form of cristobalite which produces a malignant pneumoconiosis not seen in crude diatomite workers. There is no increase in the incidence of tuberculosis in workers with this disease and there is no alteration of the course of tuberculosis.

The roentgen patterns are described as linear, nodular, or coalescent. The linear form results in accentuation of the bronchovascular pattern increasing to a reticular network of density throughout the lungs. Nodulation is very fine and granular at first; this may progress to coarse nodulation which may then progress to confluent or coalescent masses, usually appearing in the lung apices. Emphysema is often marked; bullae may rupture, leading to spontaneous pneumothorax. There is no constant progression from one stage to another as in silicosis. Hilar adenopathy is not present in this disease, and eggshell calcifications are not present in hilar nodes.

BERYLLIOSIS

Beryllium compounds are used in the manufacture of radio tubes, phosphors, fluorescent lamps, and precision instruments. Workers in these industries may be exposed to small amounts of beryllium, leading to a chronic form of beryllium granulomatosis. Workers in the beryllium extraction industries may be exposed to larger amounts, leading to an acute pneumonitis. Laboratory research workers who have been exposed have developed the pneumonitis. The disease has also been observed in people who live in the neighborhood of plants as a result of exposure to exhaust fumes that contain beryllium.

The disease produced by inhalation of dust containing beryllium might better be termed beryllium granulomatosis or beryllium poisoning because (1) the pathologic lesion that follows is a granuloma resembling that found in sarcoidosis; and (2) relatively small exposure can produce extensive disease. This is in sharp contrast to the pneumoconioses produced by silica and the silicates (asbestos and talc), which require years of continued exposure in dusty occupations. In addition to causing pulmonary disease, beryllium results in severe reaction in other organs and tissues wherever it is lodged. There is evidently a considerable factor of individual sensitivity to this metal. Two distinct types of pulmonary disease are observed, an acute beryllium pneumonitis that develops within a few days of exposure and a chronic beryllium granulomatosis that occurs after a latent period varying from 3 months to 3 years or more after exposure.

ACUTE BERYLLIUM PNEUMONITIS

This is a chemical pneumonitis resulting in pulmonary edema and hemorrhage. The onset is more insidious than other types of chemical pneumonitis and tends to develop over a period of several days to 2 or 3 weeks. Following the initial pulmonary edema, there is often an alveolar exudate made up largely of plasma cells. If the disease does not terminate fatally in 2 or 3 weeks, gradual recovery tends to occur over a period of several months and may be complete. The roentgen findings in the acute process are similar to those noted in pulmonary edema. There is diffuse symmetric increase in density that is most marked in the midlung field, with poorly defined, soft shadows noted peripherally. In other instances the densities may be smaller and more patchy and tend to simulate widespread bronchopneumonia. As the patient recovers there is gradual clearing which may be irregular, resulting in a more patchy or conglomerate nodular appearance. Complete clearing usually is slow and requires from 1 to 4 months. The history of exposure to beryllium is necessary to differentiate this disease from chemical pneumonitis and pulmonary edema resulting from other causes.

CHRONIC BERYLLIUM GRANULOMATOSIS

This condition is characterized by a long latent period of 1 to 20 years after the initial exposure to beryllium. Roentgen findings may be extensive before symptoms are marked. The roentgen findings are somewhat variable.

Fine diffuse granularity that resembles fine

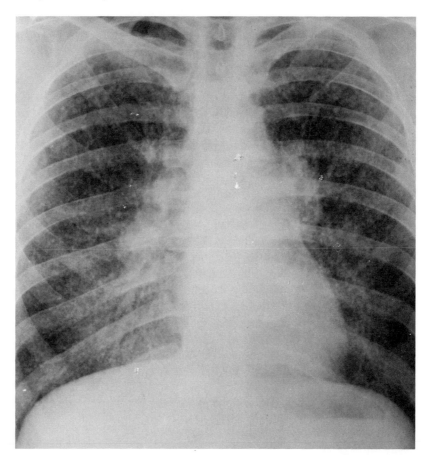

Fig. 27-6. Chronic beryllium granulomatosis. Massive hilar node enlargement is demonstrated. The parenchymal disease consists of uniform fine granulations distributed throughout both lung fields. There is some conglomeration superiorly to form nodules ranging up to 3 or 4 mm, in size.

sand may be observed (Fig. 27-6). In others there is a diffuse reticular pattern plus granularity. The hila are fuzzy and indistinct. In some the lesions are larger, and distinct nodules ranging from 1 to 5 mm in diameter, are present. Combinations may be observed. In addition, it is likely that earlier change consisting of slight increase in linear markings could be recognized if films were taken at frequent intervals following the initial exposure. Hilar enlargement is a common finding and this in part is caused by enlargement of pulmonary vessels secondary to pulmonary hypertension leading to cor pulmonale. As the fibrosis continues in the late stages there is some tendency to confluence, but this is much less than is noted in silicosis. Emphysema is found and may be severe. Spontaneous pneumothorax is common. There is no evidence of calcification in nodes and no pleural reaction. Tuberculosis is not ordinarily a complication so that cavitation is not present and the large conglomerate masses of density noted in silicosis are not common in beryllium granulomatosis. The diagnosis may be suspected on the roentgen examination but must be confirmed by adequate history of exposure. If this is lacking, or open to question, pulmonary biopsy and chemical determination of the presence of beryllium in the tissues are necessary.

THE "BENIGN" PNEUMOCONIOSES

There are a number of inorganic dusts that may be stored in the lungs following inhalation and that produce no fibrosis or other reaction. As a result there are roentgen findings in patients with no clinical evidence of disease.

SIDEROSIS. This is a benign pneumoconiosis due to accumulation of iron oxide in the lung. It is found in electric-arc and acetylene welders, silver polishers, boiler scalers, and in grinders and burners at foundries in which there is insufficient silica to produce silicosis. The iron is inhaled as small particles or in fumes containing iron oxide produced by welding. The roentgen findings are caused by the fact that the iron accumulates in the lymphatics and interstitial tissues of the lung in sufficient quantity to produce radiographic density. No fibrosis or decrease in pulmonary function is caused and there is no predisposition to tuberculosis in these patients.

The roentgen findings consist of discrete, sharply defined, granular densities (1 to 3 mm in size) scattered uniformly and symmetrically throughout both lung fields. The individual lesions are often more clearly defined than in silicosis and there is no tendency toward conglomeration. There is no reticular density extending from the hilum into the lung field in these patients and there is no hilar adenopathy such as is frequently observed in silicosis. Other features that tend to differentiate this condition from silicosis are the absence of emphysema and clinical symptoms. The densities tend to regress and may disappear when the exposure is discontinued.

BARITOSIS. This consists of deposition of barium sulfate in the lungs of workers in barium mines. The findings are similar to those in siderosis except that the density of the barium is greater and the individual lesions tend to be larger. The condition probably produces no alteration in pulmonary function. Fibrotic changes leading to diminished function have been reported, but the patients were also exposed to other dusts known to cause fibrosis.

STANNOSIS. The benign pneumoconiosis called stannosis is found in ore handlers and grinders, in tin-smelting workers, and in those who pack tin oxide into bags. It is caused by deposition of tin in the form of stannic oxide in pulmonary tissues. This results in a benign pneumoconiosis similar to baritosis.

OCCUPATIONAL DISEASES RELATED TO PULMONARY HYPERSENSITIVITY

BAGASSOSIS

Bagasse is the product remaining after extraction of the juice from sugarcane. Inhalation of this dust may cause symptomatic pulmonary disease. After an exposure of from 2 to 4 months the clinical manifestations appear in the form of an acute febrile illness with coughing and dyspnea that may become severe. A number of fungi including thermophilic actinomycetes have been found in patients with this condition. It is now believed to represent an antigen-antibody reaction with possible additional injury caused by the presence of the foreign bodies in lung tissue. The clinical findings usually disappear slowly when the patient is kept out of the dusty occupation.

Roentgen findings are those of perihilar consolidations, usually the result of prominent peribronchial markings around the hila. Occasionally a fine granular type of density is noted bilaterally and this is usually symmetric and fairly widespread. Regression is slow and the roentgen findings clear gradually in 6 to 12 months. The history of adequate exposure to the dust, along with the clinical manifestations and roentgen findings, lead to the correct diagnosis. The illness causes fever along with the nonspecific roentgen findings and must be differentiated from tuberculosis and other chronic pulmonary inflammatory diseases. Therefore it is necessary to examine and culture the sputum when there is any question as to the diagnosis.

BYSSINOSIS

This is a pulmonary disease found in cotton-mill workers. It is sometimes called "cotton-mill fever" and is believed to result from inhalation of cotton dust. Symptoms consist of sneezing and coughing along with some wheezing. They tend to come on in attacks that are related to the exposure to dust. The attacks subside when the patient is removed from the dusty atmosphere. The roentgen findings are nonspecific and consist of some accentuation of perihilar markings along with relatively symmetric distribution of irregular infiltrates in the form of patchy, poorly defined densities in the central lung fields. These findings may not appear until after a number of acute attacks. Emphysema and permanent fibrosis may result if the patient remains in the dusty occupation. This disease is believed to be caused by an antigen-antibody reaction with the target tissue principally the respiratory airways rather than the alveoli as in bagassosis.

FARMER'S LUNG

Farmer's lung or thresher's lung is a pulmonary disease that occurs in farm workers following exposure to moldy hay, grain, or silage, particularly in a closed area. It is characterized by the sudden onset of intense dyspnea, cyanosis, cough, slight fever, and night sweats that usually start a few hours after exposure to moldy material. Respirations are rapid and rales are often present but there is no typical asthmatic type of breathing. The course is one of gradual improvement of clinical and roentgen findings over a period of 6 to 8 weeks. If the patient returns and continues working in the same environment, symptoms recur. The disease varies in severity but eventually the patient is forced to stay away from the source of the dusty material that causes it. It has been demonstrated that this is an antigen-antibody reaction, with the principal antigens being thermophilic actinomycetes, i.e., *Thermopolyspora polyspora,* and to a lesser extent *Micromonospora vulgaris.* Histopathological study shows a granulomatous interstitial pneumonitis in early cases. Later interstitial fibrosis may result.

Roentgen Observations

There is a considerable variation in the roentgen findings in these patients. In the acute phase there is usually a fine granular density occupying most of both lung fields. There is some tendency to spare the apices. The involvement may be so

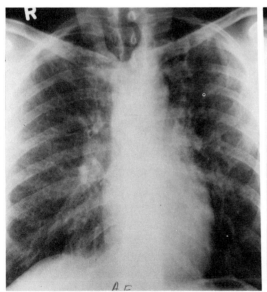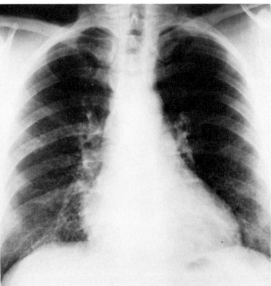

Fig. 27-7. Farmer's lung. *Left,* Patient had an acute episode of cough and fever. There is a combination of some poorly defined granular nodularity and an increase in interstitial markings which is more readily observed on the right than on the left. *Right,* The disease in this patient is manifested by numerous small granular nodules scattered in both lower lung fields with relatively small amount of interstitial change.

extensive that the small individual granular foci are obscured. The hila often appear thickened and poorly marginated. The disease regresses over a period of 6 to 8 weeks, often in an irregular manner so that the lesions become mottled and patchy; there is often some accentuation of interstitial markings extending outward from the hila for some time after the major part of the infiltrate has disappeared (Fig. 27-7). Eventually this interstitial type of density may also clear completely. Pulmonary function studies often indicate a definite decrease in pulmonary function even after all roentgen findings have disappeared.

In patients in whom there have been several attacks, permanent recognizable roentgen changes are noted. They consist of evidence of pulmonary emphysema and interstitial fibrosis. The latter is manifested by a general increase in interstitial markings extending from the hilum out to the periphery, often resulting in a rather coarse reticular appearance of the peripheral lung field. These patients may become respiratory cripples.

PIGEON BREEDER'S DISEASE

This disease occurs in pigeon handlers and appears to be caused by hypersensitivity to antigens in pigeon feathers, serum, and droppings. Roentgen findings include accentuation of interstitial markings with superimposed small nodulations. In acute or severe disease, scattered areas of poorly defined, patchy density indicating alveolar exudation are observed. On biopsy, a granulomatous interstitial pneumonitis is observed. Symptoms disappear and radiographic signs clear when the patient is removed from contact with the birds and their habitat. In some cases there is diminution in pulmonary function (diffusing capacity) which persists for a long time.

MAPLE-BARK DISEASE

This disease occurs in sawmill or papermill workers exposed to the spores of the fungus *Cryptostroma corticale* which lies deep in the bark of the maple tree. Roentgen findings are similar to those of other pulmonary hypersensitivity states, namely an increase in interstitial lung markings and nodularity producing a reticulonodular pattern in parahilar areas and lower lungs. More severe involvement results in a scattered alveolar exudate resulting in confluent pneumonia. Removal from the environment results in clearing of the process.

OTHER OCCUPATIONAL HYPERSENSITIVITY STATES

In addition to the conditions described above, a number of others have been reported in which pulmonary disease is caused by inhalation of material which evidently contains antigens to which the lungs react as a result of hypersensitivity. The radiographic findings in the lungs and the histopathologic manifestations are quite similar. Examples are: (1) Pituitary snuff users lung—inhaled posterior pituitary extracts used in treating patients with diabetes insipidus; (2) mushroom picker's disease; (3) malt-worker's lung; and (4) sequoiosis. A number of other occupational diseases have also been reported.

DISEASES CAUSED BY CHEMICAL AND PHYSICAL AGENTS

HYDROCARBON PNEUMONITIS

A number of products have been implicated in hydrocarbon ingestion or inhalation or both. They include kerosene, gasoline, furniture polish, lighter fluid, cleaning fluid, and turpentine. These products are usually ingested, but some of the irritant material is also aspirated or inhaled. The aspiration is generally the most important factor in the etiology of pneumonitis. The ingested hydrocarbon is absorbed and excreted into the lungs, adding to the pulmonary injury. If vomiting occurs, some additional hydrocarbon may be aspirated. These petroleum distillates cause an acute alveolitis with exudation of leukocytes, fluid, and fibrin and a more chronic proliferative interstitial infiltration. The pathologic findings in patients who have succumbed are those of severe hemorrhagic pulmonary edema, bronchiolar necrosis, and alveolar exudation. There are sometimes few, if any, clinical signs of pulmonary involvement despite the presence of roentgen evidence of pulmonary disease.

Roentgen Observations

There is considerable variation in pulmonary roentgen findings depending upon the severity of the injury. The manifestations are usually diffuse density, homogeneous or somewhat flocculent confined to the lower lobes, but in severe cases the diffuse density extends into the upper lung field as well. When the involvement is less marked it consists of mottled densities in one or both lung fields. The individual foci are hazy and poorly defined; there may be conglomeration in some areas (Fig. 27-8). These roentgen changes develop rapidly and can be seen as early as one-half hour following ingestion. Less frequently the changes are confined to the parahilar areas, resembling pulmonary edema. Clearing of roentgen signs usually lags behind clinical improvement. Pneumatocele formation in these patients has been reported. Rarely pleural effusion, pneumothorax, and in-

terstitial emphysema occur. The diagnosis is based on the history along with the roentgen manifestations described.

INDUSTRIAL AND WAR GASES

A number of irritant gases are capable of producing pulmonary changes that can be visualized roentgenographically. They include nitric fumes (which consist of five oxides of nitrogen), hydrogen sulphide, chlorine, phosgene, mustard gas, as well as a number of other irritating gases. All these gases produce pathologic changes in the lungs that vary with the intensity of exposure. Inflammatory changes are found in the trachea and larger bronchi with minimal exposures. As the amount of exposure increases, the damage to these structures is intensified with a tendency for the process to extend farther out into the smaller bronchi and bronchioles. This results in pulmonary edema and congestion secondary to the chemical bronchitis and bronchiolitis. If the injury is severe enough, death may result. There is often a delay in onset of clinical symptoms following

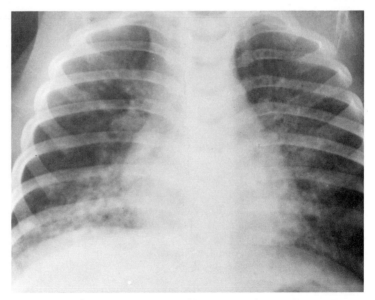

Fig. 27-8. Hydrocarbon pneumonitis (kerosene). The disease is confined to the parahilar areas and bases and is noted to be somewhat more marked on the right where there is a rather poorly defined, diffuse alveolar pneumonitis.

exposure ranging from 1 or 2 hours to as long as 36 hours. Chest pain, cough, and dyspnea are the most common symptoms.

Roentgen Observations

Roentgen findings vary with the extent and severity of the injury. They consist of a patchy mottling, usually most marked in the perihilar areas where the lesions may be confluent (Fig. 27-9). In the central and peripheral lung fields individual nodules may be visible that range up to 1 cm in size and are fluffy in appearance, with poorly defined edges resembling foci of bronchopneumonia. The periphery of the lung fields is usually spared unless the injury has been overwhelming. When the injury has not been severe, clearing occurs rather rapidly wth striking changes noted from day to day and is often complete in 10 to 14 days. During this period the lesions become more irregular and asymmetric, since small areas of atelectasis and often some patchy bronchopneumonia develop. The diagnosis is based on the history of exposure to noxious gas followed by the symptoms of cough and dyspnea plus the roentgen findings of pulmonary edema as described.

SILO-FILLER'S DISEASE

It is known that nitrogen dioxide is produced in silos within a few hours to 3 or 4 days after the silo is filled. Any person entering such a confined space and remaining there is exposed to this irritating gas. Cough and dyspnea often occur immediately. Pulmonary edema in parahilar areas and at the bases may appear in a few hours. This clears rather rapidly if the patient recovers. This may be followed by a period of relative freedom or remission of symptoms for 2 or 3 weeks. There is then a second phase of illness, characterized by fever, progressive dyspnea, cyanosis, and cough that may be fatal, or recovery may occur. The roentgen findings on films taken during the second phase consist of widespread scattered miliary densities resembling the lesions of acute miliary tuberculosis. Later these may become confluent, producing a more patchy and nodular type of appearance. The diagnosis is based upon a com-

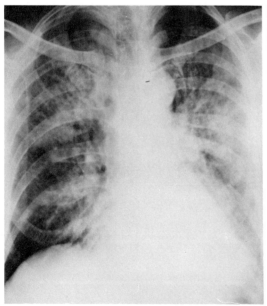 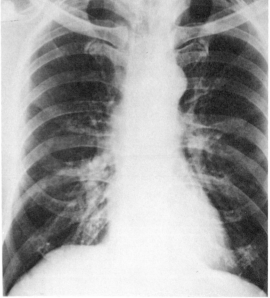

Fig. 27-9. Chemical pneumonitis. The widespread, mottled, poorly defined densities are typical, but history of exposure is necessary to differentiate this condition from others producing pulmonary edema. The changes noted in the roentgenogram on the *left* cleared completely as noted on the film on the *right* taken 3 weeks later.

bination of clinical history and roentgen findings. Patients who have died a month following exposure were found to have bronchiolitis fibrosa obliterans, with each of the small densities apparently representing the typical lesion of this condition. Another patient with a similar history of exposure died within a few hours and diffuse pulmonary edema was found similar to that which has been described in nitric-fume inhalation deaths in industry.

It is, therefore, evident that exposure to nitric fumes and oxides of nitrogen can lead to pulmonary damage sufficient to cause death within a short time of exposure or symptoms may be delayed for several weeks or months, followed by a second phase of more chronic disease. It is also likely that many of these patients recover completely with no residual illness while in others there is enough bronchial alteration to result in fibrosis and emphysema, which develop over a long period of time following the initial injury. It is also probable that other irritant gases are capable of producing a similar variety of pulmonary alteration.

RADIATION CHANGES IN THE LUNG

When tumors of the breast, lung, and mediastinum are treated with radiation, the lung tissue beneath the area being irradiated will receive radiation in varying amounts. This is capable of causing injury sufficient to be noted radiographically and pathologically. The reaction in the lung depends on a number of factors, such as variations in the rate of treatment, port size, the presence of arteriosclerosis, and individual sensitivity of the patient. These factors alter the relationship between the total dose of radiation to the lungs and the damage produced by it. Generally there is not a direct dose or dose-time relationship. As a general rule most patients develop permanent lung changes following a dose of 4500 rads and all have permanent damage when 6000 rads are delivered to the lung. The clinical symptoms are often minor and there may be considerable roentgen change with no symptoms. Cough and dyspnea may be present, however. During the acute phase there is a deposition of fibrinlike material in the alveoli to produce a hyaline membrane plus swelling, destruction of alveolar walls, and edema. These acute changes are often delayed for a month to 6 weeks, just as the severe acute skin reactions are delayed. Occasionally the findings may occur many months following completion of irradiation. The late changes are those of fibrosis, resulting in thickening of the alveolar walls and a decrease in the caliber of the vessels. In some patients an acute reaction may be superimposed on the late fibrosis when multiple courses of radiation are given.

These pathologic alterations are reflected in the radiographic findings. During the early acute phase when edema is a prominent feature there is a hazy, poorly defined increase in density, usually confined to the area of radiation but one that may extend for a short distance beyond it. Most of this is very likely caused by pulmonary edema but there is also some pleural reaction leading to a small amount of fluid and pleural thickening that very likely contributes. Pleural fluid in significant amounts is rare. After a time the density becomes somewhat more irregular and patchy. Strands of density develop that radiate from the hilum toward the periphery. These manifestations may clear gradually and disappear completely in a year or more but if the original injury was severe enough there is sufficient fibrosis to cause permanent changes. They consist of contraction of the lung and a shift of hilar and mediastinal structures to the side or area of radiation (Fig. 27-10). Pleural thickening may appear, manifested by increased density and irregularity of the pleural surface involved. Elevation of the diaphragm and tenting of its summit may occur. Severe thoracic and pulmonary distortion may occur. Chronic dry, irritating, persistent cough may be a problem in the more severely involved patients.

The diagnosis is made on the basis of the clinical history of previous radiation plus the roentgen manifestations described. There is often accompanying evidence of radiation osteitis of ribs, consisting of fractures with

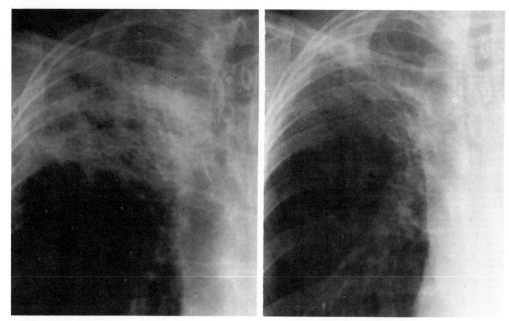

Fig. 27-10. Radiation pneumonitis. *Left,* This film was taken 5 months after completion of irradiation to the right upper thorax. There is a shift of the trachea and upper mediastinal structures to the right, elevation of the right hilum, and a rather diffuse, poorly defined density above the level of the anterior arc of the second rib. *Right,* This examination taken 2 years later shows clearing of the hazy alveolar density, more elevation of the right hilum and a rather strandlike, fibrotic appearing pulmonary process. The trachea remains deviated to the right.

demineralization of ribs in the area of fracture, and no attempt at healing for long periods of time so far as can be detected on the roentgenogram. Radiation pneumonitis must be differentiated from metastasis or recurrent tumor. This differentiation is often difficult, since the radiation is usually given for a tumor. In patients with breast tumor, the localization of the changes to the area of irradiation without lesions elsewhere is indicative of a radiation pneumonitis and not metastasis. The signs of shrinkage in lung volume noted above are not found in metastasis and it is rare for metastatic carcinoma to involve one lung to any significant degree without evidence of disease on the other side. The problem of recurrence or residual disease after heavy irradiation of the mediastinum for Hodgkin's disease offers a particularly difficult problem, because involvement of pulmonary parenchyma extending out along the lymphatics radiating from the hilum is often found in this disease. These findings

simulate the fibrotic changes resulting from radiation after treatment of hilar and mediastinal nodes. All factors, including the clinical condition of the patient, the time interval following radiation, and the progress of the lesions must be considered in these instances. Even then differentiation is sometimes impossible. The acute pulmonary reaction must be differentiated from acute pneumonitis resulting from irritants and from bacterial infections. This can be done on the basis of clinical history plus the presence of the localized radiating strands that are common in postradiation pneumonitis.

REFERENCES AND SELECTED READINGS

1. BAGHDASSARIAN, O. M., and WEINER, S.: Pneumatocele formation complicating hydrocarbon pneumonitis. *Am. J. Roentgenol. Radium Ther. Nucl. Med. 95:* 104, 1965.
2. BONTE, F. J., and REYNOLDS, J.: Hydrocarbon pneumonitis. *Radiology 71:* 391, 1958.

3. BRINGHURST, L. S., BYRNE, R. N., and GERSOHN-COHEN, J.: Respiratory diseases of mushroom workers: Farmer's lung. *JAMA 171:* 15, 1959.

4. BRISTOL, L. J.: Pneumoconioses caused by asbestos and by other siliceous and nonsiliceous dusts. *Semin. Roentgenol. II:* 283, 1967.

5. CATHCART, R. T., THEODOS, P. A., and FRAIMOW, W.: Anthrasilicosis: Selected aspects related to the evaluation of disability, cavitation, and the unusual x-ray. *Arch. Intern. Med. 106:* 368, 1960.

6. CORNELIUS, E. A., and BETLACH, E. H.: Silo-filler's disease. *Radiology 74:* 232, 1960.

7. DE NARDI, J. M., VAN ORDSTRAND, H. S., and CURTIS, G. H.: Berylliosis: Summary and survey of all clinical types in ten year period. *Cleve. Clin. Q. 19:* 171, 1952.

8. EDLING, N. P. G.: Aluminum pneumoconiosis. *Acta Radiol. 56:* 170, 1961.

9. EMANUEL, D. A., WENZEL, F. J., and LAWTON, B. R.: Pneumonitis due to *Cryptostroma corticale* (maple-bark disease). *N. Engl. J. Med. 274:* 1413, 1966.

10. ENGELSTAD, R. B.: Pulmonary lesions after roentgen and radium irradiation. *Am. J. Roentgenol. Radium Ther. Nucl. Med. 43:* 676, 1940.

11. FLETCHER, C. M.: Classification of roentgenograms in pneumoconiosis. *Arch. Indust. Health 11:* 17, 1955.

12. FRANK, R. C.: Farmer's lung. *Am. J. Roentgenol. Radium Ther. Nucl. Med. 79:* 189, 1957.

13. FRIED, J. R., and GOLDBERG, H.: Post-irradiation changes in the lung and thorax. *Am. J. Roentgenol. Radium Ther. Nucl. Med. 43:* 877, 1940.

14. GREENING, R. R., and HESLEP, J. H.: The roentgenology of silicosis. *Semin. Roentgenol. II:* 265, 1967.

15. HARDY, H. L.: Current concepts of occupational lung disease of interest to the radiologist. *Semin. Roentgenol. II:* 225, 1967.

16. HARDY, H. L., and TABERSHAW, I. R.: Delayed chemical pneumonitis occurring in workers exposed to beryllium compounds. *J. Indust. Hyg. Toxicol. 28:* 197, 1946.

17. HEACOCK, C. H.: Pneumonia in children following the ingestion of petroleum products. *Radiology 53:* 793, 1949.

18. HURWITZ, M.: Roentgenologic aspects of asbestosis. *Am. J. Roentgenol. Radium Ther. Nucl. Med. 85:* 256, 1961.

19. JACOBSON, G., FELSON, B., PENDERGRASS, E. P., FLINN, R. H., and LAINHART, W. S.: Eggshell calcifications in coal and metal miners. *Semin. Roentgenol. II:* 276, 1967.

20. JIMENEZ, J. P., and LESTER, R. G.: Pulmonary complications following furniture polish ingestion. *Am. J. Roentgenol. Radium Ther. Nucl. Med. 98:* 323, 1966.

21. KLEINERMAN, J.: The pathology of some familiar pneumoconioses. *Semin. Roentgenol. II:* 244, 1967.

22. LE MONE, D. V., SCOTT, W. G., MOORE, S., and KAVEN, A. L.: Bagasse disease of lungs. *Radiology 49:* 556, 1947.

23. LOWRY, T., and SCHUMAN, L. M.: "Silo-filler's disease": A syndrome caused by nitrogen dioxide. *JAMA 162:* 153, 1956.

24. MAHON, W. E., SCOTT, D. J., ANSELL, G., MANSON, G. L., and FRASER, R.: Hypersensitivity to pituitary snuff with miliary shadowing in the lungs. *Thorax 22:* 13, 1967.

25. NICHOLSON, D. P.: Bagasse worker's lung. *Am. Rev. Resp. Dis. 97:* 546, 1968.

26. OECHSLI, W. R., JACOBSON, G., and BRODEUR, A. E.: Diatomite pneumoconiosis: Roentgen characteristics and classification. *Am. J. Roentgenol. Radium Ther. Nucl. Med. 85:* 263, 1961.

27. RANKIN, J., KOBAYASHI, M., BARBEE, R. A., and DICKIE, H. A.: Pulmonary granulomatoses due to inhaled organic antigens. *Med. Clin. North Am. 51:* 459, 1967.

28. REED, E. S., LEIKEN, S., and KERMAN, H. D.: Kerosene intoxication. *Am. J. Dis. Child. 79:* 623, 1950.

29. REED, E. S., WELLS, P. O., and WICKER, E. H.: Coal miners' pneumoconiosis. *Radiology 71:* 661, 1958.

30. SANDER, O. A.: Berylliosis. *Semin. Roentgenol. II:* 306, 1967.

31. SANDER, O. A.: The nonfibrogenic (benign) pneumoconioses. *Semin. Roentgenol. II:* 312, 1967.

32. SMITH, A. R.: Pleural calcification resulting from exposure to certain dusts. *Am. J. Roentgenol. Radium Ther. Nucl. Med. 67:* 375, 1952.

33. TEPPER, L. B.: The work history in industrial lung disease. *Semin. Roentgenol. II:* 235, 1967.

34. THOMPSON, P. M.: Poisoning due to petroleum products. *Arch. Pediat. 72:* 35, 1955.

35. UNGER, J. DEB., FINK, J. N., and UNGER, G. F.: Pigeon breeder's disease. *Radiology 90:* 683, 1968.

36. UICC/Cincinnati classification of the radiographic appearances of pneumoconiosis. *Chest 58:* 57, 1970.

37. WARREN, S., and SPENCER, J.: Radiation reaction in the lung. *Am. J. Roentgenol. Radium Ther. Nucl. Med. 43:* 682, 1940.

38. ZUCKER, R., KILBOURNE, E. D., and EVANS, J. B.: Pulmonary manifestations of gasoline intoxication. *Arch. Indust. Hyg. Occup. Med. 2:* 17, 1950.

28

CIRCULATORY DISTURBANCES

PULMONARY EDEMA

Pulmonary edema is the term used to indicate that there is an abnormal accumulation of fluid in the extravascular pulmonary tissues. There are a number of causes which have been grouped into five major categories:[9]

1. Obstructive causes
   a. Left-sided heart failure
   b. Mechanical venous obstruction (intracardiac tumor)
   c. Lymphatic obstruction (mediastinal tumor)
2. Toxic causes
   a. Uremia
   b. Near drowning
   c. Inhalation
3. Circulatory abnormalities
   a. Overload
   b. Transfusion reaction (? hypersensitivity)
   c. Postoperative heart-lung bypass
4. Hypoxia
   a. High altitude
   b. Other
5. Neurogenic causes
   a. Epilepsy, brain tumor, brain trauma, etc.
   b. Pheochromocytoma, thyroid storm, central nervous system depressants

These various conditions disturb the balance between capillary pressure and osmotic pressure of the plasma or produce altered permeability of the capillary wall or both. There may be other factors as yet incompletely understood which are of importance in pathogenesis, particularly in the neurogenic and hypoxic groups.

Clinical symptoms are varied and depend upon the associated disease or injury. When the edema is acute there is usually severe respiratory distress but when the onset is insidious, particularly in uremia, there may be very few respiratory symptoms. There is a notable discrepancy between roentgen and physical findings in chronic pulmonary edema and in some patients with acute or subacute interstitial edema. Therefore the roentgen examination is very important in this condition. Two major roentgen patterns of edema are observed depending on the site of the transudate in relation to the pulmonary alveoli and interstitial structures, namely alveolar and interstitial.

INTERSTITIAL EDEMA

There are several signs of interstitial edema which are reliable as a group, particularly when correlated with the clinical findings. They are:

1. Appearance of septal lines.
   a. Kerley's B lines are 1.5 to 2 cm dense, horizontal lines best seen in the lower lung on oblique projections. They repre-

sent interlobular septa thickened by fluid (Fig. 28-1).

b. Kerley's A lines are longer and range in size up to 4 or 5 cm. They tend to be straight or slightly curved and extend from the hila or parahilar area toward the periphery. They are seen in the upper lobes and tend to appear in acute interstitial edema. Transudate in the septa also causes these changes.

2. Perivascular blurring or cuffing in which the margins of the vessels become indistinct and widened beginning in hilar and perihilar

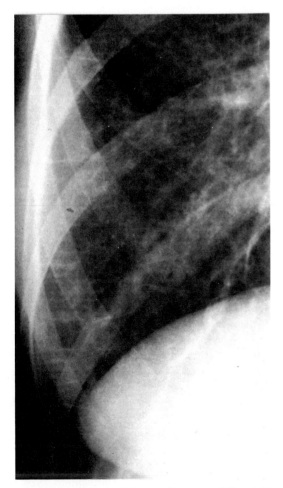

Fig. 28-1. Kerley's B lines. Close-up of the right lateral lung base in a patient with mitral stenosis and interstitial edema. The numerous transverse, short, dense lines at the periphery represent interlobular septa thickened by edema fluid.

areas and extending well out into the parenchyma.

3. "Hilar haze" refers to a loss of definition of large central pulmonary vessels with a slight general increase in density. This can often be best appreciated when an earlier film is available for comparison or when a film is taken after successful treatment of the edema.

4. Diffuse reticular pattern is visible when edema fluid widens pulmonary interstitial structures throughout the lung (Fig. 28-2).

A similar pattern may be seen in patients with widespread interstitial fibrosis, but A lines are not present in these. "Pure" interstitial edema is not as frequent as a combination with the alveolar type (Fig. 28-3). Interstitial edema probably precedes alveolar edema in these instances, but often the onset is very rapid with massive alveolar edema overshadowing all subtle signs.

ALVEOLAR EDEMA

The classic roentgen findings of alveolar pulmonary edema are those of bilateral densities that extend outward in a fan-shaped manner from the hilum on both sides. The peripheral lung fields are relatively clear. This includes the bases as well as the apices except in congestive failure, in which basal congestive changes and edema produce density there. When the edema is moderate the density is somewhat patchy and mottled but it may become quite homogeneous as the amount increases (Fig. 28-4). In the latter instance, the fluid-filled alveoli surrounding the bronchi produce contrast with the air-containing bronchi and as a result, the bronchi are visible as linear radiolucent spaces traversing the opaque edematous area (Fig. 28-5). The density is often bilaterally symmetric or nearly so. There are many exceptions to this rule and cases have been reported in which the edema was unilateral. Serial films often show rapid changes in the amount and distribution of the edema from day to day. When pulmonary edema is early and minor it may produce scat-

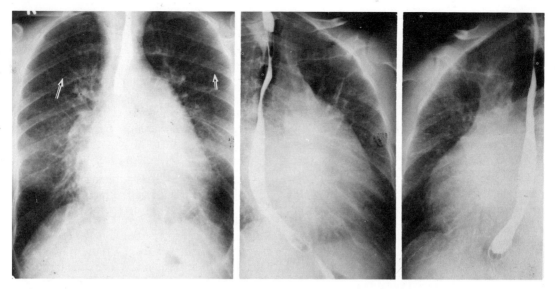

Fig. 28-2. Interstitial edema. This patient with rheumatic mitral disease and a grossly enlarged heart shows typical Kerley's B lines at both lateral bases and there are some longer, finer lines in the upper central lungs (**arrows**) which probably represent Kerley's A lines. There is a little parahilar haze noted particularly on the right side with a general increase in interstitial markings resulting in a somewhat reticular pattern noted best in the oblique projections. There is also a small amount of pleural fluid on the left.

tered localized densities that may simulate miliary or nodular disease (Fig. 28-6). Bizarre forms may also be present with large, rather rounded areas of increased density that may actually simulate tumor. As a general rule the alveolar density is hazy and poorly defined, so there is no difficulty making the diagnosis. Pleural effusion is commonly associated with edema, particularly in congestive heart failure and in uremia.

Numerous reports of unusual and asymmetric distribution of edema have led to some experimental work and much speculation as to the factors involved in the distribution of edema fluid. Gravity is undoubtedly a factor in many cases, but lateral views of patients who have been supine sometimes shows the fluid to be in anterior or lingular segments or in the middle lobe. Lack of peripheral edema is probably related to better peripheral drainage of lymphatics and to the increased respiratory motion of the peripheral lung acting to "pump" the fluid out. The relative lack of compliance in the central lung and in lung which has been previously diseased may also be involved.

There are no constantly reliable changes that will determine the cause, but in edema secondary to cardiac failure the observations of cardiac enlargement, pulmonary congestion, and pleural effusion are strong indications that the edema is the result of heart disease. Exceptions include the absence of cardiac enlargement in some patients with pulmonary edema secondary to acute coronary thrombosis, and the absence of basal congestive changes in patients with edema secondary to acute left ventricular failure. As a general rule, pulmonary edema caused by uremia (azotemic edema) produces the classic central "fluffy" density of the lungs without evidence of cardiac enlargement or pulmonary congestion. Pulmonary edema caused by inhalation of irritant gases tends to be somewhat more widespread than the other types and results in a mottled and patchy appearance extending farther to the periphery with slightly less central involvement than is seen in uremia; it also tends to be more basal. Roentgen distribution is not characteristic, however, and the history is of great importance in arriving at the diagnosis in these patients.

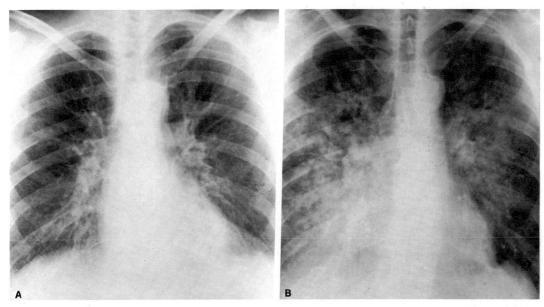

Fig. 28-3. Interstitial and alveolar edema. Patient with chronic renal disease was being carried on dialysis. *A,* Interstitial edema. There is general increase in interstitial markings, particularly at the bases and in the parahilar areas. Perivascular edema has resulted in very poor definition of the vessels. There tends to be a little parahilar haze blurring the vessels there, particularly on the right side. *B,* At this time there is noted bilateral alveolar edema. On the left side several lucent streaks representing air bronchogram are noted in the left central lung and at the right base. The unequal distribution is not uncommon.

PULMONARY THROMBOEMBOLISM AND INFARCTION

Pulmonary embolism with or without infarction is a more common lesion than is generally realized. In addition to its occurrence as a postoperative complication and in patients with cardiac disease, it occurs in a number of other medical conditions. The most common sources of pulmonary emboli are thrombi in the deep veins of the leg. When the embolus is very large and occludes the entire pulmonary arterial tree, death may occur very quickly. When the embolus is somewhat smaller it may or may not produce infarction but will often cause immediate symptoms of chest pain and dyspnea. There may be no symptoms or signs with small emboli. In addition to parts of thrombi, a number of other materials may act as emboli. Air embolism which may follow trauma is not usually demonstrated radiographically; it disappears very quickly if the patient survives. If it causes sudden death the air can be demonstrated on postmortem films. Opaque contrast materials used in hysterosalpingography and in myelography occasionally enter the bloodstream and have been demonstrated in the lungs following these procedures. A few cases of barium in the pulmonary vessels following barium enema have been reported in which fatalities have occurred during the examination.

PULMONARY INFARCTION

The incidence of infarction varies in different groups of patients with pulmonary thromboembolism. In patients with chronic heart disease and congestive failure it approaches 100 per cent, while in young, healthy individuals, complete infarct is rare unless there are complicating factors such as severe trauma. In the elderly, chronically ill who are bedridden, the incidence is in the range of 60 to 70 per cent of those who have pulmonary emboli.

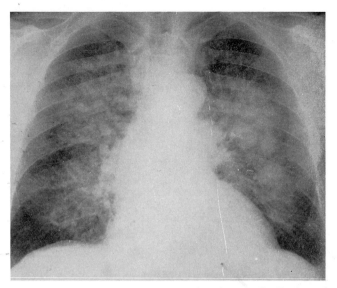

Fig. 28-4. Pulmonary edema. The fan-shaped distribution of the density in the parahilar areas and midzones of the lung fields is characteristic of alveolar edema. The patient has chronic renal disease.

The roentgenographic diagnosis is often difficult. The major error is usually failure to suspect infarction as the cause for abnormal roentgen findings in the chest. An infarct must be differentiated from pneumonia, edema, and atelectasis as well as other local conditions, such as infected cysts and abscesses. The right lower lobe is the most frequent site, but the lesion may occur in any lobe. Elevation of the diaphragm or small pleural effusion or both may be the earliest signs of infarction. At times the actual shadow of the infarct may not be visible and the effusion is the only sign. It takes from 10 to 24 hours for an infarct to evolve to the point where it is visible roentgenographically. This is probably the hazy, poorly defined, edematous lesion which requires an additional 2 to 4 days and sometimes a week to form a well-defined complete infarct. It always extends to a pleural surface but since this may be the interlobar pleura, its shadow is not necessarily peripheral as visualized in the frontal projection. The shape of the infarct is dependent upon the location. The visceral pleura always forms one side of the lesion and often two or three sides. The long axis of the

infarct is in the plane of the longest pleural surface with which it is in contact. The actual shadow may be rounded or roughly triangular. It may assume the shape of the lingula or of the right middle lobe or may fill and obliterate a costophrenic sulcus if the lateral segment of a lower lobe is involved. Oblique views aided by fluoroscopic positioning are necessary to bring out the relationship of the lesion to the pleura in many cases. The hilar aspect of the infarct is usually rounded or hump-shaped rather than resembling the apex of a triangle. The amount of associated pleural effusion is usually not great and multiple lesions may be visualized in one or both lungs (Fig. 28-7). At first the periphery of the lesion is rather hazy and poorly defined but as time goes on it becomes more sharply outlined and as it heals it gradually becomes smaller. The size of the infarct can vary greatly, from bare visibility to the greater part of a lobe. The average size is about 3 to 5 cm. The pulmonary changes resolve rather slowly. The complete hemorrhagic necrotic infarct requires 4 weeks or more for complete resolution. When infarction is incomplete, there is no necrosis, the local findings are

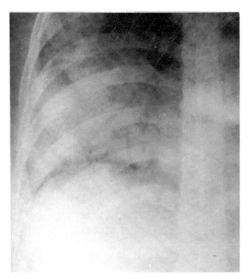

Fig. 28-5. Pulmonary edema. Closeup of the right lower lung to show air bronchogram in the otherwise dense, fluid-filled lung.

those of edema and hemorrhage. This process may clear quickly, within a week or less and leave no residue. The complete infarct slowly decreases in size. Eventually only a linear fibrous band may remain indicating the site of a previous infarct. The linear scar may be quite small and inconspicuous. There is often a small amount of localized pleural thickening associated with the linear density.

Linear densities in the lower lungs described in patients with embolism usually represent platelike or focal atelectasis caused by a combination of poor ventilation, narrowing of the bronchi, decreased compliance of the lung, and lack of surfactant, all of which occur in pulmonary embolism with infarction. Other causes include parenchymal fibrosis or scarring, thrombosed arteries or veins, and some probably represent linear shadows of pleural origin. An accessory sign that may be noted on the films is splinting secondary to the pleural involvement that may be represented by elevation of the diaphragm. At fluoroscopy this is manifested by decrease in diaphragmatic motion, particularly near the site of the infarct if the lesion is basal.

If the possibility of pulmonary infarction is

kept in mind in bedridden, debilitated, or cardiac patients with sudden pleuritic type of chest pain, the presence of one or all of the above signs should lead to the diagnosis or at least a suspicion of it in most instances. The lack of a characteristic contour cannot be overemphasized because of the wide variety of shapes, depending on location; the size also varies greatly. It is also important to remember that infarction can occur in the absence of congestive heart disease. There may be enough fluid in the pleural space to hide the pulmonary lesion and decubitus films are of value to outline the basal lung when infarction is suspected. When the diagnosis is in doubt, progress films should be taken since the shadow of the infarct cannot be visualized until hemorrhage and exudation have occurred. Lung scans with radioactive-tagged, macroaggregated, human serum albumin are helpful in the diagnosis of infarction when roentgen signs are present, but scanning is more useful when the chest roentgenogram appears normal.

EMBOLISM WITHOUT INFARCTION

Pulmonary embolism may be massive and life-threatening. Prompt diagnosis is of utmost importance in these patients. Roentgen findings are often minimal or absent in contrast to the clinical findings in a desperately ill patient. The central pulmonary arteries may be increased in size, with sharp diminution in size of branches off the hilum and relative radiolucency of the ischemic areas. If the patient happens to have had a chest film in the recent past, comparison can be very helpful (Fig. 28-8). At best, the diagnosis of massive pulmonary embolism can be suggested. Since embolectomy might be indicated when the patient is hypotensive and cyanotic, pulmonary arteriography is indicated to confirm the presence of large central emboli which can be surgically removed. The catheter is placed in the main pulmonary artery if possible, if not it can be placed in the right atrium.

As a general rule, we do not advocate pulmonary arteriography in patients in whom no surgery is contemplated. The diagnosis can be

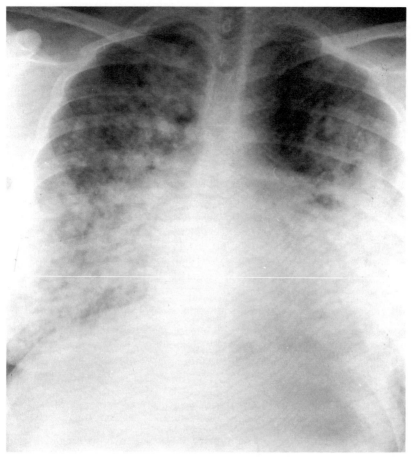

Fig. 28-6. Alveolar edema. In this patient the appearance in the right upper lung resembles rather poorly defined, large nodular disease. It was bilateral however and there was no difficulty in making the diagnosis. Patient was azotemic.

made usually using the combination of plain-film chest roentgenogram and lung scan. When serious doubt regarding the diagnosis arises following these procedures, pulmonary arteriography can be done. The major angiographic signs of pulmonary embolism are: (*1*) the demonstration of defects in the major arteries which represent the clots (Fig. 28-9); (*2*) "cut-off" of one or more large branch vessels with no opacification of the lung peripheral to them; and (*3*) absent or diminished local bloodflow usually manifested by decreased arborization or truncation.

In embolization without infarction which is not life-threatening, plain-film findings are often very subtle and sometimes absent. Dilatation of central pulmonary arteries may be present, but is difficult to assess unless a comparison film is available. This may be unilateral or bilateral and probably represents the mass of the embolus. There may be a decrease in size of the arteries peripheral to the embolus; this sign is also very difficult to evaluate on a single film. Lobar or segmental hyperlucency may be present; it, too, is very difficult to evaluate. In these patients with normal or nearly normal chest roentgenograms, the lung scan is virtually diagnostic. When antecedent

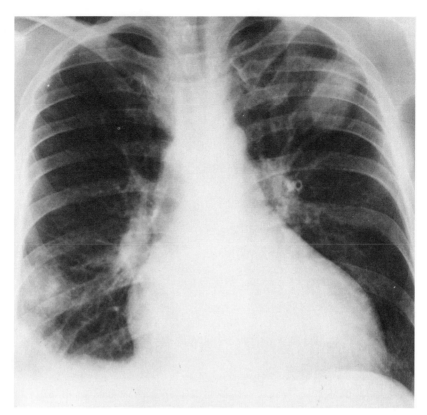

Fig. 28-7. Pulmonary infarcts. The oval density at the left apex represents an old infarct. There is a little fluid remaining in the major fissure in the region of the infarct which is now quite well circumscribed. There are two infarcts in the right base, one producing a humplike shadow obliterating the costophrenic angle and projecting above the level of the dome of the diaphragm. The other is somewhat rounded and lies above it. There is some pleural fluid as well.

or complicating lung disease is present, the scan is not as useful. It is in this situation that a pulmonary arteriogram may be necessary to confirm the diagnosis.

SEPTIC INFARCTION

When the embolus producing infarction contains or is made up of bacteria, septic infarction results, which leads to tissue breakdown and formation of cavity. These lesions may occur in subacute bacterial endocarditis or other infections in which there is septicemia. They may be single or multiple as in aseptic infarction. A cavity rarely may form in an infarcted area as the result of secondary bronchogenic infection. There may be sequestration of the necrotic center of an infarct to produce cavity without infection. Usually infection supervenes, however, and when these infarcts become infected the pneumonitis surrounding them causes further increase in density with a poorly circumscribed periphery. The roentgen appearance is that of a central cavity within a poorly defined area of increased density. When there is a typical history and other infarcts are present, the diagnosis is not difficult but in single lesions the differentiation between infarct cavity and cavity secondary to primary inflammatory disease is difficult, if not impossible.

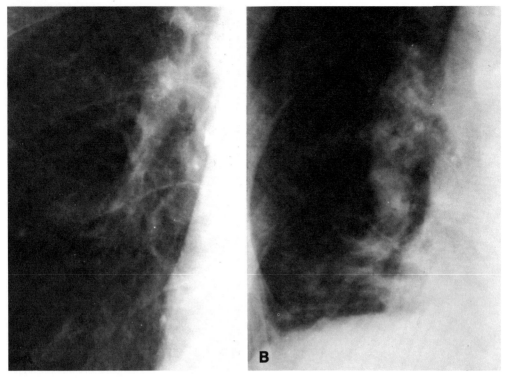

Fig. 28-8. Pulmonary embolism. Patient developed chest pain while in the hospital. *A*, Close-up of the right hilum on the admission film. *B*, Film, taken 1 week later 1 day after the onset of chest pain, shows the enlargement of the pulmonary artery which was found to be the site of a large embolus. The diaphragm is elevated with horizontal linear densities in the lung, probably secondary to poor ventilation of the lower lobe. This patient did not develop infarction which could be recognized radiographically.

POSTTRAUMATIC FAT EMBOLISM

There is experimental and some clinical evidence to show that fat embolism is very common following bone and soft-tissue injury, particularly fractures of the tibia and femur. However, despite the fact that many severely injured patients are observed, the clinical entity and pulmonary roentgen evidence of posttraumatic fat embolism is relatively rare. It is likely that small amounts of fat may form emboli without symptoms and signs. The roentgen findings are varied, but are uniformly bilateral. (*1*) Diffuse bilateral density which resembles pulmonary edema except that there is more basal involvement than is usually observed in edema and the involvement is more peripheral often with relatively little alveolar density centrally. (*2*) Bilateral, multiple small nodular densities; often more nodules are noted in the lower lungs than elsewhere. This probably represents a somewhat lesser involvement than the more confluent homogeneous edemalike pattern. (*3*) There is usually no pleural effusion or cardiac enlargement; and (*4*) The onset is delayed, usually from 1 to 3 days following trauma. This is in contrast to pulmonary contusion with hemorrhage and edema which occurs very soon after injury. The diagnosis can usually be made on the basis of the history of chest pain and cough 12 hours to several days following injury, along with chest roentgen findings as described. Resolution varies from 6 days to 2 weeks.

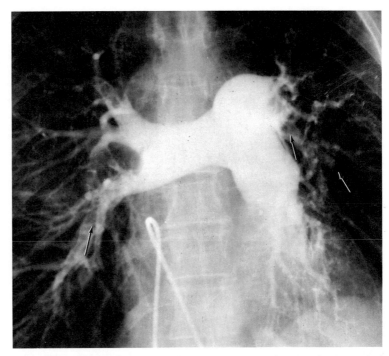

Fig. 28-9. Pulmonary emboli. This pulmonary arteriogram shows several small lucencies representing emboli in the pulmonary arteries (**arrows**).

PULMONARY HYPERTENSION

Bloodflow through the lungs and pulmonary artery pressure are dependent upon a number of factors including arterial and venous resistance, the amount of bloodflow which may be altered in various shunts, and combinations of these factors. Pulmonary hypertension may be predominantly arterial (precapillary) or venous (postcapillary) or combined. Since the roentgen changes vary with the type and the site of the major causative factors, a classification[10] of pulmonary hypertension is presented:

I. Precapillary (Arterial Hypertension)
  A. Increased resistance
    1. Obstructive: pulmonary embolism, idiopathic or primary pulmonary hypertension, pulmonary schistosomiasis, reverse shunts (ventricular septal defect, atrial septal defect, or patent ductus arteriosus)
    2. Obliterative: emphysema, diffuse interstitial diseases—fibrotic, granulomatous, neoplastic, or infectious
    3. Constrictive: anoxia
  B. Increased flow
    1. Large left-to-right shunts: PDA, VSD

II. Postcapillary (Venous Hypertension)
  A. Acute: Left ventricular failure, regardless of cause
  B. Chronic: Mitral valvular disease, left atrial myxoma, anomalous pulmonary venous return, mediastinal fibrosis

III. Combined Pre- and Postcapillary Hypertension

IV. Diffuse Pulmonary Arteriovenous Shunting Complicating Chronic Lung Disease (Simon): Emphysema—shunt syndrome

Pulmonary hypertension is defined as elevation of pressure in the pulmonary circuit above certain limits at rest or during mild exercise.

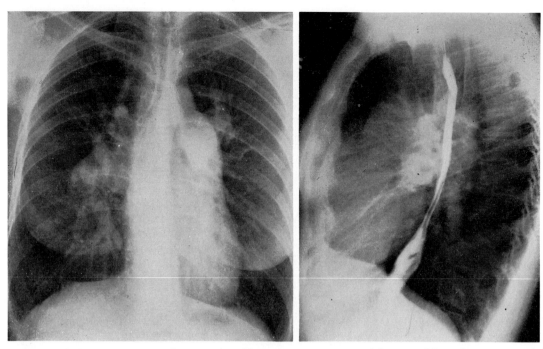

Fig. 28-10. Pulmonary arterial hypertension. The pulmonary artery and its central branches are grossly enlarged in contrast to the peripheral arteries which are small. This patient had an atrial septal defect with the pulmonary hypertension resulting in reversal of the initial left-to-right shunt.

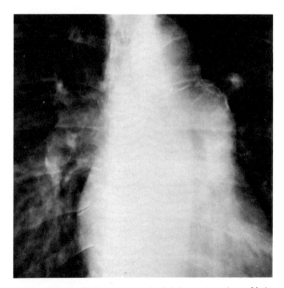

Fig. 28-11. Pulmonary arterial hypertension. Note the dense calcification in the pulmonary artery and ductus in this patient with patent ductus who had developed a reversal of the shunt as a result of pulmonary hypertension.

These limits are generally accepted as 30 mmHg systolic and 15 mmHg diastolic with a mean of 18 mmHg on the arterial side. On the venous side the upper limit is considered to be 12 mmHg; this is applied equally to the mean left atrial pressure and to the mean capillary-wedge pressure.

Most of the diseases causing pulmonary hypertension produce an increase in pulmonary vascular resistance. In the normal upright chest film, the upper zone vessels are smaller than those in the lower zones. In recumbency this difference disappears; this accounts in part for disparity between angiograms and routine films.

There are distinct radiographic differences in the pre- and postcapillary groups. The roentgen changes in pulmonary arterial (precapillary) hypertension include: Dilatation of the pulmonary artery and its central branches on either side; narrowing of the peripheral pulmonary arteries, resulting in a rather sharp fall-off in

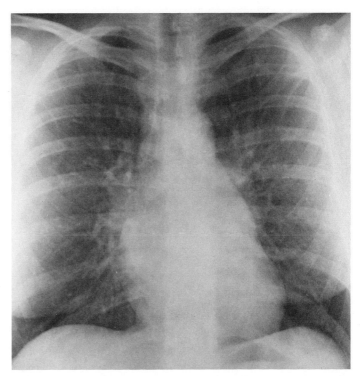

Fig. 28-12. Pulmonary venous hypertension. This patient with mitral stenosis demonstrates a little perihilar haze and basal vascular constriction so that the upper lobe vessels are more prominent than the basal vessels. There is little if any perivascular change.

size from central to peripheral arteries (Fig. 28-10); tortuosity of peripheral arteries, particularly in lower zones, observed along with a general decrease in caliber of pulmonary veins; varying enlargement of the right ventricle, depending upon severity and duration of the hypertension; and calcification observed in the pulmonary artery (Fig. 28-11). Signs of the underlying causative disease may be minimal, obvious, or absent. In general, increasing severity of the hypertension is accompanied by an increase in the roentgen signs, but there are exceptions, so caution should be observed in predicting pulmonary artery pressure ranges. The lungs are relatively clear unless the underlying disease has produced considerable change.

Another situation is one in which pulmonary arterial hypertension develops as systemic high-pressures are transmitted across congenital defects causing left-to-right shunts at the aorto-pulmonary (patent ductus) or ventricular (ventricular septal defect) level. A substantial high-pressure shunt at the aortic or ventricular level or a massive shunt at the atrial or great vein level will eventually cause a reactive sclerosis, intimal thickening, and medial hypertrophy in pulmonary arteries. This progresses to marked pulmonary arterial hypertension with resultant shunt reversal. The following roentgen signs are produced:

1. Marked enlargement of the pulmonary artery and its central branches extending out for a short distance along the lobar arteries. Calcification is occasionally observed in the pulmonary artery.

2. Constriction of segmental and peripheral arteries to normal or smaller than normal size.

3. Pulmonary veins are normal or small.

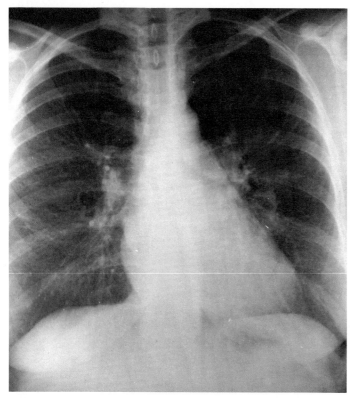

Fig. 28-13. Postcapillary (venous) hypertension. This patient with mitral valvular disease shows a general increase in interstitial markings, some constriction of basal vessels, and poor definition of vascular shadows secondary to some perivascular edema.

4. The heart shows alteration consistent with the initial defect; however, eventually the right ventricle may increase to become the predominant chamber.

Venous — Postcapillary hypertension is often accompanied by changes which cause a considerable increase in pulmonary density, e.g., edema. The roentgen findings are as follows: Slight distention of all pulmonary veins is the earliest sign, but it is very difficult to evaluate unless comparison films are available. Constriction of the pulmonary arteries and veins in the lower zones and dilatation of the arteries and veins in the upper zones occur.[10] This finding may be striking when present, but is not well defined in every patient with venous hypertension. These signs may be obliterated by pulmonary edema and congestion in left ventricular failure. An upright chest film should be obtained, since the vascular size tends to equalize in the supine position. The cause for the basal constriction remains controversial. Mild, venous hypertension shows only the vascular constriction which may be very difficult to assess (Fig. 28-12). As the venous pressure increases, additional findings of early interstitial edema can be observed; they include the appearance of Kerley's B lines and Kerley's A lines. A slight perihilar haze may be evident. Vascular margins are blurred and poorly defined and there is a general increase in interstitial markings (Figs. 28-13 and 28-14). Alveolar edema and pleural effusion appear when venous hypertension is marked and left ventricular failure occurs. Chronic postcapillary hypertension such as that found in mitral stenosis and left atrial myxoma

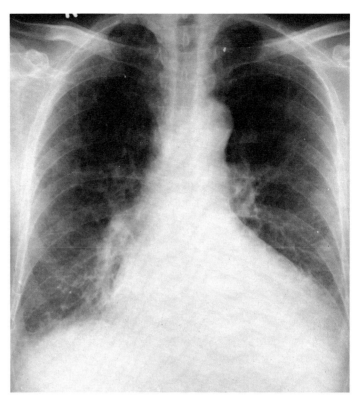

Fig. 28-14. Postcapillary (venous) hypertension. The patient had had a myocardial infarct and was in failure. Signs of interstitial edema are manifested by the Kerley's B lines best observed at the extreme right lateral base. There is also bilateral pleural effusion and considerable perivascular edema manifested by very poor definition of vessels. The interstitial markings are generally increased in the bases while there is very little interstitial edema in the upper lungs.

result in irreversible constriction of lower-zone pulmonary vessels.

When there is a combined arterial (pre-) and venous (postcapillary) hypertension, the roentgen changes depend on the sequence of events. Mitral stenosis is a good example, with venous hypertension occurring for some time being followed by arterial hypertension. The roentgen findings are then in combination and develop as the disease develops—a summation of changes.

Chronic lung diseases such as pulmonary fibrosis and emphysema cause increased pulmonary arterial resistance resulting in pulmonary arterial hypertension. Occasionally such a patient will develop general dilatation of pul-

monary arteries and veins involving all of the lung zones. This is caused by diffuse arteriovenous shunting. There may be some interstitial edema and the patients are dyspneic and cyanotic. It is postulated by Simon, Sasahara, and Cannilla,[10] that a combination of increased pulmonary resistance and left ventricular decompensation probably caused by hypoxia results in this "emphysema-shunt syndrome."

REFERENCES AND SELECTED READINGS

1. Berrigan, T. J., Jr., Carsky, E. W., and Heitzman, E. R.: Fat embolism. *Am. J. Roentgenol. Radium Ther. Nucl. Med. 96:* 967, 1966.

2. Bookstein, J. J.: Pulmonary thromboembolism

with emphasis on angiographic-pathologic correlation. *Semin. Roentgenol. V:* 291, 1970.

3. FIGLEY, M. M., GERDES, A. J., and RICKETTS, H. J.: Radiographic aspects of pulmonary embolism. *Semin. Roentgenol. II:* 389, 1967.

4. FLEISCHNER, F. G.: Roentgenology of the pulmonary infarct. *Semin. Roentgenol. II:* 61, 1967.

5. GOODWIN, J. F., STEINER, R. E., GRAINGER, R. G., and HARRISON, C. V.: Pulmonary hypertension: A symposium. *Br. J. Radiol. 31:* 174–226, 1958.

6. HEITZMAN, E. R., and ZITER, F. M., JR.: Acute interstitial pulmonary edema. *Am. J. Roentgenol. Radium Ther. Nucl. Med. 98:* 291, 1966.

7. KEATS, T. E., DREIS, V. A., and SIMPSON, E.: The roentgen manifestations of pulmonary hypertension in congenital heart disease. *Radiology 66:* 693, 1956.

8. QUINN, J. L.: Radioisotope lung scanning. *Semin. Roentgenol. II:* 406, 1967.

9. RIGLER, L. G., and SURPRENANT, E. L.: Pulmonary edema. *Semin. Roentgenol. II:* 33, 1967.

10. SIMON, M., SASAHARA, A. A., and CANNILLA, J. E.: The radiology of pulmonary hypertension. *Semin. Roentgenol. II:* 368, 1967.

11. SIMON, M., POTCHEN, E. J., and LeMAY, M.: *Frontiers of Pulmonary Radiology.* New York, Grune & Stratton, 1969.

29

TUMORS OF THE LUNGS AND BRONCHI

MALIGNANT TUMORS

CLASSIFICATION

The following is a satisfactory working classification of lung tumors, adapted from Liebow.*

I. Primary Malignant Epithelial Tumors
  A. Bronchogenic Carcinoma
    1. Epidermoid (squamous cell carcinoma) (45 to 60 per cent)
    2. Adenocarcinoma (15 per cent)
    3. Anaplastic carcinoma (30 per cent)
    4. Mixed
  B. Bronchiolar Carcinoma (Pulmonary Adenomatosis, Alveolar Cell Carcinoma)
  C. Bronchial Adenoma

II. Sarcoma
  A. Differentiated Spindle Cell Sarcoma
  B. Differentiated Sarcoma
  C. Primary Lymphosarcoma

III. Mixed Epithelial and Sarcomatous Tumor (Carcinosarcoma)

IV. Neoplasms of Reticuloendothelial System Involving the Lung

V. Metastatic Tumors of the Lung

* Mayer, E., and Maier, H. C.: *Pulmonary Carcinoma.* New York, New York University Press, 1956, p. 74. Adapted from Liebow.[10]

BRONCHOGENIC CARCINOMA

There has been an absolute as well as a relative increase in the incidence of carcinoma of the lung in the past 35 years that is reflected in the mortality rate. In white males the reported death rate from cancer of the lung is 25 times higher now than in 1914. Of all carcinomas this mortality rate is exceeded only by that of carcinoma of the stomach. Despite the advances in thoracic surgery, the overall 5-year survival rate is very low, in the range of 5 to 6 per cent. In contrast to this, the 5-year survival rate in a small series of patients with bronchogenic carcinoma discovered in a survey of asymptomatic patients was 30 per cent. This suggests that there is an opportunity to improve the high mortality rate in this type of cancer. Earlier diagnosis by means of roentgen examination is one way in which it may be accomplished.

In a series of 148 proved primary bronchogenic tumors reviewed in 1952, we found an overall ratio of 9 males to 1 female. The average age was 56.1 years and nearly all the tumors were found in patients over 40.

The epidermoid or squamous cell neoplasm occurs predominantly in males, with a ratio of 10 or 20 to 1. They make up 45 to 60 per cent of all bronchogenic tumors and tend to occur in relatively old-age groups with the peak incidence at age 60. This tumor often arises in or immediately adjacent to lobar and segmental bronchi, but is occasionally peripheral. When a primary tumor is noted to invade the thoracic wall, it is more likely to be epidermoid than any other type. Necrosis with formation of cavity is also fairly common and when a tumor of this type is found in an elderly male it is nearly always epidermoid in origin. The well-differentiated squamous cell tumor is more likely to remain confined to the bronchus of origin and adjacent nodes than the more atypical forms and the rate of growth is often less rapid in this tumor than in the others. Invasion of veins with hematogenous metastasis does occur late in the disease however.

The adenocarcinoma with an overall incidence of 15 per cent is the most common of the bronchogenic tumors found in the female. It tends to be more peripheral than the other types but may be central. The rate of growth is rapid; hematogenous and lymphogenous metastases occur early. This is the tumor most often observed peripherally in relatively young females. The anaplastic carcinoma, which makes up 30 per cent of bronchogenic tumors, often occurs centrally, with hilar enlargement and massive lymph-node metastases. This type may resemble mediastinal lymphosarcoma. It does not often form a peripheral tumor and does not usually undergo necrosis to form cavitation.

The alveolar cell carcinoma or pulmonary adenomatosis is more likely of bronchiolar than alveolar origin so the term bronchiolar carcinoma is preferable. There is some question as to whether or not it is multifocal, but some investigators believe that it begins as a single focus and spreads widely through the lymphatics. Two general gross pathologic types are described: (1) the tumorlike or nodular form, (2) the diffuse type, which may resemble pneumonic consolidation roentgenographically.

Bronchial adenoma is included in the malignant bronchogenic tumor group because this lesion metastasizes locally to nodes, but there is a marked difference in the clinical course and the prognosis between this tumor and bronchogenic carcinoma. The relatively good prognosis holds, even though hilar node metastases are found at surgery. The tumor occurs in a younger age group and is as frequent in females as in males. In contrast to the low survival rate in bronchogenic carcinoma, the 5-year survival rate is 90 per cent or more.

Roentgen Findings

The changes caused by bronchogenic carcinoma vary widely, depending upon the site of the tumor and its relation to the bronchial tree. The tumor itself may or may not be visible. When it is not visible its presence can be detected by such findings as localized emphysema, atelectasis, and inflammatory disease, all of which are secondary to the tumor within or compressing a bronchus. Each radiological sign of bronchogenic carcinoma may occur as the only evidence of tumor or several of the signs may occur in a single patient. Each of the following may occur as the initial sign of bronchogenic carcinoma: (1) Atelectasis which may be segmental or lobar; (2) unilateral hilar enlargement; (3) emphysema, obstructive in type, which may be segmental or lobar; (4) mediastinal mass, often simulating lymphoma; (5) apical pulmonary density with or without rib destruction; (6) cavitation in a solitary mass; (7) segmental consolidation, resembling local pneumonitis which does not clear or which clears incompletely; or (8) parenchymal mass, including sharply defined peripheral nodule and poorly defined irregular nodular mass which may be surrounded by abnormal thickened vessels demonstrated on tomography. Occasionally the initial sign may be a very poorly defined, irregular, nonhomogeneous density which may be linear and resemble a fibrotic scar. Therefore it is necessary to be suspicious of nearly every density in the lung which does not clear, or which appears in a patient with previously normal lungs, particularly if the patient is a male smoker over age 40.

In addition to the above findings a number of other roentgen changes may result from metastasis or local invasion. They consist of (1) pleural effusion, (2) hematogenous or lymphogenous intrapulmonary metastasis, (3) elevation of the diaphragm secondary to phrenic nerve paralysis, and (4) pleural masses with or without rib destruction.

ATELECTASIS. Atelectasis is probably the most common single roentgen sign of bronchogenic carcinoma. It may be segmental, lobar, or massive atelectasis of one lung. The radiographic signs of atelectasis resulting from tumor are no different than those resulting from endobronchial block from other causes. The amount of density produced varies with the size of the bronchus obstructed. It is not uncommon to find a combination of atelectasis and tumor (Figs. 29-1, 29-2, and 29-3). This is most readily visualized in the right upper lobe, where the atelectasis results in elevation and concavity of the secondary interlobar fissure laterally. A convexity medially with greater density there represents the tumor mass. In these patients the inferior margin of the lobe resembles the reversed letter S. A combination of pneumonitis and atelectasis may also occur, which may cause confusion. Persistence of the shadow in spite of antibiotic therapy or failure of complete disappearance of it is strong evidence of neoplasm.

UILATERAL ENLARGEMENT OF THE HILUM. This sign of bronchogenic carcinoma may be very difficult to evaluate when only a single roentgenogram is available. When there is a difference in the size of the hilum on the two sides, every effort should be made to obtain any previous roentgenograms of the patient that may be available. If a film of an earlier examination is obtained, a difference in hilar size between the two films is of particular significance. It is also of value to obtain tomograms through the hilum in question in an attempt to outline local bronchial narrowing produced by tumor. It is also helpful in detecting some blurring of hilar vascular detail which may be caused by tumor. Roentgenograms in inspiration and expiration should also be obtained when there is a question as to the significance of unilateral hilar enlargement, because a small amount of obstructive emphysema may be determined by this examination. Bronchoscopy and bronchography may also be indicated (Fig. 29-4).

LOCAL EMPHYSEMA. Bronchogenic carcinoma may not cause enough obstruction to interfere with air entering the segment, lobe, or lung supplied by the bronchus, but the slight decrease in bronchial size on expiration may result in partial obstruction to the egress of air. This causes emphysema, which may precede atelectasis by a considerable period of time. It

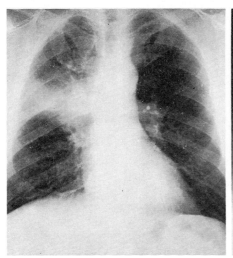
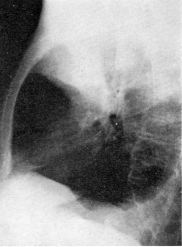

Fig. 29-1. Bronchogenic carcinoma. *Left,* Frontal view shows right hilar mass with minimal atelectasis in the anterior segment of the right upper lobe. In the lateral view (*right*) there is noted some fluid in the posterior pleural space on the right which is not visible in the frontal projection.

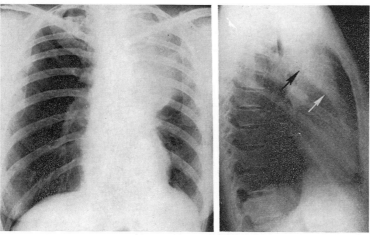

Fig. 29-2. Bronchogenic carcinoma. This tumor is associated with atelectasis of the left upper lobe. On the frontal projection (*left*) the mass obscures the upper cardiac border and aorta and fades off into the lung field. On the lateral view (*right*) the **arrows** point to the anteriorly displaced major fissure with the partially atelectatic lung anterior to it and the mass extending posteriorly toward the hilum between the **two arrows** and extending above the **black arrow.**

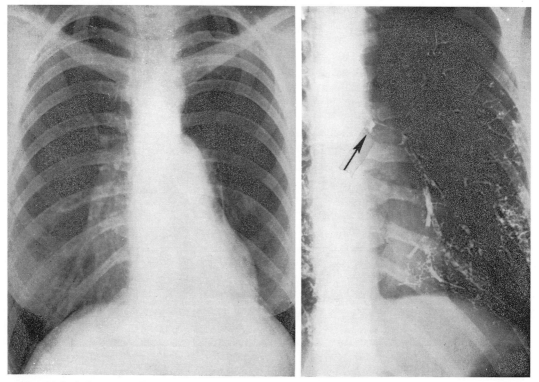

Fig. 29-3. Left lower lobe atelectasis. Note the density behind the heart which blurs the left diaphragm and extends up lateral to the hilum which is displaced downward. Elsewhere there is increased radiability of the left lung. The bronchogram showed complete obstruction of the lower lobe bronchus with a mass extending into the upper lobe bronchus (**arrow**). The tumor proved to be a bronchial adenoma (adenocarcinoma, grade 1).

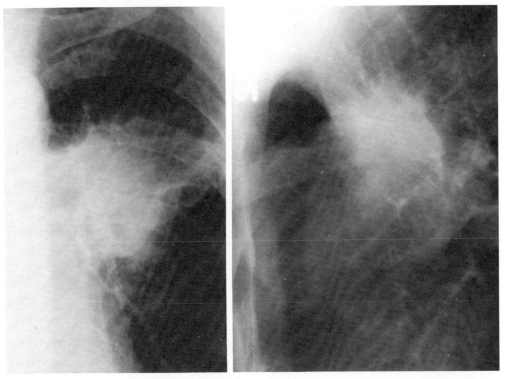

Fig. 29-4. Bronchogenic carcinoma. This large left hilar mass seen in the frontal (*left*) and lateral (*right*) projections represents bronchogenic carcinoma which surrounds the upper lobe bronchus and narrows it somewhat. There is no difficulty in diagnosis when the mass reaches this size.

is therefore an important sign of bronchogenic carcinoma. Films in inspiration and expiration and fluoroscopy accentuate the findings and verify the presence of obstructive emphysema. These studies should be done when there is a wheeze detected on auscultation or a suggestion of local emphysema on the chest roentgenogram (Fig. 29-5). When this is found in a patient past middle age, bronchogenic carcinoma should be suspected. Then further studies such as tomography and bronchography can be done.

MEDIASTINAL WIDENING. When the mediastinum is enlarged as a result of bronchogenic carcinoma, it often indicates the presence of an anaplastic type. The primary tumor is usually in a stem bronchus and rarely beyond a lobar bronchus, so that the primary tumor mass is often obscured by a large mediastinal mass.

Therefore this tumor cannot be differentiated from malignant lymphoma in some patients. The tumor is inoperable when there is mediastinal invasion but may respond to irradiation (Fig. 29-6).

APICAL DENSITY WITH OR WITHOUT RIB DESTRUCTION. This is termed a superior pulmonary sulcus tumor or Pancoast tumor. It is usually caused by a squamous cell type of bronchogenic tumor; occasionally other types of bronchogenic carcinoma may be found. The four cardinal parts of the Pancoast syndrome are: (*1*) mass in pulmonary apex, (*2*) destruction of adjacent rib or vertebra, (*3*) Horner's syndrome, and (*4*) pain down the arm. Other tumors, including metastatic carcinoma and malignant neurogenic tumor, may cause it in addition to bronchogenic carcinoma. When only a small amount of parenchymal density is

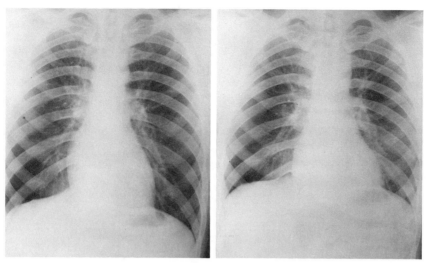

Fig. 29-5. Obstructive emphysema of the right lower lobe resulting from carcinoma of the lower lobe bronchus. *Left,* Roentgenogram in inspiration reveals slight questionable increased radiability of the right lower lung field. *Right,* Expiratory roentgenogram accentuates the contrast between the lower lungs and confirms the presence of obstructive emphysema on the right. There is no roentgenographically visible neoplasm.

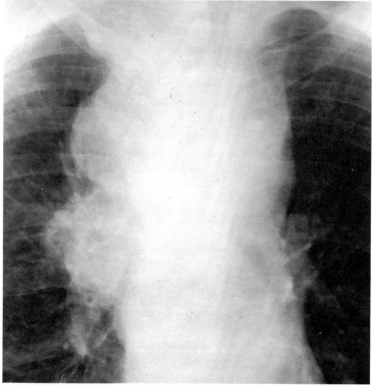

Fig. 29-6. Anaplastic bronchogenic carcinoma. Lobulated mass involving the right hilum and extending up into the superior mediastinum where it is noted to displace the trachea to the left. There is also some tumor in the superior mediastinum on the left. This type of tumor is impossible to differentiate from lymphoma on roentgen findings.

visible representing the peripheral tumor, the diagnosis of malignancy is very difficult to make because it simulates the minor amount of pleural thickening often visualized in the apex in elderly patients. The presence of pain should lead to the strong suspicion of tumor and the other clinical findings of Horner's syndrome, loss of sensation in the forearm, and atrophy of the hand muscles that are often present make the diagnosis almost certain. The tumor often grows rapidly with early destruction of the ribs (Fig. 29-7). Special films of the apex taken with techniques to show bone detail may be necessary to determine the presence or absence of rib destruction. Occasionally peripheral bronchogenic carcinoma elsewhere may spread locally to produce similar roentgen findings.

SOLITARY CAVITY. When a solitary cavity is found in an elderly male who has few if any signs of infection, the presence of bronchogenic carcinoma should be suspected. The cavity wall is usually thick and irregular, but may be very thin. If tomograms are obtained, there is almost invariably a local mass projecting from the rounded or oval cavity wall into the cavity in one or more areas. Another helpful sign is the lack of evidence of inflammatory disease in the vicinity of the solitary cavity (Fig. 29-8). The epidermoid tumor is the usual type in which cavitation occurs.

PNEUMONITIS THAT DOES NOT CLEAR. Partial obstruction of a bronchus resulting from tumor may cause inflammatory disease in the lobe or

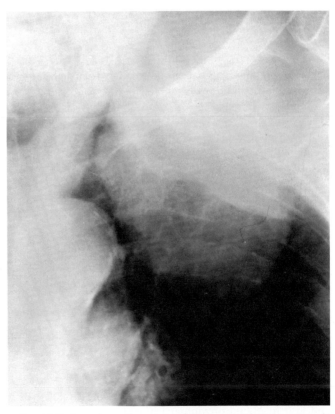

Fig. 29-7. Superior pulmonary sulcus tumor. The large mass is easily defined and there is a considerable amount of rib destruction which is common in this type of tumor.

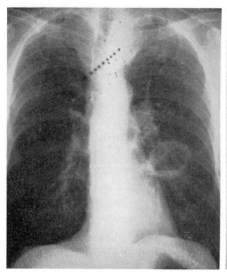 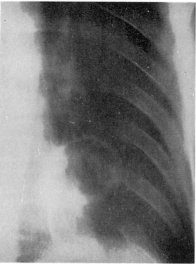

Fig. 29-8. Bronchogenic carcinoma. The cavity in the left lung below the hilum represents a bronchogenic carcinoma. Enlargement of a tomogram (*right*) shows a nodule on the medial wall of the cavity. There is no inflammatory disease surrounding the cavity but there is some enlargement of left hilar nodes. The small nodule projecting into the cavity is typical of carcinoma. There is fibronodular tuberculosis in the left apex.

segment supplied by that bronchus. On roentgen study the findings simulate those of an ordinary pneumonia localized to the area. If the process fails to resolve or clears incompletely, bronchogenic carcinoma should be suspected (Fig. 29-9). Furthermore, if the pneumonitis clears and then reappears in the same area, endobronchial tumor should also be suspected and further studies, including bronchography and tomography, done to determine the cause. The density noted in these patients with disease that resembles pneumonitis may be caused in part by tumor; tomograms will then frequently outline tumor nodulation within the area of pneumonic consolidation.

Smaller, poorly defined infiltrates resembling very small patches of inflammatory disease may actually represent the first sign of bronchogenic carcinoma. When such a minor lesion is found, particularly in an elderly male, it is important to obtain follow-up roentgenograms and also to obtain previous roentgenograms, if available, for comparison. When such a lesion does not respond to antibiotic therapy and does

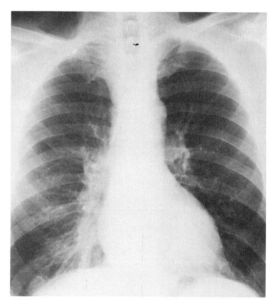

Fig. 29-9. Bronchogenic carcinoma simulating inflammatory disease. The patient was febrile when the poorly defined disease in the right lower lobe was discovered. When the acute symptoms subsided and the parenchymal disease failed to clear, thoracotomy revealed an infiltrating carcinoma in the right lower lobe.

not contain calcium, bronchogenic tumor is a distinct possibility.

LARGE PARENCHYMAL MASS. Bronchogenic carcinoma that begins as a peripheral nodule may reach very large size before causing symptoms. These large lobulated but generally rounded or oval masses may lie far out in the periphery or adjacent to the hilum. They range from 4 to 10 or 12 cm in diameter and even larger. Tomograms may show some areas of radiolucency, indicating necrosis within the mass. There is usually very little difficulty in arriving at the diagnosis of pulmonary carcinoma in these patients because any solitary mass lesion of large size in a patient in the carcinoma age period is most likely malignant and must be considered as such until disproved. There is often associated hilar node involvement resulting in unilateral hilar enlargement (Fig. 29-10).

THE SOLITARY PULMONARY NODULE. The solitary, peripheral, pulmonary, parenchymal nodule presents a diagnostic and therapeutic problem that has been extensively investigated and discussed in recent years. When such a nodule is visualized on a chest roentgenogram, the question of lung tumor always arises. These nodules may range from a few millimeters up to 4 cm or more in size. When they are more than 4 cm in size and contain no calcium, bronchogenic carcinoma is highly probable. When a small nodule is found, there are certain steps that should be taken to ascertain the nature of the lesion. If previous films are available they should be reviewed and if the lesion was not present on previous examinations made within the past 1 or 2 years in a patient (particularly if a male) over 40, malignant tumor is the first consideration and exploratory thoracotomy is indicated. Inflammatory granulomata occasionally appear in patients of middle age but this is uncommon. If the nodule in question has increased in size on review of films taken several months, or even years earlier, bronchogenic carcinoma is the first consideration in diagnosis unless calcification can be demonstrated within it. Tomography should be used in all these patients with solitary pulmonary nodules to determine the presence or absence of calcification. When calcification is present the lesion is most likely benign. The character of calcification is of significance. A central nidus, a laminated character, or both almost certainly indicate an inflammatory lesion. Calcium in a malignant nodule may be: (1) coincidental—the tumor

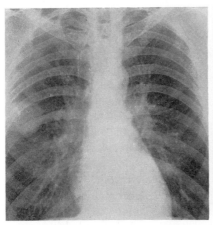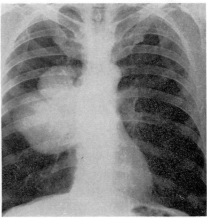

Fig. 29-10. Bronchogenic carcinoma. Chest roentgenograms on two patients, both of whom were asymptomatic. *Left,* Anaplastic bronchogenic carcinoma arising in the lower lobe. *Right,* Undifferentiated adenocarcinoma of the right lung.

grows around an old Ghon tubercle, or (2) calcification in the tumor itself—this is very uncommon. Even then the lesion should be kept under observation by means of follow-up roentgenograms. A few cases of bronchogenic carcinoma have been reported in nodules containing calcium but by far the majority of them are benign. If the lesion containing calcium continues to grow, thoracotomy with removal should be considered because of the remote possibility of carcinoma; furthermore if inflammatory, the growth indicates activity of the granulomatous process (Fig. 29-11).

When tomograms fail to show calcium within the nodule, it does not mean that it is malignant but it indicates that malignancy cannot be excluded (Fig. 29-12). Active inflammatory nodules may be irregular, and small satellite nodules are often present; however, in the absence of calcium these signs cannot be taken to exclude carcinoma. There are several additional findings which are helpful in the roentgen differentiation of benign and malignant tumor nodules. The malignant tumors often have indefinite, irregular or fuzzy borders

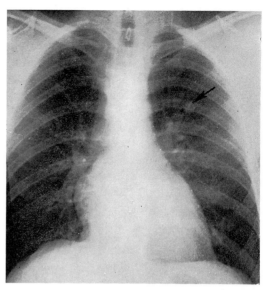

Fig. 29-12. Solitary pulmonary nodule. No calcification was demonstrated on tomography. No tumor was found elsewhere. Nodule was removed and found to be anaplastic bronchogenic carcinoma.

in contrast to the sharp borders of benign tumors. Linear densities are more often associated with inflammatory nodules than with malignant tumors. They may extend from the hilum to the nodule or from the nodule to the pleura or both. Lobulation of the nodule is more suggestive of carcinoma than of inflammation.

Roentgen Signs Indicating Metastasis or Local Invasion

PLEURAL EFFUSION. The presence of pleural effusion in a patient with a visible pulmonary tumor mass usually indicates that there is involvement of the pleura by direct extension or as the result of metastasis. At times clear fluid may indicate only that lymphatics are obstructed and is not a certain indication of spread of tumor to the pleura. However, if the fluid is bloody, involvement of the pleura by tumor is almost invariably present. Not infrequently the effusion is massive and obscures the lung. When the fluid is removed, the tumor mass or secondary signs of tumor may be visible. Bronchopleural fistula may result in

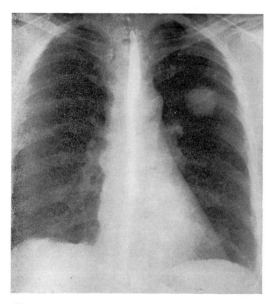

Fig. 29-11. Benign pulmonary mass simulating malignancy. Tomography revealed a small amount of mottled calcification in the mass but removal was recommended because of its size. Final diagnosis was that of tuberculoma.

pyopneumothorax and occasionally empyema occurs in patients with bronchogenic carcinoma.

HEMATOGENOUS AND LYMPHOGENOUS METAS-TASIS. Lymphogenous metastasis is the most common type of spread in bronchogenic carcinoma. The lymphatics drain toward the hilum except in the peripheral areas close to the pleura, where they follow the septal and pleural veins to the pleural surface. From there these lymphatics drain to the hilum through superficial pleural channels. This leads to lymphogenous metastasis involving the tracheal, bronchial, and mediastinal nodes. When these nodes become enlarged the local involvement may be visible roentgenographically. As a result the tumor is visualized along with enlargement of the hilum or paratracheal nodes. When this occurs, the tumor is most likely advanced and inoperable (Fig. 29-13). It is not uncommon to observe strands of density

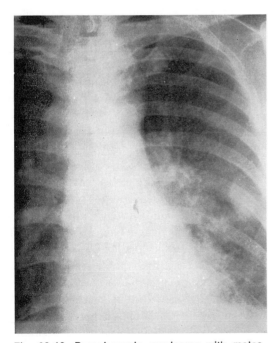

Fig. 29-13. Bronchogenic carcinoma with metastases. Note the enlarged paratracheal nodes on the right and the pleural mass along the left lateral chest wall. Large hilar tumor is seen on the left with secondary inflammatory disease below it.

extending from the peripheral or midzone type of tumor to the hilum, representing involvement of the bronchial lymphatics. Rarely, lymphogenous metastasis is widespread and results in irregular strandlike accentuation of markings extending into the lung fields from both hila. Hematogenous pulmonary metastasis occurs occasionally in bronchogenic carcinoma. There are then signs of the original tumor plus scattered parenchymal lesions that appear as rounded or oval masses of varying size, usually smaller than the primary. Massive mediastinal involvement, which is observed in anaplastic carcinoma, has been discussed earlier.

PLEURAL MASS WITH OR WITHOUT RIB DE-STRUCTION. The visceral pleura may be involved as a result of lymphogenous metastasis. Direct invasion of the parietal pleura and chest wall may result in a mass with or without destruction of the adjacent rib. This occurs in the superior pulmonary sulcus tumor and to a lesser degree with peripheral tumors elsewhere. The pleural mass is often obscured by effusion. Hematogenous metastasis to ribs may occur with destruction of bone and production of a soft-tissue mass that may extend into the thorax. The roentgen findings are similar in either type of lesion except that pleural effusion is more likely to occur in the lymphogenous type.

DIAPHRAGMATIC ELEVATION. Elevation with evidence of paresis, or paralysis, of the hemidiaphragm on the side of the tumor is another late sign and indicates involvement of the phrenic nerve. Fluoroscopy can be used to demonstrate these findings.

GENERAL CONSIDERATIONS

Various combinations of the findings given above may occur in any individual patient. Occasionally none of the characteristic findings will appear and some pulmonary malignancies cannot be identified by roentgen signs. An additional factor that makes the diagnosis difficult is the association of bronchogenic carcinoma with chronic inflammatory disease. Tuberculosis is estimated to be associated with bronchogenic carcinoma in 10 per cent of the latter. In these cases the association makes the diagnosis of carcinoma extremely difficult, since a tumor nodule may appear in or near the nodular tuberculosis or may arise in the wall of a tuberculous cavity and thus escape recognition for a long period of time. It is therefore important to keep the possibility of bronchogenic carcinoma in mind, particularly in elderly males with tuberculosis. There are several roentgen signs which are suggestive of tumor: (1) an increase in hilar size during treatment with antituberculous drugs; (2) the failure of a local lesion to respond to treatment, while in other areas the disease is regressing; and (3) increase in size of a lesion despite treatment.

The roentgen diagnosis of bronchogenic carcinoma is based on the finding of one or more of the signs described in the previous sections. In order to do this, it is necessary to obtain good films in frontal and lateral projections and in oblique or other directions, such as the lordotic view, when indicated. Examination in different phases of respiration using films and fluoroscopy must also be employed in some instances. Tomography is of particular value in the examination of solitary parenchymal nodules and of the hilum when tumor obstructing a bronchus is suspected. Bronchography is also a valuable method of examination and its use often demonstrates signs of endobronchial mass or bronchial obstruction that are highly characteristic of bronchogenic carcinoma. Bronchographic signs of carcinoma include: (1) abrupt obstruction of a bronchus, often somewhat irregular; (2) annular constriction of a bronchus, which may cause complete obstruction to produce the so-called "rat tail" appearance; (3) localized midbronchial displacement usually indicating malignancy (benign lesions may produce local masses but tend to extend around the bronchus rather than displace it); and (4) localized unilateral indentation of a bronchus caused by tumor invasion. Bronchography is particularly useful in patients wth segmental involvement in whom bronchoscopy fails to visualize the bronchus in question. It is of little value in the differential diagnosis of small peripheral pulmonary nodules. Many of the tumors are more indolent than is commonly realized, so that the importance of comparison of all available chest roentgenograms cannot be overemphasized, particularly

when a small parenchymal shadow is present or when one hilum is questionably enlarged.

The use of bronchial and intercostal arteriography in the diagnosis of bronchogenic carcinoma is advocated by some. If successful, this study may indicate the presence of spread to the chest wall and may aid in differentiation of pulmonary from pleural or chest-wall tumors. However it may be of no aid in differentiating benign and malignant tumors and inflammatory disease. At present we rarely use this procedure in patients with suspected bronchogenic carcinoma. We use a combination of superior cavography and pulmonary arteriography along with azygography in attempting to assess operability of lung tumors (Fig. 29-14).

OTHER MALIGNANT TUMORS

BRONCHIAL ADENOMA

This tumor is included under the malignant lung lesions because metastases to lymph nodes are found in approximately 20 per cent of patients. It should be recognized, however, that this tumor is relatively benign and its clinical course and prognosis are entirely different from that of bronchogenic carcinoma. There are two main pathologic types: carcinoid, which is the most common (approximately 85 per cent) and cylindroid which resembles mixed salivary gland tumors. Cylindromas tend to be more central in location and more invasive than the carcinoid type. Very few of the carcinoid tumors of the bronchus secrete serotonin, so the carcinoid syndrome is uncommon. The tumor occurs in females as frequently as in males and is found in younger age groups than is bronchogenic carcinoma. It is most often found between the ages of 20 and 40 but a number of cases have been reported in children. Our youngest patient was 12 years of age. The adeoma tends to bleed rather easily, so that repeated hemoptysis may be the major clinical finding. It grows slowly and produces slowly progressing bronchial obstruction leading to repeated attacks of pneumonitis, obstructive emphysema, and eventually to atelectasis.

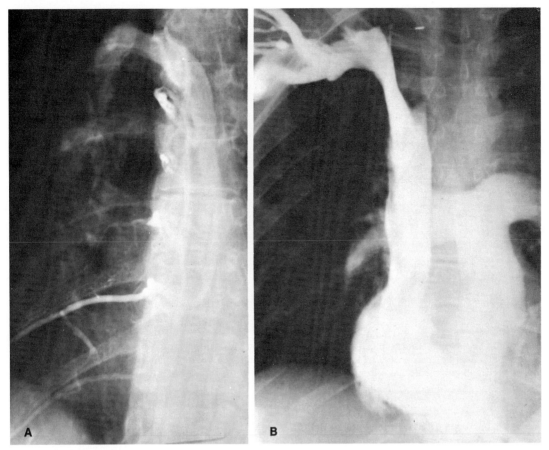

Fig. 29-14. Azygography, superior cavography and pulmonary arteriography in the study of broncho-genic carcinoma. *A,* Normal azygogram. Note the intercostal veins filling the azygos vein which empties into the superior vena cava. There is no evidence of obstruction; this is a normal examination. *B,* The superior cava is clearly defined. There is some filling of the right side of the heart and major pulmonary arteries. There is no evidence of involvement of the cava or of the pulmonary arteries by tumor. These findings indicate operability of the tumor.

Roentgen Findings

Occasionally the rounded or oval tumor may be visible as a solitary mass in the lung periphery. It usually arises in a large bronchus and is therefore near the hilum. Most frequently, however, the actual tumor mass is not visible because of its small size. The diagnosis then rests upon the manifestations of bronchial obstruction. The findings range from complete atelectasis (Fig. 29-15), to lobar or segmental obstructive emphysema when check-value stenosis is produced. Signs of pulmonary infection and bronchiectasis are not infrequent in the lobe distal to the tumor. Tomography is useful when such a lesion is suspected. The rounded tumor mass may then be visualized within a bronchus. Bronchograpy will almost invariably outline the endobronchial tumor, which produces a smoothly rounded mass resulting in partial or complete obstruction (see Fig. 29-3).

BRONCHIOLAR CARCINOMA

This is a pulmonary tumor, the origin of which has been under investigation for several

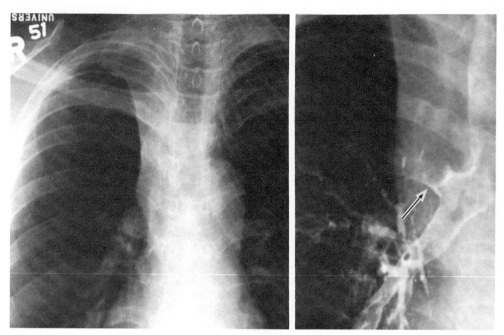

Fig. 29-15. Bronchial adenoma. *Left,* Atelectasis of the right upper lobe in a young female. *Right,* Bronchogram; **arrow** indicates the smoothly rounded defect produced by the bronchial adenoma which obstructed the upper lobe bronchus.

years. It has been called "pulmonary adenomatosis," "bronchioloalveolar," and "alveolar cell carcinoma," but most investigators now think that the cells are bronchiolar in origin, so that the term "bronchiolar carcinoma" is preferred. Despite a uniform pathologic pattern of tall columnar cells with basal nuclei producing a glandular pattern, there is a rather wide variation in the clinical course of the tumor. Progression may be exceedingly rapid or very slow. Bronchogenic spread appears to occur commonly. Some investigators believe that multicentric origin causes the disseminated form, but most believe that the origin is unicentric.

This tumor occurs with about equal frequency in males and females. Cough and dyspnea are the two most prominent symptoms. The cough may be productive of large quantities of mucoid sputum. This is an important clinical sign in the diagnosis of the disease and is found in 25 to 30 per cent of patients.

Roentgen Findings

When first observed on chest roentgenogram, this tumor may be localized or disseminated. In the local form, the most common finding is that of homogeneous density, which may vary considerably in size from a small nodule of 1 cm or less in diameter to a mass involving most of a lobe. The boundaries are hazy and poorly defined and the density resembles an area of local pneumonitis. This diagnosis is often entertained when the lesion is first observed. At times the density is more clearly outlined and resembles the solitary nodular mass observed in bronchogenic carcinoma. No evidence of atelectasis is present and the pleura is not ordinarily involved. Roentgenograms taken at intervals following the initial examination show gradual progression on the side first involved and often spread to the opposite side, where similar consolidation is observed. Eventually, there may be massive involvement of both lungs (Fig. 29-16). A less common form of the disease is one in which poorly defined nodules are scattered throughout both lungs. They are less distinct than the nodules usually observed in hematogenous metastasis. We have also observed several patients in whom the disease was disseminated widely, with tiny foci resembling miliary inflammatory disease. When the disease is extensive and resembles alveolar pneumonia, an air bronchogram is often observed. Bronchographic findings have been described by Zheutlin, Lasser, and Rigler,[19] which they believe are typical. The small bronchi are narrow, elongated, and rigid and are filled with the iodized oil rather than coated with it. In addition, the normal alveolar filling beyond the bronchi is not present. The diagnosis of this tumor can be suspected when the roentgen and bronchographic findings described are present

along with a history of cough producing large amounts of mucoid sputum. Earlier in the disease, pneumonia is usually considered but when the process gradually advances despite antibiotic therapy, the diagnosis should be suspected.

PULMONARY SARCOMA

Primary sarcoma occurring in the lung is very rare, but myosarcoma, chondrosarcoma, and fibrosarcoma have been reported. In some instances the cells are undifferentiated and difficult to classify. Occasionally they appear to be mixed, with some sarcomatous elements and some elements that resemble carcinoma. These tumors usually arise peripherally and reach large size before producing symptoms so that they may be found on routine roentgen examination of the chest. Occasionally they arise in the wall of a bronchus and then result

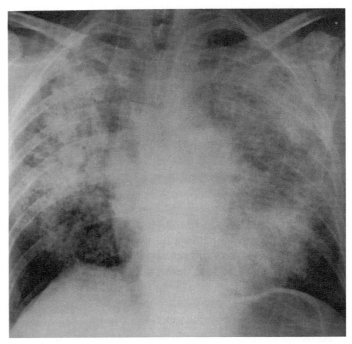

Fig. 29-16. Bronchiolar carcinoma. The disease is bilateral. There are large areas of homogeneous consolidation which resemble alveolar pneumonia but there are also numerous, widely scattered, small nodules ranging up to about 7 or 8 mm in diameter. On the initial film air bronchogram could be observed in the left base and in the right upper lung field.

in obstructive signs similar to those described earlier in other tumors.

Roentgen Findings

The roentgen findings are not characteristic but the mass is visible. It is often large and may be somewhat lobulated. Thoracotomy and biopsy or removal is necessary to ascertain the histopathologic diagnosis.

LEUKEMIA AND LYMPHOMA OF THE LUNG

The leukemias primarily involve the hilar and mediastinal nodes but occasionally pulmonary parenchymal involvement may occur. Adenopathy is more frequent in lymphatic leukemia than in the myeloid type. When the lung is involved by leukemia, there is extension of the tumor cells into the peribronchial and perivascular connective tissues of the lung. This results in strands of increased density radiating outward from the hilum on one or both sides. This is usually accompanied by recognizable enlargement of the hilar lymph nodes. The roentgen findings are not characteristic and must be correlated with the known presence of leukemia in the patient. Infections are common in leukemia and usually account for pulmonic involvement noted in this disease. Hemorrhage may also produce pulmonary densities. Pleural involvement, resulting in effusion, is somewhat more common than pulmonary leukemic infiltrates.

Lymphosarcoma may also involve the lung along with mediastinal nodes and rarely this disease may be primary in the lung. The primary form tends to be more benign than lymphosarcoma elsewhere. Roentgen findings are of a large mass, which is usually clearly defined; slight haziness and irregularity of the edges is often observed. It grows slowly and, unlike bronchogenic carcinoma, does not ordinarily invade the bronchi and cause bronchial obstruction. Mediastinal adenopathy is not a feature of this disease and pleural effusion is rare, even though the tumor extends to a pleural surface.

Secondary involvement of the lung in patients with mediastinal lymphoma is usually a late feature of the disease. This occurs in a variety of forms, resulting in a number of different roentgen manifestations: (1) direct invasion of the lung in the presence of visible mediastinal mass; (2) large lobar infiltrates associated with mediastinal mass; or (3) smaller pulmonary parenchymal infiltrates that may be well circumscribed or irregular and poorly defined. These are usually associated with hilar or mediastinal adenopathy or with disease elsewhere so that the diagnosis is not difficult to make on roentgen examination. Reticulum cell sarcoma may occasionally occur as a primary pulmonary tumor. The findings in the primary and secondary forms of this disease are similar to those of lymphosarcoma.

It is evident that roentgen manifestations are extremely variable but the presence of associated adenopathy usually makes classification of the disease into the lymphoma group possible on roentgen examination. Of the lymphomas Hodgkin's disease most commonly involves the lung secondarily (Figs. 29-17 and 29-18). Usually the parenchymal involvement is a direct extension of the mediastinal disease. The tumor advances in a compact manner and tends to destroy the tissue it invades. Bronchial obstruction is more common than in lymphosarcoma. Pleural involvement accompanied by pleural effusion is often present. Parenchymal masses, not in direct contiguity with mediastinal lesions may also be observed, however, and may be single or multiple. Occasionally the parenchymal mass in Hodgkin's disease may undergo central necrosis with cavitation and resemble tuberculosis. To be noted also is the fact that patients with Hodgkin's disease show a tendency to develop tuberculosis or fungal infections during terminal stages. Hodgkin's disease rarely, if ever, occurs as a solitary, pulmonary, parenchymal mass. This finding may be the only manifestation on the chest film, however, since the other sites may be in nodes outside of the thorax. Multiple myeloma (plasmocytoma) often invades the thorax from the ribs or spine. Rarely, a primary myeloma may arise in the lung. There is no way to

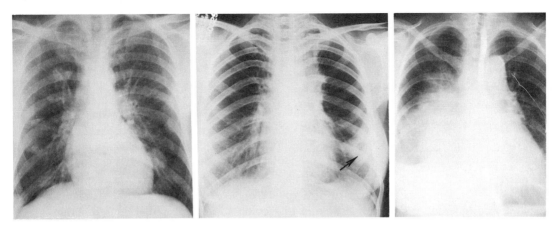

Fig. 29-17. Hodgkin's disease. *Left*, Pulmonary parenchymal nodules ranging up to 3 cm in diameter plus enlargement of right paratracheal nodes and hilar nodes. *Center*, Mediastinal node involvement with marked widening of the mediastinum on the left. The rounded parenchymal mass at the left base contains central radiolucency representing a cavity. *Right*, Massive involvement of mediastinal nodes with invasion of pulmonary parenchyma and pleura resulting in a small pleural effusion on the right.

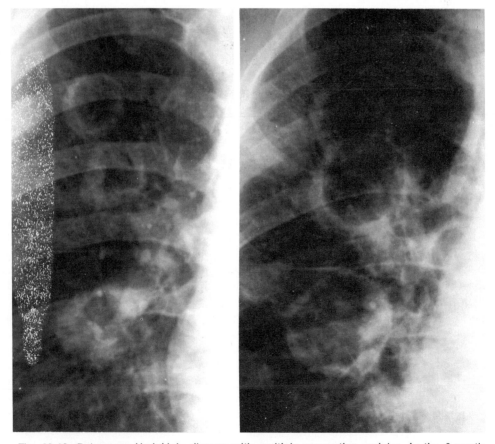

Fig. 29-18. Pulmonary Hodgkin's disease with multiple excavating nodules. In the 2-month period of observation the nodules increased in size with a loss of soft tissue in their walls.

differentiate it from bronchogenic carcinoma roentgenographically.

METASTATIC TUMORS

HEMATOGENOUS METASTASIS

Hematogenous pulmonary metastases are usually multiple and consist of smoothly rounded nodules scattered throughout both lung fields. They may be uniform in size or may vary considerably. They may range up to 10 cm or more in diameter while others in the same lung will be less than 1 cm in size. Occasionally a solitary metastasis is present and cannot be differentiated from solitary primary tumor on the basis of roentgen findings. The source of metastasis can be malignancy anywhere in the body but there are some tumors that show a marked tendency to metastasize to the lung. All the sarcomas, including osteogenic sarcoma and chondrosarcoma as well as the various soft-tissue sarcomas and malignant melanoma, frequently metastasize to the lung. Carcinoma of the breast, kidney, ovary, testis, colon, and thyroid also metastasizes frequently to the lung, while tumors of the stomach, respiratory tract, and prostate do so infrequently.

Roentgen Findings

The roentgen findings are those of multiple nodules that may be few or many in number. They may be uniform or vary considerably in size. Occasionally a solitary metastasis may be observed as a solitary parenchymal nodule that may become large without producing symptoms. A solitary metastasis may arise from any organ. However the following primary neoplasms are the more likely origins: tumors of the colon, kidney, testicle, breast, malignant melanoma and bone sarcoma. There are some differences in the roentgen findings in pulmonary metastases from different organs but these are variable and not too reliable in differential diagnosis. Renal and thyroid tumors result in metastases that are few in number and often large in size. Osteogenic sarcoma metastasizing to the lungs may result in formation of tumor bone in the metastases that may be characteristic. Calcification may occur in metastases from cystadenocarcinoma of ovary and rarely in metastases from tumors of other organs. Ovarian and testicular tumors and chorioepithelioma often result in widespread, rapidly growing, metastatic lesions (Fig. 29-19). Occasionally central necrosis with cavitation is found in metastatic nodules. We have observed this in carcinoma of the colon more frequently than in other lesions. Cavitation is rather common when metastatic pulmonary tumors respond to treatment with cytotoxic drugs.

LYMPHOGENOUS METASTASIS

In contrast to the nodular hematogenous type of pulmonary metastasis, lymphangitic metastasis tends to cause respiratory dysfunction leading to dyspnea, which may be severe. This type of metastasis is usually caused by primary tumors of the stomach, breast, pancreas, and prostate. Primary bronchogenic carcinoma and carcinoma of the colon may also result in this type of spread. The tumor cells grow within and along the lymphatic pathways spreading outward from the hila to the periphery.

Roentgen Findings

The appearance of the chest in this type of metastasis is entirely different from the appearance in the presence of hematogenous metastases, although both may occur in a single patient. There is usually enough hilar node enlargement to be recognized as such. This is particularly true if earlier roentgenograms are available for comparison. In addition to the hilar enlargement, there is an irregular strand-like network of density extending outward from the hila well into the parenchyma. When this change is early, findings are often minimal and comparison with an earlier examination is necessary to be certain of the diagnosis. Later the

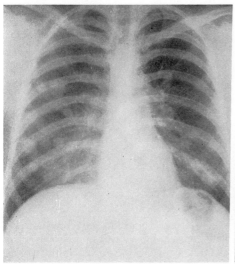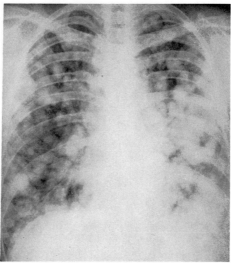

Fig. 29-19. Hematogenous pulmonary metastasis. *Left,* The metastatic nodules scattered in the lungs are clearly defined and range up to nearly 3 cm in size. *Right,* Extensive nodular pulmonary metastasis. Despite the massive involvement of the lung, the patient experienced very little dyspnea. Primary tumor was seminoma of testis.

findings become characteristic (Fig. 29-20). Unilateral or bilateral pleural effusions may also be present. Occasionally there are small granular densities associated with the reticular network of increased density extending into the parenchyma that may resemble sarcoidosis, hematogenous tuberculosis, or other inflammatory disease. Correlation of the roentgen with the clinical findings usually permits a correct diagnosis in these instances.

BENIGN TUMORS

HAMARTOMA

Hamartoma consists of a mass of tissue containing the elements of the organ within which it develops but without organization and without function. Hamartoma of the lung may contain cartilage, muscle, fibrous connective tissue, and epithelial elements. Often cartilage and fibrous connective tissue predominate. The tumor is usually peripheral in type and is found near a pleural surface. It may occur near the hilum, however. It is usually relatively small in size and grows very slowly.

Roentgen Findings

Roentgenographic findings are those of a well-circumscribed, pulmonary parenchymal nodule, usually small in size. It is clearly defined and smoothly rounded or oval but occasionally is lobulated. No satellite nodules are demonstrated in the area. Calcification is rarely present and occasionally there is ossification noted within the tumor. When calcification is present, it is scattered within the lesion; the distribution has been likened to the appearance of a popcorn ball. In our experience this is exceedingly uncommon. When such a mass is found within a lung, it is necessary to determine whether or not calcification is present. Tomography is indicated if evidence of calcium is not visible on the routine roentgenogram. If there is no calcification present, the mass cannot be differentiated from the peripheral type of primary bronchogenic carcinoma or from solitary metastasis so that thoracotomy with excision is indicated. When calcification is present it usually indicates that the lesion is benign. Bronchography is of little use in the examination of this type of tumor because the peripheral location produces no alteration in the bronchial tree other than possible slight displacement of peripheral branches. Occasionally, multiple hamartomas are present. This tumor has been observed to enlarge

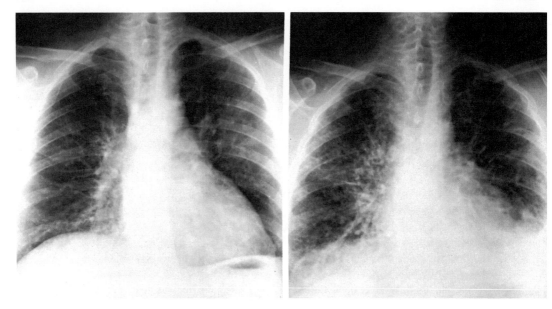

Fig. 29-20. Lymphogenous metastasis. *Left,* There is a little increase in the interstitial markings in the parahilar areas and at the bases. *Right,* Five weeks later the interstitial process has advanced considerably and there is now a moderate-sized left pleural effusion. The patient had carcinoma of the pancreas.

and if no calcification is present, it then becomes impossible to differentiate it from malignant tumor.

OTHER BENIGN TUMORS

A wide variety of tumors have been found within the lung. They include leiomyoma, fibroma, neurofibroma, hemangioma, hemangiopericytoma, and lipoma. They are usually asymptomatic when they occur peripherally and may reach large size before being discovered because of the absence of symptoms. If calcification is present within the tumor it is likely benign but if there is no calcification, malignancy cannot be excluded. Occasionally a lymphoid nodule is observed as a small nodular mass in the pulmonary parenchyma.

Roentgen Findings

Findings are similar to those described in hamartoma except that the tumors may become considerably larger. Occasionally these benign tumors may reach massive proportions and fill most of the thorax on one side. They therefore present as rounded, oval, or lobulated masses of considerable size. Tomography should be used to define them

clearly and if calcification is not present, surgery is indicated since they cannot be differentiated from carcinoma. Occasionally lipoma or fibroma may arise within a bronchus and produce symptoms as well as radiographic signs that cannot be differentiated from those of malignant endobronchial tumor.

REFERENCES AND SELECTED READINGS

1. AMERICAN CANCER SOCIETY: Cancer of the lung, an evaluation of the problem. *Proceedings of the Scientific Session, Annual Meeting, November 1953.* New York, 1956.

2. BARON, M. G., and WHITEHOUSE, W. M.: Primary lymphosarcoma of the lung. *Am. J. Roentgenol. Radium Ther. Nucl. Med. 85:* 294, 1961.

3. BOUCOT, K. R., COOPER, D. A., WEISS, W., and CARNAHAN, W. J.: Appearance of the first roentgenographic abnormalities due to lung cancer. *JAMA 190:* 1102, 1964.

4. CONDON, V. R., and PHILLIPS, E. W.: Bronchial adenoma in children. *Am. J. Roentgenol. Radium Ther. Nucl. Med. 88:* 543, 1962.

5. FLEISCHNER, F. G.: Mediastinal lymphadenopathy in bronchial carcinoma. *Radiology 58:* 48, 1952.

6. GARLAND, L. H.: A three-step method for diagnosis of solitary pulmonary nodules. *Can. Med. Assoc. J. 83:* 1079, 1960.

7. GARLAND, L. H.: The rate of growth and natural duration of primary bronchial cancer. *Am. J. Roentgenol. Radium Ther. Nucl. Med. 96:* 604, 1966.

8. GOOD, C. A., HOOD, R. T., JR., and McDONALD, J. R.: Significance of a solitary mass in the lung. *Am. J. Roentgenol. Radium Ther. Nucl. Med. 70:* 543, 1953.

9. KITTERIDGE, R. D., and SHERMAN, R. S.: Terminal bronchiolar carcinoma. *Am. J. Roentgenol. Radium Ther. Nucl. Med. 87:* 875, 1962.

10. LIEBOW, A. A.: Pathology of carcinoma of the lung as related to the roentgen shadow. *Am. J. Roentgenol. Radium Ther. Nucl. Med. 74:* 383, 1955.

11. McCORT, J. J., and ROBBINS, L. L.: Lymph node metastases in carcinoma of the lung. *Radiology 57:* 339, 1951.

12. MAYER, E., and MAIER, H. C.: *Pulmonary Carcinoma.* New York, New York University Press, 1956.

13. RIGLER, L. G.: The earliest roentgenographic signs of carcinoma of the lung. *JAMA 195:* 655, 1966.

14. ROZSA, S., and FRIEDMAN, H.: Extramedullary plasmocytoma of the lung. *Am. J. Roentgenol. Radium Ther. Nucl. Med. 70:* 982, 1953.

15. SHEINMEL, A., ROSWIT, B., and LAWRENCE, L. R.: Hodgkin's disease of the lung: Roentgen appearance and therapeutic management. *Radiology 54:* 165, 1950.

16. STEIN, J., JACOBSON, H. G., POPPEL, M. H., and LAWRENCE, L. R.: Pulmonary hamartoma. *Am. J. Roentgenol. Radium Ther. Nucl. Med. 70:* 971, 1953.

17. WEISS, L., and INGRAM, M.: Adenomatoid bronchial tumors. A consideration of the carcinoid tumors and the salivary tumors of the bronchial tree. *Cancer 14:* 161, 1961.

18. WOODRUFF, J. H., JR., OTTOMAN, R. E., and ISAAC, F.: Bronchiolar-cell carcinoma. *Radiology 70:* 335, 1958.

19. ZHEUTLIN, N., LASSER, E. C., and RIGLER, L. G.: Bronchographic abnormalities in alveolar cell carcinoma of the lung. *Dis. Chest 25:* 542, 1954.

30

MISCELLANEOUS PULMONARY CONDITIONS

PULMONARY EMPHYSEMA

The term "emphysema" is used to designate a variety of conditions in which overinflation occurs. This may involve the lungs and other tissues. Pulmonary emphysema may be on the basis of functional change such as in the compensatory type in which a portion of lung is diseased and the remainder assumes its function, or it may be associated with definite anatomic changes. Nonpulmonary emphysema may occur anywhere in the body and is usually designated by its anatomic position. In the present discussion nonpulmonary emphysema will be mentioned only in relation to the thorax, where it is usually either mediastinal or in the chest wall.

CHRONIC PULMONARY EMPHYSEMA

Chronic pulmonary emphysema is defined by the American Thoracic Society[2] as follows: "Emphysema is an anatomic alteration of the lung characterized by an abnormal enlargement of the air spaces distal to the terminal non-respiratory bronchiole, accompanied by destructive changes of the alveolar walls." Such terms as essential, substantial, alveolar, vesicular, irreversible, and obstructive have been applied to this disease. Pathogenesis is somewhat controversial but it seems to be the result of a congenital constitutional defect plus obstruction of bronchioles. Chronic bronchial infection is found in a large majority of the patients and infection probably predisposes to emphysema if it is not the cause in these patients. Emphysema also is observed in patients with bronchiectasis, severe pulmonary infections, silicosis, and other pneumoconioses.

Emphysema can be classified into selective and nonselective types (Ciba Sym.)[55] on the basis of morphology. The most important selective form is the centrilobular in which the destruction of parenchyma predominates in the central portion of the secondary lobule. Panlobular is the term used for the diffuse non-selective form of the disease in which the acinus and secondary lobule are diffusely involved without particular relationship to the respiratory bronchioles. There are also several less important as well as an unclassified group.

There is general agreement that early mild manifestations of emphysema produce no roentgen findings in most instances. Roentgen signs are related to overinflation, vascular changes, and irregular involvement or bullae. They are:

1. Low, flat diaphragm with blunting of the costophrenic angles. The diaphragm is at or below the level of the seventh rib anteriorly in deep inspiration.

2. Diaphragmatic motion is diminished,

with excursion limited to 2 or 3 cm instead of a more normal 3 to 5 cm.

3. Abnormal enlargement of the retrosternal space—between the posterior sternum and the anterior wall of the ascending aorta. Separation of the aorta from the sternum extends more inferiorly than in the normal.

4. Irregular lucency of lung fields is often detected most readily on tomograms. Clearly defined bullae may be present.

5. There is a narrow, vertical heart with a large pulmonary artery. The hilar arteries are also large.

6. There is diminution in size of peripheral vessels which can be observed to best advantage when whole-chest tomography is used. The vascular diminution is often asymmetric and, on tomography, can be observed to coincide with areas of increased lucency of the lung. Large bullae devoid of vessels may be observed.

7. An increase in bronchovascular markings has been described by several writers, presumably related to chronic infection which so frequently accompanies emphysema (see Figs. 30-1 and 30-2).

Bronchography is sometimes used to study patients with chronic infection and emphysema (Fig. 30-3). The signs of chronic bronchitis may be present (see p. 799). Findings related to emphysema are as follows:

1. Overinflation resulting in spreading of bronchi which may be irregular and asymmetric.

2. Filling of small, rounded peripheral structures which probably represent enlarged centrilobular emphysematous spaces.

3. Spider deformity of the distal bronchioles; several branching from a single point.

4. Bronchioles end abruptly, with minimal "alveolarization" of contrast.

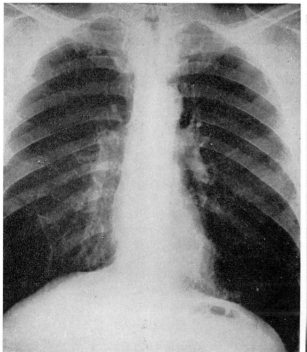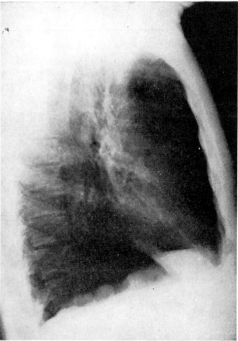

Fig. 30-1. Chronic pulmonary emphysema. The diaphragm is flat as observed in the lateral projection (*right*) and the retrosternal space is prominent. Radiability at the bases is increased and the pulmonary artery and its central branches are enlarged.

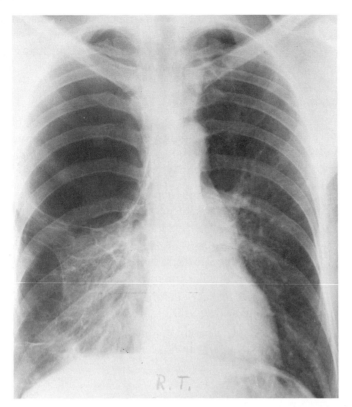

Fig. 30-2. Bullous emphysema. There are a few bullae in the left upper lung field. On the right there is a very large bulla superiorly and at least one inferolaterally. These occupy more than 50 per cent of the thoracic volume and are seen to compress the remaining lung on the right.

NONDESTRUCTIVE EMPHYSEMA

Exclusive of chronic emphysema described above associated with chronic bronchitis and defined as being accompanied by destructive changes of the alveolar walls, pulmonary emphysema may be divided into two main categories according to etiology, the obstructive and nonobstructive forms. Acute obstructive emphysema is usually caused by a foreign body in a bronchus and most often seen in children.

Nonobstructive emphysema may be divided into two general forms: (1) Compensatory emphysema, in which there is enlargement of the alveoli to meet functional space requirements when there is a loss of lung tissue elsewhere; it includes enlargement as a part of anatomic readjustment when a portion of a lung or lobe has been removed or is decreased in volume owing to disease or injury; or (2) Senile or postural emphysema, in which the enlargement of alveoli is secondary to alteration in the size and shape of the thoracic cage. A typical example is the barrel chest in which there is an increased thoracic volume because of an increased anteroposterior diameter of the chest.

ACUTE OBSTRUCTIVE EMPHYSEMA

This refers to the temporary condition observed most frequently in children, in which there is a one-way-valve type of obstruction caused by foreign body, usually in a main stem bronchus. Occasionally it may be lobar or segmental, however. The size of the foreign body

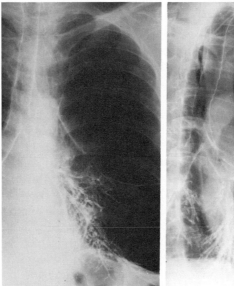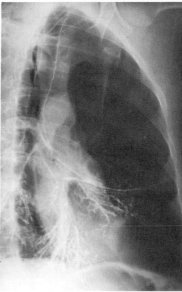

Fig. 30-3. Bullous emphysema. The bronchogram shows how the emphysema has compressed the lower lobe and the anterior and lingular segments of the upper lobe. Most of the volume of the left hemithorax is occupied by the bullae. Note that no normal markings are present in the peripheral two-thirds of the thorax.

and its situation are such that it does not completely obstruct the bronchus in which it is lodged. The normal bronchus enlarges in caliber during inspiration and narrows during expiration. Inspiration also is an active phase of respiration in which muscular action is required. Expiration is a passive phase. A foreign body that does not completely obstruct a bronchus on inspiration may do so during expiration. When this happens, air can enter the lung distal to the foreign body but cannot escape, or at least the ingress is less hampered than the egress. This situation will cause the lung, lobe, or segment distal to the foreign body to become increasingly distended until the pressure within it prevents more air from entering. This is known as a check-valve type of obstructive emphysema. In children it usually results from the aspiration of a food particle; substances such as nuts, popcorn, or other hard and small particles are the common offenders. Because most of the objects are nonopaque to roentgen rays, diagnosis depends upon the secondary changes caused by bronchial obstruction. If the

obstruction is complete so that no air can pass in either direction, there is absorption of gas from the lung distal to the obstruction, the alveoli collapse, and the lung becomes shrunken in volume and atelectatic. It is also possible for a foreign body to cause complete obstruction of one lobar bronchus and a check-valve type of obstruction of another resulting in a combination of atelectasis in one lobe and obstructive emphysema in the other.

In adults this type of emphysema either in a lobe, segment, or entire lung may be the earliest sign of carcinoma or other type of endobronchial tumor. In these instances the emphysema is more or less chronic but as the tumor increases in size complete obstruction will occur, leading to atelectasis.

Roentgen Observations

The roentgen diagnosis of acute obstructive emphysema is difficult on a single roentgenogram since there may be little change if the film is taken in complete inspiration. Therefore, it is essential that films be made in inspiration and expiration when obstructive emphysema is suspected. Fluoroscopy is an extremely valuable aid in the diagnosis. On inspiration the mediastinum moves toward the affected side in children with obstructing foreign bodies, whether atelectasis or obstructive emphysema is produced. On expiration the mediastinum shifts away from the involved side and the hemidiaphragm on the normal side tends to rise in a normal manner while the hemidiaphragm on the affected side remains more or less stationary or is limited in its motion. This is because the involved lung will remain fully aerated or hyperaerated while the normal lung deflates to become more radiopaque. In small children where the mediastinum is usually movable, it tends to swing widely away from the lesion on expiration and toward it on inspiration. These same findings are observed on inspiratory and expiratory films, but they are often difficult to obtain (Fig. 30-4). Occasionally the obstructing foreign body may be opaque to roentgen rays and thus readily identified. When the obstructive emphysema involves a single lobe the signs are similar but are less marked, and in these instances films in inspiration and expiration as well as fluoroscopy are necessary to make the diagnosis. Rarely, a foreign body becomes lodged in the trachea without causing sudden death but results in symmetric, bilateral obstructive emphysema.

INFANTILE LOBAR EMPHYSEMA (CONGENITAL LOBAR EMPHYSEMA)

Lobar emphysema is an obstructive type of emphysema usually found in young infants, often in the first few days of life. It is considered to be caused by a check-valve obstruction of the involved bronchus. Abnormality of the bronchial cartilage is found in a third of the patients; redundant bronchial mucosa, mucous plugs, and extrabronchial pressure by anomalous vessels are other possibilities and, in some instances, no cause can be found. The condition appears to involve either upper lobe or the middle lobe; the lower lobes are rarely affected. The involved lobe is greatly overexpanded. Roentgen findings consist of marked radiolucency of the involved lobe, increase in its size resulting in displacement of the mediastinum to the opposite side, depression of the diaphragm, and compression of the remaining lung. If bronchial aspiration does not relieve the obstruction, emergency surgery with removal of the overexpanded lobe may be necessary.

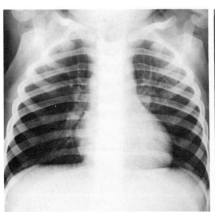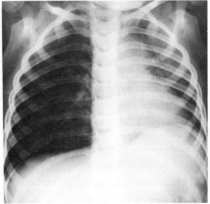

Fig. 30-4. Obstructive emphysema caused by a peanut in the right main bronchus. *Left,* Roentgenogram in complete inspiration shows only slight increase in radiability of the right lung. *Right,* Roentgenogram in expiration. The mediastinum has moved to the left and the left diaphragm has moved upward normally. The right diaphragm has remained in a position comparable to that noted on the inspiratory film and the difference in the amount of air in the lungs is now readily apparent.

UNILATERAL HYPERLUCENT LUNG

This syndrome (Swyer-James syndrome) is characterized by unilateral emphysema, hypoplasia of the pulmonary artery, and a widespread peculiar form of bronchiectasis confined to the involved lung or lobe. The roentgen findings consist of unilateral radiolucency of the lung or a lobe with no increase in volume of the lung, and failure of the involved lung to expand and contract normally on respiration. Excursion of the diaphragm and thoracic wall are limited and the mediastinum shifts away from the affected side on expiration and toward it on inspiration. The small size of the pulmonary artery and its branches on the affected side is readily visible on plain films. Bronchography shows no evidence of obstruction of major bronchi. There is a strikingly constant type of bronchiectasis consisting of moderate bronchial dilatation in an irregular beaded pattern accompanied by absence of alveolar filling. The bronchogram is of particular value in differentiating this condition from other causes of radiolucent lung. The cause is not established, but obstruction of small peripheral bronchi is thought to be most likely a result of infection. Obliterative bronchiolitis is produced which causes distal airspace distention. Perfusion of the involved lobe or lung is then decreased, resulting in the vascular findings noted above. Some authors believe that this radiographic syndrome may be the result of a number of conditions.

BULLOUS EMPHYSEMA

William Snow Miller defines a bulla as a localized vesicular emphysema within the lung substance, which may project above the surface but leaves the pleura intact. A bleb is an interstitial emphysema within the pleura producing a thin-walled prominence on the surface of the lung. When bullae constitute the major feature of the disease, the lesion is termed "bullous emphysema." The bullae vary in size from 1 or 2 cm to the size of a lobe or even larger. A single lesion may become so large that differentiation between it and pneumothorax is difficult and sometimes impossible. The cause is often obscure but most investigators believe that this disease is acquired and usually results from some lesion that produces obstruction.

The obstruction may be peripheral in type, such as that produced by any disease in which bronchiolitis is a factor. This may range from acute infections to the inhalation of various irritating gases. The causative factor usually recedes and the bullous emphysema remains as the only evidence of it. Roentgen findings are characteristic. Large, radiolucent, air-filled sacs appear at the periphery, either predominantly at the apices or at the bases. The disease may be predominantly unilateral but is usually present on both sides. When one lobe or portion of it is involved, the lobe or segment may be inflated to the point that severe respiratory embarrassment is produced by compression of the remaining relatively normal lung. In these instances surgical removal of an affected lobe is sometimes indicated. Bronchography is necessary to define the position of the bronchi and thus indicate the amount of compression and the lobe or segments that are compressed (Fig. 30-3). A study of the vascularity of the lungs also permits definition of the disease, as well as outlining distortion resulting from bullae. Tomography has been used for several years in the study of the pulmonary vessels in emphysema. The bullae are readily identified and areas of relative avascularity indicating diffuse emphysema are also clearly outlined. Angiography can also be used to study the pulmonary vascularity in this disease preliminary to surgery. Films taken at intervals usually show progression of the disease and the term "vanishing lung" is used when it is severe and progressive.

NONOBSTRUCTIVE EMPHYSEMA

COMPENSATORY EMPHYSEMA

This is physiologic alteration of a lung or portion of it in response to loss of lung tissue elsewhere. There are many causes since there are many pulmonary lesions that lead to a decrease in size of the involved areas. Whenever atelectasis occurs there is compensatory emphysema in the adjacent lung. The same is true following removal of lung tissue surgically.

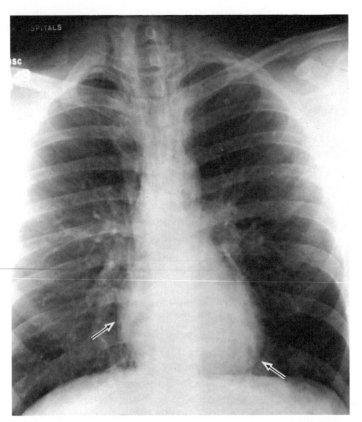

Fig. 30-5. Mediastinal and interstitial emphysema. **Arrows** indicate streaks of gas along the cardiac borders. There is also a considerable amount of streaky lucency in the superior mediastinum and in the low neck representing emphysema in these areas. These findings occurred during an acute asthmatic attack.

As in other forms of emphysema the affected area is more radiolucent than the uninvolved lung. This sign is important in detecting lobar atelectasis in patients where the atelectatic lobe has diminished so that it is difficult to define as an area of density. When pneumonectomy is done the normal lung undergoes compensatory emphysema and there is often a shift of mediastinal structures and a herniation of the lung into the opposite hemithorax that may be extreme (see Fig. 25-15). Focal compensatory emphysema occurs in relation to focal atelectasis and serves to accentuate the density produced by the small atelectatic area. There is considerable variation in the amount of compensatory emphysema in patients with lobar atelectasis, depending upon the chronicity of

the disease producing it and the mobility of the diaphragm and mediastinum.

SENILE EMPHYSEMA

This is a nonobstructive type of emphysema secondary to the degenerative changes in the dorsal spine that lead to kyphosis. It also causes an increase in the angulation between the body and manubrium of the sternum. The vertical diameter of the chest is often decreased but the increase in the anteroposterior diameter is greater, resulting in an increase in thoracic volume. This results in distention of the lungs that is usually uniform. Atrophy of the alveolar septa reduces the amount of pulmonary tissue and adds to the increased radiability of the lungs. The diaphragm is usually normally rounded and diaphragmatic motion is not impaired to any great extent. In addition to the alterations in the thorax, the roentgen finding of increased radiability of the lungs is present along with a relative prominence of vascular and interstitial markings. Roentgen diagnosis is sometimes difficult but emphysema should be suspected when the above findings are present.

MEDIASTINAL EMPHYSEMA

Pulmonary interstitial emphysema leads to mediastinal emphysema (pneumomediastinum). There are three other ways in which air may reach the mediastinum but they are much less common than the above: (1) along the fascial planes of the neck; (2) as a result of perforations of the trachea, esophagus, or main bronchus; and (3) by dissection along the retroperitoneal spaces. Pulmonary interstitial emphysema usually results from an increase in intra-alveolar pressure that is often acute and can be produced by anything that results in overinflation of the lungs. In the newborn, artificial respiration is apparently a frequent cause. When the rupture of an alveolus occurs adjacent to a vessel, air dissects along vascular

channels to the mediastinum. From there it may extend into the soft tissues of the neck or into the retroperitoneal space, or may rupture into the pleural space, producing pneumothorax. The air in the mediastinum causes increased pressure that in turn may produce venous and tracheal obstruction, leading to severe cyanosis and dyspnea; this is particularly true in the newborn. The roentgen diagnosis is usually not difficult but roentgenograms in both frontal and lateral projections are necessary. In the frontal view, streaks of radiolucency representing air are noted outlining the pericardium and extending up into the neck (Fig. 30-5). In the lateral view the air collects retrosternally and extends in streaks downward and anterior to the heart. Very small amounts are difficult to visualize, whereas a large pneumomediastinum is easily identified in either frontal or lateral projections. Both views should be obtained when it is suspected, however.

In the newborn, air may dissect from the mediastinum into the extrapleural space between the parietal pleura and diaphragm. The resultant accumulation may simulate pneumoperitoneum because the air is confined to the space over the diaphragm. However, the pleural line above it is not as thick as the normal diaphragm, and the air remains in the same place on supine, decubitus, and upright projections.

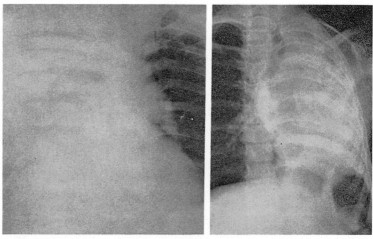

Fig. 30-6. *Left,* Postoperative atelectasis of the right lung. There is enough air remaining to produce a slight amount of radiolucency so that the diaphragm is visible and is noted to be elevated. There is also moderate shift of the heart and trachea to the right. *Right,* Atelectasis of the left lung. The lung is almost completely airless. The diaphragm is elevated and there is marked shift of mediastinal structures to the left with herniation of the right lung across the midline.

INTERSTITIAL EMPHYSEMA OF THORACIC WALLS

Thoracic interstitial emphysema is most commonly caused by thoracotomy but may also result from trauma and other causes. The amount varies considerably and when small, the gas is limited to the side of surgery or trauma. As the amount of gas increases it extends downward into the soft tissues of the abdomen and upward into the neck, and from there into the mediastinum, producing pneumomediastinum. Occasionally the amount of emphysema may be so great that tracheostomy is necessary to relieve respiratory embarrassment. Roentgen findings are similar to those in mediastinal emphysema secondary to pulmonary interstitial emphysema but in addition there is gas in the soft tissues of the neck and thoracic wall, producing linear streaks of radiolucency. There is also evidence of thoracotomy or of trauma, which usually is sufficient to indicate the cause.

ATELECTASIS

GENERAL CONSIDERATIONS

Atelectasis is a state of incomplete expansion of a lung or any portion of it. There is a decrease or absence of air in the alveoli of the involved region. Atelectasis is always a secondary lesion and is therefore a sign of disease rather than a disease in itself. The causes of atelectasis can be grouped into four general categories:

1. Bronchial obstruction. This may be intrinsic, owing to tumor, foreign body, inflammatory disease, heavy secretions, etc. Extrinsic pressure by tumor and enlarged nodes or constriction secondary to inflammatory disease may also cause it.

2. Extrapulmonary pressure. This can have a variety of causes, including pneumothorax, pleural fluid, diaphragmatic elevation regardless of cause, herniation of abdominal viscera into the thorax, and large intrathoracic tumors.

3. Paralysis or paresis resulting in inability completely to expand a lung, such as is found in poliomyelitis and other neurologic disorders. In addition to the weakness of respiratory muscles per se there is inability to raise the bronchial secretions and this may add the factor of obstruction in these patients.

4. Restriction of motion as a result of pleural disease or injury. Examples of this are chronic constrictive pleuritis, which causes decrease in volume of one hemithorax or a part thereof, so that normal expansion cannot occur. Acute conditions such as pleural infections and thoracic and upper abdominal trauma may also restrict motion and therefore produce some degree of atelectasis. In these patients there is also a factor of inability to handle secretions so that an additional obstructive element may be present.

The fundamental alteration in the thorax produced by atelectasis is a decrease in volume of the lobe, segment, or lung involved. This in turn gives the classic roentgen signs of elevation of the diaphragm, shift of mediastinum to the side of involvement, and narrowing of rib interspaces. Any of these signs may predominate in a given instance, depending on mediastinal and diaphragmatic fixation. In some patients the remaining lung on the involved side undergoes compensatory emphysema so there is no actual change in volume of the hemithorax and none of the above signs are then present. The relative airlessness of the affected portion of lung results in an area of increased density. The classic ground-glass appearance is due to the density produced by airless lung plus some air in a lobe or segment anterior or posterior to it. This appearance is noted most commonly in atelectasis of the left upper lobe. The density is uniform but has a grainy character that has been likened to the appearance of ground glass. It is usually dense medially and fades off to a lesser density laterally. When atelectasis involves the entire lung, the density is complete and homogeneous. Bronchi as well as lung become airless in atelectasis caused by obstruction, so there is usually absence of the "air bronchogram." Associated with mediastinal shift there is often herniation of the opposite lung across the midline into the involved hermithorax and in chronic long-standing atelectasis this may become extensive. When the atelectasis is on the right side the height of the diaphragm is often not ascertained. There is usually enough gas in the stomach or colon to outline the left hemidiaphragm, however. The cause of the atelectasis may be visible on the film and add to the density (Fig. 30-6).

LOBAR ATELECTASIS

LOWER LOBE ATELECTASIS

Lower lobe atelectasis is easily overlooked, particularly on the left side where the lobe may be hidden by the heart. When there are no pleural adhesions present, the involved lobe moves medially to form ultimately a rather narrow triangle with the apex at the level of the hilum and the base at the diaphragm. In the lateral projection the earliest sign of decrease in volume of a lower lobe is downward and posterior displacement of the major interlobar fissure. Later, as the amount of atelectasis increases, the density of the atelectatic lobe may obliterate the shadow of the posterior aspect of the diaphragm on the affected side. The signs of mediastinal shift, diaphragmatic elevation, and decrease in size of the bony thorax may be present to varying degrees or may be absent. If they are absent, there is usually enough compensatory emphysema of the upper lobe on the left or of the upper and middle lobes on the right to alert the observer

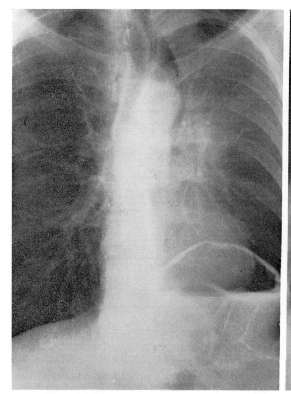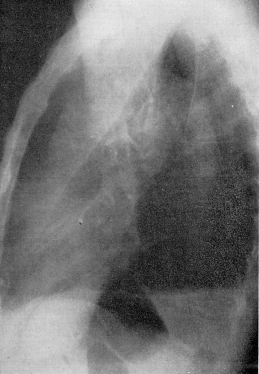

Fig. 30-7. Atelectasis of left upper lobe. There is elevation of the left hemidiaphragm, slight shift of mediastinal structures to the left, and a ground-glass density in the left upper central lung field. In the lateral (*right*) view the dense upper lobe stands out in contrast to the overexpanded lower lobe. The fissure is displaced anteriorly.

to the possibility of lobar collapse. When the roentgenogram is of sufficient penetration, the triangular shadow of the collapsed left lower lobe is usually outlined behind the heart on the frontal projection.

RIGHT MIDDLE LOBE ATELECTASIS

Right middle lobe atelectasis occurs frequently; this may be complete or incomplete. It is often caused by inflammatory disease, resulting in enlarged nodes that compress the bronchus to this lobe. The obstruction may then result in inflammatory disease within the lobe. This produces a somewhat more mottled and irregular appearance than is present in simple lobar atelectasis. When this lobe becomes atelectatic, the secondary interlobar fissure moves downward and the primary fissure can be outlined in contrast to the dense lung above it. This lobe moves upward and inward so that a triangular shadow appears just above the diaphragm. Its base is at the mediastinum and the apex points to the lateral chest wall. As atelectasis becomes complete, the lobe may shrink to a very small size and may be difficult to visualize clearly. The density caused by the atelectatic lobe blurs the right cardiac margin. When this blurring is noted the lateral view is confirmatory. In this view varying degrees of collapse are readily outlined. The appearance is that of a dense triangle, the apex of which is at or near the hilum and the base points downward and anteriorly. The outer borders of this dense triangle may be slightly concave.

UPPER LOBE ATELECTASIS

In upper lobe atelectasis the roentgen appearance depends on the presence or absence of adhesions between the visceral and parietal pleurae. When adhesions are present they hold all or part of the lobe in its normal position; when there are no adhesions the lobe tends to shrink uniformly and move toward the hilum. In right upper lobe atelectasis the first sign is elevation of the interlobar fissure. If there are lateral adhesions the inferior aspect of the lobe

becomes concave, elevating the fissure in its medial aspect, as well as producing slight increase in density of the lobe. As the amount of collapse progresses this concavity increases and the lobe shrinks to occupy the apex and upper mediastinum. Partial adherence of the lobe in one area or another may alter this general contour so that a considerable variety of form is possible. In the lateral view the major fissure tends to move anteriorly with increasing atelectasis and the upward displacement of the secondary fissure can also be outlined in this projection. The middle lobe moves upward anteriorly. The lower lobe moves upward posteriorly. Its superior segment may actually occupy the apex and rotate forward to lie in a caplike manner over the collapsed upper lobe. This is often readily outlined in the lateral projection and can be predicted by the appearance of normally aerated or hyperaerated lung at the apex above the more dense atelectatic upper lobe in the frontal projection. The signs of mediastinal and tracheal displacement toward the involved side, elevation of the right diaphragm, and decrease in size of the hemithorax, resulting in narrowing of the intercostal spaces may also occur in varying degrees; but compensatory emphysema of the middle and lower lobes may be sufficient so that none of the other signs will be present. Mediastinal displacement is usually a prominent feature when there are extensive adhesions holding the upper lobe to the lateral parietal pleura. The hilum may also be elevated and retracted to the right in such cases. When atelectasis is relatively complete and there are no adhesions, the shadow of the upper lobe tends to move toward the hilum and upper mediastinum. It may then resemble a slight mediastinal widening and occasionally may become so small that it is difficult to recognize.

Atelectasis of the left upper lobe is somewhat similar to that of the right upper lobe in that the lobe moves medially and anteriorly but early change is more difficult to recognize in the frontal projection because there is no secondary interlobar fissure. The ground-glass density is helpful if there is enough atelectasis to produce it. In the lateral view the major fissure tends to move forward and the density produced by the collapse is noted anteriorly with the lingula occupying a position similar to that of the middle lobe on the right. The density of the partially collapsed lobe tends to be narrower inferiorly owing to the smaller volume occupied by the lingula and to extend upward and toward   the periphery (Fig. 30-7). Pleural adhesions produce similar shift of the mediastinum to that noted in right upper lobe disease except that it is in the opposite direction. When atelectasis occurs in patients with chronic pulmonary inflammatory disease such as tuberculosis, there is often a considerable amount of associated pleural disease and contracting fibrosis of the lung. The lobe or segment involved is then difficult to evaluate on routine projections. In these instances bronchography is often necessary to study segmental anatomy.

SEGMENTAL ATELECTASIS

It is often possible to ascertain with a fair degree of accuracy the segment involved by segmental collapse, since the area of density produced by the atelectasis occupies the general area usually occupied by that segment in the absence of severely distorting associated pulmonary disease. By using frontal, lateral, and oblique projections as necessary, the site of the density can be clearly established and its relation to the interlobar fissures ascertained. The fissure tends to bow toward the site of the atelectasis; for example, in anterior segmental atelectasis of the right upper lobe the secondary interlobar fissure elevates centrally to indicate that the volume of this lobe has decreased and in the lateral view the density will lie anteriorly. The same rules apply for lower lobe segments but the basal segments are more difficult to identify accurately (Fig. 30-8).

FOCAL ATELECTASIS (PLATELIKE OR LOBULAR ATELECTASIS)

When there is obstruction of a small subsegmental bronchus a small area of atelectasis may result. This produces a thin horizontal or "platelike" line that is most often seen in the

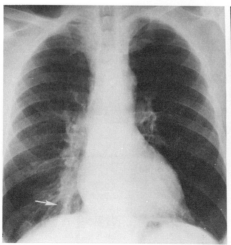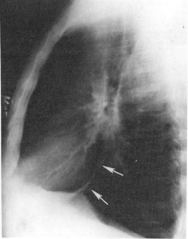

Fig. 30-8. Segmental atelectasis. There is partial atelectasis of the anterior segment of the right lower lobe. This produces irregular, poorly defined density at the right medial base noted in the frontal projection (**arrow**). In the lateral view the density is noted to be immediately posterior to the secondary interlobar fissure, which is bowed backward (**arrows**). Bronchogram revealed obstruction of the anterior basal segmental bronchus.

basal lung fields, where it occurs frequently. These small areas of atelectasis have been referred to as platelike or lobular atelectasis. They vary in size and cannot be distinguished from small areas of fibrosis in some instances. Films taken at frequent intervals will show disappearance or change in position of the linear areas of density and when this occurs, the diagnosis of focal atelectasis is confirmed. The amount of involved lung is small so that the finding is usually of no clinical significance. When it is observed postoperatively, however, it is an indication that aeration is incomplete and that there probably is an accumulation of secretions causing obstruction of some of the basal subsegmental bronchi. Restriction of diaphragmatic movement and elevation of the diaphragm are additional factors in production of this type of atelectasis (Fig. 30-9).

It is fundamental to remember that atelectasis causes an area of increased density be-cause of airlessness or relative airlessness of the involved segment, lobe, or lung and that the resultant decrease in volume must be compensated by a decrease in total volume of the involved hemithorax or by an increase in volume of the uninvolved lobe or segments.

HYALINE MEMBRANE DISEASE OF THE NEWBORN

This is a disease of newborn infants characterized by the presence of membranes lining the alveoli and sometimes the alveolar ducts, often leading to death by asphyxiation in the first 48 to 72 hours of life. In 90 per cent or more of cases it occurs either in premature infants, in infants delivered by cesarean section, or in offspring of diabetic mothers. The process is found in infants who breathe after birth, not in the stillborn. Respirations may be normal at or shortly following birth but within a few hours dyspnea and cy-

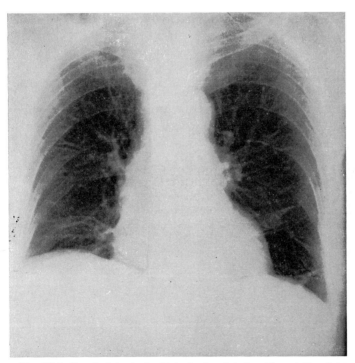

Fig. 30-9. Focal atelectasis. Note horizontal densities at the right base and a somewhat larger area of density at the extreme left lateral base. These were noted to disappear in the roentgenogram obtained a week later. At times linear fibrosis may occur in the lower lung field and simulate focal atelectasis.

anosis appear. In this disease a chest roentgenogram taken very shortly after birth may be normal, but abnormalities appear within a few hours. Whatever the underlying mechanism, the disease is the result of loss of surfactant and the inability to dispose of fibrin within the alveolar ducts and alveoli. Histopathologic findings consist of the presence of a hyaline material lining the alveoli and sometimes the alveolar ducts. This causes atelectasis of alveoli, which is accompanied by emphysema of the alveolar ducts and terminal bronchioles. Therefore the volume of the lung is not necessarily decreased, even though there is atelectasis.

Roentgen Findings

Four stages in the evolution of the disease have been described and identified radiographically. The first recognizable abnormality is an air-bronchogram pattern greater than normal. Next there is a fine miliary granularity associated with a slight increase in the reticular pattern of the lung fields. This may be so minor as to be very difficult to ascertain. The air bronchogram stands out more clearly however. The third stage is a gradual progression resulting in a confluent opacification or an unequivocal dense, reticular pattern. Infants who recover show gradual clearing which is often irregular over a period of 3 to 10 days. The fourth stage is one of confluent density that may vary in extent. It is usually bilateral but it is not unusual to note some asymmetry. The roentgen pattern does not follow the described stages in each instance. The most characteristic appearance is that of a granular pattern of marked increase in density, corresponding to stage three, above, with associated demonstrable bronchial air shadows that are sharply outlined and extend peripherally well out into the lung fields (Fig. 30-10).

In other neonatal respiratory distress syndromes caused by pulmonary disease there are usually pulmonary densities. However they tend to be coarse and irregular, often bilateral but not necessarily symmetric. This pattern is usually associated with bronchopneumonia or aspiration pneumonitis.

TRANSIENT RESPIRATORY DISTRESS (WET-LUNG DISEASE) OF THE NEWBORN

The roentgen findings in another neonatal distress syndrome, transient respiratory distress

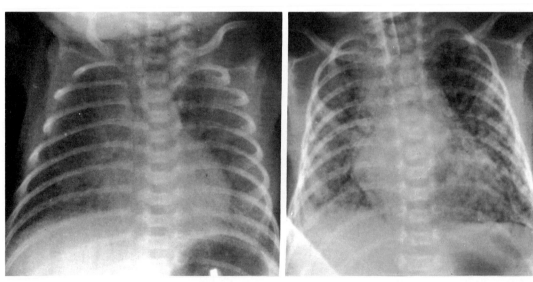

Fig. 30-10. Hyaline membrane disease. *Left,* Premature infant at 2 days of age shows a rather diffuse granular and peripheral reticular density with streaks of air representing an air bronchogram noted particularly well at the bases. *Right,* Three days later. On the fifth day of age there is an endotracheal tube in place and there is now a great deal of alveolar density interspersed with streaks of gas representing interstitial emphysema which is also noted above the dome of the left diaphragm and along the right cardiac margin. The patient did not survive.

of the newborn (TRDN), has been described by Swischuk.[71] This occurs in infants delivered of diabetic mothers, prematurity, breech deliveries, and cesarean deliveries. The distress (tachypnea) is noted early in the neonatal period and clears in 1 to 4 days. Pathogenesis appears to be incomplete or delayed clearing of alveolar fluid after birth. As a result the lungs are "wet." This is manifested radiographically by a pattern resembling alveolar edema with an air bronchogram, or in less severe cases interstitial edema, often with what appear to be Kerley's A lines and small amounts of pleural fluid. Minimal to moderate overaeration is common. At times, the roentgen findings may be similar to those of hyaline membrane disease, but in wet-lung disease there is progressive and rapid improvement (Fig. 30-11).

WILSON-MIKITY SYNDROME

This is another disease which causes the respiratory distress syndrome in the premature infant. The cause remains obscure. The roentgen features are quite distinct. There is a rather coarse reticular pattern interspersed with irregularly rounded, cystlike areas of lucency. The lungs are overdistended (Fig. 30-12). The disease tends to be chronic. Some of the babies recover over a period of months, others die of right-sided heart failure.

PNEUMOTHORAX

The presence of air or gas in the pleural cavity is termed "pneumothorax." Under normal conditions the pressure in the pleural space is less than atmospheric pressure. When this space communicates with the atmosphere either through a defect in the parietal pleura and chest wall or through a defect in the visceral pleura, air enters the pleural space. The amount of air that enters depends upon a variety of factors, including the elasticity of the lung, the presence or absence of pleural adhesions, and the type of defect in the pleura.

SPONTANEOUS PNEUMOTHORAX

This term is usually reserved for pneumothorax that occurs in an otherwise healthy individual. The air enters the pleural cavity through an opening in the visceral pleura. In many instances the cause is obscure and the site of the defect not accurately localized. In some of these, pulmonary interstitial emphysema is probably the cause. In others, subpleural blebs are visible and it is presumed that rupture of one of these may introduce the pneumothorax. Once the pneumothorax is established, the course depends upon the defect in the pleura. If it closes promptly, the air in the

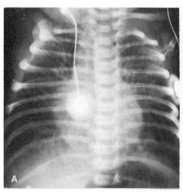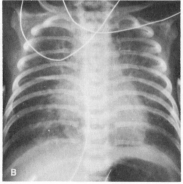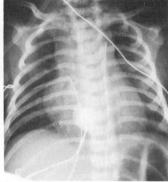

Fig. 30-11. Newborn infant with transient respiratory distress. *A*, Film taken shortly after birth shows some central alveolar density with linear interstitial densities more peripherally. *B*, One and a half hours later there has been some improvement peripherally but there is a persistent perihilar and central hazy density. *C*, Five hours later; the lungs are now clear.

pleural space is absorbed in a few days and the pneumothorax disappears. If the defect remains open in a manner that allows air to enter and leave the pleural space, the size of the pneumothorax tends to remain constant provided no complications such as infection supervene (Fig. 30-13).

TENSION PNEUMOTHORAX

Occasionally there is a check-valve or one-way-valve type of defect through which air can enter the pleural space but cannot leave it. This results in a much more serious condition known as tension pneumothorax. When this occurs there is rapid or slow accumulation of air in the pleural space, resulting in complete collapse of the lung provided there are no adhesions to hold it out. This is followed by shift of mediastinal structures away from the side of the pneumothorax as well as increase in size of the involved hemithorax and depression of the diaphragm on the side of the lesion (Fig. 30-14). This condition is particularly hazard-

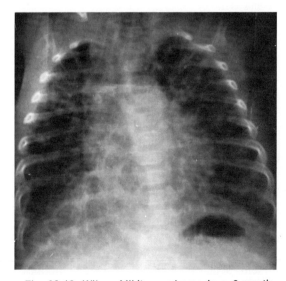

Fig. 30-12. Wilson-Mikity syndrome in a 2-month-old child shows typical coarse reticular pattern with rounded cystlike areas of radiolucency which are most clearly defined in the right lung base below the dome of the diaphragm.

ous in the newborn and, if not treated promptly, can cause death.

TRAUMATIC PNEUMOTHORAX

Air may enter the pleural space through the parietal pleura as the result of penetrating wounds of the thorax. It may also be secondary to renal surgery, sympathectomy, and other upper abdominal surgical procedures or it may be introduced through a needle at the time of thoracentesis. Trauma to the lungs or bronchi may also result in defects in the visceral pleura, causing pneumothorax. When associated with rib fractures it is often caused by a rent in the pleura produced by sharp bony spicules. There is injury to the visceral and parietal pleurae in these instances but the air usually enters through the defect in the visceral pleura. The pneumothorax commonly seen in the newborn is very likely traumatic in origin in most instances. Pneumothorax of this type may also occur as a complication in diagnostic or therapeutic pneumoperitoneum and occasionally it follows bronchoscopy. In addition to the findings of pneumothorax, the cause may be apparent on the chest roentgenogram.

BRONCHOPLEURAL FISTULA

Regardless of the cause, bronchopleural fistula results in pneumothorax that usually persists for a long period of time. Tuberculosis is a common cause and the fistula can be produced by rupture of a subpleural lesion into the pleural space or by rupture of a tuberculous empyema through the pleura into the lung with subsequent formation of a fistula. Other inflammatory diseases of the lung, both acute and chronic, may also cause bronchopleural fistula with resultant pneumothorax. Other infectious diseases of the pleura producing empyema may also result in bronchopleural fistula with rupture of the empyema through the visceral pleura leading to bronchial communication.

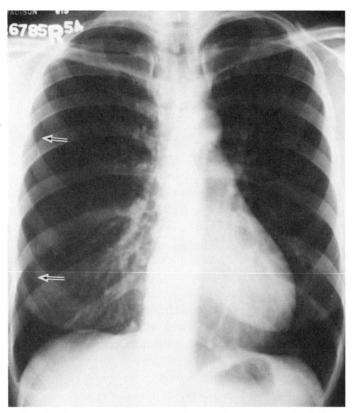

Fig. 30-13. Spontaneous pneumothorax. **Arrows** indicate the visceral pleural line of the upper and lower lobes. There is an air-fluid level in the posterior gutter which is frequently present and is a helpful sign when the pneumothorax is small.

INDUCED (ARTIFICIAL) PNEUMOTHORAX

This is usually a diagnostic procedure. In therapeutic pneumothorax the differential collapse of the tuberculous lung in contrast to the relatively good expansion of the normal lung was the basis for the use of this method of collapse therapy. This has been supplanted by antituberculous drugs. Diagnostic pneumothorax is performed usually to differentiate intrapulmonary masses from those arising from the ribs, mediastinum, or diaphragm.

ROENTGEN CONSIDERATIONS

The presence of a large pneumothorax is identified readily on roentgen examination and in many instances, where it is secondary to disease or trauma, the cause can be established. The air in the pleural space is more radiolucent than the lung adjacent to it, particularly if the lung is decreased in volume, compressed, or is involved by disease that increases its density. When pleural adhesions are present, small amounts of loculated pneumothorax may be very difficult to visualize unless lateral or oblique projections are taken. Such spaces often contain a small amount of fluid and the presence of a horizontal fluid level indicates that there is gas as well as fluid present. When the amount of pneumothorax is very small and is apical in position, its presence is indicated by visualization of a thin, smooth, curved, linear density representing the visceral pleura. Above this line no pulmonary

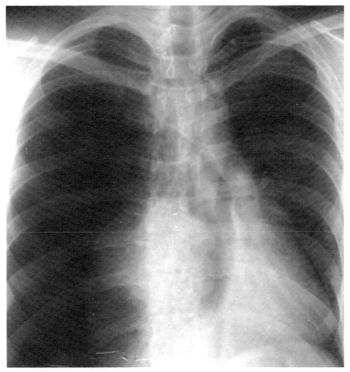

Fig. 30-14. Tension pneumothorax. Mediastinal structures are shifted to the left and the right lung is collapsed and displaced to the left with herniation across the midline. Note the absence of lung markings on the right.

markings are visible. Occasionally the pneumothorax is so small that its presence at the apex can only be suspected on the usual roentgenogram taken in deep inspiration. In these patients a roentgenogram made during maximum expiration will aid in confirming the diagnosis, since the lung then is relatively more dense than the pneumothorax. The lung decreases in volume during expiration but the pneumothorax space does not change. There is, therefore, relatively more pneumothorax in relation to lung in expiration than in inspiration. In tension pneumothorax the shift of mediastinal structures, compression of the lung and depression of the diaphragm are readily visualized.

In summary, the diagnosis of pneumothorax is usually not difficult on roentgen examination of the chest. When it is small in amount a film in expiration is often of value and occasionally when peripheral loculated pneumothorax is present, lateral and oblique views are needed to visualize it distinctly. In addition to the value of roentgenograms in making the diagnosis, progress films are used to follow its course.

DIFFERENTIAL DIAGNOSIS

Occasionally a peripheral emphysematous bleb or bulla may simulate a localized pneumothorax but in most instances the rounded or geometric form of its inner wall indicates the nature of the lesion and differentiates it from pneumothorax. When the diagnosis is particularly difficult, progress films are often of assistance since pneumothorax usually changes from day to day in contrast to emphysema, which is stable and changes little over long periods of time. Occasionally these emphysematous bullae become very large (tension bullae) and may displace the lung and mediastinum in a manner simulating displacement by tension pneumothorax. In these instances differentiation cannot be made with certainty on roentgen examination alone. In patients with far-advanced tuberculosis large peripheral cavitation, often involving the greater part of an upper lobe (usually the left), may be difficult to distinguish from pneumothorax caused by bronchopleural fistula. If serial roentgenograms are available, the progress of the lesion will indicate its nature in most instances but there are some patients in whom the nature of the lesion remains uncertain and even at autopsy or at surgery the disease may be so extensive that the visceral pleura cannot be identified. The same type of lesion may follow other pulmonary infections but is less common.

PULMONARY HEMOSIDEROSIS

In this condition macrophages filled with the iron-containing blood pigment, hemosiderin,

are deposited in the alveoli and in the interstitial tissues of the lung. The macrophages gather in clumps that become large enough to produce roentgenographically recognizable densities. This occurs in two diseases with different clinical and etiological patterns: (1) idiopathic pulmonary hemosiderosis; and (2) hemosiderosis associated with rheumatic valvular disease (mitral stenosis). The latter form is discussed on page 1020. A third form has been described in which the hemosiderosis is accompanied by glomerulonephritis. This is called Goodpasture's syndrome.

IDIOPATHIC PULMONARY HEMOSIDEROSIS

This disease is manifested by recurrent episodes of acute illness in which dyspnea, cyanosis, and weakness, along with cough, hemoptysis, and chest pain occur. The attack lasts a few days or weeks and subsides, only to recur. A second more

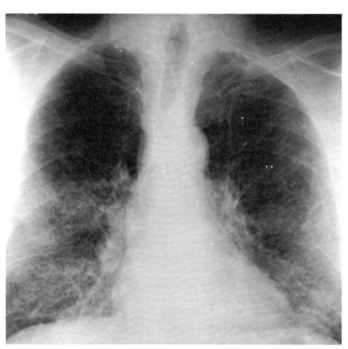

Fig. 30-15. Idiopathic pulmonary hemosiderosis. Forty-year-old male with long history of repeated hemoptysis. Note the extensive interstitial change which is linear in the upper lung fields and is associated with a reticulonodular pattern in the central and lower lung fields.

chronic form of the disease has also been described in which the acute exacerbations are minimal and the disease is chronic with ultimate formation of marked roentgen changes. The prognosis is generally poor, although the disease may progress very slowly in some instances. The disease is found more frequently in children than in adults. There is a reported slight preponderance of females in children with the disease; in adults the reverse is true, with a preponderance of males of nearly three to one.

The roentgen findings in the early acute phase are caused by multiple, small, alveolar hemorrhages, the cause for which is not clearly understood. These hemorrhages cause widespread patchy, pulmonary densities that clear gradually but tend to leave some interstitial change manifested by increase in the reticular pattern of interstitial markings. As hemorrhages are repeated, the acute mottled patchy densities again appear superimposed on the background of increased interstitial density. Eventually small granular opacities appear scattered throughout the lung fields (Fig. 30-15). The hila are usually prominent by the time this stage of the disease is reached because of deposition of blood pigment in the lymphatics in and around the hilum. The thickening is usually irregular and no clearly defined, rounded, node enlargement can be detected. The diagnosis is made by correlating the clinical history of repeated attacks with the chest roentgen changes described. This condition must be differentiated from miliary tuberculosis, widespread pulmonary sarcoidosis, and other conditions causing miliary densities in the lung fields. The rapid changes noted in the acute phase of the disease serve to differentiate it from miliary tuberculosis.

GOODPASTURE'S SYNDROME

This syndrome consists of a combination of pulmonary hemorrhage and necrotizing glomerulonephritis. In contrast to idiopathic pulmonary hemosiderosis, it occurs mainly in young adult males; we have observed this disease in young females, however. It is evidently an autoimmune disease which involves the kidneys as well as the lungs. An acute, necrotizing alveolitis causes repeated episodes of pulmonary hemorrhage. The roentgen findings are similar to those of idiopathic hemosiderosis. This syndrome should be suspected when evidence of glomerulonephritis is found in a young male with a history of recurrent pulmonary hemorrhage and roentgen signs of pulmonary hemosiderosis. The disease usually progresses rapidly and prognosis is poor.

PULMONARY CHANGES FOLLOWING HEMOPTYSIS

When hemoptysis occurs and blood is aspirated there are resultant roentgen changes. The roentgen findings indicating the presence of aspirated blood vary with the amount and distribution. The aspirated blood causes density that is comparable in degree with a patch of pneumonitis of similar size. The density is usually hazy and poorly defined and may be a single localized area or may consist of several mottled opacities. In areas where the opacity is not great a granular pattern may be seen that is somewhat more clearly defined than the more hazy density of inflammatory disease. The opacity from aspiration of blood clears within 2 or 3 days. The rapid clearing helps to differentiate it from inflammatory disease. Evidence of the disease causing the hemoptysis may or may not be present.

PULMONARY CHANGES IN ALLERGIC STATES

BRONCHIAL ASTHMA

This condition is very common, occurs at all ages, and is characterized by wheezing, prolongation of the expiratory phase of respiration, dyspnea, and cough. It tends to come on in attacks. Early in the course of the disease there are no roentgen findings in the chest between the acute episodes. During an acute asthmatic attack there is increased radiability of the lungs because of acute overdistention. Small areas of focal atelectasis often cause scattered patchy densities parallel to the bronchovascular markings. They are often widespread throughout both lung fields. The markings may also be thickened, particularly in the parahilar and central pulmonary zones. There is also depression of the diaphragm and

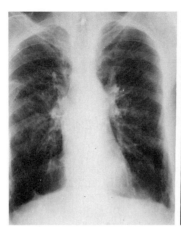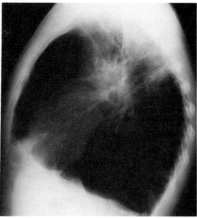

Fig. 30-16. Pulmonary changes in bronchial asthma in a 44-year-old male with long-standing asthma. Note the low flat diaphragm, deep anteroposterior diameter of the chest, and increase in interstitial markings throughout the lung fields. Hilar arteries are enlarged.

decreased diaphragmatic motion that can be detected on fluoroscopic examination. In some instances no permanent radiographic changes occur. These patients are subject to recurrent pulmonary infections leading to pulmonary fibrosis associated with the emphysema. The roentgen findings then consist of prominence of interstitial markings in a chest that is otherwise more radiolucent than normal. The anteroposterior diameter of the chest is increased, the diaphragm is low and flat, and the ribs are often more horizontal than normal (Fig. 30-16). The emphysema may become severe leading to formation of large emphysematous bullae and blebs peripherally. Mucous plug or impaction may occur in patients with asthma. The bronchial obstruction produced by the impaction may result in atelectasis or in an accumulation of secretions in the obstructed segment, and infection. Eventually, bronchiectasis may result. There appears to be some predilection for the upper lobes. Roentgen findings depend on the nature of the associated pulmonary disease and when segmental atelectasis or an apparent pneumonitis is found in an asthmatic, mucous plug or impaction should be suspected.

LÖFFLER'S SYNDROME (TRANSIENT PULMONARY INFILTRATION WITH EOSINOPHILIA)

This syndrome consists of fleeting pulmonary infiltrations associated with eosinophilia. It is usually found in allergic individuals and is believed to represent pulmonary reaction to a variety of allergens. The symptoms are usually mild and consist of cough, malaise, low-grade fever, dyspnea with occasional wheezing, mild chest pain, and metallic taste in the mouth. It is associated with an eosinophilia that ranges from 10 to 70 per cent. Leukocytosis is usually found also. The amount of pathologic material available is small since this is a benign condition, but the findings on patients who have died accidentally consist of eosinophilic pneumonia in which the involvement is interstitial as well as alveolar and there is also some associated pulmonary edema, probably secondary to hyperpermeability of capillaries.

Roentgen Findings

The infiltrations cause poorly defined densities that may be single or multiple, unilateral or bilateral. The volume of lung affected varies considerably and the individual areas of involvement are patchy in type and usually poorly outlined.

They resemble pneumonia from other causes but are unique in that rapid change is the rule. It is not unusual to observe clearing or partial clearing in one area and progression in another area of the same lung or of the opposite lung. At times the findings remain stable for several days. When such a changing infiltrate is observed and the patient is found to have eosinophilia the diagnosis of Löffler's syndrome can be made (Fig. 30-17). A minor amount of pleural reaction resulting in small amounts of pleural effusion may occur but its presence or absence is of no diagnostic significance. The administration of cortisone usually causes rapid clearing of the pulmonary infiltrates and a decrease in the circulating eosinophils.

PULMONARY INFILTRATES WITH EOSINOPHILIA (THE P.I.E. SYNDROME)

The P.I.E. syndrome[38] is similar to Löffler's except that the symptoms are prolonged and the course more malignant. Episodes of weakness, weight loss, fever, cough, dyspnea, and hemoptysis may occur. Roentgen findings consist of a variety of patterns of density, some resembling confluent pneumonia, others consist of coarse, strandlike densities which may be widespread. Changes in the pulmonary disease are common as in Löffler's syndrome. Eosinophils are found in the biopsy specimen which shows interstitial pneumonia of varying degrees of severity, sometimes associated with fibrosis. There is also an elevated eosinophil count in the circulating blood. The lesions do not respond to antibiotics, but clear dramatically on steroids.

NITROFURANTOIN SENSITIVITY

Nitrofurantoin (Furadantoin) has been used for urinary tract infections for nearly 18 years. Occasionally its administration may cause an acute reaction manifested by chills, fever, cough, dyspnea, malaise, and pleuritic pain. Eosinophilia may be present. There also appears to be a chronic form with few symptoms, but similar roentgen findings, which consist of thickening of interstitial markings in the parahilar areas and at the bases. When the drug is discontinued, clearing

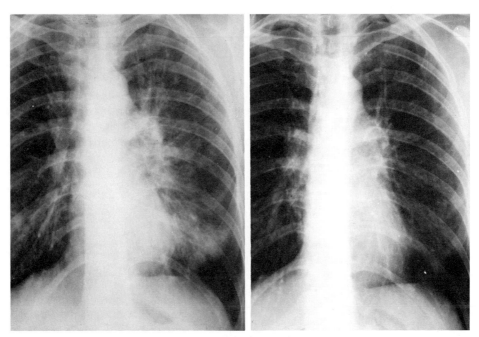

Fig. 30-17. Löffler's pneumonia. *Left,* Note the poorly defined scattered infiltrate in the left central and lower lung field. *Right,* The infiltrate has cleared completely in 15 days. The patient was allergic and had eosinophilia. Sputum also contained eosinophils.

is very rapid, suggesting that the pulmonary findings are caused by edema. It is generally agreed that the condition represents a hypersensitivity to nitrofurantoin.

SENSITIVITY TO OTHER DRUGS

A number of other drugs have been reported to cause pulmonary disease, presumably on the basis of hypersensitivity or some allergic phenomenon. Antibiotics such as Madribon (sulfadimethoxine), Prontosil (sulfachrysoindine) PAS (para-aminosalicyclic acid) and penicillin may cause an acute alveolar reaction similar to that found in nitrofurantoin sensitivity. Dilantin (Diphenylhydantoin) and Mesantoin (3-methyl 5, 5-phenyl-ethyl-hydantoin) cause hilar adenopathy and a combined alveolar and interstitial pulmonary pattern. (Fig. 30-18): Diuril (hydrochlorthiazide) and Methotrexate (peteroylglutamic acid) cause a similar pulmonary reaction without the adenopathy. Hexamethonium chloride, Inversine (mecamylamine), Myleran (busulfan) and Sansert (methysergide) may produce a chronic interstitial pulmonary pattern.

LYMPHOCYTIC INTERSTITIAL PNEUMONITIS (L.I.P.)

In 1966, Liebow and Carrington[39] described a condition manifested by disseminated pulmonary infiltrates in patients with a history of cough, dyspnea, fever, and weight loss for long periods of time (6 months to 5 years). Etiology is not clear but some type of hypersensitivity may contribute. Roentgen findings are a combination of diffuse increase of interstitial markings resulting in linear densities plus patchy nodular densities. This may be related to pseudolymphoma, which is a local, benign, lymphocytic infiltration of the lung characterized by the presence of true germinal centers in a mass of well-differentiated lymphocytes and other inflammatory cells. There is no roentgen similarity, since the pseudolymphoma presents as a large pulmonary mass which is often central. The margins are indistinct and an air bronchogram is usually present. The mass may resemble confluent pneumonia or parenchymal tumor. Biopsy is necessary to differentiate it from other lung masses.

THE "COLLAGEN" DISEASES

The collagen diseases consist of a heterogeneous group of conditions in which involvement of connective tissue, particularly the intercellular amorphous ground substance, is the common morphological feature. They appear to be related to hypersensitivity in some instances, but this is not the only cause since the tissue changes are known to be produced by a variety of dissimilar diseases. Polyarteritis (periarteritis) nodosa, rheumatic fever, rheumatoid arthritis, disseminated lupus erythematosus, and scleroderma are all members; Wegener's granulomatosis is related and is included by many in this group of conditions. These diseases are related and there is a considerable amount of overlapping in the clinical findings so that lesions that are usually predominant in one entity may be seen in another. Individual cases have been reported in which four or five varieties of involvement have been present.

POLYARTERITIS NODOSA (PERIARTERITIS)

In this disease the medium-sized arteries and their smaller branches are affected so that the lesions are often found throughout the body. Pulmonary involvement causes a variety of roentgen changes. Massive pulmonary edema may occur in patients who are acutely ill. Other pulmonary changes consist of scattered patchy densities, some of which are due to infarcts; these may excavate and cause small cavities. When present this cavitation is often multiple and it is characteristic that one cavity becomes smaller and closes while another is in the process of forming. Clearly defined or hazy nodules may appear. Some may resemble hematogenous metastases while others simulate inflammatory nodules and may raise the possibility of tuberculosis. At times the interstitial markings are increased. Basal congestion resulting in enlargement of vascular shadows and blurring of vessels is often noted and pleural effusion may occur. Enlargement of the cardiac silhouette is not uncommon. In some patients this is caused by pericardial effusion while in

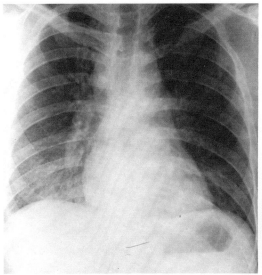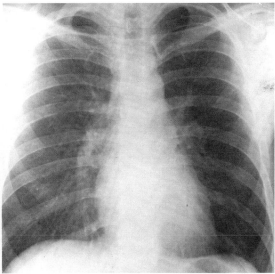

Fig. 30-18. Mesantoin sensitivity. *Left,* The patient complained of cough and fever. Note the paratracheal and hilar adenopathy as well as some basal pulmonary involvement. *Right,* Three weeks later after the drug had been discontinued. The chest now appears normal.

others there is dilatation of the heart. These pulmonary and pleural changes may undergo rapid clearing or may progress rapidly. There is nothing characteristic about the roentgen findings but in a chronically ill patient with involvement of other systems these pulmonary, pleural, and pericardial findings are suggestive of this collagen disease. The pulmonary roentgen changes usually respond rapidly and clear following institution of steroid therapy.

RHEUMATIC PNEUMONIA

Rheumatic fever is a collagen disease in which cardiac lesions are common and these may result in secondary pulmonary congestion and edema. The "pneumonia" seen in this disease is often caused by pulmonary edema and congestion and there is a considerable difference of opinion as to the incidence of actual pulmonary involvement in this collagen disease. The roentgen findings of rheumatic pneumonia simulate those of pulmonary edema and congestion and consist of hazy densities, usually in the parahilar areas and midlung fields. They may be confluent or patchy and are often associated with basal changes indicating pulmonary congestion. At times there does appear

to be involvement of lungs, so that a scattered pneumonitis in the absence of cardiac failure in a patient with rheumatic fever is most likely indicative of rheumatic pneumonia. Histopathologic study is often necessary to differentiate rheumatic pneumonia from pulmonary edema and congestion but the clinical findings, along with radiographic findings, may permit the presumptive diagnosis.

DISSEMINATED LUPUS ERYTHEMATOSUS

This disease is commonly found in young and middle-aged women. Pulmonary or pleural involvement of some type occurs in a high percentage of patients at some time in the course of the disease. The disease is chronic and usually fatal but may undergo repeated remissions and exacerbations. Pleural effusion is the most common finding. Pericardial effusion may also occur. The pulmonary parenchymal changes are varied as in polyarteritis and range from the soft, patchy density of pulmonary edema to strandlike accentuation of bronchovascular markings. Occasionally the lesions assume a nodular appearance. The pulmonary alterations tend to be basal in position (Fig. 30-19). When the pulmonary disease becomes chronic resulting in basal fibrosis, there is often elevation of the diaphragm and its motion is

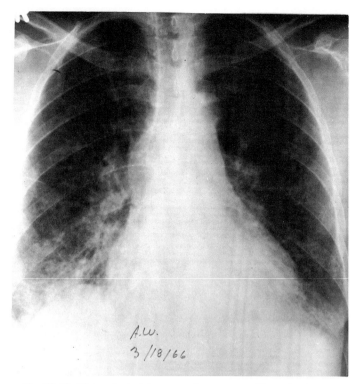

Fig. 30-19. Disseminated lupus erythematosus. Note the basal interstitial disease with a little pleural effusion on the right.

restricted. The combination of bilateral pleural effusion, pericardial effusion causing enlargement of the cardiac silhouette, and a changing bilateral pulmonary disease suggests systemic lupus erythematosus. Pulmonary changes are less frequent than pleural and cardiac involvement, but may be bizarre, with cavitation in nodules, formation of pneumatoceles, and rapid alteration. Subpleural infiltrates are common; they are probably infarcts.

SCLERODERMA

This disease is characterized by its cutaneous manifestations but the gastrointestinal tract is often involved and roentgen changes are frequently observed in the fingers. These are discussed in the sections dealing with the gastrointestinal tract and the soft tissues. Pulmonary manifestations occur in approximately 10 per cent of patients. As in the other collagen diseases a variety of lesions may be observed, but the findings tend to be more stable in this disease than in the others. The basic

lesion is fibrosis, which may take the form of accentuation of markings, usually basal at first, but with slow progression and ultimate involvement of the entire lung. There is often some scattered nodulation in the parahilar areas and in the bases as well. Pleural effusion may occur late in the disease but is not a prominent feature of the disease. In a few patients with long-standing disease, subpleural cysts have been described that are apparently caused by a disappearance of alveolar tissues. This results in small cystic spaces, surrounded by thick fibrous walls. The apices are spared in this manifestation of the disease (Fig. 30-20).

RHEUMATOID DISEASE OF THE LUNG

Rheumatoid arthritis is occasionally accompanied by pulmonary disease which is a part of the generalized involvement. Martel et al.[45] found that pulmonary lesions tend to occur in patients with high titers of rheumatoid factor and subcutaneous

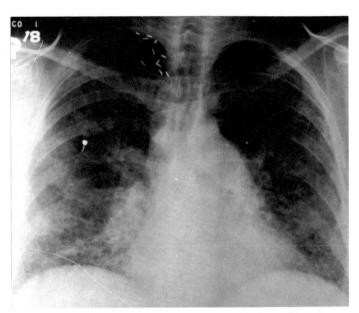

Fig. 30-20. Scleroderma. Note the extensive interstitial disease which is somewhat stringy superiorly and reticulonodular centrally with more basal involvement than there is elsewhere.

rheumatoid nodules. The most common findings in their group of 35 patients were chronic pneumonitis with interstitial fibrosis, pulmonary nodules, and pleural effusion. Pleural effusion (found in 13 patients) was minimal to moderate in amount and usually bilateral. Pulmonary nodules were found in 12 patients and confirmed histologically in six. Usually they were multiple (11 of 12), varied from a few millimeters to several centimeters in size, and were subpleural in position. Cavitation in nodules was observed in five patients. Chronic diffuse pneumonitis (noted in 21 patients) was the most common finding (Fig. 30-21). Distribution was parahilar and basal in some, and diffuse in others. In some, patchy areas resembling alveolar pneumonia were observed; in others the appearance was that of interstitial fibrosis. It is evident that there is no characteristic pattern of pulmonary involvement in rheumatoid lung disease.

WEGENER'S GRANULOMATOSIS

Midline lethal granuloma is a destructive process of unknown etiology, which some investigators believe is related to the collagen diseases. It is a fatal condition in which there is extensive de-

struction of bony structures of the nose and paranasal sinuses. When this condition is associated with generalized polyarteritis, the syndrome is known as Wegener's syndrome or necrotizing granulomatosis. The three main pathologic features are: (1) necrotizing granulomatous lesions of the upper respiratory tract, (2) necrotizing angiitis of arteries and veins, and (3) glomerulitis. The roentgen changes in the sinuses are those of soft-tissue density plus destruction of bone that cannot be differentiated from the destruction produced by malignant neoplasm. The granulomatous lesion of the lung which is characteristic of the disease may be solitary or multiple. Size varies from 1 to 8 cm in diameter; some lesions may cavitate. The cavity is usually small in relation to the size of the nodule, with an irregular inner wall, but the nodule may excavate completely leaving a thin wall, and then eventually may disappear. The outer margins of the nodules are indistinct and often have a "shaggy" appearance. When multiple, the nodules tend to be few in number, and may resemble pulmonary metastases. Other findings include areas of poorly defined consolidation resembling pneumonia. As in the other collagen diseases, there is nothing specific about the roentgen pulmonary changes. Pleural effusion may occur late in the disease.

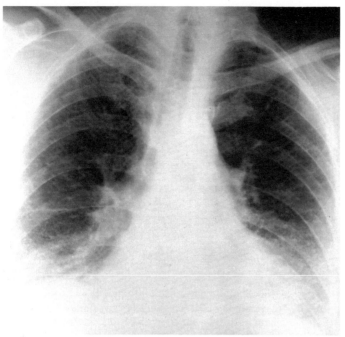

Fig. 30-21. Rheumatoid disease of the lung. There is diffuse basal change which is similar to that noted in scleroderma (Fig. 30-20).

DIFFUSE PULMONARY FIBROSIS OF UNKNOWN ETIOLOGY

Fibrosis of the lungs may result from a number of diseases. They include infections such as tuberculosis, the fungal diseases, bronchiectasis, the collagen diseases, the malignant pneumoconioses, and others. The cause can usually be ascertained in this group if clinical history, physical findings, laboratory findings and roentgen alterations are correlated. The roentgen manifestations of these diseases are discussed in the appropriate section. There is an intermediate group of patients in whom fibrosis may be localized or scattered and in whom there is no evidence of cause. In this group of patients there are some in whom histopathology reveals the cause, but in others it is a nonspecific fibrosis of obscure etiology. As more knowledge is gained regarding histopathology of the lung, however, it is likely that the number of patients placed in this category will decrease. The roentgen findings are those of an increasing thickening of interstitial lung markings which is often more prominent in the bases than elsewhere. This produces a fine reticular pattern that gradually becomes more coarse. If there is a considerable amount of associated emphysema, a honeycomb pattern may be observed. In other patients, a more linear pattern is produced which at times may be associated with a fine nodular or granular pattern. Secondary pulmonary hypertension may develop, resulting in a gradual increase in the size of the pulmonary artery and its hilar branches, as well as evidence of right ventricular enlargement. The roentgen changes develop over a period of years or many months. The etiology is never determined; even at autopsy the findings can only be described as nonspecific fibrosis (Fig. 30-22).

HAMMAN-RICH SYNDROME (DIFFUSE INTERSTITIAL PULMONARY FIBROSIS)

The disease originally described by Hamman and Rich is characterized by an insidious onset of

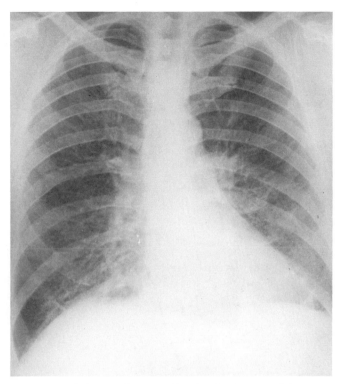

Fig. 30-22. Diffuse pulmonary fibrosis of unknown etiology was found on lung biopsy. Roentgen findings are those of general and uniform increase in interstitial markings. There was nothing in the history to indicate the cause of the widespread change.

general malaise, fever, occasional dry cough, chest pain, and dyspnea, which soon becomes severe. The patients usually die in 1 to 6 months of pulmonary insufficiency. The disease may also be subacute or chronic, with slow progression for a number of years. Respiratory insufficiency and right-sided heart failure occur and recurrent infections are common in the late stage of the disease. Microscopic examination shows marked fibroblastic proliferation in the alveolar walls often associated with edema and an infiltration of lymphocytes and plasma cells. The presence of eosinophils has been noted by several investigators. Later the fibroblastic proliferation results in extensive thickening of alveolar walls and interstitial tissues, causing severe respiratory dysfunction leading to death.

Roentgen Findings

Early in the disease there is slight increase in pulmonary markings and slight decrease in dia-phragmatic motion that can be noted fluoroscopically or on roentgenograms taken in inspiration and expiration. As the fibrosis progresses the interstitial markings become more prominent, resulting in thick linear shadows extending outward from the hila and a reticular pattern of increased density in the peripheral lung fields. The change is not necessarily symmetric but is usually bilateral. In far-advanced disease there is extensive strandlike thickening with considerable lucency surrounded by the thick strands resembling a coarse honeycomb or cystic pattern. The volume of the lung decreases progressively (Fig. 30-23). Because the roentgen findings are not characteristic, the diagnosis must be based on clinical manifestations with the history of rapidly progressing dyspnea plus failure to find any definite cause. Lung biopsy is necessary to make the diagnosis, particularly in patients with subacute or chronic disease in whom the clinical course is of no particular diagnostic value. Some investigators believe that this condition is based on sensitivity but exact etiology has

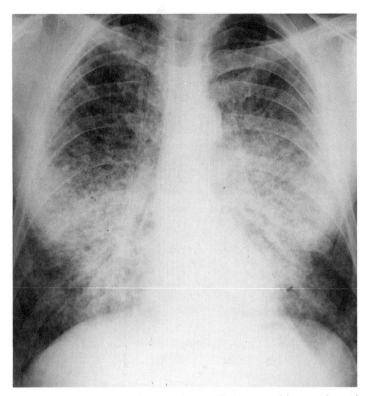

Fig. 30-23. Hamman-Rich syndrome. Pulmonary biopsy showed changes compatible with this syndrome. Roentgen changes are those that have been described in this condition and consist of marked accentuation of parenchymal markings with stringy and strandlike thickening in many areas, associated with peripheral emphysema.

not been proved. There is enough variation in the reported cases to suggest that there may be a variety of causes.

AMYLOIDOSIS

Amyloidosis is usually classified into the primary and secondary types. The secondary form of amyloidosis is found in patients with chronic inflammatory disease, such as chronic osteomyelitis, bronchiectasis and tuberculosis. Amyloid is deposited in the spleen, liver, and kidneys secondary to the chronic inflammatory disease and in conditions in which hyperglobulinemia is present, such as multiple myeloma. In the primary form of the disease no definite cause can be found and the amyloid is typically deposited in the heart, gastrointestinal tract, lungs, muscle, and skin. Primary amyloidosis is rare. The etiology

is unknown but it is probably a form of protein storage disease that is slowly progressive and is considered fatal. Amyloid is made up of a protein matrix bound by lesser protein and a sulfate bearing polysaccharide. Its chemistry is not fully understood. This material is deposited in the alveolar walls and around the interalveolar capillaries as well as in the walls of the smaller blood vessels in the lung when pulmonary involvement is present. The myocardium is affected in approximately 70 per cent of patients with the primary form of the disease. Deposits may also occur in bronchial and tracheal walls.

Roentgen Findings

The roentgen findings are of two general types. The first consists of diffuse fibrosis with radiating strands extending outward from the hilum into the central lung fields. The second results from local deposition of amyloid causing a mass density simulating primary lung tumor. In the generalized type there is often associated pleural effusion that may appear, regress, and then reappear. There is also deposition of amyloid in hilar and mediastinal nodes with a gradual increase in the hilar size and blurring of mediastinal borders. As the disease progresses, the radiating strands of fibrosis increase and in some instances fine granular or more coarse nodular lesions develop. Calcification and bone formation may be observed in the pulmonary lesions. The bone formation is peculiar and resembles spikelike pieces of broken glass. The roentgen progression is accompanied by increasing dyspnea. This generalized type of involvement must be distinguished from other chronic diseases that cause interstitial fibrosis. It may resemble sarcoidosis. The localized form of the disease consists of one or more homogeneous masses that may be somewhat lobulated and resemble primary lung tumor closely; the local form is usually found in elderly males. When amyloid disease is suspected a positive Congo red test, based on the affinity of amyloid for this dye, is considered diagnostic but a negative test is found in about 50 per cent of patients, since the chemistry of the protein is not constant.

HISTIOCYTOSIS X

Eosinophilic granuloma is the most benign of a group of diseases of unknown etiology referred to as histiocytosis X (synonyms: generalized xanthomatosis, lipid histiocytosis, lipid granulomatosis, reticuloendotheliosis). Hand-Schüller-Christian disease and Letterer-Siwe disease are closely related to eosinophilic granuloma. Letterer-Siwe disease occurs in infants; it is acute and often rapidly fatal. Hand-Schüller-Christian disease occur in older children and is more benign, while eosinophilic granuloma occurs in young adults and is often localized and benign. Niemann-Pick disease and Gaucher's disease are related and can also cause pulmonary infiltrates. Eosinophilic granuloma has been found as a lesion occurring only in the lung with increasing frequency. In some patients the typical bone lesion has been associated with the pulmonary disease, but in others the lung appears to be the sole site of involvement.

The roentgen manifestations of pulmonary histiocytosis X are of two types. In one, a solitary

dense mass is noted that resembles pulmonary neoplasm. In the other form of the disease, a more generalized involvement is noted, manifested by an increase in linear markings along with small nodular lesions on the order of 1 to 3 mm in size. These nodules are rather poorly defined, with hazy borders (Fig. 30-24). They may be scattered generally throughout the lungs but tend to be somewhat more pronounced in the upper lung fields (Fig. 30-24). The disease may regress spontaneously. It may progress, with increasing interstitial involvement. The appearance is then that of a somewhat reticular pattern of increased lung markings with small foci of cystlike rarefaction, resulting in a honeycomb lung. The small "cysts" are peripheral and are believed to be the cause of spontaneous pneumothorax which is sometimes a complication (Fig. 30-25). There is

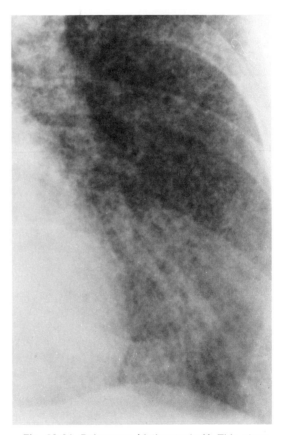

Fig. 30-24. Pulmonary histiocytosis X. This close-up of the left lower lung in a 40-year-old female with diabetes insipidus shows extensive involvement by small nodules with only a very few cystlike areas in the central lung.

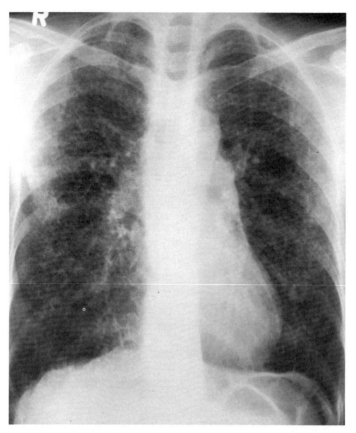

Fig. 30-25. Pulmonary histiocytosis X. This patient gave a history of having had spontaneous pneumothorax on three occasions. In addition to the scattered granular nodules there is a somewhat lacy reticular pattern resulting in the so-called "honeycomb" lung.

no hilar adenopathy and usually no pleural involvement.

In eosinophilic granuloma the patient is asymptomatic or has relatively few symptoms and the lesions clear slowly. Because the roentgen findings are not characteristic and simulate other chronic pulmonary disease, the diagnosis must be based on clinical manfestations plus the presence of the typical roentgen changes observed in bone. Lung biopsy is necessary but the diagnosis can be suspected in asymptomatic young patients with extensive pulmonary disease and no adenopathy or pleural involvement. Diabetes insipidus may be present and is helpful in the diagnosis. A history of repeated spontaneous pneumothorax in a patient with the above pulmonary findings is also suggestive of histiocytosis X.

PULMONARY TUBEROUS SCLEROSIS

Tuberous sclerosis is a hereditary disease characterized by mental deficiency, seizures, adenoma sebaceum (acneform rash) on the face with butterfly distribution, and tumors that may affect various parts of the body, including the central nervous system, liver, spleen, kidneys, and bones. The pulmonary form of tuberous sclerosis usually occurs in adults in whom there is no mental deficiency and no clinical evidence of central nervous system damage even though calcifications are noted intracranially. Several patients have been reported in whom chest roentgenograms revealed a fine netlike or honeycomb reticulation throughout both lung fields, resembling the changes noted in cystic diseases of the lungs. In some patients the reticular pattern is rather coarse and the small radiolucencies produced by the cystic lesions vary from 1 or 2 mm to 1 cm in diameter. These cysts may occur subpleurally and rupture to cause spontaneous pneumothorax.

PULMONARY ALVEOLAR MICROLITHIASIS

This rare disease is characterized by the presence of small calcium-containing bodies in the alveoli of the lung. The etiology is not known but there is a high familial incidence, indicating that there is a hereditary factor. The disease is asymptomatic for long periods of time but eventually dyspnea appears, followed by cough, cyanosis, and right-sided heart failure. Because of the late appearance of symptoms the disease is usually first discovered on routine chest roentgenography.

Roentgen Findings

The appearance of the chest in this disease is characteristic. There is widespread uniform distribution of fine sandlike particles of calcific density, which are usually less than 1 mm in diameter. They are uniform in size and there is no tendency to conglomeration. When extensive, some of the tiny calcifications may overlap and be difficult to define as individual particles. Overexposed or Bucky films are of value in visualizing them, particularly when the disease is far advanced. The density is often great enough to obscure the heart and mediastinal outlines as well as the diaphragm. There is no other disease that resembles this condition since these tiny particles are calcific and more dense than particles of comparable size in any of the miliary diseases.

FAMILIAL DYSAUTONOMIA (RILEY-DAY SYNDROME)

This syndrome results from dysfunction of the autonomic nervous system. It is a familial congenital disorder transmitted as an autosomal recessive trait that occurs in children and young adults, usually of Jewish extraction. Clinical findings consist of defective (decreased) lacrimation, excessive perspiration, blotchy skin, drooling, emotional instability, motor incoordination, hyporeflexia, and indifference to pain. Death is usually caused by pulmonary disease. The pulmonary findings are re-

lated to bronchial hypersecretion and resultant obstruction that often leads to infection. Pulmonary manifestations sufficient to produce roentgen changes on the chest film occur in approximately two-thirds of the patients. Early changes consist in diffuse accentuation of markings resulting from interstitial infiltration. Patchy bronchopneumonia is common and often persists for long periods of time. The repeated episodes of pneumonia accentuate the findings and may produce areas of homogeneous density scattered in the lung fields; these areas appear and disappear. Atelectasis of a lobe or segment is common and tends to persist for several weeks. The right upper lobe is frequently involved. Bronchiectasis is not commonly found. The pulmonary disease is usually more focal and not as widespread as in cystic fibrosis of the pancreas.

POLYCYTHEMIA

Polycythemia may be secondary to anoxia in a variety of chronic pulmonary diseases and in congenital heart disease. In these instances it is a compensatory phenomenon and there are no pulmonary roentgen findings indicating its presence. Polycythemia vera or primary polycythemia is a hematologic disorder characterized by hyperplasia of the red bone marrow, resulting in an increase in circulating red blood cells and in leukocytosis. In these patients, vascular engorgement results in prominence of vascular shadows in the lung fields. Basal fibrosis resulting in increased basal markings is sometimes noted along with changes suggesting basal congestion. Discrete rounded densities in the midzones of the lungs that are believed to represent venous thromboses have also been reported; they vary in size and appear and disappear in a few weeks. These findings are not diagnostic but when pulmonary vascular distention is present without cardiac or pulmonary disease evident to account for it, the diagnosis can be suggested.

THE AGAMMAGLOBULINEMIAS

These diseases are characterized by inability to form antibodies because of an absence or deficiency of gamma globulin. Congenital agammaglobulinemia is a sex-linked, recessive genetic defect transmitted by females to their male offspring. Hypogammaglobulinemia may be secondary to diffuse disease of the reticuloendothelial system such as multiple myeloma, leukemia, and lymphoma. Acquired and physiological forms of hypogammaglobulinemia have also been described. The patients are susceptible to infections because they lack the normal immunologic defense mechanisms. Repeated infections are commonly observed in the lungs, sinuses, mastoids, urinary tract, skin, etc. The pulmonary findings are therefore those of recurrent bronchopneumonia which may lead to postinflammatory fibrotic changes. No hilar adenopathy is present, so small hila have been reported in patients with repeated infections. The scarcity of lymphoid tissue in the pharynx results in a large pharyngeal airway, characteristic of this disease in children. This is readily observed in a lateral roentgenogram of the nasopharynx.

CHRONIC PNEUMONITIS OF THE CHOLESTEROL TYPE

This is a rare type of chronic interstitial inflammation of the lung in which the exudate consists of large mononuclear cells filled with cholesterol and cholesterol esters. These cells are noted to infiltrate the interstitial tissues and alveolar walls and to fill the alveoli. The etiology is not clear and the disease does not appear to be related to lipid pneumonia of the aspiration type. This disease is sometimes called "endogenous lipid pneumonia" and small deposits are often found associated with chronic pulmonary diseases that produce bronchial obstruction.

Roentgen Findings

This disease is characterized by a single confluent homogeneous density that may be lobar or segmental in distribution. There is usually a decrease in the volume of the lobe affected by the disease. The process extends to the pleura and the medial border is clearly defined. Hilar node enlargement is common, and pleural fluid or pleural thickening is usually present. The absence of endobronchial block and the fact that only a part of a segment is involved in the segmental type of disease are factors in favor of cholesterol pneumonitis

over tumor. It is more compact and clearly defined than lipid pneumonia and its distribution, with the lesion extending to the pleura, is unlike that in lipid pneumonia.

LIPID PNEUMONIA

Lipid pneumonia is the term used to designate the granulomatous and fibrotic changes resulting from aspiration of various organic or inorganic fatty materials. In adults, the most common cause is the use of mineral oil taken for the treatment of constipation. Frequent or continued use of oily nose drops can also cause this condition and, rarely, it occurs after bronchography. In children it is caused by aspiration of cod liver oil and in some instances milk fats probably produce the condition in infants. Lipid pneumonia also occurs in achalasia (see Ch. 15, section on achalasia). As the result of aspiration of lipid materials there is an inflammatory process produced that results in consolidation of pulmonary parenchyma. Large phagocytes containing lipid material are noted in the alveoli and in the interstitial tissues. Chronic inflammatory cells may also be present within the alveoli. As the disease progresses, a considerable amount of fibrosis develops that causes contraction of the involved lung, compression of the alveoli, and often compression and obliteration of the bronchi. These pathologic changes result in abnormalities that can be outlined on chest roentgenograms.

The roentgen findings are of two general types, diffuse and nodular. In the diffuse type there are scattered areas of increased density that are usually at the bases but may involve the right middle lobe and the superior segment of the lower lobe as well. Occasionally the condition involves the upper lobes. The individual lesions are usually poorly defined, with the density fading off into normal lung radiolucency. The lesions are not unlike those found in other types of aspiration pneumonitis but tend to be more linear with a fine granular and linear pattern (Fig. 30-26). There is also reduction in volume of the affected lobe. Serial films show that the infiltrate in this condition

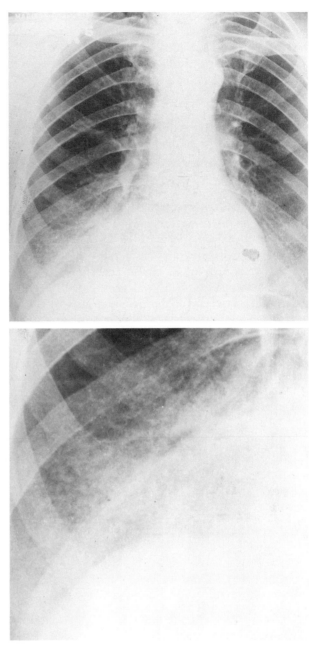

Fig. 30-26. Lipid pneumonia. *Top,* Note bilateral basal changes. *Bottom,* Enlargement of the right lower lobe to show the detail of the changes, which consist of a granular and reticular increase in density that is diffuse and relatively uniform in the area of involvement.

persists with little change over a long period of time, in contrast to the changes noted in bacterial and viral pneumonitis, which resolve leaving little, if any, residual density. In some cases, as lipid pneumonitis progresses, the area involved may decrease in size because of fibrosis. At times there may be persistent, irregular, patchy densities scattered in one or both lungs which resemble chronic nonspecific inflammatory disease. In the absence of a suggestive history, lung biopsy is the only method of diagnosis.

The nodular type of disease may also be unilateral or bilateral and probably results from a local conglomeration of the diffuse type. The area of density varies considerably in size but may reach 8 to 10 cm in diameter. It appears as a mass, usually oval or rounded in shape. The periphery of the nodule is usually irregular but occasionally becomes very smooth, so that the lesion may resemble a benign cyst or tumor (Fig. 30-27). This lesion

is also known as an oil or lipid granuloma. In some patients the right middle lobe is involved, being contracted and completely airless with its bronchus obstructed by inflammatory reaction.

Lipid pneumonitis usually produces less symptoms than comparable involvement by an infectious process. This is of help in differentiating it from infectious disease. Serial examinations also show more stability of this lesion than in most of the lesions it may simulate. The nodular disease may resemble bronchogenic carcinoma or other intrapulmonary tumor and in some instances thoracotomy and biopsy are the only methods of differentiation. If a history of ingestion of mineral oil or the use of nose drops can be obtained and the roentgen findings described are also associated with the presence of lipid-containing phagocytes in the sputum, the diagnosis can be made with a considerable degree of accuracy.

PULMONARY ALVEOLAR PROTEINOSIS

This disease was described by Rosen, Castleman, and Liebow in 1958.[59] It is characterized by the presence in the alveoli of PAS-positive (periodic acid-Schiff stain) proteinaceous material rich in lipid. The exact nature of the material has not been determined; it appears to be produced by septal lining cells which slough into the lumen and become necrotic. Cellular infiltrate and reaction is absent or minimal. The cause is not known; inhalation of some of the newer chemical agents used in sprays, etc., has been suggested, along with an infectious agent antigenically allied to pneumocystis carinii. The disease occurs in adults in the age range of 20 to 50 years but may occasionally be observed in children. It appears to be a new disease, since no examples of it were observed before 1955. It often runs an insidious course characterized by malaise, cough, dyspnea, and weight loss. Physical findings are minimal and gross roentgen abnormality may be observed in patients with few symptoms. The course of the disease may also be variable; in a few patients it is rapidly progressive, leading to pulmonary insufficiency with cyanosis, clubbing of the fingers, and death caused by the progressive loss of pulmonary function or intercurrent infection. Secondary fungal infection is the cause of most deaths

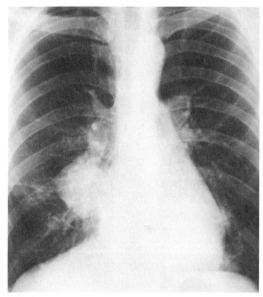

Fig. 30-27. Lipid pneumonia. This represents the nodular type of lipid pneumonia with a readily visible large mass in the region of the right middle lobe. A second mass, which is only slightly smaller, is present at the left base in the medial aspect of the left lower lobe but is not clearly defined on this roentgenogram, since it lies behind the heart.

in this disease. *Nocardia* is the most common of these organisms, but *Candida, Mucor,* and *Cryptococcus* may also be the cause. In others, the symptoms may regress, with partial clearing of pulmonary changes; occasionally the disease may clear completely. Iodides appear to be of some value in treatment. Tracheobronchial lavage of the involved lobes with heparin or other enzymes or saline has been used with definite improvement in some patients. Steroids are ineffective and are contraindicated.

The roentgen findings at the height of the disease are those of perihilar densities simulating pulmonary edema. The infiltrate appears to radiate from the hila chiefly to the bases; it is indistinct or "soft" and may have a somewhat irregular pattern resembling nodularity. There are variations of this pattern; at times the disease appears to be unilateral and it need not be perihilar; it is predominantly basal and central however. A number of cases have been reported in which distribution of the alveolar density was quite atypical, so the disease must be kept in mind when alveolar densities persist in an afebrile, relatively asymptomatic patient. (Fig. 30-28). Roentgen findings change slowly and when clearing occurs, there is often some residual fibrosis. The diagnosis can be suspected on the basis of clinical and roentgen findings, but lung biopsy is necessary to confirm it.

DESQUAMATIVE INTERSTITIAL PNEUMONIA (DIP)

This entity was described by Liebow, Steer, and Billingsley[40] in 1965. Clinical findings consist of dyspnea, usually gradual in onset, nonproductive cough, chest pain, and weight loss. It is relatively rare and is characterized by extensive desquamation of granular pneumocytes (large alveolar cells) which proliferate actively in and adjacent to the alveoli. Etiology is not certain. Roentgen findings consist of bilateral, basilar, peripheral alveolar density which tends to spare the costophrenic angles; it is hazy and has been described as having a ground glass appearance. In some patients there

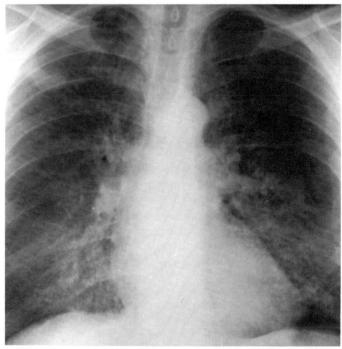

Fig. 30-28. Pulmonary alveolar proteinosis. Bilateral basal involvement which is rather typical of this disease. It tends to be confluent at the right base and is rather indistinct and poorly defined laterally. There is a lesser amount of change in the perihilar areas, slightly more prominent on the left than on the right.

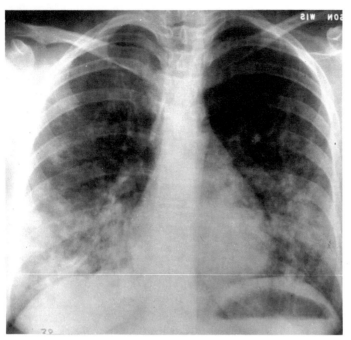

Fig. 30-29. Appearance of lungs after near drowning. Immediately following resuscitation there were no abnormalities noted on
the chest film. This examination was done about 3 hours later and
shows bilateral basal change resembling alveolar edema with
lesser change centrally and relatively clear upper lungs.

is a progressive loss of volume of the lower lobes.
Complications are unusual; they include pleural
effusion and spontaneous pneumothorax. Steroids
appear to cause remission of the process.

PULMONARY MUSCULAR HYPERPLASIA
(MUSCULAR CIRRHOSIS OF THE LUNG)

The term muscular cirrhosis of the lung was
used to describe this condition because the involved lung tissue is similar to advanced Laen-
nec's cirrhosis of the liver in its gross appearance.
The entity has also been termed lymphangiomyoma of the lung, bronchiolar emphysema, and
pulmonary myomatosis with microcyst formation.
It occurs almost exclusively in females. Microscopic findings consist of overgrowth of smooth
muscle elements, obliteration of the alveoli, fibroplasia and saccular dilatation of the respiratory
bronchioles which resemble air-filled cysts. This
causes great thickening of alveolar septa and at
times distortion of architecture by tumorlike

masses of smooth muscle. There is mediastinal and
retroperitoneal lymphatic involvement, often complicated by chylothorax. The roentgen features
are not diagnostic; they consist of diffuse coarse
accentuation of pulmonary markings interspersed
with areas of radiolucency producing a honeycomb effect in some instances. The lung bases tend
to be more markedly involved than the upper lung
fields. Hilar adenopathy has also been reported.
There appears to be an unusually high incidence of
bronchogenic carcinoma associated with this condition. In the single patient we observed the disease
resembled the basal fibrosis noted in a number of
other conditions. The disease is rare and presumably fatal. Diagnosis depends upon lung biopsy.

NEAR-DROWNING

When a patient is recovered from the water in a
state of apnea and subsequently revived, pulmonary changes occur which are evidently caused by
hypoxia. Pulmonary edema and hemorrhage have

been observed histopathologically in drowning victims, and the roentgen findings in the near-drowning patient resemble those of pulmonary edema of varying degrees of severity. There may be a delay in appearance of roentgen changes for several hours. The findings consist of bilateral, poorly defined, alveolar densities which may be very extensive and confluent, sparing the periphery (Fig. 30-29). In other patients the involvement is less marked and tends to be reticulonodular and poorly defined. Clearing is usually rapid and is complete in 2 to 6 days. As the process resolves, the appearance changes from that of alveolar edema to a pattern resembling interstitial edema. Aspiration of foreign material may complicate the picture. When recovery is delayed, pulmonary infection is usually found as a complication.

REFERENCES AND SELECTED READINGS

1. ALLEN, J. H., JR.: Agammaglobulinemia. *Am. J. Roentgenol. Radium Ther. Nucl. Med. 80:* 475, 1958.

2. AMERICAN THORACIC SOCIETY: Definitions and classification of chronic bronchitis, asthma and pulmonary emphysema. *Am. Rev. Resp. Dis. 85:* 762, 1962.

3. BAGGENSTOSS, A. H.: Loeffler's syndrome. *Arch. Path. 40:* 376, 1945.

4. BAGHDASSARIAN, O. M., AVERY, M. E., and NEUHAUSER, E. B. D.: A form of pulmonary insufficiency in premature infants. Pulmonary dysmaturity? *Am. J. Roentgenol. Radium Ther. Nucl. Med. 89:* 1020, 1963.

5. BARRETT, B., and VOLIWILER, W.: Agammaglobulinemia and hypogammaglobulinemia—The first five years. *JAMA 164:* 866, 1957.

6. BRETTNER, A., HEITZMAN, E. R., and WOODIN, W. G.: Pulmonary complications of drug therapy. *Radiology 96:* 31, 1970.

7. BRODY, J. S., and LEVIN, B.: Interlobar septa thickening in lipid pneumonia. *Am. J. Roentgenol. Radium Ther. Nucl. Med. 88:* 1061, 1962.

8. BRONSON, S. M.: Idiopathic pulmonary hemosiderosis. *Am. J. Roentgenol. Radium Ther. Nucl. Med. 83:* 260, 1960.

9. BRUTON, O. C.: Agammaglobulinemia. *Pediatrics 9:* 722, 1952.

10. BRUWER, A. J., KIERLAND, R. R., and SCHMIDT, H. W.: Pulmonary tuberous sclerosis. *Am. J. Roentgenol. Radium Ther. Nucl. Med. 75:* 748, 1956.

11. BULGRIN, J. G., DUBOIS, E. L., and JACOBSON, G.: Chest roentgenographic changes in systemic lupus erythematosus. *Radiology 74:* 42, 1960.

12. BUSH, J. K., McLEAN, R. L., and SIEKER, H. O.: Diffuse lung disease due to lymphangiomyoma. *Am. J. Med. 46:* 645, 1969.

13. DAWSON, J.: Pulmonary tuberous sclerosis. *Q. J. Med. 23:* 113, 1954.

14. DIRKSE, P. R.: Primary amyloidosis of the lungs. *Am. J. Roentgenol. Radium Ther. Nucl. Med. 56:* 577, 1946.

15. DULFANO, M. J., and DiRIENZO, A.: Laminagraphic observations of the lung vasculature in chronic pulmonary emphysema. *Am. J. Roentgenol. Radium Ther. Nucl. Med. 88:* 1043, 1962.

16. ELLMAN, P., and GEE, A.: Pulmonary hemosiderosis. *Br. Med. J. 2:* 384, 1951.

17. ESPOSITO, M. J.: Focal pulmonary hemosiderosis in rheumatic heart disease. *Am. J. Roentgenol. Radium Ther. Nucl. Med. 73:* 351, 1955.

18. FEINBERG, R.: Necrotising granulomatosis and angiitis of the lungs and its relationship to chronic pneumonitis of the cholesterol type. *Am. J. Path. 29:* 913, 1953.

19. FEINBERG, S. B., and GOLDBERG, M. E.: Hyaline membrane disease: Preclinical roentgen diagnosis. *Radiology 68:* 185, 1957.

20. FELSON, B., and BRAUNSTEIN, H.: Noninfectious necrotizing granulomatosis. *Radiology 70:* 326, 1958.

21. FLEISCHNER, F. G., and BERENBERG, A. L.: Idiopathic pulmonary hemosiderosis. *Radiology 62:* 522, 1954.

22. GAENSLER, E. A., GOFF, A. M., and PROWSE, C. M.: Desquamative interstitial pneumonia. *N. Engl. J. Med. 274:* 113, 1966.

23. GARLAND, L. H., and SISSON, M. A.: Roentgen findings in the "collagen" diseases. *Am. J. Roentgenol. Radium Ther. Nucl. Med. 71:* 581, 1954.

24. GEIST, R. M., JR., and MULLEN, W. J., JR.: Roentgenologic aspects of lethal granulomatous ulceration of the midline facial tissues. *Am. J. Roentgenol. Radium Ther. Nucl. Med. 70:* 566, 1953.

25. GENEREUX, G. P.: Lipids in the lungs: Radiologic-pathologic correlation. *J. Can. Assoc. Radiol. 21:* 2, 1970.

26. GLUECK, M. A., and JANOWER, M. L.: Nitrofurantoin lung disease. *Am. J. Roentgenol. Radium Ther. Nucl. Med. 107:* 818, 1969.

27. GÓMEZ, G. E., LICHTEMBERGER, E., SANTAMARÍA, A., CARVAJAL, L., JIMÉNEZ-PEÑUELA, B., SAAIBÍ, E., BARRERA, A. R., ORDÍEZ, E., and CORTEA-HENAO, A.: Familial pulmonary alveolar microlithiasis. *Radiology 72:* 550, 1953.

28. GREENSPAN, R. H.: Chronic disseminated alveolar diseases of the lung. *Semin. Roentgenol. II:* 77, 1967.

29. GREER, A. E.: Mucoid impaction of the bronchi. *Ann. Intern. Med. 46:* 506, 1957.

30. HAMMAN, L., and RICH, A. R.: Acute diffuse interstitial fibrosis of the lungs. *Bull. Johns Hopkins Hosp. 74:* 177, 1944.

31. HAMPTON, A. O., BICKHAM, C. E., JR., and WINSHIP, T.: Lipoid pneumonia. *Am. J. Roentgenol. Radium Ther. Nucl. Med. 73:* 938, 1955.

32. HASTINGS-JAMES, R.: Radiologic appearances following hemoptysis. *J. Fac. Radiol. 4:* 44, 1952.

33. HUTCHINSON, W. B., FRIEDENBERG, M. J., and SALTZSTEIN, S.: Primary pulmonary pseudolymphoma. *Radiology 82:* 48, 1964.

34. JENSEN, K. M., MISCOLL, L., and STEINBERG, I.: Angiocardiography in bullous emphysema: Its role in selection of the case suitable for surgery. *Am. J. Roentgenol. Radium Ther. Nucl. Med. 85:* 229, 1961.

35. KEATS, T. E., and CRANE, J. F.: Cystic changes of lungs in histiocytosis. *Am. J. Dis. Child. 88:* 764, 1954.

36. KIRKPATRICK, R., and RILEY, C. M.: Roentgenographic findings in familial dysautonomia. *Radiology 68:* 654, 1957.

37. LACKEY, R. W., LEAVER, F. Y., and FARINOCCI, C. J.: Eosinophilic granuloma of lung. *Radiology 59:* 504, 1952.

38. LEVIN, D. C.: The "P.I.E." syndrome—pulmonary infiltrates with eosinophilia; a report of 3 cases with lung biopsy. *Radiology 89:* 461, 1967.

39. LIEBOW, A. A., and CARRINGTON, C. B.: The eosinophilic pneumonias. *Medicine 48:* 251, 1969.

40. LIEBOW, A. A., STEER, A., and BILLINGSLEY, J. G.: Desquamative interstitial pneumonia. *Am. J. Med. 39:* 369, 1965.

41. LILLARD, R. L., and ALLEN, R. P.: The extrapleural air sign in pneumomediastinum. *Radiology 85:* 1093, 1965.

42. LUNDBERG, G. D.: Goodpasture's syndrome. *JAMA 184:* 915, 1963.

43. MACKLIN, C. C.: Transport of air along sheaths of pulmonic blood vessels from alveoli to mediastinum: Clinical implications. *Arch. Intern. Med. 64:* 913, 1939.

44. MARGOLIN, H. N., ROSENBERG, L. S., FELSON, B., and BAUM, G.: Idiopathic unilateral hyperlucent lung. *Am. J. Roentgenol. Radium Ther. Nucl. Med. 82:* 63, 1959.

45. MARTELL, W., ABELL, M. R., MIKKELSEN, W. M., and WHITEHOUSE, W. M.: Pulmonary and pleural lesions in rheumatoid disease. *Radiology 90:* 641, 1968.

46. MATHEWS, W. H.: Primary systemic amyloidosis. *Am. J. Med. Sci. 228:* 317, 1954.

47. MILLEDGE, R. D., GERALD, B. E., and CARTER, W. J.: Pulmonary manifestations of tuberous sclerosis. *Am. J. Roentgenol. Radium Ther. Nucl. Med. 98:* 734, 1966.

48. MILNE, E. N. C., and BASS, H.: The roentgenologic diagnosis of early chronic obstructive pulmonary disease. *J. Can. Assoc. Radiol. 20:* 3, 1969.

49. MOLOSHOK, R. E., and MOSELEY, J. E.: Familial dysautonomia: Pulmonary manifestations. *Pediatrics 17:* 327, 1956.

50. NICE, C. M., JR., MENON, A. N. K., and RIGLER, L. G.: Pulmonary manifestations in collagen diseases. *Am. J. Roentgenol. Radium Ther. Nucl. Med. 81:* 264, 1959.

51. PETERSON, H. G., JR., and PENDLETON, M. E.: Contrasting roentgenographic pulmonary patterns of the hyaline membrane and fetal aspiration syndromes. *Am. J. Roentgenol. Radium Ther. Nucl. Med. 74:* 800, 1955.

52. PREGER, L.: Pulmonary alveolar proteinosis. *Radiology 92:* 1291, 1969.

53. REID, L. M.: Correlation of certain bronchographic abnormalities seen in chronic bronchitis with pathologic changes. *Thorax 10:* 199, 1955.

54. REIMANN, H. A., SAHYOUN, P. F., and CHAGLASSIAN, H. T.: Primary amyloidosis. *Arch. Intern. Med. 93:* 673, 1954.

55. Report of the conclusions of a Ciba guest symposium: Terminology, definitions and classification of chronic pulmonary emphysema and related conditions. *Thorax 14:* 286, 1959.

56. RILEY, C. M.: Familial autonomic dysfunction. *JAMA 149:* 1542, 1952.

57. ROBBINS, L. L., and HALE, C. H.: The roentgen appearance of lobar and segmental collapse of the lung. *Radiology 45:* 23–26, 120–127, 260–266, 347, 355, 1945.

58. ROBBINS, L. L., and SNIFFEN, R. C.: Correlation between the roentgenologic and pathologic findings in chronic pneumonitis of the cholesterol type. *Radiology 53:* 187, 1949.

59. ROSEN, S. H., CASTLEMAN, B., LIEBOW, A. A. with the collaboration of ENZINGER, F. M., and HUNT, R. T. N.: Pulmonary alveolar proteinosis. *N. Engl. J. Med. 258:* 1123, 1958.

60. ROSENBAUM, H. T., THOMPSON, W. L., and FULLER, R. H.: Radiographic pulmonary changes in near-drowning. *Radiology 83:* 306, 1964.

61. ROTTENBERG, L. A., and GOLDEN, R.: Spontaneous pneumothorax: A study of 105 cases. *Radiology 53:* 157, 1949.

62. RUBIN, E. H., KAHN, B. S., and PECKER, D.: Diffuse interstitial fibrosis of the lungs. *Ann. Intern. Med. 36:* 827, 1952.

63. SALTZMAN, P. W., WEST, M., and CHOMET, B.: Pulmonary hemosiderosis and glomerulonephritis. *Ann. Intern. Med. 56:* 409, 1962.

64. SANDLER, B. P., MATTHEWS, J. H., and BORNSTEIN, S.: Pulmonary cavitation due to polyarteritis. *JAMA 144:* 754, 1950.

65. SCHECHTER, M. M.: Diffuse interstitial fibrosis of the lungs. *Am. Rev. Tuberc. 68:* 603, 1953.

66. SCHULTZE, G.: Chest film findings in neonatal respiratory distress. *Radiology 70:* 230, 1958.

67. SHEFT, D. J., and MOSKOWITZ, H.: Pulmonary muscular hyperplasia. *Am. J. Roentgenol. Radium Ther. Nucl. Med. 93:* 836, 1965.

68. SIMON, G.: Radiology and emphysema. *Clin. Radiol. 15:* 293, 1964.

69. SOSMAN, M. C., DODD, G. D., JONES, W. D., and PILLMORE, G. U.: Pulmonary alveolar microlithiasis. *Am. J. Roentgenol. Radium Ther. Nucl. Med. 77:* 947, 1957.

70. SPAIN, D. M.: Patterns of pulmonary fibrosis. *Ann. Intern. Med. 33:* 1150, 1950.

71. SWISCHUK, L. E.: Transient respiratory distress of the newborn (TRDN): A temporary disturbance of a normal phenomenon. *Am. J. Roentgenol. Radium Ther. Nucl. Med. 108:* 557, 1970.

72. WESENBERG, R. L., GRAVEN, S. N., and McCABE, E. B.: Radiological findings in wet-lung disease. *Radiology 98:* 69, 1971.

73. WOLFSON, S. L., FRECH, R., HEWITT, C., and SHANKLIN, D. R.: Radiographic diagnosis of hyaline membrane disease. *Radiology 93:* 339, 1969.

31

DISEASES OF THE PLEURA, MEDIASTINUM, AND DIAPHRAGM

THE PLEURA

PLEURAL EFFUSION

GENERAL CONSIDERATIONS

The pleural space is lined by a smooth serous membrane that is lubricated by a small amount of serous fluid. This fluid is absorbed as fast as it is secreted so that an excess does not accumulate. Except for this thin layer of lubricating fluid, the pleural surfaces are in contact; therefore the pleural space is a potential one in the normal. The formation of excess fluid is caused by many conditions, a number of which are serious diseases either involving the lungs primarily or as a secondary manifestation of systemic disease. The causes include infections by many types of bacteria of which tuberculosis is one of the most frequent. Infections caused by viruses, rickettsia, and fungi may also cause effusion. Malignant tumors of the lung, mediastinum, and chest wall and metastatic tumors may also cause pleural effusion that is often bloody or blood-tinged. Diseases that cause lymphatic obstruction and produce hypoproteinemia as well as cardiac failure and pulmonary infarction are

also accompanied by pleural effusion in many instances. Accidental and surgical trauma produce effusions that are often bloody or blood-tinged.

There is some difference of opinion as to the amount of fluid necessary in the pleural space to produce enough density to be visible on a posteroanterior roentgenogram of the chest. In the unobstructed pleural space, fluid gravitates to the lowermost portion of the thoracic cavity, which is the posterior gutter, and amounts as large as 300 to 400 cc may be present and not visible. If a lateral view is taken, smaller amounts of fluid can be detected by the characteristic appearance of obliteration of the sharp, posterior costophrenic angle by homogeneous density that is slightly concave. This concavity can be simulated by thickened pleura and adhesions. Therefore, if detection of a small amount of fluid is necessary, decubitus views may be obtained. The best method for detection of small amounts of fluid is to have the patient lie with the affected side down, following which a posteroanterior or anteroposterior film is obtained in inspiration. Small amounts of fluid will then be visible along the lateral chest wall, since the fluid produces homogeneous density that lies between the inner rib margin and the visceral pleura of the lung. If the fluid is loculated as in empyema, this shifting does not occur. If there is a question as to the presence of fluid producing obliteration of the lateral costophrenic sulcus in the frontal projection, the patient is placed in the lateral decubitus position on the side opposite the affected one and a horizontal beam is directed to take an anteroposterior or posteroanterior roentgenogram. In this instance, if fluid is present it will gravitate to the mediastinum, leaving the costophrenic sulcus sharply angulated. Large amounts of fluid in the free pleural space also gravitate with change in position and these positions can be used to demonstrate the parts of the pulmonary parenchyma that are obscured by the fluid in the routine upright frontal and lateral chest roentgenograms. The earliest roentgen sign of fluid on the routine upright chest film is obliteration of the sharp angle produced by the normal costophrenic sulcus. As the amount of fluid increases, more of the diaphragm and the basal lung become obscured by it. The superior border of the fluid is concave and often blurred, since some of the fluid extends upward into the pleural space by capillary action. If the superior pleural line is horizontal and clearly defined (i.e., the air-fluid level), it indicates that some air or gas is present along with the fluid in the pleural space. As the amount of fluid increases so that it occupies a sizable portion of the volume of the affected hemithorax there is increasing compression of the lung, depression of the diaphragm, and often a shift of the mediastinum to the opposite side. When the effusion is massive and fills one hemithorax, the mediastinal shift may become marked.

When films are taken in the supine or recumbent position, the fluid shifts to the most dependent part of the thorax. Therefore it causes a homogeneous hazy density that is uniformly distributed throughout the involved hemithorax unless there is loculation. The degree of density then varies with the amount of fluid (Fig. 31-1).

Atypical arrangements of pleural fluid may occur as a result of disease in the underlying lung. The differentiated collapse of diseased pulmonary tissue was observed in tuberculosis and was the basis for the use of therapeutic pneumothorax. The elasticity of the lung also plays an important part in distribution of fluid. When a change caused by disease modifies the

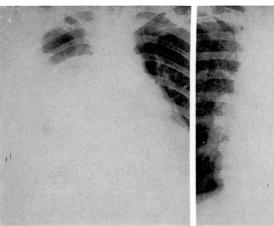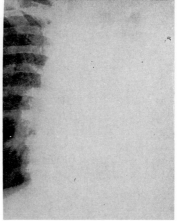

Fig. 31-1. Pleural effusion. These are examples of massive pleural effusion. *Left,* Note the homogeneous density obliterating all but the apical lung. The roentgenogram on the *right* also shows some shift of mediastinal structures to the right as a result of the massive effusion on the left.

uniform recoiling tendency of the lung, atypical distribution of fluid occurs in the absence of loculation. The presence of fluid without true loculation in these instances can be confirmed by decubitus and other views as needed.

LOCULATED PLEURAL EFFUSION

Pleural fluid in varying amounts may become loculated or encapsulated adjacent to any pleural surface, including the interlobar fissures. This occurs commonly in empyema and in patients with hemothorax. It is also seen in some patients with cardiac failure. Small amounts of fluid in the interlobar fissures are identified best in lateral and oblique views. The one exception is the secondary interlobar fissure on the right, which is readily visible in the frontal projection. The fluid causes apparent widening of the fissure, which is usually very slightly convex (Fig. 31-2). As the amount of fluid increases the convexity increases until it may become round or oval and simulate tumor. The differentiation between tumor and loculated fluid can usually be made without difficulty when oblique and lateral views are obtained, since the characteristic elongated shape tends to be more prominent in these projections than in the frontal view (Fig. 31-3). The clearly defined borders of these loculated effusions are also of differential diagnostic significance. Fluid in the major interlobar fissures often produces a poorly defined increase in density when viewed in the frontal projection and lateral views are usually needed to identify clearly the nature of the process. When fluid is loculated at the mediastinum, it produces a local or general mediastinal widening that may simulate a mediastinal or pleural tumor. When the fluid adjacent to the mediastinum simulates tumor, decubitus views to show alteration in the shape of the density are helpful in the differential diagnosis and the presence of fluid elsewhere or in the opposite hemithorax is a useful sign whenever loculated fluid simulates mass. When the fluid is located along the costal surface, it does not ordinarily present a diagnostic problem but when doubt-

ful as to the nature of the process or the type of transudate or exudate present, the lesion may be localized fluoroscopically and thoracentesis performed.

INFRAPULMONARY PLEURAL EFFUSION

Occasionally a large pleural effusion may be present in the basal hemithorax, elevating the lower lung without distorting it and simulating elevation of the diaphragm. This is observed particularly on the right side where the fluid density blends with that of the liver and diaphragm below it. In some instances the costophrenic angle appears to be preserved while in others there is slight blunting or concavity. In the latter instance, infrapulmonary effusion can be suspected, but when the lateral inferior lung margin is maintained so that a costophrenic sulcus is simulated, a high index of suspicion is necessary to make the diagnosis. When an infrapulmonary effusion is present on the left, the diagnosis is made more readily since the presence of air in the stomach usually outlines its fundus and identifies the height of the diaphragm in the routine frontal and lateral chest roentgenograms. Fluoroscopy or roentgenograms in the supine position are used to confirm the presence of infrapulmonary effusion. The fluid is then distributed in the dependent posterior hemithorax and causes a hazy density throughout. In addition, the diaphragm can be identified. Its position is noted to be lower than the density simulating diaphragm in the upright view. Lateral decubitus views may also be used as described earlier (Fig. 31-4). If loculated, pneumoperitoneum may be needed to differentiate it from other conditions.

SUMMARY

In summary, pleural fluid causes a homogeneous density that does not vary with the type of fluid. In the upright chest roentgenogram taken in the frontal projection, several hundred cubic centimeters of fluid may be present without producing any roentgen change, but much smaller amounts, ranging from 50 to 100 cc, can be detected when lateral decubitus views are taken. As the amount of fluid increases it gradually obscures the diaphragm and lower lung field and when large, tends

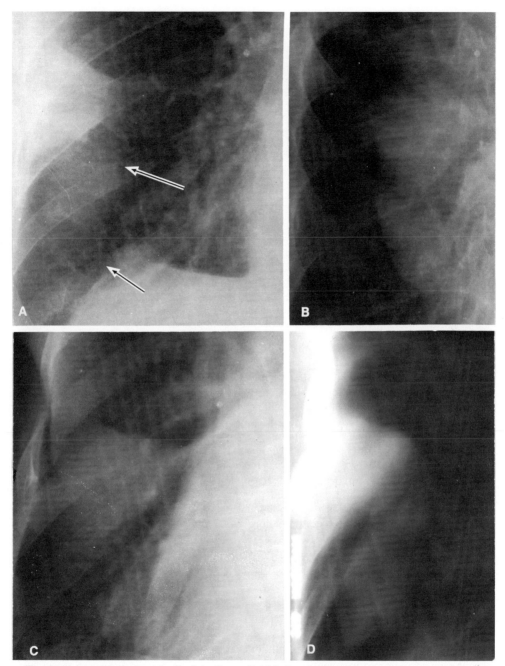

Fig. 31-2. Loculated pleural effusion. Some fluid is loculated in the lateral aspect of the secondary interlobar fissure and there is an elongated loculation in the major fissure. *A*, Frontal projection. **Arrows** outline the lower loculation. *B*, Left anterior oblique view. *C*, Right anterior oblique view. *D*, Tomogram.

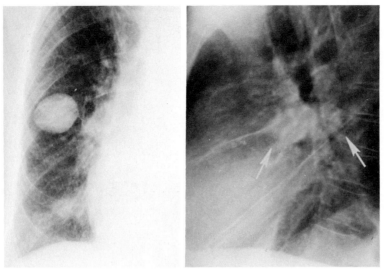

Fig. 31-3. Loculated pleural effusion simulating tumor. The oval mass in the right central lung field is noted to be rather elongated in the lateral view (**arrows**) and represents fluid in the secondary interlobar fissure. Note the extension resulting from a small amount of fluid or pleural thickening in the anterior aspect of this fissure.

to depress the diaphragm (see p. 966) and displace the mediastinum to the opposite side. Free fluid is concave superiorly, owing to capillary action, unless air or gas is present, in which case a straight, horizontal gas-fluid level is present. Loculated fluid may simulate tumor but recumbent, lateral, and decubitus views plus progress roentgenograms to show the rapid changes that often occur are usually sufficient to make the proper diagnosis. Pulmonary disease may alter pulmonary elasticity and lead to atypical accumulations of free pleural fluid.

INFLAMMATORY DISEASES

ACUTE PLEURITIS

Acute infection of the pleura results in a serofibrinous inflammatory reaction that causes some pleural thickening and edema. This produces density that can sometimes be recognized radiographically, provided that the area of involvement is situated in a region in which the thickness of the pleura can be determined. This condition is associated with considerable pain, resulting in some fixation of the thorax and decrease in diaphragmatic motion as well as elevation of the diaphragm; in some instances these may be the only roentgen signs. A correlation of history, clinical findings, and roentgen findings indicates the diagnosis. A small amount of pleural effusion may result and if it is large enough in amount, it can be recognized also. The diagnosis of acute fibrinous or serofibrinous pleurisy is not ordinarily difficult on clinical examination but chest roentgenography is of value in excluding other disease even though the small area of pleural thickening may not be visible.

CHRONIC PLEURAL THICKENING

Chronic, nonsuppurative pleural disease may be caused by a variety of bacteria; tuberculosis is among the most common causes. Pleuritis of tuberculous etiology is often localized to the apex of the lung. Chronic pleuritis results in pleural thickening manifested by soft-tissue density between the inner aspect of the ribs and the adjacent lung. The inner surface is often irregular. The amount varies from a very

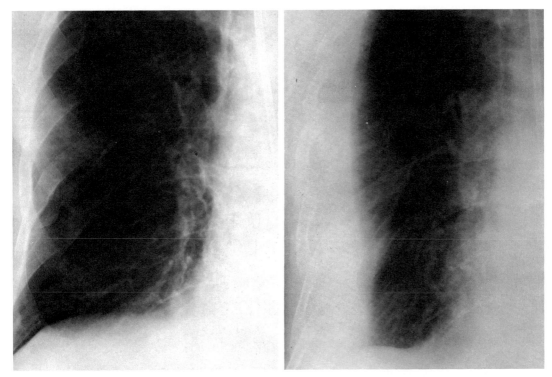

Fig. 31-4. Infrapulmonary pleural effusion. *Left,* Upright frontal projection. The right lower lung field and diaphragmatic dome are included. The costophrenic angle is clear but there is a little blurring of the cardiohepatic angle. The right diaphragm appeared high and effusion was suspected. *Right,* This right lateral decubitus projection shows a large amount of fluid along the right lateral thoracic wall.

thin linear band to a large amount of homogeneous density, representing grossly thickened fibrotic pleura. In other instances this may extend along the lateral chest wall to the base and occasionally may surround the entire lung, resulting in gradual fibrotic contraction leading to decrease in size of the involved hemithorax, along with the homogeneous density produced by the thickened fibrotic pleura. It is not uncommon to find large thick calcium plaques in the pleura in these patients. Occasionally a shell of pleural calcification may encase large portions of the lung and may also extend into the interlobar fissures. It is manifested by irregular linear plaques of density that are more opaque than the soft-tissue density produced by thick pleura alone (Fig. 31-5).

When extensive bilateral pleural thickening is present, particularly if linear calcific plaques are visible in the diaphragmatic pleura, asbes-

tosis or talcosis are nearly always the cause. Calcific plaques may also occur along the mediastinal pleura and along the lower lateral chest wall (parietal pleura) bilaterally. It is usually seen as linear or irregular plaques which are not very thick in contrast to the heavy, irregular plaques which may occur in chronic inflammatory disease. Parenchymal pulmonary involvement need not be roentgenographically visible in asbestosis.

Unilateral pleural thickening with calcification is nearly always secondary to inflammatory disease or to trauma with calcification in a hematoma.

In many instances small amounts of pleural thickening are noted along one or both thoracic walls in patients with no history of antecedent disease, so that the cause cannot be established. It is not infrequent to observe obliteration of a costophrenic sulcus in patients who

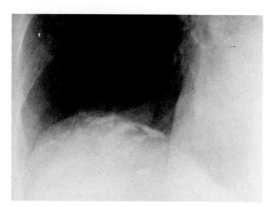

Fig. 31-5. Pleural calcification. Note dense flecks of calcium in the diaphragmatic pleura. No basal pulmonary disease is present.

have had previous pneumonia with associated pleuritis. Pleural infection results in more or less obliteration of the pleural space as a result of fibrous adhesions between the visceral and parietal layers. They are recognized roentgenographically by their effect on adjacent structures as well as by visualization of the bandlike density representing the adhesion. Adhesions over the diaphragm often produce small, local, tentlike elevations of the diaphragm. Similar distortion may be caused by contraction of local pulmonary lesions, however. Adhesions between the pleura and pericardium can sometimes be recognized roentgenographically by small spikelike irregularities of the outline of the pericardium. When sizable pneumothorax is present, the presence of adhesions can be readily detected since the lung pulls away from the parietal pleura if there are no adhesions.

EMPYEMA

Thoracic empyema, or pyothorax, is an inflammatory disease of the pleura with suppuration that results in an accumulation of pus in the pleural space. A number of organisms may cause this disease, including *Mycobacterium tuberculosis*. Staphylococcal pneumonia is frequently complicated by empyema. It is likely that any organism capable of causing pulmonary infection may also produce empyema and

the latter is usually, but not always, a complication of the former. Roentgenograms outline the empyema as a mass that may vary in size from a large lesion that obscures most of the lung to a relatively small loculated mass along the chest wall or in an interlobar fissure. Postpneumonic empyemas usually occur along the posterior pleural space or within an interlobar fissure. Anterior empyema from this cause is very rare. There need not be evidence of associated pulmonary disease. If present, the type of alteration in the lungs resulting from the disease may aid in determining the etiology of the empyema. In the acute stage there is usually some inflammation in the lung adjacent to the empyema cavity and this results in fuzzy irregularity of the margin. The fluid may not be loculated early in the disease. In the more chronic empyema the pulmonary inflammatory reaction may subside so that the mass is more clearly defined and sharply demarcated from the adjacent aerated lung (Fig. 31-6). Air or gas within the empyema causes a fluid level and

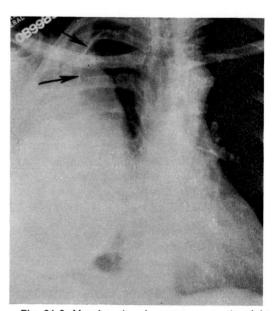

Fig. 31-6. Massive chronic empyema on the right, which is clearly defined superiorly where it is outlined against the aerated lung. There is some calcification in the pleura (**arrows**) superiorly. The lung has been compressed considerably and the greater portion of the hemithorax is obscured by the empyema.

indicates communication with a bronchus or with the skin surface. The pleural infection is usually peripheral, with one part of the empyema adjacent to the costal pleura. It can be localized roentgenographically or fluoroscopically and aspirated if there is doubt as to the diagnosis.

TUMORS OF THE PLEURA

BENIGN TUMORS

Primary benign pleural tumors are rare. They include lipoma, fibroma, hemangioma, chondroma, and neurofibroma that actually originate in the chest wall and project into the thorax. The fibrous pleural mesothelioma is the only benign tumor which originates in the pleura. It is localized and may be pedunculated and move in relationship to other thoracic structures. Otherwise, its roentgen characteristics are similar to those of the other benign pleural tumors. These tumors may become very large and produce large, smoothly rounded or lobulated densities, the internal aspects of which are clearly outlined by the air-filled lung. The outer aspects blend into the chest wall and often produce some widening of the intercostal space and rib erosion or deformity to indicate that they are primary chest-wall tumors. At times it is necessary to differentiate them from tumors arising in the lung. Diagnostic pneumothorax is then of value. It will clearly outline the relationship of the lung to the mass.

PRIMARY MALIGNANT TUMORS

Primary malignant tumors of the pleura are called mesotheliomas. They arise in the pleura, often in the interlobar fissures, and extend rapidly to involve a large part of the pleural space. The roentgen findings consist of a somewhat scalloped-appearing mass involving the pleura. It is often extensive when first observed, and may surround the entire lung (Fig. 31-7). Earlier an irregular nodular or scalloped pleural mass may be observed locally. Pleural effusion is common and may obscure the tumor. When massive effusion is present, mediastinal shift toward the contralateral side may not occur because of fixation of the mediastinum by tumor. Fluid tends to reaccumulate rapidly fol-

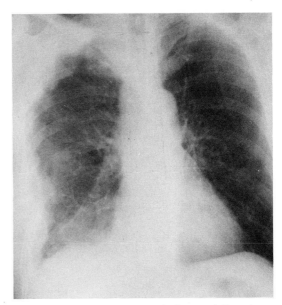

Fig. 31-7. Malignant mesothelioma of the pleura on the right. Note the extensive involvement by irregular lobulated pleural density representing the tumor. There is very little pleural effusion.

lowing thoracentesis. When extensive, these tumors may block the lymphatics sufficiently to result in accumulation of interstitial fluid in the lungs, so that severe interstitial edema is observed. The major differential problem is metastatic malignancy with extensive pleural involvement. If the fluid is drained and pneumothorax induced, the tumor may be visible. Even then, the appearance simulates that of pleural thickening and loculated fluid associated with the pleural disease so that diagnosis usually depends upon biopsy.

METASTATIC TUMORS

Metastatic pleural tumors are much more frequent than the malignant primary neoplasms. The actual pleural tumor in many instances is very small and forms tiny nodules in the visceral or parietal pleura that are not visible roentgenographically. Bloody pleural effusion is common so that the major roentgen finding is often that of pleural effusion. There may be direct extension into the pleura from a chest-wall metastasis in which rib is also involved. Then a soft-tissue, chest-wall mass and irregular rib destruction indicate that there is a malignant neoplasm present to account for the pleural effusion and mass projecting into the pleural space. The history of primary tumor elsewhere is of great importance in making the roentgen diagnosis. In our experience, breast carcinoma is the most common cause of pleural metastases.

FIBRIN BODIES

Fibrin bodies or fibrin balls are made up of masses of fibrin that resemble tumor within the pleural space. They form in patients with fibrinous pleuritis with effusion and are usually obscured by the fluid during formation, but when the fluid is removed by means of thoracentesis or is absorbed, they become apparent. They were commonly observed in pulmonary tuberculosis treated with pneumothorax and often complicated the effusion that developed during artificial pneumothorax when that was used as a method of collapse therapy. The roentgen findings are those of rounded or oval, single or multiple masses usually appearing at the base, often partially obscured by pleural effusion or becoming visible after the effusion has been drained or absorbed. Alteration of the patient's position may result in displacement of these bodies; when this is observed, the diagnosis is almost certain. They may disappear spontaneously, but may persist for years.

THE MEDIASTINUM

INFLAMMATORY DISEASES

ACUTE MEDIASTINITIS

Acute inflammations of the mediastinum most commonly arise from injury of the esophagus caused by ingestion of sharp foreign bodies that penetrate the esophagus, or instrumentation of the esophagus. Occasionally inflammation extends into the mediastinum from infections involving the sternum, spine, anterior chest wall, and mediastinal lymph nodes, and rarely from infections originating in the anterior neck and in the subdiaphragmatic area. These infections may result in abscess formation that may rupture into the esophagus, tracheobronchial tree, or pleural space. When antibiotics are given early following an esophageal injury, actual abscess formation is uncommon so that the incidence of mediastinal abscess is now relatively low. The roentgen findings are those of a diffuse increase in density and widening of the mediastinum to both sides of the midline in the region of involvement. If the process extends downward from the neck from a retropharyngeal abscess, roentgenograms of the neck taken in lateral projection often show the soft-tissue mass displacing the pharynx and trachea anteriorly.

When the infection has resulted from esophageal injury it is not uncommon to observe a small amount of mediastinal emphysema manifested by streaks of radiolucency. If an abscess becomes chronic, it may be large and clearly defined so that its appearance may simulate that of mediastinal tumor. It is not unusual to have enough pleural reaction to produce effusion (Fig. 31-8). The diagnosis is made on the basis of correlation of roentgen findings with the clinical history.

CHRONIC MEDIASTINITIS

Tuberculosis and actinomycosis may produce a chronic infection in the mediastinum or the infection may be nonspecific, such as that which follows trauma. The roentgen findings are not characteristic and may be very minor unless chronic mediastinal abscess is formed. In the latter event, the abscess produces a mass shadow that is usually found in the posterior mediastinum. This lesion may be impossible to differentiate from mediastinal tumor. Occasionally diffuse mediastinal inflammation caused by histoplasmosis results in enough fibrosis to produce obstruction of the superior or inferior vena cava and in these patients

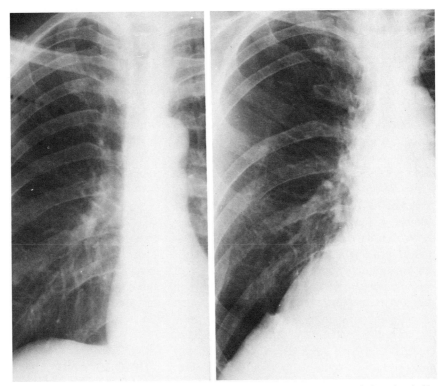

Fig. 31-8. Acute mediastinitis. *Left,* Preoperative roentgenogram of the chest. No abnormalities are noted in the mediastinum. *Right,* Roentgenogram taken 2 weeks following resection of an esophageal neoplasm. The patient developed an acute febrile illness. The mediastinal border on the right is rather indistinct superiorly as compared to the original film and the infection resulted in mediastinal pleuritis with loculated pleural effusion producing the mass density at the right medial base.

roentgen findings may be minimal. There may be an associated pulmonary involvement. Enlargement of mediastinal nodes is common early in the disease. They may decrease in size and disappear in the chronic phase, however. Occasionally, signs of superior caval obstruction will appear with no antecedent history of pulmonary, esophageal, tracheal, or pharyngeal disease. This evidently may be caused by a number of conditions, including subclinical histoplasmosis, other infections, and an idiopathic fibrosis similar to that noted in retroperitoneal fibrosis. Venography can be used to demonstrate venous obstruction. The clinical findings must be correlated with radiographic findings to arrive at the proper diagnosis. Surgical exploraton may be necessary to confirm it.

INFLAMMATORY DISEASES OF THE MEDIASTINAL LYMPH NODES

In nearly all infectious diseases of the lungs and bronchi there is histopathologic involvement of the mediastinal nodes, but most of these diseases do not usually cause enough enlargement to be of roentgen importance. There are chronic pulmonary inflammatory diseases, however, in which there is sufficient enlargement of hilar and mediastinal nodes to produce recognizable density on chest roentgenograms.

ACUTE NONSPECIFIC LYMPHADENOPATHY

Some enlargement of the hilum shadow is often present in pneumonia but is so minimal that it usually escapes detection or is obscured by the pulmonary infection. Occasionally an infected node may undergo suppuration, leading to acute mediastinitis or mediastinal abscess.

CHRONIC INFLAMMATIONS

Occasionally lymph nodes are enlarged in chronic suppurative disease of the bronchi, leading to recognizable hilar enlargement. It is often poorly defined and is associated with the accentuation of basal markings and patchy pneumonitis often found in bronchiectasis. A number of fungi are capable of producing pulmonary disease and they also involve the hilar nodes, resulting in enlargement. Adenopathy is most commonly found in the acute phase of coccidioidomycosis and histoplasmosis and may be present in other fungal diseases, such as actinomycosis and blastomycosis. In these diseases the pulmonary infection produces changes that have been described in the previous sections relating to these infections. This involvement of hilar and mediastinal nodes often leads to calcification in the nodes, which requires 1 or 2 years to develop. It is most commonly observed in histoplasmosis.

Primary tuberculosis is associated with mediastinal lymphadenopathy. The enlargement of hilar or paratracheal nodes may or may not be associated with a visible parenchymal lesion. Characteristically in primary tuberculosis a single group of nodes is involved. If more than one group is affected, one group is usually considerably larger than the other. The roentgen findings are those of a somewhat lobulated hilar enlargement with the outline of the hilum moderately fuzzy and indistinct. A visible parenchymal lesion may be present. When the acute phase is over, the borders of the hilum become more distinct and nodes gradually decrease in size. Calcification is often noted after a year or more; complete resolution may require several years.

All these chronic inflammatory diseases that involve the lungs, as well as the mediastinal nodes, must be differentiated from one another by appropriate skin tests and bacteriologic studies as indicated in Chapters 25 and 26. Node enlargement is noted in a variety of diseases of the lungs, including some of the pneumoconioses. In these patients, the pulmonary lesions are usually predominant.

Massive mediastinal, lymph-node enlargement has been reported occasionally in patients without other disease. The large nodes simulate mediastinal tumors or malignant lymphomata. Biopsy reveals a nonspecific chronic lymphadenitis.

SARCOIDOSIS

Sarcoidosis is usually associated with mediastinal lymphadenopathy sufficient to produce recognizable enlargement of hilar and mediastinal lymph nodes at some time during the disease. This is discussed in Chapter 26 under the heading "Sarcoidosis."

TUMORS AND ALLIED LESIONS

There are a number of structures within and extending through the mediastinum. Tumors and cysts may arise from any of them. There is a definite correlation between location within the mediastinum and the histologic type. Table 31-1 lists the lesions in order of incidence and site of relative frequency.

In addition to routine roentgenograms in frontal and lateral projections it is often necessary to obtain oblique films and to examine the patients fluoroscopically in order to obtain as much information as possible Esophagrams, tomograms, angiograms, or retrograde aortograms may be needed in some cases. When the mass is localized in relation to other mediastinal structures and its dynamic characteristics are determined by fluoroscopy (pulsation or lack of it, movement or lack of it on respiration and swallowing), it is often possible to be reasonably certain of the diagnosis. In other patients thoracotomy is necessary to make the histologic diagnosis as well as to remove the mass.

TABLE 31-1. Location of Tumors and Cysts in the Mediastinum

Anterior mediastinum	Superior mediastinum	Middle mediastinum	Posterior mediastinum
Thymoma	Goiter	Bronchogenic cyst	Neurogenic tumors
Teratoma	Bronchogenic cyst	Lymphomas	Fibrosarcoma
Goiter	Parathyroid adenoma	Pericardial cyst	Lymphomas
Parathyroid adenoma	Myxoma	Plasma cell myeloma	Goiter
Lymphomas	Lymphomas		Xanthofibroma
Lipoma			Gastroenteric cyst
Fibroma			Chondroma
Lymphangioma			Myxoma
Hemangioma			Meningocele
Chondroma			
Thymic cyst			
Rhabdomyosarcoma			

Adapted from Schlumberger, H. G. *Tumors of the Mediastinum.* Washington, D.C. Armed Forces Institute of Pathology, 1951.

TUMORS OF THE MEDIASTINAL LYMPH NODES

LYMPHOMA

The lymphomas commonly involve the hilar and mediastinal lymph nodes and often cause massive enlargement of them. The involvement is characteristically bilateral and the nodes affected produce mass shadows corresponding to their location. The roentgen findings vary widely with the amount and distribution of the enlargement. Often there is a single large mass projecting to both sides of the superior mediastinum with bilateral hilar enlargement. In other patients, individual nodes are outlined, resulting in a more lobulated appearance. The latter is somewhat more common in Hodgkin's disease, while the single massive enlargement is often found in lymphosarcoma. In the lateral view the masses appear in the superior, anterior, and middle mediastinum. When unilateral, the trachea may be displaced but this is not commonly noted in malignant lymphoma. It is not unusual to observe stringy densities extending outward into the pulmonary parenchyma, indicating involvement of the lungs. This results in some blurring of the hilar and mediastinal mass along its outer borders and is somewhat more frequent in Hodgkin's disease than in the others (Fig. 31-9).

METASTASES

Lymph-node metastases are usually a part of generalized lymphogenous spread to the lungs, resulting in enlargement of mediastinal nodes plus strands of density radiating outward from the hilum into the lung fields. Pleural involvement resulting in pleural effusion is commonly associated with this type of disease. Enlarged mediastinal nodes may also be associated with the multiple nodular hematogenous type of metastases. Occasionally enlarged nodes may be the only roentgen manifestation of metastatic disease in the chest. In the latter instance, differentiation between metastasis and malignant lymphoma cannot be made on the basis of roentgen findings alone. A history of primary tumor elsewhere favors metastasis while the presence of lymph-node enlargement elsewhere favors malignant lymphoma. It may be necessary to resort to thoractomy and biopsy if nodes are not available elsewhere for biopsy.

NEUROGENIC TUMORS

Ganglioneuroma and neurofibroma (neurilemmoma) are the two most common tumors of neurogenic origin found in the mediastinum. The neurofibromas arise from intercostal nerves and occur most commonly in the posterior

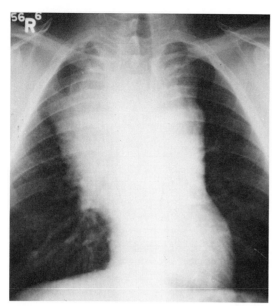

Fig. 31-9. Mediastinal Hodgkin's disease. The mass is bilateral and lobulated. It appears to involve hilar as well as anterior mediastinal nodes.

neuroma. As a general rule the neurofibroma or neurilemmoma tends to be a round mass, while the ganglioneuroma is more elongated, e.g., its vertical diameter is greater than the transverse or sagittal diameter (Fig. 31-11). These neurogenic tumors are usually fairly smooth and clearly defined but occasionally they may be lobulated. They are usually benign but occasionally a neurofibrosarcoma is found in the same location. Rarely a neurogenic tumor may arise from the vagus nerve and present as a middle mediastinal mass. Rarely neuroblastoma may involve the mediastinum. This childhood tumor tends to metastasize widely and grow rapidly. Pheochromocytoma also may occasionally originate in the posterior mediastinum. There are no distinguishing roentgen features. Paraganglioma (chemodectoma) is another rare tumor of neurogenic origin; it may arise anywhere in the mediastinum.

Pleural fluid is occasionally present in patients with neurogenic tumors and does not

mediastinum, where they produce a rounded density that may reach large size (Fig. 31-10). Some of them arise in the region of a spinal foramen and extend into the spinal canal, producing the so-called dumbbell type of tumor. This often results in pressure erosion of the adjacent pedicles and vertebral body. Oblique views are usually necessary to determine the presence or absence of bony involvement and when it is present the diagnosis of neurogenic tumor can be made with great accuracy. Ganglioneuroma arises in the sympathetic ganglia of the thoracic region and also produces a posterior mediastinal tumor mass that may become very large. Occasionally the thoracic neurofibroma may be a manifestation of multiple neurofibromatosis and is then associated with numerous subcutaneous neurofibromas. There are some slight differences which aid in the differentiation of the neurogenic tumors. The neurofibroma tends to have a narrow mediastinal base, as seen in the frontal projection, whereas the ganglioneuroma tends to have a broad mediastinal base. The angle between the tumor and the mediastinum tends to be acute in the neurofibroma and obtuse in the ganglio-

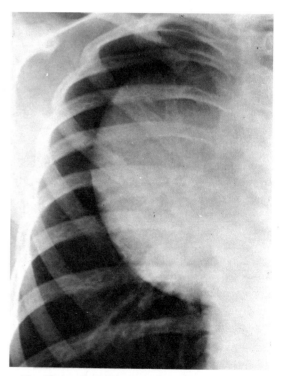

Fig. 31-11. Ganglioneuroma. Large right posterior mediastinal mass. The vertical diameter is greater than the transverse diameter.

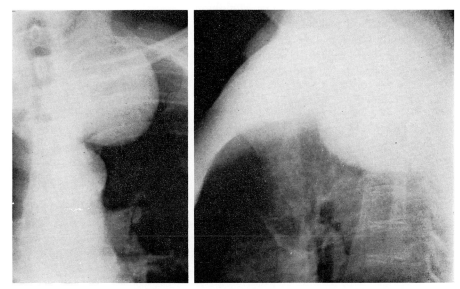

Fig. 31-10. Neurofibroma. Note the smooth outline of the tumor and its posterior location on the lateral view.

necessarily indicate malignancy. Calcification also is rarely seen in these tumors.

TERATOID TUMORS

BENIGN

Mediastinal teratoma is an anterior mediastinal lesion that grows very slowly and may reach great size before producing symptoms. When it contains only ectodermal derivatives it may be called dermoid cyst. Histologic examination usually reveals derivatives of the other germ layers so the term "teratoma" or "teratoid cyst" is more accurate. When benign, it is usually a well-encapsulated cystic tumor that is multilocular and lobulated. Calcification is often present in the wall and it is not uncommon to find calcium, bone, and poorly formed teeth within the mass. The tumor is usually found in young adults. The roentgen findings are those of an eccentric anterior mediastinal mass, the bulk of which extends to one side. Calcification in the wall and within it can be more clearly demonstrated on tomograms or overexposed roentgenograms (Fig. 31-12). It

may be round, oval, or lobulated and is usually clearly defined laterally while the medial wall blends with mediastinal structures. These cysts may become massive in size and produce very few symptoms.

MALIGNANT

This tumor also occupies the anterior mediastinum but grows rapidly and usually causes death within a year of discovery. It produces symptoms and is discovered because of them, unlike the benign teratoma that is often discovered on routine roentgen study of the chest. The roentgen findings are those of an anterior mediastinal mass that is often less clearly defined and more lobulated than benign teratoma. Extension into the lung as well as into mediastinal structures blurs the margins. Pleural extension may result in effusion.

MEDIASTINAL CYSTS

All the mediastinal cysts appear as rounded or oval mass lesions that are smooth and clearly defined. They tend to change slightly in shape with alteration in position and with respiration. Fluoroscopy is helpful in determining motion, alteration on position change, and the absence of expansile pulsations in these cysts.

BRONCHOGENIC CYST

Cysts of bronchogenic origin are lined with ciliated columnar epithelium and are usually asymptomatic. They commonly occur in the

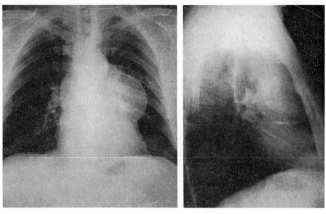

Fig. 31-12. Mediastinal dermoid cyst. *Left,* Frontal view showing large mass projecting to the left below the aortic arch. *Right,* Lateral view in which the mass is observed to lie anteriorly. Note calcification in the wall of the cyst.

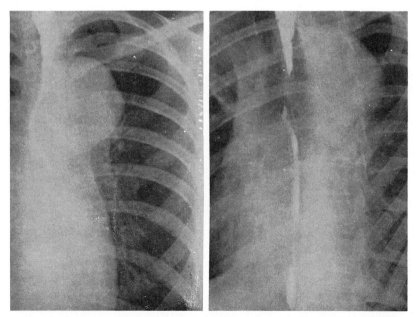

Fig. 31-13. Bronchogenic cyst. *Left,* Clearly defined mediastinal mass on the left overlying the aortic arch. *Right,* The left anterior oblique view shows the mass to be posterior to the aortic arch. Fluoroscopy was helpful in demonstrating lack of expansile pulsation.

superior and middle mediastinum near the trachea and below the carina but may be found anywhere in the mediastinum (Fig. 31-13).

GASTROENTERIC CYST (DUPLICATION)

These cysts probably represent small local duplications of the intestinal tract. They contain secretory cells and may grow to a large size early in life. They produce symptoms because of pressure on mediastinal structures and are often discovered during infancy, usually before the age of 2 years. They appear as large rounded or oval densities in the posterior mediastinum near the esophagus and usually extend to one side of the midline (Fig. 31-14).

NEURENTERIC CYST

This is a rare mediastinal cyst[21] which appears to be formed from a remnant of the neurenteric canal that forms an evanescent communication from the gut through the dorsal midline structures to the dorsal surface of the embryo. The lesion consists of a mediastinal cystic mass which may be continuous with a duplication or giant diverticulum of the intestinal tract and associated with a diaphragmatic hernia. There is also a defect in the anterior aspect of the spine and faulty vertebral development. A fibrous stalk connects the cyst to the meninges in the spinal canal. They may connect with the intestine via a tubular structure extending through the diaphragm to the jejunum.

PERICARDIAL CYST

These cysts usually arise near and are attached to the parietal pericardium. They are lined by flat cells that may be endothelial or mesothelial in origin. They contain clear fluid and are sometimes termed "clear-water" or "simple" cysts. When a small cyst of this type is found in the region of the cardiohepatic angle it may extend into the primary interlobar fissure. The interlobar portion is then "tear-drop" or pear-shaped (Fig. 31-15). The usual location of the oval mass adjacent to the heart and attached to the pericardium is helpful in diagnosis. The pericardial cyst is often basal and

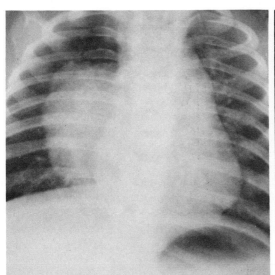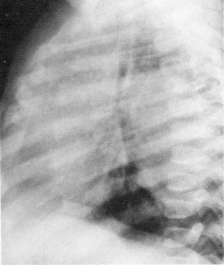

Fig. 31-14. Gastric cyst. The large posterior mediastinal mass on the right resulted in a feeding problem in this infant. It was surgically excised and the symptoms disappeared. The symptoms had been present since birth but had progressed. The infant was 3 months of age when these roentgenograms were obtained. *Left,* Posteroanterior projection. *Right,* Right lateral view shows the posterior location of the cyst.

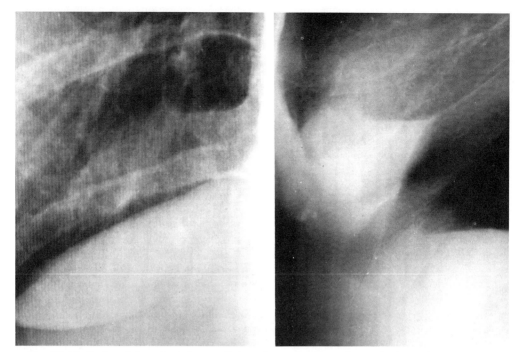

Fig. 31-15. Pericardial cyst at the cardiohepatic angle. Note the typical teardrop appearance in the lateral view.

may simulate a diaphragmatic tumor or a foramen of Morgagni hernia. Diagnostic pneumothorax or diagnostic pneumoperitoneum or both may be necessary to aid in differential diagnosis (Fig. 31-16).

OTHER TUMORS AND MASSES

CYSTIC HYGROMA (LYMPHANGIOMA)

Lymphangioma or cystic hygroma may extend into the superior mediastinum from the neck and produce a tumor mass that can be visualized radiographically. The presence of the spongy mass in the neck plus apparent continuation of it into the superior mediastinum usually permits the diagnosis. This lesion is soft and pliable, and alteration in contour may be visible in different phases of respiration on films or at fluoroscopy. Anterior mediastinal lymphangioma may also occur in the absence of a cervical mass.

INTRATHORACIC THYROID

This is a relatively common tumor noted in the anterior and superior mediastinum, which is usually connected by an isthmus of tissue to the thyroid gland in the neck. This is often wide enough to be recognized roentgenographically so that the connection between the intrathoracic mass and the thyroid is demonstrated. Even if bilateral, it is usually eccentric enough to produce tracheal deviation and often compression; this becomes a significant finding for the diagnosis of intrathoracic goiter. The lateral view often shows posterior displacement of the trachea as well. It is not uncommon to observe calcification within the mass. The intrathoracic thyroid often moves on swallowing but may be fixed. Occasionally it may produce a mass in the posterior mediastinum behind the lower trachea, almost always on the right side. The mass of thyroid tissue may also extend far downward into the inferior aspect of the anterior mediastinum. It may reach great size

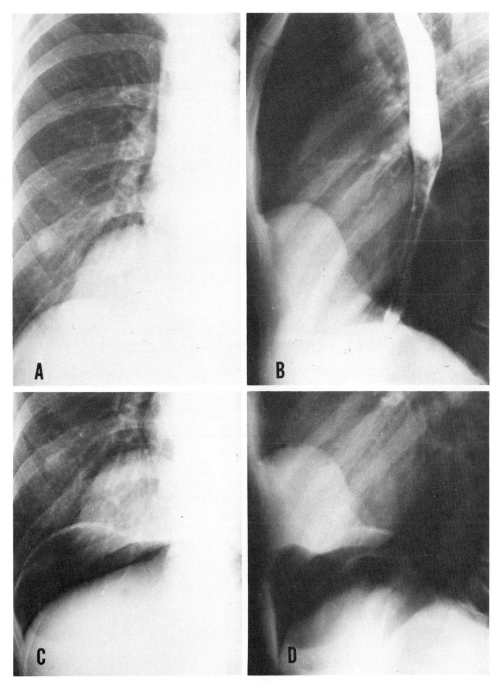

Fig. 31-16. Pericardial cyst. Mass density noted at the cardiohepatic angle inferiorly in *A* and *B*. *C*, Frontal projection of the right lower thorax and upper abdomen following diagnostic pneumoperitoneum, which shows that the mass is above the diaphragm. *D*, Right lateral projection of the same area confirms the finding and indicates that the mass originates in or above the diaphragm.

without producing symptoms. Even though the mediastinal thyroid is posterior in position, there is usually some displacement of the trachea as well as the esophagus. This is helpful in making the diagnosis (Fig. 31-17). When positive, scans using radioactive iodine (^{131}I) are diagnostic; but there may be no function, so a negative scan does not exclude intrathoracic thyroid.

PARATHYROID ADENOMA

This tumor is usually found in the anterior aspect of the superior mediastinum or in the anterior mediastinum. It is usually eccentric and presents to either side. These tumors tend to be relatively small. There is nothing diagnostic about the appearance of the mass as visualized on the roentgenogram. When renal liathiasis or bone le-

sions of hyperparathyroidism are present in association with an anterior mediastinal mass, the diagnosis of parathyroid adenoma is reasonably certain.

THYMIC TUMORS

BENIGN. The benign thymoma is located in the anterior mediastinum at the level of the junction of the heart and great vessels. It grows slowly and may become very large. At times the tumor is in the midline and may be difficult or impossible to visualize in the frontal projection, but is readily visible in oblique or lateral views. Mottled calcification is occasionally noted within it. Myasthenia gravis is found in 50 per cent of patients with thymoma. Of the patients with myasthenia gravis, about 15 per cent have thymic tumors. The patient with myas-

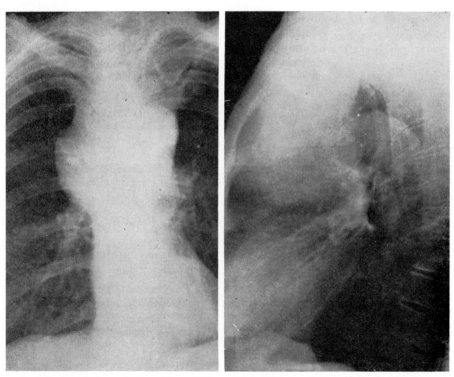

Fig. 31-17. Intrathoracic thyroid. *Left*, Note the mediastinal mass above the right hilum with some mediastinal widening extending up into the neck. The trachea is not well visualized but is deviated to the left and displaced posteriorly. *Right*, Lateral view showing that the mass is in the anterior mediastinum and extends into the anterior aspect of the superior mediastinum. The extension upward, resulting in failure to define the upper aspect of the mass, is typical of intrathoracic thyroid.

thenia gravis should be examined for thymic tumor because of this relationship.

Thymoma may be cystic and contain calcium which outlines the wall and suggests cystic nature of the tumor. Location is similar to that of the solid type of thymoma (Fig. 31-18). There is no way to be certain that a thymic mass is benign or malignant on roentgen examination, however.

MALIGNANT. Early in its development, the thymic malignancy resembles benign thymoma in appearance and location. It grows rapidly, however, and is invasive, so that the margins become blurred. It often becomes very large, extends to both sides of the midline, and then resembles malignant lymphoma. The tumor may be carcinomatous or sarcomatous.

INTRATHORACIC MENINGOCELE

This is a herniation of the meninges laterally to cause a posterior mediastinal mass. It is rare and usually mistaken for the more common posterior mediastinal neurofibroma. Diagnosis is made readily on myelography if the lesion is suspected, since the opaque medium will enter the meningocele when the patient is positioned properly. It is often associated with neurofibromatosis (von Recklinghausen's disease). There may be erosion about the intervertebral foramen through which the meninges protrude and skeletal defects are commonly associated with it. These meningoceles may be single or multiple and unilateral or bilateral. The diagnosis can be made when it is suspected and confirmed by myelography.

MEDIASTINAL LIPOMATOSIS CAUSED BY STEROIDS

The use of long-term, large-dose steroid therapy in renal transplantation and in treatment of various chronic diseases may result in deposition of fat in the mediastinum. The patients usually manifest Cushing's syndrome, often with fat deposition in supraclavicular and epicardial areas as well as in the mediastinum. This is important only in that it must be differentiated from other conditions which may cause mediastinal widening. Roentgen findings consist of mediastinal widening which is relatively radiolucent and poorly defined when compared to other superior mediastinal masses (Fig. 31-19). The trachea is not compressed or displaced, and excess epicardial fat may also be present.

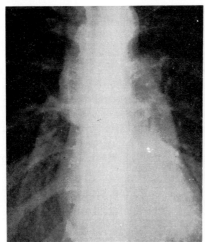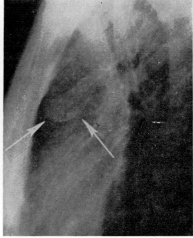

Fig. 31-18. Cystic thymoma. *Left,* The frontal projection shows a mass in the right upper mediastinum. Inferiorly it extends to a point just below the hilum. Superiorly its extent is difficult to outline. *Right,* In the lateral projection the mass is clearly defined inferiorly and posteriorly. Again its superior extent is not outlined. The mottled density noted in the lower part of the mass is caused by calcification there (**arrows**).

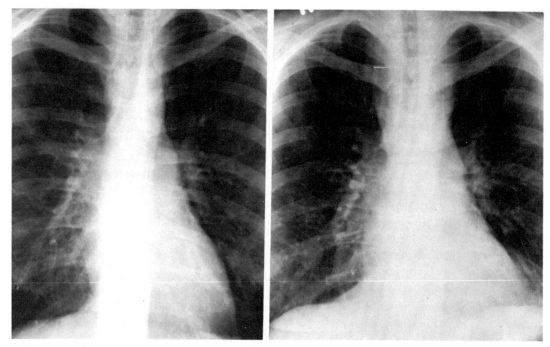

Fig. 31-19. Mediastinal lipomatosis. This 18-year-old female had a renal transplant and was on long-term steroid therapy. *Left,* Initial chest film. *Right,* Follow-up film 1 year later. There is mediastinal widening superiorly which is very poorly defined. There is also some epicardial fat at the apex and at the cardiohepatic angle.

MISCELLANEOUS MASSES

Benign tumors such as lipoma, fibroma, chondroma, and hemangioma occur rarely within the mediastinum. There is nothing characteristic about the roentgen appearance of a lipoma or fibroma. The chondroma may contain a considerable amount of irregular calcification that helps identify it. Hemangioma often is a poorly defined, widespread mass and may contain small rounded calcifications that represent phleboliths. When the latter are present, the diagnosis can be made with a reasonable degree of certainty. Most hemangiomas occur in the anterior mediastinum. They tend to be clearly defined in the anteroposterior projection but are often difficult to outline in the lateral projection. Rarely, pheochromocytoma may occur in the thorax; its posterior location is similar to that of neurogenic tumor. Otherwise unexplained hypertension plus the mass should lead to the suspicion of this tumor. Fibrosarcoma and other sarcomas arising in the mediastinal soft tissues are extremely rare and there is nothing characteristic about their radiographic appearance. Rarely "primary" seminoma or similar germinal cell tumors may occur in the anterior mediastinum. There are no roentgen signs to differentiate them from thymic malignancy or from malignant teratoma.

Extramedullary hematopoiesis may occur in a number of diseases in which there is chronic anemia. Occasionally, the heterotopic bone marrow may develop in the paravertebral region of the thorax, presenting as a posterior mediastinal mass that may be very large. It may be unilateral or bilateral and may extend for some distance along the spine in the posterior mediastinum. Lobulation is usually present. The diagnosis can be suspected if the patient has a long history of anemia.

Occasionally esophageal diverticula may attain large size and present as mediastinal masses. There is usually enough air within them so that a gas-fluid level is demonstrated, indicating the type of lesion. An esophagram will readily outline and define this type of lesion. In achalasia (cardiospasm) of the esophagus this organ becomes grossly dilated and may simulate mediastinal tumor.

Paraspinal abscess secondary to tuberculosis

or other chronic infection of the thoracic spine often produces a shadow that may simulate tumor. The abscesses are usually somewhat spindle-shaped and the density produced merges with the normal paraspinal shadow above and below the mass. Lateral and oblique projections that outline the vertebral bodies and intervertebral discs usually indicate the cause for the lesion, since varying amounts of destruction of one or more vertebral bodies, along with narrowing of the intervening intervertebral disc space, are common findings. There is also calcification within the abscess in many instances. Tumors of the thoracic spine may produce masses but their location is usually clearly defined in lateral views so that there is no difficulty in differentiation between these lesions and mediastinal tumor.

Mediastinal hematoma may also produce a mediastinal mass. Usually there is a history of trauma or of recent surgical procedure so that presumptive diagnosis can be made. Rapid changes in the size of the mass are characteristic when they occur. This is discussed further in Chapter 32 under the heading "Traumatic Aneurysm or Hematoma."

Cardiac disease and lesions of the great vessels within the mediastinum are discussed in the chapter on cardiovascular diseases. Mediastinal emphysema and mediastinal pleural effusion are discussed in the sections on emphysema and on pleural effusion respectively.

THE DIAPHRAGM

The diaphragm is a muscle of respiration that separates the thorax from the abdominal cavity. Its position is described in Chapter 22. There are a number of openings in it through which structures such as the esophagus and aorta pass to enter the abdomen (Fig. 31-20). The superior surface of the diaphragm is readily visualized in the roentgenogram of the normal chest because it is clearly outlined by the radiolucent lung above it. Its lower margin is often visible on the left, at least in part, because there is usually some gas in the fundus of the stomach and gas or fecal material in the splenic flexure of the colon that define its undersurface. On the right side, the liver is of comparable density so that the undersurface of the diaphragm cannot be visualized unless pneumoperitoneum is present. The right diaphragm is usually one interspace higher than the left. In full inspiration the dome of the right leaf of the diaphragm is at the approximate level of the tenth rib posteriorly, the left is at the level of the eleventh rib posteriorly. Using the anterior ribs as landmarks, the dome of the right diaphragm lies between the level of the fifth rib and the level of the sixth interspace measured on the standard 6-foot roentgenogram taken in moderately deep inspiration. It tends to be higher in hypersthenic and in obese patients and may be lower in asthenic subjects. The height of the diaphragm appears to be related to the position of the apex of the heart rather than to the position of the liver; e.g., the low hemidiaphragm is on the side of the heart.

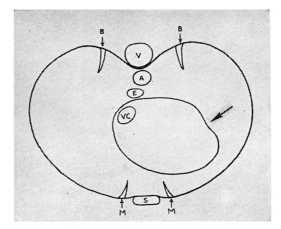

Fig. 31-20. Diagram to show the normal openings and areas of potential weakness in the diaphragm. Sketch is drawn viewing the diaphragm from above downward. The vertebral body (V) and the sternum (S) are labeled for orientation purposes. The letters represent the following: B, foramen of Bochdalek; A, aorta; E, Esophageal hiatus; VC, the opening for the inferior vena cava; M, foramen of Morgagni. The attachment of the pericardium to the diaphragm is also sketched (arrow).

FUNCTIONAL DISTURBANCES OF THE DIAPHRAGM

The most common disturbance is hiccough (singultus). This consists of sudden diaphragmatic contraction associated with closure of the glottis. It is either local in origin, caused by irritation of the diaphragm, or central, in which case it may be produced by encephalitis, uremia, or brain tumor. Occasionally it is hysterical in origin. Attacks are usually very short but occasionally paroxysms may last for months or years. Radiography is of indirect value only since it may serve to identify the irritating lesion producing the contraction. Fluoroscopy can be used to determine the severity of the contraction and to determine whether one or both hemidiaphragms are involved.

Tonic contraction or splinting of the diaphragm often results when basal pleuritis, subphrenic abscess, or trauma has produced diaphragmatic injury. In these instances there is greater or less elevation of the diaphragm, which may be bilateral but is usually unilateral, and may be confined to one portion of a hemidiaphragm. Chest roentgenography outlines the height of the diaphragm and fluoroscopy will reveal the amount and location of the limitation of motion.

PARALYSIS AND PARESIS OF THE DIAPHRAGM

When the diaphragm is paralyzed, it is elevated by intra-abdominal pressure that is greater than the thoracic pressure. The amount of elevation varies considerably and it may be unilateral or bilateral. When paralysis is complete on one side, paradoxical motion is usually visible at fluoroscopy. This means that during inspiration the paralyzed hemidiaphragm rises while the normal hemidiaphragm descends; during expiration the normal hemidiaphragm rises and the paralyzed one descends. This paradoxical motion can be accentuated by having the patient sniff. This causes a rapid but shallow inspiration. In paresis of the diaphragm there may or may not be elevation visible on chest roentgenograms but a lag in contraction of the involved hemidiaphragm is readily visible fluoroscopically and this is also accentuated by having the patient sniff. Normally there may be a slight difference in motion on the two sides. In our experience, the left diaphragm moves slightly more rapidly than the right on deep, rapid inspiration. When there is much difficulty in determining relative diaphragmatic motion on the two sides, fluoroscopy in the lateral decubitus position is helpful, since motion on the dependent side is augmented and comparison is easier with greater excursion.

EVENTRATION OF THE DIAPHRAGM

Eventration of the diaphragm is the term used to describe an abnormal elevation of the diaphragm. It is thought to result from a deficiency of muscular development which may be general or local. The local form may be bilateral, but bilateral general eventration is very rare. There is some difference of opinion as to the cause of eventration. Some observers believe that there is a deficiency of nervous as well as of muscular tissue. The diagnosis is based upon observation of the elevated diaphragm on a chest roentgenogram. There is no disease or tumor visible to produce the elevation and at fluoroscopy the hemidiaphragm involved is usually observed to move. The movement may be normal or diminished and paradoxical motion can be observed on rapid inspiration in some instances. It is often difficult to differentiate from hernia and phrenic paralysis or paresis. When eventration is left-sided, the fundus of the stomach or the splenic flexure of the colon lies adjacent to the undersurface of the diaphragm in both frontal and lateral projections (Fig. 31-21). There is often a long fluid level in the gastric fundus in the upright position. The afferent and efferent limbs of the stomach or colon are widely sepa-

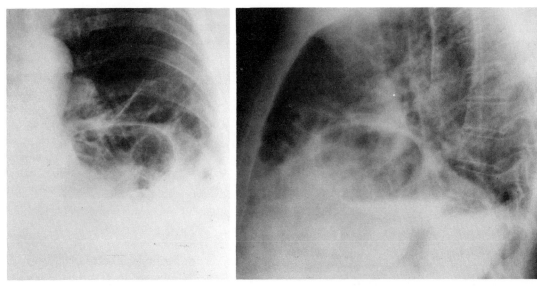

Fig. 31-21. Eventration of the diaphragm. The dome of the left diaphragm is difficult to visualize in the frontal projection (*left*) because of changes in the basal lung on the left. It is more clearly defined in the lateral view (*right*) and is noted to be elevated considerably and generally. The patient experienced respiratory symptoms secondary to poor diaphragmatic function. Surgical repair was done and the diagnosis of congenital eventration was confirmed.

rated in eventration, but are together or nearly so in congenital or acquired hernia, being constricted at the hernial opening.

LOCALIZED EVENTRATION

Local weakness of the diaphragm with upward protrusion of the liver is the most common manifestation of localized eventration. It usually occurs on the anteromedial aspect of the right diaphragm through which a portion of the right lobe of the liver bulges. This has been termed the anteromedial hump of the liver. The smoothly rounded appearance of the bulge is usually characteristic but if it simulates tumor, pneumoperitoneum or preferably liver scan will differentiate. In our experience, primary or metastatic hepatic tumor does not cause this type of local elevation. Local eventrations may occur elsewhere, particularly posteriorly, where upward displacement of the kidney may produce a rounded mass density simulating tumor. This probability should be considered when the mass is comparable in size to the upper pole of

the kidney. When suspected, intravenous urography can be used to outline the kidney and determine its relationship to the diaphragm.

DIAPHRAGMATIC DISPLACEMENTS

In addition to the elevation of the diaphragm noted in eventration, paralysis, and paresis, a number of intrathoracic and intrabdominal conditions may result in elevation of the diaphragm. On the right side, tumors and cysts of the liver, subphrenic abscess, and right renal tumors may elevate the diaphragm generally or locally. On the left side the causes include enlargement of the spleen, left renal tumors, dilatation or tumors of the stomach, and of the splenic flexure of the colon. Ascites, obesity, large intra-abdominal tumors, and pregnancy may result in bilateral elevation. Intrathoracic diseases that decrease pulmonary volume cause elevation on the side involved. This includes pulmonary fibrosis, chronic pleural disease, and atelectasis. The elevation may be relatively uniform or rather irregular. The amount depends upon the severity of the lesion producing it.

Irregularity of the diaphragm superiorly is often secondary to previous pulmonary inflammatory disease. This is termed "tenting" or "adhesive tenting" and is often associated with basal pulmonary fibrosis and obliteration of the costophrenic sulcus.

The diaphragm is displaced downward by lesions that produce an increase in thoracic volume, such as large intrathoracic neoplasms, massive pleural effusion, pulmonary emphysema, and tension pneumothorax. Massive pleural effusion may actually cause inversion of the left diaphragm, displacing the kidney, spleen, and stomach downard. This inversion may produce a pseudomass in the left upper abdominal quadrant which disappears when thoracentesis and removal of pleural fluid is accomplished. Fig. 31-22.

DIAPHRAGMATIC MASSES, INCLUDING HERNIAS

TUMORS

Primary diaphragmatic tumors are rare and may be benign or malignant. The most common benign tumor is lipoma but numerous other benign tumors have been reported; they include fibroma, chondroma, and angioma as well as congenital cysts. The malignant tumors are all sarcomas; fibrosarcoma is the most common. These tumors produce basal masses that usually project above the normal rounded density produced by the diaphragm. They may be smooth or lobulated and vary considerably in size. When the tumor is on the left it may project downward to encroach on the gastric air bubble. The limits of the tumor may then be outlined inferiorly as it projects into the stomach and superiorly as it projects above the diaphragm. It is often necessary to use diagnostic pneumoperitoneum to differentiate a tumor of the diaphragm from an intra-abdominal mass and diagnostic pneumothorax to differentiate it from a mass arising in the basal lung. Roentgen studies serve only to identify a mass, since the various cell types produce no characteristic findings,

therefore surgical exploration is usually indicated when a tumor is found in the diaphragm.

ESOPHAGEAL HIATAL HERNIA

Herniation of all or part of the stomach through the esophageal hiatus into the thorax produces a mass shadow at the left medial base that is often visible on the frontal roentgenogram. Not infrequently, gas and fluid within the thoracic portion of the stomach make the diagnosis apparent on plain-film roentgenograms; if not, the lesion can be readily identified by means of a barium swallow. This examination also serves to identify the occasional diverticulum of the esophagus in this region and to differentiate the esophageal lesions from pulmonary cyst or abscess as well as from diaphragmatic tumor.

FORAMEN OF MORGAGNI HERNIA

This is a rare diaphragmatic hernia that may result in a basal mass shadow, usually in the region of the cardiohepatic angle (Fig. 31-23). This type of hernia is usually small and often contains omentum, but occasionally a portion of bowel may lie within the hernial sac. In the latter instance, the diagnosis may be possible on routine chest roentgenograms but further studies are usually required in the smaller hernias. This includes barium enema examination, which may show upward angulation of the midtransverse colon when the hernial sac contains omentum. The pyloric end of the stomach and proximal duodenum may also be displaced upward toward the diaphragm. In some instances pneumoperitoneum may be necessary to make a diagnosis. Rarely, the liver may herniate through the foramen of Morgagni into the thorax in infants and young children. This is usually accompanied by partial obstruction of the inferior vena cava. Inferior vena cavography demonstrates the kinking and partial obstruction.

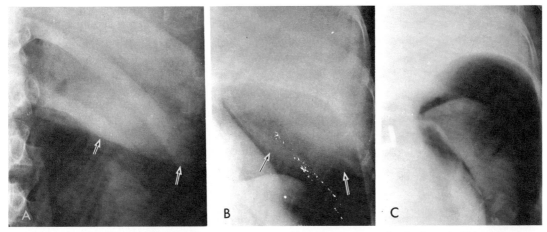

Fig. 31-22. Inversion of the diaphragm caused by massive left pleural effusion. *A,* This film shows the mass in the left upper quadrant which was continuous with the massive left pleural effusion (**arrows**). *B,* Pneumoperitoneum shows the inverted diaphragm projecting downward into the abdominal cavity (**arrows**). *C,* Pneumoperitoneum following thoracentesis showing the diaphragm to have assumed its normal upward convexity.

OTHER DIAPHRAGMATIC HERNIA

Herniation through the pleuroperitoneal foramen of Bochdalek is often large, and loops of bowel can be visualized and identified so that differential diagnosis is not difficult. When the hernia is smaller and does not contain gas filled bowel, the diagnosis is more difficult. Occasionally the left kidney projects upward through a weak area in the posterior portion of the left hemidiaphragm and may be mistaken for tumor. The high position of the kidney can sometimes be determined on the chest roentgenogram; if not, intravenous urography can be used to make the diagnosis.

Congenital defects of the diaphragm may be large or small, with absence of most of one diaphragmatic leaf or a part of it. The larger defects may be associated with herniation of a large proportion of abdominal viscera into the thorax. This may cause acute respiratory insufficiency in the newborn, making it a surgical emergency. The roentgen findings vary with the amount of herniation. Gas-filled bowel is recognized within the thorax when the defect is on the left. The liver may also extend into the thorax when the defect is on the right. The remaining diaphragm is often visible; oblique

and lateral views will often demonstrate the site of the defect.

Traumatic hernia of the diaphragm usually results from severe crushing types of injury to the abdomen, thorax, or both. The diaphragm may be ruptured completely with defects in the parietal pleura and peritoneum. Then there is no hernial sac. In other instances either the pleura or peritoneum may form a sac. The left diaphragm is involved in 95 per cent of cases. There may not be immediate herniation of abdominal viscera into the thorax, so serial films are sometimes necessary. Occasionally the traumatic rupture of the diaphragm is followed years later by a traumatic hernia. The roentgen findings are similar to those in the congenital defects with herniation. Oblique and lateral views often permit localization of the defect. If necessary, a barium enema or barium meal may be given to identify the parts of the gastrointestinal tract within the hernia.

EPICARDIAL FAT PADS

Localized fat deposits are often present at the cardiac apex and in the cardiohepatic angle. Those at the apex are usually readily

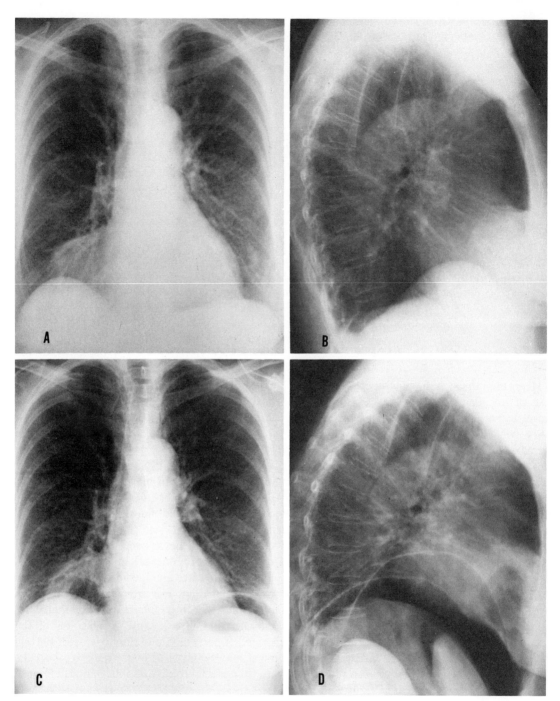

Fig. 31-23. Foramen of Morgagni hernia. *A,* Frontal projection showing mass at the cardiohepatic angle. *B,* Lateral projection showing the mass to be anterior. *C,* Frontal projection following diagnostic pneumoperitoneum showing a small amount of gas between the diaphragm and the liver, and the somewhat larger amount of gas extending up into the cardiohepatic mass. *D,* Left lateral view of the upper abdomen and lower thorax following larger pneumoperitoneum, showing a considerable amount of gas below the diaphragm on both sides and a moderate amount of it extending up through the foramen of Morgagni into the hernial sac, which presents as a cardiohepatic mass.

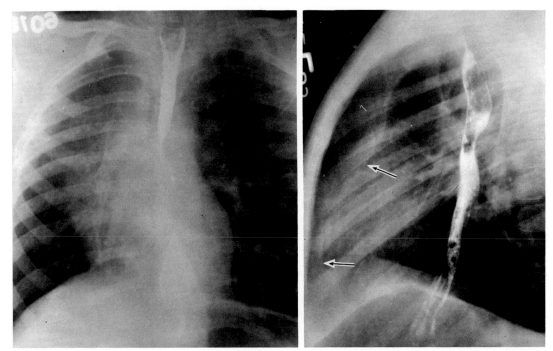

Fig. 31-24. Accessory diaphragm on the right. *Left,* Note the mediastinal shift to the right with poor definition of mediastinal structures on the involved side. There is also hazy density in the medial lung in the upper half of the right hemithorax. *Right,* Lateral projection showing a somewhat curved line resembling an anteriorly displaced major fissure except that it extends down to the diaphragm anteriorly **(arrows)**. An aortogram of this patient showed an anomalous artery originating below the diaphragm supplying a portion of the right lower lobe.

identified. When the amount of fat is unusually great it can produce a mass in the cardiohepatic angle that simulates foramen of Morgagni hernia or diaphragmatic tumor. Deposits of fat are usually of less density than the adjacent heart and diaphragm but this difference in density is small and not entirely reliable since the omentum, frequently present in foramen of Morgagni hernia, is of similar density. It is probable that small foramen of Morgagni hernia is sometimes the cause of the shadow, but it is usually asymptomatic and the differentiation is then of no clinical importance. The fat pads tend to occur in obese patients and when a fat pad is present in the cardiohepatic angle, there is usually a fat pad at the cardiac apex. The association of these densities is of some diagnostic importance.

ACCESSORY DIAPHRAGM

This anomaly, sometimes termed duplication of the diaphragm, is very rare and usually occurs on the right side. It consists of a sheet of fibrous and muscular tissue extending from the anterior aspect of the normal diaphragm, upward and posteriorly to insert along the fifth to seventh rib. It parallels the major fissure, usually extends into it to separate the lower lobe from the upper and middle lobes. It is usually attached to the pericardium medially and has a medial hiatus. Pulmonary anomalies associated with accessory diaphragm include partial fissure anomalies, aplasia or hypoplasia of a lobe, partial division of the lower lobe by the anomalous diaphragm, and anomalous pulmonary vascular supply including lower lobe venous drainage into the inferior vena cava and anomalous arterial supply to the lower lobe from the aorta.

Roentgen findings include shift of mediastinum to the involved side because of hypoplasia, lack of clarity of the mediastinum on the same side with hazy density of the central lung field. On the lateral view the accessory diaphragm may be visible; it resembles the major fissure but extends to the diaphragm and is more anterior in position than the normal fissure (Fig. 31-24). Bronchography may show the lobar hypoplasia and angiography the anomalous arterial supply and venous drainage that often accompanies this anomaly.

REFERENCES AND SELECTED READINGS

1. BERNE, A. S., and HEITZMAN, E. R.: The roentgenologic signs of pedunculated pleural tumors. *Am. J. Roentgenol. Radium Ther. Nucl. Med.* 87: 892, 1962.

2. CAMPBELL, J. A.: The diaphragm in roentgenology of the chest. *Radiol. Clin. North Am.* 1: 395, 1963.

3. DAVIS, V. E., and SALKIN, D.: Intrathoracic gastric cysts. *JAMA* 135: 218, 1947.

4. DAVIS, W. S., and ALLEN, R. P.: Accessory diaphragm: Duplication of the diaphragm. *Radiol. Clin. North Am.* VI: 253, 1968.

5. FINBY, N., and STEINBERG, I.: Roentgen aspects of pleural mesothelioma. *Radiology* 65: 169, 1955.

6. FLEISCHNER, F. G.: Atypical arrangement of free pleural effusion. *Radiol. Clin. North Am.* 1: 347, 1963.

7. FRIEDMAN, R. L.: Infrapulmonary pleural effusions. *Am. J. Roentgenol. Radium Ther. Nucl. Med.* 71: 613, 1954.

8. HANSEN, K. F.: Idiopathic fibrosis of the mediastinum as a cause of superior vena caval syndrome. *Radiology* 85: 433, 1965.

9. HESSEN, I.: Roentgen examination of pleural fluid. *Acta Radiol. Suppl. 86,* 1951.

10. HUTCHINSON, W. B., and FRIEDENBERG, M. J.: Intrathoracic mesothelioma. *Radiology* 80: 937, 1963.

11. INADA, K., KAWAI, K., KATSUMURA, T., and NAKANO, A.: Giant lymph node hyperplasia of the mediastinum. *Am. Rev. Tuberc.* 79: 232, 1959.

12. KATZ, S., and REED, H. R.: Unusual pleural effusions. *Radiology* 45: 147, 1945.

13. KEEGAN, J. M.: Hemangioma of the mediastinum. *Am. J. Roentgenol. Radium Ther. Nucl. Med.* 69: 66, 1953.

14. KEIRNS, M. M.: Tumors of the diaphragm. *Radiology* 58: 542, 1952.

15. KIRKLIN, B. R., and HODGSON, J. R.: Roentgenologic characteristics of diaphragmatic hernia. *Am. J. Roentgenol. Radium Ther. Nucl. Med.* 58: 77, 1947.

16. LAXDAL, O. E., McDOUGALL, H., and MELLEN, G. W.: Congenital eventration of the diaphragm. *N. Engl. J. Med.* 250: 401, 1954.

17. LEIGH, T. F.: Mass lesions of the mediastinum. *Radiol. Clin. North Am.* 1: 377, 1963.

18. LULL, G. F., JR., and WINN, D. F., JR.: Chronic fibrous mediastinitis due to *Histoplasma capsulatum. Radiology* 73: 367, 1959.

19. MAIER, H. C.: Lymphatic cysts of the mediastinum. *Am. J. Roentgenol. Radium Ther. Nucl. Med.* 73: 15, 1955.

20. MEIGS, J. V., and CASS, J. W.: Hydrothroax and ascites in association with fibroma of the ovary. *Am. J. Obstet. Gynecol.* 33: 249, 1937.

21. NEUHAUSER, E. B. D., HARRIS, G. B. C., and BERRETT, A.: Roentgenographic features of neurenteric cysts. *Am. J. Roentgenol. Radium Ther. Nucl. Med.* 79: 235, 1958.

22. PAUL, L. W.: Basal mass shadows in chest roentgenograms. *Tex. Med.* 52: 1, 1956.

23. PAUL, L. W.: Diseases of the mediastinum. *Radiology* 40: 10, 1943.

24. PRICE, J. E., JR., and RIGLER, L. G.: Widening of the mediastinum resulting from fat accumulation. *Radiology* 96: 497, 1970.

25. ROSENBLUM, D., NUSSBAUM, A., and SCHWARTZ, S.: Partial obstruction of the inferior vena cava by herniation of the liver through the foramen of Morgagni. *Radiology* 68: 399, 1957.

26. SENGPIEL, G. W., RUZICKA, F. F., and LODMELL, E. A.: Lateral intrathoracic meningocele. *Radiology* 50: 515, 1948.

27. SWINGLE, J. D., LOGAN, R., and JUHL, J. H.: Inversion of the left hemidiaphragm. *JAMA 208:* 863, 1969.

28. THOMPSON, J. V.: Mediastinal tumors and cysts. *Int. Abst. Surg.* 84: 195, 1947.

29. WEISS, W., BOUCOT, K. R., and GEFTER, W. I.: Localized interlobar effusion in congestive heart failure. *Ann. Intern. Med.* 38: 1177, 1953.

32

THE CARDIOVASCULAR SYSTEM

METHODS OF EXAMINATION

Roentgen study of the heart and great vessels is an essential part of the examination of patients suspected of having disease involving these structures. In some conditions the diagnosis can be made by means of roentgen methods alone, but it is important to recognize that roentgenographic and fluoroscopic studies form only a part of the complete examination and that the findings must be correlated with clinical history, physical findings, and electrocardiographic and catheterization studies to obtain a complete picture of cardiovascular disease. On roentgen examination, the size and shape of the heart can be determined in various projections and diseases of the pulmonary artery and aorta may be visualized. In addition, the roentgenogram furnishes a permanent record of the cardiac size and shape.

ROENTGENOGRAPHY

Roentgen examination of the heart requires a minimum of four projections: Posteroanterior, left anterior oblique at approximately 60°, right anterior oblique at approximately 45°, and lateral. The films are taken at a 6-foot distance, in the upright position, and in moderately deep inspiration. Magnification resulting

from divergent distortion is minimized by taking anterior oblique views to place the heart closer to the film (with the anterior chest adjacent to film) in addition to the posteroanterior position for the frontal projection. A left lateral view (with the left side adjacent to film) also tends to minimize magnification. We use a suspension of micronized barium to outline the esophagus as an aid in determining position and size of the aortic arch and left-sided heart chambers.

FLUOROSCOPY

Fluoroscopy is another method for examination of the heart. It is useful for determination of the amplitude and direction of pulsation in varying degrees of rotation. The presence of calcification within the heart can be determined more readily by fluoroscopy than by any other means. Examination of the pulmonary vessels can also be accomplished. The examination is used only when it is important to study motion of the heart or great vessels, and to determine the presence of calcification in the heart.

The procedure used in fluoroscopy varies with the indication for the examination as well as with the individual examiner. The examination should be systematic and the patient should be examined in frontal, both oblique, and lateral projections. It is sometimes of value to fluoroscope patients in recumbency as well as in the upright position; a thick, micronized barium suspension can be used to outline the esophagus.

There are several disadvantages in cardiac fluoroscopy, one of the most important of which is the amount of radiation to which the patient is exposed. This can be kept to a minimum by observing the rules described in Chapter 22. The second disadvantage is distortion. Because the distance between the target of the x-ray tube and the patient is short, there is considerable enlargement of the cardiac silhouette and distortion of other thoracic structures. This can be decreased by using longer distances between target and the patient and by using a small shutter opening, producing the central beam effect. The third disadvantage is lack of permanent record. This is obviated to a certain extent by the use of spot films taken during fluoroscopy and by roentgenograms taken following this procedure. We prefer to study roentgenograms on each patient before doing fluoroscopy, in order to thoroughly understand the diagnostic problems involved and to save fluoroscopic time.

ANGIOCARDIOGRAPHY

This method of contrast cardiac visualization has been used widely for examination of all types of cardiac and pulmonary diseases (Fig. 32-1). The technique and indications are discussed briefly in Chapter 22. The method is used in the diagnosis of acquired cardiac disease and congenital cardiac malformations. Selective angiocardiography in which a small amount of opaque medium (an organic iodide) is injected into the desired chamber or vessel during cardiac catheterization is also used extensively.

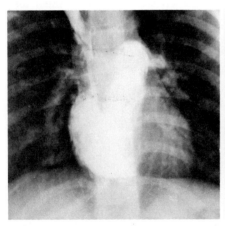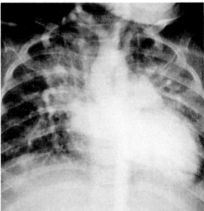

Fig. 32-1. Normal angiocardiogram. *Left,* Filling of the right side of the heart. Some medium is in the superior vena cava and can be seen entering the right atrium. The right ventricle is partially obscured by the atrium. Note the relative radiolucency of the left side of the heart. The pulmonary outflow tract and artery are well visualized but there is no opacification of the branches of the pulmonary artery as yet. *Right,* This is a later phase in a younger child to show filling of the left side of the heart. The left ventricle is clearly defined, making up the left lower cardiac border; the aorta and its major thoracic branches are clearly outlined. The left atrium is also fairly well filled and is noted to overlie the root of the aorta. The atrial appendage projects to the left above the left ventricle. A considerable amount of opaque material remains within the pulmonary system. Detail is obscured so that pulmonary veins are not clearly defined.

CORONARY ARTERIOGRAPHY

Selective catheterization of the coronary arteries followed by injection of a contrast medium (one of the organic iodides) is used in combination with cineradiography or rapid filming to visualize the coronary arteries. Arterial structures are more clearly outlined than in the method of injecting the contrast medium into the supravalvular region of the aorta. Details of technique are beyond the scope of this volume.

RETROGRADE AORTOGRAPHY

This examination consists of the injection of one of the organic iodides into the aorta via a catheter introduced into one of its major branches. The examination has a place in the investigation of patients with certain diagnostic problems relating to the aortic arch. Coronary arteriography can be done by variations of this method.

It is used in infants with congestive heart failure in whom there is evidence of a left-to-right shunt and in whom patent ductus arteriosus is suspected. Coarctation of the aorta in infancy may also cause congestive heart failure and the lesion can be defined by aortography. In adults it is used to define anomalies of the aortic arch and its branches as well as in the study of the aortic valve and the coronary arteries.

TOMOGRAPHY

This method of examination has also been described in Chapter 22. Its use in the study of the heart and great vessels is limited. Calcification in coronary vessels has been identified and calcification in the mitral valve has also been visualized on tomograms. The method has recently been used in the study of coarctation of the aorta. All these studies have been on an investigative basis and the examination is not generally used in clinical study of the cardiovascular system.

DETERMINATION OF CARDIAC SIZE

The size of the heart is related to body weight and height as well as to surface area, sex, and age. A number of methods of correlation of these factors with cardiac size, as measured on the roentgenogram, have been described. It is unfortunate that in the borderline cases where determination of possible cardiac enlargement is most needed, the mathematical formulas are most faulty since there is a normal variation of approximately plus or minus 10 per cent. Numerous factors such as thoracic deformities, pulmonary diseases, and abdominal diseases that elevate or depress the diaphragm affect the size of the cardiac silhouette. Because the line between the normal and the abnormal size cannot be sharply drawn in an individual patient, most of the methods of measurement are chiefly of statistical value. These methods are usually based on direct measurement on teleoroentgenograms. The most commonly used are: (1) measurement of transverse diameters; (2) measurement of surface area; and (3) cardiothoracic ratio. The transverse diameter of the heart is the sum of the maximum projections of the heart to the right and to the left of the midline, using care not to include epicardial fat or other noncardiac structures in the measurement (Fig. 32-2). The diameter can then be compared with the theoretical transverse diameter of the heart for various heights and weights as described by Ungerleider and Clark.[60] Surface area estimations based on artificial construction of the base of the heart and of the diaphragmatic contour of the heart have been worked out by Hodges and Eyster.[21] Nomograms showing relationship of the frontal area of the heart as predicted by height and weight to the measured area using the long and broad diameters of the heart have been published by Ungerleider and Gubner.[61] A nomogram used for measuring children's hearts has been published by Meyer.[41] The cardiothoracic ratio is the ratio between the transverse cardiac diameter and the greatest internal diameter of the thorax, measured on the frontal teleoroentgenogram.

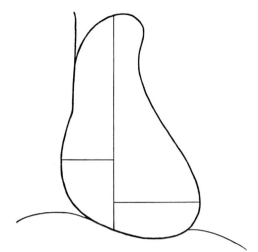

Fig. 32-2. Sketch showing method of measuring transverse diameter of the heart. The sum of the length of the horizontal projections from the vertical line is the transverse diameter.

This is the easiest and quickest method of measurement of cardiac size; an adult heart that measures more than one-half of the internal diameter of the chest is considered enlarged. The method is gross and inaccurate, since the cardiothoracic ratio varies widely with variations in body habitus. It can be used as a rough estimate of cardiac size, however.

These are a few of the many methods described; there are a number of objections to each of them. The objections are largely to the use of such methods in borderline cases, because the numerical exactness of the various measurements is not matched by the reliability of the method. Most of the measurements are relatively simple and easy to apply and do serve as a basis for discrimination between hearts that are obviously normal and those obviously enlarged. They are accurate enough for most statistical studies.

THE NORMAL HEART

THE ADULT HEART

The heart and its major vessels occupy the middle mediastinum and produce a uniform density that is readily recognized on the roentgenogram. The density of the great vessels and of the blood within the heart is comparable, so that the contours of the silhouette are visible in contrast to the adjacent radiolucent lungs. The inferior cardiac border is of density comparable to that of the diaphragm and often is not clearly defined. On the right side the shadow of the liver below the diaphragm blends into that of the heart but on the left side there is often enough air in the stomach immediately below the dome of the diaphragm to outline the left inferior border of the heart. Marked individual variations are noted in the relationships inferiorly so that in some patients the inferior border is difficult or impossible to define while in others it is clearly outlined. The heart lies two-thirds to the left of the midline and one third to the right in the average normal.

THE POSTEROANTERIOR PROJECTION

In this projection the right side of the heart border is divided into two segments. The lower segment is usually convex and represents the lateral border of the right atrium. This segment is often separated from the upper border by an indentation. The upper segment is nearly vertical in the young adult and is usually formed by the superior vena cava. In older adults, the aorta tends to dilate and elongate so that the right upper border becomes more convex. The convexity represents the right lateral aspect of the ascending aortic arch. In asthenic patients with vertical heart, it is sometimes possible to outline the reflection of the pericardium down to the inferior vena cava. It appears as a small straight or slightly concave downward continuation of the convex shadow of the right atrium. On the left side there are usually three visible segments. The uppermost is rounded and convex laterally. It represents the aortic knob, or transverse aortic arch. The descending aorta may also form a portion of the left border, particularly in the patients with vertical hearts. The left lateral wall of the aorta can often be followed downward in the left paraspinal area nearly to the diaphragm, particularly on overpenetrated films. Immediately below this is another short segment, the contour of which varies considerably. It represents the pulmonary artery and occasionally its left main branch. In most normal adults it is straight or slightly convex. Considerable prominence of the pulmonary artery is a common finding in normal young females and should not be considered abnormal. The left pulmonary artery passes over the lower portion of the left main bronchus and the main pulmonary artery arises just below this bronchus as a general rule. There is some variability, but the left auricular appendage usually forms a short segment of the left border of the heart below the pulmonary artery. It is likely that in some patients a portion of the distal right ventricular outflow tract may be border-forming in this area. The left ventricle forms the remainder of the left cardiac margin, by far the largest segment of it, including the apex. The contour of this border is usually dependent upon the habitus of the patient. It tends to be relatively straight and descends sharply in the asthenic individual while in the hypersthenic person it is convex and angles outward considerably. There is then a considerable range between these two extremes of vertical and transverse cardiac configuration. There is some difference of opinion, but the wide use of angiocardiography has demonstrated rather clearly that the left auricular appendage does not project beyond the left ventricle along the left border of the heart in the normal. In patients with disease resulting in enlargement of the left atrium, the appendage does project to the left of the ventricle and usually produces a convexity immediately below the level of the pulmonary artery. The amount of this change varies with the amount and type of left atrial enlargement. These various segments can usually be identified on the roentgenogram, and at fluoroscopy the difference in pulsations is an additional aid in the identification of the chambers and segments. The cardiac apex usually forms the lower left border of the heart and is usually at or near the level of the dome of the diaphragm; it is somewhat angular, with the apex of the angle rounded (Fig. 32-3). A shadow that is less than the density of the heart often extends lateral to it. This represents the apical fat pad.

THE RIGHT ANTERIOR OBLIQUE PROJECTION

In this projection the patient is rotated to his left 45° so that the right anterior chest wall is nearest the cassette and the left posterior chest wall is nearest the tube. In this projection the left or most anterior cardiac border consists of the ascending aortic arch, the pulmonary artery, pulmonary conus,* right ventricle, and a portion of the left ventricle, from above downward. If the patient is rotated more than 45°, an increasing amount of the left border is made up of right ventricle accompanied by a decrease in the left ventricular contribution to this border. The posterior (right) contour in this projection is formed by the left atrium, right atrium, and a short segment of the inferior vena cava from above downward. These contours are outlined in Fig. 32-4. This projection is useful in detecting enlargement of the left atrium and in determining the prominence of the pulmonary outflow tract and artery.

THE LEFT ANTERIOR OBLIQUE PROJECTION

In this position the patient is turned to his right about 60° so the left anterior chest is nearest the cassette while the right posterior chest is nearest the tube. In this projection the anterior (right) contour is formed by the ascending aorta, the right atrial appendage, right atrium, and the right ventricle from above downward. In some instances the right atrium forms much of the lower anterior border in this projection, however. The posterior (left) contour is formed by the left atrium above and the left ventricle below. Occasionally the shallow indentation representing the atrioventricular groove can be outlined in this projection. The contours are indicated on Fig. 32-5. The left

---

* The terms "pulmonary conus" and "infundibulum" are used interchangeably to indicate the infundibular portion (conus infundibularis) or outflow tract, of the right ventricle.

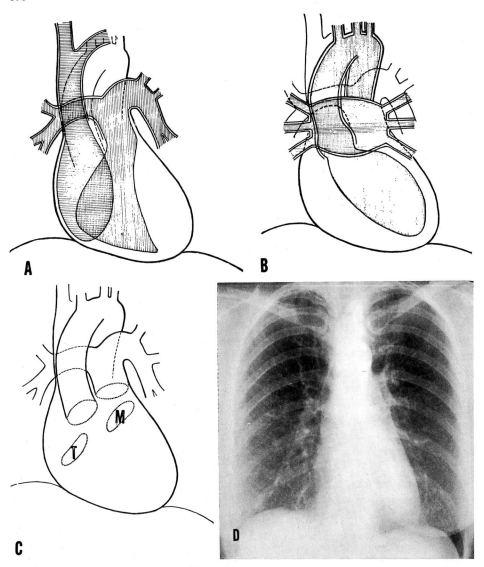

Fig. 32-3. The normal heart, frontal projection. *A,* Diagram to show the relative position of the right heart chambers in the anteroposterior projection. **Horizontal lines** outline the vena cava and right atrium. Vertical lines outline the right ventricle, pulmonary artery, and its major branches. The aortic arch is also indicated. *B,* The left side of the heart in frontal projection. Note that the left ventricle forms most of the left border of the heart. The position of the left atrium in the diagram is slightly above its usual position. *C,* Sketch to show approximate position of valves in the posteroanterior projection. **M,** Mitral valve; **T,** tricuspid valve. Aortic and pulmonic rings noted at root of these arteries. *D,* Roentgenogram showing the normal cardiovascular silhouette. There are many variations as indicated in the text. (Redrawn from Dotter, C. T., and Steinberg, I.[7])

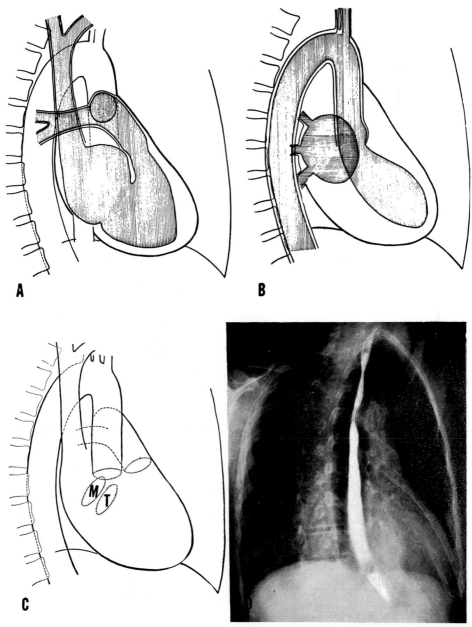

Fig. 32-4. The normal heart. Right anterior oblique projection. *A,* The right side of the heart. The vena cava, right side of the heart, and the pulmonary artery are outlined by vertical lines. *B,* The left side of the heart. Note that the left atrium forms the left upper posterior contour, and the apex of the left ventricle forms the lower anterior contour. *C,* Sketch to show the approximate position of the valves in the right anterior oblique position. **M,** Mitral valve; **T,** Tricuspid valve. Aortic and pulmonic rings noted at roots of these arteries. *D,* Roentgenogram in the right anterior oblique projection showing the normal cardiac configuration. Barium in esophagus shows no displacement of it. (Redrawn from Dotter, C. T., and Steinberg, I.[7])

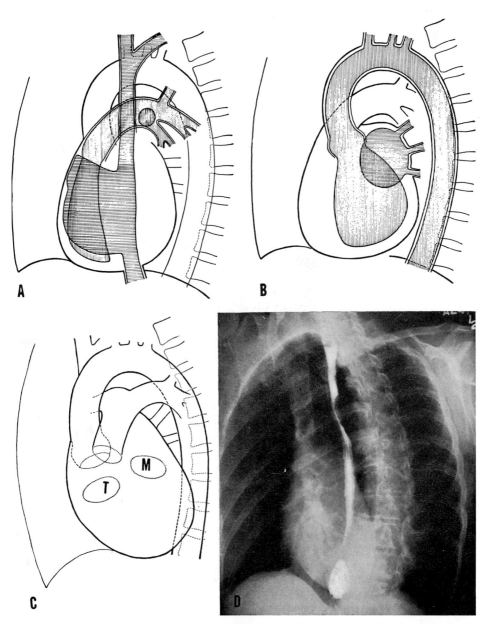

Fig. 32-5. The normal heart. Left anterior oblique projection. *A,* The right side of the heart. The vena cava and the right atrium are outlined by horizontal lines. The right ventricle and outflow tract, along with the pulmonary artery, are outlined by vertical lines. The aortic arch is also indicated. The diagram is a somewhat exaggerated left oblique projection. Note that the anterior contour is made up of the right atrium and ventricle. *B,* The left side of the heart. The left atrium is outlined by horizontal lines, the left ventricle and aorta by vertical lines. The pulmonary artery is also indicated. *C,* Sketch to show approximate position of the valves in the left anterior oblique position. **M,** Mitral valve; **T,** tricuspid valve. Aortic and pulmonic rings noted at roots of these arteries. *D,* The left anterior oblique roentgenogram showing the normal cardiac contour in this projection. Normal esophageal relationships outlined by barium within the esophagus. (Redrawn from Dotter, C. T., and Steinberg, I.[7])

anterior oblique view is also used in examination of the aorta, since the arch is "opened," with very little overlapping.

THE LATERAL PROJECTION

In this view the anterior contour of the cardiovascular silhouette is formed by the ascending aorta, the pulmonary artery, the pulmonary conus, and the right ventricle from above downward. The posterior silhouette is formed by the left atrium and left ventricle from above downward. The contours are indicated in Figure 32-6, except that slight rotation into the lateral projects the right ventricle anteriorly to form the lower anterior contour (Fig. 32-6).

THE HEART IN INFANCY AND CHILDHOOD

At birth the right ventricle is relatively large and is approximately the same size as the left ventricle. During early life the left ventricle

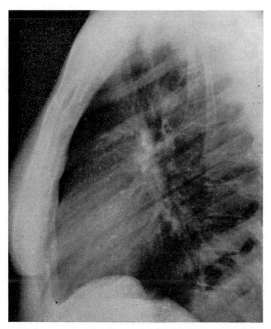

Fig. 32-6. The normal heart shown in lateral roentgenogram. Contours are described in text and are similar to those of Figure 32-5.

grows more rapidly than the right and its wall becomes thicker. The heart is globular in shape in the newborn and extends to the right almost as far as it does to the left in contrast to the adult heart, two-thirds of which lies to the left of the midline in the average normal. In addition to the globular shape noted on the frontal projection in infancy, the chambers and great vessels are not clearly defined. There is great variability in the size and shape of the heart in the newborn and during the first few weeks of life. Therefore the diagnosis of cardiac enlargement should be made with caution. There is often more prominence in the region of the pulmonary artery and right ventricular outflow tract than in the adult and the aortic knob is not readily visible in the newborn and in the young infant. There is frequently enough thymic enlargement so that the cardiac base and great vessels are obscured. As a rule the heart maintains its globular shape for the first 6 months of life. Then it begins to descend in the thorax and as it does, the long axis shifts from horizontal to a more oblique and then to an obliquely vertical position. This is a gradual process and at 5 to 7 years of age the silhouette approaches that of the adult heart, although the ascending aortic arch and knob are not as prominent as they later become. As in the adult, the general contour of the heart is related to body habitus. This becomes apparent in the 5- to 10-year-old child.

Measurements of cardiac size in children show that the size of the heart in relation to the thoracic size is somewhat greater than in adults. This is particularly true when the cardiothoracic ratio is used as an indication of relative heart size. The long axis of the heart tends to be more horizontal in infants and children than in adults so the cardiothoracic index ranges from an upper limit of 0.65 in the first year to 0.50 in the fifth year and from then on until the early teens the ratio is in the range of 0.50. Measurements of the heart in childhood are subject to the same errors as indicated in the discussion on heart size in the adult, and there is the additional factor of inability to control the depth of respiration in infants and young children.

THE NORMAL AORTA

The border-forming contours of the aorta have been mentioned above and are outlined in Figures 32-3 through 32-5. The right lateral contour of the ascending aorta is partially border-forming in adults with aortic dilatation or elongation. The medial border of the ascending aorta is not visible in the frontal projection but the superior and lateral borders of the aortic knob are visualized as the upper left margin of the cardiovascular shadow and in older adults a portion of the descending aorta may be border-forming just below the aortic knob. It is often possible to outline the descending aorta even though it is not border-forming. It appears as a slightly convex, linear shadow extending downward, overlying the left upper cardiac silhouette. In the right anterior oblique view the upper anterior portion of the cardiovascular silhouette is formed by the ascending aorta. In this view the descending arch and part of the thoracic aorta can often be outlined posterior to the cardiac silhouette. In the left anterior oblique view the aortic arch is more clearly defined. Again the ascending arch forms the upper anterior portion of the cardiovascular silhouette and the transverse and descending portions of the arch, as well as the remaining thoracic aorta, are often visible in this projection. The aorta is often clearly defined in older adults in whom arteriosclerotic changes have resulted in deposition of calcium in the aortic walls. With the development of arteriosclerosis associated with advancing age the aorta becomes elongated so that the ascending arch becomes more prominent and its silhouette more convex. The aortic knob also becomes prominent and larger in diameter and there is often considerable tortuosity of the aorta, which is the result of elongation.

Numerous methods of aortic measurement have been described. They are subject to the same errors as the various mathematical formulas used in determining cardiac size. The measurements are most faulty in the borderline group in which accurate determination is most necessary. There is a gradual decrease in diameter of the aorta as it is more distant from the heart so that the ascending portion of the arch is the widest, followed by the transverse, the descending, and the lower thoracic aorta. Dotter and Steinberg[7] measured the inner diameter of the aorta by means of angiocardiography and observed a wide range. In 100 patients the diameter of the ascending aorta ranged from 16 to 38 mm with an average of 28.6 mm. Measurements elsewhere showed comparable wide ranges.

In addition to visualization of the aorta on roentgenograms taken in various projections, this structure is occasionally studied by means of fluoroscopy. It is usually not difficult to identify because of its typical pulsation and appearance. Aortography is often used when localized density continuous with the aorta cannot be differentiated from aortic aneurysm on the roentgenograms.

THE PERICARDIUM

The pericardium is a closed endothelium-lined sac that envelops the heart. It consists of a visceral layer covering the heart and a parietal layer reflected to form a continuous sac. It contains 15 to 25 cc of clear fluid. The parietal pericardium fuses with the diaphragm below and the mediastinal pleura laterally and anteriorly except in the sternal area, where there is no pleura. The reflection of the parietal pericardium occurs in a line that begins at the superior vena cava above its junction with the right atrium on the right side and continues to the left over the anterior aspect of the ascending aorta to the pulmonary artery, which is covered by pericardium nearly to the level of the ligamentum arteriosum. Posteriorly the pericardium extends up as far as the proximal superior vena cava and down to the inferior vena cava. The pericardium cannot be visualized roentgenographically in the normal. The apical fat pad frequently seen at the left cardiodiaphragmatic angle lies between the parietal pericardium and a reflection of the parietal pleura as it extends downward and laterally to cover the diaphragm in this region. A similar situation exists on the right and a fat pad is occasionally noted in the cardiohepatic angle.

ENLARGEMENT OF THE HEART

GENERAL CARDIAC ENLARGEMENT

General cardiac enlargement may be caused by disease that produces a toxic effect on the myocardium and weakens it, and by conditions that cause an increase in the work load on the heart. This load is usually on a single chamber at first, and when it fails a second chamber becomes enlarged; eventually all chambers may be enlarged. In the latter type of disease, therefore, single or double chamber enlargement may predominate while in the conditions producing toxic myocarditis there is more likely to be uniform generalized cardiac enlargement.

The roentgen appearance of the heart in generalized myocardial disease varies considerably but the lateral contours on both sides often become more convex inferiorly and the normal slight alterations in the contour indicating the various segments are often effaced. The transverse diameter is usually increased more than the vertical diameter. Evidence of pulmonary congestion manifested by prominence and poor definition of pulmonary basal vascular markings may also be present. At fluoroscopy, pulsations are diminished and in extreme cases are so poor as to be difficult to define. When single or multiple chamber enlargement is present, the cardiac contour often shows characteristic changes that can be recognized roentgenographically.

LEFT VENTRICULAR ENLARGEMENT

When there is an increased work load on a cardiac chamber, the muscle fibers elongate in response to the added work and dilatation results. When this load is maintained over a period of time the dilatation is followed by hypertrophy, which is represented by actual increase in the size of the individual muscle fibers. The initial dilatation that precedes hy-

pertrophy is the means by which heart muscle increases its ability to work. When the work load becomes great there is secondary dilatation that results from failure of the heart muscle to do its work adequately. This type of dilatation indicates cardiac decompensation and failure. Hypertrophy of the heart muscle is a clearly defined pathologic finding, but the roentgen changes are often minimal or absent, making it difficult to determine in many instances. Hypertrophy may cause alteration in cardiac shape, however. This is usually a rounding of the contour of the ventricle involved. Little if any change in size results when hypertrophy is present without dilatation. On the other hand, dilatation causes an increase in size and may also alter the shape of the cardiac silhouette. The ventricles may be divided into two functional components, the inflow tract and the outflow tract. The blood flows into the left ventricle from the left atrium through the mitral valve that lies posterior and somewhat caudad to the aortic valve. The inflow tract extends from the valve along the posterior wall of the left ventricle and posterior half of the septum to the apex. The outflow tract is anterior and extends from the apex along the anterior half of the septum and anterior portion of the lateral ventricular wall. Any disease that causes an increased work load on the left ventricle may cause enlargement of this chamber. This is manifested first by elongation of the outflow tract. This produces an increase in the length of the left ventricular segment making up the left lateral cardiac contour as visualized roentgenographically. The second sign of enlargement of this tract is rounding of the contour of the left ventricle. As a result of this enlargement downward and to the left, the cardiac apex may extend below the dome of the diaphragm. Enlargement of the inflow tract of the left ventricle, which follows that of the outflow tract, produces posterior enlargement best outlined on the roentgenogram taken in the left anterior oblique projection. This posterior enlargement has led to the use of the angle of clearance between the left ventricle and spine in the left anterior oblique position as a criterion for left ventricular enlargement.

The angle of clearance of the left ventricle is the angle through which the patient must be rotated to his right from the posteroanterior position into the left anterior (or right posterior) oblique position to clear the posterior silhouette of the left ventricle from the thoracic spine. The angle is measured at the point where these structures do not quite overlap. There is so much normal variation, however, that the specific angle of 55°, which is often quoted, is very likely too high in some individuals and too low in others. In addition to the enlargement downward and to the left as well as posteriorly, disease resulting in increased left ventricular work may result in concentric hypertrophy of this chamber. This indicates that the ventricle is hypertrophied without significant dilatation so that there is very little actual enlargement. It is manifested roentgenographically by rounding of the left ventricular contour and apex as visualized in the frontal projection. Enlargement of the left ventricle is demonstrated in the posteroanterior, lateral, and left anterior oblique projections.

The most marked enlargement of the left ventricle is caused by hypertension and aortic insufficiency. Other lesions that produce enlargement of this chamber are aortic stenosis, mitral insufficiency, coarctation of the aorta, arteriovenous shunts that may be intracardiac or extracardiac, arteriosclerotic cardiovascular disease, and hyperthyroidism.

RIGHT VENTRICULAR ENLARGEMENT

Enlargement of the right ventricle is found in diseases that increase the work of this chamber. This includes a number of pulmonary diseases as well as primary vascular disease in the pulmonary arteries that results in pulmonary hypertension. Stenosis of the pulmonary valve or infundibulum and other congenital cardiac lesions, such as truncus arteriosus and septal defects, may also result in enlargement of this ventricle. Mitral valvular disease is also a common cause. When enlargement occurs, the outflow tract is the site of the earliest

dilatation. This extends from the apex of the right ventricle to the pulmonic valve and includes the anterior wall along with the upper half of the interventricular septum. The inflow tract that extends from the tricuspid valve to the apex includes the lower half of the interventricular septum, the diaphragmatic wall of this ventricle inferiorly, and the lower part of its outer wall anteriorly. Enlargement of the outflow tract of the right ventricle results in lengthening of the anterior ventricular wall, which is manifested radiographically by prominence of the pulmonary conus resulting in an anterior bulge in the upper anterior cardiac contour just below the pulmonary artery noted in the right anterior oblique projection. There is often associated enlargement of the pulmonary artery, which adds to the anterior prominence of the upper border of the heart in this projection. When this occurs there is more prominence and convexity of the pulmonary artery segment in the frontal projection than in the normal. This results in straightening or convexity of the left upper cardiac contour below the aortic knob. When the enlargement of the right ventricle becomes greater, the heart tends to be rotated to the left so that the conus of the right ventricle may become border-forming, and in the right anterior oblique projection the anterolateral bulge in the region of the outflow tract of the right ventricle reduces the size of the retrosternal space between the upper cardiac border and the sternum. The pulmonary artery also contributes to this narrowing. There is also noted a fullness superiorly in the retrosternal space in the lateral projection. When the inflow tract of the right ventricle enlarges, the diaphragmatic portion of this ventricle is increased in length and this results in an anterior rounding or bulge in the right ventricular area as visualized in the left anterior oblique projection. This enlargement may also displace the left ventricle posteriorly and elevate the cardiac apex. The latter is a common finding in infants and children with congenital cardiac disease resulting in right ventricular enlargement. When right ventricular dilatation is associated with enlargement of the left ventricle, the differentiation and evaluation of the relative size of each chamber is often very difficult.

LEFT ATRIAL ENLARGEMENT

Rheumatic mitral valvular disease is the most common cause of left atrial enlargement. It also occurs in other diseases such as congenital cardiac lesions resulting in intracardiac shunts, and in left ventricular failure. This chamber lies posteriorly and does not form any part of the cardiac contour as visualized in the frontal projection in the normal. Small amounts of enlargement are often entirely posterior and the earliest radiologic sign is displacement of the esophagus posteriorly and slightly to the right. This can be demonstrated by administration of barium orally to outline the esophagus on the chest film. In the normal, the esophagus is relatively straight as visualized in this right anterior oblique projection and a small amount of atrial enlargement produces a localized posterior bulge in the region of the atrium that lies just below the level of the carina. As this chamber becomes larger, it enlarges to the right and left as well as posteriorly. The left auricular appendage may then project beyond the left ventricle to produce a localized convexity or straightening of the left cardiac border just below the pulmonary artery segment. The enlargement to the right may be sufficient to make the right border of this chamber extend beyond the upper aspect of the right atrium and the superior vena cava, resulting in a double contour on the right as visualized in the frontal projection. Elevation of the left main bronchus may also be visible and when the enlargement reaches this stage, the mass of this chamber is often large enough to produce an oval localized density that can be seen through the heart in the frontal projection. When enlargement is massive, the left atrium may form most of the right cardiac contour and part of the left upper cardiac contour in the frontal projection. Rarely the left atrium projects only to the left when it enlarges.

RIGHT ATRIAL ENLARGEMENT

This chamber is enlarged in atrial septal defect, tricuspid stenosis and insufficiency, and in right ventricular failure. The right auricular appendage enlarges first and enlargement of the right atrium can be suspected when there is a bulge or prominence in the right atrial segment in the left anterior oblique projection. This bulge represents the auricular appendage and occasionally enlargement of this appendage produces actual angulation between it and the right ventricle in the left oblique projection. When the body of the atrium enlarges, it produces enlargement of the lower right cardiac contour to the right with increased convexity of this contour. Marked increase of this chamber produces great enlargement to the right in the frontal projection and a local prominence to the right and posteriorly as visualized in the right anterior oblique projection. In this view the local enlargement lies just above the diaphragm and below the area in which the left atrium is visible when it is increased in size.

CONGENITAL HEART DISEASE

Accurate diagnosis of the nature of congenital cardiac malformations is now imperative because surgical techniques are available for the cure of a number of lesions and palliation of others. The radiographic methods are a very important part of the examination of patients with congenital defects but accurate diagnosis depends upon correlation of all clinical and laboratory findings. There are wide variations in the roentgen findings in any single defect because of the wide range of severity of single or multiple defects. For example, septal defects may be small and produce little shunting of blood and very little alteration in the appearance of the cardiovascular silhouette; they may be very large and accompanied by a large shunt and marked changes in the cardiovascular silhouette. The same is true of the defects that produce cyanosis and a broad spectrum of physiologic and anatomic alteration is possible for each defect. The typical findings in the various defects will be described. The differential diagnosis of many of these lesions is difficult and it is helpful to classify the defects into those that produce cyanosis and those that do not. These can then be subdivided according to the radiographic appearance of the pulmonary vessels and to the presence or absence of cardiac enlargement. These differentiations are listed in Table 32-1. By using this approach, each defect can be placed in a relatively small group and special studies can then be done to differentiate the members of that group. Selective angiocardiography is the most useful radiologic method in the diagnosis of the congenital cardiac diseases.

CYANOTIC DEFECTS

TETRALOGY OF FALLOT

This anomaly consists of two fundamental defects, (*1*) pulmonic stenosis and (*2*) high interventricular septal defect. The third and fourth alterations described in tetralogy are secondary to these and consist of the aorta overriding the ventricular septum with dextroposition, and hypertrophy of the right ventricle.

TABLE 32-1. Common Congenital Cardiac Defects

Cyanotic	Noncyanotic
Increased pulmonary vascularity	
Transposition of great vessels	Patent ductus arteriosus
Patent ductus (malignant) with reversed flow	Interventricular septal defect
Eisenmenger's complex	Interatrial septal defect
Interatrial septal defect with reversed flow	Lutembacher's syndrome
Decreased pulmonary vascularity	
Tetralogy of Fallot	Isolated pulmonary stenosis
Truncus arteriosus	Ebstein's anomaly
Pulmonary stenosis plus interatrial septal defect	
Tricuspid atresia	
Normal pulmonary vascularity	
	Coarctation of the aorta
	Pulmonary stenosis—occasionally
	Aortic stenosis
	Endocardial fibroelastosis
	Ebstein's anomaly
Heart enlarged	
Transposition of great vessels	
Eisenmenger's complex	Coarctation (infantile type in failure)
Truncus arteriosus	Interatrial septal defect
Tricuspid atresia	Interventricular septal defect
Pulmonary stenosis with interatrial septal defect	Fibroelastosis
Ebstein's anomaly	
Heart not enlarged or slightly enlarged	
Tetralogy of Fallot	Patent ductus
Tricuspid atresia	Pulmonary stenosis
	Aortic stenosis
	Variable
	Interatrial septal defect
	Interventricular septal defect

The pulmonic stenosis causes an elevation of pressure in the right ventricle; the septal defect and overriding of the aorta allow blood from the right ventricle (venous blood) to be shunted directly into the general circulation. This right-to-left shunt from the right ventricle into the aorta results in cyanosis owing to unsaturation of the arterial blood. In addition to the abnormalities originally described, other anomalies often occur in combination. The most common is a patent foramen ovale. True atrial septal defect is less common; when this defect is present, the term pentalogy of Fallot is sometimes used. A right-sided aortic arch is present in about 20 per cent of patients with tetralogy. Extracardiac anomalies consisting of malformations of the aortic arch system are also common. Rarely such abnormalities as stenosis of peripheral pulmonary arteries, partial anomalous venous return, absence or hypoplasia of the pulmonary valve, persistent common atrioventricular canal, and tricuspid insufficiency may be associated with tetralogy of Fallot. The pulmonic stenosis is usually infundibular in type. The infundibulum is usually constricted into a long, narrow channel and there may be an associated valvular stenosis. Valvular stenosis alone is unusual in tetralogy however. When this occurs there may be some poststenotic dilatation of the pulmonary artery which alters the configuration of the left cardiovascular border. Occasionally the stenosis is localized to the proximal infundibulum, the ostium infundibuli. When this occurs the infundibulum dilates to a greater or lesser extent, forming a "third" ventricle. The degree of stenosis varies from a very slight narrowing to pulmonary atresia. In the latter instance, which is very rare, the aorta forms a pseudotruncus and the pulmonary blood supply is through the bronchial arteries or through a patent ductus arteriosus and pulmonary arteries. The roentgenographic findings vary with the degree of pulmonic stenosis and the amount of shunt.

Roentgen Findings

HEART SIZE. The heart is usually within the normal limits of size and may appear to be somewhat smaller than the average normal. Appreciable cardiac enlargement in this condition is unusual unless the patient survives into adult life. The right ventricle hypertrophies, but usually does not dilate.

PULMONARY ARTERY. The pulmonary artery segment, as visualized in the frontal projection, is small and this results in concavity of the upper left cardiac margin in the region of this segment. The degree of concavity is dependent upon the degree of stenosis and varies from marked concavity to a pulmonary artery segment that cannot be distinguished from the normal. In the occasional patient with stenosis of the ostium infundibuli the dilated infundibulum may produce a convexity in the left side of the heart border at and just below the level of the left main bronchus, which represents the distal right ventricle. When poststenotic dilatation of the pulmonary artery is present, there is slight convexity rather than concavity in the region of this artery.

PULMONARY VASCULARITY. There is a decrease in pulmonary vascularity, resulting in decrease in the size of the vessels making up the hilum on both sides, and relative avascularity of the lung fields. This is an indication of decreased pulmonary bloodflow. In severe stenosis and in patients with pseudotruncus, the branching of the dilated bronchial arteries may produce a brushlike appearance, with small vessels of uniform caliber in contrast to the decreasing caliber of pulmonary arteries usually noted. In patients with minimal defects resulting in the so-called "acyanotic" tetralogy, the vascularity is normal or nearly so.

HEART SHAPE. The enlargement of the right ventricle results in elevation of the apex and a rounded configuration of the lower left cardiac margin. The appearance resembles a boot. In the left anterior oblique projection the right ventricular enlargement produces rounding of the anterior cardiac contour and when the enlargement is great, the left ventricle is elevated and displaced posteriorly so that the left or posterior cardiac border has a convex prominence in its central portion well above the diaphragm. This represents the left ventricle in an abnormal position, sometimes termed the "left ventricular cap." There is also noted unusual radiolucency in the region of the pulmonary artery that lies below and within the arch of the aorta. This is sometimes termed the "aortic window." In the right anterior oblique projection there may be rounding of the anterior cardiac contour in the region of the right ventricle, with decrease in the region of the distal pulmonary outflow tract and pulmonary artery segment. In the lateral view there is anterior and upward bulging of the heart, tending to fill the retrosternal space superiorly.

THE AORTA. The findings in the right aortic arch that occur in approximately 20 per cent of patients consist of absence of aortic shadow on the left and presence of a vascular shadow on the right at the aortic level. This is readily detected in adults and older children, but in infants the aortic arch may not be visible. The superior vena cava is displaced laterally, however, and the resulting convex density in the right upper mediastinum may suggest the aortic position. Sometimes barium in the esophagus is helpful along with visualization of the trachea, where an indentation on the right may identify the site of the aortic arch. The aorta is enlarged in rough proportion to the amount of right-to-left shunt.

OTHER FINDINGS. Occasionally there is poststenotic dilatation of the main pulmonary artery, as indicated above, so that the pulmonary artery is normal or slightly larger than normal. Also the presence of a "third" ventricle may alter the silhouette as noted previously. It is apparent then that the appearance of the heart in tetralogy varies from one in which there is very little deviation from the normal to one in which there is marked alteration (Figs. 32-7 through 32-9).

ANGIOCARDIOGRAPHY. Angiocardiography outlines the right ventricle and shows immediate filling of the aorta from the right ventricle, often with little if any shunt into the left ventricle. The site of stenosis is usually outlined, particularly in the right anterior oblique or lateral view. Pulmonary artery size is also defined.

PULMONARY STENOSIS WITH INTACT VENTRICULAR SEPTUM AND ATRIAL RIGHT-TO-LEFT SHUNT (TRILOGY OF FALLOT)

In this entity the atrial defect is usually a patent foramen ovale. Cyanosis appears when right atrial pressure has increased enough to cause a right-to-left shunt through the patent foramen ovale or atrial septal defect. This often occurs early in life but may be delayed.

Roentgen Findings

HEART SIZE. The heart is moderately to markedly enlarged, with elevation of the apex indicating right ventricular enlargement. The aorta is usually normal in size and the arch is on the left side.

PULMONARY ARTERY. Poststenotic dilatation of the pulmonary artery results in prominence of the pulmonary artery segment in the frontal and oblique projections but is not always present. Poststenotic dilatation occurs with valvular stenosis, which usually occurs in this condition. Infundibular stenosis may result as a secondary change when muscular hypertrophy occurs in the infundibulum, or it may be primarily responsible for the high right ventricular pressure which occurs in an estimated 10 per cent of patients. If stenosis is of infundibular type, there is a small pulmonary artery distal to the narrowing (Fig. 32-10).

PULMONARY VASCULARITY. Pulmonary vascularity tends to be decreased but may appear normal when the stenosis is not marked.

HEART SHAPE. The silhouette is that of right atrial and right ventricular enlargement; poststenotic dilatation results in prominence of the pulmonary artery. The left atrium may be enlarged. The apex is elevated and the right

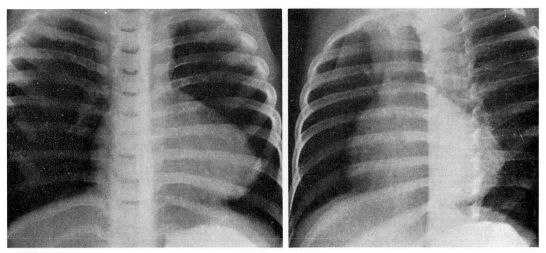

Fig. 32-7. Tetralogy of Fallot. Child, 6 months of age, with severe tetralogy. Note the concavity in the left upper cardiac border, the elevation of the apex, and the relative avascularity of the hila and lung fields. The roentgenogram on the *right* is taken in the left anterior oblique projection and shows the prominence of the right heart chambers as well as the elevation of the apex and avascularity.

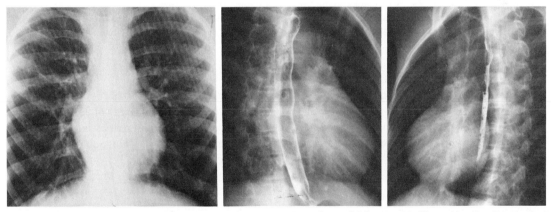

Fig. 32-8. Tetralogy of Fallot. Moderately severe tetralogy in a child, age 11. Note the round apex and the prominence of the right heart border in the left anterior oblique projection. The diminution of vascularity is minimal.

ventricle prominent in the left anterior oblique and frontal projections.

ANGIOCARDIOGRAPHY. Angiocardiography is a valuable examination in this condition and films taken in rapid succession after caval or right atrial injection will show the defect at the atrial level, with a jet of opaque material propelled through the defect rapidly filling the left atrium, left ventricle and then the aorta. This results in rapid opacification of the left atrium and ventricle along with opacification of the right chambers and simultaneous, or nearly simultaneous, opacification of the pulmonary artery and aorta. The pulmonary stenosis may be directly visible in some cases. The post-stenotic dilatation frequently present is also readily recognized on the angiocardiogram. Selective right ventricular injection is best to show the enlarged right ventricle associated with muscular hypertrophy. The pulmonary valve is usually thickened and often dome-

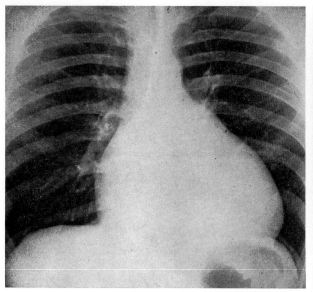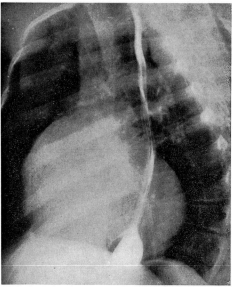

Fig. 32-9. Tetralogy of Fallot. Male, aged 35, with moderate cyanosis. *Left,* Note that the heart is enlarged in this patient but the hilar vessels are small and the peripheral vascularity very scanty. There is no concavity in the region of the pulmonary artery segment, however. *Right,* In this left anterior oblique projection, the marked prominence of the cardiac silhouette anteriorly indicates the right-sided enlargement. The apex appears to be elevated to some extent.

shaped, with a jet of opaque medium crossing the valve into a moderately dilated pulmonary artery. The infundibulum is long and smooth and shows rather marked change in diameter from systole to diastole in contrast to the findings in tetralogy of Fallot.

COMPLETE TRANSPOSITION OF THE GREAT VESSELS

The relative positions of the pulmonary artery and the aorta are reversed in complete transposition. This would result in two closed circulations because the blood from the lungs enters the left atrium via the pulmonary veins and goes from there into the left ventricle and through the pulmonary artery back to the lungs. The systemic venous return enters the right atrium, goes into the right ventricle, and out through the aorta back into the systemic circulation. Since this situation is incompatible with life, complete transposition must be accompanied by other anomalies allowing intra or extracardiac shunts. These consist of patent ductus arteriosus, interatrial and interventricular septal defects. Ventricular septal defect occurs in less than one-half of patients while some type of interatrial defect is usually present. It may be a small atrial septal defect or a patent foramen ovale. The ductus arteriosus may be patent. Rarely anomalous pulmonary venous return shunts blood from the lungs to the right side of the heart.

This anomaly is more frequent in males than females in a ratio of two or four to one. Prognosis is poor, with an estimated 90 per cent mortality in the first year of life.

Roentgen Findings

HEART SIZE. The heart size is usually increased and may be greatly enlarged. The enlargement may not be apparent at birth but is usually present by the age of 2 months.

HEART SHAPE. Both ventricles are enlarged and the general shape of the heart is oval or egg-shaped. The right ventricle is usually en-

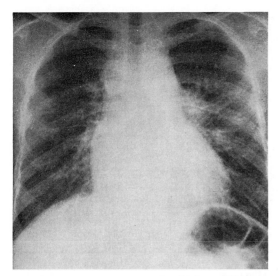

Fig. 32-10. Pulmonary stenosis with interatrial septal defect. The stenosis was severe and the lungs were supplied by the bronchial arteries to a great extent. This accounts for the absence of normal hilar vessels, noted particularly on the right, and the brushlike character of the arteries that are visualized.

larged to a greater extent than the left. The shape of the heart in the lateral and left anterior oblique positions tends to be round, and as the obliquity is increased, the vascular pedicle tends to become larger in its transverse diameter. In the frontal projection, however, the base usually produced by the great vessels is narrow. Furthermore, the absence of normal thymic tissue accentuates this finding. The thymus may also be small or absent in other severe congenital heart conditions and in infants with severe, stressful, noncardiac disease.

PULMONARY ARTERY AND AORTA. There is narrowing of the shadow of the great vessels in the frontal projection, the result of a more anteroposterior course of the aorta that arises anteriorly and tends to course directly backward. This produces a widening of the shadow of the great vessels in the oblique projections, because the vessels that are superimposed in the frontal projection are separated by the obliquity. Since the pulmonary infundibulum is not normally formed and the pulmonary artery lies nearer the midline than normal, the con-

vexity usually formed by the infundibulum and pulmonary artery is not present, and in some instances a distinct concavity is noted in the left upper cardiac border. The outline of the aortic arch is absent. (Fig. 32-11.)

PULMONARY VASCULARITY. Pulmonary vessels are enlarged and prominent and may pulsate in a hyperactive manner as visualized fluoroscopically. Rarely there is pulmonic stenosis associated with transposition. This results in a decrease in size of the pulmonary vessels.

ANGIOCARDIOGRAPHY. Venous angiocardiographic findings consist of filling sequentially of the right atrium, the right ventricle, and of an anteriorly placed aorta from the right ventricle. There is usually very poor opacification of the pulmonary artery and the shunt that makes this condition compatible with life may be visualized. If an atrial septal defect is present it is usually apparent, with rapid opacification of the left atrium. Patent ductus may be demonstrated. Interventricular septal defect is very difficult to define. The enlargement of the right-sided heart chambers can also be noted on the angiocardiogram. There tends to be some difference in relationship of the great vessels, ranging from a pulmonary artery that lies posterior and slightly to the left of the aorta to one which lies directly posterior or rarely directly to the left of the aorta.

Selective, right-ventricular angiocardiography is somewhat more satisfactory than a venous injection, particularly in outlining ventricular septal defect and the pulmonary artery.

TRICUSPID ATRESIA

Tricuspid atresia with hypoplasia or aplasia of the right ventricle is associated with several other malformations in order that circulation may be sustained. The tricuspid valve is atretic and there is hypoplasia or absence of the right ventricle. Edwards et al.[9] classify these anomalies based on the relationship of great vessels and the presence or absence of pulmonary stenosis. In Type I the great vessels are normally related and there are: (1) coexistent tricuspid and pulmonary atresia;

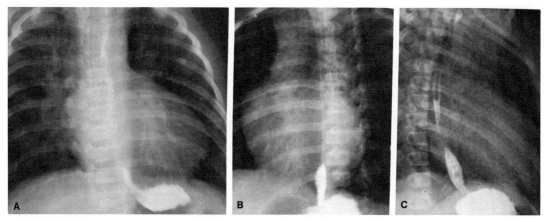

Fig. 32-11. Transposition of the great vessels. *A*, Frontal projection. *B*, Left anterior oblique. *C*, Right anterior oblique. There is cardiac enlargement. The large pulmonary vessels are best seen in the right hilum and central lung. The apex is elevated, indicating right ventricular enlargement. The vascular pedicle is narrow in the frontal projection and rather broad in both oblique views.

(*2*) a narrow septal defect between the left ventricle and the infundibular portion of the right ventricle, a small vestigial right ventricle, and a small pulmonary artery (this is the most common form); or (*3*) a large interventricular septal defect with valvular stenosis and normal pulmonary artery. Rarely, transposition of great vessels occurs in this form. In Type II, transposition of the great vessels without pulmonic stenosis occurs, and there is essentially a common ventricle. Rarely, this anomaly is found without transposition. As indicated, in Type I, there is some type of right ventricular or pulmonary artery obstruction. In these patients, an atrial septal defect is present so that the blood flows into the right atrium, is shunted across the septal defect to the left atrium, and then to the left ventricle. The blood is then distributed to the lungs via an interventricular septal defect and hypoplastic right ventricle through the pulmonary artery to the lungs. If the right ventricle or pulmonary artery is atretic, then the blood must get to the lungs via a patent ductus.

TRICUSPID ATRESIA WITH PULMONARY STENOSIS

Roentgen Findings

HEART SIZE. The heart is usually enlarged, but there is considerable variation; at times the enlargement is slight and in others it is marked.

HEART SHAPE. The heart is often boot-shaped and may resemble the silhouette of tetralogy of Fallot. The pulmonary artery segment is concave. The left atrium may be enlarged; when present, this is a helpful diagnostic sign. The right atrium is usually somewhat enlarged and may be markedly enlarged. Evidence of left ventricular preponderance on the electrocardiogram is often necessary to make certain that the left ventricle is enlarged, because right ventricular enlargement can rotate the heart and produce a similar silhouette. The left side of the heart border is rounded with apparent elevation of the apex, simulating the elevation associated with right ventricular enlargement. The change in the contour of the heart commonly described to indicate absence or hypoplasia of the right ventricle is not often found in this condition. This change consists of diminished convexity or actual concavity of the right lower heart border in the frontal projection and of the anterior inferior border in the left anterior oblique view. The reason for the absence of this sign is that the right atrium enlarges to the extent that it fills the deficit resulting from right ventricular absence or hypoplasia.

PULMONARY ARTERY. There is concavity in the region of the main pulmonary artery in the frontal projection. It may be extreme, so that the junction between the aorta and the upper left ventricular silhouette is angular.

PULMONARY VASCULARITY. Pulmonary vascularity is usually decreased, unless there is complete transposition of the great vessels. When that is present, vascularity is normal or increased.

THE AORTA. The aorta is generally enlarged.

ANGIOCARDIOGRAPHY. This examination is useful in establishing the anatomic diagnosis in tricuspid atresia. The findings are those of large right atrium below which is a triangular radiolucent notch, representing the defect caused by absence of filling of the right ventricle. A shunt from the right to the left atrium is observed, resulting in rapid opacification of the left side of the heart. The size of the pulmonary vessels is demonstrated, but the root of the pulmonary artery, the site of stenosis, and the right ventricular chamber may be difficult to outline.

TRICUSPID ATRESIA WITHOUT PULMONARY STENOSIS

As indicated above, this form of the anomaly is usually associated with transposition of the great vessels and a common ventricle.

Roentgen findings consist of gross cardiac enlargement, narrowing of the great vessels at the base indicating transposition and some left atrial enlargement. Pulmonary vascularity is greatly increased. Correlation with electrocardiographic findings of left ventricular preponderance in a cyanotic child with hypervascularity is very suggestive of the diagnosis.

TRICUSPID STENOSIS

Congenital tricuspid stenosis is very rare and is usually combined with other congenital cardiac defects. The only consistent roentgen finding is hypovascularity of the lung fields. The enlargement of the right atrium present in these patients may not be readily recognized. In some cases, the appearance simulates that of tetralogy of Fallot. No consistent roentgen appearance has been described.

EBSTEIN'S ANOMALY

This malformation consists of downward displacement of the tricuspid valve far into the right ventricle. The upper portion of the right ventricle is incorporated into the right atrium. As a result the ventricle is small and the atrium is large. The myocardium proximal to the abnormally placed valve is thin and the large right atrium is unable to empty itself properly. Cyanosis is often present in this disease because venous blood is shunted from the right to the left atrium through an interatrial septal defect which is usually present. If there is no intracardiac shunt no cyanosis is produced.

Roentgen Findings

The heart is usually greatly enlarged and the lung fields are hypovascular. The right atrium and ventricle are the chambers involved. Enlargement to the right with a shoulderlike prominence of the right upper cardiac enlargement is characteristic. There is often enlargement of the left upper cardiac contour in a more sloping manner, caused by enlargement of the outflow tract of the right ventricle. This gives the heart a square or boxlike shape (Fig. 32-12). When this is found, along with hypovascularity of the lung fields and a small aorta, the roentgen diagnosis can be made with reasonable certainty, particularly when correlated with electrocardiographic findings. Therefore angiocardiography may not be needed. On venous angiocardiography, the large right atrium fills and empties slowly through the foramen ovale into the left atrium and through the tricuspid valve into the right ventricle. The right side of the heart remains opacified for an unusually long period of time. Selective injection of contrast medium into the right ventricle will identify the level of the tricuspid valve and will show tricuspid insufficiency when present. Occasionally there is an associated pulmonic valvular stenosis which is defined in this examination.

TOTAL ANOMALOUS PULMONARY VENOUS RETURN

In this anomaly the pulmonary veins empty into the right atrium by one of several pathways. The most common is a left innominate vein. Others empty (1) directly into the coronary sinus, (2) directly into the right atrium, (3) through a large vein into the right superior vena cava, (4) into a persistent left superior vena cava, (5) into the portal vein, ductus venosus or inferior vena cava below the diaphragm, and (6) occasionally in-

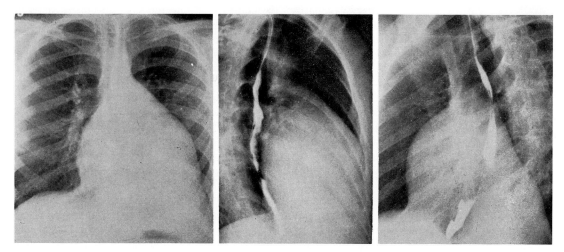

Fig. 32-12. Ebstein's anomaly. The heart is enlarged and rather square in contour. In the left oblique projection (*right*) the right atrium is noted to be prominent. Enlargement of the right heart is also noted in the right anterior oblique view (*center*).

to the azygos vein or hepatic vein. The latter type occurs predominantly in males. In the patients with the persistent left superior vena cava or vertical vein the blood flows upward in this vein for a short distance to the level of the superior aspect of the aortic arch and then flows to the right, in the left innominate vein, which unites with the superior vena cava on the right. When all the pulmonary venous blood is returned to the right side of the heart, a right-to-left shunt is needed to be compatible with life. The most common anomaly is atrial septal defect or patent foramen ovale. As a result of this combination of defects, the right heart is overloaded and becomes enlarged while the left heart and aorta are relatively small. Cyanosis is usually present but may not be severe. When partial anomalous pulmonary venous return is present there may be no symptoms and very few signs. Single anomalous pulmonary veins are not infrequently found associated with other defects.

Roentgen Findings

The heart is enlarged. The enlargement is right-sided although this may not be readily apparent. Pulmonary vessels are prominent, owing to the increased bloodflow in the lesser circulation. When there is a persistent left vena cava, or left vertical vein with total anomalous pulmonary venous connection to the left innominate vein, there is characteristic figure-of-eight deformity of the cardio-

vascular silhouette. The upper limbs of the eight are formed by the vena cavae on both sides that are markedly dilated and form convexities on either side above the heart (Fig. 32-13). In the occasional patient in whom the veins drain into the right superior or inferior vena cava, they may be visualized on the plain-film roentgenogram. Tomography will often outline the abnormal vessel to good advantage. The aorta is small and hypoplastic and the pulmonary artery is often enlarged to the extent that its upper border forms a horizontal shelf immediately below the hypoplastic aortic arch. Angiocardiography can be used to establish the diagnosis but when the figure-of-eight is present along with the evidence of enlargement of pulmonary vessels the diagnosis can be made with reasonable certainty on plain films alone. The thymic shadow may produce a figure-of-eight sign and must be differentiated. Most of the other sites of return show no characteristic vascular pattern, but since there is a bidirectional shunt, cyanosis and pulmonary hypervascularity are both present. There is right-sided cardiac enlargement with no evidence of left atrial enlargement.

Total anomalous pulmonary venous return below the diaphragm presents a different roentgen picture. The heart is usually normal in size and shape, but the lungs are abnormal. The findings are of pulmonary vascular congestion and edema. The vascular changes resemble those seen in adults with venous hypertension secondary to mitral val-

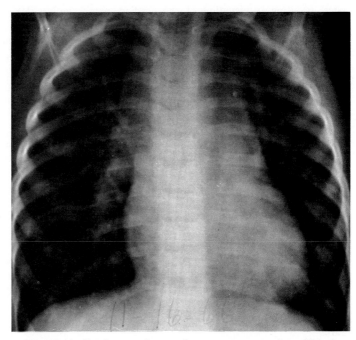

Fig. 32-13. Total anomalous pulmonary venous return. This is a reasonably typical example of the figure-of-8 deformity with the large veins forming a convexity on either side in the upper mediastinum. The pulmonary vascularity is increased.

vular disease, except that the hilar vessels are not prominent in these infants. This association of normal-sized heart and roentgen and clinical evidence of congestive failure in a cyanotic male infant with no heart murmurs is highly suggestive of the diagnosis. Angiocardiography can then be used to demonstrate the draining vein extending below the diaphragm.

PARTIAL ANOMALOUS VENOUS RETURN

The most common partial anomalous venous connection is to the right atrium. This results in a left-to-right shunt of modest proportions which usually does not cause symptoms and is often found upon study of patients with atrial septal defect. Roentgen findings are similar to those of atrial septal defect and include pulmonary arterial enlargement and hypervascularity related to the size of the shunt. A rare combination of hypoplasia of the right lung and anomalous right pulmonary venous return into the inferior vena cava is termed the "scimitar syndrome" because the anomalous vein is visible as a curved shadow in the right lower lung.

PERSISTENT TRUNCUS ARTERIOSUS

In this anomaly, which is rare, there is only one large arterial trunk that overrides the ventricular septum. The pulmonary artery may arise as a branch of the common trunk. A second form consists of separate origin of pulmonary arteries from the dorsal wall of the truncus. In a third form, one or both pulmonary arteries arise independently from either side of the truncus. In these anomalies, the pulmonary vascularity is usually increased. A fourth form consists of absence of the pulmonary artery with a truncus arteriosus that supplies the lungs via the bronchial arteries or other collateral vessels. There is marked decrease in pulmonary vascularity in this type.

Roentgen Findings

The truncus is usually large and produces a convexity in the region of the ascending arch. There is often prominence of the peripheral pulmonary vessels despite a concavity in the region of the main pulmonary artery. The heart is usually enlarged. Right ventricular enlargement predominates, resulting in elevation of the cardiac apex that may be striking, so that the silhouette resembles that of severe tetralogy of Fallot except that it tends to be larger in the truncus. In the fourth type and in pseudotruncus the ascending aortic arch is prominent and the pulmonary artery segment is concave but the pulmonary vascularity is markedly diminished and the bronchial arteries that supply the lungs are visualized as small vessels extending outward in a fine brushlike pattern from the hila on both sides. The comma-shaped pattern of the pulmonary arteries is absent in these patients. The shape of the heart is often significant in the frontal position. There is a sharp right-angled junction between the vascular pedicle on left and the upper left ventricular border, or an acute angle may be present. Angiocardiography demonstrates opacification of the large truncus from the large right ventricle and shows the pulmonary artery filling after the truncus has filled. In the fourth type and in pseudotruncus the appearance is similar to that in severe tetralogy on the angiocardiogram.

OTHER CYANOTIC DEFECTS

TRANSPOSITION OF THE TAUSSIG-BING TYPE

This is a variant of transposition in which the aorta arises from the right ventricle while the pulmonary artery overrides the ventricular septum. A high ventricular septal defect is present. When this defect is above the crista supraventricularis and is closely applied to the origin of the pulmonary trunk, it represents the Taussig-Bing type of transposition. Another type is one in which the ventricular septal defect is below the crista supraventricularis, remote from the pulmonary valve. In the latter, the left ventricular bloodstream is directed toward the aorta, while in the Taussig-Bing type the left ventricular bloodstream is directed to the pulmonary artery. This results in enlargement of the right ventricle and atrium. The pulmonary artery is dilated but its branches are often diminished in size as compared to the large main vessels. This is the result of vascular changes that cause pulmonary hypertension.

Roentgen Findings

There is cardiac enlargement, primarily owing to the enlarged right ventricle. This is associated with enlargement of the pulmonary artery segment and hilar vessels. The mid zone pulmonary vascular channels may be full but become small when pulmonary hypertension develops. There may be left atrial and left ventricular enlargement as well. On plain films the two types cannot be differentiated. In the Taussig-Bing type, angiocardiography shows immediate filling of the aorta from the right ventricle with relatively poor filling of the pulmonary artery and its branches from this chamber. The pulmonary trunk is wider than the aorta. The aortic and pulmonary valves are at the same horizontal level and are superimposed in the lateral view.

When the septal defect is below the crista supraventricularis there is better filling of the pulmonary artery from the right ventricle. The valves are on the same horizontal plane or the pulmonary valve may be slightly higher than the aortic. Similar lateral superimposition is noted.

OTHER ANOMALIES

A number of other rare anomalies may be associated with cyanosis. They include the trilocular heart, the bilocular heart, atrioventricularis communis, and a number of others, often associated with obstruction to pulmonary flow. The roentgen findings are not characteristic in these conditions, but the heart is usually enlarged in all of them.

NONCYANOTIC DEFECTS

The cardiovascular anomalies to be discussed in this section consist of defects that cause left-to-right shunts under ordinary circumstances and of other anomalies, chiefly involving the valves. The shunting of blood from left to right is dependent upon the pressure gradient across the defect. The pressure is usually higher on the left side so that the shunt is maintained from left to right, but when pulmonary hypertension is caused by the lesion, the pressure in the right-sided heart chambers may exceed that on the left. Then the shunt is reversed and cyanosis or arterial unsaturation develops. The roentgen diagnosis of this group of congenital anomalies often rests in part upon differentiation between right and left ventricular enlargement. The criteria for enlargement of these chambers described in the sections on "left ventricular enlargement" and "right ventricular enlargement" may be useless in these patients because enlargement of one chamber may simulate that of another. Therefore differentiation cannot be made on plainfilm study alone and radiographic findings must be correlated with clinical, electrocardiographic, angiocardiographic, and catheterization data. In patients with left-to-right intracardiac shunts pulmonary inflammatory disease is common. Obstruction with lobular, segmental, and even lobar atelectasis may be found. These findings may be of significance when the cardiac silhouette does not suggest the type of congenital anomaly.

PATENT DUCTUS ARTERIOSUS

The ductus arteriosus serves to shunt blood into the systemic circulation from the pulmonary artery in intrauterine life and is patent at birth. Functionally the ductus apparently closes very early in life and anatomic closure is usually complete in 2 months but is sometimes delayed up to 6 months and rarely for a year. The ductus arises near the origin of the left pulmonary artery and empties into the aorta just distal to the left subclavian artery. Occasionally a right-sided ductus is found.

Roentgen Findings

The findings on the routine frontal, oblique, and lateral roentgenograms are not always diagnostic, particularly in infants and young children, and must be correlated with clinical data. The left atrium and left ventricle are enlarged and there is enlargement of the aorta proximal to the ductus. The pulmonary artery and pulmonary vessels in the lung fields are enlarged. The findings are roughly parallel to the amount of left-to-right shunt. In patients with small shunts, no detectable cardiovascular abnormalities may be noted radiographically.

HEART SIZE. Slight cardiac enlargement is present in about half the patients; in large shunts,

a considerable amount of enlargement may be present.

HEART SHAPE. There may be enough left atrial enlargement to produce recognizable displacement of the esophagus in the right anterior oblique projection. Left ventricular enlargement is also present, causing elongation of the left border of the heart in the frontal view and rounding of the left ventricular silhouette in the left anterior oblique projection. Continued increase in pulmonary bloodflow may result in some degree of pulmonary hypertension, which in turn causes right ventricular enlargement.

PULMONARY ARTERY. The most consistent finding in patent ductus arteriosus is enlargement of the pulmonary artery segment. This produces convex prominence in the region of the segment in the frontal projection (Fig 32-14).

PULMONARY VASCULARITY. The vascularity in the hila and lung fields is increased. The amplitude of pulsation of these vessels may be recognizably increased at fluoroscopy.

THE AORTA. The aorta is often enlarged (Fig. 32-15). There may be a slight bulge of the left aortic wall below the prominent knob indicating minor enlargement in this region. This represents the infundibulum of the patent ductus. It is not a frequent sign in children and is not diagnostic, since similar slight convexity can occur in patients without patent ductus. Rarely there is calcification at the aortic end of the ductus in adults; it has not been reported in children. Occasionally the ductus itself is visible as a small convexity between the aortic knob or transverse arch and the pulmonary artery.

ANGIOCARDIOGRAPHY. This examination is often disappointing but may show reopacification of the pulmonary artery from the aorta and slight enlargement of the left heart chambers. The demonstration of the local aortic enlargement at the site of the ductus or of a ductus diverticulum is helpful but not conclusive. A transient local defect in the opacifica-

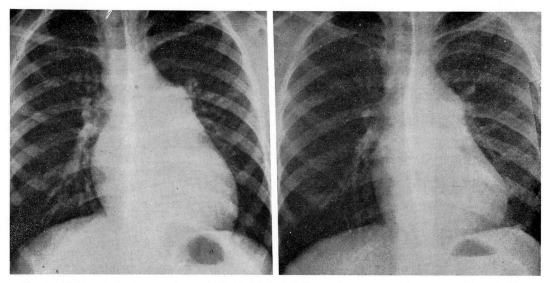

Fig. 32-14. Patent ductus arteriosus. *Left,* Moderate cardiac enlargement with considerable prominence of the pulmonary artery segment, resulting in convexity of the left upper border just below the aortic arch. There is also evidence of hypervascularity, noted best in the right hilum and parahilar area. The left lateral border appears elongated, indicating left ventricular enlargement. *Right,* Roentgenogram taken nearly 1 year later and 8 months following ligation of the ductus. There has been slight decrease in the cardiac size and in pulmonary vascularity. Enlargement of the pulmonary artery has decreased very little.

tion of the pulmonary artery at the site of the ductus, owing to a jet of nonopacified blood shunted through the ductus, is diagnostic when visualized.

RETROGRADE AORTOGRAPHY. This examination is much more useful. The opaque material is injected directly into the aorta and the opacified blood traverses the ductus and outlines the pulmonary artery and its branches.

PATENT DUCTUS WITH RIGHT-TO-LEFT SHUNT

This is sometimes termed a malignant ductus. The flow is reversed when the pulmonary arterial pressure exceeds that in the aorta. Normally the pulmonary arterial systolic pressure is much lower than systemic arterial pressure. In wide patent ductus arteriousus the pulmonary and systemic arterial pressures are equal. Equalization depends on a large-volume, left-to-right shunt. Pulmonary arterial disease may

eventually develop to the point where pulmonary arterial resistance is greater than systemic resistance. When this degree of pulmonary hypertension is reached, the ductus acts as a safety valve for the lesser circulation. A right-to-left shunt is created so that cyanosis becomes apparent in the lower extremities but may not be present in the upper extremities. As a result of the pulmonary hypertension, the right ventricle becomes enlarged and the main pulmonary artery is often increased further in size along with the vessels in the hila, while the vessels in the central and peripheral lung fields are relatively small. This difference in size of proximal and peripheral pulmonary vessels is reliable only when it is unequivocal, however.

INTERATRIAL SEPTAL DEFECT

Atrial septal defects are among the most frequent congenital heart lesions. There are several types. The most common is a patent foramen ovale that is large enough to result in a

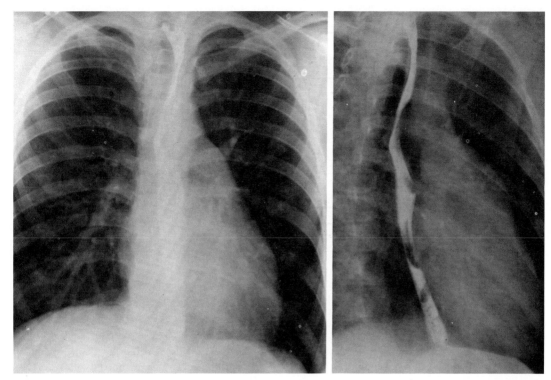

Fig. 32-15. Patent ductus arteriosus in a 12-year-old boy. The aorta is large and indents the esophagus which contains barium in both the frontal (*left*) and oblique (*right*) views. The main pulmonary artery is enlarged and there is moderate hypervascularity. The slight indentation of the esophagus below the carina noted in the oblique view indicates left atrial enlargement and there is probably a little left ventricular enlargement as well.

shunt. When there is a defect at the fossa ovalis, it may be termed an ostium secundum defect. Persistent ostium primum is a defect at the base of the atrial septum. There may also be a high atrial septal defect which is usually associated with anomalous pulmonary venous return from the right lung. As a result of the defect there is free communication between the two atria, permitting a shunt. The anatomic location of the defect is not as important as its size and the difference in atrial pressures; these factors determine the amount of blood shunted across the defect. Since left atrial pressure is usually higher than the pressure in the right atrium, the shunt is from left to right. As a result, the pulmonary bloodflow is increased and this increases the amount of right ventricular work.

Roentgen Findings

HEART SIZE. The heart is usually slightly enlarged, but may be normal in size.

HEART SHAPE. Enlargement of the right ventricle and atrium occurs and may be typical enough to be recognized, but differentiation between right and left ventricular enlargement is not always possible. The left atrium is not enlarged.

THE PULMONARY ARTERY. This artery is enlarged and may be markedly increased in size, causing a large convexity that may partially obscure the smaller aortic knob. The size of the pulmonary artery segment in this anomaly is usually larger than in the other two common anomalies that produce left-to-right shunts, patent ductus arteriosus, and ventricular septal defect (Fig. 32-16).

PULMONARY VASCULARITY. The hilar and pulmonary vascularity is also increased and at fluoroscopy the increased amplitude of pulsation of the pulmonary artery and its branches may be noted.

THE AORTA. The shunting of blood away from the left side of the heart into the lesser circulation results in decreased flow through the aorta, and it tends to be smaller than normal in size. This may readily be visualized, particularly in adults, but in infants and small children aortic size is often difficult to determine.

ANGIOCARDIOGRAPHY. Angiocardiography is used occasionally to visualize the shunt and indicate its size and location.

ATRIAL SEPTAL DEFECT WITH RIGHT-TO-LEFT SHUNT

Pulmonary hypertension may occur, causing a reversal of the shunt when the right atrial pressure exceeds that in the left atrium. It is caused by organic changes in pulmonary arteries resulting in increasing vascular resistance. Arterial unsaturation occurs and cyanosis may then be observed. The right-sided heart chambers become more enlarged, particularly the right ventricle. The pulmonary artery also increases in size and there may be a marked decrease in arterial size between central hilar vessels and peripheral pulmonary arteries, a sign of pulmonary hypertension.

ATRIAL SEPTAL DEFECT WITH MITRAL STENOSIS (LUTEMBACHER'S SYNDROME)

This rare condition consists of atrial septal defect combined with either congenital or acquired mitral stenosis. It results in a greater increase in right ventricular work load than an uncomplicated atrial septal defect of similar size. It causes extreme enlargement of the pulmonary artery; this is the characteristic feature noted on the roentgenogram. The heart is generally enlarged and pulmonary vascularity is increased. At fluoroscopy the increased amplitude of pulsation is noted in the large pulmonary artery and its branches. The right ventricle and atrium are considerably enlarged and there may be some enlargement of the left atrium.

Angiocardiographic findings in this condition are similar to those in atrial septal defect. A jet of opaque medium crossing the plane of the septum from the left atrium to the right atrium is diagnostic of atrial septal defect. There are other indirect angiocardiographic signs that may aid in the diagnosis. They consist of (1) enlargement of the right atrium and ventricle along with the pulmonary artery, (2) reopacification of the right side of the heart following left-sided opacification, and (3) dilution in the right atrium when a large shunt is present.

VENTRICULAR SEPTAL DEFECT

This is the most common of the congenital cardiac diseases. Defects may occur low in the septal wall but more commonly the defect is high. When the opening occurs high and adjacent to the mitral and tricuspid valves, it may involve the atrial septum and result in the defect known as atrioventricularis communis. Ventricular septal defect results in a left-to-right shunt because the left ventricular pressure is usually higher than the pressure in the right ventricle. As in the atrial septal defects, the size of the shunt is determined by the relationship of pressures on the two sides of the shunt and the size of the defect. There may be very little change in the size and shape of the heart when the defect is small and there is not much shunt. If a sizable shunt is present, there will be alterations that can be visualized on the chest roentgenogram.

Roentgen Findings

The left ventricle and left atrium are enlarged, along with the right ventricle. The right ventricle increases in size as pulmonary arterial pressure rises. It is often difficult to determine which ventricle predominates. The aorta is normal in size.

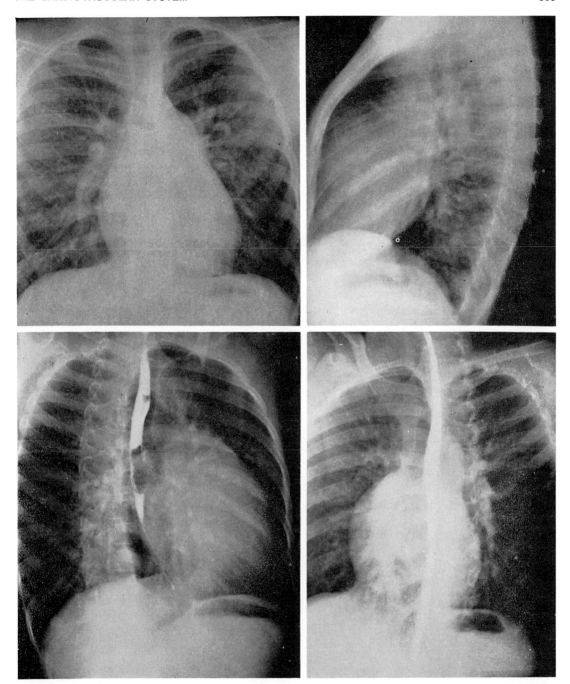

Fig. 32-16. Atrial septal defect. Note the enlargement of the right ventricle and pulmonary artery; the lung fields are hypervascular.

HEART SIZE. The heart may be normal in size but is often enlarged.

HEART SHAPE. Ventricular work is increased on both sides so that both ventricles may enlarge. The left ventricle often enlarges first. There may be left atrial enlargement resulting in recognizable displacement of the esophagus by this chamber in the right oblique and lateral projection (Fig. 32-17).

THE PULMONARY ARTERY. This vessel is enlarged and prominent.

PULMONARY VASCULARITY. Hilar and peripheral pulmonary vascularity is increased when the shunt is large.

THE AORTA. The aorta is normal in size.

ANGIOCARDIOGRAPHY. Angiocardiography shows a shunt of opaque material across the defect from the left into the right ventricle. Cardiac catheterization is a reliable diagnostic method in the study of this anomaly. Selective angiocardiography can be used to localize the site of the defect.

VENTRICULAR SEPTAL DEFECT WITH RIGHT-TO-LEFT SHUNT

Occlusive pulmonary vascular changes develop in patients with ventricular septal defect, leading to reversal of the shunt when the pulmonary arterial pressure exceeds the systemic pressure. The term, Eisenmenger's complex has been used in the past to indicate this complication of shunt reversal with cyanosis developing in adolescence or adult life.

Roentgen findings are those of cardiac enlargement, usually biventricular and moderate in amount. The pulmonary artery segment and central hilar vessels are very large, with disproportionate decrease in midzone and peripheral arteries indicating pulmonary hypertension. (Fig. 32-18). When there has been a right-to-

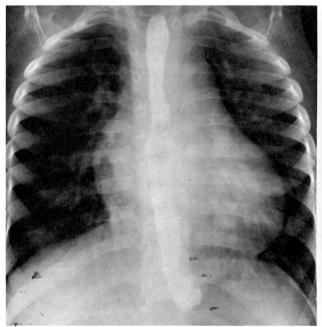
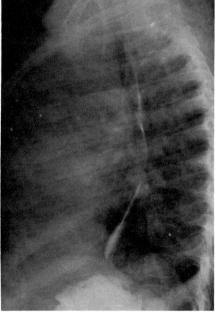

Fig. 32-17. Ventricular septal defect in a 16-month-old child. The heart is enlarged and there is some hypervascularity in the lung fields. The posterior displacement of the midesophagus indicates some left atrial enlargement. Aortic size is very difficult to assess in a child of this age.

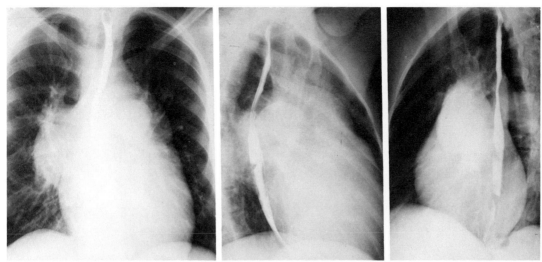

Fig. 32-18. Ventricular septal defect with right-to-left shunt and evidence of pulmonary hypertension. The heart is generally enlarged and there is great enlargement of the pulmonary artery and central hilar arteries in contrast to peripheral hypovascularity. The right ventricle is enlarged. This is manifested by the prominence of the distal right ventricle in the right anterior oblique projection and of the right side of the heart in the left anterior oblique projection.

left shunt from early childhood, the heart is not as large and the arterial disproportion is minimal. The latter type may show very minor roentgen changes.

PERSISTENT COMMON ATRIOVENTRICULAR CANAL (A–V COMMUNIS)

This defect may vary from the complete form in which there is a low atrial septal defect, a high ventricular septal defect and clefts in mitral and tricuspid valves to a lesser form in which the tricuspid valve is normal, or one in which the ventricular septum is intact and the tricuspid valve normal.

As in other left-to-right shunts, the roentgen findings depend upon the magnitude of the shunt and the presence or absence of pulmonary hypertension. Cardiac enlargement, usually biventricular, is present along with hilar prominence and peripheral hypervascularity. As a rule the heart is larger than in patients with atrial or ventricular septal defect. (Fig. 32-19.) There may be left atrial enlargement. The aorta tends to be small. If pulmonary hyperten-

sion develops, the changes are similar to those noted in ventricular septal defect with right-to-left shunt.

PULMONIC STENOSIS

The term is usually used to refer to the two types, namely valvular and infundibular stenosis. Of the two, the former is the more frequent when pulmonary stenosis occurs as a single lesion. Occasionally supravalvular stenosis may occur. Isolated pulmonic stenosis is a more common lesion than had been suspected before cardiac catheterization was used widely in the diagnosis of congenital heart disease.

Roentgen Findings

In a number of patients no recognizable abnormality is noted. The characteristic findings in valvular stenosis are right ventricular enlargement and prominence of the pulmonary artery in a patient with normal or slightly decreased peripheral pulmonary vascularity. The right atrium is sometimes enlarged. Isolated infundibular stenosis is rare.

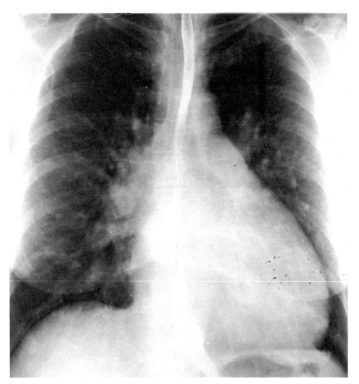

Fig. 32-19. Persistent common atrioventricular canal. Note the gross cardiac enlargement and hypervascularity, particularly marked in the central lung fields. The enlargement appears to be biventricular.

HEART SIZE. The heart may be normal in size but is enlarged in about half of the patients.

HEART SHAPE. The enlargement is right-sided and results in a rounded, right lower cardiac contour in the frontal projection and rounding of the right upper cardiac border in the left anterior oblique projection. The apex may be elevated and blunted. The outflow tract of the right ventricle is often prominent in the right anterior oblique projection.

PULMONARY ARTERY. The most characteristic finding is enlargement of the main pulmonary artery, resulting in convexity of the left upper cardiac margin below the aortic knob. This enlargement of the main pulmonary artery is due to poststenotic dilatation. The dilatation involves the pulmonary artery and the left pul-

monary artery which result in prominence of the arterial silhouette in the left hilum. The right pulmonary artery may be dilated, but this vessel is hidden by mediastinal density. Therefore, the size of hilar vessels tends to be asymmetric in contrast to the symmetry often observed in pulmonary hypertension, and is a helpful differential diagnostic sign. Poststenotic dilatation occurs in valvular stenosis (Fig. 32-20). In infundibular and supravalvular stenosis, the pulmonary artery is not prominent, and there may be no roentgen findings indicating cardiovascular disease.

PULMONARY VASCULARITY. The large main artery is associated with normal to decreased size of the vessels in the lung fields and in the right hilum. The pulsation in the left pulmonary artery may be increased as observed fluoroscop-

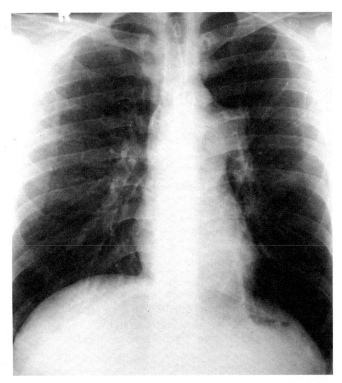

Fig. 32-20. Valvular pulmonic stenosis in a 23-year-old male. Note the great enlargement of the pulmonary artery and the proximal aspect of the left pulmonary artery so that the left hilar vessels are large in contrast to the small hilar vessels on the right. There is general hypovascularity elsewhere.

ically, while pulsation in the right pulmonary artery is usually decreased.

ANGIOCARDIOGRAPHY. Angiocardiography may demonstrate enlargement of the right atrium and ventricle, as well as outline the actual site and degree of pulmonic stenosis along with the poststenotic dilatation of the pulmonary artery.

AORTIC STENOSIS

Congenital aortic stenosis may be valvular, supravalvular or subvalvular. The valvular type of stenosis is more common than subaortic stenosis of the ventricular outflow tract, and supravalvular stenosis is quite rare. The valve may be bicuspid, but more commonly, there is a single cusp with a single commissure. Usually the bicuspid valve is not stenotic, but there is a tendency to acquire calcification and to become stenotic.

Roentgen Findings

Poststenotic dilatation of the aorta usually occurs in valvular stenosis. The dilatation is characteristically located in the ascending aorta and results in increased convexity of the right lateral aspect of the ascending aorta. It may be more clearly defined in the left anterior oblique than in the frontal projection. The transverse arch or aortic knob is not enlarged. Left ventricular hypertrophy and dilatation also occurs in this condition and results in increased prominence of the left ventricle in the left oblique projection and enlargement of the heart downward and to the left. The heart is usually not greatly enlarged. In nearly half of our patients (in whom the stenosis was minimal to moderate) no detectable roentgen abnormalities were found except for the slight prominence of the ascending aorta. When present, the findings are characteristic. Subaortic stenosis is particularly difficult to diagnose roentgenographically because there is no poststenotic dilatation and the left ventricular hypertrophy is often minimal. The pulmonary artery, right side of the heart, and pulmonary vascularity are normal.

CORRECTED TRANSPOSITION OF THE GREAT VESSELS

There are two major components in this anomaly: (1) transposition of the origins of the aorta and pulmonary artery, so that the aortic root is anterior and to the left of the pulmonary artery; (2) inversion of the ventricles with their accompanying atrioventricular valves. There is also inversion of the coronary arteries. Venous blood then enters the right atrium, flows through a bicuspid (mitral) valve into the anatomic left ventricle and to the lungs via the posteriorly placed pulmonary artery. Arterial blood returns from the lungs into the left atrium, flows through a tricuspid valve into the anatomic right ventricle and to the general circulation via an anteriorly placed left-sided aorta.

When this lesion occurs alone, no functional circulatory abnormality is present and no symptoms occur. In the majority of patients, however, there is an associated cardiovascular anomaly. Septal defects, especially ventricular, are the most common of these, and mitral valve anomalies are common. Pulmonic stenosis is also frequent.

The roentgen appearance depends on the associated defects. However, there are signs caused by the anomalous position of the great vessels which may be quite characteristic. The ascending aorta often forms the upper left border of the heart and may produce a slight convexity, a long straight line, or a very slight concavity of this border (Fig. 32-21). The pulmonary artery does not form a part of the left border, but may indent the esophagus below the normal position of the aortic indentation. Angiocardiography can be used to confirm the diagnosis. The anomalous position of the great vessels is readily determined.

ENDOCARDIAL FIBROELASTOSIS

Endocardial sclerosis, congenital subendothelial myofibrosis, congenital idiopathic hypertrophy of the heart, prenatal fibroelastosis, fetal endocarditis, endocardial dysplasia, and elastic tissue hyperplasia are synonyms. This is a disease that is probably congenital or developmental in origin,

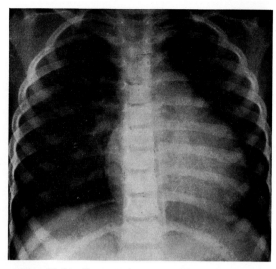

Fig. 32-21. Corrected transposition of the great vessels. Note the slight convexity of the left upper cardiovascular border produced by the ascending aorta. No aortic shadow is noted on the right. There was an associated atrial septal defect with a small left-to-right shunt.

although the etiology is not definitely known. It is manifested by marked endocardial thickening that involves the left side of the heart more frequently than the right. The endocardium is thickened by fibrous and elastic tissue without evidence of inflammation. Valves are often involved by contracture, thickening, and sometimes adhesions of the leaflets. The mitral valve is the most commonly and the most severely affected. The patients usually show no evidence of heart disease at birth and may develop normally for a variable period of time. Then symptoms begin and progress rapidly. They consist of dyspnea and evidence of congestive failure that may lead to death in a very short time. In others the process appears to develop more slowly and the patient survives for some length of time.

Roentgen Findings

The heart is usually enlarged and may be markedly so. It tends to be globular in shape and there is often evidence of pulmonary congestion indicating failure. The involvement of the mitral valve often results in insufficiency that produces left atrial and ventricular enlargement. This can be recognized by the characteristic posterior displacement of the esophagus, bulging of the left upper cardiac border, double contour on the right, and enlargement of the left ventricle downward and to the left. Pulmonary venous congestion may also be present. When the history is reasonably typical and these radiographic findings are noted, the diagnosis is fairly certain. In many instances it is made largely by the exclusion of other diseases (Fig. 32-22). A difference in pulsation may be observed fluoroscopically as a result of the predominant left ventricular involvement. The right ventricle pulsates normally, whereas the left ventricular pulsation is decreased or absent.

COARCTATION OF THE AORTA

This congenital malformation consists of an area of constriction in the aorta. It varies in degree from slight stenosis to atresia. The most commonly associated abnormality is bicuspid aortic valve, which is found in about 85 per cent of patients with coarctation. Two general types, or groups, are recognized. The most common is the type in which the site of constriction is at or distal to the ductus arteriosus. The constriction develops early in intrauterine life, resulting in stimulus to the formation of collateral circulation to the lower body. As a result the infant is born with some collaterals

and there is no change in the circulation when the ductus closes. The other general group, termed the preductal type, consists of constriction proximal to the ductus. The coarcted segment is usually longer than in the other form and this lesion is often associated with other congenital cardiovascular anomalies. In this type there is no stimulus to the development of collateral circulation for the lower extremities during intrauterine life because blood from the pulmonary circulation is shunted into the descending aorta through the ductus. After birth the ductus closes and the pulmonary bloodflow to the descending aorta is shut off, causing a sudden increase in left ventricular work. This often results in decompensation before collaterals are developed. If the patent ductus persists in coarctation of the preductal type, it results in cyanosis of the lower extremities with normal oxygenation of the head and upper extremities. Associated cardiac anomalies may result in intracardiac right-to-left shunt; then desaturation is generalized. In the infantile type the roentgen findings are not characteristic. The heart is often grossly enlarged and there is evidence of pulmonary congestion. When coarctation results in congestive cardiac failure in

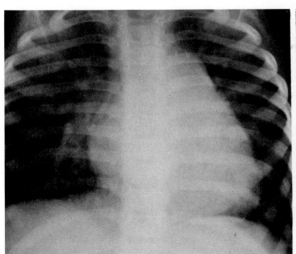 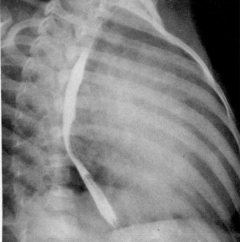

Fig. 32-22. Endocardial fibroelastosis. *Left,* Anteroposterior projection showing general cardiac enlargement with some pulmonary congestion. The large vessels are best outlined in the right parahilar region and at the right medial base. *Right,* Left anterior oblique projection. In addition to the generalized backward displacement of the esophagus by the large heart there is localized displacement caused by left atrial enlargement. The patient was found to have mitral valvular involvement producing stenosis.

infants, the roentgen and clinical findings are usually not diagnostic. Then retrograde aortography may be used to make the diagnosis.

Roentgen Findings

The signs are usually characteristic enough to permit the diagnosis of coarctation on routine roentgen studies.

RIB NOTCHING. Rib notching is an important radiologic sign. It is caused by dilatation and tortuosity of the intercostal arteries which serve as collaterals between the proximal aorta via the internal mammary, and the aorta distal to the coarctation. It is almost universally present in adults but may not be demonstrated in children in the first 5 or 6 years of life. The sign consists of an irregular, scalloped appear-

ance of the inferior margins of the ribs that is usually most common and readily outlined in the fourth through the eighth ribs. The third rib is sometimes involved but the first and second are rarely notched. The irregularity is usually bilateral but it is not necessarily symmetric (Fig. 32-23). A number of other causes for rib notching have been described. They include subclavian artery obstruction, superior caval obstruction with long-standing venous engorgement, arteriovenous fistula of the intercostal vessels, aortic valvular disease, and tetralogy of Fallot. In this group of diseases the rib notching is often local and almost invariably unilateral.

THE AORTA. The appearance of the aorta may be characteristic. The ascending arch is wide, producing convexity on the right side while the

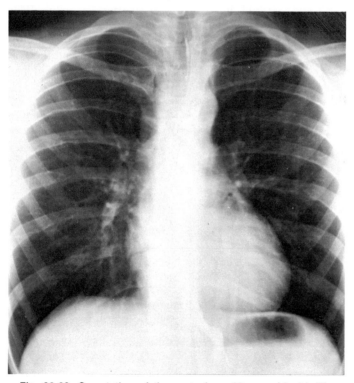

Fig. 32-23. Coarctation of the aorta in a 10-year-old girl. There is very clearly defined rib notching which is extremely helpful for diagnosis in this patient since the site of the coarctation is not demonstrated nor is there a very clearly defined area of poststenotic dilatation.

aortic knob or transverse aortic arch is small. Normally the left contour of the descending aorta can be visualized as a straight or gently convex line extending downward from the knob until it is obscured by the shadow of the heart below the hilum. In coarctation, a small indentation may be visible just below the knob that represents the actual site of coarctation. This is often associated with convexity below the coarctation site representing poststenotic dilatation. The appearance is that of two convexities, one representing the aortic knob and the second representing the dilated aorta distal to the coarctation. In other patients the actual indentation is not visible but the normal, clearly visualized, left aortic border is discontinuous. There is often enough dilatation of the left subclavian artery to result in convexity or prominence of the left superior mediastinal contour; this is often noted to be continuous with the shadow of the aortic knob. In the left

anterior oblique projection, the notch and dilatation below it may be visible and the esophagus is often displaced by the dilated aorta immediately below the coarctation. This displacement is to the right and slightly anteriorly and is definitely below the transverse aortic arch (Fig. 32-24). Congenital nonstenotic "kinking" of the aorta has also been described that may cause roentgen changes in this artery resembling those of coarctation. The other roentgen findings are absent, however, and there is no clinical evidence of coarctation.

HEART SIZE AND SHAPE. The heart may be normal in size and shape but the left ventricular work load is increased; eventually left-ventricular hypertrophy and dilatation result in enlargement of this chamber. The left atrium may also be enlarged. In infants with coarctation and cardiac failure the heart is relatively larger and there is evidence of pulmonary con-

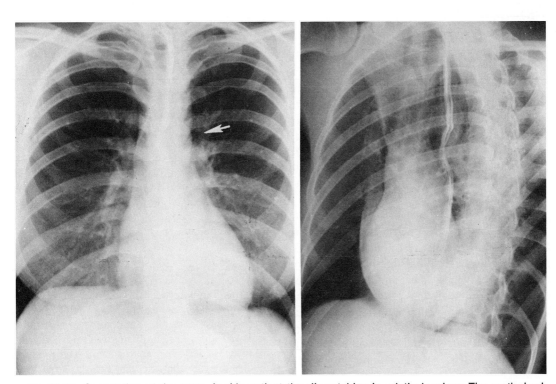

Fig. 32-24. Coarctation of the aorta. In this patient the rib notching is relatively minor. The aortic knob is small but there is a dilatation below it representing slight poststenotic enlargement of the aorta (retouched) (**arrow**). Note that the esophagus is displaced slightly in the left anterior oblique projection (*right*) by the dilated aorta below the coarctation.

gestion. These patients often have an associated anomaly such as patent ductus arteriosus or interventricular septal defect resulting in a left-to-right shunt. These defects cause hypervascularity and it is difficult to ascertain how much of the change is secondary to shunting and how much to congestive failure. As a general rule, when infants with coarctation develop venous congestion, an additional anomaly is usually present.

ANGIOCARDIOGRAPHY. This method is not ordinarily employed for the diagnosis of coarctation.

RETROGRADE AORTOGRAPHY. This examination is more useful than angiocardiography and clearly defines the coarcted segment as well as the aorta and its branches above and below it.

KINKING OF THE AORTIC ARCH (PSEUDOCOARCTATION)

Kinking or buckling of the aortic arch is sometimes termed pseudocoarctation because it simulates coarctation roentgenographically. No aortic constriction is present, however. The abnormality is presumably caused by a short, taut ligamentum arteriosum; but this does not account for the elongation of the arch that may be observed in this condition so a more likely cause is variation in normal differential growth rate of the aortic arch segments in early development.

Roentgen findings are somewhat variable, depending on the amount of elongation. The high aortic arch casts a round or crescentic shadow projecting to the left in the superior mediastinum, which may simulate a mediastinal tumor. Below this a second convexity projects to the left. The latter represents the arch at and distal to the kink and may be more dense than the upper shadow. In other patients the appearance is that of an unusually large aortic knob with an abrupt indentation at its inferior margin and a second convexity immediately below it caused by actual dilatation of the aorta distal to the kink. Either or both of the shadows may indent the esophagus. The left anterior oblique and lateral views are usually diagnostic, since the indentation at the site of buckling can usually be identified (Fig. 32-25). Tomograms in these projections may aid in the diagnosis. There is no left ventricular enlargement or rib notching.

ANEURYSM OF THE SINUS OF VALSALVA

The aortic sinuses are three dilatations in the root of the aorta just above the aortic valves. They are named according to their corresponding aortic valve cusps, the right, left, and posterior. The right and left coronary arteries originate in or above the corresponding sinus of Valsalva and the posterior sinus is sometimes termed the noncoronary sinus. Aneurysm is a rare congenital anomaly, usually involving the right aortic sinus. This sinus lies adjacent to the ventricular septum and occasionally a fistulous tract develops into the right ventricle. Rupture into the right atrium has also been reported. Rarely, aneurysmal dilatation of all the sinuses of Valsalva may be associated with coarctation of the aorta. Aneurysm also occurs in patients with Marfan's syndrome.

Roentgen Findings

The most common finding is a localized convex bulge of the right lower anterolateral cardiac contour. At fluoroscopy this region exhibits an increased amplitude of pulsation. In some patients, no abnormalities are observed on plain films of the chest because the lesion is small and located in an intracardiac position. Retrograde aortography can be used to define clearly the localized aneurysmal dilatation.

ANOMALOUS LEFT CORONARY ARTERY

In this anomaly the blood supply to the myocardium is affected because the left coronary artery arises from the pulmonary artery. As a result the left ventricle dilates early in life, leading to marked cardiac enlargement. The roentgen findings are not characteristic but the large heart is visualized and there is often evidence of pulmonary congestion. Although the left ventricle is enlarged, the signs commonly associated with enlargement of this chamber are not necessarily

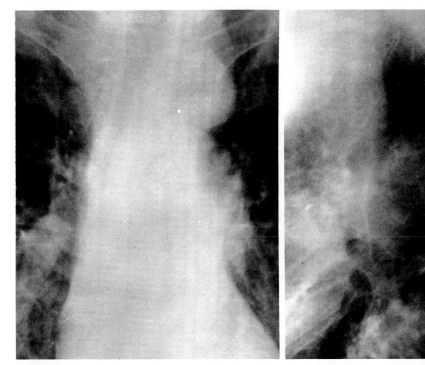

Fig. 32-25. Pseudocoaractation of the aorta. The transverse aortic arch is high and there is a very large, broad convexity of the aorta to the left below the arch. In the lateral view (*right*) the severe kinking is demonstrated (**arrows**).

present. When a large collateral forms, the blood flows into the pulmonary artery via the anomalous coronary, a left-to-right shunt. Angiocardiography is necessary to make the diagnosis.

ROTATION ANOMALIES OF THE HEART

The literature on classification and descriptions of various rotation and alignment anomalies is voluminous and somewhat confusing. Rosenbaum's classification[48] of cardiac alignments based on patterns of bloodflow is presented because of its consistency with current embryological thought, and its relative simplicity and precision. His definitions are indicated in Table 32-2. The possible courses of bloodflow are given in Figure 32-26.

Using these definitions and combining them with the positional designations, a description of cardiac alignment includes designation of the ventriculotruncal alignment (e.g., isolated ventricular inversion, inverted transposition, etc.), and a secondary indication of: (*1*) the presence of situs solitus or situs inversus and, (*2*) a left-sided or right-sided heart. The abdominal visceral situs

TABLE 32-2. Definitions

Right and left ventricles and atria	Denotes morphology only; no functional or positional connotation
Inversion	Relationship between ventricles and feeding atria
	Noninverted: RV* fed by RA, and LV fed by LA
	Inverted: RV fed by LA, and LV fed by RA
Transposition	Aorta arises from RV anterior to pulmonary artery which arises from the LV

* RV, right ventricle; LV, left ventricle; RA, right atrium; LA, left atrium.

From Rosenbaum, H. D.[48]

(situs solitus indicates the stomach is on the left; situs inversus indicates the stomach is on the right) indicates the position of the atria according to Rosenbaum[48] except in rare instances of isolated gastric inversion. Elliott, Jue, and Amplatz,[10] and others believe that atrial position is more consistent with the side of the aortic arch. If the right atrium

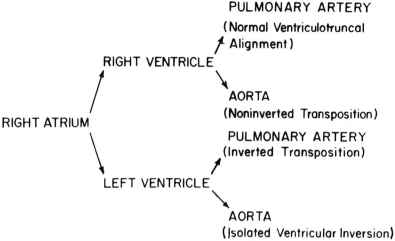

Fig. 32-26. Possible courses of bloodflow from the right atrium. (From Rosenbaum, H. D.[48])

is on the side opposite the stomach and on the same side as the liver, nearly all of the possible alignments can be determined with good biplane angiocardiograms. A few exceptions include the abnormalities associated with asplenia and polysplenia as well as some cases of common atrium. Although Rosenbaum's classification is not in common use, it is valuable in defining the four fundamental ventriculotruncal alignments (Fig. 32-27). Fig. 32-28 outlines the possible variations in abdominal situs and cardiac position and their relation to ventriculotruncal alignments.

Dextrocardia with situs solitus is nearly always associated with severe congenital cardiac malformation. Dextrocardia which is a part of complete situs inversus, a mirror image of the normal, nearly always has a normal ventriculotruncal alignment. When the heart is right-sided as a result of pulmonary, diaphragmatic, or spinal abnormalities, there are usually no associated cardiac malformations.

ANOMALIES OF THE AORTIC ARCH AND ITS LARGE BRANCHES

The embryologic development of the aortic arch and its branches is complex. Six pairs of aortic arches develop in the embryo of man but not all are present at the same time. They originate anteriorly in the aortic sac, which represents the proximal portion of the developing aortic arch. They course backward on both sides to join the dorsal aorta, which is bilateral. The arches develop in the fifth week and their transformation occupies the sixth and seventh weeks of fetal development. The first and second arches disappear early. The dorsal aorta at these levels persists as part of the internal carotid and the third arch persists as the proximal part of the common carotid artery on either side. The external carotid arteries arise as separate buds from the aortic sac and later transfer their origins onto the third arches. The fourth arch persists on both sides. The left forms the permanent or left-sided aortic arch while the right side forms the innominate artery. The fifth arches are transitory and disappear without a trace. The sixth arches arise from each dorsal aorta and extend across to the primitive pulmonary artery on either side to form the ductus arteriosus. The connection is lost on the right but persists on the left until after birth, when it closes to form the ligamentum arteriosum. Early in development the dorsal aorta fuses below the arch to form a single descending aorta.

RIGHT AORTIC ARCH

The most common aortic anomaly is right aortic arch with left descending aorta in which

VENTRICULOTRUNCAL ALIGNMENTS

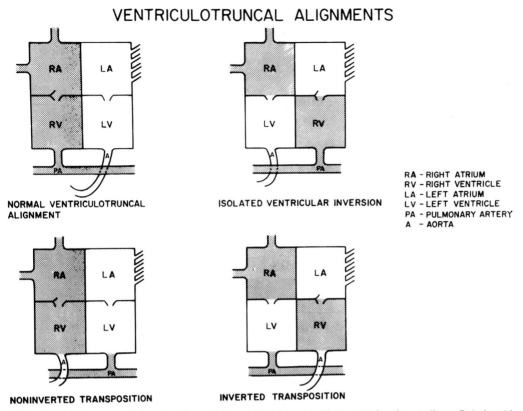

NORMAL VENTRICULOTRUNCAL
ALIGNMENT

ISOLATED VENTRICULAR INVERSION

RA – RIGHT ATRIUM
RV – RIGHT VENTRICLE
LA – LEFT ATRIUM
LV – LEFT VENTRICLE
PA – PULMONARY ARTERY
A – AORTA

NONINVERTED TRANSPOSITION

INVERTED TRANSPOSITION

Fig. 32-27. Diagrams of four fundamental ventriculotruncal alignments in situs solitus. Relationships are reversed in situs inversus. (From Rosenbaum, H. D.[48])

the arch crosses behind the esophagus and indents it posteriorly. It is of no clinical significance when it occurs as an isolated anomaly. Right aortic arch with right descending aorta is not as common and may be complicated by a left retroesophageal subclavian artery. Right aortic arch with right descending aorta is the type frequently associated with tetralogy of Fallot; it is also associated with tricuspid atresia and transposition of the great vessels. A rare anomaly included in this group is a right descending aorta in which the arch is left-sided but curves backward and to the right behind the esophagus.

Roentgen Findings

On the frontal projection a prominent aortic mass is noted on the right side with absence of the convex shadow of the aortic knob on the left. The right arch tends to be higher in position than the left. An esophagram outlines the retroesophageal aorta, which produces a rounded indentation on the posterior aspect of the esophagus if the descending aorta is on the left (Fig. 32-29). It does not ordinarily cause any symptoms. When the descending aorta is on the right the esophagram reveals slight indentation in the right lateral aspect of the esophagus. The soft-tissue density produced by the aorta can often be outlined descending on the right side.

OTHER ANOMALIES

The innominate artery may arise more distally than normal and cross anterior to the trachea from left to right. It produces slight indentation and occasionally may cause respi-

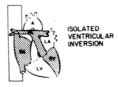
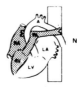

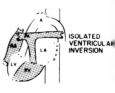

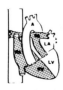
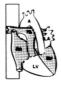
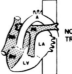
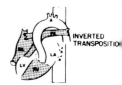

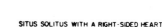

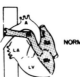
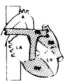

SITUS SOLITUS WITH A LEFT-SIDED HEART

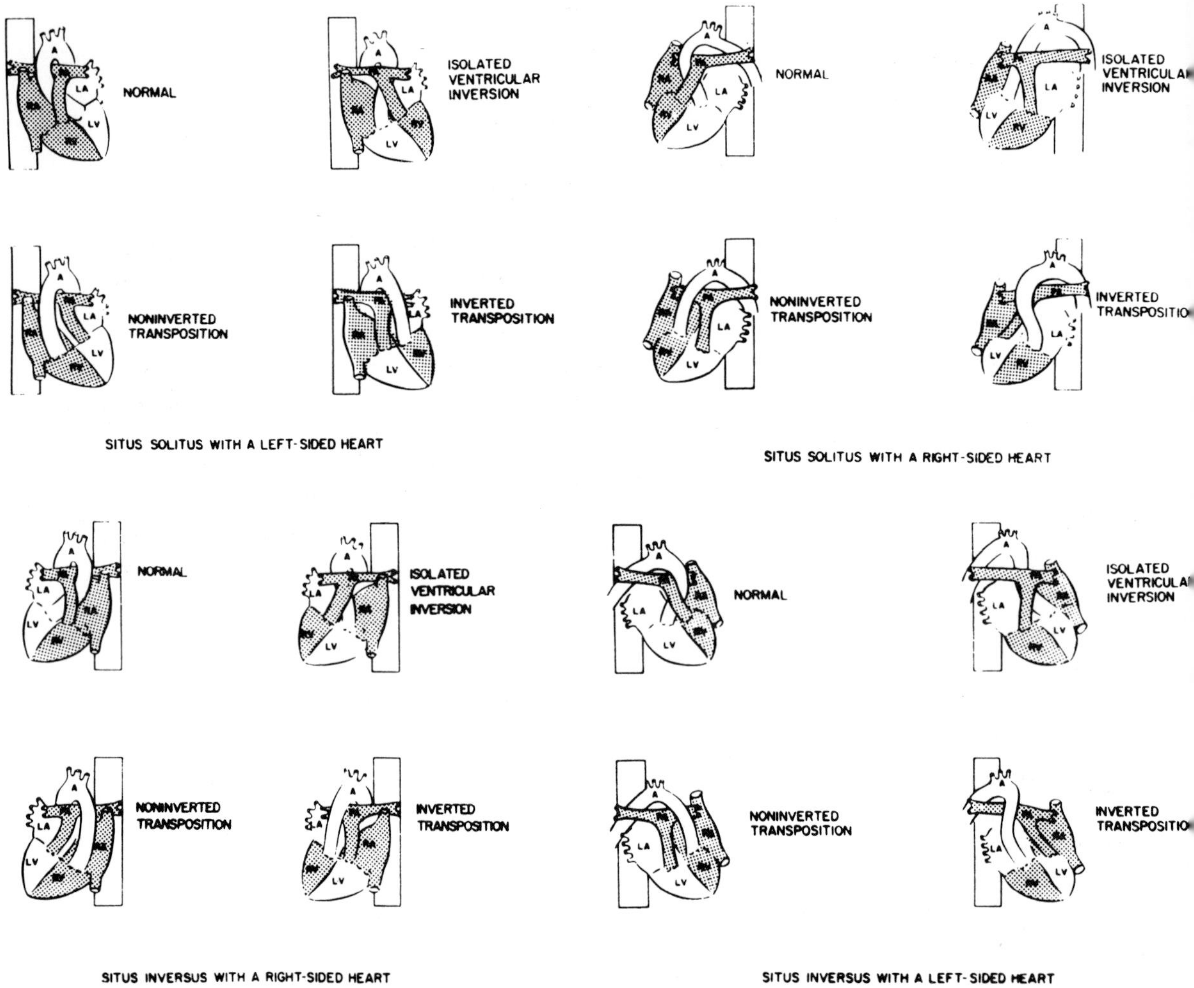

SITUS SOLITUS WITH A RIGHT-SIDED HEART

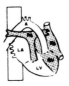
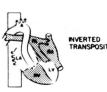

SITUS INVERSUS WITH A RIGHT-SIDED HEART

SITUS INVERSUS WITH A LEFT-SIDED HEART

Fig. 32-28. The four fundamental ventriculotruncal alignments in situs solitus and situs inversus, both with a right-sided heart and with a left-sided heart. Please note that the alignments of situs solitus with a right-sided heart are identical to those seen with situs solitus and a left-sided heart. The only difference is the location of the cardiac apex. Similarly, the alignments for situs inversus and a left-sided heart are identical to those seen in situs inversus with a right-sided heart. (From Rosenbaum, H. D.[48])

ratory distress in infants. Similar anterior indentation and compression may be caused by the left carotid artery when it arises more proximally than normal and must cross from right to left anterior to the trachea.

ANOMALIES FORMING VASCULAR RINGS

DOUBLE AORTIC ARCH. The double aortic arch comprises a large group of anomalies in which

there are many variants. The fundamental defect results from persistence of both the right and the left aortic arches that encircle the trachea and esophagus and often produce partial obstruction of these structures. Either or both of the arches may function and may be comparable in size or one may be larger than the other. The aorta may descend on either the right or the left side and anomalous origins of one or more of the great vessels often accompany this anomaly. The roentgen and fluoro-

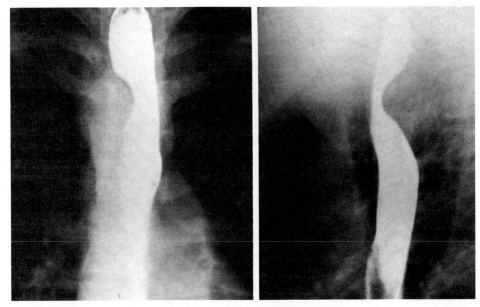

Fig. 32-29. Right aortic arch. In the frontal view (*left*) no arch is noted on the left and there is a vascular shadow on the right resembling the transverse aortic arch which indents the esophagus. In the lateral view (*right*) there is posterior indentation of the esophagus indicating that the arch turns to the left and in this patient descends on the left.

scopic findings consist of evidence of compression of the trachea and esophagus by an encircling vascular ring. The double arch produces densities on either side of the mid line that may be symmetric. Angiocardiography has limited value but if necessary, aortography can be used to define the vascular ring.

RIGHT AORTIC ARCH WITH LEFT LIGAMENTUM ARTERIOSUM OR PATENT DUCTUS ARTERIOSUS. This is a rare cause of vascular ring that often results in enough tracheal and esophageal obstruction to produce symptoms in early childhood. If the ligamentum or ductus is relatively long the condition may go unrecognized. In this anomaly the aorta descends on the right and the ligamentum arteriosum extends from the pulmonary artery backward and to the right behind the esophagus, where it joins the distal aortic arch. In the common variety of right aortic arch, the ligamentum arteriosum usually lies on the same side as the upper portion of the descending aorta and does not produce a ring.

The roentgen findings are similar to those found in double aortic arch but there is often enough difference to suspect the diagnosis that can be confirmed by retrograde aortography if necessary. Frontal roentgenograms show that the major mass of the aorta and aortic arch lie to the right of the midline and the right descending aorta may also be visible. The barium-filled esophagus is indented on the right by the arch and a transverse or slightly oblique defect is visible on the posterior aspect of the esophagus just below the level of the aortic arch. The obliquity is downward and to the left from the region of the right aortic arch. Occasionally there is a shallow defect along the left lateral aspect of the esophagus, made by the ligamentum as it extends from the pulmonary artery backward and toward the right along the left esophageal margin. The left subclavian artery arises to the right of the midline in these patients with a right aortic arch and courses upward and to the left behind the esophagus. It may also produce a very slight indentation on the posterior esophageal wall (Fig. 32-30).

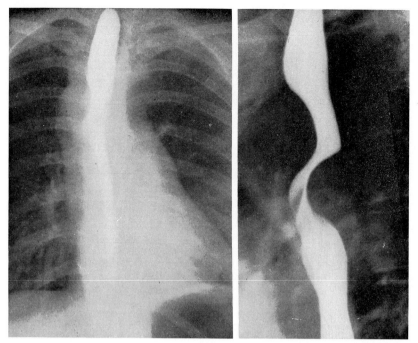

Fig. 32-30. Right aortic arch with left patent ductus forms a vascular ring, resulting in moderate dysphagia. *Left,* In the frontal projection the aortic knob is absent on the left and the aorta is noted on the right where it indents the right lateral aspect of the esophagus. It also descends on the right. Some indentation is noted on the left lateral aspect of the esophagus slightly below the level of the aorta. The roentgenogram on the *right* is an enlarged view of a spot film taken during fluoroscopy. The patient was in the left anterior oblique position. The narrowing of the esophagus is clearly defined. The ductus arteriosus crossed behind the esophagus from below upward, producing the well-marked posterior indentation noted. The ductus was ligated and sectioned, relieving the patient's symptoms.

ABERRANT RIGHT SUBCLAVIAN ARTERY

This is the most common of the anomalies of the great vessels. The right subclavian originates as the most distal of the branches of the arch and reaches the right side by coursing obliquely upward and to the right, usually behind the esophagus. This defect is often asymptomatic but may be associated with other cardiovascular anomalies. The major roentgen finding is an oblique indentation of the posterior aspect of the esophagus above the aortic arch, which extends upward and to the right. It is usually outlined best in the lateral and left anterior oblique projections. Fluoroscopic examination with barium swallow will outline this defect and its effect on the esophagus, and the pulsation of the anomalous artery is usually apparent.

CONGENITAL ANOMALIES OF THE PULMONARY ARTERY AND ITS BRANCHES

AGENESIS OF THE PULMONARY ARTERY

This is an uncommon anomaly in which there is absence of one pulmonary artery. It is associated with an anomalous systemic arterial blood supply to the lung that arises either from the aorta or from one of its major branches. The anomaly is often associated with other congenital anomalies of the cardiovascular system. Occasionally the systemic artery supplying the involved lung is very large; this results in a large arteriovenous shunt that may eventually cause cardiac failure. The high pressure in this anomalous system is believed to be the cause of hemoptysis, the most common symptom of the condition.

Roentgen Findings

The roentgen findings are characteristic enough to make the diagnosis or strongly suspect it in most instances. The involved hemithorax is smaller in size than the normal. In addition to the difference in size of the bony thorax, the hemidiaphragm is often elevated and mediastinal structures are shifted to the affected side. There is often some herniation of the normal lung across the midline anterior to the aorta. The normal shadows of the pulmonary arterial branches in the hilum and in the lung are absent and the vessels that are visible form a relatively fine reticular vascular pattern caused by the branching bronchial arteries. The result is an absence of the hilum shadow or an inconspicuous one. Tomography is very useful to define clearly the difference in the hilar vessels on the two sides. Bronchography outlines the normally branching bronchial tree and excludes atelectasis, while angiocardiography can be used to define the main pulmonary artery and its remaining branch and to show the lack of filling on the opposite side (Fig. 32-31). Agenesis of a lobe, or lobes, may occur in conjunction with agenesis of the pulmonary artery. Hypoplasia of one pulmonary artery may result in similar but somewhat less marked roentgen findings. Unless the hypoplasia is relatively severe, however, it is unlikely that the diagnosis can be made without the use of angiocardiography.

PULMONARY ARTERIOVENOUS MALFORMATIONS

This is a congenital vascular anomaly, sometimes termed a fistula or aneurysm (we prefer the term "arteriovenous malformation") through which a relatively large amount of nonoxygenated blood flows; therefore the lesion represents a right-to-left shunt and is associated with varying degrees of unsaturation of the arterial blood. The malformations are usually multiple and occur more frequently in the lower lobes than elsewhere. Because the caliber of the vessels within the mass varies, there is

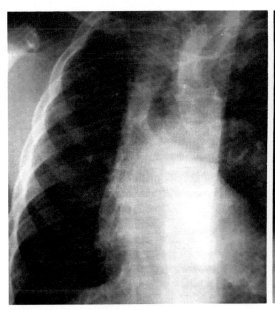 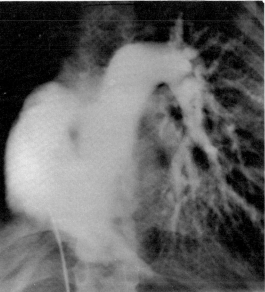

Fig. 32-31. Agenesis of the right pulmonary artery. *Left,* Frontal chest film shows rather marked shift of the heart and mediastinal structures to the right. The branches of the right pulmonary artery are absent so that no hilar vessels are visible and the entire right lung shows very little vascularity. *Right,* The angiocardiogram shows the main pulmonary artery and its left branch. Note that the right pulmonary artery is absent.

no quantitative correlation between the size of the anomaly and the amount of shunt. The pulmonary lesions may be accompanied by hemangiomas or telangiectases elsewhere and are then a part of a generalized angiomatous process. Since these are right to left shunts which may be quite large, the filtering effect of the pulmonary capillary circulation is lost and any embolic process arising in the systemic venous system may result in systemic embolization. For example, brain abscess is among the complications.

Roentgen Findings

The malformation is represented by a round, oval, or lobulated mass or several masses, usually in the lower lobes. The lesion is clearly defined and it is often possible to see a large pulmonary artery extending from the hilum to the lesion and another vessel, the pulmonary vein, extending from it to the region of the left atrium. If large vessels can be demonstrated going to it and draining it, the diagnosis should be strongly suspected. Tomograms are useful in outlining the blood supply and in clearly defining the lesions. When one is visualized, it is wise to look carefully for others since they are often multiple. At fluoroscopy active pulsations may be visible in the angioma itself as well as in the pulmonary artery supplying it. It may be possible to demonstrate a decrease in size during the Valsalva experiment (expiration against closed glottis) and an increase in size of the lesion when the intrathoracic pressure is reduced (Müller maneuver). Pulmonary arteriography is used to confirm the finding before surgical removal and also to determine the presence of smaller lesions that cannot be outlined on routine roentgenograms (Fig. 32-32).

PULMONARY ARTERY COARCTATIONS

A wide variety of pulmonary coarctations have been reported. The stenosis may involve the pulmonary artery above the valve and either or both of its main branches. Multiple peripheral stenoses involving many segmental arterial branches may also occur. The stenosis may be sharply localized or involve a relatively long segment of the affected artery. The coarctation may be unilateral or bilateral and is associated with valvular pulmonic stenosis in 60 per cent of patients.

Roentgen findings are varied and depend upon the location of the stenotic lesion, its length, and the presence or absence of poststenotic dilatation. In the central types, poststenotic dilatation may

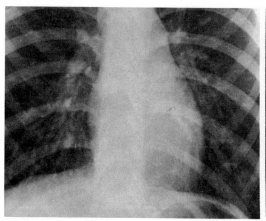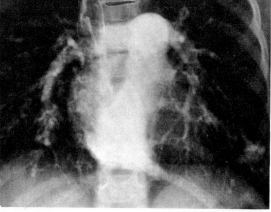

Fig. 32-32. Multiple pulmonary arteriovenous malformations. *Left,* In the frontal chest film there are numerous large vessels extending from the hila downward to the bases with an irregularly lobulated, clearly defined mass noted in the left base just above the diaphragm. At the right medial base there are many vessels resulting in considerable increase in density. The right side of the heart and pulmonary arteries are filled on the angiogram (*right*) clearly defining the large basal arteriovenous malformations bilaterally.

result in an increase of the hilar vascular shadow. When the stenosis involves a long segment of either the right or left pulmonary artery or both, the hilar vascular shadow may be decreased, often with distinct increase in vessel size a short distance from the central hilum. In patients with multiple peripheral stenoses, the poststenotic dilatations may produce a nodular vascular pattern in the parahilar region unilaterally or bilaterally. When such findings are present, the diagnosis can be suspected. Pulmonary arteriography is needed for definitive diagnosis, however. The coarctations are readily demonstrated when the vessels are opacified.

ABERRANT LEFT PULMONARY ARTERY

The left pulmonary artery arises from the right in this rare anomaly, and courses usually between the trachea and the esophagus to the left lung. It produces a posterior tracheal and an anterior esophageal indentation and can be positively identified on pulmonary arteriography.

IDIOPATHIC ENLARGEMENT OF THE PULMONARY ARTERY

Dilatation of the pulmonary artery in diseases of the heart and lungs has been described. Occasionally marked dilatation of the pulmonary artery occurs as an isolated finding. This is sometimes termed "congenital aneurysm." The dilatation may extend into the left main branch for a short distance and occasionally into the right branch. All clinical and laboratory studies, including cardiac catheterization, fail to demonstrate a cause so occasionally this enlargement probably represents a true congenital aneurysm. The diagnosis is made by exclusion, however, since there are many known cardiac and pulmonary diseases that can result in considerable dilatation of the pulmonary artery. The only roentgenographic finding is prominence in the region of the artery, resulting in convexity and enlargement of the artery segment as seen in the frontal projection. The enlargement can also be observed in oblique and lateral views. The diagnosis is made with caution since it is one of exclusion and cannot be made on the basis of roentgenographic findings alone.

The pulmonary artery is often prominent in childhood and early adult life. The convexity produced by the pulmonary artery is moderately enlarged, with no sign of cardiac or pulmonary

disease on roentgenographic examination. Examination reveals no cause for it and the vessel evidently decreases in size because the finding is uncommon in older adults.

ACQUIRED VALVULAR CARDIAC DISEASE

MITRAL VALVULAR DISEASE

MITRAL STENOSIS

Acquired mitral valvular disease usually results from rheumatic heart disease. Mitral stenosis is most common but there is often some degree of mitral insufficiency. The left atrium must empty itself against increased resistance caused by the mitral stenosis and the chamber enlarges. The increased pressure is reflected back through the lesser circulation to the right ventricle. This results in changes in the pulmonary vessels and in the right side of the heart.

Roentgen Findings

The appearance of the cardiovascular silhouette in mitral valvular disease is often characteristic (Fig. 32-33). There are alterations caused by left atrial enlargement. This may be the only change in the cardiac silhouette for some time. There is often enough stenosis to ultimately cause right ventricular enlargement and enough insufficiency to cause some left ventricular enlargement. There are also pulmonary vascular alterations which will be described. The signs of left atrial enlargement are: (1) Convexity of the left upper cardiac margin below the level of the left main bronchus. This represents enlargement of the auricular appendage (Fig. 32-34). In patients with a transverse heart the only alteration may be a straightening of the left upper cardiac margin in contrast to its usual slight concavity below the pulmonary artery. (2) A double contour or double convexity occurs on the right. The atrium may be large enough to be border-forming on the right side in which case a double convexity is visible. When it is not border-

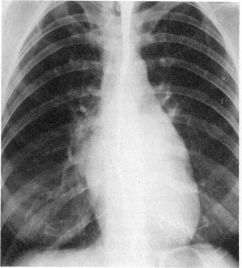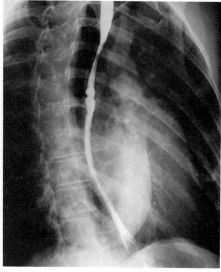

Fig. 32-33. Mitral stenosis. *Left,* The frontal view shows a double convexity on the right and a prominence of the left upper cardiac border below the left bronchus. These signs indicate left atrial enlargement. The overall cardiac size is normal. Note the scarcity of pulmonary vessels at the bases despite sizeable hilar arteries. *Right,* The right anterior oblique view shows posterior displacement of the esophagus by the large left atrium. There is also noted some prominence of the outflow tract of the right ventricle manifested by some convexity of the upper cardiac border on the left.

forming it is often of sufficient density to be identified within the right atrial border, forming a more dense convexity within the longer, right atrial convexity. (*3*) There is often a sufficient posterior enlargement of this chamber to recognize it as an area of increased density within the cardiac margins on either side below the level of the carina. (*4*) The left main bronchus may be elevated. The findings through 4 are observed in the frontal projection. (*5*) In the lateral and right anterior oblique projections barium is given to outline the esophagus which is displaced posteriorly and sometimes slightly to the right by the enlarged atrium. This results in a posterior convexity of the esophagus in this region.

Calcium is often deposited in the mitral valve and in the mitral annulus. This may be somewhat difficult to demonstrate on roentgenograms of the chest but is usually easily seen fluoroscopically. The valvular calcification usually indicates mitral stenosis while calcium in the mitral annulus may not necessarily be asso-

ciated with valvular abnormality. The latter has a somewhat elliptical shape.

Calcification in the left atrium is occasionally observed in patients with mitral stenosis. The calcium may be in the atrial wall or within a thrombus attached to the wall. When calcification in the atrium is suspected but not positively identified on the chest film, fluoroscopy can be used to confirm the diagnosis.

If the disease results in pulmonary arterial hypertension, eventually the right ventricle enlarges and the signs of an increase in size of this chamber are observed. Enlargement of the central pulmonary arteries is helpful in calling the attention of the observer to the likelihood of right ventricular enlargement.

As indicated above, there are alterations in pulmonary vascular pressure which tend to cause progressive pulmonary changes. Initially there is some venous hypertension. The first sign is that of slight general venous distintion or engorgement which is difficult to assess. It is most readily identified when earlier films are

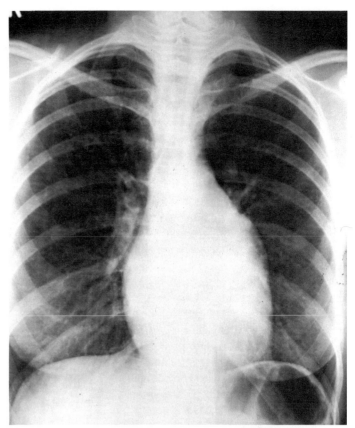

Fig. 32-34. Mitral stenosis. In this patient the left atrium is very large and the appendage produces a marked local bulge below the left pulmonary artery in the upper left cardiac margin. *The* vessels are approximately equal in the upper and lower lung fields.

available for comparison. As the hypertension becomes more marked there is constriction of the lower lobe arteries and veins and distention of the upper lobe vessels resulting in a reversal of the usual pattern in which the lower lobe vessels are more prominent (Fig. 32-35). Most of the blood flow is then maintained through the upper lobes. This alteration in the vascular pattern is usually readily identified early but in long-standing chronic venous hypertension there may be enough interstitial change to obscure the vascular findings. As the venous pressure increases more fluid escapes into the perivascular tissues and the lymphatics become dilated. This causes the appearance of Kerley's B lines which are short, dense lines representing interlobular septa extending to the pleural surface. They are observed in the lower lung fields and are at right angles to the pleural surface (Fig. 32-36). They do not bifurcate and are often observed best on oblique films. It is likely that interstitial edema fluid as well as lymphatic distention contributes to the density. The deep septal lines, Kerley's A lines, may also become visible. They are about 2- to 5-inches long, tend to be straight and extend outward and upward in a somewhat fanlike manner from the upper hilar area into the periphery of the upper lung field. Kerley's C lines also represent interstitial structures or lymphatics within the interstitial structures. They tend to be transient and difficult to visualize but cause a fine spider-web or reticular pattern throughout the lung. In chronic venous

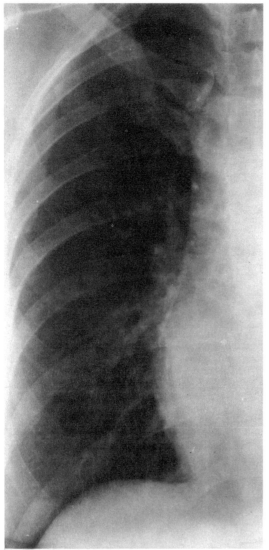

Fig. 32-35. Pulmonary vessels in mitral stenosis. The lower lung vessels are constricted and appear smaller in size than the upper lung vessels.

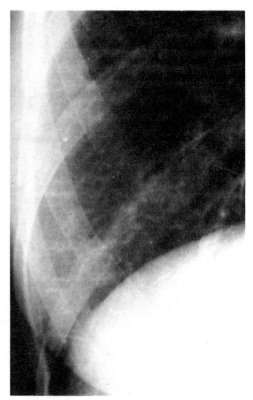

Fig. 32-36. Kerley's B lines. This close-up view of the right lateral base in a patient with mitral stenosis shows short, horizontal dense lines representing interstitial edema and dilatation of the lymphatics.

hypertension associated with chronic passive congestion deposits of hemosiderin are added to the other causes for prominence of the septal lines.

Eventually pulmonary arterial hypertension may occur. This results in dilatation of the main pulmonary artery and its branches centrally, which is associated with a constriction of arteries in the midlung and peripheral lung zones. These findings are then superimposed on those of chronic venous hypertension.

Pulmonary hemosiderosis secondary to mitral disease is a frequent pathologic finding but is not commonly recognized as such on chest films. It consists of a deposition of blood pigments in the interstitial tissues. When the amount is sufficient the deposits are visible roentgenographically as fine granular or miliary shadows throughout the lungs (Fig. 32-37). They may become large enough to produce nodular densities ranging from 2 to 5 mm in diameter. Then the appearance of the lungs may resemble that noted in miliary tuberculosis or early nodular silicosis. The associated findings of mitral disease are usually obvious however so that there is no difficulty in making the differential diagnosis.

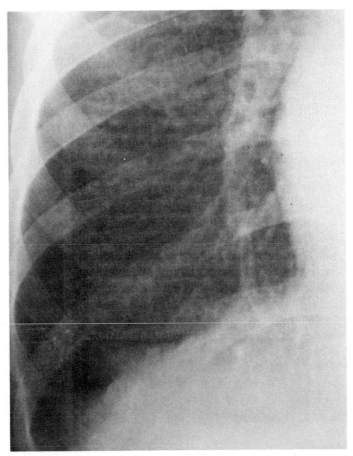

Fig. 32-37. Hemosiderosis in a patient with mitral stenosis. Close-up view of the right lower lung field shows numerous small, granular-appearing nodules which developed over several years of observation.

Pulmonary ossification or calcification is an uncommon finding in mitral stenosis. It is usually found in the lower lobes and produces multiple opacities resembling the calcified lesions of histoplasmosis scattered widely in the lung bases (Fig. 32-38).

MITRAL INSUFFICIENCY

Mitral insufficiency is often associated with mitral stenosis. This valvular defect increases the left ventricular work load and leads to dilatation and hypertrophy of this chamber. It is manifested by enlargement of the heart downward and to the left with lengthening and rounding of the left lower cardiac contour. The left atrium is also enlarged and causes the signs described above for enlargement of this chamber. Pulmonary congestion develops as in mitral stenosis. Often it is impossible to differentiate mitral stenosis and insufficiency. Relative mitral insufficiency commonly occurs in diseases which produce left-ventricular dilatation. Its presence, although suspected, may be difficult to detect radiographically in many of these cases.

COMBINED MITRAL DISEASE

In many instances there are gross changes indicating a double lesion, while in others the findings are sufficiently characteristic to war-

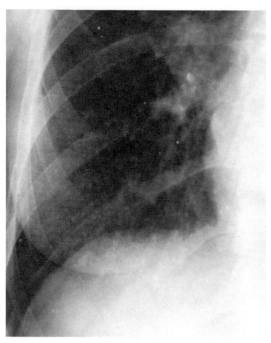

Fig. 32-38. Scattered pulmonary calcifications in mitral stenosis. This close-up view of the right lower lung field shows scattered calcifications ranging up to about 2 mm in diameter. These were also noted at the left base with very few calcified nodules in the upper lung fields.

rant the diagnosis of mitral stenosis without significant regurgitation. There is a third group in which differential diagnosis is difficult on roentgen study. As a rule, the left atrium is larger in combined stenosis and insufficiency. There should be left ventricular enlargement when insufficiency is present, but this may be very difficult to detect. The posterior curve of the enlarged left atrium in the right anterior oblique projection tends to be longer in insufficiency than in isolated stenosis. Rheumatic heart disease also causes aortic stenosis and insufficiency that result in left ventricular enlargement. These lesions must be kept in mind in addition to mitral insufficiency when left ventricular enlargement is present (Fig. 32-39). When surgery is contemplated in patients with mitral valve disease, cardiac catheterization is used to assess pulmonary arterial and venous pressures as well as to define the amount of stenosis or insufficiency or both

present. Selective angiocardiography may be used in conjunction with catheterization to assess the amount of regurgitation, the severity of the stenosis, and the pliability of the valve.

AORTIC VALVULAR DISEASE

AORTIC STENOSIS

Rheumatic heart disease is the most common cause of acquired aortic stenosis. Occasionally it may develop as a degenerative process in patients with bicuspid aortic valves, leading to a calcified valve with stenosis. This lesion causes increased work load on the left ventricle and results in hypertrophy. As a result there is rounding of the left lower cardiac border. Hypertrophy is usually present without dilatation (concentric hypertrophy), the heart is within normal limits of size and the only finding is rounding of the apex. When dilatation occurs, the left border elongates, moving the apex downward and to the left. The aortic knob is normal in size and the ascending aortic arch is enlarged, resulting in convexity of the right upper cardiac margin. This may be observed best in the left anterior oblique projection. This enlargement represents poststenotic dilatation. There may be a considerable amount of calcification in the aortic valve. This is usually readily visible fluoroscopically but is difficult to see in the frontal roentgenogram because the valve is projected over the shadow of the spine. It is often visible in the right and left oblique positions, however, and is a valuable sign of acquired aortic stenosis (Fig. 32-40). The roentgen findings in aortic stenosis may be diagnostic, but in some cases must be supported by clinical findings to make the diagnosis. As a general rule left ventricular enlargement is found late in the disease as a result of dilatation in left ventricular failure.

AORTIC INSUFFICIENCY

Aortic insufficiency may be caused by rheumatic fever (rheumatic valvulitis), and less often by syphilis and arteriosclerosis. Incom-

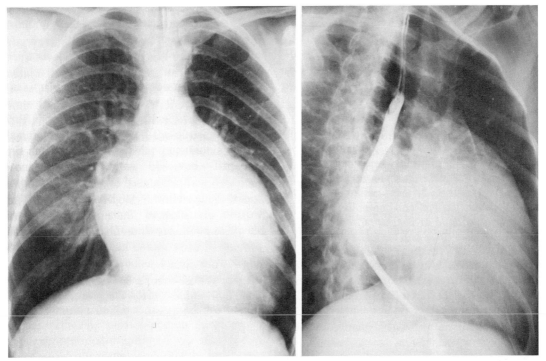

Fig. 32-39. Combined mitral stenosis and insufficiency. Marked cardiac enlargement with massive enlargement of the left atrium noted on the frontal (*left*) and right anterior oblique (*right*) projections. There is also marked prominence of the pulmonary outflow tract. Note paucity of basal vessels.

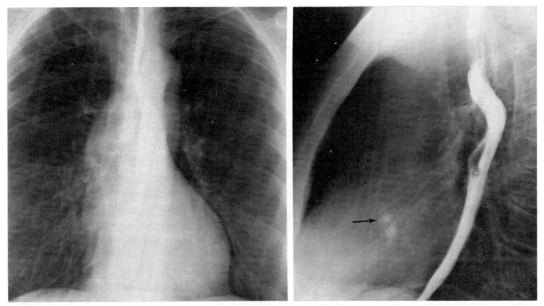

Fig. 32-40. Calcific aortic stenosis. *Left,* In the frontal projection note the marked dilatation of the ascending aorta producing a convexity to the right. The apex is rounded indicating left ventricular hypertrophy. On the lateral view (*right*) the **arrow** indicates calcium in the aortic valve.

petence of the aortic valve results in dilatation of the left ventricle along with hypertrophy. The outflow tract of this chamber is the first to enlarge, resulting in an increase in length of the left lower cardiac contour that represents the ventricular segment. The apex then extends below the dome of the diaphragm. The lower left ventricular contour is also rounded. As enlargement progresses with involvement of the inflow tract, the left ventricular segment increases further and the upper left contour tends to become more rounded. There is then evidence of posterior enlargement with rounding of the lower posterior cardiac margin as visualized in the left anterior oblique projection (Fig. 32-41). The aorta is occasionally dilated, resulting in convexity of the aortic segment comprising the upper right cardiovascular margin and the aortic knob is often prominent. The enlargement of the heart may be extreme in aortic regurgitation and when massive left ventricular enlargement occurs, the term "cor bovinum" is sometimes used to describe it. Combined stenosis and regurgitation may be present but there is no way to ascertain the predominant lesion on roentgen study. Fluo-

roscopy is useful; the marked increase in pulse pressure is reflected in an increased amplitude of pulsation of the aorta when aortic regurgitation is present. When aortic valvular disease results in cardiac failure, the signs of pulmonary congestion develop along with the appearance of relative mitral insufficiency resulting in left atrial enlargement.

In rheumatic valvular disease both the aortic and mitral valves are often involved and there may be massive generalized cardiac enlargement along with enlargement of the chambers in which work is increased. At times it is possible to determine the predominant defect but this is not always the case. When a proximal valve (such as the mitral) is involved by stenosis and insufficiency it becomes very difficult to assess change in the distal (aortic) valve by roentgen means short of angiocardiography and aortography.

PULMONARY VALVULAR DISEASE

Pulmonary stenosis is usually a congenital anomaly; the roentgen findings produced by

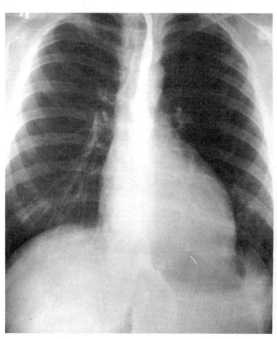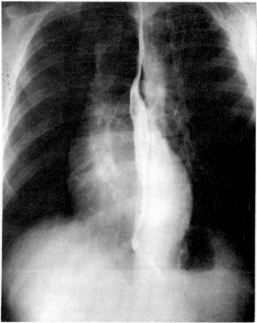

Fig. 32-41. Aortic insufficiency. The left ventricle is considerably enlarged and there is no dilatation of the aorta.

this lesion have been described in the section on pulmonic stenosis.

Pulmonary insufficiency is rare but is usually acquired. It usually results from endocarditis of the valve that is septic in character. This causes repeated pulmonary emboli. Right ventricular enlargement accompanied by enlargement of the pulmonary artery may be recognized.

TRICUSPID VALVULAR DISEASE

Acquired tricuspid valvular disease is uncommon but this valve may be involved by rheumatic disease. Relative tricuspid insufficiency is also caused by excessive dilatation of the right ventricle. Disease involving this valve is manifested by enlargement of the right atrium, which may be extreme. The enlargement causes widening of the heart to the right and increased convexity of the right lower cardiac margin. In the left anterior oblique and frontal views there may be a shoulder-like projection of the right auricular appendage producing a sharp angulation between it and the ascending aorta; this indicates marked right atrial enlargement and is suggestive of tricuspid disease. The superior and inferior venae cavae tend to be enlarged and, in tricuspid insufficiency, pulsation of the great veins may be recognized. Since tricuspid disease tends to decrease the load on the lesser circulation, unusual clarity of the lung fields has been described. Mitral defects result in dilatation of the right atrium, owing to retrograde stasis, so in the presence of mitral disease the roentgen diagnosis of tricuspid insufficiency is difficult. Therefore, the roentgen signs of tricuspid valvular disease may only be suggestive and not diagnostic.

MISCELLANEOUS CARDIAC CONDITIONS

HYPERTENSIVE CARDIOVASCULAR DISEASE

Persistent systemic arterial hypertension results in an increased work load on the left ventricle. Since the disease varies from a relatively benign form that causes little or no alteration in the cardiac silhouette to severe long-standing disease that produces marked

changes, it is evident that the degree of roentgen change varies greatly. The heart may remain normal in size and shape for some time but in patients with persistent high pressures, left ventricular hypertrophy develops. The earliest change is rounding of the left lower cardiac border caused by concentric hypertrophy. The heart then enlarges downward and to the left with lengthening of the left ventricular contour and rounding of the apex, resulting in displacement of the apex below the dome of the diaphragm in many instances. This enlargement also causes posterior convexity noted in the lateral and left anterior oblique projections. These latter changes indicate dilatation in addition to the hypertrophy which preceded it. The cardiac silhouette is similar to that seen in aortic insufficiency. It is important to remember that in transient hypertension and in the early stages of essential hypertension no roentgen abnormalities are recognized. In addition to the alteration in the size and shape of the heart, there are aortic changes as a result of this disease. There is dilatation of the aorta which may be sufficient to produce convexity of the aortic segment of the right upper cardiovascular silhouette and enlargement of the aortic knob (Fig. 32-42).

When hypertension is relieved the heart may decrease in size. This represents a decrease in the amount of dilatation. In many instances irreversible changes have occurred so that the heart does not regain its normal contour following surgical or medical correction of the underlying disease. When decompensation occurs, there is often relative mitral insufficiency resulting in left atrial enlargement, pulmonary congestion, edema, and pleural effusion.

ARTERIOSCLEROTIC CARDIOVASCULAR DISEASE

GENERAL ARTERIOSCLEROTIC (ISCHEMIC) DISEASE

Arteriosclerotic disease is probably the cause of cardiac failure in the elderly patient with normotensive, nonvalvular heart disease.

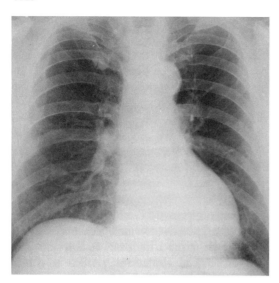

Fig. 32-42. Hypertensive cardiovascular disease. There is moderate cardiac enlargement and rounding of the apex, indicating concentric hypertrophy of the left ventricle. The aortic knob is prominent and there is a calcific plaque noted in the transverse arch. The patient had long-standing hypertension. The aortic calcification indicates arteriosclerosis.

Most of them will be found to have moderate to severe coronary sclerosis, which presumably causes myocardial changes leading to eventual failure. Ischemia is the likely cause, so "ischemic heart disease" is probably a better term.

Arteriosclerotic changes in the aortic valve may produce stenosis or insufficiency, resulting in some enlargement of the left ventricle. The changes in the heart are accompanied by changes in the aorta that result from arteriosclerosis. They consist of dilatation and elongation of the aorta, resulting in enlargement and tortuosity. Calcific plaques are often present, particularly in the transverse arch.

The roentgen findings of ischemic cardiovascular disease vary considerably with the severity and duration. They consist of cardiac enlargement, which is left ventricular in type and is usually moderate in degree. Dilatation is more prominent than hypertrophy so there is less rounding of the ventricle than in hypertensive disease. The two diseases are often combined, however. Calcification may be noted in the annulus fibrosus. The aortic knob is promi-

nent and may contain calcium. It is often dilated. In the left oblique and lateral views the aorta is noted to curve forward more than in the normal and extends farther upward, resulting in elongation of the vertical diameter of the silhouette. When decompensation occurs, generalized cardiac enlargement follows along with pulmonary congestive changes described previously (Fig. 32-43).

CORONARY ARTERY DISEASE

Roentgen examination in sclerotic disease of the coronary arteries is usually not helpful since marked clinical and electrocardiographic signs of coronary insufficiency may be present without any alteration noted on the roentgenogram. Occasionally there is enough calcification in the coronary arteries to be visualized on roentgenograms of good quality. Fluoroscopy or cine with an image intensifier may also permit visualization of calcified vessels. The circumflex and anterior descending branches of the left coronary artery are most often visible and appear as linear streaks of calcification, usually along the left margin of the heart below

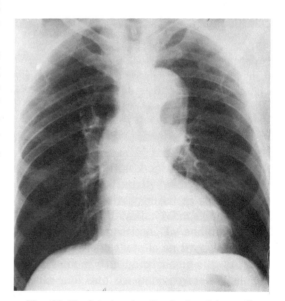

Fig. 32-43. Arteriosclerotic (ischemic) cardiovascular disease. There is moderate cardiac enlargement which is largely left ventricular. The aorta is dilated, elongated, and tortuous.

the pulmonary artery segment. Right coronary artery calcification may also be seen in oblique or lateral cine; the calcification can be seen to move horizontally with a windshield-wiperlike motion. Selective coronary arteriography demonstrates stenosis and occlusion of major vessels and outlines the collateral circulation. Further discussion of the various findings is beyond the scope of this book.

CORONARY ARTERY OCCLUSION

Coronary occlusion resulting in myocardial infarction may produce cardiac failure and lead to generalized cardiac enlargement. Not infrequently, however, a chest roentgenogram taken within a few hours of a coronary occlusion will not show significant enlargement but it is not unusual to see some degree of pulmonary edema. When the infarct heals, the scar may be large enough to produce changes that can be recognized fluoroscopically and on kymography. The area of scar does not contract and therefore does not pulsate normally. This lack of pulsation is local. Occasionally there is some slight paradoxical pulsation that can be recognized fluoroscopically and recorded on the roentgenkymogram. Later, following a myocardial infarct, there may be calcification in the myocardial scar or in the adjacent pericardium.

VENTRICULAR ANEURYSM

The most common cause of ventricular aneurysm is coronary occlusion. Rarely, trauma or inflammation may produce a cardiac aneurysm. As a result of weakening of the myocardial wall at the site of infarct, a local bulge develops. It is most often noted at the left lower cardiac margin near the apex since this is the most common site of the infarct causing it. The roentgen findings are those of localized or somewhat diffuse bulge along the left lower heart border that results in a bizarre silhouette (Fig. 32-44). Fluoroscopically a paradoxical pulsation can sometimes be recognized and occasionally calcification is visible in the wall of the aneurysm. Ciné of the heart or video-tape recording of motion may be used when there is question regarding paradoxical motion. Similar bizarre masses may be caused by tumor arising in the myocardium or metastatic to the myocardium, but if paradoxical pulsation can be demonstrated, the diagnosis is

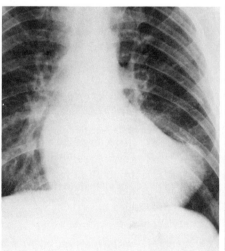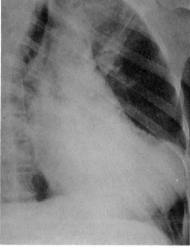

Fig. 32-44. Ventricular aneurysm. *Left,* Frontal projection. Note the localized bulge of the left lower cardiac margin. *Right,* Right anterior oblique projection. The localized aneurysm extends anterolaterally and is more clearly defined in this projection than in the frontal view.

fairly certain. Occasionally coronary artery aneurysms may develop and produce masses simulating ventricular aneurysms.

THE HEART AND LUNGS IN CONGESTIVE FAILURE

In cardiac failure there is nearly always dilatation of one or more cardiac chambers, resulting in cardiac enlargement. The generalized enlargement may obscure the single-chamber enlargement that has been present earlier. The transverse diameter of the heart usually increases while the vertical diameter may actually decrease in the upright position, since the cardiac muscle may be weakened to the extent that it does not maintain the normal cardiac contour against the pull of gravity. There is one general exception to the rule that the heart in failure is considerably enlarged and that is in acute left ventricular failure secondary to coronary thrombosis. In these patients there may be marked pulmonary congestion and edema with very little cardiac enlargement. In ischemic cardiovascular disease where there is a considerable amount of coronary involvement, failure may also occur with less enlargement than in other diseases.

When the left ventricle fails to expel blood at the same rate as the right side of the heart, left ventricular failure is said to occur. In this situation, left atrial pressure increases resulting in an increase in pulmonary venous pressure and finally pulmonary congestion and edema result. The roentgen findings consist of dilatation of the pulmonary veins, causing accentuation of vascular markings. In some patients, the veins in the upper zones are noted to be more prominent than at the bases. The individual vessels often appear blurred and less distinct than in the normal, indicating perivascular edema. Interstitial markings throughout the lungs also become increasingly prominent as fluid accumulates there. Kerley's B and A lines may become visible. Small amounts of pleural effusion producing basal densities obliterating the costophrenic sulci and often extending into the interlobar fissures are also

present in many instances. In acute left ventricular failure alveolar pulmonary edema is common. This produces bilateral parahilar and basal density that may be diffuse or patchy but is poorly defined in either instance. Effusion and edema may become marked depending upon the severity of the failure (Fig. 32-45).

In right ventricular failure the blood accumulates on the venous side of the major circulation and dependent edema as well as congestion of the abdominal viscera occurs. The lungs may be relatively clear. Usually right ventricular failure is secondary to left ventricular failure, so the findings mentioned in the previous paragraph may predominate.

COR PULMONALE

"Chronic cor pulmonale" is the term used to indicate the right ventricular hypertrophy leading to right-sided heart failure produced by any disease or abnormality (exclusive of primary cardiac disease) that results in increased pressure in the lesser circulation. Numerous pulmonary diseases can cause cor pulmonale. They include congenital and acquired alterations in the thorax such as kyphoscoliosis and thoracoplasty, pulmonary artery disease such as arteriosclerosis that elevates the pressure, chronic pulmonary inflammatory disease such as pulmonary tuberculosis, the pneumoconioses, and such suppurative diseases as chronic bronchiectasis. Pulmonary emphysema of the chronic type is also a common cause. Usually the diseases cause changes in peripheral arteries and arterioles or there is a primary disease of these vessels which leads to pulmonary hypertension. There is some controversy regarding pathogenesis in some of the conditions. In addition to the findings given below, pulmonary changes caused by the underlying disease may be present.

Roentgen Findings

The heart is not necessarily enlarged and in the frontal projection is often vertical in type and appears small and round. There is promi-

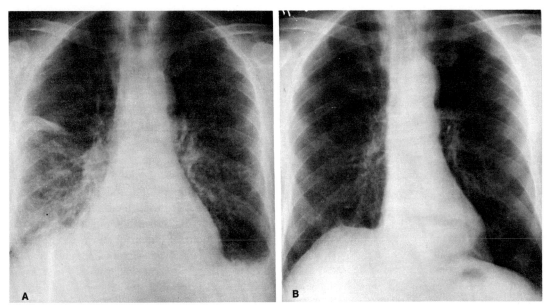

Fig. 32-45. Congestive heart failure. *A,* The heart is enlarged. There is some pleural effusion bilaterally producing a hazy density at the bases and obscuring the costophrenic angles. There is also some fluid in the secondary fissure on the right. The basal vessels are poorly defined and on the right side there is considerable basal density, some of which is interstitial and some very likely alveolar, indicating edema. *B,* Follow-up film taken 2 weeks later. There is no longer evidence of edema, congestion, or pleural effusion and the heart has decreased in size.

nence of the pulmonary artery segment in the left upper silhouette along with prominence of the arteries in the hilum on both sides. The pulmonary infundibulum is enlarged along with the pulmonary artery. This is manifested by convex prominence of the pulmonary outflow tract and infundibular segment noted in the right anterior oblique projection. There is a discrepancy between the caliber of pulmonary arteries; the hilar arteries are enlarged and the midzone and peripheral arteries are either normal or smaller than normal in diameter. In some instances there is a rapid and striking diminution in caliber of arteries in the parahilar areas. Not infrequently, the vascular changes must be used to suggest the diagnosis, since the cardiac silhouette may not be typical. When right ventricular hypertrophy is marked, there may be some increased convexity of the lower right anterior cardiac silhouette noted in the left anterior oblique projection and the apex may be elevated and rounded. There is no enlargement of the left atrium or left ventricle

in this condition. Pulmonary emphysema is often present and may be severe. When the ventricular enlargement becomes great there may be sufficient anterior protrusion and convexity to result in decrease in the retrosternal space anterior to the base of the heart as viewed in the lateral or extreme left anterior oblique projection. In addition, marked enlargement of the pulmonary outflow tract may produce a longer convexity in the region of the pulmonary artery segment than is normally outlined.

In patients with severe thoracic deformities or marked pulmonary disease, the disease causing the increase in pulmonary artery pressure may distort the heart to the point where chamber enlargement cannot be ascertained but the enlargement of the pulmonary artery is usually visible. In order to make the diagnosis, correlation with clinical history, physical findings, and electrocardiographic findings should be made, but when they are typical the roentgen findings are reasonably reliable.

Acute cor pulmonale is found in massive pulmonary embolism, pulmonary edema, tension pneumothorax, and other conditions which cause acute hypoxia or anoxia. The various conditions are discussed under the pulmonary disease in question.

THE HEART IN THORACIC DEFORMITIES

KYPHOSCOLIOSIS

The heart is usually displaced to the side opposite the convexity of the dorsal spine and when the convexity is to the right, the right side of the heart border is often obscured by the shadow of the lower thoracic vertebrae. When the thoracic deformity is marked there is often rotation and torsion sufficient to interfere with cardiac function. In these patients there is so much deformity of the heart produced by the thoracic change that normal landmarks are altered and evaluation of chamber size and identification of chambers is very difficult.

FUNNEL CHEST (PECTUS EXCAVATUM)

This deformity consists of depression of the sternum, which may be severe, and results in displacement of the heart backward and to the left. On the lateral view the position of the sternum is easily recognized so that the diagnosis is made without difficulty in this projection. In the frontal view that are several radiographic signs that are diagnostic when present. They consist of the following: (1) Sharp downward angulation of the anterior arcs of the ribs with the degree of slant roughly proportional to the amount of depression. (2) Displacement of the cardiac shadow to the left with some convexity in the left upper border so that the silhouette suggests mitral disease with enlargement and prominence of the left auricular appendage. (3) The right side of the heart border is indistinct and often obscured by the thoracic spine. (4) The density of the heart may be decreased with more severe deformity,

owing to the decrease in its anteroposterior diameter. In these patients the lower thoracic spine is more readily visible than in the normal. (5) Increased density and cloudiness of the medial aspect of the right lung base. This is caused by some compression of the underlying lung and is accentuated by the visibility of pulmonary vessels that are often hidden by the right lower cardiac border. (6) The normal rounded curve of the thoracic spine may be somewhat straightened or actually reversed in some instances. (7) The heart is occasionally displaced backward and compressed between the sternum and thoracic spine so that there is actual widening with an increase in the transverse diameter to the right as well as to the left. Most of these signs are usually present so that the diagnosis of this deformity in the frontal projection is not difficult. The differentiation from mitral valvular disease in this projection is important, however (Fig. 32-46).

DISEASES OF THE MYOCARDIUM

MYOCARDIOPATHY

Myocardial damage may occur in a number of generalized diseases with a wide variety of causes. Inflammatory diseases such as rheumatic myocarditis and the toxic myocarditis found in diphtheria as well as toxic changes secondary to sepsis and to ingested toxins are among the conditions that may cause acute myocarditis. Chronic myocardiopathy can be caused by myxedema, beriberi, alcoholism, amyloidosis, glycogen and other storage diseases, chronic cardiac involvement associated with collagen diseases, muscular dystrophy, and many others. There are no roentgen changes which permit differentiation of them in the absence of associated pulmonary findings.

The roentgen manifestations of these diseases are not specific but there is usually cardiac enlargement that may be massive. The enlargement is usually caused by dilatation of all the chambers. The contractility of the heart is decreased so that at fluoroscopy, marked diminution of pulsation is noted. The transverse diameter often increases more than the longitudinal diameter. The heart appears broad and normal contours are effaced.

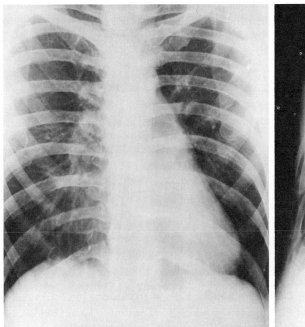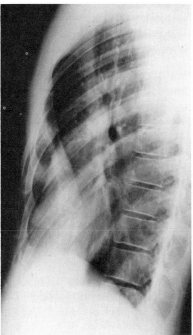

Fig. 32-46. Funnel chest deformity. Most of the roentgen signs described in the text are present, including prominence of the left cardiac border, shift of the heart to the left, slight increase in density below the right hilum along the mediastinum, failure to visualize the right border of the heart, and accentuation of the downward angulation of ribs. *Right,* The lateral view shows the marked posterior displacement of the lower sternum.

Even though the heart may be markedly enlarged, there may be no signs of failure. In these patients the differentiation from pericardial effusion is often difficult.

THE HEART IN BERIBERI

Vitamin B₁ deficiency resulting in beriberi is uncommon in the United States but is occasionally encountered. The roentgen findings are those of cardiac dilatation that may be diffuse and symmetric producing generalized enlargement of the cardiac silhouette. The right ventricle is occasionally damaged more markedly than the myocardium elsewhere, resulting in dilatation of the pulmonary artery and of the right ventricle and atrium. Pericardial effusion may be present and contribute to the enlargement of the cardiac shadow. Some people believe that pericardial effusion accounts for all of the roentgen findings in this disease.

THE HEART IN DISEASES OF THE THYROID

HYPOTHYROIDISM. Hypofunction of the thyroid gland resulting in myxedema causes general dilatation of the cardiovascular silhouette. Pericardial effusion is common in myxedema and may contribute part, if not all, of the increase in cardiac size. Some patients with "myxedema heart" have been shown to have massive pericardial effusions that have contributed most of the cardiac enlargement but some myocardial damage may also be present, resulting in slight cardiac dilatation. In treated patients, the heart returns to normal.

HYPERTHYROIDISM. The heart in hyperthyroidism is hyperactive. The pulse pressure is usually high, resulting in an increased amplitude of pulsation as visualized fluoroscopically. The cardiac configuration is not characteristic but cardiac enlargement is frequently present. The enlargement may be left ventricular with rounding and elongation of the left ventricular border; at times the pulmonary artery and right ventricular outflow tract are enlarged. Some investigators believe that right ventricular enlargement is more characteristic of this disease than left ventricular enlargement. It is generally agreed that there is cardiac enlargement in severe hyperthyroidism and that the size of the heart decreases when the disease is controlled.

CARDIAC INJURIES

Many cardiac injuries result in death before the patient can be treated but occasionally various types of wounds result in hemopericardium without enough tamponade to cause immediate death. The roentgen signs are similar to those of pericardial effusion described in the section on diseases of the pericardium. In addition, the injury that produces the hemopericardium may cause hemothorax or pneumothorax. Occasionally metallic foreign bodies such as bullets can penetrate the heart wall or actually go through it into one of the cardiac chambers without causing death. They are readily visualized and may be localized by fluoroscopy. The motion of the opaque foreign body can be used as an aid in identifying its position. When the projectile is within a cardiac chamber, a considerable amount of movement is usually visualized in a somewhat irregularly circular or pendulous type of motion while a projectile imbedded in the myocardium moves in a more uniform manner. Whenever foreign bodies are found within the heart or in its wall, study of the heart shortly before surgery is important since the foreign body may move out through the aorta into the systemic circulation when on the left side or into the lesser circulation when on the right. Occasionally small opaque foreign bodies such as lead shot have been observed to move through the venous system to the heart.

TUMORS OF THE HEART

Primary cardiac tumors are rare. Benign and malignant neoplasms can occur, however, and such tumors as fibroma, myxoma, rhabdomyoma, and rhabdosarcoma have been described, along with primary tumors of vascular origin. The most common benign tumor is the myxoma. It arises from the atrial septum near the foramen ovale. It is found in the left atrium in about 75 per cent of cases and most of the remainder arise in the right atrium. Ventricular myxoma is rare. The tumor is usually pedunculated and may cause intermittent obstruction at the mitral valve. When it occurs in the right atrium, it may obstruct the tricuspid valve. Roentgen findings in myxoma may then resemble those of mitral or tricuspid stenosis, depending upon the site of origin. Left atrial myxoma can be suspected when there is roentgen evidence of mitral stenosis, and no previous history of rheumatic fever, an inconstant and changing murmur, and embolic phenomena occurring without atrial fibrillation (Fig. 32-47). Right atrial myxoma results in roentgen findings suggesting tricuspid stenosis or Ebstein's anomaly; here, too, the murmur is inconstant and embolic (pulmonary) phenomena occur. About 10 per cent of atrial myxomas calcify enough to be visible at fluoroscopy. Right atrial myxoma does not interfere with valvular function as often as myxoma of the left atrium. Therefore the right atrial tumor tends to be larger than the left before causing symptoms. Angiocardiography is useful in outlining the intracardiac tumor. The other benign tumors tend to be intramural and include fibroma, hamartoma, rhabdomyoma, and lipoma. Most involve the left ventricular wall. They tend to produce cardiac enlargement, to calcify (20 per cent) and usually occur in children.

Malignant tumors such as rhabdomyosarcoma or fibrosarcoma are very rare and usually arise in the ventricular walls, while angiosarcoma apparently arises most commonly in the right atrial wall. Angiocardiography is required to make the diagnosis. Masses projecting from the outer cardiac surface may produce bizarre cardiac shapes, so the diagnosis may be suspected on roentgen examination, however. Diagnostic pneumopericardium or pneumothorax may be of value in demonstrating the site of a bizarre mass that appears to be intimately associated with the heart.

Metastatic myocardial tumors are much more common than the primary tumors. Cardiac involvement by lymphoma and various carcinomas often results in pericardial effusion. Therefore the roentgen findings may be caused by hemopericardium. An irregular cardiac mass occurring alone (or associated with hemopericardium) in a patient with known Hodgkin's disease, lymphoma, or carcinoma, virtually indicates myocardial metastasis.

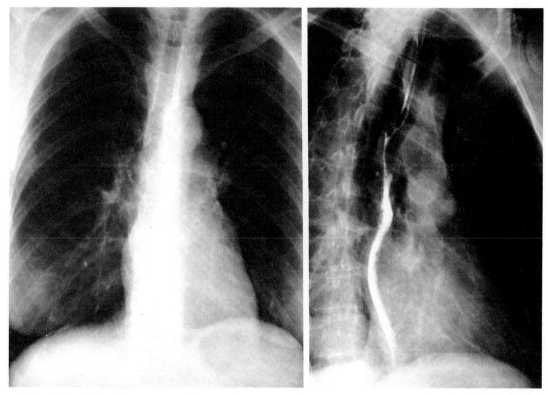

Fig. 32-47. Left atrial myxoma. The cardiovascular silhouette is remarkably similar to that of mitral stenosis including slight constriction of basal vessels in the lungs.

ACQUIRED DISEASES OF THE AORTA

ARTERIOSCLEROSIS OF THE AORTA

A certain amount of alteration in the appearance of the aorta with advancing age is secondary to loss of elasticity. The change consists of elongation and dilatation; it eventually occurs in all patients who live long enough. As a result of these anatomic changes, the configuration of the aortic arch changes roentgenographically. The ascending arch becomes more prominent, resulting in more convexity of the right upper cardiac margin. The aortic knob on the left side becomes more prominent and somewhat enlarged. The descending aorta curves to left in the posteroanterior view and then back to midline or even to the right side before passing through the diaphragm. In the left oblique view and in the lateral projection, the arch of the aorta is noted to swing in a wider arc so that it often angles forward and upward, then backward, resulting in widening of the area between the limbs of the arch, which is termed the "aortic window." The descending aorta may curve far backward to overlie the thoracic spine in the lateral view.

In arteriosclerotic disease of the aorta, the manifestations of elongation and dilatation occur earlier in life and plaques of calcium are often visualized in the transverse aortic arch. The amount of calcification varies considerably. The plaques are noted as dense linear shadows and are most commonly seen in the aortic knob but may be extensive throughout the aorta distal to the transverse arch, so that the entire wall of this structure may be outlined by calcium in extreme instances (Fig. 32-48). Aortic arteriosclerotic disease per se may not be significant unless complicated by dissection or aneurysm, but it is often associated with

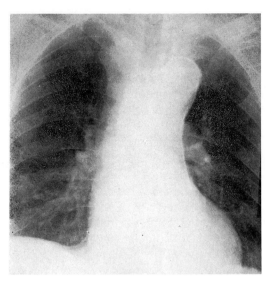

Fig. 32-48. Arteriosclerotic disease of the aorta. Note calcification in the arch and uniformly throughout the thoracic aorta below the arch. The aorta is elongated, tortuous, and slightly dilated. The patient had extensive generalized arteriosclerosis.

arteriosclerotic disease elsewhere, e.g., in the carotid, renal, and coronary arteries, which may cause morbidity and mortality.

SYPHILITIC AORTITIS

Luetic aortitis produces alterations that can often be recognized radiographically before clinical signs of specific aortic involvement are present. Circumscribed dilatation of the ascending aortic arch may occur and be recognized as enlargement of this portion of the aorta before the signs of aneurysm appear but similar dilatation may occur in arteriosclerosis so that this finding is not pathognomonic. The dilatation in arteriosclerotic disease is usually more diffuse. Calcification in the wall of the ascending aortic arch is a more reliable sign of luetic aortitis. It is manifested by a thin, curvilinear shadow of calcific density in the outer wall of the ascending aorta that may be visible in the frontal projection but is often more readily visualized in the left anterior oblique and lateral positions. This is in contrast to the calcification in arteriosclerotic disease that is

noted in the transverse aortic arch. Calcification may occur in the ascending aortic arch in arteriosclerosis, but this is usually found in elderly patients in whom the disease is severe. Furthermore, the plaques are thicker and more irregular than the somewhat thin linear shadows noted in syphilis. On pathologic examination of the aorta in arteriosclerosis, calcification is often found in the ascending aorta but it is most prominent in the inner wall of the arch and is not often roentgenographically visible. Aneurysms of the ascending aorta are frequently found in vascular syphilis.

AORTIC ANEURYSM

An aneurysm is a circumscribed area of localized widening in the wall of a blood vessel. Some dilatation of the aorta occurs in arteriosclerosis and there is no sharply limited differentiation between simple dilatation and an aneurysm. The latter term is usually reserved for a clearly defined local area of cylindrical or saccular enlargement. Aneurysms involving the ascending aortic arch are usually of syphilitic origin, particularly when they are saccular in type, but connective-tissue disorders may also be associated with aneurysm. Aneurysms of the descending aorta may be arteriosclerotic in origin. Rarely aneurysms are mycotic, traumatic, or congenital in origin. Roentgen and fluoroscopic study usually is sufficient to make the diagnosis.

Roentgen Findings

Aneurysm results in a mass shadow continuous with the aortic silhouette that varies considerably in size and shape from one patient to another. It is not unusual to note widening of the superior mediastinum above the arch on the right when the aneurysm involves the ascending aorta, caused by aneurysm of the innominate artery. The mass of the aneurysm in the ascending aortic arch usually projects to the right while that of the descending arch projects to the left in the frontal plane. Occasionally the communication between the aorta and the aneurysm is very narrow (pedunculated aneurysm). Then the aneurysm may project in a direction not usually observed in the more common saccular lesion. The relationships should be studied in the lateral and in the oblique projections. Barium in the esophagus is used to show the relationship of the aortic mass to the esophagus in fluoroscopic and roentgen examinations. The lesion is most clearly defined in the left anterior oblique position in the usual instance. Occasionally there may be more than one saccular aneurysm with an area of fusiform dilatation between them. It is often possible to make the diagnosis of aneurysm on roentgenograms alone, but fluoroscopy is useful in detecting the amount of pulsation. When the differentiation between aortic aneurysm and mediastinal mass owing to other cause cannot be made roentgenographically, fluoroscopy is of value in demonstrating the relationship of the mass to the heart and aorta and determining the presence of expansile pulsation that usually indicates that the lesion is an aneurysm. Occasionally, however, a tumor may partially surround the aortic arch in such a manner that it may actually exhibit expansile pulsation. Furthermore, when there is a considerable amount of thrombus within an aneurysm, pulsation may be markedly dampened or absent. When there is any doubt in such a patient, retrograde aortography can be used to make the differential diagnosis. Arteriosclerotic aneurysms usually occur in the abdominal aorta but may occur in the arch and descending portion of the thoracic aorta. They are generally smaller than those of leutic origin and often show calcification. Rarely there may be erosion of bone secondary to aortic aneurysm. When the ascending arch is involved the erosion occurs along the posterior aspect of the sternum; erosion through this bone has been described. Aneurysms of the distal arch may erode one or more of the dorsal vertebral bodies. The bone erosion is a manifestation of the syphilitic type of aneurysm in most, if not all, instances. The vertebrae involved have a scalloped appearance because the discs resist the erosion. The vertebral bodies are then con-

cave anteriorly. Retrograde aortography may be necessary to differentiate aneurysm from other mediastinal masses (Fig. 32-49).

TRAUMATIC ANEURYSM OR HEMATOMA

Rupture of all layers of the aorta caused by trauma usually leads to exsanguination and sudden death. When the adventitia is spared and rupture is incomplete, the patient may survive. Survival in others is evidently dependent upon mediastinal hematoma which may temporarily prevent exsanguination. Thrombus may then dissect the adventitia from the media, creating a false aneurysm with a connective tissue wall. The usual site of such rupture is in the aortic arch, immediately distal to the left subclavian artery at the site of the ligamentum arteriosum. The disruption is often circumferential and the ruptured layers may retract. The roentgen findings in the acute phase consist of hematoma in the vicinity of the aortic arch, resulting in widening of the mediastinum in that area which also obscures the aorta. This is an important finding in this condition. Slight deviation of the trachea also appears to be a significant finding; it was present in all eight patients at our hospital reported by Flaherty et al.,[15] including one in whom the mediastinum did not appear to be widened. Hemorrhage into the pleural space and lung is common and there may be evidence of rib or sternal fracture. Pneumomediastinum and pneumothorax may occur but are not of particular diagnostic significance. When these signs are present in a patient who has suffered severe thoracic trauma, traumatic aortic fracture should be suspected. Angiography can be used to confirm the diagnosis (Fig. 32-50). Surgical repair may then be done. When no corrective measures are taken and the patient survives, in time the diffuse mediastinal density clears leaving a more or less clearly defined mass which represents the false aneurysm adjacent to the aortic knob. Calcification develops in the wall in most of the lesions as they become chronic. Expansile pulsation is not necessarily present, be-

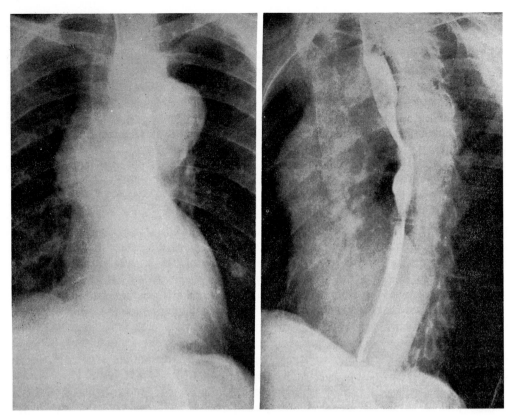

Fig. 32-49. Aortic aneurysms. Note fusiform dilatations of the ascending and transverse arches. *Left,* Frontal projection. *Right,* Left anterior oblique projection.

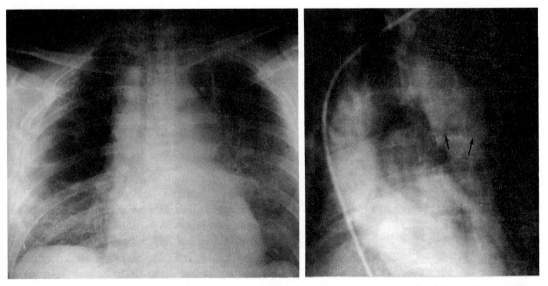

Fig. 32-50. Traumatic fracture of the aorta. *Left,* This film, taken a few hours after injury, shows widening of the superior mediastinum, loss of clear definition of the transverse aortic arch on the left, deviation of the trachea to the right, and probable downward displacement of the left main bronchus. *Right,* Forward aortogram shows aortic dilatation distal to left subclavian artery. There is some infolding of the disrupted aortic wall (**arrows**) below which the caliber is normal.

cause of the organized thrombus in the wall. The diagnosis can usually be made on the basis of the roentgen findings in a patient who has a history of previous thoracic trauma. Aortography can then be used to confirm the diagnosis and localize the site of origin (Fig. 32-51).

DISSECTING ANEURYSM

In this condition blood splits or dissects the media, separating the inner and outer layers to form a second channel surrounding the lumen of the aorta. This condition usually results from medial necrosis. Transverse defects or tears in the intima may then occur, allowing blood under systemic pressure to further dissect the media. The common sites of the intimal defects are in or adjacent to the sinus of Valsalva and in the descending aorta near the ligamentum arteriosum. Dissection or rupture may also start at the site of an atheromatous

plaque, and in this instance the abdominal aorta is the more common site. The condition ends fatally in a few hours or days in most patients. In about 10 per cent, there is a "reentry" into the abdominal aorta at the bifurcation or into one of the iliacs. This permits the dissection to decompress and the patient may live for months or years. The roentgen diagnosis is often difficult and the findings must be correlated with the clinical history of severe pain that usually occurs at the site of dissection, along with pallor and, often shock. There is widening of the aorta extending from the site of dissection distally and, occasionally, proximally. This can be most readily appreciated when a chest roentgenogram taken prior to dissection is available for comparison. Roentgenograms taken on successive days may show extension of the area of widening and when this occurs in a patient with a typical clinical history and findings, the diagnosis is almost certain. In the patients with extensive arteriosclerosis in whom calcification in atheromatous

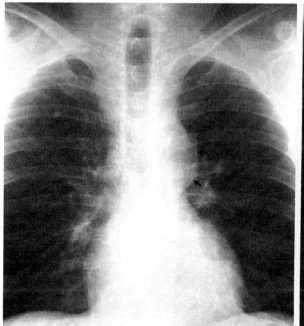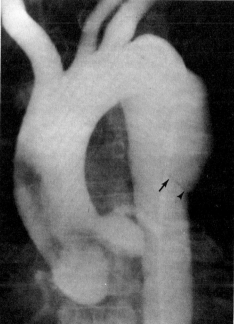

Fig. 32-51. Chronic traumatic fracture of the aorta. *Left,* **Arrows** indicate the mass in the vicinity of the transverse and upper descending aorta. Note the thin curvilinear calcification in the wall of the mass. *Right,* Aortogram shows the false aneurysm and there is a thin infolding of the aortic wall (**arrows**).

plaques is visible, it is often possible to outline the inner wall of the aorta by means of this calcification and note the great thickening formed by the dissecting aneurysm because the outer wall is readily visible against the radiolucency of the lung. Pleural effusion is a common accessory finding. It usually occurs on the left side. Occasionally recognizable enlargement of the branches of the aorta can be demonstrated, since dissection not infrequently extends into the walls of these vessels. When this is present it is of considerable diagnostic significance. The patients are often desperately ill and roentgen examination is difficult to obtain, so the use of this method is limited in many instances. In patients in whom the diagnosis is suspected early in the course of the disease, surgical measures may be warranted. In these instances, aortography may be used to confirm the diagnosis.

DISEASES OF THE PERICARDIUM

PERICARDIAL EFFUSION

The pericardium is a thin membrane that is not ordinarily recognized as a separate structure since it is of the same density as the adjacent heart. It is relatively inelastic and conditions that produce rapid accumulation of fluid within it may compress the heart enough to produce severe alteration of cardiac function leading to death. This occurs most commonly as the result of hemorrhage secondary to trauma. Roentgenograms are not usually obtained during this acute situation.

In chronic or subacute pericardial effusion there are roentgen changes produced when the amount of fluid reaches 400 or 500 ml. Smaller effusions up to 300 ml are not ordinarily diagnosed, since they produce no significant alteration in the contour of the cardiovascular silhouette. This slow accumulation of fluid may reach massive proportions without producing tamponade.

Roentgen Findings

There is an increase in size of the cardiac silhouette that depends upon the amount of fluid present. The shape of the cardiovascular silhouette is also altered. With moderate amounts of fluid, the enlargement is generalized and the cardiohepatic angle appears more acute than in the normal. As the amount of fluid increases there tends to be disproportionate enlargement of the heart inferiorly in the transverse diameter as compared to the increase in the vertical diameter. Demonstration of rapid progression, or regression, of these findings is a most valuable sign in roent-

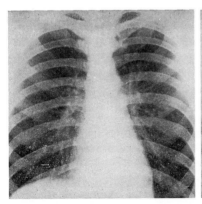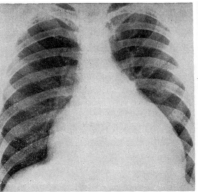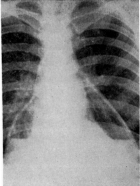

Fig. 32-52. Pericardial effusion. *Left,* Chest shows normal heart before onset. *Center,* Two months later, note gross increase in transverse diameter of the heart. *Right,* Diagnostic pneumopericardium. Fluid level is demonstrated and the heart is outlined by air within the pericardial sac. Note thickening of parietal pericardium.

gen diagnosis (Fig. 32-52). At fluoroscopy the pulsations are dampened or obliterated and there is some alteration in contour of the heart noted between the upright and the recumbent positions. This finding is often equivocal, however. Large effusions also tend to obliterate the normal segments noted on either side and the cardiac enlargement is noted to extend to the right as well as to the left. Dilatation of the heart in myocardial failure can produce a silhouette that simulates that of pericardial effusion. Furthermore, in these patients the amplitude of pulsation is also small owing to the myocardial weakness so that differentiation is very difficult. Mellins, Kottmeier, and Kiely[40] found experimentally on dogs that fluid accumulated anteriorly, laterally, and superiorly, but not posteriorly in the pericardial space. As a result pericardial fluid dampened the cardiac pulsations anteriorly but not posteriorly. This sign was noted on a few patients and may be of value. Roentgenkymography or cineradiography in the lateral projection may show

dampened or absent anterior pulsations and normal pulsations manifested by motion of the barium-filled esophagus posteriorly. There is a layer of epicardial fat beneath the visceral pericardium which may be visible and thus outline the cardiac borders. In our experience, this is most frequently seen over the lower two-thirds of the left cardiac margin extending over the inferior aspect of the heart, but usually not to the right of the midline (Fig. 32-53). We use a combination of fluoroscopy with image intensification and cine. If fat can be demonstrated, this finding is of definite value but a negative result is of no assistance. When differentiation between pericardial effusion and enlargement resulting from other cause cannot be determined in any other way, angiocardiography can be used to define the inner wall of the cardiac chambers and thus indicate the presence of effusion. Other methods include the instillation of carbon dioxide intravenously while the patient is in the left lateral decubitus position to outline the right lateral wall of the right atrium.

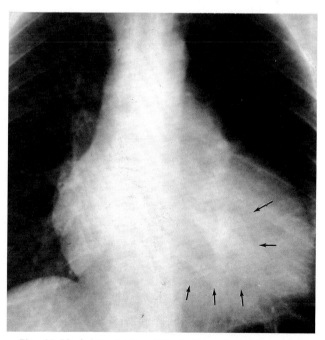

Fig. 32-53. Large pericardial effusion. Epicardial fat line was easily observed at fluoroscopy and on cine. The **arrows** show its position on this film. This indicates that the heart is not enlarged and that there is a large effusion.

A horizontal beam is used when taking the film. Venous angiocardiography may be used in a similar manner. A measurement of the combination of right atrial wall and pericardial thickness over 5 mm should indicate the presence of effusion. Blood-pool scanning using technetium[99]-labeled albumin may be used, but this method is not as accurate as venous angiocardiography or the carbon dioxide method. Thickening of the right atrial wall may result in a falsely positive result for pericardial fluid in these methods, however. Pericardial tap can also be done as a diagnostic and therapeutic procedure and if necessary air can be injected to determine the thickness of the parietal pericardium as well as the actual heart size. Films can then be taken in various projections to outline the heart borders and pericardium.

Echocardiography - 1st choice.

ADHESIVE AND CONSTRICTIVE PERICARDITIS

Adhesive pericarditis without constriction is usually of little clinical significance. Adhesions between the pleura and pericardium may result in some irregularity of the cardiac silhouette in the neighborhood of the adhesions. The cause of constrictive pericarditis is often obscure although a number of possiblities exist, including infection and trauma. Whatever the cause, the amount of pericardial fibrous-tissue reaction may reach the point where constriction occurs. The visceral and parietal pericardium is adherent and also contracted. The basic abnormality is the inability of the ventricles to fill normally, resulting in diminution of stroke volume. Venous pressure is elevated. When this occurs there may be severe clinical symptoms but the radiographic changes are minimal. The heart is often normal or small, and engorgement of the great veins may be evident. At fluoroscopy the diminished pulsations may be apparent. Calcific plaques often occur in the thickened pericardium and are readily visible. At times the heart is nearly encased in a calcific shell. Occasionally there is actually ossification that follows the calcification. When cal-

cification is present in a patient with clinical signs of constrictive pericarditis, the diagnosis is not difficult; but when there is no calcification present, roentgen findings are often equivocal. Calcification is present in about 50 per cent of patients with constrictive pericarditis. However, the presence of pericardial calcification does not necessarily indicate significant constriction. The classic finding is that of a quiet heart with clinical signs of failure. The heart may be enlarged, however. Hepatic enlargement and ascites may be evident on abdominal examination.

PERICARDIAL TUMORS

The most common mass lesion of the pericardium is the pericardial or clear-water cyst that has been described in Chapter 31 under the heading "Pericardial Cyst." Primary pericardial tumors are rare and produce localized enlargements of various sizes and shapes that cannot be differentiated from cardiac tumors unless pneumopericardium is used. Occasionally sarcoma or mesothelioma arising in the pericardium can surround the cardiac shadow and produce enlargement of it. The pericardium is much more frequently involved by metastatic tumor and the presence of pericardial and pleural effusion may obscure the actual lesion. Hodgkin's disease not infrequently involves the pericardium and malignant melanoma occasionally metastasizes to the heart and pericardium. The associated presence of masses elsewhere in the thorax is helpful in making the diagnosis. In the presence of a solitary pericardial or cardiac mass, thoracotomy is often necessary to confirm the diagnosis.

"SPONTANEOUS" PNEUMOPERICARDIUM

This is a rare condition for which there are a number of causes. Left subphrenic abscess may penetrate the pericardial portion of the diaphragm, resulting in infection with pus and often gas within the pericardial sac. Direct extension of esophageal carcinoma may produce a similar situation. Occasionally congenital diaphragmatic hernia may occur through a defect in the pericardial portion of the diaphragm. In this situation, gas-filled loops of bowel may be noted within the pericardial sac.

Traumatic hernia of abdominal contents into the pericardial sac has also been reported. Gas-filled loops of intestine may also be visible within the pericardium in this condition.

CONGENITAL PERICARDIAL DEFECTS

The majority of congenital pericardial defects are on the left side. They vary from a small defect overlying the pulmonary artery to absence of the pericardium on the left. The parietal pleura is also involved, so that there is no barrier between the heart and the left lung. The roentgen findings in complete absence of the left pericardium are characteristic enough to make the diagnosis or strongly suggest it. The heart is shifted to the left. The left border of the heart is flattened as the heart extends to the left over the dome of the diaphragm. The pulmonary artery segment is long and more sharply defined than usual and there is a radiolucent portion of lung between the aorta and pulmonary artery which provides the contrast necessary for the clear definition. The left ventricular segment is also distinct and clearly defined. In the lateral view the pulmonary artery or aortic root if the defect is on the right may be more distinct than usual. Diagnostic pneumothorax can be used to confirm the diagnosis; the air extends into the pericardial sac. Small defects may permit herniation of the left auricular appendage to produce a bizarre appearance of the left upper cardiac silhouette. Right-sided defects permit unusually clear visualization of the great vessels; lung tissue may herniate medial to the superior vena cava to clearly outline this vessel. Protrusions of the heart, usually the atria, through surgical defects in the pericardium are not uncommon. This possibility must be kept in mind when an unusual bulge or protrusion is noted in the postoperative period.

REFERENCES AND SELECTED READINGS

1. ABRAMS, H. L., and KAPLAN, H. S.: *Angiocardiographic Interpretation in Congenital Heart Disease.* Springfield, Ill., Thomas, 1956.

2. AMPLATZ, K., LESTER, R. G., SCHIEBLER, G. L., ADAMS, P., JR., and ANDERSON, R. C.: The roentgenologic features of Ebstein's anomaly of the triscupid valve. *Am. J. Roentgenol. Radium Ther. Nucl. Med. 81:* 788, 1959.

3. BLOUNT, S. G., JR., McCORD, M. C., KOMESN, S., and LANIER, R. R.: Roentgen aspects of iso-lated valvular pulmonic stenosis. *Radiology 62:* 337, 1954.

4. BRUWER, A. J.: Posteroanterior chest roentgen-ogram in two types of anomalous pulmonary venous connection. *J. Thorac. Surg. 32:* 119, 1956.

5. CAREY, L. S., and EDWARDS, J. E.: Roentgeno-graphic features in cases with origin of both great vessels from the right ventricle without pulmonary stenosis. *Am. J. Roentgenol. Radium Ther. Nucl. Med. 93:* 269, 1965.

6. DAVIS, G. D., KINCAID, O. W., and HALLERMANN, F. J.: Roentgen aspects of cardiac tumors. *Semin. Roentgenol. IV:* 384, 1969.

7. DOTTER, C. T., and STEINBERG, I.: "Angiocardiography," in *Annals of Roentgenology.* New York, Harper & Row, 1951, vol. 20.

8. DUISENBERG, C. E., and ARISMENDI, L.: Demonstration of pulmonary arteriovenous fistula. *Radiology 53:* 66, 1949.

9. EDWARDS, J. E., CAREY, L. S., NEUFELD, H. N., and LESTER, R. G.: *Congenital Heart Disease.* Philadelphia, Saunders, 1965.

10. ELLIOTT, L. P., JUE, K. L., and AMPLATZ, K.: A roentgen classification of cardiac malpositions. *Invest. Radiol. 1:* 17, 1966.

11. ELLIS, K., LEED, N. E., and HIMMELSTEIN, A.: Congenital deficiencies in the parietal pericardium. *Am. J. Roentgenol. Radium Ther. Nucl. Med. 82:* 125, 1959.

12. EPSTEIN, B. S.: Calcification of the ascending aorta. *Am. J. Roentgenol. Radium Ther. Nucl. Med. 77:* 281, 1957.

13. EYLER, W. R., ZIEGLER, R. F., SHEA, J. J., and KNABE, G. W.: Endocardial fibroelastosis: Roentgen appearance. *Radiology 64:* 797, 1955.

14. FIGLEY, M. M.: Accessory roentgen signs of coarctation of the aorta. *Radiology 62:* 671, 1954.

15. FLAHERTY, T. T., WEGNER, G. P., CRUMMY, A. B., FRANCYK, W. P., and HIPONA, F. A.: Nonpenetrating injuries to the thoracic aorta. *Radiology 92:* 541, 1969.

16. GAY, B. B., JR., FRANCH, R. H., SHUFORD, W. H., and ROGERS, J. V., JR.: The roentgenologic features of single and multiple coarctations of the pulmonary artery and branches. *Am. J. Roentgenol. Radium Ther. Nucl. Med. 90:* 599, 1963.

17. GOETZ, A. A., and GRAHAM, W. H.: Aneurysm of the sinus of Valsalva. *Radiology 67:* 416, 1956.

18. GOTT, V. L., LESTER, R. G., LILLEHEI, C. W., and VARCO, R. L.: Total anomalous pulmonary return. An analysis of thirty cases. *Circulation 13:* 543, 1956.

19. HARRIS, E. J.: Aneurysms of the sinus of Valsalva. *Am. J. Roentgenol. Radium Ther. Nucl. Med. 76:* 767, 1956.

20. HARRIS, G. B. C., NEUHAUSER, E. B. D., and GIEDION, A.: Total anomalous pulmonary venous return below the diaphragm. *Am. J. Roentgenol. Radium Ther. Nucl. Med. 84:* 436, 1960.

21. HODGES, P. C., and EYSTER, J. A. E.: Estimate of transverse cardiac diameter in man. *Arch. Intern. Med. 37:* 707, 1926.

22. JÖNSSON, G., and SALTZMAN, G. F.: Infundibulum of patent ductus arteriosus—Diagnostic sign in conventional roentgenograms. *Acta Radiol. 38:* 8, 1952.

23. KEATS, T. E., KREIS, V. A., and SIMPSON, E.: The roentgen manifestations of pulmonary hypertension in congenital heart disease. *Radiology 66:* 693, 1956.

24. KEATS, T. E., and STEINBACH, H. L.: Patent ductus arteriosus. A critical evaluation of its roentgen signs. *Radiology 64:* 528, 1955.

25. KERLEY, P.: Lung changes in acquired heart disease. *Am. J. Roentgenol. Radium Ther. Nucl. Med. 80:* 256, 1958.

26. KIRKLIN, J. W., and CLAGETT, O. T.: Vascular "rings" producing respiratory obstruction in infants. *Mayo Clin. Proc. 25:* 360, 1950.

27. KLATTE, E. C., CAMPBELL, J. A., and LURIE, P.R.: Aortic configuration in congenital heart disease. *Radiology 74:* 555, 1960.

28. KRABBENHOFT, K. L., and EVANS, W. A.: Some pulmonary changes associated with intracardiac septal defects in infancy. *Radiology 63:* 498, 1954.

29. LESTER, R. G., ANDERSON, R. C., AMPLATZ, K., and ADAMS, P.: Roentgenologic diagnosis of congenitally corrected transposition of the great vessels. *Am. J. Roentgenol. Radium Ther. Nucl. Med. 83:* 985, 1960.

30. LEVENE, G., and KAUFMAN, S. A.: The roentgen diagnosis of pericardial effusion. *Radiology 57:* 373, 1951.

31. LEVIN, B., and BORDEN, C. W.: Anomalous pulmonary venous drainage into the left vertical vein. *Radiology 63:* 317, 1954.

32. LEVIN, B., and RIGLER, L. G.: Rib notching following subclavian artery obstruction. *Radiology 62:* 660, 1954.

33. LEVIN, B., and WHITE, H.: Total anomalous pulmonary venous drainage into the portal system. *Radiology 76:* 894, 1961.

34. LODWICK, G. E.: Dissecting aneurysms of the thoracic and abdominal aorta. *Am. J. Roentgenol. Radium Ther. Nucl. Med. 69:* 907, 1955.

35. LODWICK, G. S., and GLADSTONE, W. S.: Correlation of anatomic and roentgen changes in arteriosclerosis and syphilis of the ascending aorta. *Radiology 69:* 70, 1957.

36. MADOFF, I. M., GAENSLER, E. A., and STRIEDER, J. W.: Congenital absence of right pulmonary artery. *N. Engl. J. Med. 247:* 149, 1952.

37. MARDER, S. N., SEAMAN, W. B., and SCOTT, W. G.: Roentgenologic considerations in the diagnosis of congenital tricuspid atresia. *Radiology 61:* 174, 1953.

38. MARKS, M. O., and ZIMMERMAN, H. A.: Roentgen and differential diagnosis of chronic cor pulmonale. *Am. J. Roentgenol. Radium Ther. Nucl. Med. 66:* 9, 1951.

39. McCORD, M. C., and BAVENDAM, F. A.: Unusual causes of rib notching. *Am. J. Roentgenol. Radium Ther. Nucl. Med. 67:* 405, 1952.

40. MELLINS, H. Z., KOTTMEIER, P., and KIELY, B.: Radiologic signs of pericardial effusion. *Radiology 73:* 9, 1959.

41. MEYER, R. R.: A method for measuring children's hearts. *Radiology 53:* 363, 1949.

42. NEUHAUSER, E. B. D.: Roentgen diagnosis of double aortic arch and other anomalies of the great vessels. *Am. J. Roentgenol. Radium Ther. Nucl. Med. 56:* 1, 1946.

43. NEUHAUSER, E. B. D.: Tracheo-esophageal constriction produced by right aortic arch and left ligamentum arteriosum. *Am. J. Roentgenol. Radium Ther. Nucl. Med. 62:* 493, 1949.

44. PAUL, L. W., and RICHTER, M. R.: Funnel chest deformity and its recognition in posteroanterior roentgenograms of the thorax. *Am. J. Roentgenol. Radium Ther. Nucl. Med. 46:* 619, 1941.

45. REICH, N. E., and WITTER, M.: Roentgenographic visualization of the coronary arteries. *Am. J. Roentgenol. Radium Ther. Nucl. Med. 77:* 274, 1951.

46. ROEHM, T. U., JR., JUE, K. L., and AMPLATZ, K.: Radiographic features of the scimitar syndrome. *Radiology 86:* 856, 1966.

47. RONDEROS, A.: Endocardial fibroelastosis. *Am. J. Roentgenol. Radium Ther. Nucl. Med. 84:* 442, 1960.

48. ROSENBAUM, H. D.: The roentgen classification and diagnosis of cardiac alignments. *Radiology 89:* 466, 1967.

49. SCATLIFF, J. H., KUMMER, A. J., and JANZEN, A. H.: The diagnosis of pericardial effusion with intracardiac carbon dioxide. *Radiology 73:* 871, 1959.

50. SCHINZ, H. R., BAENSCH, W. E., FROMMHOLD, W., GLAUNER, R., UEHLINGER, E., and WELLAUER, J.: *Roentgen Diagnosis*, 2nd ed. Ed. by L. G. Rigler. New York, Grune & Stratton, 1970, vol. IV.

51. SCHWEDEL, J. B.: *Clinical Roentgenology of the Heart.* New York, Harper & Row, 1946.

52. SLOAN, R. D., and COOLEY, R. N.: Coarctation of the aorta. *Radiology 61:* 701, 1953.

53. SNOW, P. J. D.: Tricuspid atresia: New radioscopic sign. *Br. Heart J. 14:* 387, 1952.

54. STEINBERG, I.: Anomalies (pseudocoarctation) of the arch of the aorta. *Am. J. Roentgenol. Radium Ther. Nucl. Med. 88:* 73, 1962.

55. STEINBERG, I., and FINBY, N.: Roentgen manifestations of unperforated aortic sinus aneurysms. *Am. J. Roentgenol. Radium Ther. Nucl. Med. 77:* 263, 1957.

56. STEVENS, G. M.: Buckling of the aortic arch (pseudocoarctation, kinking): A roentgenographic entity. *Radiology 70:* 67, 1958.

57. SUSSMAN, M. L., and JACOBSON, G.: Critical evaluation of roentgen criteria of right ventricular enlargement. *Circulation 11:* 391, 1955.

58. SWISCHUK, L. E.: *Plain Film Interpretation in Congenital Heart Disease.* Philadelphia, Lea & Febiger, 1970.

59. TORRANCE, D. J.: Demonstration of subepicardial fat as an aid in the diagnosis of pericardial fluid or thickening. *Am. J. Roentgenol. Radium Ther. Nucl. Med. 74:* 850, 1955.

60. UNGERLEIDER, H. E., and CLARK, C. P.: Study of transverse diameter of heart silhouette, with prediction table based on teleroentgenogram. *Am. Heart J. 17:* 92, 1939.

61. UNGERLEIDER, H. E., and GUBNER, R.: Evaluation of heart size measurements. *Am. Heart J. 24:* 494, 1942.

62. WILLIAMS, R. G., and STEINBERG, I.: The value of angiocardiography in establishing the diagnosis of pericarditis with effusion. *Am. J. Roentgenol. Radium Ther. Nucl. Med. 61:* 41, 1949.

63. WITTENBORG, M. H., NEUHAUSER, E. B. D., and SPRUNT, W. H.: Roentgenographic findings in congenital tricuspid atresia with hypoplasia of the right ventricle. *Am. J. Roentgenol. Radium Ther. Nucl. Med. 66:* 712, 1951.

64. WYMAN, S. M.: Congenital absence of a pulmonary artery. *Radiology 62:* 321, 1954.

65. WYMAN, S. M.: Dissecting aneurysm of the thoracic aorta: Its roentgen recognition. *Am. J. Roentgenol. Radium Ther. Nucl. Med. 78:* 247, 1957.

Section VI

THE FACE, MOUTH, AND JAWS

33

THE ORBIT AND EYE

Roentgen examination of the orbit and eye is used to detect and localize foreign bodies, to detect the presence of tumor within the orbit, and to determine what effect, if any, this tumor has on the bony orbital wall. The optic foramen is examined to determine its size in the presence of alteration caused by disease or by tumor involving the optic nerve. Examination in orbital trauma is discussed in Chapter 35 in the section entitled "Orbital Fractures."

ROENTGEN METHODS

The actual positioning and radiographic technique cannot be considered here. As a general rule the orbits are examined by means of stereoscopic posteroanterior and lateral views (Fig. 33-1). Additional projections may be used, depending upon the problem. If the presence of an opaque foreign body is suspected, localizing procedure usually is preceded by a scout roentgenogram in frontal and lateral projection to determine the presence of the suspected foreign body and its general location. Bone-free films are sometimes made, using small dental films to outline foreign bodies in the anterior chamber of the globe. The simplest method to determine whether a foreign body is intra- or extraocular is to make a double exposure in the lateral projection with the patient looking up and down. If the head is immobilized properly, a double image of the foreign body on the film is presumptive evidence that it is in the globe. Slight motion is possible if it is lodged in one of the ocular muscles. Therefore, the method carries some chance for positive error but is simple and in the absence of suitable localizing equipment, is useful. The optic foramina are examined by means of a specialized technique. Views of both foramina are obtained in order to compare the two sides. An example of the projection is shown in Figure 33-2. Tomography of the optic foramina is useful in patients with suspected disease in this region. It is also used in the diagnosis of destructive, sclerotic, or traumatic changes in the orbital walls.

ORBITAL PNEUMOGRAPHY. In patients with proptosis or other signs of intraorbital mass, several special examinations may be used. Orbital pneumography consists of the injection of 15 to 20 ml of air into the retrobulbar space. Water-soluble organic iodides are also used for orbitography; 20% dilutions in 3- to 5-ml amounts are injected. In addition to roentgenograms in frontal and lateral projections, tomography may be used in conjunction with orbitography.

ORBITAL VENOGRAPHY. The ophthalmic veins are opacified by hand injection of an organic iodide into the frontal vein, angular veins, or via retrograde catheterization of the inferior petrosal sinus. Serial filming in frontal, lateral, and basal projections then outlines the ophthalmic veins. They are more constant in location than the arteries, so venography is more accurate in localizing intraorbital masses than is arteriography.

OPHTHALMIC ARTERY ANGIOGRAPHY. This is probably used more frequently than venography in the study of intraorbital structures. The contrast

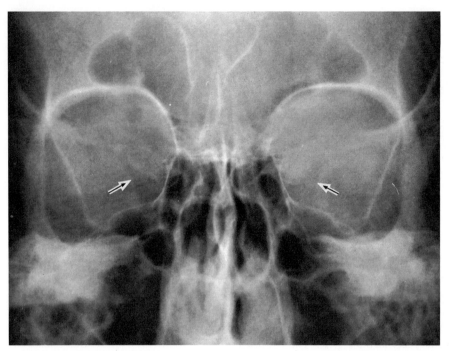

Fig. 33-1. Normal orbit. The bony orbital rims are clearly defined. The bony walls of the orbit are thin, resulting in relative radiolucency. The superior orbital fissures are indicated by **arrows.**

medium is injected selectively into the internal carotid artery and the examination is timed for best visualization of ophthalmic arteries, capillaries, and veins. In some departments, both examinations are used. Venography seems to be more promising for localizing intraorbital masses than arteriography and will probably be used more extensively in the future than it is now. Subtraction techniques are very helpful in the study of ophthalmic vessels.

MEASUREMENT OF INTERORBITAL DISTANCE. The interorbital distance in the growing child as well as in the adult is of some importance, since there are a number of congenital disorders in which ocular hypertelorism or hypotelorism are an important part. Hansman[9] has presented standards for interorbital distances in males and females to age 24 (Tables 33-1 and 33-2). The distance was measured on sinus films taken on an angle board with the patient's nose and forehead touching the cassette and the tube in a vertical position. Focal film distance was 28 inches. The subjects were healthy and presumably normal.

In addition to Greig's syndrome, hypertelorism is found in a number of conditions including craniostenosis, craniofacial dysostosis, mandibulofacial dysostosis, achondroplasia, Bonnevie-Ullrich syndrome, and in some patients with cleft palate. Hypotelorism may be found in such disorders as arrhinencephaly and Marchesani's syndrome.

INTRAOCULAR FOREIGN BODIES

Before any special methods are used to localize radiopaque foreign particles in the eye, roentgenograms in frontal and lateral projections are necessary to make sure that the foreign material is visible and can be identified on the radiographic localization films. If the presence of a foreign body is detected on the scout films; then special localization can be done. The most common method in use in this country is the method of Sweet[19] for which special apparatus as well as charts are available. It is a triangulation method, the details of which are

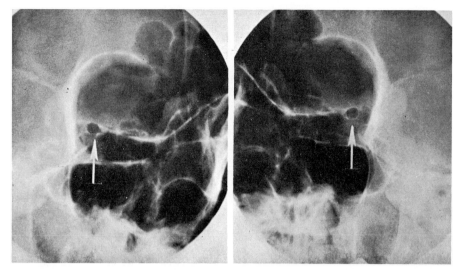

Fig. 33-2. Normal optic canals. These special views outline the optic foramina, which are indicated by **arrows.**

available in standard texts dealing with roentgen technique. Semiopaque materials such as glass can sometimes be visualized on roentgenograms of good quality. When a small, semiopaque, foreign body is suspected in the anterior chamber, the bone-free type of examination can be used.

CALCIFICATIONS WITHIN THE ORBIT AND GLOBE

HYPERCALCEMIA

Calcification within the conjunctiva and cornea has been described in patients with hyperparathyroidism and hypervitaminosis D, evidently secondary to the associated hypercalcemia. Radiographically, these calcifications appear as faint annular shadows that can be localized to the cornea and conjunctiva in tangential views of the anterior globe. The bone-free type of examination can be used to demonstrate the calcium.

RETINOBLASTOMA

Retinoblastoma is a glioma of the retina that occurs chiefly in infants and children. There are other diseases, including inflammations, which simulate this tumor clinically and make its differentiation difficult. Early removal of the eye is necessary to effect cure in retinoblastoma, so roentgen signs that assist in making the diagnosis are important. There is stippled or mottled calcification in the globe which is almost pathognomonic of retinoblastoma. It is found in approximately 75 per cent of patients so that its absence does not exclude retinoblastoma. Calcifications have also been reported in intracerebral metastases from retinoblastoma. In addition to the calcification, a soft-tissue mass may be noted within the orbit. The tumor may extend along the optic nerve to produce enlargement of the optic foramen, which can be visualized roentgenographically and when the tumor spreads beyond the nerve, irregular erosion of the optic foramen may develop.

OTHER CALCIFICATIONS

1. Calcium deposits occasionally occur in the cornea, associated with degenerative processes there.

2. In hypermature cataracts, calcification may be visualized in the lens. This results in a typical, small, rounded, calcific density located within the

TABLE 33-1. Percentile Standards for Interorbital Distance as Measured on Sinus Roentgenograms for Girls

Age	N	Minimum	10th	25th	50th	75th	90th	Maximum
0–6	95	1.200	—	—	—	—	—	2.160
1–0	96	1.230	—	—	—	—	—	2.270
1–6	100	1.290	1.514	1.632	1.733	1.854	1.988	2.290
2–0	99	1.330	1.567	1.682	1.784	1.905	2.039	2.330
2–6	100	1.340	1.616	1.726	1.823	1.949	2.084	2.370
3–0	98	1.360	1.657	1.764	1.859	1.992	2.130	2.390
3–6	100	1.430	1.696	1.801	1.892	2.032	1.173	2.450
4–0	102	1.460	1.729	1.837	1.929	2.070	2.215	2.480
4–6	98	1.570	1.763	1.873	1.968	2.109	2.252	2.523
5–0	97	1.620	1.790	1.906	2.007	2.146	2.288	2.530
5–6	97	1.650	1.817	1.936	2.043	2.183	2.324	2.560
6–0	98	1.690	1.842	1.964	2.078	2.218	2.362	2.636
6–6	98	1.730	1.868	1.992	2.111	2.254	2.398	2.680
7–0	96	1.750	1.896	2.021	2.144	2.288	2.431	2.703
7–6	94	1.770	1.923	2.053	2.174	2.320	2.459	2.730
8–0	94	1.790	1.949	2.087	2.207	2.352	2.487	2.758
8–6	92	1.830	1.970	2.118	2.237	2.379	2.513	2.803
9–0	89	1.860	1.989	1.140	2.270	2.409	2.542	2.840
9–6	89	1.860	2.015	2.159	2.292	2.433	2.568	2.880
10–0	88	1.880	2.044	2.180	2.313	2.458	2.596	2.900
10–6	89	1.900	2.076	2.207	2.332	2.481	2.620	2.940
11–0	84	1.930	2.102	2.234	2.359	2.510	2.649	2.998
11–6	82	1.940	2.128	2.262	2.389	2.541	2.679	3.000
12–0	82	1.980	2.148	2.284	2.419	2.573	2.710	3.050
12–6	80	1.990	2.174	2.308	2.445	2.602	2.742	3.110
13–0	76	2.020	2.196	2.328	2.466	2.623	2.766	3.110
13–6	74	2.050	2.216	2.350	2.484	2.638	2.782	3.130
14–0	73	2.080	2.228	2.363	2.498	2.646	2.786	3.130
14–6	71	2.080	2.235	2.375	2.513	2.656	2.792	3.150
15–0	68	2.100	2.243	2.385	2.524	2.668	2.803	3.150
15–6	66	2.115	2.255	2.399	2.538	2.683	2.820	3.150
16–0	64	2.120	2.275	2.416	2.547	2.693	2.833	3.150
16–6	59	2.080	2.293	2.430	2.556	2.699	2.841	3.155
17–0	58	2.130	2.306	2.442	2.563	2.704	2.847	3.160
17–6	51	2.135	2.309	2.448	2.573	2.714	2.856	3.165
18–0	49	2.140	2.309	2.453	2.581	2.724	2.865	3.170
18–6	47	2.140	2.310	2.457	2.587	2.733	2.874	3.175
19–0	46	2.140	2.314	2.459	2.588	2.738	2.882	3.180
19–6	43	2.135	2.314	2.459	2.587	2.742	2.887	3.191
20–0	42	2.130	2.318	2.460	2.587	2.743	2.890	3.200
20–6	37	2.136	2.323	2.462	2.585	2.740	2.889	3.200
21–0	35	2.143	2.333	2.466	2.584	2.738	2.888	3.200
21–6	32	2.149	2.332	2.463	2.583	2.733	2.884	3.200
22–0	32	2.120	2.326	2.458	2.579	2.722	2.869	3.200
22–6	28	2.138	2.312	2.450	2.573	2.707	2.842	3.200
23–0	24	2.148	2.293	2.444	2.569	2.693	2.814	2.880
23–6	20	2.142	2.270	2.439	2.573	2.690	2.802	2.886
24–0	19	2.141	2.256	2.437	2.583	2.698	2.806	2.898
24–6	18	2.143	—	—	—	—	—	2.912
25–0	18	2.145	—	—	—	—	—	2.915

From Hansman, C. F.[9]

TABLE 33-2. Percentile Standards for Interorbital Distance as Measured on Sinus Roentgenograms for Boys

Age	N	Minimum	10th	25th	50th	75th	90th	Maximum
0–6	91	1.230	—	—	—	—	—	2.160
1–0	94	1.230	—	—	—	—	—	2.270
1–6	95	1.250	1.524	1.651	1.773	1.920	2.063	2.290
2–0	95	1.270	1.578	1.700	1.822	1.971	2.114	2.360
2–6	96	1.290	1.631	1.748	1.866	2.013	2.157	2.390
3–0	92	1.350	1.680	1.795	1.909	2.056	2.201	2.393
3–6	93	1.400	1.725	1.839	1.953	2.099	2.246	2.470
4–0	95	1.420	1.760	1.877	1.994	2.143	2.292	2.530
4–6	95	1.420	1.795	1.916	2.035	2.187	2.337	2.570
5–0	94	1.450	1.830	1.952	2.073	2.229	2.382	2.620
5–6	93	1.520	1.864	1.989	2.110	2.270	2.427	2.650
6–0	91	1.520	1.896	2.022	2.143	2.308	2.466	2.730
6–6	91	1.560	1.925	2.050	2.173	2.342	2.501	2.750
7–0	89	1.570	1.957	2.076	2.199	2.371	2.537	2.840
7–6	91	1.620	1.991	2.103	2.226	2.400	2.573	2.890
8–0	93	1.640	2.025	2.132	2.256	2.429	2.607	2.860
8–6	92	1.680	2.049	2.161	2.284	2.456	2.634	2.950
9–0	92	1.720	2.069	2.187	2.310	2.480	2.656	2.950
9–6	93	1.730	2.089	2.211	2.333	2.506	2.685	2.990
10–0	92	1.750	2.114	2.236	2.357	2.534	2.716	3.080
10–6	89	1.800	2.139	2.262	2.385	2.564	2.752	3.080
11–0	88	1.920	2.164	2.288	2.412	2.592	2.780	3.160
11–6	86	1.870	2.191	2.315	2.440	2.617	2.807	3.180
12–0	84	1.860	2.220	2.344	2.468	2.643	2.834	3.100
12–6	78	2.000	2.251	2.375	2.498	2.674	2.868	3.123
13–0	78	2.050	2.278	2.405	2.529	2.704	2.904	3.160
13–6	78	2.050	2.304	2.433	2.560	2.735	2.938	3.220
14–0	74	2.080	2.328	2.460	2.590	2.760	2.964	3.250
14–6	70	2.090	2.353	2.489	2.622	2.789	2.993	3.250
15–0	70	2.180	2.374	2.515	2.650	2.817	3.024	3.320
15–6	69	2.180	2.392	2.537	2.672	2.847	3.059	3.330
16–0	68	2.190	2.407	2.553	2.697	2.868	3.084	3.372
16–6	66	2.180	2.422	2.570	2.713	2.884	3.096	3.390
17–0	65	2.180	2.438	2.586	2.723	2.894	3.101	3.430
17–6	64	2.205	2.447	2.599	2.733	2.903	3.107	3.464
18–0	62	2.230	2.454	2.608	2.741	2.915	3.119	3.490
18–6	56	2.230	2.454	2.612	2.750	2.924	3.131	3.505
19–0	55	2.230	2.456	2.616	2.759	2.937	3.148	3.520
19–6	50	2.230	2.463	2.622	2.768	2.952	3.169	3.535
20–0	45	2.230	2.469	2.629	2.778	2.971	3.196	3.550
20–6	40	2.230	2.468	2.633	2.788	2.993	3.224	3.560
21–0	37	2.230	2.461	2.638	2.806	3.014	3.247	3.570
21–6	33	2.230	2.460	2.643	2.822	3.033	3.265	3.570
22–0	29	2.370	2.470	2.653	2.830	3.041	3.269	3.570
22–6	28	2.384	2.477	2.651	2.835	3.043	3.271	3.573
23–0	26	2.400	2.479	2.651	2.836	3.043	3.269	3.577
23–6	23	2.400	2.476	2.647	2.839	3.053	3.276	3.580
24–0	23	2.400	2.472	2.647	2.843	3.059	3.273	3.583
24–6	22	2.400	—	—	—	—	—	3.587
25–0	21	2.400	—	—	—	—	—	3.590

From Hansman, C. F.[9]

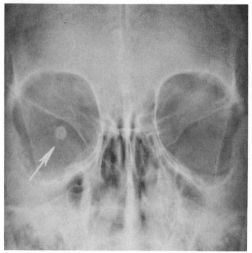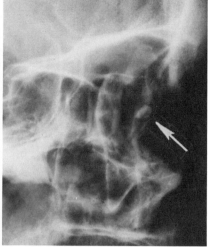

Fig. 33-3. Cataract on the right. Roentgenogram of the orbit in frontal and lateral projections reveals small rounded calcific density representing calcification in the lens **(arrows)**.

globe in the position of the lens (Fig. 33-3). Calcification may also occur in congenital cataract and, therefore, may be seen in children.

3. Intraorbital hemangioma and orbital varices may be recognized by the presence of round, calcified phleboliths.

4. Calcification also occurs in intra- and extra-orbital hemorrhage following trauma.

5. Retrolental fibroplasia may also cause calcification in the globe.

6. Calcification and ossification may occasionally occur in degenerative diseases of the choroid and produce a curvilinear density conforming to the shape of the globe.

7. Rarely, calcification and ossification may occur in the vitreous, producing a localized central shadow or a diffuse or irregular shadow of calcific density peripherally in the globe.

8. Globe degeneration, phthisis bulbi, may be accompanied by nodules and plaques of calcium in the lens and globe (Fig. 33-4).

9. Ocular phacoma may contain nodular calcification.

THE OPTIC CANAL

GENERAL CONSIDERATIONS

The canals are examined by means of special posteroanterior projections in which the beam is parallel to the long axis of the canal. Both canals are examined for comparison in most instances. Special devices are available to hold the head and to insure proper angulation, which is about 37° off the sagittal plane toward the side examined and 31° caudad to a line from the outer canthus of the eye to the external auditory meatus. Tomography may be of value in patients in whom no abnormality is visible on the standard projection. Films can be taken perpendicular to the long axis of the canal or in the axial projection, parallel to it, using the basal (submentovertex) position, or both of these may be used if necessary. The canal is approximately 7 mm in length. The canals are not always bilaterally symmetric but they are usually nearly the same size. Their margins are very clearly defined. The normal optic canal measures approximately 5 mm in its greatest diameter on the roentgenogram. Any diameter over 6 mm or under 4 mm is considered abnormal. The canal attains its adult size early in life, between the ages of 3 and 5 years. The canal is slightly oval at either end, the long axis is roughly horizontal at the cranial end and vertical at the orbital end, and the midportion is round. In the standard view, the orbital end is visible, since its walls are more dense. Rarely, the canal is divided, with

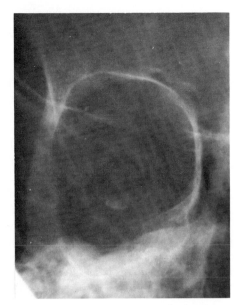

Fig. 33-4. Phthisis bulbi. There is a local plaque of calcium inferiorly with faintly visualized, curvilinear calcifications extending to either side which appear to be in the wall of the globe.

an upper opening for the optic nerve and a lower one for the ophthalmic artery. Narrowing of the canal may be congenital in patients with craniofacial dysostosis (Crouzon's disease) and oxycephaly; the deformity may be so severe as to cause blindness in some patients. Acquired narrowing may be caused by Paget's disease, fibrous dysplasia, or may be secondary to trauma, osteopetrosis, or pycnodystosis.

TUMORS

Tumors usually cause enlargement of the optic foramina. In neurofibromatosis, involvement of the optic nerve on one side or the other may result in marked enlargement of the optic foramen. The walls are usually smooth, even when considerable enlargement is present. Retinal glioma may extend posteriorly along the optic nerve to enlarge the optic foramen. A normal-sized foramen does not exclude the presence of a tumor involving the nerve, however. Glioma arising in the brain and extending anteriorly along the optic nerve may also enlarge this foramen. Meningioma may extend

from the globe into the cranial vault, or vice versa, resulting in enlargement of the optic foramen. In addition, meningioma usually evokes a hyperostotic response and causes a dense bony thickening which may actually narrow the foramen.

THE SUPERIOR ORBITAL (SPHENOIDAL) FISSURE

This fissure is bounded below by the greater sphenoid wing and above by the lesser sphenoid wing. It is bounded medially by the body of the sphenoid and the orbital plate of the frontal bone laterally. It is usually readily visualized in standard posteroanterior views of the orbits. It is oblique; its wide medial end is posterior and the more narrow lateral end is anterior and slightly superior to the medial end. The wide end is at the apex of the orbital pyramid, and is below and lateral to the optic canal. The third, fourth, and sixth nerves, the ophthalmic division of the fifth, the ophthalmic veins, the nasociliary nerve, and the sympathetic root of the ciliary ganglion all pass through the wide medial portion of the fissure. All of these structures may be involved by a disease process in this region. Infection, tumor arising locally such as orbital tumors, meningioma, metastatic tumor, and aneurysm of the anterior half of the intracavernous portion of the carotid artery are among the conditions which may affect the orbital apex.

THE INFERIOR ORBITAL FISSURE

This fissure forms an angle with the superior orbital fissure which is open laterally. It lies between the greater sphenoid wing superiorly and the orbital surface of the maxilla inferiorly and connects the orbit with the pterygopalatine fossa. The orbital branches of the sphenopalatine ganglion and a venous plexus extend through it. This is not often examined by roentgen methods, but a special view taken posteroanteriorly at 25° caudad to the canthomeatal line with the central ray on the glabella will outline the fissure adjacent to the postero-superior aspect of the maxillary sinus on either side.

TUMORS OF THE ORBIT

A number of tumors and inflammatory lesions may result in intraorbital mass that may produce some radiographic changes in the bony walls of the orbit. Plain films may then be sufficient to determine the site and cause of the mass (Fig. 33-5). When there are clinical signs of an intraorbital mass, including proptosis, orbitography using diatrizoate (or other opaque media) or gas may be used to outline the globe and abnormal masses within the orbit. Tomograms may be used in conjunction with this study. More often, orbital venography and arteriography are used. These intraorbital masses often are difficult clinical problems and require cooperative effort of the ophthalmologist, the neurosurgeon, and the radiologist in the complete study of the patient.

Among the masses which may produce proptosis without bone changes are lacrimal gland tumors, hemangioma, inflammatory granuloma, neurofibroma, orbital varices, metastases, melanoma, lymphosarcoma, histiocytosis X, psuedotumor, pseudolymphoma, meningioma, and fibroma. Many of them may cause bone changes early, however, and others cause bone changes late in their development.

There are other masses which usually cause bone change which can be recognized radiographically; in some instances the diagnosis can be made on plain-film study with reasonable certainty. Among the diseases which usually cause bone changes are inflammatory disease of paranasal sinuses with spread to the orbit, mucocele of frontal sinus with orbital involvement, carcinoma of sinus with orbital spread, meningioma, dermoid cyst, aneurysm, ossifying fibroma, fibrous dysplasia, posttraumatic meningocele, various sarcomas and, in some instances, neurofibromatosis. The tumors listed exhibit changes in the orbital walls similar to those produced in other areas. The hyper-

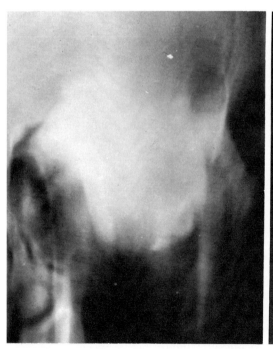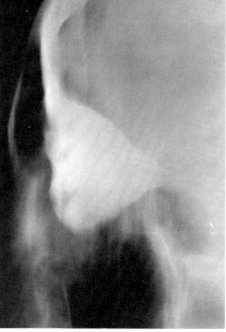

Fig. 33-5. Orbital osteoma. Note the large, dense tumor mass arising in the roof of the left orbit and projecting downward. It is well defined on tomography, particularly in the lateral projection.

ostotic changes in meningioma are characteristic of that type of tumor. In neurofibroma,
enlargement of the optic foramen is a helpful
diagnostic sign; this tumor is also capable of
producing great orbital enlargement and distortion. Dermoid cyst or cholesteatoma may also
result in orbital enlargement and distortion as
well as erosion and decalcification of the bony
orbital walls. When malignant tumor is present,
bone invasion may result in destruction of
orbital walls; this is particularly true of carcinoma extending from adjacent sinuses. The
destruction is manifested by disappearance of
bone in an irregular manner without sclerosis.
Tumors of the lacrimal gland may cause erosion or destruction of bone in the orbital roof
adjacent to the gland, which lies in a shallow
fossa that indents the superior aspect of the
orbit laterally. Slowly expanding benign tumors
may enlarge the fossa without invasion of
bone. Malignant tumors tend to invade and
either destroy the bone or cause sclerosis of the
fossa and adjacent orbital rim.

THE LACRIMAL PASSAGES

The lacrimal passages extend from the
puncta in the medial aspect of the eyelids to
the inferior nasal meatus. Radiographic methods may be used to study them. An iodine-
containing contrast material is injected into the
lower canaliculus and films are taken in frontal
and lateral projections. The water-soluble
media are now preferred over Lipiodol which
was used for a number of years. The examination is used chiefly in localizing the site of
obstruction of the nasolacrimal duct. Tomography may be useful in the examination of
fine bony structures in this area. The anatomy
in this area is beyond the scope of this volume.

REFERENCES AND SELECTED READINGS

1. BERTELSON, T. I., and PETERSEN, O.: Orbital
   pneumography. *Acta Radiol. 47:* 426, 1957.

2. BINET, E. F., KIEFFER, S. A., MARTIN, S. H., and
   PETERSON, H. O.: Orbital dysplasia in neurofibromatosis. *Radiology 93:* 829, 1969.

3. DAVIS, L. A., and DIAMOND, I.: Metastatic retinoblastoma as a cause of diffuse intracranial calcification. *Am. J. Roentgenol. Radium Ther. Nucl.
   Med. 78:* 437, 1957.

4. ETTER, L. E.: Detailed roentgen anatomy of the
   orbits. *Radiology 59:* 489, 1952.

5. EVANS, R. A., SCHWARTZ, J. F., and CHUTORIAÑ,
   A. M.: Radiologic diagnosis in pediatric ophthalmology. *Radiol. Clin. North Am. I:* 459, 1963.

6. FLEISCHNER, F. G., and SHALEK, S. R.: Conjunctival and corneal calcification in hypercalcemia:
   Roentgenologic findings. *N. Engl. J. Med. 241:*
   863, 1949.

7. HANAFEE, W. N., SHIU, P. C., and DAYTON, G. O.:
   Orbital venography. *Am. J. Roentgenol. Radium
   Ther. Nucl. Med. 104:* 29, 1968.

8. HANAFEE, W. N., and DAYTON, G. O.: The roentgen diagnosis of orbital tumors. *Radiol. Clin.
   North Am. VIII:* 403, 1970.

9. HANSMAN, C. F.: Growth of interorbital distance
   and skull thickness as observed in roentgenographic measurements. *Radiology 86:* 87, 1966.

10. HARTMANN, E., and GILLES, E.: *Roentgenologic
    Diagnosis in Ophthalmology.* Philadelphia, Lip-
    pincott, 1959.

11. INGALLS, R. G.: *Tumors of the Orbit and Allied
    Pseudo Tumors.* Springfield, Ill., Thomas, 1953.

12. LOMBARDI, G.: Orbitography with water-soluble
    contrast media. *Acta Radiol. 47:* 417, 1957.

13. MERRILL, V.: *Atlas of Roentgenographic Posi-
    tions.* St. Louis, Mosby, 1967, vol. II.

14. MINTZ, M. J., and MATTES, M. W.: Detection of
    foreign bodies in the anterior chamber of the
    bulbus oculi. *Radiology 75:* 612, 1960.

15. NEWTON, T. H.: Roentgen appearance of lacrimal
    gland tumors. *Radiology 79:* 598, 1962.

16. POTTER, G. D., and TROKEL, S.: Tomography of
    the optic canal. *Am. J. Roentgenol. Radium Ther.
    Nucl. Med. 106:* 530, 1969.

17. ROBERTS, W. E.: The roentgenographic demon-
    strations of glass fragments in the eye. *Am. J.
    Roentgenol. Radium Ther. Nucl. Med. 66:* 44,
    1951.

18. SCHINZ, H. R., BAENSCH, W. E., FROMMHOLD, W.,
    GLAUNER, R., UEHLINGER, E., and WELLAUER, J.:
    Roentgen Diagnosis, 2nd ed. Ed. by L. G. Rigler.
    New York, Grune & Stratton, 1969, vol. III.

19. SWEET, W. M.: Improved apparatus for localizing
    foreign bodies in the eyeball by the roentgen rays.
    Arch. Ophthalmol. 38: 623, 1909.

20. WHEELER, E. C., and BAKER, H. L., JR.: The
    ophthalmic arterial complex in angiographic diag-
    nosis. *Radiology 83:* 26, 1964.

34

THE SINUSES AND MASTOIDS

THE PARANASAL SINUSES

The roentgen examination of the paranasal sinuses is an essential part of the study of these structures. Diseases affecting them cause alterations in the normal radiolucency of the sinuses which can be detected on roentgenograms.

METHODS OF EXAMINATION

STANDARD POSITIONS

There are a number of special views for demonstrating the various paranasal sinuses. The actual techniques are described in the text on radiographic technique[11] and will not be discussed here. If possible, roentgenograms of the sinuses should be obtained in the upright position in order to demonstrate fluid levels when they are present. Techniques for the various projections should be standardized so that films of comparable density are obtained. Some techniques call for a stationary grid or Potter-Bucky diaphragm while others specify a nongrid technique with cones to confine the beam to the area of the sinuses. The standard positions we use are: (1) The occipitomental or Waters' projection in which the maxillary antra are particularly well defined. This view is also used in trauma cases for examination of the facial bones (Fig. 34-1); (2) The occipitofrontal or Caldwell position, which is of particular value for visualiz-

ing the frontal and ethmoid sinuses. The upper aspect of the maxillary antra is also well outlined. (Fig. 34-2); (3) The lateral position, chiefly for viewing the sphenoid and frontal sinuses (Fig. 34-3); and (4) The occipitosubmental position with the mouth open, primarily used to demonstrate disease in the sphenoid sinuses but maxillary and frontal sinuses are also fairly well visualized (Fig. 34-4). The submentovertical with 15° cephalad angulation gives a clear definition of the sphenoid and posterior antra (Fig. 34-5). A number of other projections may be used to solve problems in any patient.

SPECIAL METHODS

CONTRAST STUDIES. Dionosil, oily may be introduced into the paranasal sinuses by the displacement technique of Proetz or it can be injected by direct antral puncture. The latter method is preferred. Once the iodized oil is within the desired sinus or sinuses, roentgenograms can be taken in the routine projections and in any additional views deemed necessary to obtain desired information. This method is used to outline masses within a sinus and to estimate the thickness of the lining membrane. The examination has few indications and is not used commonly.

TOMOGRAPHY. This method is used extensively in the examination of paranasal sinuses to outline foreign bodies, to determine the presence and extent of bone involvement by tumor, and to de-

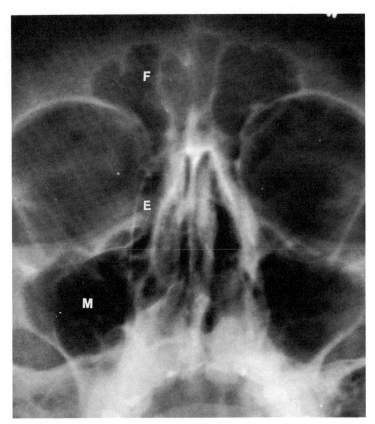

Fig. 34-1. Normal sinuses as seen in Waters' projection. **F,** Frontal sinus; **E,** ethmoid cells; **M,** maxillary sinus.

termine the extent and location of fractures of the bony walls of the sinuses and nasal bones.

THE NORMAL SINUSES

The paranasal sinuses are paired cavities lined by mucous membrane (mucoperiosteum) that arise as outpouchings from the nasal fossa and extend into the maxillary, ethmoid, sphenoid, and frontal bones. They are named according to the bones in which they develop.

MAXILLARY

The maxillary antra are the first of the paranasal sinuses to appear in fetal life. They arise as outpouchings from the anterior recess of the middle meatus. At birth they are small, vertically ovoid cavities located in the maxilla on either side of the midline. They usually contain a jellylike material and are not clearly defined roentgenographically at birth. Aeration is often incomplete for a week or 10 days after birth and may be incomplete for a month or more. At times, aeration is not complete for 6 months after birth. These sinuses develop gradually and at 1 year the outer wall of the antrum is medial to the infraorbital foramen; at 2 years it extends to the level of the foramen. The growth in the transverse diameter is nearly completed at 8 years of age and most of the later growth takes place in the vertical and anteroposterior diameters. Growth is usually complete at 12 years. When fully developed, the sinus is shaped by the body of the maxillary bone. It is considered to have a roof, a floor, and three walls—the nasal, facial, and infratemporal.

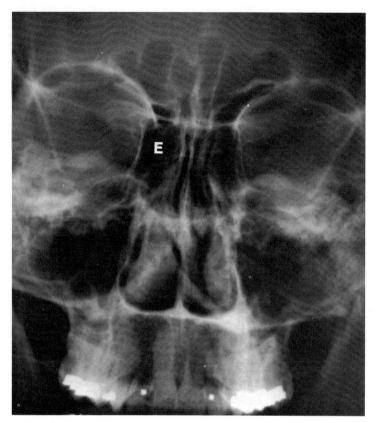

Fig. 34-2. Normal sinuses as seen in the occipitofrontal or Caldwell position. **E** indicates the ethmoid cells on the right.

The floor is often irregular since the alveolar process of the maxilla is immediately below the sinus and some of the teeth may project with their bony and periosteal coverings into the floor of the sinus. Complete or incomplete bony or membranous septa occasionally divide the antrum into two or more compartments.

FRONTAL

The frontal sinuses are usually present at birth but cannot be identified because they are incompletely aerated and lie adjacent to the anterior ethmoid cells in the orbital plate of the frontal bone. They communicate with the middle nasal meatus by means of the nasofrontal duct. These sinuses can usually be identified by the end of the first year but may not be visible until 2 years of age, when they have extended up into the vertical plate of the frontal bone. They can then be differentiated from the anterior ethmoid cells. These sinuses are often asymmetric and vary widely in size. They may extend high into the vertical portion of the frontal bone and backward into the orbital plate. They gradually increase and reach their extent of growth at 10 to 12 years of age. Complete and incomplete division into compartments by septa is common.

ETHMOID

The ethmoid sinuses consist of two groups of cells lying on either side of the midline in the ethmoid bone, where they form the medial wall of the orbit and the lateral wall of the upper half of the nasal cavity. They vary from three or four up to 18 or more in number. The

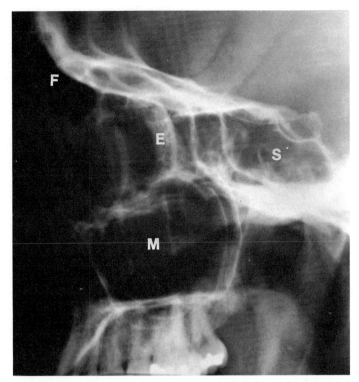

Fig. 34-3. Normal sinuses on lateral view. **F,** Frontal sinuses; **E,** ethmoid cells; **S,** sphenoid sinus; **M,** maxillary antra.

frontal anterior ethmoids open into the frontal recess, the infundibular anterior cells into the ethmoid infundibulum, and the bullar anterior cells open above the ethmoidal bulla. The posterior ethmoid cells usually communicate with the superior or supreme nasal meatus. The ethmoids may extend into the adjacent maxillary, frontal, sphenoid, and palatine bones; their distribution varies considerably. Some of the ethmoid cells are present at birth but are often poorly aerated and difficult to visualize. These sinuses develop at the same rate as the maxillary antra and are usually fully developed at 10 to 12 years of age.

SPHENOID

The sphenoid sinuses lie in the body of the sphenoid bone and communicate with the sphenoethmoid recess in the posterior superior portion of the nasal cavity. They are not ordinarily visible at birth. Pneumatization begins anteriorly in the third or fourth year and progresses posteriorly into the sphenoid bone below the sella turcica. The sphenoid sinuses not infrequently extend posterior to the sella turcica upward into the dorsum. These sinuses, although superimposed, are most readily outlined in the lateral projection. Their development is somewhat slower than that of the remaining sinuses and their growth continues into young adult life. In the first 4 years of life these sinuses develop in the cupolar recess of the nasal cavity. Pneumatization extends posteriorly in the next 8 years, and from age 12 to 20 the migration extends posteriorly to the level of the dorsum sellae and sometimes extends into it.

NORMAL ROENTGEN APPEARANCE

The normal sinuses are radiolucent because of the air content; the radiability of the maxillary antra is usually comparable to that of the

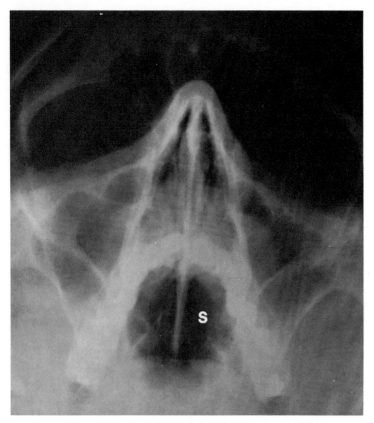

Fig. 34-4. Normal sinuses. The occipitosubmental open mouth position. **S**, Sphenoid sinuses. The maxillary antra are also well visualized.

orbits. Variations in thickness of the bony walls of the sinuses may alter the density to a moderate degree. This is particularly true of the frontal sinuses where the frontal bone may be relatively dense. In the interpretation of roentgenograms of the sinuses the variation in bone density and in thickness of overlying soft tissues must be considered. The normal lining membrane of the sinuses is invisible on the roentgenogram and the bony walls are distinct and clearly defined. Any increase in density involving one or more sinuses must be examined carefully to exclude changes caused by normal soft-tissue structures. Care must be taken in interpreting variations of aeration in the sinuses in infancy because the mucosa is often redundant and aeration incomplete in the normal, particularly in the infant under 1

month of age. Furthermore, the frequent asymmetry of the sinuses must be kept in mind.

INFLAMMATORY DISEASES

ACUTE SINUSITIS

Acute inflammatory disease involving the paranasal sinuses results in swelling of the lining membrane. There is often retention of fluid in the sinus also. The maxillary antra are most commonly affected and in the presence of disease affecting the other sinuses, the changes in the antra are often more marked than those elsewhere. The disease may be unilateral or bilateral. Fluid is manifested by fluid levels when roentgenograms are made with the pa-

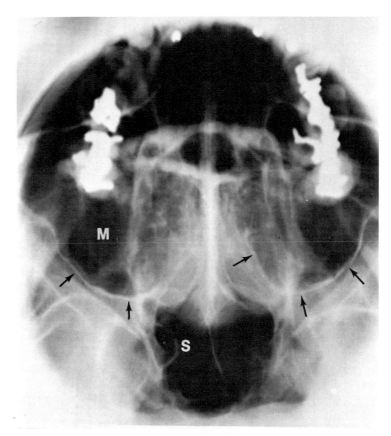

Fig. 34-5. Normal sinuses, the submentovertical view. **M**, Maxillary sinus; **S**, sphenoid sinus. **Arrows** outline posterior walls of the maxillary sinuses which are particularly well visualized in this projection.

tient upright (Fig. 34-6). The levels are noted particularly in the maxillary antra and frontal sinuses and occasionally in the sphenoids. In patients who cannot assume an upright position, horizontal beam films may be taken in appropriate projections in order to define fluid levels. A diffuse clouding is observed as the result of thickening of the lining membrane and the presence of inflammatory exudate. The mucosal swelling may be manifested by a soft-tissue density lining the bony walls of the sinus if it is not sufficient to cause complete diffuse type of density. In the acute disease there is no alteration in the bony walls. The roentgen findings should be correlated with clinical findings in these patients because some swelling of the lining membrane may persist after an infection

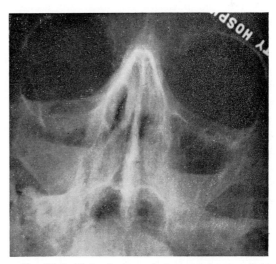

Fig. 34-6. Waters' view of sinuses showing fluid levels in the maxillary antra.

has subsided. It is also possible to have an acute process with very little swelling of the mucosa so that no detectable roentgen findings may be present.

CHRONIC SINUSITIS

Chronic sinusitis may follow the acute phase or represent a more slowly developing process that is subacute or chronic from its inception. The roentgen findings are due to thickening of the mucosa that results in soft-tissue density of varying thickness lining the sinus or sinuses involved. Fluid levels may also be present in the patients with chronic sinus disease. The thickening of the membrane is usually more clearly defined and less hazy than in more acute disease. In chronic sinusitis the additional finding of some thickening or sclerosis of the bone forming the wall of the sinus may be observed (Fig. 34-7). This is found more commonly in the frontal sinuses than elsewhere. In chronic sinusitis, as a general rule the maxillary antra are the most commonly affected; the ethmoids are often involved as well. When the frontal sinuses are infected there is almost invariably sinusitis affecting the ethmoid cells, but the ethmoids may be infected without involvement of the frontal sinuses. The sphenoids are less frequently the site of disease but when they are, the posterior ethmoids are almost invariably involved. Rarely, infection may lead to osteomyelitis of the sinus wall. It is more commonly associated with involvement of the maxillary antrum secondary to dental infection than it is with sinusitis. When this occurs there is usually clouding of the sinus and an irregular moth-eaten type of destruction of the bony sinus wall in the area of involvement; dense sequestra are often present. Prior to the use of antibiotics, acute frontal sinusitis occasionally led to the development of acute osteomyelitis of the frontal bone. This is a rare lesion at the present time.

Occasionally the sinuses may be involved by such chronic inflammatory diseases as tuberculosis, syphilis, actinomycosis, and other bacterial and fungal infections. The roentgen find-

ings are not specific. There is evidence of chronic sinus disease in these patients, with or without destruction of bony walls. Occasionally it is possible to suspect certain organisms, e.g., *Actinomyces, Mucor,* and other fungi, because they characteristically cross tissue boundaries and destroy bone. Diagnosis of the specific organism is made on bacteriologic study of material from the infected sinus.

SCLEROMA (RHINOSCLEROMA)

This rare disease is evidently caused by *Klebsiella rhinoscleromatis;* it often starts in the nose and progresses down the respiratory tract. Roentgen findings are those of thickening of the nasal septum and intranasal soft-tissue masses which often occlude the nares. Sinuses are often opaque and in advanced disease, extensive destruction of the bony sinus walls may be present.

CYSTS AND TUMORS

MUCOUS CYST (RETENTION CYST)

This is a secretory retention cyst caused by obstruction of a mucous gland, usually within the maxillary antrum. This results in gradual enlargement with formation of a cyst most often in or near the floor of the antrum but it may be formed anywhere in the sinuses. It appears as a smooth, rounded soft-tissue opacity usually projecting from the floor of the antrum. It is usually small but rarely may become large enough to occupy most of the sinus (Fig. 34-8).

SEROUS (NONSECRETING) CYST

This cyst arises in the connective tissue of the sinus mucosa. It has no epithelial lining and usually lies on the floor of the maxillary antrum. It is the most common antral cyst and is usually not associated with other abnormality of the affected sinus. Like the mucous reten-

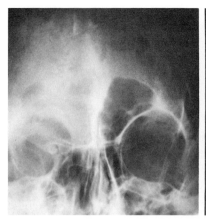
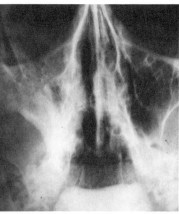

Fig. 34-7. Chronic right frontal and maxillary sinusitis. *Left,* Occipito-frontal projection showing clouding in the right frontal sinus along with considerable sclerosis of its bony walls. Note the normal radiolucency and normal bony walls of the left frontal sinus. *Right,* Open mouth occipito-submental view. There are changes in the right maxillary antrum similar to those in the right frontal sinus, with clouding and considerable sclerosis. Note the normal appearance of the left maxillary antrum.

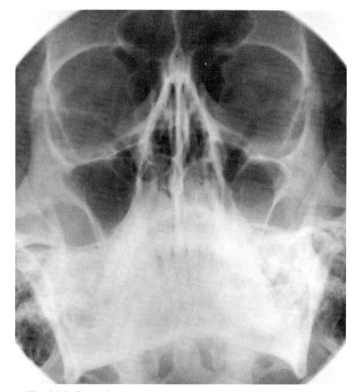

Fig. 34-8. Retention cyst in the floor of the left maxillary antrum. Note the clearly defined, smoothly rounded superior border silhouetted against the air in the maxillary sinus.

tion cyst, it is usually small and never enlarges to the point where it erodes the sinus walls. Roentgenographically it cannot be differentiated from mucous retention cyst.

MUCOCELE

Mucocele consists of a fibrous tissue sac lined by low cuboidal or stratified columnar epithelium. It is produced by obstruction of a sinus ostium. It occurs commonly in the frontal sinuses and with somewhat less frequency in the ethmoids. It is rare in the maxillary antra and in the sphenoids.

Roentgen Findings

The increased pressure within the mucocele caused by accumulation of secretions results in enlargement of the sinus, causing gradual erosion of bony walls. As a result of the destruction of bone, the mucocele is often as radiolucent as an air-filled sinus. The degree of radiolucency of the lesion depends upon the

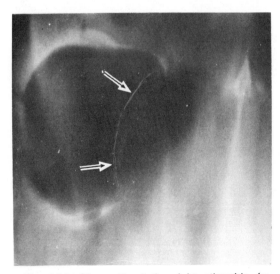

Fig. 34-9. Mucocele of the right ethmoids (retouched). This tomogram shows a large radiolucency in the ethmoid area on the right in which no cell walls are visible. The mucocele has enlarged into the medial aspect of the orbit where the thin wall is outlined by **arrows.**

degree of destruction of bony sinus walls (Fig. 34-9). The enlargement of the sinus as a result of the expanding mucocele causes loss of the normal scalloped sinus margin and the normal soft tissue making up the wall of the sinus is obliterated. The lesion is usually unilateral and the difference between the normal and abnormal sinus is readily apparent. Mucocele of the sphenoid sinus is rare, but the enlargement of this sinus may erode the sellar floor, extend anteriorly into the ethmoid area, erode the superior orbital fissure or optic canal. This makes accurate diagnosis very important. Tomography is of particular value in mucocele of the sphenoid or ethmoid areas, since the thin expanded wall may be clearly defined (Fig. 34-9).

Rarely there is a sclerotic change in the bone forming the margins of the mucocele. Calcification in a mucocele is sometimes found and may be very dense, but this is also rare.

POLYPOSIS AND ALLERGIC DISEASE

Allergic conditions which involve the upper respiratory tract are often associated with polyposis. Polyps consist of edematous masses of mucous membrane with some myxomatous changes; most of them are secondary to allergy. They are usually found in the nasal cavity and when present are often associated with polyps in the maxillary antra. They may also occur in sphenoids, ethmoids, and frontals but are more difficult to demonstrate roentgenographically in these locations. In the antra they produce soft-tissue densities projecting from the sinus wall that may be single or multiple and may fill the entire sinus, causing general cloudiness. The density caused by these masses is similar to that caused by mucous retention cysts but polyps are often associated with polyps in the nose so that there is loss of aeration of the nasal cavities. As a general rule, both maxillary sinuses are involved with multiple, small mucosal masses. There is often some associated thickening of the mucosal lining of the antra and sometimes the frontal sinuses. It is not unusual to have complete clouding of one or both antra, and fluid levels may be present. The roentgen observations should be correlated with the clinical findings in these patients.

BENIGN TUMORS

TUMORS OF SOFT-TISSUE ORIGIN

Fibroma, neurofibroma, papilloma, and angioma may occur in the wall of the maxillary antrum. They are rare, usually small, and cannot be differentiated from cysts. Epidermoid tumor may rarely arise in the frontal or maxillary sinuses. Pathogenesis is somewhat controversial, but most are evidently acquired. Occasionally they become large and their slow growth gradually expands the sinus. This produces atrophy and sometimes complete destruction of one or more bony walls in a manner similar to that caused by mucocele. When this occurs, the tumor may resemble mucocele to the point where they cannot be differentiated

roentgenographically. Similar gross enlargement is sometimes seen with other benign tumors; biopsy is necessary to differentiate them.

TUMORS OF BONY ORIGIN

Osteoma is a relatively common tumor that usually arises in the frontal and much less frequently in the ethmoid sinuses. Rarely it is found in the maxillary or sphenoid sinuses. The roentgen findings are characteristic and consist of a rounded or lobulated mass of bony density. It is usually small but may become moderately large and is readily recognized because of its ivorylike density similar to that of cortical bone (Fig. 34-10). Occasionally osteochondroma may arise in the wall of the sinus; this tumor may become large, resulting in pressure with erosion and atrophy of bone. If calcification does not occur within the tumor it cannot be distinguished from other slowly growing soft-tissue masses such as a large fibroma or mucocele; however, calcification is

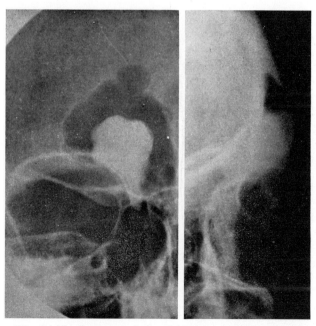

Fig. 34-10. Osteoma of the right frontal sinus. Note the ivorylike density of the mass in the floor of the right frontal sinus. *Left,* Occipitofrontal projection. *Right,* Lateral projection.

often present within it. The calcification has a mottled appearance similar to calcification occurring in osteochrondroma elsewhere. If this is visible, the diagnosis can be made with a reasonable degree of certainty. Occasionally a hemangioma occurs in the wall of a sinus and the appearance resembles the striated appearance of hemangiomata occurring in the bones of the cranial vault. Paget's disease of the skull may extend to involve sinus walls, and fibrous dysplasia may also involve sinus walls as well as other facial bones. These lesions are discussed more fully in Chapters 2 and 8.

MALIGNANT TUMORS

SARCOMA

Fibrosarcoma occasionally occurs in the sinuses, usually in the maxillary antrum, and causes destruction of the walls of the sinus in addition to the production of a soft-tissue mass. From the radiographic standpoint it cannot be distinguished from carcinoma.

CARCINOMA

Carcinoma may arise in any of the paranasal sinuses but is much more common in the maxillary antrum than elsewhere. Occasionally the ethmoids are the site of origin while the frontal and sphenoid sinuses are rarely involved. The roentgen findings are caused by the dense appearance of the mass of the tumor plus irregular destruction of bone. The tumor may be very large, obliterating the airspace and causing soft-tissue density beyond the sinus. The destruction of bone is irregular with no evidence of sclerosis (Fig. 34-11). It is entirely different from the smooth, pressure atrophy type of defect that results when large benign soft-tissue tumors involve the sinuses. Tomography is of value in outlining the extent of destruction. We

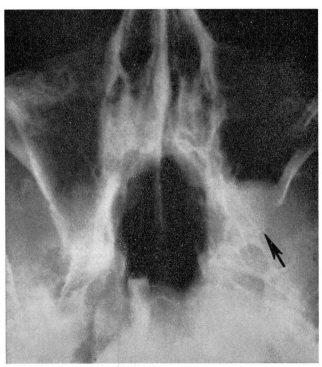

Fig. 34-11. Carcinoma of the left maxillary antrum. Note the soft-tissue mass in the floor of the left maxillary antrum with destruction of the bony wall of the floor (**arrow**).

use tomography in addition to the standard projections in virtually every patient with clinical findings suggesting sinus carcinoma (Fig. 34-12).

When a carcinoma arising in a sinus extends into the nasal cavity it may occlude the ostia of the other sinuses and lead to infection involving them. A malignant tumor primary in the nasal cavity is prone to obstruct the ostia of the sinuses on that side. In either event, the roentgen signs of uniformly clouded sinuses on one side (unilateral pansinusitis) with normal sinuses on the other may be encountered. This observation always raises the question of a tumor as the causative agent and necessitates careful clinical and additional roentgen investigation for such a lesion.

MISCELLANEOUS TUMORS

Plasmocytoma or plasma cell myeloma may arise in the sinuses producing bone destruction and soft-tissue mass similar to that caused by carcinoma. Metastatic tumors may involve the bones of the sinuses and produce destruction and soft-tissue mass that is visible radiographically. Tumors of the pituitary, as well as chordoma that may arise in the region of the clivus, may project into the sphenoid sinus and produce soft-tissue density there. The appearance of the sella and of the clivus usually indicates the site of primary disease. Cysts and tumors of dental origin involve the lower jaw as well as the floor of the maxillary sinuses and are discussed in Chapter 35.

MISCELLANEOUS CONDITIONS

SYNDROMES WITH SINUS ABNORMALITY

Gorlin and Sedano[8] have tabulated a number of syndromes involving the paranasal sinuses which are listed briefly below, since the roentgen examination of the sinuses may suggest the diagnosis:

GARDNER'S SYNDROME. This syndrome includes (1) multiple polyposis of the colon; (2) multiple osteomas in sphenoid and ethmoid sinuses, frontal bone, maxilla, and mandible as well as the cal-

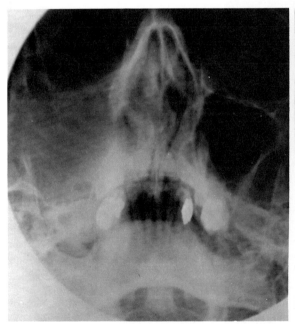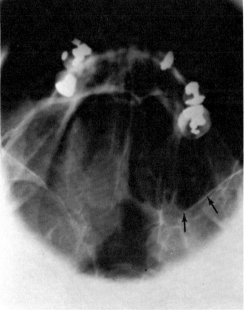

Fig. 34-12. Carcinoma of the right maxillary antrum. *Left,* Waters' view shows a soft-tissue mass filling the antrum and destroying its walls. *Right,* Submentovertical view shows the mass on the right. **Arrows** indicate normal lucency of the left maxillary antrum in contrast to the right antrum, which contains a dense mass.

varium; and (3) epidermoid inclusion cysts of the skin and fibromas, lipomas, and desmoid tumors of the skin.

CLEIDOCRANIAL DYSOSTOSIS. The following are present: Aplasia or hypoplasia of clavicles; the paranasal sinuses are often absent or underdeveloped; anomalies of teeth and calvarium occur.

MAXILLONASAL DYSPLASIA. Aplasia or hypoplasia of anterior nasal spine of maxilla occurs, and uni- or bilateral hypoplasia of frontal sinuses is found.

PYCNODYSOSTOSIS. Sinus films may show frontal sinuses absent, other sinuses are hypoplastic or absent, and increased radiopacity is evident at the base of the skull. Dwarfism, osteopetrosis, partial agenesis of terminal phalanges, cranial anomalies such as persistence of fontanelles and open cranial sutures, frontal and occipital bossing, and hypoplasia of the angle of the mandible are also found.

PROGERIA. Sinus examination shows hypoplasia of maxilla and mandible with crowded teeth, the frontal sinuses often are absent, and the other sinuses are hypoplastic.

CRANIOMETAPHYSEAL DYSOSTOSIS AND CRANIODIAPHYSEAL DYSOSTOSIS. In both of these conditions there is severe overgrowth of bone in the frontal bone, maxillae, and basal skull resulting in encroachment upon, or obliteration of paranasal sinuses. There are differences in the long bone involvement in the two conditions, but both show considerable sclerosis of long bones.

MIDLINE LETHAL GRANULOMA

This disease is often associated with generalized periarteritis. The etiology is not definite but it is most likely a hyperimmune reaction involving the nose and paranasal sinuses. Visceral changes may or may not be present. There are granulomatous

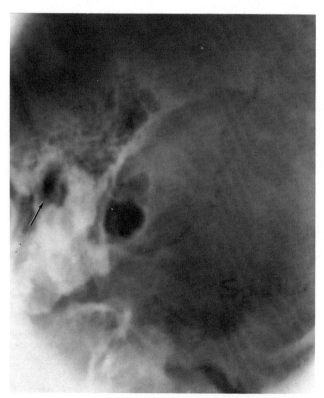

Fig. 34-13. Normal mastoid as seen in the Schüller projection. The external auditory canal (**arrow**) lies directly posterior to the mandibular condyle and fossa.

masses in the nose and sinuses that result in roentgen clouding and complete obliteration of the airspace; this is followed in time by extensive destruction of bone. The maxillary antra are most frequently involved but the remaining sinuses may also be affected. When there is associated visceral disease, the changes often progress more rapidly than when the midline facial tissues are the only site of involvement.

There is some confusion in the literature regarding the relationship of this disease to Wegener's granulomatosis. They both appear to be allergic or autoimmune in origin and are probably related. Wegener's syndrome includes pulmonary and renal lesions in addition to the involvement of the upper respiratory tract.

TRAUMA

Fractures of the bony walls of the paranasal sinuses are not uncommon and are usually associated with fractures of the other facial bones and base of the skull. The signs of fracture are irregular linear defects, often with jagged overriding edges and depression or displacement of bony walls. The involved sinus is usually clouded, with loss of aeration secondary to edema and hemorrhage into the lining membrane or into the sinus itself. Facial bone fractures are discussed at greater length in Chapter 35.

FOREIGN BODIES

Foreign bodies may gain access to the sinuses by direct trauma such as gunshot wounds. Dental roots may be displaced into the antrum during extraction. Roentgenograms taken in various projections or tomograms will outline the foreign body and ascertain its relationship to the sinus. Foreign bodies within the nasal cavities can also be localized provided they are dense enough to be visible on the roentgenogram.

THE MASTOIDS

The roentgen examination of the temporal bone in which the mastoid cells are located is

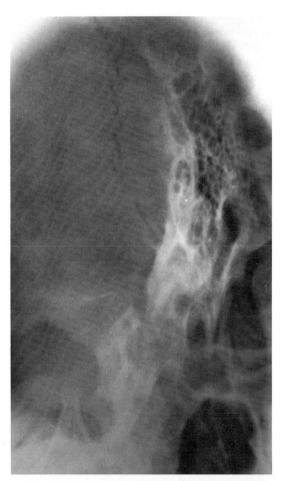

Fig. 34-14. Normal mastoid as seen with patient in the Mayer position. In this projection the bony bridge adjacent to the mastoid aditus is clearly defined.

important in the diagnosis of inflammatory diseases. Prime prerequisites for roentgen interpretation of mastoid disease are films of good technical quality in proper projections.

METHODS OF EXAMINATION

There are several projections used in the examination of the mastoids. They should be standardized technically so that films of good quality are available on each patient. There have been numerous projections described; most are useful if properly taken. We use the following in our routine examination of the mastoids:

1. Schüller (or Runstrom), a lateral taken with the tube angled 30° caudad.

2. Mayer, an axial projection in which the head is angled 45° toward the side to be examined and the tube is angled 45° caudad.

3. Chamberlain-Towne, an anteroposterior projection in which the tube is angled caudad (we use a 30° angle).

4. Chausse III, an anteroposterior projection with the head rotated 15° away from the side to be examined and the tube rotated 30° caudad.

On all of the anteroposterior projections the caudad angles are in relation to the canthomeatal line. Good coning is essential to quality examinations. Both mastoids are always included on the examination so the two sides can be compared. Tomography is of considerable value in examining the mastoid. The ossicles of the middle ear can also be studied by means of tomography.

When we refer to tomography of the mastoid and petrous pyramid, we mean that multidirectional equipment is essential. We use equipment capable of circular and elliptical motion in addition to linear and zonographic technics. Hypocycloidal motion perhaps is a bit superior, but depends on an excellent technologist. As a rule we begin with sections taken at 2-mm intervals, and after the radiologist has checked these, we take as many intermediate 0.5- or 1.0-mm films as needed. These methods are used in trauma as well as in disease of the middle ear. McGann[10] has developed a multiscreen cassette which is capable of holding four films at approximately 1-mm intervals. This saves time and radiation exposure. The published tomograms are of good quality, however we have had no experience with this cassette.

THE NORMAL MASTOIDS

The temporal bone is an extremely complex structure that contains the external auditory canal, the middle and internal ear as well as the vestibular apparatus. The bone consists of three parts: (1) The squamous or squamozygomatic, (2) the tympanic, and (3) the petrous or petromastoid. Mastoid cells are found in the squamous as well as in the petrous portion of the temporal bone. The relationship of the mastoid cells to the adjacent structures is illustrated in Figures 34-13 through 34-16.

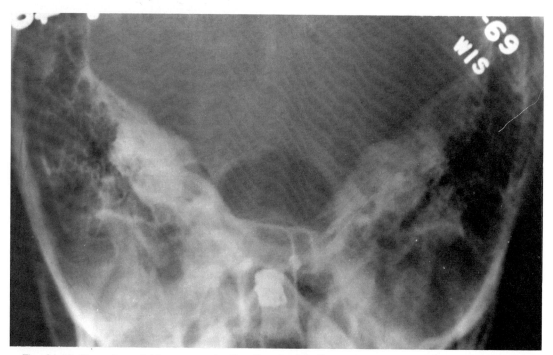

Fig. 34-15. Normal mastoids as seen in the Chamberlain-Towne projection. In this projection the internal auditory canals and petrous pyramids are well visualized.

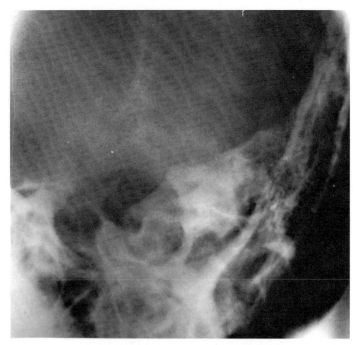

Fig. 34-16. Normal mastoid as seen with patient in the Chausse III position. The petrous pyramid and tip are well outlined in this projection.

DEVELOPMENT OF THE MASTOIDS

The mastoid cells develop as saclike extensions from the mastoid antrum. The process begins in the first year of life and is usually complete by the end of the fourth to sixth year. There is considerable variation in the amount of pneumatization in the normal. When pneumatization is complete and involves the mastoid process, the lateral aspect of the petrous, and the squamous portion of the temporal bone, the mastoid is called pneumatic in type. When pneumatization is incomplete with only small, thick-walled cells formed immediately above and posterior to the tympanic cavity the mastoid is diploic in type (Fig. 34-17). The mastoid is sclerotic in type when there is no pneumatization and the bone is dense and eburnated. Intermediate degrees of pneumatization are frequent.

In addition to the parts of the ear, there are vascular and nerve structures that can be visualized. Their location is of considerable importance if surgery is necessary. The lateral venous sinus forms a groove that curves downward posterior to the mastoid. When the mastoid is diploic or sclerotic in type, this groove is well outlined; but when it is pneumatic in type the sinus groove is some-

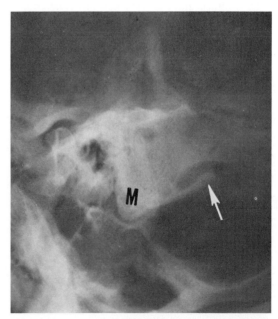

Fig. 34-17. Diploic mastoid. Very few cells are visible adjacent to the mastoid antrum. Elsewhere the mastoid is diploic. **Arrow** indicates emissary vein. **M,** Mastoid process is dense because of lack of pneumatization but there is no sclerosis. This type should not be mistaken for a diseased mastoid.

times difficult to define. The location of emissary vessels if present is also important. The mastoid emissary vein is commonly seen and is usually found midway between the mastoid tip and the genu, or curve, of the lateral sinus (see Fig. 34-17). Using tomography in both sagittal and frontal planes, the facial canal through which the seventh nerve courses, can be seen. This is important in trauma, tumors, and infection in the region of the middle ear.

INFLAMMATORY DISEASES

ACUTE MASTOIDITIS

Mastoid infection usually follows otitis media and is secondary to the middle ear infection. In early otitis media it may be possible to observe a slight increase in haziness or density in the middle ear cavity. When the infection extends to the mastoid the normal translucency of the mastoid air cells is slightly decreased, resulting in slight cloudiness unless the infection is minor and recovery is rapid. The change is minor and this diagnosis should be made with great caution. When the infection in the mastoid continues for a time edema and hyperemia result in thickening of the lining of the

cells in the region of the mastoid antrum. This is noted radiographically as a loss of the normal clear outline of the cells plus a slight increase in density. The change at this stage is minor, and comparison with the normal side is the basis of the diagnosis. The disease may spread to the remaining cells so that the process becomes more generalized. The roentgen findings are then more generalized, with poor definition of all the mastoid cells. The next change is absorption of bone that is manifested radiographically by loss of some of the cell walls with thinning and poor definition of others. The earliest signs of bone destruction are usually observed in the cells surrounding the attic. If the process continues further with suppuration and complete breakdown of cell walls, a mastoid abscess is formed. This is manifested by an area of radiolucency which begins in the epitympanic recess (attic) above and posterior to the tympanic cavity. The abscess may also extend to the tip of the mastoid process and from there into the soft tissues in the posterior aspect of the neck (Bezold's abscess). The infection may spread upward and medially into the petrous portion of the temporal bone or to the tegmen tympani and occasionally may destroy the tegmen to form an

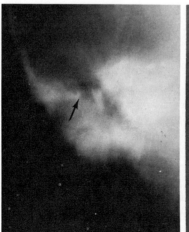 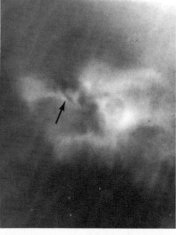

Fig. 34-18. Early osteitis and cholesteatoma. *Left,* Tomogram shows destruction of the spur (**arrow**). Note the wide separation between the ossicles and the base of the spur which remains. *Right,* Tomogram of the opposite ear (reversed for easy comparison) showing normal spur (**arrow**) and the relationship of this structure to the ossicles.

epidural abscess. Acute mastoid abscess is an uncommon finding now that a number of antibiotics are available for treatment of acute otitis media. These antibiotics may mask symptoms in some patients in whom roentgen examination shows that the destructive inflammatory process is advancing. It is, therefore, important to correlate the clinical and roentgen findings.

CHRONIC MASTOIDITIS

The changes in the mastoid are similar to those in other bony structures involved by infection. When the disease is low-grade and of long duration, bone production causes thickening and sclerosis of mastoid cell walls. When the infection is of suppurative type the cell walls are destroyed and an abscess is formed.

Roentgen Findings

The affected mastoid is dense and the few cells that may be visible in the region of the antrum often have thickened bony walls. The marked density in chronic low-grade infections may obscure the radiolucency caused by an abscess; tomograms are indispensable in the examination of densely sclerotic mastoids in which abscess is suspected. When abscess is present, it produces an area of poorly defined radiolucency in a mastoid in which there is evidence of sclerotic change elsewhere. The defect caused by cholesteatoma is similar and at times cannot be differentiated from that of an abscess. The clinical history and examination must be correlated with roentgen findings in these situations.

CHOLESTEATOMA

Cholesteatoma is an accumulation of cellular debris in the mastoid that develops when the tympanic membrane is perforated and the epithelium of the external auditory canal extends into the middle ear. It is the result of chronic mastoid disease. The accumulated material tends to destroy cell walls and create an irregularly rounded or oval cavity within the sclerotic infected mastoid. The patients usually give a history of long-continued discharge of pus from the ear.

Roentgen Findings

The cholesteatoma is noted radiographically as an area of radiolucency that may be very

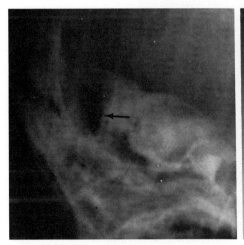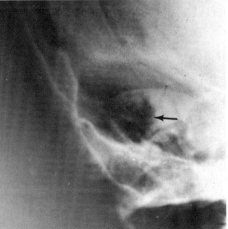

Fig. 34-19. Cholesteatoma. *Left,* Chamberlain-Towne view showing defect in the mastoid antrum caused by a large cholesteatoma (**arrow**). *Right,* Coned Stenvers projection of the same patient; the defect is more clearly defined (**arrow**).

large. There is evidence of chronic mastoid infection with sclerosis and thickening of any cell walls that may be visible. Tomography is essential in the examination of the middle ear when cholesteatoma is suspected. The early lesion begins in the region of the attic. Its inferolateral wall, the "spur" is usually the site of the earliest evidence of bone destruction in osteitis and cholesteatoma (Fig. 34-18). As the cholesteatoma enlarges, it causes an enlarging cavity in the mastoid antrum (Fig. 34-19). Occasionally there is an unusually large mastoid antrum in the normal which may be unilateral. On standard projections differentiation from cholesteatoma may be very difficult, but on tomography, destruction of ossicles, and the inferolateral wall of the attic will not be present in the normal. The cholesteatoma usually has a smooth wall which may be very clearly defined, however (Fig. 34-20).

PETROSITIS

The pneumatization of the mastoid often extends well into the petrous portion of the temporal bone. Therefore, the cells in the petrous apex may be infected along with cells in the mastoid process and those adjacent to the tympanic cavity. The roentgen findings in the early stages of petrositis are similar to that of acute mastoiditis. This consists of loss of clear bony detail. Positive diagnosis cannot be made at this stage and must await evidence of decalcification and destruction of bone in the petrous tip. At times, the petrous tip may be completely destroyed. Petrositis may follow mastoidectomy and should be kept in mind in a postmastoidectomy patient in whom symptoms recur. Occasionally the infection is chronic and low-grade; then the roentgen findings simulate those of chronic sclerotic type of mastoiditis with increase in density of the tip of the petrous bone. The basal and Stenvers' views are of particular value in addition to tomography in this condition and the abnormal side can then be compared with the normal. The disease is uncommon (Fig. 32-21).

THE POSTOPERATIVE MASTOID

The interpretation of disease in the mastoid following mastoidectomy is difficult. Cell walls

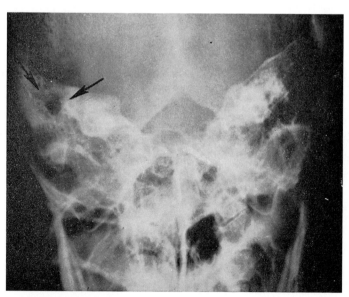

Fig. 34-20. Cholesteatoma. **Arrows** indicate area of destruction of cell walls at the site of the cholesteatoma. Elsewhere there is a moderate amount of sclerosis.

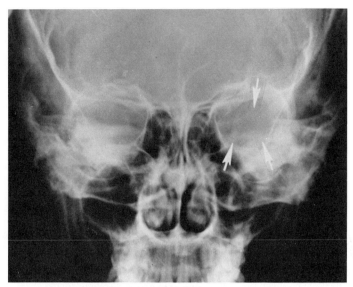

Fig. 34-21. Petrositis. The right side is normal. On the left side there is extensive destruction of the petrous tip as the result of infection involving it (**arrows**).

may be partially removed and still be visible so that residual disease in intact cells is simulated. The postoperative absence of cells may also closely resemble cholesteatoma. It is essential, therefore, that the radiologist be advised of previous surgical procedures on the mastoid in order to avoid unnecessary error in interpretation of findings.

FRACTURES OF THE TEMPORAL BONE

Fractures of the temporal bone can be classified into longitudinal (parallel to the long axis of the pyramid) and transverse (perpendicular to the long axis of the pyramid). Occasionally there are combined fractures. The longitudinal fracture is about four times more frequent; it results when force is applied to the mandibular condyle or to the temporoparietal portion of the skull. It originates in temporal squamosa, extends medially along the external auditory canal into the tegmen tympani, then anteriorly along the carotid canal to the foramen lacerum. This is usually associated with bleeding from the ear, otorrhea, and conductive hearing loss. It may originate posteriorly in the occipital bone, cross the petrous pyramid through the jugular fossa, the labyrinthine capsule, and the carotid canal. In this type, there is neurosensory hearing loss and facial paralysis caused by eighth nerve or labyrinthine trauma. Although standard views of the mastoid should be made, it is always advisable to take tomograms in the patient with suspected fracture of the petrous pyramid. As a rule, lateral tomograms are of more value than frontal views in longitudinal fracture, so they should be obtained first (Fig. 34-22 *A* and *B*). We usually get frontal tomograms as well, particularly if no fracture can be seen on the lateral tomograms or on the standard films. The transverse fractures which are much less common are usually visualized best on anteroposterior tomograms (Fig. 34-22*B*).

Ossicle dislocations, which are often associated with longitudinal temporal bone fracture, are best seen on the lateral projection. Lateral tomography is necessary in order to confirm an abnormality suspected on the standard projections, or to detect dislocations not visible on other films. Rarely we use submentovertex tomograms in suspected fracture.

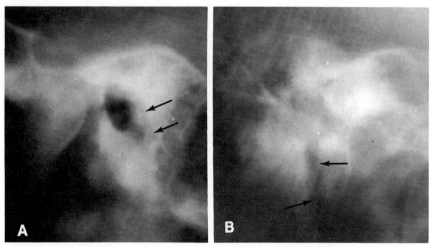

Fig. 34-22. *A*, Longitudinal fracture of the temporal bone. Lateral tomogram shows the fracture line in the anterior wall of the external auditory canal; posterior continuation courses downward and slightly posteriorly (**arrows**). *B*, Transverse temporal bone fracture. Frontal tomogram shows the wide fracture line (**arrows**). Both of these patients had seventh nerve involvement with recovery after surgery.

TUMORS

BENIGN TUMORS

Benign tumors of the middle ear and mastoid are rare. Occasionally osteoma arises in the mastoid process and results in radiographic findings of a dense mass of solid cortical bone in or attached to the mastoid process. Hemangiomas rarely arise in the middle ear and result in destruction of mastoid cells because of pressure erosion. This results in radiolucency in the region of the tumor. Evidence of hypervascularity in the area, consisting of prominent vascular channels in the bone adjacent to the mastoid process and enlargement of the emissary vein, may suggest the diagnosis. The glomus jugulare tumor (chemodectoma) is the most common benign soft-tissue tumor arising in the temporal bone. It arises in the vicinity of the tympanic branch of the ninth cranial nerve in the adventitia of the jugular bulb. Its counterpart, the chemodectoma of the middle ear, is called glomus tympanicum. The radiographic findings are not typical. The tumor grows slowly and destroys the cell walls by pressure erosion. When this occurs, radiolucency can be outlined at the site of involvement. Angiography may be helpful in localization and retrograde injection of the jugular vein may help to determine jugular bulb involvement

MALIGNANT TUMORS

Carcinoma occasionally arises in the middle ear or in the external auditory canal and extends into the antrum and mastoid process. The roentgen findings are those of destruction of bone, which is similar to bone destruction by malignant invasion elsewhere (Fig. 34-23). The process is one of osteolysis without reactive sclerosis; the soft-tissue mass associated with it can also be demonstrated on the roentgenogram.

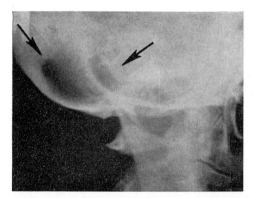

Fig. 34-23. Carcinoma that arose in the middle ear on the right and has destroyed much of the bone in the mastoid process as well as in the petrous pyramid (**arrows**).

Metastases may occasionally involve the temporal bone in the region of the middle ear and mastoid. Tumors are usually those which ordinarily metastasize to bone such as kidney, lung, breast, and prostate carcinomas. Roentgen signs are similar to those of osseous metastases elsewhere.

REFERENCES AND SELECTED READINGS

1. BECKER, J. A., and WOLOSHIN, H. J.: Mastoiditis and cholesteatoma: A roentgen approach. *Am. J. Roentgenol. Radium Ther. Nucl. Med. 87:* 1019, 1962.

2. BRÜNNER, S.: Infection of the temporal bone and its complications, including cholesteatoma. *Semin. Roentgenol. IV:* 129, 1969.

3. COMPERE, W. E., and VALVASSORI, G.: *Radiographic Atlas of the Temporal Bone.* St. Paul, Minn., American Academy of Ophthalmology and Otolaryngology, 1964.

4. ETTER, L. E.: Opacification studies of normal and abnormal paranasal sinuses. *Am. J. Roentgenol. Radium Ther. Nucl. Med. 89:* 1137, 1963.

5. ETTER, L. E.: *Roentgenography and Roentgenology of the Middle Ear and Mastoid Process.* Springfield, Ill., Thomas, 1965.

6. FELDMAN, F., SEAMAN, W. B., and BAKER, D. C., JR.: The roentgen manifestations of scleroma. *Am. J. Roentgenol. Radium Ther. Nucl. Med. 101:* 807, 1967.

7. GEIST, R. M., and MULLEN, W. H.: Roentgenologic aspects of lethal granulomatous ulceration of midline facial tissues. *Am. J. Roentgenol. Radium Ther. Nucl. Med. 70:* 566, 1953.

8. GORLIN, R. J., and SEDANO, H. O.: Syndromes involving the sinuses—congenital and acquired. *Semin. Roentgenol. III:* 133, 1968.

9. KASEFF, L. G.: Tomographic evaluation of trauma to the temporal bone. *Radiology 93:* 321, 1969.

10. McGANN, M. J.: Plesiosectional tomography of the temporal bone: A new multi-screen cassette. *Am. J. Roentgenol. Radium Ther. Nucl. Med. 88:* 1183, 1962.

11. MERRILL, V.: *Atlas of Roentgenographic Positions.* St. Louis, Mosby, 1967, vol. III.

12. POTTER, G. D.: Chausse III position. *Semin. Roentgenol. IV:* 116, 1969.

13. POTTER, G. D.: Trauma to the temporal bone. *Semin. Roentgenol. IV:* 143, 1969.

14. ROBINSON, A. E., MEARES, B. M., and GOREE, J. A.: Traumatic sphenoid sinus effusion. An analysis of 50 cases. *Am. J. Roentgenol. Radium Ther. Nucl. Med. 101:* 795, 1967.

15. ROSENDAL, T., and EWERTSEN, H.: Roentgen examination of the temporal bone for cholesteatoma. *Acta Radiol. 37:* 431, 1952.

16. RUNSTROM, G.: Roentgenological study of acute and chronic otitis media. *Acta Radiol. Suppl. 17,* 1933.

17. SAMUEL, E.: Inflammatory diseases of the nose and paranasal sinuses. *Semin. Roentgenol. III:* 148, 1968.

18. SHARP, G. S., BULLOCK, W. K., and HAZLET, J. W.: *Oral Cancer and Tumors of the Jaws.* New York, McGraw-Hill, 1956.

19. TARP, O.: Tomography of the temporal bone with the polytome. *Acta Radiol. 51:* 105, 1959.

20. WIGH, R.: Mucoceles of frontoethmoidal sinuses; analysis of roentgen criteria. *Radiology 54:* 579, 1950.

21. ZIMMER, J.: Planigraphy of the temporal bone. *Acta Radiol. 37:* 419, 1952.

22. ZIZMOR, J., and NOYEK, A. M.: Cysts and benign tumors of the paranasal sinuses. *Semin. Roentgenol. III:* 172, 1968.

23. ZIZMOR, J., and NOYEK, A. M.: Tumors and other osseous disorders of the temporal bone. *Semin. Roentgenol. IV:* 151, 1969.

35

THE TEETH, JAWS, AND FACIAL BONES

The roentgen examination of the teeth is used by the medical profession largely to determine the presence or absence of infection involving the teeth and jaws. There are certain changes in the alveolus that result from generalized disease, and examination of the teeth is helpful in these conditions as well. Tumors arising on the alveolar ridge, tongue, or other intraoral sites may involve the bony alveolus. Roentgen examination is used to look for and follow the progress of such tumors.

Specific techniques for dental radiography cannot be discussed here but are described in the texts listed in the References. Two general intraoral methods of examination are used, the intraoral dental and occlusal. The standard intraoral films are placed in position and held there by the patient while the exposure is being made. A total of 14 of these small films are taken as a complete dental survey. These films should include the crowns and roots of all the teeth. The occlusal film is larger and is also employed as an intraoral film. It is used most widely in patients who are edentulous in a search for retained root fragments or local infection of the alveolus. It is also useful in the examination of small cysts or tumors of the alveolar ridge and jaw. There are two special devices which are now used for examination of the teeth and jaws. The Panoramix machine or device has a small tube, the target end of which can be placed in the mouth. The film is held

against the part to be examined, such as the mandible or maxilla, a single exposure is made to include the teeth, most of the mandible, and the alveolus of the maxilla. This device can also be used for special views of the mandibular condyles in trauma and for a number of problems in roentgenography of extremities. The second device is the Panorex (*see* Fig. 35-11) or a more sophisticated unit, the Orthopantomograph. These devices rotate during filming around a fixed head position. A single exposure may be used to survey all of the teeth as well as the jaws. In our experience, dental detail is not as good as in dental films, so we use the two types of devices more often for the examination of the mandible and maxilla than for the teeth. The mandible is examined by means of special views in frontal and lateral oblique projection. The temporomandibular joints also require special techniques and are examined with the mouth opened and closed. Films of the normal as well as the abnormal joint are usually made for comparison purposes. Tomography is of considerable value in the examination of the temporomandibular joints.

THE NORMAL TEETH

The teeth appear in two sets. The first are termed deciduous or temporary teeth. There are 20 deciduous teeth, 10 in each jaw and five in each quadrant. They are named from the midline as follows: central incisor, lateral incisor, cuspid, first molar (premolar) and second molar (premolar). In the adult jaw there are normally 32 teeth; eight in each quadrant named as follows from the midline: central incisor, lateral incisor, cuspid, first bicuspid, second bicuspid and first, second, and third molar. Examples of these teeth are shown in Figures 35-1 through 35-3.

Each tooth consists of a crown and a root. The junction between them is called the neck or cervix. The roots lie in sockets in the alveolar process of the jaw and are attached by alveolar periosteum. There are a number of variations in density noted on dental radiographs. Listed in decreasing order of density they are as follows: (*1*) metal crowns and fillings, (*2*) enamel of the teeth, (*3*) dentine, (*4*) cementum, (*5*) cortical bone, (*6*) cancellous bone; and (*7*) medullary spaces, canals, foramina, and soft tissues. The crown of the tooth is therefore slightly more dense than the root and within each tooth is a narrow radiolucency termed the root canal. Immediately surrounding each tooth is a radiolucent space representing the alveolar periosteum (periodontal membrane). Adjacent to this is a thin, dense structure composed of compact bone called the lamina dura (Fig. 35-4).

The mandible or lower jaw is composed of two equal halves united at the symphysis anteriorly. Each half consists of a body extending from the midline backward in a roughly horizontal direction and a ramus at somewhat less than a right angle so that the ramus is nearly vertical. It articulates with the base of the skull by means of a condylar process that projects upward from the posterior aspect of the ramus. The other upward projection anteriorly is termed the coronoid process. The lower teeth are set in the alveolar process. The upper teeth are set in the alveolar process of the maxilla. The lower aspect of the maxillary antrum is visible on dental films of the upper teeth. The mental foramen appears as a radiolucency be-

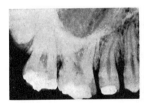 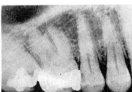 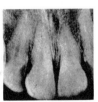

Fig. 35-1. Examples of normal teeth. Upper jaw. From *left* to *right:* partially visualized unerupted third molar tooth, second molar, first molar, second bicuspid, first bicuspid. Partially visualized second molar, first molar, second bicuspid, first bicuspid, lateral incisor, and central incisor. Note radiolucency above the molars that represents the maxillary antrum.

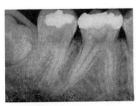 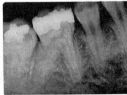 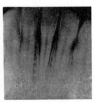

Fig. 35-2. Examples of lower teeth. From *left* to *right:* Partially visualized and unerupted third molar, second molar, first molar, partially visualized second bicuspid, partially visualized second molar, first molar, second bicuspid, partially visualized first bicuspid, lateral incisor, central incisor, central incisor, lateral incisor, cuspid.

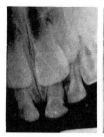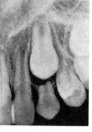

Fig. 35-3. Examples of developing teeth. Unerupted permanent teeth are noted above the deciduous teeth. Note the resorption of the root of the deciduous cuspid on the right.

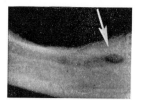

Fig. 35-5. Mental foramen. Roentgenogram of the left lower jaw, which is edentulous. **Arrow** indicates the mental foramen; the mandibular canal is the radioluency extending posteriorly from the foramen.

marginated and occasionally appearing somewhat bilobed. The radicular cyst, from which it must be differentiated, maintains its relation to the dental root in contrast to the foramen (see page 1081).

DENTAL INFECTIONS

DENTAL CARIES

The presence of a cavity may escape detection by clinical methods of examination and yet be readily visible on a roentgenogram. Regardless of etiology, dental caries may lead to foci of infection involving the periapical tissues of the jaw and are, therefore, important lesions. On the roentgenogram a carious area is radiolucent and appears as an area of decreased density that is usually slightly irregular and may occur anywhere on the crown of a tooth or in its neck (Fig. 35-6).

PERIAPICAL INFECTIONS

All the periapical inflammatory lesions represent chronic disease when they are ad-

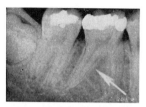

Fig. 35-4. Lower molar teeth. **Arrow** indicates the lamina dura surrounding the dental root. The bony alveolus extends to the neck of the tooth. The crown is above it and the roots are in the bony alveolus. The dental root canal is represented by the thin radiolucent line extending into the roots of the teeth. The alveolodental periosteum (periodontal membrane) forms the radiolucent zone between the lamina dura and the dental root.

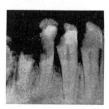

Fig. 35-6. Dental caries. Note multiple radiolucent defects in all the teeth. The distal half of the crown of the molar tooth has been destroyed, leaving root snags without a crown.

low and between the lower bicuspids. The mandibular canal extends forward, parallel to the alveolar ridge, and is a radiolucency that should not be mistaken for disease (Fig. 35-5). There are a few structures in the maxilla that should also be mentioned. The intermaxillary suture is observed in children and often in young adults. It appears as a midline radiolucent suture extending from the alveolar crest between the upper central incisors back to the posterior aspect of the palate. It may be interrupted in some areas. It has cortical margins which are smooth or slightly irregular. Usually there is no difficulty differentiating it from a fracture. The incisive foramen (anterior palatine foramen) varies in size from a slit near the sagittal plane of the maxilla near the level of the apices of the central incisors to a rather large round or oval foramen, usually clearly vanced enough to produce roentgen changes. Chronic infection around the apex of a dental root is manifested by several changes that can be recognized and classified. At times the division into the various types of roentgen pattern is difficult. The lesions may occur in the absence of clinical signs, which makes radiographic examination doubly important. Usually the infection follows the death of the pulp; bacteria pass through the root canal into the periapical tissues.

CHRONIC ALVEOLODENTAL PERIOSTITIS. This condition may be caused by occlusal trauma as well as by infection. It results in some thickening of the periosteum at the apex of the root and is manifested on the roentgenogram by increased width of the radiolucent space between the lamina dura and the dental apex. The lamina dura is usually intact but may be thinned (Fig. 35-7A).

CHRONIC RAREFYING OSTEITIS AND GRANULATION TISSUE (PERIAPICAL "GRANULOMA"). This represents the second stage of periapical infection in which there is destruction of bone adjacent to the apex of the tooth. The resultant space is filled with granulation tissue. Roentgenographically there is a radiolucent zone, usually with clearly defined margins, which is located at the dental root apex. The lamina dura is usually destroyed but the bony margin of the radiolucent zone is clearly outlined (Fig. 35-7B).

CHRONIC RAREFYING OSTEITIS WITH ABSCESS (PERIAPICAL ABSCESS). This is the stage of the disease in which there is actual suppuration. A radiolucent zone is noted around the apex of the tooth in this condition and the margin is somewhat irregular and poorly defined but may be sclerotic in disease of long duration. The lamina dura is destroyed in the area of the disease (Fig. 35-7C).

CHRONIC RAREFYING OSTEITIS WITH CYST FORMATION (RADICULAR OR ROOT CYST). Proliferation of squamous cells frequently found in granulation tissue about a dental root apex is stimulated by chronic inflammation. This mass of epithelial cells breaks down to form a cystlike cavity that gradually enlarges, owing to slow constant pressure produced by the cellular proliferation. Eventually a cyst wall is formed by dense fibrous tissue. Roentgen findings are those of a radiolucent area around the apex of one or more teeth, which may be rather large. The margins are clearly defined, often with a thin layer of compact bone clearly outlining the cyst. A large cyst may expand the bone and displace contiguous teeth (Fig. 35-8).

At times the various manifestations of periapical infection are difficult to classify into one of the groups named above, but should be recognized as lesions caused by infection. That is, they represent a focus of infection that must be managed by dental surgery.

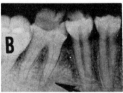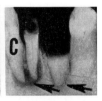

Fig. 35-7. Periapical infections. *A,* Alveolodental periostitis. **Arrow** indicates the increase in radiolucency between the dental apex and lamina dura. The tooth is also carious. *B,* Chronic osteitis with granulation tissue. **Arrow** indicates destruction of bone adjacent to the apex of the root of the first molar. Note that its crown is carious. *C,* Periapical abscess. **Arrows** indicate abscess resulting in considerable destruction of bone around the apices of the involved teeth.

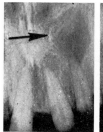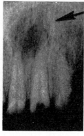

Fig. 35-8. Radicular (root) cyst. Note the large rarefied area extending into the alveolus from the root of the right lateral incisor. The cyst is moderately well circumscribed with a clearly defined margin. In the view on the right the cyst overlaps the apex of the adjacent cuspid.

ALVEOLAR (PERIODONTAL) INFECTIONS

The earliest clinical manifestation of infection involving the alveolar tissues surrounding the teeth is that of gingivitis. The infection progresses to the alveolodental periosteum, where chronic periostitis is produced. This results in absorption and destruction of bone surrounding the teeth (alveolar recession) (periodontitis). When the process involves a single tooth and extends downward toward or to the apex it is called the vertical type of alveolar periostitis. If it is more generalized and results in destruction of the alveolar septum between several teeth, it is termed the horizontal type of periostitis (alveolar recession) (periodontitis).

Roentgen Findings

The roentgen changes parallel the destructive process. At first there is some widening of the radiolucency between the root and the lamina dura at the neck associated with some loss of the alveolar process. In the vertical type, the radiolucency around a single tooth increases, leading to loss of bony support and loss of the lamina dura. In the horizontal type, the alveolar ridge gradually disappears between the teeth until there is loss of bony support for several teeth. From the roentgen standpoint, the presence of pus in these pockets of infection cannot be ascertained but when the alveolar destruction is marked there usually is a

considerable amount of local sepsis. Dense projections often appear at the neck of the affected teeth which represent calculus. Occasionally root resorption occurs, resulting in loss of the root in one or more areas. This is manifested on the roentgenogram by an area of irregular radiolucency indenting the normally smooth surface of the involved root (Fig. 35-9*A*, *B*, and *C*).

HYPERCEMENTOSIS (EXOSTOSIS OF THE DENTAL ROOT). Cementum which is somewhat more dense than cortical bone is produced and accumulates around the root of an affected tooth, usually a permanent one, to cause this abnormality. The upper bicuspids and lower first molar are the most commonly affected. Roentgen findings are those of an enlarged, bulbous, dense root which may be rather bizarre in shape. The relationship of the lamina dura to the root does not change; it covers the abnormal root as in the normal.

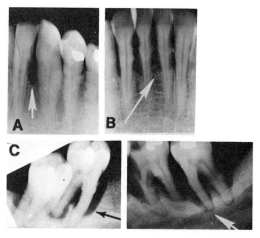

Fig. 35-9. *A*, Vertical alveolar periostitis (periodontitis). Note loss of bone of the alveolar process extending downward between the roots of the lateral incisor and cuspid of the right lower jaw. The process is localized in this patient. *B*, Horizontal alveolar periostitis (periodontitis). The alveolus has been destroyed to a comparable extent throughout the incisor area. The density surrounding the necks of the teeth represents calculus. *C*, Examples of severe alveolar periostitis (periodontitis) with pockets extending nearly to the apices of the involved teeth.

DENTAL MANIFESTATIONS OF GENERALIZED DISORDERS

Intraoral dental films in addition to outlining the teeth also include the alveolar process of the mandible, which may reflect changes in certain systemic diseases.

ENDOCRINE AND METABOLIC DISORDERS

HYPOPITUITARISM. Delayed dentition along with delay in osseous development is characteristic of hypopituitarism and dental films will show the delay in development as well as the small underdeveloped jaw.

HYPERPITUITARISM. In acromegaly and giantism there is an overgrowth of the mandible so the teeth are more widely separated than normal. Roentgen study is helpful in differentiating this type of overgrowth from that associated with other conditions that produce abnormal enlargement of the jaw.

HYPOTHYROIDISM (CRETINISM). Delayed development of the teeth that occurs in this condition is manifested on dental roentgenograms.

HYPOPARATHYROIDISM. Hypoplasia of the enamel occurs when the onset of the disease is early in life, before the enamel is completely formed. Hypoplasia of the dentine may also occur if the hypoparathyroidism occurs before the dental roots are developed. This is manifested by short underdeveloped roots.

HYPERPARATHYROIDISM. There is loss of the lamina dura noted on dental roentgenograms along with marked decalcification of the alveolus. Dental films of the upper jaw also demonstrate a loss of the clearly defined outline of the bony floor of the maxillary antrum that is also a result of decalcification (Fig. 35-10). In severe disease, cystlike rarefactions may appear in the mandible. Following successful removal of the tumor causing the parathyroid hyperfunction, the alveolus tends to return to normal and the lamina dura reappears.

CUSHING'S SYNDROME. Moderate decalcification of the alveolus is noted on the dental roentgenogram in this condition along with partial loss of the

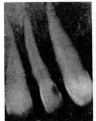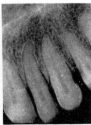

Fig. 35-10. Hyperparathyroidism. Note absence of the lamina dura of the teeth on the *left* along with decalcification of the alveolus and some alveolar periostitis. The teeth on the *right* are for comparison, showing the normal alveolar density and lamina dura.

lamina dura. As a result this structure is sometimes difficult to outline, but there are usually some areas in which it can be observed.

DIABETES MELLITUS. In severe diabetes, particularly in children, dental infection is a problem so that periapical as well as periodontal disease is commonly present and may be severe. These changes are readily outlined on dental roentgenograms.

HYPOPHOSPHATASIA. There is loss of alveolar bone, enlargement of pulp chambers of root canals, and a decrease in thickness of the enamel and dentine. As a result the roots are thin with wide, pulp cavities. Deciduous teeth are lost early because of absence of cementum without early eruption of permanent teeth (Fig. 35-11). Mild forms of the disease may have no dental findings.

DEVELOPMENTAL DISORDERS

MIDLINE FACIAL CLEFTS. In cleft lip and cleft palate, there are dental anomalies ranging from deformity and malposition of some upper central teeth, to the presence of supernumerary teeth, to absence of a number of teeth. The films outline the osseous deformity as well as the dental alterations. A number of other isolated anomalies of the jaws and teeth are clearly defined on occlusal films or on special films of mandible and maxilla. They include congenital hypoplasia and hyperplasia of the mandible, and unilateral hypoplasia of the face.

OSTEOGENESIS IMPERFECTA. The characteristic dental alteration in this condition is replacement

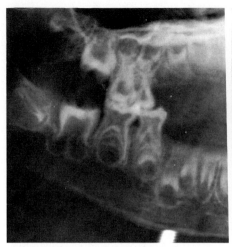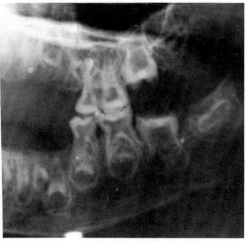

Fig. 35-11. Hypophosphatasia in a child aged 2. Panorex film of the teeth and jaws. All deciduous teeth have been lost except the premolars. The roots are small and the pulp cavities very large.

of the pulp canals by dentine, resulting in teeth that are uniformly dense. The finding of absent root canals is first observed in the incisor and the first molar teeth, which are the earliest to develop completely.

OSTEOPETROSIS. The dense, ivorylike bone characteristic of this disease is noted in the alveolus; the roots of the teeth are often incompletely developed.

ACHONDROPLASIA. There is delay in dental development in this condition that is readily observed on roentgenograms of the teeth. Many of the teeth remain unerupted into adult life.

ECTODERMAL DYSPLASIA. This disease is characterized by partial or complete absence of hair, sweat glands, and teeth. The degree of dental abnormality ranges from complete dental aplasia to congenital absence of a few of the teeth.

CHONDROECTODERMAL DYSPLASIA (ELLIS-VAN CREVELD). This disorder is characterized by dysplasia of fingernails, short stature caused by shortening of the tubular bones, polydactyly, carpal fusion, and dental abnormalities. Congenital cardiac abnormality may also be present. There is usually a decreased number of teeth which are widely spaced and peg-shaped.

CLEIDOCRANIAL DYSOSTOSIS. Abnormal dentition and abnormality of the jaws is very frequent in this condition. There is often a delay in appearance of the teeth, with numerous supernumerary teeth. Permanent teeth are frequently malposed and fail to erupt. There is absence of or hypoplasia of the clavicles and anomalies of the cranial bones; numerous wormian bones are common.

UNILATERAL HYPERPLASIA OF THE FACE. The teeth develop prematurely on the hyperplastic side of the face so that films of the jaws showing the difference in development of the teeth may permit early diagnosis of this rare condition.

MANDIBULOFACIAL DYSOSTOSIS (TREACHER-COLLINS SYNDROME). The teeth may be malposed and malocclusion is common in this syndrome in which there is hypoplasia of the facial bones, particularly the zygoma and mandible. Cleft palate, absence of palatine bones, and underdevelopment of paranasal sinuses and mastoids may also be observed on roentgenograms of the facial bones.

OTHER ANOMALIES. There are a number of other developmental disorders in which abnormality occurs, but most are very rare. They include Rutherfurd's syndrome in which deciduous teeth are unerupted and absorb with permanent teeth visible below them. This is evidently caused by gingival hyperplasia to an extent that eruption of the teeth is prevented. Dentinogenesis imperfecta is a local process in which dental roots are small and conical, necks are narrow, root canals are narrow, and pulp is absent or nearly so. Teeth are short and square. Dyscephalia mandibulo-oculo-fascialis (Hallermann-Streiff syndrome) is another rare condition in which teeth are malformed, erupt early and irregularly, and may be erupted at birth.

Dental and jaw abnormalities may also occur in achondroplasia, the mucopolysaccharidoses, chondrodystrophia calcificans congenita, hypotelorism, hypertelorism, Marchesani's syndrome, Marfan's syndrome, and in mental deficiences of various types including mongolism. The list is virtually inexhaustible; it is beyond the scope of this book to include all of them.

MISCELLANEOUS DISORDERS

Eosinophilic Granuloma (Histiocytosis X) of Bone. This lesion not infrequently involves the jaw, resulting in destruction of the area of bone affected, with no visible reaction. It is not unusual to observe the bone destroyed so completely that teeth are left with no bony supporting structure; the so-called "floating" teeth. The bony lesions may be solitary or multiple within the mandible and may involve other bones. There are several other diseases which may destroy the mandible in a similar way; they include reticulum cell sarcoma, lymphosarcoma, metastatic neuroblastoma and Ewing's tumor. The teeth may appear to "float," but there are often soft-tissue changes and other signs which tend to make the diagnosis.

Acrosclerosis and Scleroderma. There is an increase in the thickness of the alveolodental membrane, resulting in uniform widening of the radiolucent space between the dental roots and the lamina dura. The uniform widening of this space in all the teeth differentiates it from inflammatory disease of the alveolus.

Osteomalacia. The decalcification caused by this disease is noted in the alveolus. The lamina dura is also involved and is absent in some areas but can usually be visualized in others.

Rickets. A deficiency of vitamin D may cause dental disturbances as well as the classic skeletal abnormalities. Hypoplasia of the enamel is frequently observed, since the disease usually occurs in young children and infants. When the onset is late as in rachitis tarda, the development of the dental roots may be retarded. This is caused by defective dentine and cementum which may result in poor attachment of the teeth and lead to periodontal infection. The pulp chambers are abnormally large.

Renal Osteodystrophy. The dental findings are similar to those of hyperparathyroidism, with demineralization of the alveolus and loss of the lamina dura. In the child, delayed dental development is also observed.

Infantile Cortical Hyperostosis. This disease frequently involves the mandible. It is described in Chapter 8, under the heading "Infantile Cortical Hyperostosis."

CYSTS AND TUMORS OF THE JAW

DENTAL CYSTS

Radicular or Dental Root Cysts. These cysts are the result of chronic periapical infection and have been described in the section on "Periapical Infections." The cystic cavity is clearly defined and usually unilocular. The relationship of the radiolucent cystic structure to the dental root is important in the differential diagnosis. This is the most common "cyst" of the jaw, all others are relatively rare.

Follicular Cysts. This type of cyst arises in relation to a tooth follicle. Three forms may occur, depending upon the cyst content. These are the (1) dentigerous, (2) simple follicular (primordial), and (3) cystic odontoma. The most common type of follicular cyst is the dentigerous cyst formed about the crown of a tooth. It develops about an unerupted, malposed tooth. Characteristically, it produces a sharply marginated, expansile, rarefied area with a formed or incompletely formed tooth projecting into the cavity along one side. Roentgen examination shows the large rarefaction, usually in the molar area, which causes expansion of the mandible. Its edges are clearly

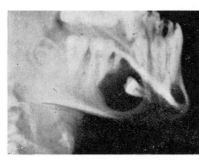

Fig. 35-12. Dentigerous cyst. Note the clearly defined radiolucent cyst in the mandible that has resulted in erosion of the root of the second bicuspid and first molar. The small tooth projecting into it is typical of this cyst.

defined and there is a tooth or a part of a tooth projecting into the radiolucent cyst (Fig. 35-12). They may occur in the maxilla as well as in the mandible.

The *simple follicular* (*primordial*) *cyst* is rare; it arises from the epithelium of the enamel before development of the tooth, so that it is roentgenographically similar to the dentigerous cyst, except that there is no tooth associated with it. Since these follicular cysts are related to the developing teeth, they are usually found in patients under the age of 15. They tend to occur in the third molar region of the mandible.

Cystic odontoma is a follicular cyst that contains a mass of rudimentary teeth or a mass of very dense material that may be amorphous.

BASAL CELL NEVUS SYNDROME. This is an hereditary disorder manifested by multiple, basal cell epitheliomas of the skin, cysts of the jaws, and skeletal anomalies which include short fourth metacarpal, rib anomalies, vertebral anomalies, and ectopic calcifications in soft tissues. The cysts in the jaw are usually symptomatic before the skin changes are noted and appear to be simple follicular or dentigerous cysts.

DENTAL TUMORS

Zizmor and Noyek[12] classify dental tumors as follows:

Epithelial:

1. Ameloblastoma—without inductive connective tissue change.
2. Complex and compound odontoma—with inductive connective tissue change.

Mesodermal:

1. Odontogenic fibroma
2. Cementifying fibroma

AMELOBLASTOMA (ADAMANTINOMA): The adamantinoma is a slowly growing tumor that is malignant, since local recurrence with eventual widespread local involvement may occur. It arises from the anlage of the enamel organ. The tumor is usually found in young adults; the age range varies from 10 to 35 years. It may occur in either jaw but is more common in the mandible than the maxilla. The tumor may be divided into numerous compartments by bony septa. The roentgen findings are those of a central tumor producing destruction of bone and the dental roots as well as expansion of the cortex through which numerous complete or incomplete trabeculations pass to give the appearance of multicystic mass (Fig. 35-13).

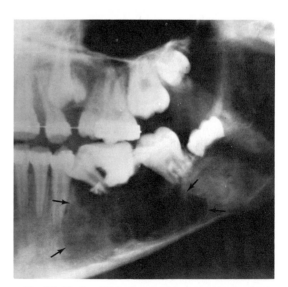

Fig. 35-13. Ameloblastoma. This tumor in the body of the mandible is reasonably well defined (**arrows**). It has destroyed the bone in the premolar and molar areas and appears to be somewhat multicystic anteriorly.

Occasionally it is unilocular with no trabeculation. There is no attempt at new bone formation but the mass is clearly defined by a smooth-appearing bony wall. The recurrent or more malignant form is more invasive and its limits are not clearly defined. The unilocular adamantinoma may resemble a radicular cyst or simple follicular cyst. The polycystic type may resemble a central giant cell tumor and radiographic differentiation is not absolute.

COMPLEX (COMPLEX COMPOSITE) ODONTOMA. This is a single mass made up of two or more of the solid dental tissues, including enamel, dentin, pulp and cementum. Roentgenographically it is a densely opaque mass of malformed dental elements in either jaw, surrounded by a thin radiolucent line similar to the periodontal membrane. There is condensation of bone surrounding the mass resulting in an encapsulated appearance. The most common sites are the upper central incisor and the lower molar areas. They are usually found in childhood, are asymptomatic except as a mass is produced, and may become very large.

COMPOUND (COMPOUND COMPOSITE) ODONTOMA. This is similar to the complex odontoma except that the dense mass is composed of a bundle of dwarfed misshapen teeth, which are recognizable as teeth. It is found most often in the cuspid area with equal frequency in maxilla and mandible.

ODONTOGENIC FIBROMA (FIBROMYXOMA). This evidently arises from dental tissue and may be associated with an unerupted tooth. Radiographically it is a multicompartmented, cystlike rarefaction, with fine trabeculations which may be angular. Thinning of the cortex is present in large lesions. At times the lesion is unilocular and associated with an unerupted tooth. Then it cannot be differentiated from dentigerous cyst since roentgen appearances are identical.

CEMENTIFYING FIBROMA (CEMENTOMA). There is confusion in the literature regarding this benign tumor. It usually occurs in the mandible and is often multiple. It begins in the periapical region with proliferation of connective tissue of the periodontal membrane; in this stage it resembles a periapical granuloma or root cyst. The second stage is one in which the fibrous tissue is converted into a calcified cementumlike substance. This dense mass then develops within the cystlike space. There may be some associated hypercementosis of the adjacent dental root.

NONODONTOGENIC CYSTS AND TUMORS

INCISIVE FORAMEN CYST (ANTERIOR PALATINE FORAMEN CYST). As indicated earlier, the normal incisive foramen may vary considerably in size, so that the roentgen diagnosis must be made on the basis of the clinical history of a slowly enlarging mass either in the anterior palate or protruding into the nose, associated with a midline cyst which usually has clearly defined borders of condensed bone. They are benign, so they can be followed if there is any doubt as to the diagnosis. Rarely, a median mandibular cyst may occur; the appearance is similar except for location.

SOLITARY BONE CYST OF THE MANDIBLE. This cyst is probably caused by trauma to the developing mandible. It is lined by connective tissue and may contain blood, serosanguineous fluid, or blood clot. The roentgen findings are those of a radiolucency which may be quite large, but poorly defined and with an irregular wall. There may be thinning and expansion of the cortex. They arise in the cancellous bone of the medullary canal. In the posterior mandible the large cysts tend to extend into the alveolus between the dental roots. They occur in young adults and appear to regress spontaneously. The relationship of this lesion to *aneurysmal bone cyst* is not clear.

ANEURYSMAL BONE CYST. This condition is very rare in the mandible. As in aneurysmal bone cyst elsewhere, it tends to be a cortical lesion which expands the bone locally. It has the appearance of a trabeculated lytic cavity projecting blisterlike from the bone in a manner that may suggest a soap-bubble. There may be marked expansion and thinning of the cortex. Its relation to trauma is not entirely clear, nor is its relationship to reparative giant cell granuloma.

BENIGN GIANT CELL REPARATIVE GRANU-LOMA (BENIGN GIANT CELL TUMOR). There is controversy as to how this lesion should be classified, but it is probably a nontumorous reparative process. The origin may be central or peripheral; the latter originates in the alveolar soft tissue and may produce a smooth, pressure defect of the bone on the alveolar crest, but does not invade bone. The central type may be unilocular, expansile, and resemble a large cyst, except that there is no condensation of bone forming the wall of the defect. The other form is multilocular. It may also expand the cortex and deform and displace adjacent teeth. The borders are not clearly defined by condensation of bone; this type cannot be differentiated from ameloblastoma.

FIBROUS DYSPLASIA OF THE JAW. The alveolar areas of one or both jaws may be involved by fibrous dysplasia as local or as part of general disease. This is not a true tumor but does cause expansion of the cortex in the area involved. It characteristically involves a considerable extent of bone and may occur in both the mandible and maxilla in the same patient. The roentgenographic finding is that of a radiolucent defect that is widespread and results in expansion of bone. There are often irregular trabeculations giving the lesion a multicystic appearance. At times the disease may be localized, with a reasonably well-circumscribed area of mandibular expansion in which are mottled areas of density and rarefaction.

CEMENTOMA (PERIAPICAL OSTEOFIBROSIS). This lesion was also described in the section on "Odontogenic Tumors," but its histopathology is such that it is considered by some to be a form of fibrous dysplasia or ossifying fibroma. The origin of this condition is uncertain. The tooth is viable and nonsymptomatic. The term "periapical osteofibrosis" is preferred, since cementum forms only a portion of the lesion.

OTHER BENIGN TUMORS

CHERUBISM. This is a familial disease characterized by symmetric swellings of the mandible caused by a rather massive, fibrous tissue proliferation which expands the cortex. It is centered in the region of the angle and extends to the ramus and body. The maxilla may also be involved occasionally. Roentgen findings consist of expansive areas in the mandible which are bilaterally symmetric. The cortex may be very thin and there are no teeth in the involved areas. (See also Chapter 2.)

TORUS PALATINUS. This is an exostosis arising at the margins of the palatal processes at the median palatal suture, usually bilaterally. The radiographic signs are those of a moderately flat mass of cortical bone density projecting downward from the palate, often somewhat lobular with a midline groove (Fig. 35-14). *Torus mandibularis* is a similar dense exostosis projecting from the medial aspect of the anterior mandible. It is usually bilateral and there may be multiple masses with a somewhat lobulated appearance. The torus is signficant only if it becomes large enough to interfere with speech or with dental function.

Osteoma of the jaw may occur and resemble osteoma elsewhere. Multiple osteomas are not uncommon. As in other bones, they may be flat and broad-based, or somewhat pedunculated and are more common in the mandible than in the maxilla. Osteomas of the jaws and other bones are associated with multiple polyposis of the colon, multiple epidermoid cysts, and desmoid tumors in Gardner's syndrome, a rare familial condition. Occasionally *ossifying fibroma* may occur in the mandible or in the maxilla in the region of the maxillary antrum. The roentgen findings are those of large radiolucent expanding lesion, which is usually found in young patients ranging from 10 to 30 years of age. At first the lesions are usually entirely destructive and therefore radiolucent. The wall

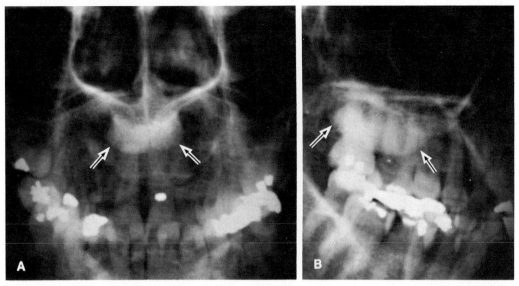

Fig. 35-14. Torus palatinus. *A,* Frontal projection showing the dense bone forming the torus extending downward from the palate. **Arrows** outline the lesion. There is a poorly defined midline groove. *B,* Lateral projection. **Arrows** outline the somewhat elongated bony mass in the hard palate.

is clearly defined. Later some calcification is noted within the tumor. *Osteoid osteoma* may occasionally involve the mandible, where its typical roentgen appearance is usually diagnostic. *Hemangioma* of the jaw also presents an appearance typical of this lesion in other flat bones.

MALIGNANT TUMORS

Osteogenic sarcoma and chondrosarcoma rarely occur in the jaw and the appearance there is similar to the appearance of these tumors elsewhere. Ewing's tumor is also found occasionally. The appearance of this tumor is similar to its appearance elsewhere (see Chapter 7).

Carcinoma of the alveolar ridge or carcinoma arising in the maxillary antrum may involve the alveolus by direct extension. This results in destruction of bone in an irregular manner with no clearly defined wall and often with evidence of an associated soft-tissue mass (Fig. 35-15). In patients with carcinoma involving the alveolar ridge, there is often ulceration, and infection may involve the bone. Infection is characterized by sequestrum formation

(Fig. 35-16). Fragments of devitalized bone separating or separated from the area of disease always are highly suggestive of osteomyelitis (see Chapter 6). Differentiation between infection and actual carcinomatous destruction of bone is sometimes difficult; biopsy is then required to make the diagnosis. Occasionally

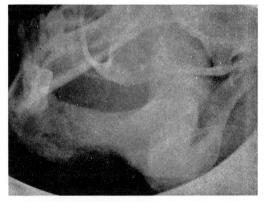

Fig. 35-15. Carcinoma eroding mandible. Note the irregular destructive lesion on the inferior aspect of the body of the right mandible. This resulted from direct extension of a squamous cell carcinoma in the submandibular region.

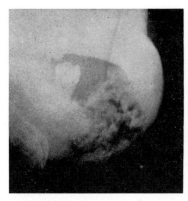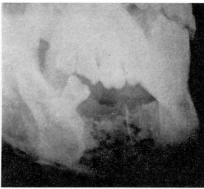

Fig. 35-16. Osteomyelitis of the jaw. Note the irregular destruction of bone in the left mandible with a number of moderately dense sequestra forming a mosaic pattern in the area of disease.

metastatic malignancy may involve the jaw and, in widespread multiple myeloma, lesions caused by this tumor may be visible. The manifestations are those of multiple areas of destruction without reaction.

THE TEMPOROMANDIBULAR ARTICULATION

This articulation is examined with the mouth open and closed by the use of special projections and by means of tomography. Both joints are usually examined so that one can be compared with the other. Occasionally we also use fluoroscopy and cinefluorography or video tape to study joint motion in certain patients with pain in the joints and normal roentgenograms. Normally the articular surfaces are smooth and the mandibular condyle moves forward out of the glenoid fossa when the mouth is opened. The range of motion in the normal is similar on the two sides and the appearances are similar but not necessarily identical (Fig. 35-17). There are variations in the formation of the glenoid fossa ranging from a flat appearance to a deeply concave fossa. Pain upon motion of the jaw along with crepitation and limitation of motion are often secondary to dental disease and malocclusion, and may not be accompanied by radiographic change. Effusion in the joint is manifested by widening of the joint space. Degenerative changes are similar to those noted in other joints, with some eburnation of joint surfaces and narrowing of the radiographic joint space. Rheumatoid arthritis may involve these articulations, resulting in loss of joint space, irregularity, poor definition of joint surfaces and destruction of subchondral bone. This disease may also lead to fibrous and occasionally to bony ankylosis. Fibrous ankylosis may also result from trauma and may be incomplete so that the range of motion is markedly diminished. Occasionally bony ankylosis occurs, usually following septic arthritis. Roentgenograms show the continuity of bone between the condyle and glenoid fossa in this condition.

THE SALIVARY GLANDS

Roentgen methods are used to study the salivary glands in patients with suspected calculi. The calculi are usually very dense and visualization is largely a matter of proper technique. Submaxillary glands and ducts are examined by placing an occlusal film in the mouth and using a submentovertex type of projection. Parotid calculi may be in the gland or duct. Intraoral, lateral extraoral, and anteroposterior or tangential, extraoral films are needed. Sialography can be used for localization if needed.

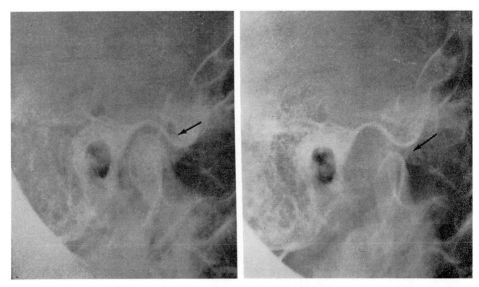

Fig. 35-17. The normal temporomandibular joint. *Left,* **Arrow** indicates mandibular condyle. Note fossa with normal joint space. *Right,* Same patient with mouth open. The mandibular condyle has moved forward normally (**arrow**).

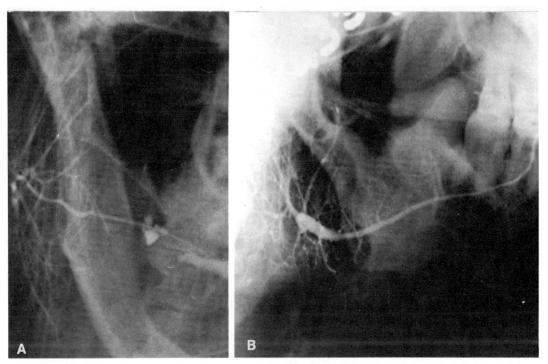

Fig. 35-18. Normal parotid sialogram. *A,* Frontal projection showing the treelike branching of the ducts which are normal in caliber. *B,* Oblique projection. The findings are similar.

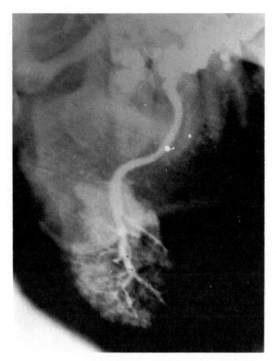

Fig. 35-19. Submandibular sialogram. The duct is somewhat overdistended and there is considerable amount of opaque medium outlining the gland, indicating that there was more pressure used than necessary. Otherwise the examination is normal.

SIALOGRAPHY. This examination consists of filling the salivary ducts of the parotid or submaxillary glands with an opaque medium; we use Pantopaque. A preliminary film is taken to check for calcification. The duct is entered with a fine, silver-tipped probe dilator. Then a small polyethylene catheter is introduced for a distance of 1 to 3 cm using a guide wire. The catheter can be kept in place during the exposure. Some prefer using a blunt-tipped cannula which can also be taped in place. Local anesthesia (Xylocaine) may be used if necessary. When the parotid is to be examined, Stensen's duct can be probed for a short distance without much difficulty in most patients. Approximately 1 to 2 cc of Pantopaque is injected under very low pressure and films are made of the parotid gland and duct area in lateral and frontal projections with the catheter left in place (Fig. 35-18). The examination is best

completed under fluoroscopic control, then spot films can be obtained in suitable projections. We examine the submandibular gland much less frequently, and the injection of Wharton's duct is more difficult (Fig. 35-19). A fine dilator and a thin polyethylene catheter with guide wire are used; the catheter may be introduced for a distance of 2 to 5 cm and injection of 1 to 2 cc of an opaque medium is made under fluoroscopic control. It is important to correlate the sialogram with the clinical findings. Ducts may be incompletely filled when obstructed by calculus; tumors in and adjacent to the parotid may displace the ducts; malignant tumor within the parotid gland characteristically causes irregular filling of the ducts. Normally the glands empty in 30 minutes. Follow-up films can be taken if desired, to study emptying of the gland.

THE FACIAL BONES

The roentgen examination of the facial bones is used extensively for the diagnosis of fracture in patients who have had head and facial trauma. Inflammatory disease and tumor may also involve these structures. A number of different views are used, including those described for examination of the paranasal sinuses. The projections needed depend upon the problem (Fig. 35-20). Tomography is of definite value in the examination of the facial bones.

FRACTURES

Fractures of the bones of the face are commonly caused by direct trauma and may be severe and extensive. The roentgen signs of fracture of facial bones are comparable to those described for fractures elsewhere.

NASAL BONE FRACTURES. A minimum of a lateral and an occlusal view are necessary in examination of the nose. Fractures of the nasal bones are commonly in the anterior half; both bones are usually involved (Fig. 35-21). The

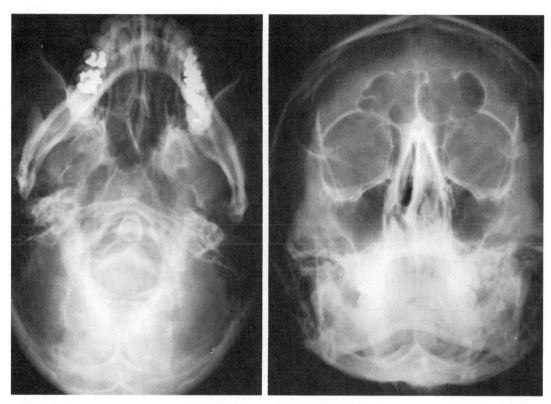

Fig. 35-20. The facial bones. *Left,* Basal view of the skull and facial bones. *Right,* Waters' view of the facial bones. This is a good projection when zygomatic and facial bone fractures are suspected.

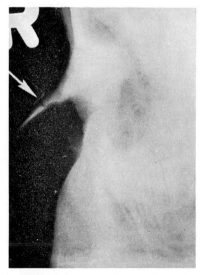

Fig. 35-21. Fracture of the nasal bones. **Arrow** indicates fracture line. There is no significant displacement.

fragments are depressed and displaced laterally in most instances. It is important not to mistake suture lines between the nasal bones and the frontal and maxillary bones for fractures. Diastasis of these sutures may occur however. It is important to check the anterior nasal spine of the maxilla since it may be fractured when the nose is injured. Unless the trauma is very local, it is also wise to get a Waters view to check for adjacent facial bone injury which may be manifested by fluid or soft-tissue swelling in either antrum.

MAXILLARY FRACTURES. When there has been severe facial injury with suspected maxillary fracture, there are often injuries elsewhere which make roentgen examination difficult or may delay it for a time. We try to use a more or less standard set of exposures in these situa-

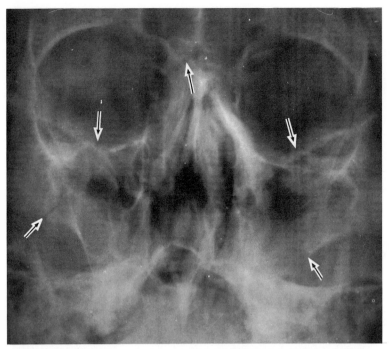

Fig. 35-22. Facial bone fractures (LeFort II). **Arrows** indicate the maxillary and orbital fracture sites. The fracture at the base of the nose is well defined on the right (**arrow**) but not on the left.

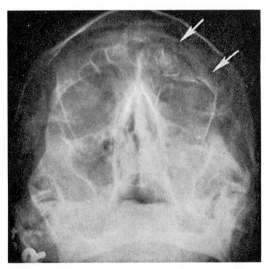

Fig. 35-23. Multiple fractures. **Arrows** indicate comminuted fractures in the left frontal bone extending into the roof of the orbit. The left zygomatic arch is fractured and depressed. Compare it with the right. The roof and lower lateral wall of the left maxillary antrum is also fractured and this antrum is clouded as a result of hemorrhage and edema.

tions which includes a Waters view (stereo if possible), lateral, posteroanterior, and basal (submentovertical) stereo. A brow-up lateral view is useful if basal fracture is suspected to determine the presence of sphenoid sinus fluid. Then additional views are taken if necessary after the initial films are checked. We depend upon tomography to a large extent in the more complex injuries and usually start with anteroposterior films at 5-mm intervals and obtain other sections as needed without moving the patient. There are numerous classifications of maxillary fractures; one of the oldest is the Le Fort (Table 35-1) which is still useful in describing these fractures.

Obviously there are many variations, and unilateral fractures often occur. The alveolar processes may be involved without injury elsewhere. Dental fractures may occur. Clouding of maxillary sinuses is often present in fractures of the maxilla. As indicated above, we try to tailor the examination to the observed injury, using tomography very frequently.

TABLE 35-1. Classification of Maxillary Fractures
(Le Fort)

LE FORT I. This is a transverse fracture through the maxillary sinus walls above the teeth; posteriorly it extends through the junction of the middle and lower third of the pterygoid processes of the sphenoid.

LE FORT II. This is a pyramidal fracture extending through the maxillary sinus in an oblique fashion to include the lower lateral sinus wall, the inferior orbital margin, the nasal bones in the region of the nasofrontal suture then downward and laterally in a similar fashion on the opposite side. Posteriorly the fracture terminates in the midportion of the pterygoid process (Fig. 35-22).

LE FORT III. This severe fracture extends from the region of the nasofrontal suture across the frontal processes of the maxillae, lacrimal bones, ethmoids, medial aspect of the inferior orbital fissure to the base of the pterygoid processes.

ZYGOMATIC FRACTURES. Injury in the zygomatic area may range from a local depressed fracture of the arch to a combination of injuries involving the frontozygomatic suture, the lateral wall and floor of the orbit, lateral wall of the maxillary sinus and the region of the zygomatic-maxillary junction. Depression, comminution and sutural separation are common (Fig. 35-23). The submentovertical view in addition to a tangential is useful in detecting depression of the zygomatic arch. Antral clouding is common in this group of injuries.

ORBITAL FRACTURES. Fractures of the medial or inferior orbital rim may be associated with fracture of the orbital floor, the so-called "blowout" fracture. The thin fragments of the orbital floor are displaced downward to encroach on the superior aspect of the maxillary sinus. A Waters view may show the bony fragments displaced downward or a similar displacement of the soft tissues of the floor of the orbit into the upper antrum. A "half" Waters view taken at 20° rather than at 37° is useful in this injury, since the central ray parallels the orbital floor and the small blowout fragments may be visualized (Fig. 35-24A). At times the fragments may be easily seen on a lateral view. If the antrum is opacified by

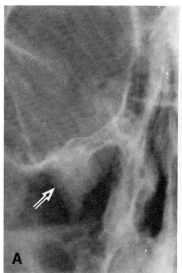
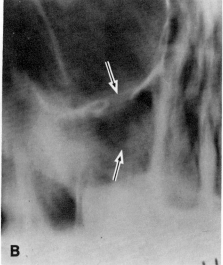

Fig. 35-24. Blow-out fractures of the orbit. A, Half Waters' view to show the pseudopolypoid mass extending downward into the right maxillary antrum from the floor of the orbit (arrow). B, Tomogram of another patient showing bone deficit in the orbital floor and a soft-tissue mass extending into the antrum (arrows).

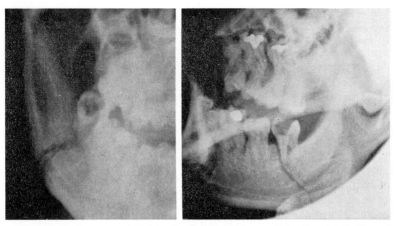

Fig. 35-25. Fracture of the body of the right mandible. Frontal (*left*) and lateral (*right*) projections clearly show the fracture line extending to the alveolus at the level of the second molar tooth.

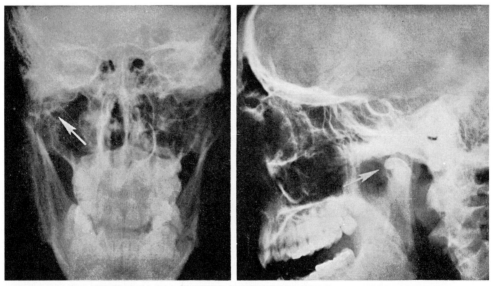

Fig. 35-26. Fracture dislocation of the right mandibular condyle. There is also a fracture of the body of the mandible on the left side. *Left,* **Arrow** indicates mandibular condyle displaced downward and medially. The fracture line is not clearly identified in this projection. *Right,* **Arrow** indicates mandibular condyle, which is rotated and displaced anteriorly and downward.

disease or trauma, tomography is needed to outline the fragments and make the diagnosis. We take the initial tomograms at 5-mm intervals, check them, and add more levels if needed. There is usually no difficulty in making the diagnosis if proper films are available (Fig. 35-24*B*). There may be associated fractures elsewhere in the orbit or facial bones, so further roentgen examination may be needed. If orbital emphysema is present, fracture extending into the ethmoids or maxillary antrum is likely. Enophthalmos, which ultimately results, is not apparent in the immediate posttraumatic period because of edema and hemorrhage. Diplopia may be present to suggest the possibility of alteration in position of the globe in these patients.

MANDIBULAR FRACTURES. The mandible is the facial bone most frequently fractured. Direct trauma is the cause in most instances. Multiple fractures are common; when one fracture is visualized, the remainder of the mandible should be examined closely. The most common fracture site is in the body of the mandible in the region of the cuspid tooth. When there is not much displacement the fracture line may not be visible in one plane, therefore two views should always be obtained at a 90° angle if possible (Fig. 35-25). The neck of the condylar process is particularly difficult to visualize in some patients. If a fracture in this area is suspected, special views used to visualize temporomandibular joints are sometimes of value in addition to the routine frontal and lateral projection. We use a combination of Panorex examination and sometimes Panoramix along with routine mandibular projections in patients with jaw injury. Occasionally tomograms are used when the area cannot be clearly visualized in any other manner. There is often dislocation of the condyle, associated with fracture of the neck of the condylar process (Fig. 35-26).

CYSTS AND TUMORS

Cysts and tumors involving the facial bones are those that are found in the sinuses and jaws and have been discussed under those headings.

REFERENCES AND SELECTED READINGS

1. BECKER, M. H., KOPF, A. W., and LANDE, A.: Basal cell nevus syndrome: Its roentgenologic significance. *Am. J. Roentgenol. Radium Ther. Nucl. Med. 99:* 817, 1967.

2. EINSTEIN, R. A. J.: Sialography in the differential diagnosis of parotid masses. *Surg. Gynecol. Obstet. 122:* 1079, 1966.

3. FREIMANIS, A. K.: Fractures of the facial bones. *Radiol. Clin. North Am. IV:* 341, 1966.

4. HOEFNAGEL, D., and BENERSCHKE, K.: Dyscephalia mandibulo-oculo-facialis (Hallermann-Streiff syndrome). *Arch. Dis. Child. 40:* 57, 1965.

5. HOUSTON, I. B., and SHOTTS, N.: Rutherfurd's syndrome. A familial oculo-dental disorder. *Acta Paediat. Scand. 55:* 233, 1966.

6. MERRILL, V.: *Atlas of Roentgenographic Positions.* St. Louis, Mosby, 1967, vol. II.

7. PAVSEK, E. J.: Mandibulofacial dysostosis (Treacher Collins syndrome). *Am. J. Roentgenol. Radium Ther. Nucl. Med. 79:* 598, 1958.

8. STAFNE, E. C.: Dental roentgenologic manifestations of systemic disease. *Radiology 58:* 9–22, 507–516, 820–827, 1952.

9. STAFNE, E. C.: *Oral Roentgenographic Diagnosis,* 3rd ed. Philadelphia, Saunders, 1969.

10. UNGER, J. D., and UNGER, G. F.: Fractures of the pterygoid processes accompanying severe facial bone injury. *Radiology 98:* 311, 1971.

11. WORTH, H. M.: *Principles and Practices of Oral Radiologic Interpretation.* Chicago, Year Book, 1963.

12. ZIZMOR, J., and NOYEK, A. M.: Cysts and benign tumors of the paranasal sinuses. *Semin. Roentgenol. III:* 172, 1968.

13. ZIZMOR, J., SMITH, B., FASANO, C., and CONVERSE, J. M.: Roentgen diagnosis of blow-out fractures of the orbit. *Am. J. Roentgenol. Radium Ther. Nucl. Med. 87:* 1009, 1962.

INDEX

Abdomen, 411–464
abscesses of, 439–441
ascites in, 438–439
calcification in, 428–434
examination of, 411
foreign bodies in, 441–442
gallbladder, 466–486
hernias in, 593–594
lipomas, retroperitoneal, 464
liver, 454–458
mesenteric cysts, 463–464
normal, 411–412
pancreas, 443–454
pneumoperitoneum, 434–438
pregnancy in, 726
pseudomyxoma, peritonei, 462–
463, 638–639
spleen, 458–462
Abdominal aortography, 328
Abscess
appendiceal, 637–638
Bezold, in acute mastoiditis, 1072
of bone, 176–177
acute, 176
Brodie, 177
chronic, 176–177
tuberculous, 180
of brain, 381
pineal displacement in, 355
dental, periapical, 1081
epidural, 407
intra-abdominal, 439–441
of liver, 456
of lung, 791–794
in mastoiditis, 1072
in mediastinitis, acute, 950
paraspinal, differential diagnosis
of, 962–963

Abscess (continued)
perirenal, 671–672
psoas, 672
renal, 670–671
of spine, in tuberculosis, 266,
268
subdiaphragmatic, 440–441
Accessory bones and ossification
centers, 66–70
Acetabular angle
increased, 89–90
in trisomy 21 syndrome, 98
Acetabulum, 68–69
protrusion of, 297
in osteomalacia, 115
in rheumatoid arthritis, 272
Achalasia, 504–506
differential diagnosis of, 511, 962
pulmonary complications of,
505–506
Achondroplasia, 34–38
cone-shaped epiphyses in, 64
differential diagnosis of, 30, 31,
34, 37–38, 39, 40, 42, 44
long tubular bones in, 36
pelvis in, 35–36
ribs in, 64
short tubular bones in, 36–37
skull in, 35
teeth in, 1084
vertebrae in, 35
Acoustic neuroma, 374–375
Acrocephalosyndactylism, 75
Acromegaly, 24–26, 369
long bones in, 25
skull in, 24–25
spine in, 25–26
teeth in, 1083

Acromioclavicular joint, dislocation or subluxation of,
160–161
Acropachy, thyroid, 316–317
Acrosclerosis, 314
teeth in, 1085
Actinomycosis
of bone, 181–182
differential diagnosis of, 180
of lungs, 826–827
mediastinal lymph nodes in, 952
and mediastinitis, 950
of spine, 269
Adamantinoma, of jaw, 1086–1087
Addison's disease, and calcification
in adrenal glands, 431,
711
Adenocarcinoma
of appendix, 638, 639–640
of kidney, 695–697
of uterus, 732
See also Carcinoma
Adenoma
bronchial, 882, 892–893
of colon, 613
villous, 619
of gallbladder, 478
gastric, villous, 536
of kidney, 693
parathyroid, in mediastinum,
960
pituitary, 354, 368–370
of small intestine, 578
Adenomatoid malformation of
lung, cystic, 777
Adenomatosis
of colon, familial, 615
pulmonary, 882, 894

Adenomyoma, of gallbladder, 478
Adenomyomatosis, of gallbladder, 478, 479
Adenopathy, lymphangiography in, 333
Adhesions
    arachnoid, 382–383, 403–404
    of gallbladder, 479
    between gallbladder and duodenum, 470
    and pericarditis, 1040
    periduodenal, 566
    pleural, 948
Adrenal glands, 710–712
    bone growth in hyperfunction of, 26
    calcification in, 430–431, 710–711
    carcinoma of, calcification in, 433
    and Cushing's syndrome, 107–109
    cysts of, 711
        calcification of, 431
    neuroblastoma of, 712
    tumors of
        cortical, 711
        medullary, 712
Aerosol-foam enema, 599
Agammaglobulinemia, lung changes in, 933–934
Aganglionosis, 606–608
Air-bronchogram, in alveolar disease, 754
Albers-Schönberg disease, 46–48
Albright's syndrome, 53
Alcoholism, and ischemic necrosis of bone, 243
Alkaline phosphatase. *See* Phosphatase
Allergic states
    and polyposis of paranasal sinuses, 1064–1065
    pulmonary changes in, 921–924
    pulmonary hypersensitivity and occupational diseases, 858–860
Allison-Johnstone anomaly, 492
Alveolar cell carcinoma, 882, 894
Alveolar process of jaw, 1079
    infections of, 1082
Alveolodental periostitis, chronic, 1081
Alveolus, pulmonary
    disease of, 754
    edema of, 867–868
    microlithiasis of, 933
    proteinosis of, 936–937

Alzheimer's disease, 376
Amebiasis
    colon in, 612, 628–631
    lungs in, 838
Amebic abscess, of liver, 456
Ameboma, 612, 628, 630
Ameloblastoma, of jaw, 1086–1087
Aminoaciduria, and rickets, 115
Amniography
    in fetal death diagnosis, 725
    for placental localization, 729
Amyloidosis
    bone lesions in, 222–223
    lungs in, 930–931
    of small intestine, 588
Anemia
    bone changes in, 253–258
    sickle cell. *See* Sickle cell anemia
Anencephaly, 76
Anesthesia, in bronchography, 745
    reactions to, 746–747
Aneurysm
    aortic, 1034–1038
    arteriography of, 330
    intracranial, 347–348
        angiography in, 359
    of renal artery, 688
    of splenic artery, calcified, 429
    of Valsalva sinus, 1008
    ventricular, 1027–1028
Aneurysmal bone cyst, 197–198
    of mandible, 1087–1088
Angiocardiography, 972
    in atrial septal defect, 998
        with pulmonary stenosis, 987–988
    in coarctation of aorta, 1008
    in Ebstein's anomaly, 991
    in patent ductus arteriosus, 995
    in pulmonic stenosis, 1003
        with atrial septal defect, 987–988
        with tricuspid atresia, 991
    in tetralogy of Fallot, 986
    in transposition of great vessels
        complete, 989
        Taussig-Bing type, 994
    in tricuspid atresia, with pulmonary stenosis, 991
    in truncus arteriosus persistence, 994
    venous, in pericardial effusion, 1040
    in ventricular septal defect, 1000
Angiography, 328–331
    abdominal, in gastrointestinal bleeding, 517
    adrenal, 711

Angiography (*continued*)
    bronchial, 750
        in bronchogenic carcinoma, 892
    cardiovascular, 972
    cerebral, thorium dioxide in, 456
    coronary, 973
    duodenal, 553
    intercostal, in bronchogenic carcinoma, 892
    intracranial, 359–362
        in subdural hematoma, 379
        thorium dioxide in, 456
    of liver, 457–458
    mesenteric, 599
    ophthalmic artery, 1047–1048
    of pancreas, 453–454
    pelvic, 731–732
    placental, 729
    pulmonary, 750
        in bronchogenic carcinoma, 892
    in pulmonary embolism, 872
    renal, 648
    small intestine studies, 572
    splenic, 461
Angioma. *See* Hemangioma
Angiomyolipoma, of kidney, 693
    in tuberous sclerosis, 349, 682
Angiosarcoma
    of bone, 213
    of heart, 1032
Ankle
    accessory bones in, 66–68
    fractures of, 165–166
Ankylosing spondylitis, 273–275
Ankylosis
    in pyogenic arthritis, 263
    in rheumatoid arthritis, 272–273
        of spine, 275
    of spine
        in rheumatoid arthritis, 275
        in tuberculosis, 268
    in Still's disease, 276
Anthrax, pneumonia in, 786
Anticholinergic drugs, effects of, 517
Anus, imperforate, 419, 604–605
Aorta, 980
    acquired diseases of, 1033–1038
    aneurysm of, 1034–1038
        abdominal, and stomach displacement, 543
        dissecting, 1037–1038
        traumatic, 1035
    arteriosclerosis of, 1033–1034
    ascending, 980
        in atrial septal defect, 998

Aorta (*continued*)
  calcification in, 428–429
    differential diagnosis of, 452
  coarctation of, 1005–1008
    pseudocoarctation, 1008
  descending, 980
  in patent ductus arteriosus, 995
  syphilitic aortitis, 1034
  in tetralogy of Fallot, 986
  in transposition of great vessels
    complete, 988–989
    corrected, 1004
    Taussig-Bing type, 994
  in tricuspid atresia, with pulmo-
    nary stenosis, 991
  in ventricular septal defect, 1000
Aortic arch
  anomalies of, 1010–1013
  ascending, 758
    in advancing age, 771
  double, 1012–1013
  kinking of, 1008
  right, 1010–1011
    with left ligamentum arteri-
      osum, 1013
Aortic valve
  insufficiency of, 1022–1024
  stenosis of, 1003–1004, 1022
Aortitis, syphilitic, 1034
Aortography
  abdominal, 328
  retrograde, 973
    in aortic aneurysm, 1035
    in coarctation of aorta, 1008
    in patent ductus arteriosus,
      996
  translumbar, 648
Apert's syndrome, 75
  cone-shaped epiphyses in, 64
Aplasia, of lungs, 773
Appendices epiploica
  calcifications in, differential
    diagnosis of, 668
  inflammation of, 632
Appendicitis, 637
  differential diagnosis of, 591
  sentinel loops in, 427
Appendix, 601, 636–641
  abscess of, 637–638
  adenocarcinoma of, 638, 639–
    640
  fecaliths in, 430, 637
  mucocele of, 638–639
    calcification in, 431
    ruptured, and pseudomyxoma
      peritonei, 462–463
  stump defect of, 640–641
  tumors of, 638–640
Arachnodactyly, 60

Arachnoiditis, adhesive, 382–383,
    403–404
Arteries. *See* Vascular conditions
Arteriography, 328–331
  See also Angiography
Arteriosclerosis, 307
  of aorta, 1033
  arteriography in, 330
  cardiovascular, 1025–1026
  intracranial, 347, 383–384
    angiography in, 361–362
  and renal artery obstruction, 691
Arteriovenous malformations
  fistula, arteriography of, 330
  intracranial, 348
    angiography in, 359
  pulmonary, 1015–1016
  of spinal cord, 404
Arthritis
  gouty, 283–285
  hypertrophic. *See* Joint disease,
    degenerative
  infectious, 262–269
  Marie-Strümpell, 273–275
  mutilans, 272
  periarthritis, 287
  in pseudogout syndrome, 294
  and psoriasis, 276–277
  pyogenic, 262–263
    differential diagnosis of, 266
  in Reiter's disease, 294
  rheumatoid, 269–276
    differential diagnosis of, 266,
      285
    lung disease with, 926–927
    of sacroiliac joints, 274, 296–
      297
    of spine, 273–275
    and Still's disease, 275–276
  and scleroderma, 276–277
  syphilitic, 269
  traumatic, 145, 282–283
  tuberculous, 180, 264–269
    and caries sicca, 266
    differential diagnosis of, 266
    of peripheral joints, 264–266
Arthrodysplasia, hereditary, and
    dystrophy of nails, 96
Arthrography, 300–301
Arthropathy. *See* Joint disease
Asbestosis, 849–854
Ascites, 438–439
Aspergillosis, lungs in, 833–836
Asphyxiating thoracic dystrophy,
    64
  differential diagnosis of, 38
Aspiration
  emphysema from, obstructive,
    905

Aspiration (*continued*)
  pneumonia from, 783
    lipid, 934–936
Asthma, lungs in, 921–922
Astragalus
  fracture of, 167
    ischemic necrosis after, 244
  secondary, 67
Astrocytoma, 364–365, 372
  calcification in, 351
Atelectasis, 910–914
  in carcinoma, bronchogenic, 883
  in emphysema, obstructive, 905
  focal, 913–914
  general considerations in, 910–
    911
  lobar, 911–913
    lower lobe, 911
    right middle lobe, 912
    upper lobe, 912–913
  in middle lobe syndrome, 795
  in pneumonia
    pneumococcal, 781
    primary atypical, 788
  segmental, 913
  in tuberculosis, 812
Atherosclerosis. *See* Arterioscle-
    rosis
Atresia
  of colon, 605
  of duodenum, congenital, 554
  of esophagus, congenital, 494–
    496
  of small intestine, congenital,
    574–575
  tracheal, congenital, 777
  tricuspid, 989–991
Atrioventricularis communis, 998,
    1001
Atrium
  enlargement of
    left, 983
    right, 983
  myxoma of, 1032
  septal defects, 996–998
    with mitral stenosis, 998
    with pulmonary stenosis, 986–
      988
    with right-to-left shunt, 998
Atrophy of brain, 376–377
  congenital, 350
Avulsion
  of cervical roots, 406–407
  fractures, 131
Axillary vein, venography of, 327
Azygography, 750–751
  in bronchogenic carcinoma, 892
Azygos lobe, 773–774
Azygos lymph node, 756

Bagassosis, 858
Baker's cyst, 296
Baritosis, 858
Barium, in bronchography, 745
Barium enema examination, 487
  of appendix, 636
  of colon, 596–598
    in functional disturbances, 633
    in Hirschsprung's disease, 607–
      608
  of intestinal tract, 414, 487
  mixtures for, 597
  postoperative, 634–636
  of small intestine, 572
    in intussusception, 589–590
  technique of, 597–598
Barium meal examination, 487
  of colon, 596
    in functional disturbances, 633
  of esophagus, 488–489
  of intestinal tract, 414, 487
  in pancreatitis, acute, 446
  postoperative, 547–551
  of small intestine, 571
  of stomach, 515–516
Barrett's esophagus, 492, 500
Basal angle of skull
  normal, 76
  in osteomalacia, 115
Basal cell nevus syndrome, and
    cysts in jaw, 1086
Basal ganglia, symmetric calci-
    fication of, 350–351
Basilar invagination, in skull, 76
Bathrocephaly, 78
Battered child syndrome, 169
Bauxite fibrosis, pulmonary, 854–
  855
Beaded esophagus, 493
Bennett's fracture, 156
Beriberi, heart in, 1031
Berylliosis, 856–857
Bezoars, 540
Bezold's abscess, in acute mas-
    toiditis, 1072
Bile, milk-of-calcium, 479–480
Bilharziasis
  bladder in, 705
  lungs in, 840–841
Biliary tract
  cholangiography of, 450, 481–
    486
  common bile duct
    cholangiography of, 450
    cyst of, 481
    lithiasis in, differential diag-
      nosis of, 668
    in pancreatic enlargement,
      449–450

Biliary tract (*continued*)
  fistula in, 468
  gas in, 468–469
  sclerosing cholangitis of, 481
  See also Gallbladder
Biologic effects of radiation, 5–6
Biopsy of lung
  bronchial brush method, 752–
    753
  needle aspiration for, 753
Bismuth poisoning, bone changes
    in, 247
Bladder, 412, 702–710
  anatomy of, 652
  calculi in, 703–704
  carcinoma of, 708–709
    calcification in, 433
  congenital anomalies of, 702–
    703
  cystography of, 649–650, 655
    voiding, 649
  diverticulum of, 707
  duplication of, 703
  enlargement of, congenital, 703
  exstrophy of, 702
  foreign bodies in, 709–710
    and calculi formation, 704
  gas in wall of, 322
  infections of, 704–705
  megacystis syndrome, 708
  neurogenic, 707–708
  obstruction of, 705–707
  rhabdomyosarcoma of, 709
  in schistosomiasis, 705
  trauma of, 709
  tumors of, 708–709
  vesicoureteral reflux, 664, 708
"Bladder ears," 703
Blastomycosis
  of bone, 181–182
    differential diagnosis, 180
  lungs in, 832–833
  mediastinal lymph nodes in, 952
  of spine, 269
Block vertebra, 80
Blood pressure, increased. *See*
    Hypertension
Blood vessels. *See* Vascular con-
    ditions
Blount's tibia vara, 93, 95–96
  differential diagnosis of, 101
Bochdalek foramen, hernia
    through, 967
Boeck's sarcoid. *See* Sarcoidosis
Bones. *See* Osseous system
Bowlegs
  in Blount's disease, 93, 95–96
  physiologic, of infancy, 93

Bowlegs (*continued*)
  in rickets, 112
    vitamin D-refractory, 117
Brachycephaly, 74
Brain, 337–385
  See also Intracranial diseases
Breast
  calcification in, 319–320, 325
  in chest films, 755
  mammography of, 325–326
  nipple shadows in, 755
Breschet, veins of, 338
Brittle bones, 45–46
Brodie's abscess of bone, 177
Bronchi, 757–758
  adenoma of, 882, 892–893
  bronchiectasis, 801–803
  bronchitis, 799–801
  brush biopsy of, 752–753
  cysts of, 777
    congenital, 803–805
  diseases of, 799–806
  obstruction of
    and emphysema, 904–905
    and middle lobe syndrome,
      794–796
    by tumors, 781
  stenosis of, in tuberculosis, 818–
    819
  supernumerary, 774–775
Bronchial arteries, angiography of,
    750
  in bronchogenic carcinoma, 892
Bronchiectasis, 801–803
  bronchography in, 744
  cylindrical, 801
  cystic, 802, 806
  in middle lobe syndrome, 795
  reversible, 803
  saccular, 802
  tomography in, 749
  in tuberculosis, 815–816
Bronchiolar carcinoma, 882, 893–
  895
Bronchiolectasia, 800
Bronchiolitis, acute, 801
Bronchitis, 799–801
  acute, 799
  chronic, 799–801
Bronchogenic carcinoma. *See*
    Lungs, carcinoma of
Bronchogenic cysts, mediastinal,
    956–957
Bronchogram, air, in alveolar dis-
    ease, 754
Bronchography, 743–747
  anesthesia for, 745
    reactions to, 746–747
  in bronchial adenoma, 893

Bronchography (*continued*)
  in carcinoma, bronchogenic, 892
  contraindications to, 744
  in emphysema, 903
  hazards in, 746–747
  indications for, 744
  iodized oil in, 745
    reactions to, 747
  in middle lobe syndrome, 795–
    796
  technique of, 744–745
Bronchopleural fistula, and
    pneumothorax, 917
Bronchopneumonia, 782–783
Bronchus. See Bronchi
"Brown tumors," in hyperpara-
    thyroidism, 119, 121
  differential diagnosis of, 201
Brucellosis, lungs in, 785
Brunner's glands, hypertrophy of,
    566
Bubonic plague, pneumonia in, 786
Buckling fractures, 133–134
Budd-Chiari syndrome, 462
Bulbar palsy, swallowing difficulty
    in, 513
Bullous emphysema, 806, 907,
    919–920
Bursae, distention of, 296
Bursitis, 287, 317
Butterfly, vertebra, 82
Byssinosis, 858–859

Cafe-au-lait spots
  in Albright's syndrome, 26, 53
  in neurofibromatosis, 56
  in tuberous sclerosis, 348
Caffey's disease, 249–250
Caisson disease, 299–300
  infarction of diaphysis in, 244
  ischemic necrosis of bone in, 243
Calcaneonavicular bar, 87–88
Calcaneus
  fractured, 166–167
  ischemic necrosis of apophysis
    of, 238
  secondarius, 67
Calcification
  in abdominal cysts, 431–432
    differential diagnosis, 668, 678
  in adrenal glands, 430–431, 710–
    711
    in carcinoma, 433
  in aorta, differential diagnosis of,
    452
  in aortic stenosis, 1022

Calcification (*continued*)
  and appendiceal fecaliths, 430,
    637
  arterial, 307
  articular and periarticular, 294,
    317–318
  of basal ganglia, symmetric,
    350–351
  in bladder carcinoma, 433
  in breast, 319–320, 325
  of cartilage, 294
    in rheumatoid arthritis, 272
  of celiac axis, differential diag-
    nosis of, 452
  of chondromas, 245
  of choroid plexus, displacement
    of, 342, 355
  in coronary arteries, 1026
  in costal cartilage, 755
  of dura mater, 343
  enteroliths, 430
  of fetus, 726
  after fractures, 138
  in gallbladder wall, 466–467
  in gastric neoplasms, 531
  in gastrointestinal carcinoma,
    433
  in hyperparathyroidism, 121
  and interstitial calcinosis, 312–
    314
  of intervertebral discs, in child-
    hood, 297–298
  intra-abdominal, 428–434
  intracranial
    physiologic, 339–343
    in tumors, 351, 355–356
  in liver, 430, 456
  in lungs, 430
  of lymph nodes, 318
    differential diagnosis of, 451–
      452, 704
    mesenteric, 428
  in meconium peritonitis, fetal,
    433–434
  of mediastinal teratoid cyst, 954
  of mesenteric lymph nodes, 428
  in mitral stenosis, 1018, 1021
  in myositis ossificans, progres-
    sive, 310, 318
  in neuroblastoma, 432–433
  in orbit and globe, 1049–1052
  in osteochondroma of paranasal
    sinuses, 1065–1066
  of ovary, 731
    in cystadenocarcinoma, 432
  of pacchionian bodies, 343
  Pellegrini-Stieda, 318–319
  pelvic, female, 731
  pericardial, 1040

Calcification (*continued*)
  periosteal, 314–317
  phleboliths, 429
    See also Phleboliths
  pineal gland, displacement of,
    340, 354, 355
  and pleural thickening, 947
  provisional, zone of, 17, 18
  psammoma, in ovarian tumors,
    733
  in pulmonary artery, in pulmo-
    nary hypertension, 877
  of pulmonary nodules
    in aspergillosis, 834
    in bronchogenic carcinoma,
      889–890
    in histoplasmosis, 830
    in silicosis, 848
  in renal carcinoma, 433
  in small intestine duplications,
    573
  in soft tissues, 307–321
    in Ehlers-Danlos syndrome,
      311
    parasitic, 310
    after spinal cord injury, 312
    after trauma, 310–311
  of spinal ligaments, in rheuma-
    toid arthritis, 275
  in spleen, 430, 460
  of thymoma, 960
  in tumors, 311–312, 432–433
    intracranial, 351, 355–356
  in uterine arteries, 433
  in uterine leiomyoma, 432
  in vas deferens, 433, 710
  vascular, intra-abdominal, 428–
    430
  of veins, 307–309
    See also Calculi
Calcinosis
  circumscripta, 313–314
  with dermatomyositis, 313
  interstitial, 312–314
  with Raynaud's phenomenon,
    314
  renal, 669–670
  with scleroderma, 312–313, 314
  tumoral, 320–321
  universalis, 312–313
Calcitonin, effects of, 124
Calcium
  in gallstones, 467, 475
  hypercalcemia, idiopathic
    bone changes in, 248
    intracranial calcification in,
  milk-of-calcium bile, 479–480
  in tuberculous nodules, 816
    352

Calculi
    alveolar microlithiasis, pulmonary, 933
    broncholithiasis, in tuberculosis, 819
    enteroliths, 430
    in fallopian tube, 731
    fecaliths, appendiceal, 430, 637
    gallstones, 467–468
        See also Gallstones
    in pancreas, 44, 446, 450–452
    phleboliths. *See* Phleboliths
    renal, in hyperparathyroidism, 119
    ureteral, differential diagnosis, 429
    in urinary tract, 666–669
        See also Urinary tract, calculi
    vesical, 703–704
Callus
    endosteal, in fractures, 141
    osteoid, in fractures, 138, 139
    periosteal, in fractures, 140–141
        absence of, 144
Calvarium, diffuse hyperostosis of, 352
Calvé's vertebra plana, 226, 239
Calycine cysts, renal, 686
Candidiasis, lungs in, 836
Carbuncle, renal, 670
Carcinoid syndrome, 578
Carcinoid tumors
    of appendix, 640
    of bronchus, 892
    of small intestine, 578
Carcinoma
    adrenal, calcification in, 433
    of bladder, 708–709
        calcification in, 433
    of breast, calcification in, 319, 325
    bronchiolar, 882, 893–895
    bronchogenic. *See* Lungs, carcinoma
    of colon, 608–613
    of duodenum, 564–565
    of esophagus, 498–501
    of gallbladder, 478–479
    gastrointestinal, calcification in, 433
    of jaw, 1089
    of mastoids, 1076
    metastatic. *See* Metastasis
    of pancreas, 452–453
    of paranasal sinuses, 1066–1067
    renal, calcification in, 433
    of stomach, 527–531
Cardia, of stomach, 492, 519
Cardioesophageal relaxation, 506

Cardiohepatic angle
    fat deposits in, 967–969
    pericardial cyst in, 957
Cardiomegaly. *See* Heart, enlargement of
Cardiospasm, 504–506
    See also Achalasia
Cardiothoracic ratio, 973
    in childhood, 979
Cardiovascular system, 971–1041
    aberrant right subclavian artery, 1014
    angiocardiography, 972
    anomalous left coronary artery, 1008–1009
    anomalous pulmonary venous return
        partial, 993
        total, 991–993
    aorta, 980
        acquired diseases of, 1033–1038
    aortic arch anomalies, 1010–1013
    aortic valve disease, 1022–1024
    aortography, retrograde, 973
    arteriosclerosis, 1025–1026
    atrial septal defects, 996–998
        with mitral stenosis, 998
    atrioventricularis communis, 998, 1001
    coarctation of aorta, 1005–1008
        pseudocoarctation, 1008
    congenital anomalies of, 983–1017
        cyanotic, 984–994
        of heart, 983, 1010
        noncyanotic, 994–1010
    cor pulmonale, 1028–1030
    coronary arteriography, 973
    coronary artery disease, 1026–1027
    ductus arteriosus patency, 995–996
    Ebstein's anomaly, 991
    endocardial fibroelastosis, 1004–1005
    examination of, 971–974
    fluoroscopy of, 971–972
    heart, 974–979
    hypertension, 1025
    mitral valve disease, 1017–1022
    myocardial diseases, 1030–1032
    pericardium, 980, 1038–1041
    pulmonary artery anomalies, 1014–1017
    pulmonary valvular disease, 1024–1025
    roentgenography of, 971

Cardiovascular system (*continued*)
    rotation anomalies of heart, 1009–1010
    size of heart, determination in childhood, 979
    tetralogy of Fallot, 984–986
    tomography, 973
    transposition of great vessels
        complete, 988–989
        corrected, 1004
        Taussig-Bing type, 994
    tricuspid valvular disease, 1025
    truncus arteriosus persistence, 993–994
    Valsalva sinus aneurysms, 1008
    valvular disease, acquired, 1017–1025
    ventricular aneurysm, 1027–1028
    ventricular septal defects, 998–1001
Caries
    dental, 1080
    sicca, 266
Carotid arteries
    aneurysms of, 347
    angiography of, 359
    left, anomalous position of, 1012
Carpal scaphoid, divided, 69
Cartilage
    bone formation in, 15
    calcification of, 294
        in rheumatoid arthritis, 272
    formation after fractures, 138
    in tuberculous arthritis, 265
Cartilage-hair dysplasia, 38–39
    differential diagnosis of, 37
Cartilaginous tumors, of joints, 291–292
Cataracts, calcification in, 1049
Cathartics, affecting colon, 634
Caudal dysplasia syndrome, 85–86
Caustics
    esophagitis from, 501
    gastritis from, 538–539
Cavitation of lungs
    in abscess, 791–794
    in carcinoma, 887
    in coccidioidomycosis, 828
    in silicotuberculosis, 849
    in tuberculosis, 814–815
        cavity drainage of, 824
Cavography, superior, in bronchogenic carcinoma, 892
Cecum, 601
    lipomas of, 613
    tuberculosis of, differential diagnosis, 612
    volvulus of, 424–425

Celiac axis
  arteriography of, 572
  calcification in, 429
    differential diagnosis of, 452
  catheterization of
    in duodenal arteriography, 553
    in gastrointestinal bleeding, 517
    in liver angiography, 457
    in pancreatic angiography, 453
    in splenoportography, 462
Celiac disease, 586
Cementoma, 1088
  of jaws, 1087
Cementum, accumulations of, 1082
Cephalhematoma, 149
Cephalic index, 74
Cephalometry, fetal, 719–721
Cerebellopontine angle tumor, 374–375
Cerebellum, tumors of, 372–373
  ventricular system in, 358
Cerebral tumors. *See* Intracranial disease, tumors
Cerebrocranial cicatrix, in skull fractures, 148
Cerebro-hepato-renal syndrome, 29
Cerebrospinal fluid
  and hydrocephalus, 381–382
  increased pressure of, 352–355
Cerebrovascular ferrocalcinosis, idiopathic, 350
Cerebrum. *See* Intracranial disease
Cervical nerve roots, avulsion of, 406–407
Cervical ribs, 85, 772
Cervico-occipital fusion, 76, 80–81
Cervico-occipital meningocele, 70
Chalasia, of esophagus, 506
Chalk gout, 314
Chamberlain's line, 81
Charcot joint, 286
Chemodectoma
  of mastoids, 1076
  of mediastinum, 954
Cherubism, 55, 1088
Chest, 741–1041
  accessory lobes and fissures in, 773–775
  in advancing age, 770–771
  alveolar disease, 754
  angiography, pulmonary, 750
  azygography, 750–751
  azygos lobe, 773–774
  biopsy
    with bronchial brush method, 752–753
    with needle aspiration, 753

Chest (*continued*)
  bony thorax, 755
    congenital malformations of, 771–773
  bronchi, 757–758
    diseases of, 799–806
  bronchography, 743–747
  cardiothoracic ratio, 973
    in childhood, 979
  cardiovascular system, 971–1041
  congenital variations in, 86–97, 771–778
  diaphragm, 768–769, 963–970
  dystrophy, asphyxiating, 64
    differential diagnosis of, 38
  examination of, 741–753
  fluoroscopy of, 742–743
  heart in thoracic deformities, 1030
  in infancy and childhood, 770, 979
  interstitial disease of, 754
  laryngography, 747
  lungs, 761–768
  mediastinum, 756–761, 950–963
  normal chest, 753–770
    in adults, 755–769
  pleura, 769, 942–950
  pneumomediastinography, diagnostic, 752
  pneumothorax, diagnostic, 751–752
  roentgenkymography of, 751
  roentgenography of, 741–742
  silhouette sign in, 754
  soft tissues in, 755–756
  thoracic muscle, internal, 760
  thoracoplasty, in tuberculosis, 824
  thymus, 758
  tomography of, 747–750
  trachea, 757
Chickenpox, and pneumonia, 790
Childhood conditions. *See* Pediatrics
Chip fractures, 131
Cholangiography, 450, 481–486
  intravenous, 483–485
  operative, 482
  oral, 483–485
  percutaneous transhepatic, 450, 485–486
  postoperative, T-tube, 483
  transjugular, 486
Cholangitis, sclerosing, 481
Cholecystitis
  acute, sentinel loops in, 427
  chronic, with gallstones, 476

Cholecystitis (*continued*)
  emphysematous, 322, 469
  glandularis proliferans, 479
Cholecystoduodenal fistula, 468
Cholecystography, 470–481
  physiology of procedure, 472
  technique of, 470–472
Cholecystokinin, 473
Cholecystoses, hyperplastic, 478, 479
Choledochus. *See* Biliary tract
Cholelithiasis. *See* Gallstones
Cholesteatoma
  intracranial, 228–229, 371–372
  in mastoids, 1073–1074
  of orbit, 1055
Cholesterol, in gallstones, 467
Cholesterol-type of pneumonitis, chronic, 934
Cholesterolosis, of gallbladder, 477
Cholografin, in cholangiography, 475, 477, 483
Chondroangiopathia calcarea seu punctata, 28
Chondroblastoma, 202–203
  differential diagnosis, 199
Chondrocalcinosis, 294
Chondrodysplasia, deforming, hereditary, 33
Chondrodystrophia calcificans congenita, 28
Chondroectodermal dysplasia, 62–64
  differential diagnosis of, 126
  teeth in, 1084
Chondroma, 191
  calcified, 245
  central, 191
  of diaphragm, 966
  of joints, 291
  juxtacortical, 194
  mediastinal, 962
Chondromyxoid fibroma, 203–204
  differential diagnosis of, 199
Chondro-osteodystrophy, 40
Chondrosarcoma, 209–212
  central, 210–211
  of jaw, 1089
  of joints, 291
  peripheral, 211–212
Chordoma, 79, 229–230, 375
Chorioepithelioma, of uterus, 732
Choroid plexus, 341–343
  calcified, displacement of, 342, 355
Chromosomal abnormalities, 97–101
  trisomy 13–15 syndrome, 101
  trisomy 18 syndrome, 98–101

Chromosomal abnormalities
  (*continued*)
 trisomy 21 syndrome, 98
 Turner's syndrome, 101
Cinefluorography
 of esophagus, 489
 of gastrointestinal tract, 488
 of stomach, 517
Circulatory disturbances, pulmonary, 866–879
Cirrhosis
 of liver, splenoportography in,
  462
 of lung, muscular, 938
Clavicle
 in cleidocranial dysostosis, 61
 fractures of, 161
 in hyperparathyroidism, 121
 rhomboid fossa of, 92, 755
 supraclavicular border, 766
Clefts, facial, teeth in, 1083
Cleidocranial dysostosis, 60–62
 paranasal sinuses in, 1068
 teeth in, 1084
Clinodactyly, 93
Cloverleaf skull, 74
Clubbing of digits, in hypertrophic
  osteoarthropathy, 298
Clysodrast, in barium mixture, 597
Coal worker's pneumoconiosis, 855
Coarctation
 of aorta, 1005–1008
  pseudocoarctation, 1008
 of pulmonary artery, 1016–1017
Coccidioidomycosis
 of bone, 181–182
 lungs in, 827–829
 mediastinal lymph nodes in, 952
 of spine, 269
Coccyx, dislocation of, 162
Codman's triangles, 206
 in tumors of bone, 179
Codman's tumor, 202–203
Colitis
 granulomatous, 579, 626–628
  differential diagnosis of, 612
 ulcerative, 622–626
  arthritis in, 277
  barium enema studies of, 597
  and carcinoma, 625–626
  differential diagnosis of, 616
  early changes in, 623–625
  hypoproteinemia in, 591
  later changes in, 625
  and pseudopolyposis, 625
Collagen diseases
 arthritis with, 277
 lungs in, 924–928
 in Marfan's syndrome, 60
Colles fracture, 154–155

Colon, 596–641
 adenoma of, 613
  villous, 619
 in amebiasis, 612, 628–631
 ameboma of, 612, 628, 630
 anastomosis of, end-to-end, 635–
  636
 anatomy and physiology of,
  599–603
 ascending, 601
 atresia and stenosis of, 605
 carcinoma of, 608–613
  differential diagnosis of, 612–
  613, 621–622
  infiltrating or annular, 610
  inflammatory changes in, 611
  intussusception in, 611–612
  obstructive, 610–611
  polypoid or fungating, 608–
  610
  sinus tracts and fistulas in,
  611
  and ulcerative colitis, 625–626
 cathartics affecting, 634
 congenital malformations of,
  603–608
 in Cronkhite-Canada syndrome,
  617
 descending, 601–602
 dilatation of, toxic, 624
 diseases of, 608–641
 diverticula of, 619–622
  differential diagnosis of, 615
 diverticulitis, 620–622
 diverticulosis, 620
 divisions of, 600–602
 duplication of, 604
 endometriosis of, 619
 examination of, 596–599
 fibrosis of, after radiation, 631
 functional disturbances of, 633–
  634
 in Gardner's syndrome, 616
 gastrocolic fistula in, 549–550
 haustral sacculations in, 602–603
 hemorrhage in, intramural, 632
 hernias affecting, 632–633
 imperforate anus, 604–605
 ischemia of, segmental, 592,
  631–632
 lipomas of, 618
 lymphogranuloma venereum of,
  632
 lymphoid hyperplasia in, nodular, 616–617
 lymphosarcoma of, 618–619
  differential diagnosis of, 616
 megacolon, 605–608
 movements of, 603
 necrotizing enterocolitis, 631

Colon (*continued*)
 normal, 559–603
 obstruction of, 422–425
 in Peutz-Jeghers syndrome, 616
 polyposis of, familial, 615–617
  differential diagnosis of, 583
 polyps of, 613–618
  barium enema studies of, 598
  differential diagnosis of, 612,
  615
  juvenile, 617–618
  roentgen findings in, 613–614
  postoperative studies of, 634–636
  pseudopolyps of, 615, 616
   and ulcerative colitis, 625
 resection of, 636
 rotation errors of, 603–604
 sigmoid, 602
  volvulus of, 421, 424
 taeniae coli, 602
 transverse, 601
  mass in, and stomach displacement, 543
 tuberculosis of, 628
  differential diagnosis of, 612,
  630
 tumors of, 608–619
  intramural, 613, 615, 618
 ulcerative colitis, 622–626
Colostomy, barium enema after,
  634–635
Compact islands, 52
Compression fractures, 133
 vertebral, 150–151
  differential diagnosis, 268–269
Cone-shaped epiphyses, 63–64
Conradi's disease, 28
Conray, in excretory urography,
  646
Contraction ring, in lower esophagus, 512
Contractures, in rheumatoid
  arthritis, 272
Contrast media. *See specific agents*
Convolutional impressions, cranial,
  72
 increased, 354–355
Cooley's anemia, bone changes in,
  253–256
Coproliths, appendiceal, 430, 637
Cor pulmonale, 1028–1030
Corkscrew esophagus, 493
Corner fractures, 131
Corner sign, in scurvy, 109
Coronary arteries
 angiography of, 973
 anomalous left artery, 1008–
  1009
 diseases of, 1026–1027
 occlusion of, 1027

Cortical hyperostosis, infantile, 249–250
Corticosteroid therapy, ischemic necrosis of bone after, 243
Costal cartilage, calcifications in, 755
 differential diagnosis of, 668
Costophrenic angle, 768
 in pleural effusion, 943
Costovertebral joints, rheumatoid arthritis of, 275
Cough fractures, 162
Coxa plana, 232
Cranial nerve palsies
 in metaphyseal dysplasia, 49
 in osteopetrosis, 47
Cranium. *See* Skull
Cretinism, 21–22
 differential diagnosis of, 31
 teeth in, 1083
Crohn's disease, 579
 of colon, 626
 of duodenum, 565–566
 of ileum, 579–580
 of jejunum, 580–581
 of stomach, 539
Cronkhite-Canada syndrome, 533
 colon in, 617
 hypoproteinemia in, 591
Crouzon's disease, 74
 optic canal in, 1053
Crush fractures, 132
Cryptococcosis, lungs in, 832
Cuboideum secondarium, 68
Curling phenomenon, esophageal, 493, 507
Cushing's disease
 ischemic necrosis of bone in, 243
 osteoporosis in, 107–109
 teeth in, 1083
Cyanotic defects, congenital, 984–994
Cylindromas, bronchial, 892
Cyst(s)
 of adrenal glands, 711
 in astrocytomas, 364
 Baker's 296
 of bone, 195–198
  in mandible, 1087–1088
 bronchial, 777
  congenital, 803–805
 choledochal, 481
 in degenerative joint disease, 279
 dentigerous, 1085
 dermoid. *See* Dermoid cysts
 and duplications. *See* Duplications
 echinococcus. *See* Echinococcus cyst

Cyst(s) (*continued*)
 esophageal, and duplications, 496
 of facial bones, 1097
 gastroenteric, affecting mediastinum, 957
 of incisive foramen, 1087
 intra-abdominal, calcification in, 431–432
 intracranial
  dermoid, 372
  epidermoid, 228–229, 371–372
  of third ventricle, 371
 of jaw, 1085–1087
 of joints, 296
 of lung, 777, 805–806
  congenital, 803–805
 mediastinal, 955–958
 mesenteric, 463–464
 neurenteric, mediastinal, 957
 ovarian, 733
 of pancreas, 453
 of paranasal sinuses, 1062–1064
 pelvic, 731
 pericardial, 957–958, 1040
 in pneumatosis cystoides intestinalis, 435, 547
 pyelitis cystica, 676
 radicular, 1081, 1085
  differential diagnosis of, 1080
 renal cystic diseases, 679–688
 of spinal cord, 404–406
 of spleen, calcified, 460
 teratoid, mediastinal, 954–955
 urachal, 663
 ureteritis cystica, 676
Cystadenocarcinoma of ovary, calcified, 432
Cystic duct, calculi of, differential diagnosis of, 668
Cystic fibrosis of pancreas
 lungs in, 796–797
 and meconium ileus, 418
Cystic hygroma, mediastinal, 958
Cysticercosis
 calcification in, 310
 intracranial, 346
 lungs in, 840
Cystine storage disease, and rickets, 115
Cystitis, 704–705
 emphysematous, 705
Cystography, 649–650
 normal, 655
 voiding, 649
Cystourethrography, voiding, 649
Cytomegalic inclusion disease
 bone changes in, 259
 cerebral lesions in, 349
 differential diagnosis of, 346–347

Dactylitis, syphilitic, differential diagnosis of, 180
Deafness, in osteogenesis imperfecta, 45
Decalcification. *See* Osteoporosis
Degenerative diseases
 of brain, 350
 of joints, 277–283
Demineralization. *See* Osteoporosis
Dental conditions. *See* Teeth
Dentigerous cyst, 1085
Dentinogenesis imperfecta, 1085
Dermatomyositis
 arthritis in, 277
 calcinosis with, diffuse, 313
 small intestine in, 588
Dermoid cysts
 intracranial, 372
 of mediastinum, 954–955
 of orbit, 1055
 of ovary, 733
  calcified, 432
Dermoid tumors, of scalp, 77
Dextrocardia, 1010
Dextroposition of stomach, 521
Diabetes
 bronze, 456
 insipidus
  and histiocytosis X, 932
  hydronephrosis in, 664
 mellitus
  arthropathy in, 286
  gangrene of foot in, 321
  osteoporosis in, 109
  teeth in, 1083
Diaphragm, 768–769, 963–970
 accessory, 969–970
 in advancing age, 771
 in bronchogenic carcinoma, 891
 in childhood, 770
 congenital defects of, 967
 displacements of, 965–966
 eventration of, 964–965
 functional disturbances of, 964
 hernias of, 966–967
 paralysis and paresis of, 964
 trauma of, 967
 tumors of, 966
Diaphysis, 18, 28
 infarction of, 244–245
 sclerosis of, 50
  multiple, hereditary, 50–51
Diastatic fracture of skull, 147
Diastematomyelia, 85
Diatomite pneumoconiosis, 855–856
Dilatation
 of bladder, congenital, 703
 of bronchi, 801–803
 of colon, toxic, 624

Dilatation (*continued*)
  of renal pelvis and calyces. *See* Hydronephrosis
  of small intestine, in sprue, 586
Dionosil, in bronchography, 744–745
Diploic veins, 338–339
Disaccharidase deficiency, in small intestine, 593
Discitis, juvenile, 179
Discography, 392
Dislocation
  of acromioclavicular joint, 160–161
  of ankle, 165–166
  at elbow joint, 157–158
    congenital, 91
  of hip, 164
    congenital, 88–91
  of humerus, 159–160
  lunate and retrolunar, 156
  of sacrum, 162
  in shoulder area, 159–161
  vertebral, 151
Displacements
  of calcified choroid plexus, 342, 355
  of calcified pineal gland, 340, 354, 355
  diaphragmatic, 965–966
  esophageal, in hyperparathyroidism, 121
  of fat pads at elbow, 157
  of femur, lateral, 90
  gastric, 447, 542–543
Distortion of images, 8–9
Distraction of fracture fragments, 143
Diverticulitis, of colon, 620–622
Diverticulosis
  of colon, 620
  of esophagus, intramural, 497
  of small intestine, 591
Diverticulum
  of bladder, 707
  of colon, 619–622
  of duodenum, 561–563
  of esophagus, 496–498
  Meckel's, 574
  of stomach, 540–541
Dolichocephaly, 72, 74
Down's syndrome, 98
Drowning, revival from, lungs in, 938–939
Ductus arteriosus patency, 995–996
  with right aortic arch, 1013
  with right-to-left shunt, 996

Ductus arteriosus patency (*continued*)
  in rubella syndrome of infancy, 259
  in trisomy 18 syndrome, 100
Dumping syndrome, 548
Duodenitis, 565–566
  regional, 565–566
Duodenography, hypotonic, 448–449, 553
Duodenum, 553–568
  adhesions, periuodenal, 566
  anatomy and physiology of, 553–554
  anomalies of, 554–557
  carcinoma of, 564–565
  cholecystoduodenal fistula, 468
  diseases of, 557–568
  diverticula of, 561–563
    intraluminal, 563
  duodenitis, 565–566
  duplications of, 556–557, 564
  examination of, 553
  in gallbladder disease, 470
  gas in, resembling gallstones, 474–475
  hematoma of, intramural, 567–568
  hypertrophy of Brunner's glands in, 566
  inversum, 556
  obstruction of, congenital, 554–556
  in pancreatic enlargement, 446, 447–449
  in pancreatitis, acute, 446
  peptic ulcer of, 557–561
    bleeding, examination in, 559
    crater in, 557–558
    differential diagnosis of, 566
    healing of, 560–561
    marginal deformity in, 558
    obstruction from, 559–560
    perforation of, 560
    postbulbar, 557, 558–559
  peritoneal bands in, congenital, 555
  polyps of, 563
  prolapse of gastric mucosa through pylorus, 566–567
  redundancy of superior portion, 556
  right-sided, 556
  tumors of, 563–565
Duografin, in cholangiography, 485
Duplication
  of bladder, 703
  of colon, 604
  of diaphragm, 969

Duplication (*continued*)
  of duodenum, 556–557, 564
  of esophagus, 496
  gastroenteric, affecting mediastinum, 957
  of renal pelvis, 660–661
  of small intestine, 572–573
  of stomach, 521–522
  of ureters, 660–661
Dura mater, calcification of, 343
Dwarfing of extremities
  in epiphyseal dysplasia, multiple, 29
  in rickets, vitamin D-refractory, 117
  in stippled epiphyses, 28, 29
Dwarfism
  in achondroplasia, 34, 36
  in adrenocortical hyperfunction, 26
  in Albright's syndrome, 26
  in cartilage-hair dysplasia, 38
  diastrophic, 33–34
    differential diagnosis of, 38
  in hypophosphatasia, 118
  metatropic, 39–40
    differential diagnosis of, 38
  in osteodystrophy, renal, 123
  pituitary, 23, 26
  in spondyloepiphyseal dysplasia, 31
  thanatophoric, 34
    differential diagnosis of, 38
  ribs in, 64
Dysautonomia, familial, lung changes in, 933
Dyscephalia mandibulo-oculo-facialis, 1085
Dyschondrosteosis, 58–60, 94
Dysgammaglobulinemia, and lymphoid hyperplasia in small intestine, 582
Dysostosis
  cleidocranial, 60–62
    paranasal sinuses in, 1068
    teeth in, 1084
  craniodiaphyseal, 1068
  craniofacial, 74
    optic canal in, 1053
  craniometaphyseal, 1068
  mandibulofacial, 75–76
    teeth in, 1084
  metaphyseal, 39
    differential diagnosis of, 37
  peripheral, 63–64
    differential diagnosis of, 126
  pycnodystosis, 48–49
Dysphagia
  from pharyngeal paralysis, 513

Dysphagia (*continued*)
  in Plummer-Vinson syndrome,
    510
Dysplasia
  achondroplasia, 34–38
  arthrodysplasia, hereditary, and
    dystrophy of nails, 96
  cartilage-hair, 38–39
  caudal, 85–86
  chondroectodermal, 62–64
    differential diagnosis of, 126
    teeth in, 1084
  cleidocranial dysostosis, 60–62,
    1068, 1084
  craniometaphyseal, 49
  diaphyseal sclerosis, 50
  diastrophic dwarfism, 33–34
  dyschondrosteosis, 58–60
  ectodermal, teeth in, 1084
  enchondromatosis, 32–33
  epiphyseal
    hemimelica, 31
    hyperplasia, 31, 64
    multiple, 21, 29–31
      pseudoachondroplastic
        form, 30, 37
      tarda form, 30
    punctate, 28
      differential diagnosis of, 38
    stippled epiphyses, 28–29
  fibromuscular, renovascular,
    691–692
  fibrous, 53–55
    in Albright's syndrome, 26
    of jaws, 1088
      hereditary, 55
    optic canal in, 1053
    and osteosarcoma, 205
    paranasal sinuses in, 1066
    pseudofractures in, 136
  of hip joint, 88
    in adult, 90–91
  in Hurler's disease, 42–44
  in Marfan's syndrome, 60
  maxillonasal, 1068
  melorheostosis, 51–52
  metaphyseal, 49
    dysostosis, 39
  metatropic dwarfism, 39–40
  in Morquio's disease, 40–42
  in mucopolysaccharidoses, 40–44
  multiple exostoses, hereditary, 33
  neurofibromatosis, 55–58
  oculoauriculovertebral, 75
  osseous, 28–64
  osteogenesis imperfecta, 45–46
  osteopathia, striata, 53
  osteopetrosis, 46–48
  osteopoikilosis, 52

Dysplasia (*continued*)
  peripheral dysostosis, 63–64
  pycnodysostosis, 48–49
  renal, 679–680
  in Ribbing's disease, 50–51
  spondyloepiphyseal, 31–32
    congenita, 31, 40
    pseudoachondroplastic, 31, 37
    tarda, 31, 32
  thanatophoric dwarfism, 34
  thoracic dystrophy, asphyxiating,
    64
Dystrophies
  muscular, 304–306
  of nails, and hereditary arthro-
    dysplasia, 96
  thoracic, asphyxiating, 64
    differential diagnosis of, 38

Ebstein's anomaly, 991
Eburnation
  in degenerative joint disease, 278
  of fracture fragments, 144
Echinococcus cyst
  in abdomen, calcified, 431–432
  of liver, 456
  of lungs, 840
  renal, 688
  of spleen, 460
Ectodermal dysplasia, teeth in,
    1084
Ectopic pregnancy, 726
Ectopy of kidney, crossed, 658–659
Edema, 306–307
  alveolar, 867–868
  intestinal, in hypoproteinemia,
    591
  lymphangiography in, 333
  pulmonary, 866–868
Effusions
  in joints, in tuberculous arthritis,
    264–265
  pericardial, 1038–1040
  pleural, 942–950
  subdural, 380
Ehlers-Danlos syndrome, 311
Eisenmenger complex, 1000
Elbow
  accessory bones in, 69
  dislocations of, 157–158
    congenital, 91
  fractures of, 158–159
Electrical circuits, 6–7
Ellis-van Creveld disease, 62–64
  cone-shaped epiphyses in, 63, 64
  differential diagnosis of, 37, 125
  teeth in, 1084

Embolism, pulmonary, 869–874
Emissary vein, mastoid, 1072
Emphysema
  bronchiolar, 938
  interstitial, of thoracic walls, 910
  mediastinal, 909
    in acute mediastinitis, 950
  orbital, 1096
  pulmonary, 902–910
    acute obstructive, 904–906
    in asbestosis, 854
    in bauxite fibrosis, 855
    in berylliosis, 857
    in bronchogenic carcinoma,
      883–885
    bullous, 806, 907
      differential diagnosis of,
        919–920
    centrilobular, 902
    chronic, 902–903
    compensatory, 904, 907–908
    in diatomite pneumoconiosis,
      856
    and hyperlucent lung, uni-
      lateral, 907
    lobar, infantile, 906
    in mucoviscidosis, 797
    nondestructive, 904–907
    nonobstructive, 904, 907–910
    panlobular, 902
    and pulmonary hypertension,
      879
    senile, 904, 908–909
    in talcosis, 854
    subcutaneous, 321
Emphysematous conditions
  cholecystitis, 322, 469
  cystitis, 705
  gastritis, 547
  pyelonephritis, 670
Empyema, thoracic, 948–949
Encephalitis, toxoplasmic, 346–
    347, 349
Encephalogram. *See* Pneumoen-
    cephalography
Enchondroma, 191
  calcified, 245
  and chondrosarcoma, 210
Enchondromatosis, 32–33, 191
Endocardial fibroelastosis, 1004–
    1005
Endochondral ossification, 14, 18
Endocrine disorders
  osseous system in, 104–126
  teeth in, 1083
Endometriosis, of colon, 619
Endosteal callus, in fractures, 141
Enema
  aerosol-foam, 599

Enema (*continued*)
  barium. *See* Barium enema ex-
      amination
  water, 599
Engelmann's disease, 50
Enophthalmos, in orbital fractures,
    1096
Enteritis, regional, 579–581
  hypoproteinemia in, 591
  See also Crohn's disease
Enterocolitis, necrotizing, 631
Enteroliths, 430
Eosinophilia
  pulmonary infiltrates with, 923
    transient, 922–923
  tropical, lungs in, 841
Eosinophilic granuloma
  of bone, 224–225, 226
    vertebra plana in, 226, 240
  of lungs, 931–932
  of stomach, 535
  teeth in, 1085
Ependymomas
  intracranial, 366, 373
    calcification in, 351
  of spinal cord, 401–402
Epicardial fat pads, 967–969
Epidermoid cysts, intracranial,
    228–229, 371–372
Epidermoid tumors
  bronchogenic, 881–882
  of paranasal sinuses, 1065
Epiphyseal plate, 16, 18, 28
Epiphyseolysis, 239–240
  in cretinism, 21
  in pituitary hypofunction, 23
  in thyroid hypofunction, 21, 22
Epiphyses, 15, 18, 28
  ball and socket, 63
  cone-shaped, 63–64
    in pseudohypoparathyroidism,
      125
  dysplasia of
    hemimelica, 31
    hyperplasia, 31, 64
    multiple, 21, 29–31
      pseudoachondroplastic
        form, 30, 37
      tarda form, 30
    punctate, 28
      differential diagnosis of, 38
  fractures of, 134–135
  hyperplasia of, 31
    cone-shaped epiphyses in, 64
  as indicators of skeletal age, 15,
      17
  ischemic necrosis of, 232–241
  for metatarsal V, 67, 168–169

Epiphyses (*continued*)
  ossification centers in, 15, 18
    accessory, 66–70
    delayed in femoral head, 90
  pseudoepiphyses for metacarpals
      and metatarsals, 92–93
  slipping of capital femoral
      epiphysis. *See* Epiphyse-
      olysis
  stippled, 28–29
    differential diagnosis of, 38
Epiphysitis, vertebral, 405
Epipyramis, 70
Epispadias, pubic bones in, 702
Equipment for radiology, 6–8
Erosions of bone, marginal
  in rheumatoid arthritis, 270
  in tuberculous arthritis, 265
Erythroblastosis fetalis, 726
  intrauterine transfusions in, 730–
      731
Esophageal lip, 491
Esophagitis, 501–503
  chemical, 501
  fibrosing, chronic, 502–503
  and hiatal hernia, 503, 504, 546
  terminal, 501
  ulcerative, acute, 502
Esophagogastric junction, 493, 519,
    543
Esophagus, 487–513
  achalasia of, 504–506
    differential diagnosis of, 511,
      962
    pulmonary complications of,
      505–506
  anatomy of, 489–490
  atresia of, congenital, 494–496
  Barrett's, 492, 500
  beaded, 493
  carcinoma of, 498–501
  cardia of, 492, 519
  chalasia of, 506
  congenital anomalies of, 494–
      496
  corkscrew, 493
  curling phenomenon in, 493, 507
  diseases of, 496–513
  displacement of, in hyperpara-
      thyroidism, 121
  diverticula of, 496–498
    differential diagnosis of, 962
    epiphrenic, 497
    Zenker's type, 496, 498
  diverticulosis of, intramural, 497
  duplication of, 496
  esophagitis, 501–503
  examination of, 487–489

Esophagus (*continued*)
  foreign bodies in, 509–510
    complications of, 510
    impacted bone, 509–510
    metallic, 509
    nonopaque, 509
  gastroesophageal reflux, 494
  hiatal hernia of, 543–546, 966
    See also Hernia, hiatal
  hiatal insufficiency of, 544–545
  lower portion of, 492–493, **512**
  normal, 489–490
  peptic ulcer of, 504
  phrenic ampulla of, 491
    differential diagnosis of, 545
  in Plummer-Vinson syndrome,
      510
  polyps of, 510
  presbyesophagus, 491
  pseudodiverticula of, 494
  resection of, 548
  rupture of, spontaneous, 512–513
  spasm of, 507
  in scleroderma, 511
  strictures of
    in chemical esophagitis, 501
    congenital, 496
    in swallowing act, 490
  trauma of, and acute medias-
      tinitis, 950
  tumors of, 498–501, 510
  varices of, 508–509
Ethmoid sinus, 1058–1059
Eunuchoidism, 26
Eventration of diaphragm, 964–965
Ewing's tumor, 213–214
  differential diagnosis of, 179,
      220, 226
  of jaw, 1089
Exostosis, 191–192
  of dental root, 1082
  multiple hereditary, 33, 192
    and chondrosarcoma, 210
    cone-shaped epiphyses in, 64
    differential diagnosis of, 126
  subungual, 192
Exstrophy of bladder, 702
Extremities, congenital variations
    in, 86–97
Eye. *See* Orbit and eye

Fabella, 68
Face
  bones of, 1092–1097
    congenital variations in, 70–78
  clefts of, teeth in, 1083

Face (*continued*)
cysts and tumors of
in facial bones, 1097
in jaw, 1085–1090
fractures of, 1092–1097
mandibular, 1097
maxillary, 1093–1095
nasal, 1092–1093
orbital, 1095–1097
zygomatic, 1095
hyperplasia of, teeth in, 1084
mastoids, 1069–1077
orbit and eye, 1047–1055
salivary glands, 1090–1092
sinuses, paranasal, 1056–1069
teeth, 1078–1085
temporomandibular articulation,
1090
Fahr's disease, 350
Fallopian tubes
calculi in, 731
gas injected into, and pneumoperitoneum, 436
hysterosalpingography, 734–736
Fallot
pentalogy of, 985
tetralogy of, 984–986
trilogy of, 986
Fanconi syndrome, 115
Farmer's lung, 859–860
Fat embolism, pulmonary, posttraumatic, 874
Fat pads
at elbow, displacement of, 157
epicardial, 967–969
Fatigue fractures, 136–137
Fecal lumps, differential diagnosis
of, 615
Fecaliths
appendiceal, 430, 637
of sigmoid colon, differential
diagnosis of, 704
Feet
accessory bones in, 66–68
in acromegaly, 25
in Apert's syndrome, 75
in cleidocranial dysostosis, 61
in diastrophic dwarfism, 34
in enchondromatosis, 32
exostosis of, subungual, 192
fatigue fractures of, 136–137
flatfoot, rigid, 88
fractures, 165–169
march foot, 137
measurement of heel-pad thickness, 25
in Morquio's disease, 41
in pseudohypoparathyroidism,
125

Feet (*continued*)
in sarcoidosis, 189
tarsal coalition in, 88
Felty's syndrome, 276
Femoral artery
arteriography of, 329
percutaneous puncture of, 648
in gastrointestinal bleeding,
517
in liver angiography, 457
in pancreatic angiography, 453
for placental localization, 729
in renovascular hypertension,
691
Femur
delayed ossification of epiphysis,
90
displacement of, lateral, 90
fractures of
condylar, 164
at upper end, 162–164
ischemic necrosis of
in epiphysis, 232–236
in head, 242–243
in Cushing's syndrome, 108
linea aspera of, 317
in osteochondromatosis, 33
slipping of epiphysis. *See*
Epiphyseolysis
Ferrocalcinosis, cerebrovascular,
idiopathic, 350
Fetus, 721–727
abnormalities of, 725–727
death of, diagnosis of, 723–725
in ectopic pregnancy, 726
erythroblastosis fetalis, 726, 730
estimation of age of, 721–723
meconium peritonitis of, calcification in, 433–434
papyraceous, 726
presentation and position of,
727
skull measurements of, 719–721
transfusions for, intrauterine,
730–731
Fibrin bodies, pleural, 950
Fibroblastoma, perineural, intracranial, 374–375
Fibroelastosis, endocardial, 1004–
1005
Fibrolipomatosis, of kidney, 693
Fibroma
of bone, nonossifying, 202
cementifying, in jaw, 1087
chondromyxoid, 203–204
differential diagnosis of, 199
of diaphragm, 966
of heart, 1032
of jaw, 1087, 1088

Fibroma (*continued*)
of kidney, 693
of lungs, 900
mediastinal, 962
odontogenic, 1087
ossifying, of jaw, 1088
of paranasal sinuses, 1065
of small intestine, 578
Fibromuscular dysplasia, renovascular, 691–692
Fibromyxoma, odontogenic, 1087
Fibroplasia, retrolental, 1052
Fibrosarcoma
of bone, 212–213, 228
of diaphragm, 966
of heart, 1032
mediastinal, 962
of paranasal sinuses, 1066
of soft tissues, 323–324
Fibrosing esophagitis, chronic,
502–503
Fibrosis
cystic, of pancreas
lungs in, 796–797
and meconium ileus, 418
intestinal, from radiation, 631
myelofibrosis
differential diagnosis of, 258,
259
with osteosclerosis, 221–222
pulmonary. *See* Lungs, fibrosis
retroperitoneal, 702
Fibrositis, 287
Fibrous cortical defect, of bone,
201–202
Fibrous dysplasia, 53–55
See also Dysplasia, fibrous
Fibroxanthoma of bone, 202
Fibula, fusion with tibia, 87
Fingers. *See* Hand
Fissures
orbital
inferior, 1053–1054
superior, 1053
pulmonary, 761
absence of, 775
Fistula
arteriovenous, arteriography of,
330
biliary, 468
bronchopleural, and pneumothorax, 917
in carcinoma of colon, 611
cholecystoduodenal, 468
gastrocolic, 549–550
tracheoesophageal, congenital,
777
Flake fractures, in ankle area, 167–
168

Flat bones. *See* Pelvis; Ribs
Flatfoot
    rigid, 88
    spastic, peroneal, 88
Flatworm infestation, lungs in,
        840–841
Fluid accumulation
    in ascites, 438–439
    in pancreatitis, acute, 445
    in pleural space. *See* Pleura,
        effusions
Flukes, lung disorders from, 840–
        841
Fluorescence, 4
Fluorine intoxication, bone changes
        in, 247–248
Fluoroscopes, 7–8
    and photofluorography, 7
Fluoroscopy
    of aorta, 980
    of chest, 742–743
    of colon, 597–598
    of esophagus, 489
    of fractures, 129–130
    of heart, 971–972
    and image intensification, 8
    in pericardial effusions, 1039
    precautions with, 12, 130
    of small intestine, 571
    of stomach, 516
Foot conditions. *See* Feet
Foramen ovale patency
    in pulmonary stenosis with atrial
        septal defect, 986
    in tetralogy of Fallot, 985
Forearm, fractures of, 157
Foreign bodies
    in bladder, 709–710
    in esophagus, 509–510
    in eye, 1048–1049
    in gastrointestinal tract, 441–442
    in paranasal sinuses, 1069
    in stomach, 539–540
    in vagina, 736
Forestier's disease, 282
Fractures, 128–170
    of ankle, 165–166
    of astragalus, 167
    avulsion, 131
    in battered child syndrome, 169
    Bennett, 156
    buckling, 133–134
    of calcaneus, 166–167
    calcification after, 138
    chip, 131
    of clavicle, 161
    closed, 130
    Colles, 154–155
    comminuted, 132
        vertebral, 151–152

Fractures (*continued*)
    complete, noncomminuted, 130–
        131
    compound, 130
    compression, 133
        vertebral, 150–151
        differential diagnosis of,
            268–269
    and congenital indifference to
        pain, 169–170
    corner, 131
    cough, 162
    crush, 132
    in Cushing's syndrome, 108
    and decalcification of fragment
        ends, 140
    differentiation from anomalous
        bones, 66
    distraction of fragments in, 143
    and disuse osteoporosis, 105,
        144–145
    eburnation of fragments in, 144
    of elbow, 158–159
    endosteal callus in, 141
    epiphyseal, 134–135
    of facial bones, 1092–1097
    fatigue, 136–137
        in foot, 136–137
        in ribs, 161, 162
    of femur
        condylar, 164
        at upper end, 162–164
    in fibrous dysplasia, 53
    flake fractures in ankle area,
        167–168
    fluoroscopy of, 129–130
    of foot, 165–169
    of forearm, 157
    and granulation tissue formation,
        138
    greenstick, 132–133
    of hand and wrist, 154–157
    of humerus, 161
        supracondylar, 158–159
    in hyperparathyroidism, 121
    impacted, 133
    incomplete, 132–134
    infected, 145
    and infarctions, 133
    and ischemic necrosis, 242–244
    of knee, 164–165
    late joint changes in, 145
    of malleolus, 165–166
    mandibular, 1097
    maxillary, 1093–1095
    of metatarsals, 168–169
    Monteggia, 157
    motion between fragments of,
        144
    multiple, 131

Fractures (*continued*)
    of nasal bones, 1092–1093
    nonunion of, 142–144
        roentgen evidence of, 143–144
    oblique, 130
    occult, 129
    open, 130
    orbital, 1095–1097
    in osteogenesis imperfecta, 45,
        46
    osteoid callus in, 138, 139
    in osteopetrosis, 46, 47
    in Paget's disease, 252
    of paranasal sinuses, 1069
    of patella, 165
    pathologic, 135–136
    of pelvis, 162
    penetrating, 134
    periosteal callus in, 140–141
        absence of, 144
    in postmenopausal osteoporosis,
        106
    pseudarthrosis in, 144
    pseudofractures, 136
    in pycnodysostosis, 49
    from radiation, 250
    and reformation of trabecular
        bone, 141–142
    of ribs, 161–162
    in rickets, infantile, 112
    roentgenograms of, 128–129
    of scapula, 161
    in shoulder area, 161
    of skull, 145–149
    smoothness of fragment ends in,
        143
    spiral, 130
    of sternum, 161
    and Sudeck's atrophy, 144–145
    in syphilitic osteomyelitis, 184
    of tarsus, 166–168
    of temporal bone, 1075
    terminology in, 129
    of tibia, at upper end, 165
    transverse, 130
    union of, 137–142
        delayed, 142–144
        roentgen evidence of, 138–142
    vertebral, 149–152
    zygomatic, 1095
Fragilitas ossium congenita, 45–46
Friedländer's pneumonia, 783
Frontal bone, hyperostosis of, 352
Frontal lobe, glioblastoma multi-
        forme of, 363
Frontal sinus, 1058
Fundus of stomach, 518–520
Fungus infections
    of bone, 181–182
        differential diagnosis of, 180

Fungus infections (*continued*)
of lungs, 826–838
and alveolar proteinosis, 936–937
mediastinal lymph nodes in, 952
of spine, 269
Funnel chest, 772–773, 1030
Furadantoin sensitivity, pulmonary changes in, 923–924
Fusion
cervico-occipital, 76, 80–81
congenital synostosis, 86–88, 91
of cranial sutures, premature, 71–75
kidney anomalies in, 658–659
of vertebrae, 80–81
in Klippel-Feil syndrome, 81, 95

Gallbladder, 466–486
absence of, 481
adenoma of, 478
adenomyoma of, 478
adenomyomatosis of, 478, 479
adhesions in, 479
calcifications in wall of, 466–467
carcinoma of, 478–479
cholangiography of, 481–486
cholecystography of, 470–481
in choledochal cyst, 481
cholesterol polyp of, 477, 478
cholesterolosis of, 477
congenital anomalies of, 480–481
double, 480
and duodenal lesions, 470
emphysematous cholecystitis, 322, 469
fixed defects in, 477–479
gallstones, 467–468
See also Gallstones
gas in, 468–469
hourglass, 480
hydrops of, 479
hyperplastic cholecystoses, 478, 479
intrahepatic, 481
left-sided, 480–481
milk-of-calcium, 479–480
nonfunctioning, 475–476
normally functioning
with stones, 474–475
without stones, 472–473
papilloma of, 478
phrygian cap, 480
porcelain, 467
Rokitansky-Aschoff sinuses of, 479

Gallbladder (*continued*)
sclerosing cholangitis, 481
scout roentgenograms of, 466–469
and stomach lesions, 470
subnormally functioning, 476–477
Gallstones, 467–468
in Cooley's anemia, 256
differential diagnosis of, 451, 668
in intestines, 430
and nonfunctioning gallbladder, 475
and normally functioning gallbladder, 474–475
in sickle cell anemia, 258
small intestine obstruction from, 417–418
Ganglion cells, absence of, 606
Ganglioneuroma
adrenal, 712
of mediastinum, 953–954
Gangrene, gas, 321–322
Gardner's syndrome, 616
differential diagnosis of, 582
and osteoma of jaw, 1088
paranasal sinuses in, 1067–1068
Gargoylism, 42–44
See also Hurler's disease
Garre's sclerosing osteitis, 177–178
Gas
in abscess cavity, subdiaphragmatic, 441
bacillus infections, 321–322
in biliary ducts, 468–469
in duodenum, resembling gallstones, 474–475
in fetal circulatory system, 723–724
in gallbladder, 468–469
in gastrointestinal tract, 413–414
intramural, 422, 428, 442–443
injected into fallopian tubes, and pneumoperitoneum, 436
in joints, 300
in peritoneal cavity, 434–438
in portal veins, 443, 456–458, 469
in mesenteric vascular occlusion, 592
in necrotizing enterocolitis, 631
in soft tissues, 321–322
in stomach wall, 547
Gases, irritant, affecting lungs, 861–862
Gastrectomy
partial, 548
total, 648
Gastric conditions. *See* Stomach

Gastrin, in achalasia, 505
Gastritis, 536–539
antral, 538
atrophic, chronic, 536
chemical, 538–539
emphysematous, 547
hypertrophic, chronic, 536
mucosal folds in, 536–537
Gastrocolic fistula, 549–550
Gastroenterostomy, posterior, 547–548
Gastroesophageal junction, 493, 519, 543
Gastrografin, in gastrointestinal tract examination, 487, 515
in small intestine studies, 571
Gastrointestinal tract
appendix, 636–641
carcinoma of, calcification in, 433
colon, 596–641
duodenum, 553–568
enteroliths, 430
esophagus, 487–513
examination of, 487–489
with barium sulfate, 414, 487
with water-soluble iodinated compounds, 487
fecaliths, appendiceal, 430, 637
foreign bodies in, 441–442
gas accumulations in, 413–414
intramural, 422, 428, 442–443
gastrocolic fistula, 549–550
hemorrhage in
abdominal arteriography in, 517
and detection of duodenal ulcer, 559
in hiatal hernia, 545
mesenteric cysts, 463–464
mesenteric vascular occlusion, acute, 427–428
obstruction in
of colon, 422–425
of small intestine, 414–422
See also Ileus
pneumatosis cystoides intestinalis, 435–436, 442, 547
rupture of, and pneumoperitoneum, 434–435
sentinel loops in, 427
small intestine, 569–594
See also Small intestine
stomach, 515–551
volvulus
of cecum, 424–425
of sigmoid colon, 421, 424
Gaucher's cells, 222

Gaucher's disease, 931
  bone changes in, 222
  epiphyseal ischemic necrosis in,
    241
Genetic effects of radiation, 10–11
Genitography, 737
Genitourinary tract. See Gynecol-
    ogy; Urinary tract
Geophagia, 442
Geotrichosis, lungs in, 836–837
Ghon tubercle, 811
Giant cell tumor
  of bone, 198–201
    subperiosteal, 197–198
  of joints, 290–291
Giantism. See Gigantism
Giardiasis
  differential diagnosis of, 593
  of small intestine, 582
Gigantism, 26
  from pituitary adenoma, 369
  teeth in, 1083
Glioblastoma multiforme, 362–364
  calcification in, 351
  ventricular system in, 358
Gliomas, 362–366, 372
  calcification in, 351
  optic nerve in, 371, 1053
Glomus of choroid plexus, 341–342
  calcified, displacement of, 342,
    355
Glomus jugulare tumor, 1076
Glomus tympanicum, 1076
Goiter, intrathoracic, 958
Goldenhaar's syndrome, 75–76
Gonadal aplasia, 101
Gonadal secretions, deficiency of,
    26
Goodpasture's syndrome, lungs in,
    921
Gout
  and calcification of articular
    cartilage, 294
  chalk, 314
Gouty arthritis, 283–285
Granulation tissue formation
  dental, periapical, 1081
  after fractures, 138
Granuloma
  dental, periapical, 1081
  eosinophilic
    of bone, 224–225, 226
      vertebra plana in, 226, 240
    of lungs, 931–932
    of stomach, 535
    teeth in, 1085
  midline lethal, 1068–1069
    and Wegener's granulomatosis,
      927, 1069

Granuloma (continued)
  oil or lipid, 936
Granulomatosis
  beryllium, chronic, 856–857
  Wegener
    lungs in, 927
    and midline lethal granuloma,
      927, 1069
Granulomatous colitis, 579, 626–
    628
Granulomatous diseases, chronic,
    171
  in childhood, 797
Granulosa cell tumor of ovary,
    bone growth in, 26
Greenstick fractures, 132–133
Greig's syndrome, 75, 1048
Growth disturbances, 15–27
Growth lines in bone, in thalas-
    semia, 254
Growth plate, 16, 18, 28
Gynecography, 732
Gynecology, 731–737
  calcifications in pelvic area, 731
  cysts and tumors, pelvic, 731–
    734
  genitography, 737
  hysterosalpingography, 734–736
  vagina, 736–737
  vaginography, 737
  See also Ovary; Uterus

Hallermann-Streiff syndrome, 1085
Halo sign, in fetal death, 724–725
Hamartoma
  of heart, 1032
  of kidney, 682, 693
  of lung, 899–900
Hamman-Rich syndrome, 928–930
Hampton's line, in gastric ulcer,
    522
Hand
  accessory bones in, 69–70
  in achondroplasia, 37
  in acromegaly, 25
  in Apert's syndrome, 75
  in cleidocranial dysostosis, 61
  clubbing of digits in, 298
  degenerative joint disease of
    fingers, 279–280
  in diastrophic dwarfism, 34
  dystrophy of nails, and hered-
    itary arthrodysplasia, 96
  in enchondromatosis, 32
  fractures of, 154–157
    Bennett's, 156
    Colles, 154

Hand (continued)
  fractures of (continued)
    lunate and retrolunar, 156
    navicular, 155–156
  in hyperparathyroidism, 120
  Kirner's deformity of, 93
  in Marfan's syndrome, 60
  in Morquio's disease, 41
  in pseudohypoparathyroidism,
    125
  in pycnodysostosis, 49
  rheumatoid arthritis of, 270
  in sarcoidosis, 189
Hand-foot syndrome, in sickle cell
    anemia, 244, 257
Hand-Schüller-Christian disease,
    931
  bone lesions in, 223–226
  vertebra plana in, 240
Haustra of colon, 602–603
Hazards of radiation, 5–6, 10–12
Heart, 974–979
  in adults, 974–979
    lateral projection of, 979
    left anterior oblique projection
      of, 975
    posteroanterior projection of,
      974–975
    right anterior oblique projec-
      tion of, 975
  in beriberi, 1031
  congenital disease of, 983–1010
    classification of, 984
    cyanotic, 984–994
    noncyanotic, 994–1010
    dextrocardia, 1010
  enlargement of, 981–983
    general, 981
    left atrial, 983
    left ventricular, 981–982
    right atrial, 983
    right ventricular, 982
  examination of, 971–974
  failure, congestive, 1028
  in infancy and childhood, 979
  in kyphoscoliosis, 1030
  metastasis to, 1032
  rotation anomalies of, 1009–
    1010
    classification of, 1009
  shape of
    in atrial septal defect, 997
    in coarctation of aorta, 1007–
      1008
    in patent ductus arteriosus,
      995
    in pulmonic stenosis, 1002
      with atrial septal defect,
        986

Heart (*continued*)
  shape of (*continued*)
    in tetralogy of Fallot, 985–986
    in transposition of great vessels, complete, 988–989
    in tricuspid atresia with pulmonary stenosis, 990
    in ventricular septal defect, 1000
  size of
    in atrial septal defect, 997
    in coarctation of aorta, 1007–1008
    determination of, 973–974
      in childhood, 979
    in patent ductus arteriosus, 995
    in pulmonic stenosis, 1002
      with atrial septal defect, 986
    in tetralogy of Fallot, 985
    in transposition of great vessels, complete, 988
    in tricuspid atresia with pulmonary stenosis, 990
    in ventricular septal defect, 1000
    See also Heart, enlargement of
  in thoracic deformities, 1030
  in thyroid disease, 1031–1032
  trauma of, 1032
  tumors of, 1032
Heberden's nodes, 278, 279
Heel-pad thickness, measurement of, 25
Helminthiasis, lungs in, 840–841
Hemangioblastoma, intracranial, 372–373
Hemangioendothelioma of bone, malignant, 213
Hemangioma
  of bone, 201
  cavernous, 324
    of liver, 455, 458
    of spinal cord, 404
  cerebral, capillary and venous, 348
  of diaphragm, 966
  intraorbital, 1052
  of jaw, 1089
  of joints, 293
  of kidney, 693
  of lungs, 900
  of mastoids, 1076
  mediastinal, 962
  of paranasal sinuses, 1066
  of small intestine, 575
  of spinal cord, 404
  of trachea, 777–778

Hemangiopericytoma, of lungs, 900
Hematoma
  in aortic aneurysm, traumatic, 1035
  calcified, 310
  of duodenum, intramural, 567–568
  epidural, 380–381
    in skull fractures, 149
  intracerebral, calcified, 345
  mediastinal, 963
  placental, 730
  subdural, 377–379
    acute, 379
    arteriography in, 379
    bilateral, 378
    calcified, 345
    chronic, 379
    encephalography and ventriculography in, 378–379
    pineal gland displacement in, 355
    in skull fractures, 149
    unilateral, 379
  subperiosteal, ossifying, differential diagnosis of, 209
Hematopoiesis, extramedullary, mediastinal mass with, 962
Hemivertebra, 81–82
Hemochromatosis
  liver density in, 456
  spleen density in, 459
Hemophilia
  arthropathy in, 288
  pseudotumor of, 288
Hemophilus influenzae, pneumonia from, 786
Hemoptysis
  bronchography in, 744
  lung changes after, 921
Hemorrhage, 306–307
  in colon, intramural, 632
  gastrointestinal
    abdominal arteriography in, 517
    and detection of duodenal ulcer, 559
    in hiatal hernia, 545
  orbital, 1052
  renal and perirenal, 679
Hemosiderosis, pulmonary, 920–921
  in mitral stenosis, 1020
Hepatic artery
  catheterization of, in duodenal arteriography, 553
  opacification of, 457
Hepatoma, 455, 458

Hernia
  in Bochdalek foramen, 967
  colon affected by, 632–633
  diaphragmatic, 966–967
  hiatal, 543–546, 966
    complications of, 545–546
    and esophagitis, 503, 504, 546
    and hiatal insufficiency, 544–545
    paraesophageal, 543
    short esophagus type, 544
    sliding, 543
    and thoracic stomach, 544
  of intervertebral disc, posterior, 392–398
  intra-abdominal, 593–594
  of Morgagni foramen, 966
  differential diagnosis of, 969
Hiatal hernia, 543–546, 966
Hiccough, 964
Hilum enlargement, pulmonary, in carcinoma, 883
Hip
  accessory bones in, 68–69
  degenerative joint disease of, 280
  dislocations of, 164
    congenital, 88–91
      and delayed ossification of femoral epiphysis, 90
      and disruptions of Shenton's line, 90
      increased acetabular angle in, 89–90
      later stages of, 90
      and lateral displacement of femur, 90
    in diastrophic dwarfism, 34
  dysplasia of, 88
    in adult, 90–91
  synovitis of, transient, 233
Hippel-Lindau disease, 373
Hirschsprung's disease, 606–608
  differential diagnosis of, 419
Histiocytosis X
  bone lesions in, 223–226
  lungs in, 931–932
  teeth in, 1085
Histoplasmosis
  liver calcification in, 456
  lungs in, 829–832
  lymph nodes in, mediastinal, 952
  mediastinal involvement in, 832, 952
  and mediastinitis, 950
  of small intestine, and hypoproteinemia, 591
  and spleen calcification, 430
Hodgkin's disease
  bone lesions in, 219–220

Hodgkin's disease (*continued*)
  differential diagnosis of, 843, 844
  heart in, 1032
  lungs in, 896
  mediastinal lymph nodes in, 953
  pericardium in, 1040
  small intestine in, 579
  stomach in, 536
Homocystinuria, 60
Honeycomb lungs, 806
Horseshoe kidney, 658
Hourglass gallbladder, 480
Humerus
  dislocations of, 159–160
  fractures of, 161
    supracondylar, 158–159
  supracondylar process of, 91–92
Hunter's syndrome, 44
Hurler's disease, 42–44
  flat bones in, 44
  long bones in, 43–44
  short tubular bones in, 44
  skull in, 43
  vertebrae in, 44
Hutchinson-Gilford syndrome, 97
Hyaline membrane disease of new-
      born, 914–915
Hydatid cysts. *See* Echinococcus
      cyst
Hydatid mole, uterus in, 732
Hydramnios, diagnosis of, 726
Hydrocarbons, pneumonitis from,
      860–861
Hydrocephalus, 381–382
  acquired, 381
  congenital, 382
  external, 380, 381
  ex vacuo, 381
Hydrocolpos, 737
Hydronephrosis, 664–666
  acquired, 665–666
  congenital, 665
  nonobstructive, 664–665
  urography in, 665
Hydrops
  fetal, diagnosis of, 726
  of gallbladder, 479
Hygroma
  cystic, mediastinal, 958
  subdural, 380
Hypaque
  in excretory urography, 646
  in gastrointestinal tract examina-
      tion, 487, 515
Hypernephroma, 695–697
  differential diagnosis of, 693,
      695–696
Hyperostosis
  calvariae diffusa, 352

Hyperostosis (*continued*)
  corticalis
    deformans juvenilis, 118
    generalisata, 118
    infantile, 249–250
  frontalis interna, 352
  in meningiomas, 357, 367
Hyperplasia
  epiphyseal, 31
    cone-shaped epiphyses in, 64
  of face, teeth in, 1084
  fibromuscular, renovascular,
      691–692
  of kidney, 658
  of lymphoid follicles, in small
      intestine, 581–582
  of prostate, 705–706
  pulmonary muscular, 938
Hypersensitivity, pulmonary, and
      occupational diseases,
      858–860
Hypertelorism, 75, 1048
  in metaphyseal dysplasia, 49
  in trigonocephaly, 74
Hypertension, 1025
  in mitral stenosis, 1019, 1020
  pulmonary, 875–879
    classification of, 875
    combined arterial and venous,
      879
    postcapillary, 878–879
    precapillary, 876–878
  renovascular, 689–693
Hypertrophy of heart muscle. *See*
      Heart, enlargement of
Hypochondroplasia, 38
  differential diagnosis of, 37
Hypogonadism, 26
Hypoplasia
  of kidney, 657–658
  of lungs, 773
Hypotelorism, 75, 1048
  in trisomy 21 syndrome, 98
Hysterosalpingography, 734–736

Ileitis, regional, 579–580
  differential diagnosis of, 584, 585
Ileocecal valve, 569, 600
Ileum
  ischemia of, segmental, 592
  obstruction in, 416
  peristalsis in, 570
  regional ileitis, 579–580
    differential diagnosis of, 584,
      585
  See also Small intestine

Ileus
  adynamic or paralytic, 425–427
    combined with dynamic ileus,
      426
    differential diagnosis of, 416
    and intra-abdominal abscesses,
      439
    in pancreatitis, 445
    with peritonitis, 426
    without peritonitis, 425
  of colon, 422–425
  differential diagnosis of, 426–427
  localized, sentinel loops in, 427,
      444–445
  mechanical
    combined with adynamic ileus,
      426
    differential diagnosis of, 416
  meconium, 418–420, 423
    equivalent of, 420
  in mesenteric vascular occlusion,
      428
  in small intestine, acute, 414–422
    closed-loop, 420–422
    from gallstone, 417–418
    without gas distention, 418
    method of examination in,
      414–415
    simple, 415–420
    from tumors, 576
Iliac angle, 90
Iliac arteries, calcification in, 429
Iliac bones, osteitis of, 296–297
Iliac index, 98
Iliac horns, in hereditary arthro-
      dysplasia, 96
Image intensification, 8
Immobilization of bone, and dis-
      use osteoporosis, 105, 144
Impacted fractures, 133
Imperforate anus, 419
Inca bone, 70
Incisive foramen, 1080
  cyst of, 1087
Incisurae
  in duodenal ulcers, 558
  in gastric ulcer, 524–525
Infarction
  of bone, in sickle cell anemia,
      244, 257
  of diaphysis, 244–245
  pulmonary, 869–871
  splenic, 460
Infections
  and arthritis, 262–269
  of bone, 171–190
  of fractures, 145
Influenza, and pneumonia, 789–790

Infractions, 133
  Kohler-Freiberg, 237
Innominate artery, anomalous position of, 1011–1012
Intensification of fluoroscopic image, 8
Intercostal spaces, 755
Interorbital distances, measurement of, 1050–1051
Interstitial diseases
  calcinosis, 312–314
  in chest, 754
Intestines. *See* Gastrointestinal tract
Intracranial diseases, 337–385
  abscess of brain, 381
    pineal gland displacement in, 355
  aneurysms, 347–348
    angiography in, 359
  angiomas, capillary and venous, 348
  arachnoiditis, adhesive, 382–383, 403–404
  arteriosclerosis, 347
  arteriovenous malformations, 348
    angiography in, 359
  atrophy of brain, 376–377
    congenital, 350
  basal ganglia calcification, 350–351
  cyst(s)
    dermoid, 372
    epidermoid, 228–229, 371–372
    of third ventricle, 371
  cysticercosis, 346
  degenerative lesions, 350
  hematoma
    calcified, 345
    epidural, 380–381
    subdural, 377–379
  hydrocephalus, 381–382
  hygroma, subdural, 380
  hyperostosis frontalis interna, 352
  inflammatory lesions, 349–350
  lipomas, 372
  occlusive vascular disease, 383–384
  parasitic lesions, 346–347
  pneumoencephalography in, 357–359, 376
  toxoplasmosis, 346–347
  trichinosis, 346
  tuberous sclerosis, 348–349
  tumors, 353–376
    acoustic neuroma, 374–375
    angiography in, 359–362

Intracranial disease (*continued*)
  tumors (*continued*)
    astrocytoma, 364–365, 372
    calcification of, 351, 355–356
    and changes in cranial bones, 353–357
    chordoma, 79, 229–230, 375
    craniopharyngioma, 370
    and displacement of calcified pineal gland, 340, 354, 355
    ependymoma, 366, 373
    glioblastoma multiforme, 362–364
    gliomas, 362–366, 372
    hemangioblastoma, 372–373
    increased intracranial pressure in, 352–355
    localizing evidence of, 355–357
    medulloblastoma, 373
    meningiomas, 366–368
    metastatic, 375–376
    oligodendroglioma, 365–366
    optic nerve, 371
    pineal gland, 371
    pituitary adenomas, 368–370
    in and near sella, 368–370
    spongioblastoma, polar, 373–374
    subtentorial, 372–375
    supratentorial, 362–372
    ventriculography in, 357–359
Intracranial pressure, increased, 352–355
Intussusception
  of appendiceal mucocele, 639
  in colonic carcinoma, 611–612
  jejunal, postoperative, 550–551
  of small intestine, 589–590
  in sprue, transient, 587
Iodinated compounds, water-soluble, for gastrointestinal tract examination, 487, 515
  in small intestine studies, 571–572
Iodipamide methylglucamine, in cholangiography, 475, 477, 483
Iodized oil
  in bronchography, 745
    reactions to, 747
  for esophageal examination, 489, 495
Iopanoic acid. *See* Telepaque
Ipodate sodium, in cholecystography, 471, 473

Iron deficiency anemia, bone changes in, 258
Ischemia, segmental
  of colon, 631–632
  of small intestine, 592
Ischemic necrosis of bone, 232–245
  in astragalus, 244
    in fractures, 167
  in calcaneal apophysis, 238
  epiphyseal
    in adults, 241–244
    in children, 232–241
    secondary to other disease, 240–241
  and epiphyseolysis, 239–240
  at femoral head, 242–243
    differential diagnosis of, 222
  and osteochondritis dissecans, 238–239
  in second metatarsal head, 237
  in tarsal scaphoid, 236
  in tibial tuberosity, 236–237
  in vertebral epiphyses, 237
Isotopes, radioactive, for placental localization, 729

Jaws
  in acromegaly, 24
  ameloblastoma of, 1086–1087
  carcinoma of, 1089
  cementoma of, 1087, 1088
  in cherubism, 55, 1088
  in cretinism, 21
  cysts of
    in basal cell nevus syndrome, 1086
    dental, 1085–1086
    follicular, 1085
    nonodontogenic, 1087–1088
    radicular, 1080, 1081, 1085
    solitary, of mandible, 1087
  fibroma of
    odontogenic, 1087
    ossifying, 1088
  fibrous dysplasia of, 1088
    hereditary, 55
  hemangioma of, 1089
  incisive foramen of, 1080
    cyst of, 1087
  mandible, 1079
  maxilla, 1080
  odontoma, compound, 1087
  osteoid osteoma of, 1089
  osteoma of, 1088
  sarcoma of, osteogenic, 1089

Jaws (*continued*)
  temporomandibular articulation,
    1090
  torus mandibularis, 1088
  tumors of
    dental, 1086–1087
    giant cell, 1088
    nonodontogenic, 1087–1088
Jejunum
  diverticulosis of, 591
  enteritis of, 580–581
  intussusception of, postoperative,
    550–551
  ischemia of, segmental, 592
  obstruction in, 416
  peristalsis in, 569
  ulcer of, postoperative, 549
  See also Small intestine
Joint diseases, 261–301
  arthritis. *See* Arthritis
  arthrography in, 300–301
  in caisson disease, 299–300
  calcification in, 317–318
    of articular cartilages, 294
    of intervertebral discs, in
      childhood, 297–298
  classification of, 261
  cysts, 296
  degenerative, 277–283
    of fingers, 278, 279–280
    of hip, 280
    of knee, 280–281
    roentgen findings in, 278–279
    of spine, 281–282
    and traumatic arthritis, 282–
      283
  hemophiliac arthropathy, 288
  hip synovitis, transient, 233
  hypertrophic osteoarthropathy,
    298–299
  late changes after fractures, 145
  loose bodies, 279, 292, 293
  neurotrophic arthropathy, 285–
    287
  in ochronosis, 293–294
  osteitis condensans ilii and pubii,
    296–297
  periarticular disease, 287–288
  pigmented villonodular syno-
    vitis, 290
  protrusion of acetabulum, 115,
    272, 297
  Reiter's disease, 294
  tumors, 288–293
    cartilaginous, 291–292
    giant cell and xanthomatous,
      290–291
    hemangioma, 293
    synovioma, 289–290
  and vacuum phenomenon, 300

Kartagener's triad, 802
Kerkring, folds of, 553, 569
Kerley's lines, 866–867
  in congestive heart failure, 1028
  in mitral stenosis, 1019
Kerosene, pneumonitis from, 860–
  861
Kidneys, 412
  abscess of, 670–671
    perirenal, 671–672
  anatomy of, 650–651
  angiography, renal, 648
  angiomyolipoma of, 682, 693
    in tuberous sclerosis, 682
  anomalies of, 655–660
  arterial and venous impressions
    in 654–655
  backflow in, 653–654
    pyelointerstitial, 654
    pyelotubular, 654
  calculi in, 666–669
    See also Urinary tract, calculi
  carbuncle of, 670
  carcinoma of, calcification in,
    433
  crossed ectopy of, 658–659
  cyst puncture, percutaneous, 697
  cystic disease, 679–688
    calcification in, 431
    classification of, 680
    cortical, 681–683
    differential diagnosis of, 695–
      969
    echinococcal, 688
    extraparenchymal, 686–687
    medullary, 683–686
    multilocular, 683
    multiple, 679–680
    parapelvic, 686–687
    perinephric, 687
    pyelogenic or calycine, 686
    simple, 682–683
    in tuberous sclerosis, 681–682
    See also Kidneys, polycystic
      disease
  duplication of pelvis, 660–661
  dysplasia of, 679–680
  enlargement of, and stomach dis-
    placement, 542
  fusion anomalies, 658–659
  horseshoe, 658
  hydronephrosis, 664–666
  hypernephroma, 695–697
    differential diagnosis of, 693,
      695–696
  hyperplasia of, 658
  in hypophosphatemic vitamin D-
    refractory rickets, 115
  hypoplasia of, 657–658
  in leukemia, 700

Kidneys (*continued*)
  lipomatosis of renal sinus, 693–
    694
  in lymphoma, malignant, 700–
    701
  medullary sponge kidney, 683–
    684
  necrosis of
    bilateral cortical, 675–676
    papillary, 674–675
  nephrocalcinosis, 119, 669–670
  nephronophthisis, 684–686
  nephroptosis, 660
  nephrotomography, 648–649
  osteodystrophy, renal, 121, 122–
    124
  in polyarteritis nodosa, 688
  polycystic disease, 680–681
    adult, 680–681
    differential diagnosis of, 693
    infantile, 680
  position anomalies, 659–660
  pseudotumor of, 694–695
  "putty kidney" formation, 677
  pyelitis of pregnancy, 673–674
  pyelonephritis
    acute, 670
    chronic, 672
    xanthogranulomatous, 673
  renovascular hypertension, 689–
    693
    in atherosclerosis, 691
    in fibromuscular dysplasia,
      691–692
  sarcoma of, 699–700
  single, 657
  squamous metaplasia of pelvis,
    699
  supernumerary, 657
  trauma of, 678–679
  in trisomy 18 syndrome, 100–101
  tuberculosis of, 676–678
    differential diagnosis of, 678
    pathology of, 676–677
    roentgen findings in, 677–678
  tumors of, 693–701
    benign, 693–695
    malignant, 695–701
    in pelvis, 698–699
  vascular abnormalities of, 688–
    693
    See also Renal arteries
  Wilms' tumor, 698
    differential diagnosis of, 712
Kienbock's malacia, 244
Kirner's deformity, 93
Klebsiella pneumonia, 783
Kleeblattschädel syndrome, 74
Klippel-Feil syndrome, 81
  and Sprengel's deformity, 95

Knee
accessory bones in, 68
cysts of semilunar cartilage, 296
degenerative joint disease of, 280–281
fractures of, 164–165
Köhler's disease, 236
Köhler-Freiberg infraction, 237
Kümmell's disease, 152–153, 244
Kyphoscoliosis, heart in, 1030
Kyphosis, congenital, 773

Lacrimal gland, tumors of, 1055
Lacrimal passages, 1055
Lactase deficiency, in small intestine, 593
Lacuna skull, 71
Laminagraphy, 747
Laparotomy, pneumoperitoneum after, 436
Laryngography, 747
Lead poisoning, bone changes in, 245–246
Leather-bottle stomach, 529
Legg-Calvé-Perthes disease, 21, 232
Leiomyoma
of kidney, 693
of lungs, 900
of small intestine, 575, 576–577
of stomach, 533
of uterus, 732
calcified, 432
differential diagnosis of, 704
Leiomyosarcoma, of uterus, 732
Leontiasis ossea, 49, 54
Leprosy, bone changes in, 190
Leptospirosis, lungs in, 838
Letterer-Siwe disease, 931
bone lesions in, 223
Leukemia
acute, bone changes in, 220–221
chronic myeloid, bone changes in, 221
kidney in, 700
lungs in, 896
from radiation, 10
Leukoplakia, of renal pelvis, 699
Ligamentum arteriosum, left, with right aortic arch, 1013
Limbus vertebra, 86
Lindau's disease, 372
Linea aspera, of femur, 317
Lines
Chamberlain, 81
extraperitoneal fat line, 412
growth, in thalassemia, 254
Hampton, in gastric ulcer, 522
Kerley, 866–867, 1019, 1028

Lines (continued)
McGregor, 81
mediastinal, anterior, 759
Perkins, 90
pleural, 759
Shenton, disruption of, 90
Voorhoeve, 53
Linitis plastica, 529
Lipid pneumonia, 934–936
Lipomas
of cecum, 613
of colon, 618
of diaphragm, 966
of duodenum, 563
of heart, 1032
intracranial, 372
of kidney, 693
of lungs, 900
mediastinal, 962
retroperitoneal, 464
of small intestine, 578
of spine, 406
of stomach, 533
subcutaneous, 323
Lipomatosis
mediastinal, from steroids, 961
of renal sinus, 693–694
Lipomucopolysaccharidosis, 44
Liposarcoma
retroperitoneal, 464
of soft tissues, 323
Lissencephaly, 350
Lithopedion, 736
Liver, 411–412, 454–458
abscess of, 456
angiography of, 457–458
calcification in, 430, 456
cysts of, calcification in, 431
enlargement of, stomach displacement by, 542
and gas in portal veins, 456–458, 469
increased density of, 456
intrahepatic gallbladder, 481
portal veins. See Portal veins
Riedel's lobe of, 454
size of, 455
splenoportography of, 457, 461–462
tumors of, 455–456
Loeffler's syndrome, lungs in, 922–923
Long bones
in achondroplasia, 36
in acromegaly, 25
in epiphyseal dysplasia, multiple, 29
in Hurler's disease, 43–44
in Morquio's disease, 41
in Ollier's disease, 32

Long bones (continued)
in osteogenesis imperfecta, 45–46
in Paget's disease, 251–252
Loose bodies in joints, 293
in degenerative diseases, 279
in osteochondromatosis, 292
Looser zones, 136
in rickets, 112, 117
Lorain type of pituitary dwarfism, 23
Lowe's disease, 115
Lückenschädel, 71
Lumbar spine, herniation of intervertebral discs in, 392
Lungs, 761–768
abscess of, 791–794
accessory lobes in, 774–775
in achalasia, 505–506
actinomycosis of, 826–827
acute infections of, 780–797
classification of, 780
adenomatoid malformation of, cystic, 777
in advancing age, 771
in agammaglobulinemia, 933–934
agenesis of, 773
in allergic states, 921–924
in amebiasis, 838
in amyloidosis, 930–931
apices of, 766–768
in asbestosis, 849–854
aspergillosis of, 833–836
in asthma, 921–922
atelectasis of, 910–914
in bagassosis, 858
in baritosis, 858
bauxite fibrosis of, 854–855
in berylliosis, 856–857
biopsy of, 752–753
blastomycosis of, 832–833
in bronchiolar carcinoma, 882, 893–895
in brucellosis, 785
in byssinosis, 858–859
calcification in, 430
carcinoma of, 881–892
apical density in, 885–887
atelectasis in, 883
bronchography in, 744
cavity in, solitary, 887
diaphragmatic elevation in, 891
differential diagnosis of, 794, 796
emphysema in, local, 883–885
general considerations in, 891–892
hilum enlargement in, unilateral, 883

Lungs (*continued*)
  carcinoma of (*continued*)
    mediastinal widening in, 885
    metastasis of, 890–891
    parenchymal mass in, 889
    pleural effusion in, 890
    pleural mass in, 891
    pneumonitis in, 887–889
    ribs in, 885, 891
    roentgen findings in, 882–890
    solitary pulmonary nodule in, 889–890
    tomography in, 749
    and tuberculosis, 810, 892
  cavitation of. *See* Cavitation of lungs
  chemical agents causing diseases in, 860–863
  in childhood, 770
  cholesterol type of chronic pneumonitis, 934
  circulatory disturbances in, 866–879
  in coal worker's pneumoconiosis, 855
  coccidioidomycosis of, 827–829
  in collagen diseases, 924–928
  in cor pulmonale, 1028–1030
  cryptococcosis of, 832
  cystic disease of, 777, 805–806
    congenital, 803–805
  in cysticercosis, 840
  in diatomite pneumoconiosis, 855–856
  drug sensitivity affecting, 923–924
  in dysautonomia, familial, 933
  in echinococcosis, 840
  edema of, 866–868
    alveolar, 867–868
    interstitial, 866–867
  embolism, 869–874
    fat, posttraumatic, 874
    with infarction, 869–871
    without infarction, 871–873
  emphysema, 902–910
    See also Emphysema
  in eosinophilia, tropical, 841
  farmer's lung, 859–860
  fibrosis of
    in amyloidosis, 931
    in asbestosis, 853–854
    from bauxite, 854–855
    in Hamman-Rich syndrome, 928–930
    idiopathic, 928
    and pulmonary hypertension, 879
    from radiation, 863
    in silicotuberculosis, 849

Lungs (*continued*)
  fissures of, 761
    absence of, 775
  fungal diseases of, 826–838
    and alveolar proteinosis, 936–937
    mediastinal lymph nodes in, 952
  gases affecting, irritant, 861–862
  geotrichosis of, 836–837
  in Goodpasture's syndrome, 921
  in granulomatous disease of childhood, chronic, 797
  hamartoma of, 899–900
  in Hamman-Rich syndrome, 928–930
  in heart failure, congestive, 1028
  after hemoptysis, 921
  hemosiderosis of, 920–921
    in mitral stenosis, 1020
  in histiocytosis X, 931–932
  histoplasmosis of, 829–832
  honeycomb, 806
  hyaline membrane disease, 914–915
  in hydrocarbon pneumonitis, 860–861
  hyperlucent, unilateral, 907
  hypertension in, 875–879
  hypogenesis of, 773
  infarction of, 869–871
    septic, 873
  in leptospirosis, 838
  lipid pneumonia, 934–936
  lobar and segmental anatomy of, 761–762
  in Loeffler's syndrome, 922–923
  in lupus erythematosus, 925–926
  lymphangiectasis, 777
  lymphocytic interstitial pneumonitis, 924
  in maple-bark disease, 860
  metastasis to, 898–899
  microlithiasis, alveolar, 933
  middle lobe syndrome, 794–796
  moniliasis of, 836
  mucormycosis of, 838
  in mucoviscidosis, 796–797
  muscular hyperplasia of, 938
  mycetoma in, 836
  myeloma of, 896
  in near-drowning, 938–939
  in nitrofurantoin sensitivity, 923–924
  nocardiosis of, 827
  nodules in
    in aspergillosis, 834
    in coccidioidomycosis, 829
    in histiocytosis X, 931
    in histoplasmosis, 830

Lungs (*continued*)
  nodules in (*continued*)
    in silicosis, 848
    solitary, in bronchogenic carcinoma, 889–890
    tuberculous, 817
      calcium in, 816
  occupational diseases of, 847–860
  Pancoast tumor of, 885
  in pancreatitis, acute, 445–446
  in paragonimiasis, 840
  penicilliosis of, 837–838
  in pigeon breeder's disease, 860
  pneumatocele, 804–805
  in pneumocystis carinii pneumonia, 839–840
  pneumonia, 780–791
    See also Pneumonia
  pneumothorax, 916–920
  in polyarteritis nodosa, 924–925
  in polycythemia, 933
  in proteinosis, alveolar, 936–937
  protozoal infections, 838–840
  radiation changes in, 863–864
  resection of, 822–824
  respiratory distress in newborn, transient, 915–916
  in rheumatic fever, 925
  rheumatoid disease of, 926–927
  roentgen features of, 762–766
  in roundworm infestation, 841
  in sarcoidosis, 841–845
    differential diagnosis of, 843–845
  sarcoma of, 895–896
  in schistosomiasis, 840–841
  in scleroderma, 926
  sequestration of, 775–777
    extralobar, 776–777
    intralobar, 775–776
  in siderosis, 858
  in silicosis, 847–849
  in silo-filler's disease, 862–863
  spirochetal infections of, 838
  sporotrichosis of, 837
  in stannosis, 858
  in syphilis, 838
  in talcosis, 854
  in toxoplasmosis, 838–839
  tuberculosis, 808–824
    See also Tuberculosis
  in tuberous sclerosis, 932–933
  tumors of
    benign, 899–900
    classification of, 881
    malignant, 881–898
    metastatic, 898–899
  vanishing lung, 907

Lungs (*continued*)
vascularity of
in atrial septal defect, 998
in patent ductus arteriosus, 995
in pulmonic stenosis, 1002
with atrial septal defect, 986
with tricuspid atresia, 991
in tetralogy of Fallot, 985
in transposition of great vessels, complete, 989
in ventricular septal defect, 1000
in Wegener's granulomatosis, 927
in Wilson-Mikity syndrome, 916
Lupus erythematosus
arthritis in, 277
lungs in, 925–926
Lutembacher's syndrome, 998
Lymph nodes
calcification in, 318
differential diagnosis of, 451–452, 704
mediastinal, 756
inflammation of, 951–952
tumors of, 953
mesenteric, calcification of, 428
metastatic enlargement of, and stomach displacement, 543
Lymphangiectasia
intestinal, 588–589
hypoproteinemia in, 591
pulmonary, 777
Lymphangiography, 331–333
Lymphangioma, of mediastinum, 958
Lymphocytic interstitial pneumonitis, 924
Lymphogranuloma venereum, colon in, 632
Lymphoid hyperplasia
in colon, 616–617
in small intestine, 581–582
Lymphomas, malignant
heart in, 1032
kidney in, 700–701
lungs in, 896
mediastinal lymph nodes in, 953
stomach in, 535–536
Lymphosarcoma
of bone, 219
of colon, 618–619
differential diagnosis of, 616
intestinal, and hypoproteinemia, 591
lungs in, 896
mediastinal lymph nodes in, 953
of small intestine, 577–578

Madelung's deformity, 58, 94–95
and Turner's syndrome, 101
Maffuci's syndrome, 32
Magnification of images, 8–9
Malabsorption syndromes, 585–589
differential diagnosis of, 578
and diverticulosis, 591
from parasitic disease, 593
Malacia, Kienbock's, 244
Malleolus, fractures of, 165–166
Malnutrition, and osteoporosis, 109–110
Mammography, 325–326
Mandible, 1079
fractures of, 1097
temporomandibular articulation, 1090
See also Jaws
Mandibulofacial dysostosis, 75–76
teeth in, 1084
Maple-bark disease, 860
Marble bones, 46–48
March foot, 137
Marfan's syndrome, 60
Marie-Strümpell arthritis, 273–275
Maroteaux-Lamy syndrome, 44
Mastocytosis, systemic, 258–259
small intestine in, 582
Mastoiditis
acute, 1072–1073
chronic, 1073
Mastoids, 1069–1077
in acromegaly, 24
acute mastoiditis, 1072–1073
cholesteatoma of, 1073–1074
chronic mastoiditis, 1073
in cretinism, 21
development of, 1071–1072
examination of, 1069–1070
and fractures of temporal bone, 1075
inflammatory diseases of, 1072–1075
in metaphyseal dysplasia, 49
normal, 1070
in osteopetrosis, 47
and petrositis, 1074
postoperative appearance of, 1074–1075
in pycnodysostosis, 49
tumors of, 1076–1077
Maturation, disturbances in, 15–27
Maxilla, 1080
fractures of, 1093–1095
classification of, 1094
See also Jaws
Maxillary sinus, 1057–1058
Maxillonasal dysplasia, 1068
McGregor's line, 81

Measles, and pneumonia, 790
Meckel's diverticulum, 574
Meconium ileus, 418–420, 423
equivalent of, 420
Meconium peritonitis, 419–420
calcification in, fetal, 433–434
Meconium plug syndrome, 420
Mediastinitis
acute, 950
chronic, 950–951
Mediastinum, 756–761, 950–963
acute mediastinitis, 950
in advancing age, 770
anatomic divisions of, 756, 760
in bronchogenic carcinoma, 885
chronic mediastinitis, 950–951
cystic hygroma of, 958
cysts of, 955–958
bronchogenic, 956–957
gastroenteric, 957
neurenteric, 957
pericardial, 957–958
emphysema of, 909
in acute mediastinitis, 950
in emphysema, obstructive, 906
extramedullary hematopoiesis in, 962
hematoma of, 963
in histoplasmosis, 832
inflammatory diseases of, 950–952
intrathoracic meningocele in, 961
intrathoracic thyroid in, 958–960
lipomatosis of, from steroids, 961
lymph nodes of, 756
inflammations of, 951–952
tumors of, 953
lymphoma of, lungs in, 896
miscellaneous masses in, 962–963
parathyroid adenoma in, 960
thymic tumors in, 960–961
tumors of, 952–963
neurogenic, 953–954
teratoid, 954–955
Mediterranean anemia, bone changes in, 253–256
Medullary defects in bone, calcified, 245
Medullary sponge kidney, 683–684
Medulloblastoma, intracranial, 373
Megacolon
congenital, 606–608
functional, 606
organic, 605–606
Megacystis syndrome, 708
Meglumine, in excretory urography, 646
Meigs' syndrome, 734

Melanoma, malignant
  metastasis to small intestine, 579
  pericardium in, 1040
Melorheostosis, 51–52
Menetrier's disease, 537
  hypoproteinemia in, 591
Meningeal arteries, 337–338
Meningeal cysts, 405–406
Meningiomas
  differential diagnosis of, 54
  intracranial, 338, 366–368
    calcification in, 351
    and changes in cranial bones,
      356
    erosion of bone in, 357
    en plaque, 367
    proliferative response in, 357
    vascularity of bone in, 356
    ventricular system in, 358
  optic nerve in, 1053
  of orbit, 1055
  of spinal cord, 400–401
Meningocele
  intrathoracic, 961
  in neurofibromatosis, 56
  sacral, 406
  of skull, 70
Meniscus sign, in gastric ulcer, 526
Menopause, osteoporosis after,
      106–107
Mesenteric artery
  arteriography of, 572, 599
  catheterization of
    in gastrointestinal bleeding,
      517
    in pancreatic angiography, 453
  superior, 553–554
Mesenteric cysts, 463–464
  and stomach displacement, 543
Mesenteric lymph nodes, calcifica-
      tion of, 428
Mesenteric small intestine, 569–594
  See also Small intestine
Mesenteric vascular occlusion, 592
  acute, 427–428
Mesonephron, 656
Mesothelioma
  of pericardium, 1040
  of pleura, 949
Metabolic disorders
  of bone, 104–126
  teeth in, 1083
Metacarpals
  Bennett's fracture of, 156
  pseudoepiphyses for, 92–93
  in Turner's syndrome, 101
Metaphysis, 18, 28
  dysostosis of, 39
    differential diagnosis of, 37

Metaphysis (continued)
  dysostosis of (continued)
    Jansen type of, 39
    Schmidt type of, 39
  dysplasia of, 49
  in rickets, 112
Metaplasia, squamous, of renal
      pelvis, 699
Metastasis
  to bone, 214–217
    mixed form, 216
    osteoblastic, 216
    osteolytic, 215–216
  of bronchogenic carcinoma, 890–
      891
  to heart, 1032
  intracranial, 375–376
  to jaw, 1090
  to lungs, 898–899
  to mastoids, 1077
  to mediastinal lymph nodes, 953
  of osteogenic sarcoma, 207–208
  to paranasal sinuses, 1067
  to pleura, 949–950
  to small intestine, 579
  to spinal cord, 402
Metatarsals
  epiphysis for metatarsal V, 67,
      168–169
  fractures of, 168–169
  ischemic necrosis of second
      metatarsal head, 237
  pseudoepiphyses for, 92–93
Metoclopramide, in small intestine
      studies, 571
  in duodenal examination, 553
Metrocolpos, 737
Meyerding classification of spondy-
      lolisthesis, 83
Microcephaly, 72
Microlithiasis, pulmonary alveolar,
      933
Milk-alkali syndrome, 317
  differential diagnosis of, 321
Milk-of-calcium gallbladder, 479–
      480
Milk-drinker's syndrome, 317
  differential diagnosis of, 321
Milkman's syndrome, 114–115, 136
Mitral valve
  acquired disease of, 1017–1022
  atrial enlargement in diseases of,
      983
  insufficiency of, 1021
    with stenosis, 1021–1022
  stenosis of, 1017–1021
    with atrial septal defect, 998
    with insufficiency, 1021–1022

Mitral valve (continued)
  ventricular enlargement in dis-
      eases of, 982
Mönckeberg arteriosclerosis, 307
  intracranial, 347
Mongolism, 98
Moniliasis, lungs in, 836
Monteggia fracture, 157
Morgagni foramen, hernia in, 966
  differential diagnosis of, 969
Morgagni syndrome, 352
Morquio's disease, 21, 40–42
  differential diagnosis of, 31, 32,
      44
  flat bones in, 41
  long bones in, 41
  short tubular bones in, 41
  vertebrae in, 40–41
Mosaic skull, 45
Moulage sign, in sprue, 587
Mucocele
  of appendix, 638–639
    calcification in, 431
    rupture of, and pseudomyxoma
      peritonei, 462–463
  of paranasal sinuses, 1064
Mucoperiosteum, 1057
Mucopolysaccharidoses, 40–44
Mucormycosis, lungs in, 838
Mucosal folds of stomach, 519–520
Mucoviscidosis, lungs in, 796–797
Müller experiment, 743, 1016
Muscular dystrophies, 304–306
Muscular paralysis, pseudohyper-
      trophic, 304
Myasthenia gravis
  swallowing difficulty in, 513
  thymic tumor with, 960–961
Mycetoma, 836
Mycobacteria, atypical, 821–822
Mycobacterium tuberculosis, 808
Mycoplasma pneumoniae, 787–789
Mycotic infections. See Fungus in-
      fections
Myelofibrosis
  differential diagnosis of, 258, 259
  with osteosclerosis, 221–222
Myelography, 386–392
  in meningioma, 401
  in neurofibroma, 399–400
  oil, 387–392
    artifacts in, 390–392
    normal results with, 389–390
    technique of, 387–389
  in posterior herniation of inter-
      vertebral disc, 395–397
  postoperative, 398
Myeloma
  of lung, 896

Myeloma (*continued*)
multiple, 217–218
differential diagnosis of, 215
jaw lesions in, 1090
solitary, 218–219
Myocardiopathy, 1030–1031
Myositis ossificans
differential diagnosis of, 209
progressive, 310, 318
traumatic, 310
Myxoma, atrial, 1032

Nails
dystrophy of, and hereditary
arthrodysplasia, 96
exostosis, subungual, 192
Nasal bone fractures, 1092–1093
Nasal sinuses. *See* Sinuses, paranasal
Navicular bone of hand, fractured,
155–156
Necrosis
of bone. *See* Ischemic necrosis of
bone
intestinal
intramural gas in, 428, 442–
443
and pneumatosis intestinalis,
592
renal
bilateral cortical, 675–676
papillary, 674–675
Necrotizing enterocolitis, 631
Nemathelminth infestation, lungs
in, 841
Neostigmine, in small intestine
studies, 571
Nephrocalcinosis, 669–670
in hyperparathyroidism, 119
in osteodystrophy, renal, 123
Nephronophthisis, 684–686
Nephroptosis, 660
Nephrotomography, 648–649
Neural arch defects, 82–83
Neurenteric cyst, mediastinal, 957
Neuroblastoma
abdominal, calcified, 432–433
adrenal, 712
metastasis to bone, 216–217
differential diagnosis of, 220
Neurofibroma
bone lesions in, 226–227
of lungs, 900
of mediastinum, 953
optic foramen in, 371
of orbit, 1055
of paranasal sinuses, 1065
of spinal cord, 398–400

Neurofibroma (*continued*)
of stomach, 533
Neurofibromatosis, 55–58, 322–323
and intrathoracic meningocele,
961
optic nerve in, 1053
pseudarthrosis in, 57–58
skeletal lesions in, 56–57
Neurogenic bladder, 707–708
Neuroma, acoustic, 374–375
Neurotrophic arthropathy, 285–287
Neutrophil dysfunction syndromes,
171
Nevus syndrome, basal cell, and
cysts in jaw, 1086
Niemann-Pick disease, 931
bone changes in, 222
Nipple shadows, 755
Nitric fumes, pulmonary damage
from, 861, 863
Nitrofurantoin sensitivity, pulmonary changes in, 923–924
Nocardiosis, lungs in, 827
Nodular lymphoid hyperplasia
of colon, 616–617
of small intestine, 581–582
Nodules
pancreatic
in duodenum, 564
in stomach, 534–535
pulmonary. *See* Lungs, nodules
Nose
fractured, 1092–1093
sinuses of. *See* Sinuses, paranasal
Notochord, 78–79
and chordoma, 229–230, 375
Nutritional deficiency, and osteoporosis, 109–110

Obstetrics, 716–731
fetus, 721–727
intrauterine fetal transfusions,
730–731
pelvis, 716–719
placenta, 727–731
pyelitis of pregnancy, 673–674
radiology in pregnancy, 10, 12
roentgen diagnosis in, 716
rubella in pregnancy, and bone
lesions in infants, 259
ultrasound in, 731
Obstruction
of bladder, 705–707
bronchial
and emphysema, 904–905
and middle lobe syndrome,
794–796
by tumors, 781

Obstruction (*continued*)
from carcinoma of colon, 610–
611
of colon, 422–425
See also Ileus
duodenal, congenital, 554–556
gastric, in hiatal hernia, 545–546
pyloric, from duodenal ulcer, 559
of small intestine, acute, 414–
422
See also Ileus
ureteropelvic, 665
of vena cava, in mediastinitis,
950–951
Occipital emissary foramen, enlargement of, 353–354
Occipital lobe tumors, pineal gland
displacement in, 355
Occipitocervical fusion, 76, 80–81
Occipitocervical meningocele, 70
Occlusive vascular disease
of coronary arteries, 1027
of mesenteric vasculature, 427–
428, 592
of renal artery , 688–689
See also Arteriosclerosis
Occupational diseases, pulmonary,
847–860
pneumoconioses, 847–858
and pulmonary hypersensitivity,
858–860
Ochronosis, 293–294
Oculoauriculovertebral dysplasia,
75
Oculocerebrorenal syndrome, 115
Oddi sphincter, patulous, 468, 469
Odontoid process, fracture-dislocation of, 151–152
Odontoma
compound, 1087
cystic, 1086
Oligodendroglioma, 365–366
calcification in, 351
Ollier's disease, 32–33, 191
Omovertebral bone, 95
Ophthalmic artery, angiography of,
1047–1048
Optic canal, 1052–1053
Optic nerve, tumors of, 371
Oragrafin, in cholecystography,
471, 473
Orbit and eye, 1047–1055
angiography of ophthalmic
artery, 1047–1048
calcifications in, 1049–1052
examination of, 1047–1048
foreign bodies in, 1048–1049
fractures of orbit, 1095–1097
in hypercalcemia, 1049

Orbit and eye (*continued*)
in hypertelorism, 49, 75, 1048
in hypotelorism, 75, 1048
in trisomy 21 syndrome, 98
inferior orbital fissure, 1053–
1054
lacrimal passages, 1055
measurement of interorbital distance, 1048, 1050–1051
in metaphyseal dysplasia, 49
optic canal, 1052–1053
pneumography of, 1047
retinoblastoma, 1049
superior orbital fissure, 1053
tumors of, 1054–1055
venography, orbital, 1047
Ornithosis, 789
Orthopantomograph, 1078
Os
acetabuli. *See* Acetabulum
acromiale, 69
calcis. *See* Calcaneus
centrale, 69
intermetatarseum, 67
peroneum, 66–67
radiale externum, 69
styloideum, 70
subfibulare, 68
subtibiale, 68
sustentaculi, 67
tibiale externum, 66
triangulare, 69–70
trigonum, 66
vesalianum
manus, 70
pedis, 67
Osgood-Schlatter disease, 236–237
Osseous ridges, normal, 317
Osseous system, 15–334
abscess of bone, 176–177
acute, 176
Brodie, 177
chronic, 176–177
tuberculous, 180
accelerated maturation of, 26
accessory bones and ossification
centers, 66–70
in adrenal cortex hyperfunction,
26
in Albright's syndrome, 26
in alkaline phosphatase disturbances, 115, 117–119
in amyloidosis, 222–223
in anemia, 253–258
anomalies and syndromes of, 66–
101
cholesteatoma of, 228–229
chondroblastoma of, 202–203
chondroma of, 191, 194

Osseous system (*continued*)
chondromyxoid fibroma of, 203–
204
chondrosarcoma of, 209–212
in chordoma, 229–230
in chromosomal abnormalities,
97–101
congenital variations in
in extremities, thorax and
pelvis, 86–97
in skull, 70–78
in spine, 78–86
cysts of, 195–198
aneurysmal, 197–198
differential diagnosis of, 203
latent, 198
in mandible
aneurysmal, 1087–1088
solitary, 1087
posttraumatic, 198–199
solitary, 195–196
in cytomegalic inclusion disease,
259
dysplasias of, 28–64
Ewing's tumor of, 213–214
exostosis of, 191–192
fibroma of, nonossifying, 202
fibrosarcoma of, 212–213, 228
fibrous cortical defect in, 201–
202
fungal infections of, 181–182
differential diagnosis of, 180
in Gaucher's disease, 222
giant cell tumors of, 198–201
differential diagnosis of, 203
subperiosteal, 197–198
in granulosa-cell tumor of ovary,
26
growth and maturation disturbances in, 15–27
hemangioendothelioma, malignant, 213
hemangioma of, 201
in histiocytosis X, 223–226
in Hodgkin's disease, 219–220
in hypogonadism, 26
indicators of skeletal age, 15, 17
in infancy and childhood, 16–18
infarction of diaphysis, 244–245
inflammations and infections of,
171–190
ischemic necrosis of, 232–245
See also Ischemic necrosis of
bone
joint diseases, 261–301
leprosy of, 190
in leukemia, 220–221
lymphosarcoma of, 219
in mastocytosis, systemic, 258–
259

Osseous system (*continued*)
metabolic and endocrine disorders of, 104–126
metastatic carcinoma of, 214–
216
metastatic neuroblastoma of,
216–217
myelofibrosis with osteosclerosis,
221–222
myeloma of
multiple, 217–218
solitary, 218–219
in neurofibroma, 226–227
in Niemann-Pick disease, 222
normal osseous ridges, 317
osteoblastoma, 204
osteochondroma, 191–192
osteoid-osteoma, 194–195
osteolysis, massive, 201
osteoma, 192–194
osteomalacia, 110–117
osteomyelitis, 171–180
osteoporosis, 104–110
Paget's disease of, 251–253
in parathyroid disorders, 119–
126
Perthes' disease, 232–236
in pineal tumors, 26
in pituitary disorders, 22–26
acromegaly, 24–26
gigantism, 26
hyperfunction, 24–26
hypofunction, 22–23
poisoning affecting, 245–249
postoperative infections of, 185–
187
radiation affecting, 250–251
reticulum cell sarcoma of, 220
in rubella syndrome, 259
sarcoidosis of, 188–190
sarcoma of
osteogenic, 204–208
parosteal, 208–209
and soft tissues, 303–333
syphilis of, 182–184
teratoma of, 229
thorax, 755
in thyroid disorders, 21–22
cretinism, 21–22
hyperfunction, 22
juvenile hypothyroidism, 22
traumatic lesions of, 128–170
See also Dislocation; Fractures
tuberculosis of, 180–181
tumors of, 191–230
benign, 191–204
differential diagnosis of, 179–
180
malignant, 204–217

Osseous system (*continued*)
zone of provisional calcification
in, 17, 18
Ossification of skeleton, 15–18
endochondral, 15, 18
epiphyseal centers in, 15, 18
accessory, 66–70
delayed, in femoral head, 90
intramembranous, 15, 18
time tables for
female, 19
male, 20
in vertebral bodies, 80
Osteitis
condensans ilii, 187, 296–297
condensans pubii, 188, 296
deformans, 251–253
See also Paget's disease of
bone
dental, periapical, 1081
fragilitans, 45–46
Garre's sclerosing, 177–178
pubis, 185–187
tuberculosa cystoides, 180–181,
188
Osteoarthritis. *See* Joint disease, degenerative
Osteoarthropathy, hypertrophic,
298–299
differential diagnosis of, 315
Osteoarthrosis. *See* Joint disease,
degenerative
Osteoblast(s), 17, 137
Osteoblastoma, 204
Osteochondritis
deformans, 232
dissecans, 238–239
and patella cubiti, 69
in syphilis, 184
Osteochondroma, 191–192
differential diagnosis of, 209
and osteosarcoma, 205
of paranasal sinuses, 1065
Osteochondromatosis, 33, 192
of joints, 292
Osteochondrosis, 21, 232
deformans tibiae, 95–96
Osteodystrophy, renal, 121, 122–
124
teeth in, 1085
Osteofibrosis, dental, periapical,
1088
Osteofragilitis osseum, 46–48
Osteogenesis imperfecta, 45–46,
107
flat bones in, 46
long bones in, 45–46
pseudofractures in, 136
short bones in, 46
skull in, 45

Osteogenesis imperfecta
(*continued*)
teeth in, 1083–1084
vertebrae in, 46
Osteoid formation, 17, 18
in fractures, 138, 139
Osteoid-osteoma, 194–195
differential diagnosis of, 177, 179
giant, 204
of jaws, 1089
Osteolysis
massive, 201
in metastatic carcinoma of bone,
215
in osteosarcoma, 206
Osteoma, 192–194
of jaw, 1088
of mastoids, 1076
osteoid. *See* Osteoid-osteoma
of paranasal sinuses, 1065
Osteomalacia, 113–115
basilar invagination in, 76
infantile. *See* Rickets
and pancreatitis, chronic, 452
pseudofractures in, 136
teeth in, 1085
Osteomyelitis, 171–180
acute, 172–173
chronic, 174–176
differential diagnosis of, 179–
180, 184, 214
of pelvis, 178
in sickle cell anemia, 257
of skull, 176
syphilitic, 184
tuberculous, 180
vertebral, 178–179
postoperative, 187
pyogenic, 269
Osteopathia
condensans disseminata, 52
striata, 53
Osteopetrosis, 46–48
cone-shaped epiphyses in, 64
skull in, 47
teeth in, 1084
vertebrae in, 47
Osteopoikilosis, 52
Osteoporosis, 104–110
circumscripta, 251
in Cushing's syndrome, 107–109
of disuse, 105–106
after fractures, 144–145
in malnutrition, 109–110
postmenopausal, 106–107
in rheumatoid arthritis, 270, 272
of spine, 275
in scurvy, 109–110
of sella turcica, 345
senile, 107

Osteoporosis (*continued*)
and Sudeck's atrophy, 105–106
in tuberculous arthritis, 265
Osteopsathyrosis idiopathica, 45–46
Osteosarcoma, 204–208
differential diagnosis of, 214, 220
and Paget's disease, 252–253
parosteal, 208–209
Osteosclerosis
in hyperparathyroidism, 121
with myelofibrosis, 221–222
in osteodystrophy, renal, 124
Otitis media, and mastoid infection,
1072
Otto's pelvis, 297
in rheumatoid arthritis, 272
Ovary
calcification of, 731
cyst(s) of, 733
calcified, 432
and stomach displacement,
543
cystadenocarcinoma of, calcified, 432
granulosa cell tumor of, bone
growth in, 26
in Meigs' syndrome, 734
tumors of, 733–734
granulosa-cell, bone growth in,
26
psammoma calcification in,
733
Oxycephaly, 72
optic canal in, 1053

Pacchionian bodies, 338
calcification of, 343
Pachydermoperiostosis, 299
Pad sign, pancreatic, 450, 543
Paget's disease of bone, 251–253
basilar invagination in, 76
juvenile, 118
optic canal in, 1053
and osteogenic sarcoma, 205,
252–253
paranasal sinuses in, 1066
pseudofractures in, 136, 252
Pain, congenital indifference to,
169–170
Palate, torus of, 1088
Palatine foramen, anterior, 1080
cyst of, 1087
Pancoast tumor, 885
Pancreas, 412, 443–444
aberrant nodules of
in duodenum, 564
in stomach, 534–535

Pancreas (*continued*)
  acute pancreatitis, 444–446
  angiography of, 453–454
  annular, duodenal obstruction
      from, 555–556
  calculi in, 444, 450–452
    in acute pancreatitis, 446
    differential diagnosis of, 668
  carcinoma of, 452–453
    differential diagnosis of, 453
    duodenum in, 446
  chronic pancreatitis, 452
  cystic fibrosis of
    lungs in, 796–797
    and meconium ileus, 418
  cysts of, 453
  enlargement of, 446–450
    cholangiography in, 450
    common bile duct in, 449–450
    and duodenal loop enlarge-
        ment, 446
    duodenography in, hypotonic,
        448–449
    and forward displacement of
        stomach, 447
    pad sign in, 450
    reverse figure 3 sign in, 449
  lesions of, and stomach displace-
      ment, 447, 453
  pad sign of, 450, 543
  roentgen anatomy of, 443–444
Pancreatitis
  acute, 444–446
    barium meal examination in,
        446
    fluid accumulations in, 445
    ileus in, 445
    lung changes in, 445–446
    sentinel loops in, 427, 444–445
  chronic, 452
  and ischemic necrosis of bone,
      243
Pannus
  in rheumatoid arthritis, 270
  in tuberculous arthritis, 264
Panoramix machine, 1078
Pantopaque
  in myelography, 387
  in sialography, 1092
Papilla of Vater, 553
  enlargement in acute pan-
      creatitis, 446
Papilloma
  of gallbladder, 478
  of paranasal sinuses, 1065
Paracentesis, abdominal, pneumo-
    peritoneum after, 436
Paracuneiform bone, 68

Paraganglioma, of mediastinum,
    954
Paragonimiasis, lungs in, 840
Paralysis
  of diaphragm, 964
  pharyngeal, and dysphagia, 513
  pseudohypertrophic muscular,
      304
Paraplegia, and calcification of soft
    tissue, 312
Parasitic disease
  calcification in, 310
  intestinal, 592–594
  intracranial, 346–347
  lungs in, 840–841
Parathyroid gland
  adenoma of, in mediastinum, 960
  hyperparathyroidism, 119–122
    brown tumor of, 119, 121
      differential diagnosis of, 201
    and calcification of articular
        cartilage, 294
    calcium deposits in, 121
    chondrocalcinosis in, 294
    destructive lesions in, 121
    differential diagnosis of, 121–
        122, 321
    esophageal and tracheal dis-
        placement in, 121
    fractures in, 121
    generalized demineralization
        in, 120
    osteosclerosis in, 121
    secondary, 121, 122
    subperiosteal resorption in,
        120–121
  hypoparathyroidism, 124–125
    basal ganglia calcification in,
        350–351
    pseudohypoparathyroidism, 125,
        351
      cone-shaped epiphyses in, 64
    pseudo-pseudohypoparathyroid-
        ism, 125
    teeth in diseases of, 1083
Paresis, of diaphragm, 964
Parietal bones, thinning of, 77–78
Parietal foramina, congenital, 70
Parietal lobe tumors, pineal gland
    displacement in, 355
Parosteal sarcoma, 208–209
Patella
  bipartite, 68
  cubiti, 69
  in epiphyseal dysplasia, multiple,
      29
  fractures of, 165
Pectus excavatum, 772–773, 1030

Pediatric conditions
  acceleration of skeletal matura-
      tion, 26
  calcification of intervertebral
      discs, 297–298
  chest in, 770
  cortical hyperostosis, infantile,
      249–250
  cretinism, 21
  elbow fractures, 158–159
  epiphyseal ischemic necrosis,
      232–241
  granulomatous disease, chronic,
      797
  heart in, 979
  hyaline membrane disease, 914–
      915
  hyperthyroidism, 22
  hypogonadism, 26
  hypothyroidism, 22
  lobar emphysema, infantile, 906
  osseous dysplasia, 28–64
    See also Dysplasia
  osseous system development, 16–
      18
  periosteal stripes in infants, 315–
      316
  pituitary disorders, 22–26
  pneumonia, staphylococcal, 784
  polycystic kidney, infantile, 680
  polyps of colon, 617–618
  respiratory distress syndromes,
      914–916
  rickets, 111–113
  rubella syndrome, bone lesions
      in, 259
  scurvy, 109
  spondylarthritis, juvenile, 179
  Still's disease, 275–276
  thymus in, 758, 770
  urography, excretory, 646
  Wilson-Mikity syndrome, 916
Pellegrini-Stieda calcification, 318–
    319
Pelvic veins, phleboliths in, 308,
    429
Pelvimetry, roentgen, 718–719
Pelvis
  in achondroplasia, 35–36
  calcifications in, 731
  in cleidocranial dysostosis, 61
  congenital variations in, 86–97
  cysts and tumors of, 731–734
  female, 716–719
    android, 717
    anomalous types of, 717
    anthropoid, 717
    classification of types of, 716–
        717

Pelvis (*continued*)
 female (*continued*)
  and fetal skull measurements,
   719–721
  generally contracted, 717
  gynecoid, 716–717
  obliquely contracted, 717
  pelvimetry of, 718–719
  platypelloid, 717
  rachitic flat, 717
  roentgen measurements of,
   717–720
  transversely contracted, 717
 fractures of, 162
 in Hurler's disease, 44
 in Morquio's disease, 41
 in osteomalacia, 115
 osteomyelitis of, 178
 Otto's pelvis, 272, 297
 in Paget's disease, 252
 in trisomy 21 syndrome, 98
Penicilliosis, lungs in, 837–838
Peptic ulcer. *See* Ulcer, peptic
Periarthritis, 287
Periarticular disease, calcification
 in, 317
Pericarditis
 adhesive, 1040
 constrictive, 1040
Pericardium, 980
 congenital defects of, 1041
 cyst of, 957–958, 1040
 effusions in, 1038–1040
 pneumopericardium, spontaneous, 1040–1041
 tumors of, 1040
Perichondrium, 261
Periodontal infections, 1082
Periodontal membrane, 1079
Periosteal calcification, 314–317
 in fractures, 140–141
  absence of, 144
Periosteal stripes, in infants, 315–
 316
Periosteum, function of, 138
Periostitis
 alveolodental, chronic, 1081
 in rheumatoid arthritis, 270
 in syphilis, congenital, 182–183
Peristalsis
 in colon, 603
 duodenal, 553
 gastric, 520–521
 in gastric ulcer, 525
 in ileum, 570
 in jejunum, 569
 in kidney, 653
 and swallowing, 490
 ureteral, 653

Peritoneal bands, and duodenal obstruction, 555
Peritoneal cavity
 fluid accumulation in, 438–439
 gas in, 434–438
 pseudomyxoma peritonei, 462–
  463
Peritoneoscopy, pneumoperitoneum
 after 436
Peritoneum, 412
Peritonitis
 and ileus, adynamic, 426
 meconium, 419–420
  calcification in, fetal, 433–434
 and pneumoperitoneum, 435
 signs of, 422
Perkin's line, 90
Peroneal sesamoid bone, 66–67
Peroneal spastic flatfoot, 88
Perthes' disease, 232–236
 differential diagnosis of, 31, 222,
  239, 241, 243, 257
Pertussis, pneumonia in, 785–786
Petroclinoid ligaments, 343
Petroleum distillates, pneumonitis
 from, 860–861
Petrositis, 1074
Peutz-Jeghers syndrome, 578–579
 colon in, 616
 differential diagnosis of, 582
Pfeiffer's bacillus, pneumonia from,
 786
Phacoma, ocular, 1052
Pharynx, paralysis of, and
 dysphagia, 513
Phenacetin abuse, and renal papillary necrosis, 674
Pheochromocytoma, 712
 intrathoracic, 962
Phlebectasia, 339
Phleboliths, 308–309, 429
 differential diagnosis of, 668–669
 in mediastinal hemangioma, 962
 and small intestine hemangioma,
  575
 in splenic veins, 460
Phosphatase, alkaline
 hyperphosphatasia, 118–119
 hypophosphatasia, 117–118
  teeth in, 1083
 hypophosphatemic vitamin D-
  refractory rickets, 115–
  117
Phosphorus poisoning, bone
 changes in, 246
Photofluorography, 7
Photographic effect of roentgen
 rays, 4

Phrenic ampulla, 491
 differential diagnosis of, 545
Phrygian cap gallbladder, 480
Phthisis bulbi, 1052
Phycomycosis, lungs in, 838
Physis, 16, 18, 28
Phytobezoars, 540
Pick's disease, 376
Pigeon breast, 772
Pigeon breeder's disease, 860
Pigmented villonodular synovitis,
 290
Pineal gland, 340–341
 calcified, displacement of, 340,
  354, 355
 tumors of, 371
  bone growth in, 26
Pirie's bone, 67
Pituitary gland
 acromegaly, 24–26
 adenoma of, 354, 368–370
  basophilic, 370
  chromophobe, 368–369
  eosinophilic, 369–370
 gigantism, 26
 hyperfunction of, bone growth
  in, 24–26
 hypofunction of, bone growth
  in, 22–23
 teeth in disorders of, 1083
 tumors of, pneumoencephalography in, 358
Placenta, 727–731
 localization of, 729
 praevia, 727–729
 premature separation of, 730
Placentography, arteriographic,
 729
Plagiocephaly, 73
Planigraphy, 747
Plasmocytoma, of paranasal sinuses, 1067
Platybasia, 76–77, 80
 in osteomalacia, 115
Platyhelminth infestation, lungs in,
 840–841
Platyspondyly, 86
 in Morquio's disease, 40
Pleura, 769, 942–950
 acute pleuritis, 946
 bronchopleural fistula, and
  pneumothorax, 917
 effusions in, 942–950
  in bronchogenic carcinoma,
   890
  general considerations in,
   942–944
  infrapulmonary, 944

Pleura (*continued*)
  effusions in (*continued*)
    loculated, 944
    in mediastinitis, acute, 950
    in pneumonias, 784, 788
    in subdiaphragmatic abscess, 441
    in tuberculosis, 812, 818
  in empyema, 948–949
  fibrin bodies in, 950
  inflammatory diseases of, 946–949
  metastases to, 949–950
  thickening of, 767
    in asbestosis, 854
    chronic, 946–948
    from radiation, 863
  tumors of, 949–950
Pleuritis
  acute, 946
  chronic, 946–948
Pleuroperitoneal foramen of Bochdalek, hernia through, 967
Plombage, in tuberculosis, 824
Plummer-Vinson syndrome, 510–511
Pneumatization, mastoid, 1071
Pneumatocele, 804–805
  in primary atypical pneumonia, 788
  in staphylococcal pneumonia, 784
Pneumatosis cystoides intestinalis, 435–436, 442, 547
Pneumatosis intestinalis, 592
  in scleroderma, 588
Pneumocephalus, in skull fractures, 148–149
Pneumococcal pneumonia, 780–782
Pneumoconiosis
  asbestosis, 849–854
  baritosis, 858
  bauxite fibrosis, 854–855
  benign, 858
  berylliosis, 856–857
  coal worker's, 855
  diatomite, 855–856
  malignant, 847–857
  mediastinal lymph nodes in, 952
  roentgen classification of, 838, 850–851
  siderosis, 858
  silicosis, 847–849
  stannosis, 858
  talcosis, 854
Pneumocystis carinii pneumonia, 839–840

Pneumoencephalography, 357–359, 376
  in atrophy of brain, 376
  in hydrocephalus, 382
  in subdural hematoma, 378–379
Pneumography
  extraperitoneal, 650
  orbital, 1047
  pelvic, 732
  retroperitoneal, in adrenal tumors, 711
Pneumomediastinography, diagnostic, 752
Pneumomediastinum, and emphysema, 909
Pneumonia, 780–791
  alveolar, 780
  aspiration, 783
  bacterial, 780–786
  from bronchial obstruction by tumor, 781
  bronchopneumonia, 782–783
  and brucellosis, 785
  chickenpox with, 790
  desquamative interstitial, 937–938
  Friedländer, 783
  and influenza, 789–790
  Klebsiella, 783
  lipid, 934–936
  lobar, 780
  measles with, 790
  mycoplasmal, 787–789
  pertussis, 785–786
  pneumococcal, 780–782
  pneumocystis carinii, 839–840
  primary atypical, 786–789
  Pseudomonas aeruginosa, 786
  and psittacosis, 789
  rare causes of, 786
  rheumatic, 925
  rickettsial, 790–791
  staphylococcal, 783–784
  streptococcal, 785
  tuberculous, 808
  tularemic, 785
  viral, 786–790
Pneumonitis
  in achalasia, 505
  beryllium, acute, 856
  in bronchogenic carcinoma, 887–889
  cholesterol type, chronic, 934
  from hydrocarbons, 860–861
  lymphocytic interstitial, 924
  and middle lobe syndrome, 794–796
  radiation, 863–864
Pneumopericardium, spontaneous, 1040–1041

Pneumoperitoneum, 434–438
  diagnostic and therapeutic, 436
  in duodenal ulcer perforation, 560
  from gas injected into fallopian tubes, 436
  idiopathic spontaneous, 436–437
  after laparotomy, 436
  in peritonitis, 435
  in pneumatosis cystoides intestinalis, 435–436
  roentgen findings in, 437–438
  from rupture of stomach or intestine, 434–435
Pneumothorax, 916–920
  and bronchopleural fistula, 917
  differential diagnosis of, 919–920
  in histiocytosis X, 931
  induced, 918
    diagnostic uses of, 751–752
  roentgen findings in, 918–919
  spontaneous, 916–917
  tension, 917
  traumatic, 917
  tuberculous, 819
Podagra, 284
Poisonings, bone changes in, 245–249
Polyarteritis nodosa
  lungs in, 924–925
  renal aneurysms in, 688
Polycystic disease of kidney, 680–681
  differential diagnosis of, 693
Polycythemia vera, lung changes in, 933
Polyp(s)
  cholesterol, of gallbladder, 477, 478
  of colon, 613–618
  of duodenum, 563
  of esophagus, 510
  gastric, 531–533
Polypoid carcinoma, of colon, 608–610
Polyposis
  of colon, familial, differential diagnosis of, 582
  of paranasal sinuses, and allergic disease, 1064–1065
Pons, spongioblastoma of, 373
Popliteal cyst, 296
Porcelain gallbladder, 467
Porencephaly, 76
Porphyria, acute intermittent, 426–427
Portal veins
  gas in, 443, 456–458, 469
    in mesenteric vascular occlusion, 592

Portal veins (*continued*)
  gas in (*continued*)
    in necrotizing enterocolitis,
      631
    splenoportography, 457, 461–462
Positions, standard, 9–10
Potter-Bucky grid, 5
Precocious development, 26
Pregnancy. *See* Obstetrics
Presbyesophagus, 491
Pro-Banthine
  anticholinergic effects of, 517
  in duodenography, hypotonic,
    448
Progeria, 97
  paranasal sinuses in, 1068
Prolapse of gastric mucosa,
    through pylorus, 566–567
Proptosis, in tumors of orbit, 1054
Prostate
  calculi in, differential diagnosis
    of, 704
  hyperplasia of, 705–706
  infections of bone after surgery
    of, 185–187
Protein, deficiency of
  enteropathies with, 591
  in intestinal lymphangiectasia,
    589
  osteoporosis in, 109
Proteinosis, pulmonary alveolar,
    936–937
Protozoal infections, pulmonary,
    838–840
Protrusio acetabuli, 297
  in osteomalacia, 115
  in rheumatoid arthritis, 272
Psammoma calcification, in ovarian
    tumors, 733
Pseudarthrosis
  in fractures, 144
  in neurofibromatosis, 57–58
Pseudocyst
  in meconium ileus, 419
  in pancreatitis, acute, 445
  pararenal, 687
Pseudodiverticula, of esophagus,
    494
Pseudoepiphyses, for metacarpals
    and metatarsals, 92–93
Pseudofractures, 136
  in Paget's disease, 136, 252
  in rickets, 112, 117
Pseudogout syndrome, 294
Pseudohypertrophic muscular pa-
    ralysis, 304
Pseudohypoparathyroidism, 125,
    351
  cone-shaped epiphyses in, 64

Pseudomonas aeruginosa, pneumo-
    nia from, 786
Pseudomyxoma peritonei, 462–463,
    638–639
Pseudopolyp of colon, 615, 616
Pseudopolyposis, and ulcerative
    colitis, 625
Pseudotumor
  of hemophilia, 288
  in intra-abdominal abscesses, 439
  renal, 694–695
  in small intestine obstruction,
    420, 421
Pseudoxanthoma elasticum, 318
Psittacosis, 789
Psoas abscess, 672
Psoas muscles, 412
Psoriasis, and arthritis, 276–277
Pubic bones
  osteitis condensans pubii, 296
  postoperative infections of, 185–
    187
Pulmonary artery (arteries), 759,
    762
  agenesis of, 1014–1015
  angiography of, 750
    in bronchogenic carcinoma,
      892
  in atrial septal defect, 997–998
  calcification in, in pulmonary hy-
    pertension, 877
  coarctation of, 1016–1017
  idiopathic enlargement of, 1017
  left, aberrant, 1017
  in patent ductus arteriosus, 995
  in pulmonic stenosis, 1002
  stenosis of
    with atrial septal defect, 986–
      988
    with tricuspid atresia, 990–991
    in tetralogy of Fallot, 985
    in transposition of great vessels
      complete, 988–989
      corrected, 1004
      Taussig-Bing type, 994
    in truncus arteriosus persistence,
      993
    in ventricular septal defect, 1000
Pulmonary arteriovenous malfor-
    mations, 1015–1016
Pulmonary conditions. *See* Lungs
Pulmonary valve
  insufficiency of, 1025
  stenosis of, 1001–1003, 1024
Pulmonary veins, 759, 762
  anomalous return
    partial, 993
    total, 991–993
Pycnodysostosis, 48–49
  paranasal sinuses in, 49, 1068

Pyelitis
  cystica, 676
  of pregnancy, 673–674
Pyelogenic cysts, 686
Pyelokon, in retrograde urography,
    647
Pyelonephritis
  acute, 670
  chronic, 672
  emphysematous, 670
  xanthogranulomatous, 673
Pyeloureteritis cystica, 676
Pyle's disease, 49
Pylorus
  obstruction from duodenal ulcer,
    559
  prolapse of gastric mucosa
    through, 566–567
  stenosis of, hypertrophic, 541–
    542
    adult type, 541–542
    infantile, 541
Pyogenic conditions
  arthritis, 262–263, 266
  osteoarthritis of spine, 269
Pyothorax, 948–949

Q fever, pneumonia in, 790

Rachitic conditions. *See* Rickets
Radiation. *See* Roentgen rays
Radicular cyst, 1081, 1085
  differential diagnosis of, 1080
Radioisotopes for placental local-
    ization, 729
Radius
  fractures of
    at head, 157
    midshaft, 157
  fusion with ulna, 87, 91
Rathke's pouch tumor, 370
Raynaud's phenomenon, calcinosis
    with, 314
Recklinghausen's disease, 55–58,
    322–323
  and intrathoracic meningocele,
    961
Reflux
  gastroesophageal, 494
  vesicoureteral, 708
Reiter's disease, 294
Renal artery (arteries)
  aneurysm of, 688
    in polyarteritis nodosa, 688
  calcification in, 429
  occlusion of, 688–689

Renal vein, thrombosis of, 689
Renografin
  in cholangiography, 482
  in excretory urography, 646
Renovascular hypertension, 689–
    693
Renovist, in excretory urography,
    646
Resorption, subperiosteal, in hyper-
    parathyroidism, 120–121
Respiratory distress in newborn
  in hyaline membrane disease,
    914–915
  transient, 915–916
  in Wilson-Mikity syndrome, 916
Reticuloendotheliosis, 223
Reticulosis, 223
Reticulum cell sarcoma
  of bone, 220
  lungs in, 896
Retina, glioma of, optic nerve in,
    1053
Retinoblastoma, 1049
Retrografin, in retrograde urog-
    raphy, 647
Retrolental fibroplasia, 1052
Retropaque, in retrograde urog-
    raphy, 647
Retroperitoneal area
  fibrosis in, 702
  pneumography of, 650
  sarcoma of, and stomach dis-
    placement, 543
Rhabdomyoma, of heart, 1032
Rhabdomyosarcoma
  of bladder, 709
  of heart, 1032
Rheumatic fever, lungs in, 925
Rheumatic heart disease
  and aortic stenosis, 1022
  and mitral stenosis, 1017
  and tricuspid valvular disease,
    1025
Rheumatoid diseases
  arthritis, 269–276
  of lung, 926–927
Rhomboid fossa of clavicle, 92,
    755
Ribbing's disease, 50–51
Ribs, 755
  in achondroplasia, 64
  in advancing age, 770
  beading of, in rickets, 112
  in bronchogenic carcinoma, 885,
    891
  calcification of costal cartilage,
    755
  differential diagnosis of, 668
  cervical, 85, 772

Ribs (continued)
  congenital abnormalities of, 771–
    772
  costophrenic angle, 768
    in pleural effusion, 943
  costovertebral joints, rheumatoid
    arthritis of, 275
  fenestrated first rib, 91
  forked, 91
  fractures of, 161–162
  fusion of, 86–87
  in Hurler's disease, 43
  intrathoracic, 772
  in Morquio's disease, 41
  in neurofibromatosis, 57
  notching of, in coarctation of
    aorta, 1008
  in Paget's disease, 252
  in thanatophoric dwarfism, 64
  in thoracic dystrophy, asphyxiat-
    ing, 64
Rickets, 110–117
  with aminoaciduria, 115
  and cystine storage disease, 115
  differential diagnosis of, 39, 93,
    183, 184
  with hyperglycinuria, 115
  infantile, 111–113
  in Lowe's disease, 115
  rachitic rosary, 112
  rachitis tarda, 115
  renal, 122
  teeth in, 1085
  vitamin D-resistant, 115
    hypophosphatemic, 115–117
Rickettsial pneumonias, 790–791
Ridges, osseous, normal, 317
Ridging of intervertebral disc, pos-
    terior, 392, 397–398
Riedel's lobe, 454
Riley-Day syndrome, 933
Rocky Mountain spotted fever,
    pneumonia in, 791
Roentgen rays
  biologic effects of, 5–6
  characteristics of, 4–6
  definition of, 1–2
  discovery of, 1
  equipment for, 6–8
  fluorescence of, 4
  hazards from, 10–12
    bone changes, 250–251
    intestinal fibrosis, 631
    lung changes, 863–864
    osteosarcoma, 205
  and magnification and distortion
    of images, 8–9
  photographic effect of, 4
  positions used with, 9–10

Roentgen rays (continued)
  production of, 2–4
  scattering of, 5
  terminology of, 9
Roentgenkymography of chest, 751
Rokitansky-Aschoff sinuses, 479
Rotation errors
  in colon, 603–604
  in heart, 1009–1010
  in kidney, 659
  in small intestine, 573–574
Roundworms, 592
  lungs in, 841
Rubella, maternal, and bone lesions
  in infants, 259
Rupture
  of bladder, 709
  of esophagus, 512–513
  gastrointestinal, and pneumo-
    peritoneum, 434–435
  of intervertebral disc, posterior,
    392–398
  of spleen, 460–461
Rutherford's syndrome, 1084

Sacral spine
  agenesis of, 85–86
  cysts of, 406
Sacroiliac joints, rheumatoid arthri-
    tis of, 274, 296–297
Salivary glands, 1090–1092
  sialography of, 1092
Salmonella infections, pneumonia
    in, 786
Salpix in hysterosalpingography,
    735
SanFilippo syndrome, 44
Sarcoidosis
  lungs in, 841–845
    differential diagnosis of, 843–
      845
  mediastinal lymph nodes in, 952
  osseous system in, 188–190
Sarcoma
  chondrosarcoma, 209–212
  of diaphragm, 966
  epidural, 408
  of jaw, 1089
  of kidney, 699–700
  mediastinal, 962
  osteogenic, 204–208
    differential diagnosis of, 214,
      220
    of jaw, 1089
    metastasis of, 207–208
    mixed form, 207
    osteolytic, 206

Sarcoma (*continued*)
  osteogenic (*continued*)
    and Paget's disease, 252–253
    parosteal, 208–209
    sclerosing, 206–207
  of paranasal sinuses, 1066
  of pericardium, 1040
  pulmonary, 895–896
  reticulum cell
    of bone, 220
    lungs in, 896
  synovial, 289–290
Scalp, dermoid tumors of, 77
  See also Skull
Scaphocephaly, 72–73
Scaphoid
  carpal, divided, 69
  tarsal
    fracture of, 155
    ischemic necrosis of, 236
Scapula
  fractures of, 161
  Sprengel's deformity of, 95
Scattering, of roentgen rays, 5
Scheie syndrome, 44
Scheuermann's disease, 237, 405
  differential diagnosis of, 101
Schistosomiasis
  bladder in, 705
  lungs in, 840–841
Schmorl nodes, 79–80
  in Scheuermann's disease, 237
Schwannoma, 374–375
Scleroderma
  arthritis with, 276–277
  calcinosis with, 312–313, 314
  esophagus in, 511
  lungs in, 926
  pneumatosis intestinalis in, 588
  small intestines in, 587–588
  teeth in, 1085
Scleroma, of paranasal sinuses,
    1062
Sclerosing osteitis of Garre, 177–
    178
Sclerosis
  acrosclerosis, 314, 1085
  diaphyseal, 50
    multiple, hereditary, 50–51
  multiple, atrophy of brain in,
    376
  tuberous, 348–349
    differential diagnosis of, 346
    pulmonary, 932–933
    renal cortical cysts in, 681–682
Scoliosis, congenital, 773
Scout roentgenograms
  of abdomen, 411
  of esophagus, 488

Scout roentgenograms (*continued*)
  of gallbladder, 466–469
  in pancreatitis, acute, 444–446
  of small intestine, 570–571
  of stomach, 515
  of urinary tract, 645
Scurvy, 109–110
  corner sign of, 109
  differential diagnosis of, 184, 220
Scurvy zone, 109
Seldinger percutaneous femoral
    artery puncture, 453, 457
Sella turcica, 343–345
  in acromegaly, 24
  decalcification and erosion of,
    354
  in pituitary hypofunction, 23
  tumors in, 368–370
Semilunar cartilage of knee, cyst
    of, 296
Seminal vesicles, calculi in, dif-
    ferential diagnosis of, 704
Seminal vesiculography, 710
Seminoma, in mediastinum, 962
Senile osteoporosis, 107
Sentinel loops, in localized ileus,
    427, 444–445
Septal defects
  atrial, 996–998
  ventricular, 998–1001
Septic pulmonary infarction, 873
Sequestration, pulmonary, 775–777
Sesamoid bone, peroneal, 66–67
Shagreen patch, in tuberous scle-
    rosis, 348
Shaver's disease, 854–855
Shenton's line, disruption of, 90
Shoulder
  accessory bones in, 69
  dislocations of, 159–161
    fractures with, 160
  fractures of, 161
Sialography, 1092
Sickle cell anemia
  bone changes in, 256–258
  epiphyseal ischemic necrosis in,
    241
  hand-foot syndrome in, 244, 257
  infarction of diaphysis in, 244
  ischemic necrosis of bone in, 243
  and renal papillary necrosis, 674
Siderosis, 858
Silhouette sign, thoracic, 754
Silicosis, 847–849
  and tuberculosis, 849
Silo-filler's disease, 862–863
Singultus, 964
Sinografin, in hysterosalpingo-
    graphy, 734–735

Sinus pericranii, 77
Sinuses, paranasal, 1056–1069
  in acromegaly, 24
  acute sinusitis, 1060–1062
  carcinoma of, 1066–1067
  chronic sinusitis, 1062
  in cleidocranial dysostosis, 1068
  in Cooley's anemia, 254
  in craniometaphyseal or cranio-
    diaphyseal dysostosis,
    1068
  in cretinism, 21
  cysts of, 1062–1064
  ethmoid, 1058–1059
  examination of, 1056
  foreign bodies in, 1069
  frontal, 1058
  in Gardner's syndrome, 1067–
    1068
  inflammatory diseases of, 1060–
    1062
  maxillary, 1057–1058
  in maxillonasal dysplasia, 1068
  in metaphyseal dysplasia, 49
  in midline lethal granuloma,
    1068–1069
  mucocele of, 1064
  normal, 1057–1060
  osteochondroma of, 1065–1066
  in osteopetrosis, 47
  polyposis of, and allergic disease,
    1064–1065
  in progeria, 1068
  in pycnodysostosis, 49, 1068
  roentgen appearance of, 1059–
    1060
  sarcoma of, 1066
  scleroma of, 1062
  sphenoid, 1059
  trauma of, 1069
  tumors of, 1065–1067
Sinusitis
  acute, 1060–1062
  chronic, 1062
Situs inversus, 1009
  totalis, 521
Skeletal growth and maturation,
    disturbances of, 15–27
  See also Osseous system
Skull
  in achondroplasia, 35
  in acromegaly, 24–25
  anencephaly, 76
  in Apert's syndrome, 75
  basal angle of, 76
    in osteomalacia, 115
  bathrocephaly, 78
  blood vessel markings in, 337–
    339

Skull (*continued*)
    brachycephaly, 74
    calcification in, physiologic, 339–
        343
    cephalic index, 74
    cholesteatoma of, 228–229
    in cleidocranial dysostosis, 60–61
    cloverleaf, 74
    congenital variations in, 70–78
    in Cooley's anemia, 254
    craniodiaphyseal dysostosis, 1068
    craniofacial dysostosis, 74
        optic canal in, 1053
    craniometaphyseal dysostosis,
        1068
    craniometaphyseal dysplasia, 49
    craniopharyngioma, 370
        calcification in, 351
    craniosynostosis, 71–75
        in hypophosphatasia, 118
    in cretinism, 21
    Crouzon's disease of, 74
    dermoid tumors of, 77
    dolichocephaly, 72, 74
    facial bones in. *See* Face
    fetal, measurements of, 719–721
    in fibrous dysplasia, 53–54
    foramina of, 345
    fractures of, 145–149
        basal, 147–148
        cerebrocranial cicatrix in, 148
        depressed, 147
        diastatic, 147
        healing of, 148
        hematomas in, 149
        linear, 145–147
        pneumocephalus in, 148–149
    in Hand-Schüller-Christian dis-
        ease, 225
    hemangioma of, 201
    in Hurler's disease, 43
    in hyperparathyroidism, 120
    hypertelorism, 49, 74, 75, 1048
    in hypoparathyroidism, 125
    intracranial conditions. *See* In-
        tracranial diseases
    in iron-deficiency anemia, 258
    lacuna, 71
    mandibulofacial dysostosis, 75–
        76
    in Marfan's syndrome, 60
    meningoceles in, 70
    metabolic craniopathy, 352
    in metaphyseal dysplasia, 49
    microcephaly, 72
    mosaic, 45
    neuroblastoma of, 216, 221
    normal, 337–345
    in osteogenesis imperfecta, 45

Skull (*continued*)
    osteoma of, 192–194
    osteomyelitis of, 178
    in osteopetrosis, 47
    parietal foramina, congenital, 70
    parietal thinning of, 77–78
    in pituitary hypofunction, 23
    plagiocephaly, 73
    platybasia, 76–77, 80
    porencephaly, 76
    in pseudohypoparathyroidism,
        125
    in pycnodysostosis, 48–49
    in rickets, infantile, 112
    in rubella syndrome of infancy,
        259
    scaphocephaly, 72–73
    sinus pericranii, 77
    sutures in
        premature fusion of, 71–75
        widening of, 353
    in syphilis, 184
    trigonocephaly, 73–74
    in trisomy 21 syndrome, 98
    turricephaly, 72
    wormian bones in, 70
Small intestines, 569–594
    adenoma of, 578
    amyloidosis of, 588
    anatomy and physiology of,
        569–570
    anomalies of, 572–575
    arteriography of, 572
    atresia of, congenital, 574–575
    carcinoid tumors of, 578
    disaccharidase deficiency in, 593
    diseases of, 575–594
    diverticulosis of, 591
    duplications of, 572–573
    examination of, 570–572
    fibromas of, 578
    hemangioma of, 575
    hernias affecting, 593–594
    in Hodgkin's disease, 579
    in hypoproteinemia, 589, 591
    intussusception of, 589–590
    leiomyoma of, 575, 576–577
    lipomas of, 578
    lymphangiectasia of, 588–589
    lymphoid hyperplasia of, nodu-
        lar, 581–582
    lymphosarcoma of, 577–578
    malabsorption syndromes, 585–
        589
    Meckel's diverticulum of, 574
    mesenteric vascular occlusion in,
        592
    metastasis to, 579

Small intestines (*continued*)
    obstruction of, acute, 414–422
        See also Ileus
    parasitic diseases of, 592–593
    in Peutz-Jeghers syndrome, 578–
        579
    regional enteritis in, 579–581
        jejunal, 580–581
        prestenotic phase, 580
        stenotic phase, 580
        string sign in, 580
    rotation errors in, 573–574
    in scleroderma, 587–588
    segmental ischemia of, 592
    in sprue, 586–587
    tuberculosis of, 583–585
    tumors of, 575–579
        filling defect in, 576
        obstruction from, 576
    in Whipple's disease, 587
Soft tissues, 303–333
    arteriography of, 328–331
    calcification in, 307–321
        in Ehlers-Danlos syndrome,
            311
        parasitic, 310
        after spinal cord injury, 312
        after trauma, 310–311
    edema and hemorrhage in, 306–
        307
    gas in, 321–322
    lymphangiography of, 331–333
    mammography of, 325–326
    in muscular dystrophies, 304–
        306
    in pyogenic arthritis, 262
    in rheumatoid arthritis, 269
    thoracic, 755–756
    tumors of, 322–325
    venography of, 326–328
Spalding's sign, 723
Spasm
    esophageal, 507
    gastric, in peptic ulcer, 525
Sphenoid sinus, 1059
Sphenoidal fissure, 1053
Spherocytosis, hereditary, bone
        changes in, 258
Spina bifida
    manifesta, 82
    occulta, 82
Spine and spinal cord, 386–408
    abscess of
        differential diagnosis of, 962–
            963
        epidural, 407
    in achondroplasia, 35
    in acromegaly, 25–26

Spine and spinal cord (*continued*)
arachnoiditis, adhesive, 382–383, 403–404
arteriovenous malformations in, 404
avulsion of cervical roots, 406–407
block vertebra, 80
butterfly vertebra, 82
calcification in
after cord injuries, 312
of intervertebral discs, in childhood, 297–298
Calve's vertebra plana, 226, 239
chordoma, 79, 229–230, 375
in cleidocranial dysostosis, 61
congenital variations in, 78–86
in cretinism, 21
cysts of
epidural, 405–406
meningeal, 405–406
perineural, 404–405
sacral, 406
degenerative joint disease of, 281–282
development of, 78–80
diastematomyelia, 85
discography of, 392
epiphysitis, vertebral, 405
fractures of, 149–152
comminuted, 151–152
compression, 150–151, 268–269
in vertebral proceses, 152
fungal infections of, 269
fusion of vertebrae, 80–81
hemangioma of, 201, 404
hemivertebra, 81–82
herniation of intervertebral discs, posterior, 392–398
in Hurler's disease, 44
ischemic necrosis of epiphyses, 237
in Klippel-Feil syndrome, 81, 95
Kümmel's disease of, 152–153, 244
kyphosis, congenital, 773
limbus vertebra, 86
lipomas of, 406
in Marfan's syndrome, 60
meningioma of, 400–401
metastasis to, 402
midline clefts in, 82
in Morquio's disease, 40–41
myelography of, 386–392
neural arch defects in, 82–83
neurofibroma of, 398–400
in neurofibromatosis, 56–57

Spine and spinal cord (*continued*)
occipitocervical fusion, 76, 80–81
in osteogenesis imperfecta, 46
osteomyelitis of, 178–179
postoperative, 187
pyogenic, 269
in osteopetrosis, 47
in Paget's disease, 252
phantom disc in, 282, 300
platyspondyly, 86
in pycnodysostosis, 49
rheumatoid arthritis of, 273–275
ridging of intervertebral disc, posterior, 392, 397–398
roentgenograms of, 386
rugger jersey
in hyperparathyroidism, 121
in osteopetrosis, 47
sacral agenesis, 85–86
sandwich vertebra
in hyperparathyroidism, 121
in osteopetrosis, 47
sarcoma, epidural, 408
scoliosis, congenital, 773
in sickle cell anemia, 257
in spondyloepiphyseal dysplasia, 31
spondylolisthesis, 83, 282
spondylolysis, 83
transitional vertebra, 84–85
tuberculosis of, 266–269
anterior, 268
central, 268
differential diagnosis of, 268–269
intervertebral, 266–268
tumors of, 269, 398–403
intramedullary, 401–402
unfused center for articular process, 83–84
whiplash injury of, 153
Spirochetal infections, pulmonary, 838
Spleen, 412, 458–462
arteriography of, 461
calcification in, 430, 460
cysts of, calcified, 431, 460
enlargement of, 459–460
and stomach displacement, 542
increased density of, 456, 459
rupture of, 460–461
spontaneous, 461
splenoportography, 457, 461–462, 509
Splenic arteries, calcification in, 429
Splenic veins, phleboliths in, 460

Splenoportography, 457, 461–462
in esophageal varices, 509
Spondylarthritis, juvenile, 179
Spondylitis
ankylosing, 273–275
nonspecific, 179
Spondyloepiphyseal dysplasia, 31–32
Spondylolisthesis, 83, 282
Spondylolysis, 83
Sponge kidney, medullary, 683–684
Spongioblastoma, polar, 373–374
Sporotrichosis, lungs in, 837
Spot films
of colon, 598
of intestinal tract, 488
of stomach, 516–517
Sprengel's deformity, 95
Sprue, 586–587
differential diagnosis of, 452, 587
hypoproteinemia in, 591
idiopathic, differential diagnosis of, 452
osteomalacia from, 113
Spurring, in degenerative joint disease, 278
Squamous cell carcinoma, bronchogenic, 881–882
Stannosis, 858
Staphylococcal pneumonia, 783–784
Steatorrhea, 585
pancreatic, 452
Stenosis
aortic, 1003–1004
of aortic valve, 1022
bronchial, in tuberculosis, 818–819
of colon, 605
of duodenum, congenital, 554
mitral, 1017–1021
pulmonary artery. *See* Pulmonary artery
of pulmonary valve, 1001–1003, 1024
pyloric, hypertrophic, 541–542
renal artery, 689–693
of trachea, congenital, 777
tricuspid, 991
Stensen's duct, sialography of, 1092
Sternocleidomastoid muscle, 766
Sternum
deformities of, 772–773
fractures of, 161
Stewart-Morel syndrome, 352
Stierlin's sign, 584
Still's disease, 275–276
Stippled epiphyses, 28–29
differential diagnosis of, 38

Stomach, 515–551
    aberrant pancreatic nodules in,
        534–535
    adenoma of, villous, 536
    anatomy and physiology of, 518–
        521
    anticholinergic drugs affecting,
        517
    arteriography of abdominal ves-
        sels, 517
    carcinoma of, 527–531
        calcification in, 531
        fungating, 528
        infiltrating, 528–530
        mixed types of, 531
        recurrent, after surgery, 551
        scirrhus, 529
        superficial spreading, 529–530
        ulcerating, 530–531
    cardia of, 492, 519
    cascade, 518, 546
    congenital anomalies of, 521–
        522
    Crohn's disease of, 539
    Cronkhite-Canada syndrome,
        533
    cup and spill form, 518, 546
    delayed emptying of, postopera-
        tive, 550
    dextroposition of, 521
    diseases of, 522–551
    displacement by extrinsic masses,
        542–543
        in pancreatic enlargement, 447
    diverticula of, 540–541
    dumping syndrome, 548
    duplications of, 521–522
    eosinophilic granuloma of, 535
    in esophageal hiatal hernia, 543–
        546
        See also Hernia, hiatal
    after esophageal resection, 548
    esophagogastric junction, 492,
        493
    examination of, 515–517
    foreign bodies in, 539–540
    form and position of, 518
    fundus of, 518–520
    in gallbladder disease, 470
    gas in wall of, 547
    gastrectomy, 548
    gastritis, 536–539
    gastrocolic fistula, 549–550
    gastroenterostomy, posterior,
        547–548
    gastroesophageal reflux, 494
    hiatal insufficiency, 544–545
    in Hodgkin's disease, 536

Stomach (*continued*)
    hypertrophy or rugae, giant, 537
    leather-bottle, 529
    lymphomas of, malignant, 535–
        536
    Menetrier's disease of, 537
    motility of, 521
    mucosal folds of, 519–520
    peptic ulcer of, 522–527
        collar-button type of, 522
        differential diagnosis of benign
            and malignant ulcers,
            526–527
        gastric retention in, 525–526
        incisura of, 524–525
        meniscus sign in, 526
        mucosal folds in, 525
        palpable mass in, 525
        peristalsis in, 525
        spasm in, 525
        ulcer niche in, 522–524
    peristalisis in, 520–521
    polyps of, 531–533
    postoperative conditions, 547–
        551
    prolapse of gastric mucosa
        though pylorus, 566–567
    pyloric stenosis, hypertrophic,
        541–542
        See also Pylorus
    rupture of, and pneumoperi-
        toneum, 434–435
    stomal pouches in, postoperative,
        550
    thoracic, 544
    tone of, 521
    tumors of, 527–536
    after vagotomy, 548–549
    volvulus of, 546–547
    in Zollinger-Ellison syndrome,
        539
Strain of bone, chronic, 316
Stratigraphy, 747
Streptococcal pneumonia, 785
Stress, chronic, fractures from,
    136–137
Strictures of esophagus
    in chemical esophagitis, 501
    congenital, 496
Strongyloidiasis, differential diag-
    nosis of, 593
Sturge-Weber syndrome, 348
    differential diagnosis of, 350, 351
Subclavian artery, right, aberrant,
    1014
Subclavian steal syndrome, 384
Subclavian veins, venography of,
    327

Subluxations
    of acromioclavicular joint, 160–
        161
    in degenerative joint disease, 279
    in rheumatoid arthritis, 272
    in Still's disease, 276
    vertebral, 151
Subperiosteal resorption, in hyper-
    parathyroidism, 120–121
Sudeck's atrophy, 105–106
    after fractures, 144–145
Supranavicular bone, 67
Sutures of skull
    premature fusion of, 71–75
    widening of, 353
Swallowing, mechanisms in, 490
    See also Dysphagia
Swyer-James syndrome, 907
Syndactyly, in Apert's syndrome,
    75
Synostosis
    congenital, 86–88, 91
    craniosynostosis, 71–75
Synovioma, 289–290
Synovitis
    of hip, transient, 233
    pigmented villonodular, 290
Syphilis
    and aortitis, 1034
    dactylitis in, differential diag-
        nosis of, 180
    of joints, 269
    lungs in, 838
    osseous, 182–184
        acquired, 184
        congenital, 182–184
            latent, 184
        differential diagnosis of, 180,
            184
        and osteochondritis, 184
        and osteomyelitis, 184
        and periostitis, 182–183
        skull changes in, 184

Tabes dorsalis, arthropathy in, 286
Taenia solium, calcification of, 310
Taeniae coli, 602
Talcosis, 854
Tapeworms, 592–593
    calcification in, 310
    lungs in, 840
Tarsal scaphoid, ischemic necrosis
    of, 236
Tarso-epiphyseal aclasis, 31
Tarsus
    coalition of, 88
    fracture of, 166–168

Taussig-Bing type of transposition of great vessels, 994
Teeth, 1069–1077
  in achondroplasia, 1084
  in acrosclerosis and scleroderma, 1085
  caries of, 1080
  in cleidocranial dysostosis, 62, 1084
  in cortical hyperostosis, infantile, 1085
  in cretinism, 21
  in Cushing's syndrome, 1083
  in diabetes mellitus, 1083
  in dyscephalia mandibulo-oculo-fascialis, 1085
  in ectodermal dysplasia, 1084
  in Ellis-Van Creveld syndrome, 1084
  in generalized disorders, 1083–1085
  in histiocytosis X, 1085
  in Hurler's disease, 44
  hypercementosis of, 1082
  in hyperparathyroidism, 120
  in hyperplasia of face, unilateral, 1084
  in hypophosphatasia, 1083
  in hypothyroidism, 1083
  infections of, 1080–1082
  in mandibulofacial dysostosis, 1084
  in midline facial clefts, 1083
  normal, 1078–1080
  osteitis of, chronic rarefying, 1081
  in osteodystrophy, renal, 1085
  in osteogenesis imperfecta, 45, 46, 1083–1084
  in osteomalacia, 1085
  in osteopetrosis, 47, 1084
  in parathyroid disorders, 1083
  periapical infections of, 1080–1081
  periodontal infections of, 1082
  in pituitary disorders, 23, 1083
  in pseudohypoparathyroidism, 125
  radicular cyst, 1081, 1085
    differential diagnosis of, 1080
  radiography of, 1078
  in rickets, 1085
  in Rutherford's syndrome, 1084
  in trisomy 21 syndrome, 98
Telepaque
  in cholangiography, 450, 485
  in cholecystography, 470, 472
  multiple doses of, 476
Temporal bone. See Mastoids

Temporal lobe, glioblastoma multiforme of, 363
Temporomandibular articulation, 1090
Tendinitis, 287, 317
Teniae coli, 602
Teratoid cyst, mediastinal, 954–955
Teratoma
  bone in, 229
  calcification in, 351
  mediastinal, 954–955
  of ovary, 733
Tetany, parathyroid, 124
Tetralogy of Fallot, 984–986
Thalassemia, bone changes in, 253–256
Thiamine deficiency, heart in, 1031
Thoracic muscle, internal, 760
Thoracoplasty, in tuberculosis, 824
Thorax. See Chest
Thorium dioxide retention
  in liver, 456
  in spleen, 459
Thromboembolism, pulmonary, 869–874
Thrombosis
  arteriography in, 331
  of renal vein, 689
  venography in, 327
  venous, calcification of, 308–309
Thymus, 758, 770
  tumors of, in mediastinum, 960–961
Thyroid gland
  diseases of
    acropachy in, 316–317
    bone growth in, 21–22
    cretinism, 21–22
    heart in, 1031–1032
    teeth in, 1083
  intrathoracic, 958–960
Tibia
  fractures at upper end, 165
  fusion with fibula, 87
  ischemic necrosis of tuberosity, 236–237
  vara, 93, 95–96
    differential diagnosis of, 101
Tomography
  in bronchial adenoma, 893
  cardiovascular, 973
  of chest, 747–750
  of kidney, 648–649
  of lacrimal passages, 1055
  of mastoids, 1070
  in maxillary fractures, 1094
  of optic canal, 1052

Tomography (continued)
  in orbital fractures, 1096
  of paranasal sinuses, 1056
Tophi, in gout, 284, 314
Torsion, of stomach, 546
Torulosis, lungs in, 832
Torus
  mandibularis, 1088
  palatinus, 1088
Toxic agents, affecting bone, 245–249
Toxoplasmosis
  intracranial, 346–347, 349
  lungs in, 838–839
Trabecular bone reformation, after fractures, 141–142
Trachea, 757
  atresia of, congenital, 777
  displacement in hyperparathyroidism, 121
  hemangioma of, 777–778
  stenosis of, congenital, 777
Tracheobronchial, lymph nodes, 756
Tracheoesophageal fistula, congenital, 777
Transfusions, fetal, intrauterine, 730–731
Transitional vertebra, 84–85
Transposition of great vessels
  complete, 988–989
  corrected, 1004
  Taussig-Bing type, 994
Trauma
  aortic aneurysm in, 1035
  and arthritis, 145, 282–283
  battered child syndrome, 169
  of bladder, 709
  bone cysts after, 198–199
  of bones and joints, 128–170
    See also Dislocations; Fractures
  calcification after, 310–311
  and congenital indifference to pain, 169–170
  of diaphragm, 967
  fat embolism after, pulmonary, 874
  of heart, 1032
  intracranial, calcified hematomas in, 345
  of kidney, 678–679
  and myositis ossificans, 310
  of paranasal sinuses, 1069
  pneumothorax from, 917
Treacher-Collins syndrome, 75
  differential diagnosis of, 76
  teeth in, 1084
Treitz, angle of, 443, 553

Trichinosis
  calcification in, 310
  intracranial, 346
Trichobezoars, 540
Tricho-rhino-phalangeal syndrome, 64
Tricuspid valvular disease, 1025
  atresia, 989–991
    with pulmonary stenosis, 990–991
    without pulmonary stenosis, 991
  in Ebstein's anomaly, 991
  stenosis of, 991
Trigonocephaly, 73–74
Trisomy 13–15 syndrome, 101
Trisomy 18 syndrome, 98–101
Trisomy 21 syndrome, 98
Truncus arteriosus, persistence of, 993–994
Tuber-joint angle, 167
Tubercle bacillus, 808
Tuberculoma, 816–817
  of brain, 349
Tuberculosis
  of adrenal glands, calcification in, 711
  and arthritis, 264–269
  of bone, 180–181
    abscess in, 180
    differential diagnosis of, 179, 180
    osteitis tuberculosa cystoides, 180–181, 188
    and osteomyelitis, 180
  and calcification
    in adrenal glands, 711
    in liver, 456
    in spleen, 430
  of colon, 628
  mediastinal lymph nodes in, 952
  and mediastinitis, 950
  pulmonary, 808–824
    atelectasis in, 812
    bronchiectasis in, 815–816
    and bronchogenic carcinoma, 892
    bronchogenic spread of, 808, 814
    bronchography in, 744
    broncholithiasis in, 819
    bronchostenosis in, 818–819
    and calcium in nodules, 816
    cavitation in, 814–815
    cavity drainage in, 824
    classification of, 809
    complications of, 812, 818–819
    differential diagnosis of, 843, 920

Tuberculosis (*continued*)
  pulmonary (*continued*)
    dissemination of, 808, 819
    early infiltrate in, 813–814
    extent of disease, 809–811
    healing of, 817–818
    hematogenous, 808, 812, 819–821
    miliary, 819–821
    pleural effusion in, 812, 818
    pleural thickening in, 767
    plombage in, 824
    pneumothorax in, 819
    primary, 811–812
    pulmonary resection in, 822–824
    reinfection, 812
    and silicosis, 849
    surgery in, 822–824
    thoracoplasty in, 824
    and tuberculoma, 816–817
  renal, 676–678
  of small intestine, 583–585
  of spine, 266–269
Tuberous sclerosis. *See* Sclerosis, tuberous
Tularemia, pneumonia in, 785
Tumor(s)
  adrenal, 711–712
  of appendix, 638–640
  of bladder, 708–709
  of bone, 191–230
  bronchial obstruction from, 781
  "brown tumors" in hyperparathyroidism, 119, 121, 201
  calcification in, 311–312, 432–433
  and calcinosis, 320–321
  chordoma, 79, 229–230, 375
  of colon, 608–619
  of diaphragm, 966
  of duodenum, 563–565
  of esophagus, 498–501, 510
  of facial bones, 1097
  of gallbladder, 478–479
  of heart, 1032
  intracranial, 353–376
  of jaws, 1085–1090
  of joints, 288–293
  of kidney, 693–701
  of lacrimal gland, 1055
  of liver, 455–456
  of lungs and bronchi, 881–900
  of mastoids, 1076–1077
  of mediastinum, 952–963
  of optic canal, 1053
  of orbit, 1054–1055
  of ovary, 733–734
  Pancoast, 885
  of paranasal sinuses, 1065–1067

Tumor(s) (*continued*)
  pelvic, 731–734
  pericardial, 1040
  pineal, bone growth in, 26
  of pleura, 949–950
  retinoblastoma, 1049
  of scalp, dermoid, 77
  of small intestine, 575–579
  of soft tissues, 322–325
  of spine, 269, 398–403
  of stomach, 527–536
  thymic, in mediastinum, 960–961
  of ureter, 701–702
  of uterus, 732
  Wilms', 698, 712
  See also specific tumor sites
Tumor vessels, in liver, 458
Turner's syndrome, 101
  differential diagnosis of, 125, 126
Turret head, 72
Turricephaly, 72
Typhoid fever, pneumonia in, 786
Typhus, pneumonia in, 791

Ulcer, peptic
  abdominal arteriography in, 517
  duodenal, 557–561
  and esophagitis and hiatal hernia, 503, 504, 546
  of esophagus, 504
  gastric, 522–527
  jejunal, postoperative, 549
  pneumoperitoneum in, 434
  in Zollinger-Ellison syndrome, 539
  See also specific ulcer sites
Ulceration, in gastric carcinoma, 530–531
Ulcerative colitis, 622–626
Ulcerative esophagitis, acute, 502
Ulna
  fractures at midshaft, 157
  fusion with radius, 87, 91
Ultrasound, in obstetrics, 731
Umbauzonen, 136
Umbilical vein, in portography, 462
Urachus, patent, 663
Ureter(s)
  anatomy of, 651–652
  anomalies of, 655–656, 660–663
  calculi in, 666–669
    differential diagnosis of, 429
    See also Urinary tract, calculi
  duplication of, 660–661
  jet phenomenon in, 661
  obstruction of, 665
  orifice anomalies of, 661
  retrocaval, 661–662

Ureter(s) (*continued*)
  tumors of, 701–702
  vesicoureteral reflux, 664, 708
Ureteritis cystica, 676
Ureterocele, 662–663
Urethra, posterior valves of, 710
Urethrography, 710
Urinary tract, 645–712
  and adrenal glands, 710–712
  anatomy of, 650–655
  angiography, renal, 648
  anomalies of, 655–664
    fusion, 658–659
  in number, 657
  in position, 659–660
  in size and form, 657–658
  aortography, translumbar, 648
  bladder, 652, 702–710
  calculi in, 666–669
    differential diagnosis of, 429,
      668–669
    roentgen findings in, 666–667
    staghorn, 666
  cystography of, 649–650
    voiding, 649
  examination of, 646–650
  infections of, 670–678
  kidney, 650–651
  nephrotomography, 648–649
  patent urachus, 663
  pneumography, extraperitoneal,
    650
  in retroperitoneal fibrosis, 702
  scout films of, 645
  seminal vesiculography, 710
  trauma of, 678–679
  tumors of, 693–702
  ureters, 651–652
  urethrography, 710
  urography
    excretory, 645–647
    retrograde, 647–648
  vas deferens calcification, 710
Urinoma, 687
Urography
  in calculi, 666
  excretory, 645–647
    contraindications to, 646
    contrast media for, 645–647
    preparation of patient for, 645
    in renovascular hypertension,
      690–691
    technique of, 647
    treatment of reactions to, 646–
      647
  in hydronephrosis, 665
  normal, 652–653
  retrograde, 647–648
Urticaria pigmentosa, 258

Uterine arteries, calcification in,
  433
Uterus
  hysterosalpingography, 734–736
  leiomyoma of
    calcified, 432
    differential diagnosis of, 704
  tumors of, 732

Vacuum phenomenon, of joints,
  300
Vagina, 736–737
  foreign bodies in, 736
  hydrocolpos, 737
  metrocolpos, 737
Vaginography, 737
Vagotomy, stomach after, 548–549
Valley fever, 827
Valsalva maneuver, 743, 1016
Valsalva sinus, aneurysm of, 1008
Valves, urethral, posterior, 710
Valvulae conniventes, 416, 553,
  569
Valvular disease, cardiac, 1017–
  1025
  See also specific valves
Van Buchem's disease, 118–119
Varices
  of esophagus, 508–509
  orbital, 1052
Varicose veins, 306
  calcification in, 309
    periosteal, 315
  phleboliths in, 308
Vas deferens, calcification in, 433,
  710
Vascular conditions
  arteriography, 328–331
    See also Angiography
  calcification of arteries, 307
    intra-abdominal, 428–430
  cardiovascular system. *See*
    Cardiovascular system
  mesenteric occlusion, acute, 427–
    428
  occlusive disease. *See* Arterio-
    sclerosis
  renal abnormalities, 688–693
  venous conditions. *See* Veins
  See also specific vessels
Vater papilla, 553
  enlargement of, in acute pan-
    creatitis, 446
Veins
  of Breschet, 338
  calcification of, 307–309
    phleboliths, 308–309
    See also Phleboliths
  diploic, 338–339

Veins (*continued*)
  stasis in
    periosteal calcification in, 315
    subcutaneous calcification in,
      309
  varicose, 306
    See also Varicose veins
Vena cava, superior
  cavography of, in bronchogenic
    carcinoma, 892
  obstruction of, in mediastinitis,
    950–951
Venography, 326–328
  azygos, 750–751
  orbital, 1047
Venous lakes, cranial, 338
Ventricles, cardiac
  aneurysm of, 1027–1028
  enlargement of
    left, 981–982
    right, 982
  septal defects, 998–1001
    with right-to-left shunt, 1000–
      1001
    in tetralogy of Fallot, 985
    in trisomy 18 syndrome, 100
Ventriculography, 357–359
  in subdural hematoma, 378–379
Vertebrae. *See* Spine
Vesicoureteral reflux, 708
  and hydronephrosis, 664
Vesiculography, seminal, 710
Villonodular synovitis, pigmented,
  290
Viral pneumonia, 786–790
Vitamin A hypervitaminosis, bone
  changes in, 248–249
Vitamin B_1 deficiency, heart in,
  1031
Vitamin C deficiency, osteoporosis
  in, 109
Vitamin D
  deficiency of, and osteomalacia,
    110–117
    See also Rickets
  hypervitaminosis
    bone changes in, 248
    differential diagnosis of, 321
    falx and tentorium calcifica-
      tion in, 352–353
    periarticular calcification in,
      317
Volvulus
  of cecum, 424–425
  and meconium ileus, 419
  of sigmoid colon, 421, 424
  of stomach, 546–547
Von Recklinghausen's disease. *See*
  Recklinghausen's disease
Voorhoeve's lines, 53

Water enema, 599
Water-siphonage test, in gastro-
    esophageal reflux, 494
Webs, esophageal, in Plummer-
    Vinson syndrome, 510
Wegener's granulomatosis
    lungs in, 927
    and midline lethal granuloma,
        927, 1069
Werner's syndrome, 313
Wet-lung disease of newborn, 915–
    916
Wharton's duct, sialography of,
    1092
Whiplash injury, 153

Whipple's disease, 587
    arthritis in, 277
    hypoproteinemia in, 591
Willis circle, aneurysms of, 347
Wilms' tumor, 698
    differential diagnosis of, 712
Wilson-Mikity syndrome, 916
Wolffian ducts, mesonephric, 656
Wolman's disease, and calcification
        in adrenal glands, 431
Wormian bones, 70
Wrist
    accessory bones in, 69–70
    fractures of, 154–157
    Madelung's deformity in, 58, 94–
        95, 101

Xanthoma tuberosa, 189, 291
Xanthomatous tumors, of joints,
    290–291

Zenker's diverticulum, of esoph-
    agus, 496, 498
Zollinger-Ellison syndrome, 539
    hypoproteinemia in, 591
Zonography, 747
Zygomatic fractures, 1095

Design of text and cover by Maria S. Karkucinski

Composition in Times Roman, linotype, by American Book–Stratford Press
Plates and Printing by Pearl Pressman Liberty, Philadelphia

Harper & Row, Publishers

72 73 74 75 76 10 9 8 7 6 5 4 3 2 1